Fundamentals of Nursing

Fundamentals of Nursing

Second Edition

BT Basavanthappa MN PhD
Professor
and
Retired Principal
Government College of Nursing
Fort, Bengaluru, Karnataka, India
PhD Guide (Recognized by INC and Indian Universities)
Examiner for UG, PG and Doctoral Courses in Nursing
Ex-Programme In-charge, IGNOU, BSc Nursing Course

Life Member
Trained Nurses Association of India, New Delhi
Government Nurses Association of Karnataka, Bengaluru
Academy of Nursing Studies, Hyderabad, India
United Writers Association of India, Chennai
Nursing Research Society of India, New Delhi

President
RGUHS Nursing Teachers Association, Karnataka

Winner
Bharat Excellence Award and Gold Medal
Vikas Ratan Gold Award
UWA Lifetime Achievement Award
Shree Veeranjaneya Srujanashree Award

Author
Ten Texts on Nursing

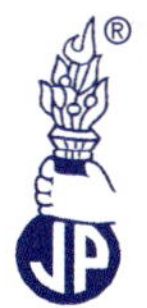

JAYPEE BROTHERS MEDICAL PUBLISHERS (P) LTD

New Delhi • Ahmedabad • Bengaluru • Chennai • Hyderabad
Kochi • Kolkata • Lucknow • Mumbai • Nagpur • St Louis (USA)

Published by

Jitendar P Vij

Jaypee Brothers Medical Publishers (P) Ltd

Corporate Office

4838/24 Ansari Road, Daryaganj, **New Delhi** - 110 002, India
Phone: +91-11-43574357

Registered Office

B-3 EMCA House, 23/23B Ansari Road, Daryaganj, **New Delhi** 110 002, India
Phones: +91-11-23272143, +91-11-23272703, +91-11-23282021,
+91-11-23245672, Rel: +91-11-32558559 Fax: +91-11-23276490, +91-11-23245683
e-mail: jaypee@jaypeebrothers.com, Website: www.jaypeebrothers.com

Branches

- 2/B, Akruti Society, Jodhpur Gam Road Satellite
  Ahmedabad 380 015 Phones: +91-79-26926233, Rel: +91-79-32988717
  Fax: +91-79-26927094 e-mail: ahmedabad@jaypeebrothers.com

- 202 Batavia Chambers, 8 Kumara Krupa Road, Kumara Park East
  Bengaluru 560 001 Phones: +91-80-22285971, +91-80-22382956, +91-80-22372664
  Rel: +91-80-32714073, Fax: +91-80-22281761 e-mail: bangalore@jaypeebrothers.com

- 282 IIIrd Floor, Khaleel Shirazi Estate, Fountain Plaza, Pantheon Road
  Chennai 600 008 Phones: +91-44-28193265, +91-44-28194897,
  Rel: +91-44-32972089 Fax: +91-44-28193231 e-mail: chennai@jaypeebrothers.com

- 4-2-1067/1-3, 1st Floor, Balaji Building, Ramkote Cross Road
  Hyderabad 500 095 Phones: +91-40-66610020, +91-40-24758498, Rel:+91-40-32940929
  Fax:+91-40-24758499 e-mail: hyderabad@jaypeebrothers.com

- No. 41/3098, B & B1, Kuruvi Building, St. Vincent Road
  Kochi 682 018, Kerala Phones: +91-484-4036109, +91-484-2395739, +91-484-2395740
  e-mail: kochi@jaypeebrothers.com

- 1-A Indian Mirror Street, Wellington Square
  Kolkata 700 013 Phones: +91-33-22651926, +91-33-22276404, +91-33-22276415
  Rel: +91-33-32901926, Fax: +91-33-22656075, e-mail: kolkata@jaypeebrothers.com

- Lekhraj Market III, B-2, Sector-4, Faizabad Road, Indira Nagar
  Lucknow 226 016 Phones: +91-522-3040553, +91-522-3040554
  e-mail: lucknow@jaypeebrothers.com

- 106 Amit Industrial Estate, 61 Dr SS Rao Road, Near MGM Hospital, Parel
  Mumbai 400012 Phones: +91-22-24124863, +91-22-24104532, Rel: +91-22-32926896
  Fax: +91-22-24160828 e-mail: mumbai@jaypeebrothers.com

- "KAMALPUSHPA" 38, Reshimbag, Opp. Mohota Science College, Umred Road
  Nagpur 440 009 (MS) Phone: Rel: +91-712-3245220,
  Fax: +91-712-2704275 e-mail: nagpur@jaypeebrothers.com

USA Office

1745, Pheasant Run Drive, Maryland Heights (Missouri), MO 63043, USA, Ph: 001-636-6279734
e-mail: jaypee@jaypeebrothers.com, anjulav@jaypeebrothers.com

Fundamentals of Nursing

This book has been published in good faith that the material provided by author is original. Every effort is made to
ensure accuracy of material, but the publisher, printer and author will not be held responsible for any inadvertent
error(s). In case of any dispute, all legal matters to be settled under Delhi jurisdiction only.

First Edition: 2002
Reprint: 2004
Second Edition: **2009**

ISBN 978-81-8448-610-0

Typeset at JPBMP typesetting unit
Printed at Replika Press Pvt. Ltd.

To
Nursing Profession
and
My Dear Students
and
In Loving Memory of
My Father

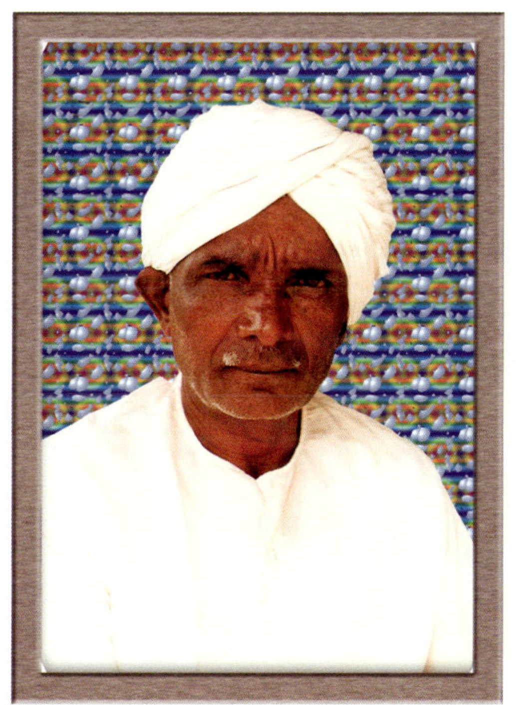

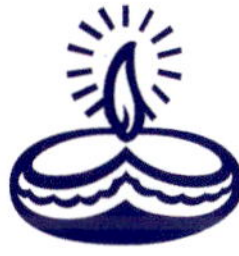 **Sri Thukkappa** 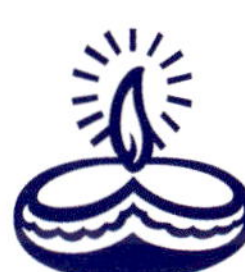

(1918-2008)

Preface to the Second Edition

It gives me an immense pleasure and satisfaction to introduce and present the second edition of my title *"Fundamentals of Nursing"*. Nursing continues to be challenged and rewarded by both new and changing opportunities and constraints. During these changing trends I have been pleased with the utilization of my titles—*Fundamentals of Nursing,* (1st edition), *Medical Surgical Nursing, Community Health Nursing* (2nd edition), *Midwifery and Reproductive Health Nursing, Paediatric/ Child Health Nursing, Psychiatric/Mental Health Nursing, Nursing Education, Nursing Administration, Nursing Research* (2nd edition) and *Nursing Theories*.

Nurses today must be able to grow and evolve in order to meet the demands of dramatically changing health care system. They need to think critically and be creative in implementing nursing strategies with clients of diverse cultural background in increasing variety of settings—hospitals, nursing homes, clinics, etc. Now we are moving in era of accelerating change in all walks of life and also moving towards newer activities based on the knowledge of nursing science and technology. Keeping in view of these changes, in this edition, every chapter has been extensively revised. The content has been updated to reflect the latest advancement. I must be appreciative of the many helpful comments, critiques and suggestions from faculty and students about my title and those are incorporated in this revised edition. The care has been taken at my best knowledge to cover almost all the contents in the revised edition of *"Fundamentals of Nursing"* as required by the respective Nursing Councils, Boards of Nursing and also Universities, which are imparting Degrees, Diplomas in Nursing at all levels.

And this text presents contents that represent the most accurate, current and clinically relevant information that is clearly written in easily read manner. I hope that this edition of *"Fundamentals of Nursing"* continue to make a contribution to nursing profession as regard and pursue new goals in the advancement of nursing as scholarly discipline.

I am aware that for manifold reasons, errors might have crept in and shall feel oblige, if such errors are brought to my notice. I sincerely welcome constructive criticism from readers that would help me to enrich myself and good suggestions will be incorporated in the next edition.

And now I invite you to open the pages beneath your finger and join me in a world of new ideas, challenging beliefs and expanding competencies for improving standards in nursing.

BT Basavanthappa

Preface to the First Edition

It gives me immense pleasure and satisfaction to introduce *"Fundamentals of Nursing"* to nursing community.

Nursing is a noble profession. Nurses constitute a major force in the health care delivery system. To maintain nobility of the profession in the new millennium, it needs new efforts to reform health care. Both high quality and cost-effective care are radically transforming the culture of care giving. Although nurses need to reassure the essence of nursing and what has traditionally served nursing well, they also need to change healthcare culture.

The goals of nursing education is to prepare today's student nurses to meet tomorrow's challenges. Nursing as a science, is characterized by growing body of knowledge that links technical and interpersonal interventions to desired client outcome; as an art nursing demands of its practitioners sufficient competency to creatively designed individual strategies to assist client (Patient). The art and science of professional nursing practice continue to evolve and expand. The growing body of nursing research and the explosion of technological advances challenge and stimulate nurses to acquire knowledge and refine critical thinking skills.

In this changing world on health care delivery system, nurses will need a broad knowledge from which to provide the expert care needed in nursing profession. The students first master theories and skills and then develop and refine ability to apply analytical thinking to each clinical situation. I believe that the changes in health care present exciting challenges to nurses and it is felt that there is a need for good nursing text of Indian origin to assist nurses to meet these challenges in the Indian context, since there is obvious need for nursing text to fit the Indian situation.

This book on *"Fundamentals of nursing"* has been designed to provide today's students with solid foundations of nursing principles to prepare them to meet the challenges of tomorrow. The comprehensive coverage of this book provides concepts and components of nursing skills and techniques of nursing practice and firm foundation of nursing. And also, it presents the theoretical and practical information necessary to make sound clinical judgement while emphasizing cognitive, affective and psychomotor skill needed to carry out fundamentals of nursing activity.

I am aware that for manifold reasons, errors might have crept in and shall feel obliged, if such errors are brought to my notice. These suggestions for improvement would be gratefully accepted. I sincerely welcome constructive criticisms from both teachers and students that would help me to enrich myself.

BT Basavanthappa

Acknowledgements

I owe a great deal of thanks to many who encouraged and supported me with their time and encouragement throughout.

- Shri G Basavannappa, Former Minister of Karnataka for having initiated and supported me to take up this "Noble Nursing Profession" as my career.
- Dr (Mrs) Manjula K Vasundhra, Former Professor and HOD of Community Medicine, Bangalore Medical College, who continuously encouraged me to write texts in the field of Nursing since nursing is a major force in Medical and Health Services.
- My Father Sri Thukkappa, who continues to grace for the progress of my career and all-round development of my personality for the welfare of the community.
- My Mother Smt Hanumanthamma, who continues to be a bright spot in the lives of all who knew her and whose grace gave me strength to progress in my life.
- My Wife Smt Lalitha, who gives meaning to my life in so many ways. She is the one whose encouragement keeps me motivated, whose support gives me strength and whose gentleness gives me comfort.
- My lovely children BB Mahesh and BB Gaanashree, for all the joy they provided me and all the hope that they instill in me and who bear with patience throughout my works of the nursing texts. They keep me young at heart.
- Finally, my warmest appreciation goes to M/s Jaypee Brothers Medical Publishers (P) Ltd, New Delhi, for sharing my vision for this book and giving me the chance to turn vision into reality.

Contents

1. Concepts of Health and Illness 1
2. Concepts of Nursing and its Profession 35
3. Ethical Aspects of Nursing 63
4. Cultural Aspects of Nursing 87
5. Legal Aspects of Nursing 99
6. Communication in Nurse–Patient Relationship 127
7. Health Promotional Nursing 157
8. Hospital Admission, Transfer, Discharge and Documentation 187
9. Health Assessment 201
10. Nursing Process 237
11. Basic Nursing Skills 311
12. Safety, Comfort and Body Mechanics 353
13. Maintaining Personal Hygiene 395
14. Promoting Sleep and Rest 447
15. Meeting Nutritional Needs/Nutrition in Nursing 461
16. Management of Bowel Elimination 501
17. Management of Urine Elimination 517
18. Management of Fluid, Electrolyte and Acid-base Balance 539
19. Management of Oxygenation 569
20. Administration of Medication 593
21. Infection Control Measures in Nursing 663
22. Biomedical Waste Management 691
23. Role of Nurses in Diagnostic Examination 709
24. Management of Stress 775
25. Perioperative Nursing and Bandaging 799
26. Management of Pain 849
27. First Aid in Emergencies 873
28. Rehabilitation/Rehabilitative Nursing 925
29. Management of Unconscious Patient 935
30. Management of Patient with Fever 941
31. Management of Patient with Shock 947
32. Management of Patient with HIV/AIDS 951
33. Management of Loss, Grief and Death 959

Glossary..**971**

Appendices
Appendix 1: Normal Reference Laboratory Values 999
Appendix 2: Calculations in Nursing.. 1008
Appendix 3: General Instruments Used in Nursing 1017
Appendix 4: Nursing Trays Used during Emergency 1022
Appendix 5: Operation Theatre Instruments 1023

Index.. 1033

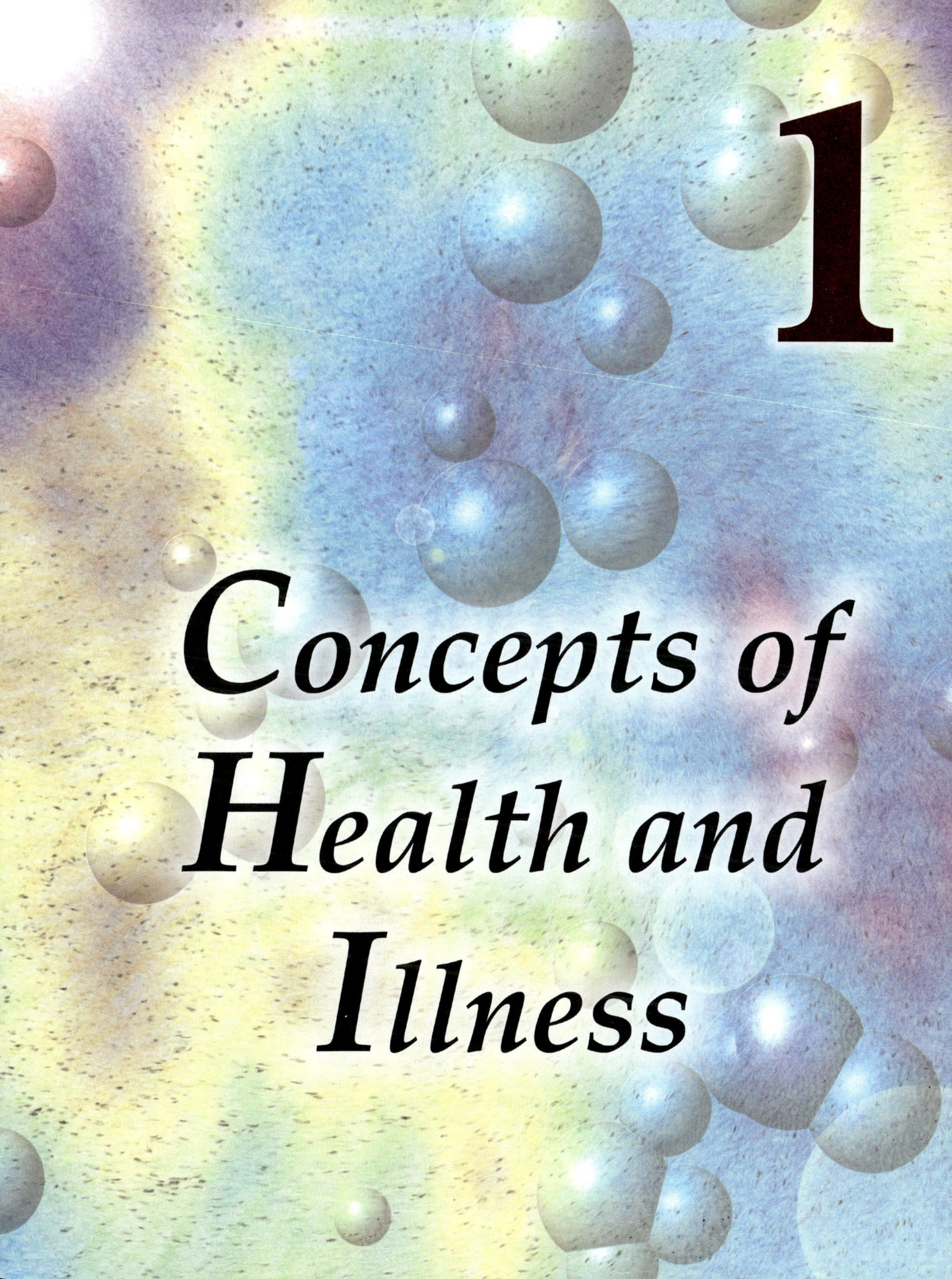

Concepts of Health and Illness

Health is an ideal state of physical and mental well-being; something to strive for, but never to attain. Good health is always around the corner but never actually reached, because there is always something more to be achieved. In this view, health is a goal itself, the end instead of one of the means of fulfilling life's purposes. True health is the strength to live, the strength to suffer, and the strength to die. Health is not a condition of the body; it is the power of the soul to cope with varying condition of that body.

Health as a "state of complete physical, mental and social well-being and not merely the absence of disease or infirmity" (WHO, 1948). Indian medicine system describes health as the trinity of body, mind and spiritual awareness (Gorine and Arnold, 1998). Florence Nightingale believed that health was prevention of disease through the use of fresh air, pure water, efficient drainage, cleanliness, and light (1859).

It has been believed that health implies at least three elements:
- A high level of overall physical, mental and social functioning;
- A general adaptive-maintenance level of daily functioning;
- The absence of illness or the presence of efforts that leads to its absence (Jean Watson, 1979).

To Watson, health is a matter of perception. Even an individual with terminal illness may be considered healthy if he has a high level of functioning, is coping with the diagnosis, and is actively making efforts to improve his status.

Views of Health

Good health is a prerequisite of human productive and developmental process. It is essential to economic and technological development. Health is the condition of being sound by body, mind or spirit, especially free from physical disease or pain. Soundness of body or mind, that condition in which their functions are duly and efficiently discharged (Webster and Oxford dictionary). The concept of health has been defined in a variety of ways. Historically, health and illness were viewed as extremes on a continuum, with the absence of clinically recognizable disease being equated with presence of health. World Health Organization (1974) defined health in terms of wellbeing and discouraged the conceptualization of health as simply the absence of disease.

Health has been viewed by different experts to their own field of interest as follows:
- *Biomedical scientists*—stresses is on germ theory, i.e. disease or ill health caused due to disease causing organism. The individual was considered to be healthy only if he was free from disease. This concept has been rejected by other scientists because it will not help to solve some other major health problems where primarily not due to disease causing organism like malnutrition, chronic diseases, accidents, drug abuse, mental illness, environment pollution, population explosion, etc.
- *Ecologists*—viewed health as a harmonious equilibrium between man and his environment and disease as a maladjustment of the human organism to the environment. This environment includes air, water, and other necessary things needed to human being for their life. For example, environmental pollution leads to health problem.
- *Sociologists*—visualizes health is not only a biomedical phenomena but that it is also influenced by various factors like social, psychological, cultural, economical and political. These factors are essential in defining and measuring health. All these factors and status help to determine and maintain health status of the population.
- *Holistic view*—is a synthesis of the views of the all experts. According to these concepts health is viewed as a multidimensional process involving the wellbeing of the whole person in the context of his environment.

Good health or wellness is not merely the absence of illness. Defining good health is difficult because each person has a personal concept of health. Health is a state of being that people define in relation to their own values.

Definitions of Health

1. About 500 BC **Pericles** defined health as 'that state of moral, mental and physical wellbeing which enables a person to face any crisis in life with utmost grace of God and facility.'
2. **HS Hayman** defines health as 'a state of feeling sound in body, mind and spirit with a sense of reserve power.' This perception of health is based on normal functioning of the body's physiological process, understanding the principles of healthful living and attitude that regards health not an end of survival and self fulfillment and a rich, fuller life as measured in constructive service of mankind.
3. **H Blum** defines health as 'person's capacity to function in a way to maximize potential; to maintain a balance appropriate to age and social needs; to be reasonably free of gross dissatisfaction, discomfort, disease or disability and to behave in ways that promote survival as well as self fulfillment or engagement'.
4. **R Dubiois** views health as 'adaption, a function of adjustment'.
5. **E Rathbone and F Rathbone** formulates health as 'a wholeness of function, movements toward self actualization, relating effecting, creative use of potential, realistic interpretation of experience and co-ordination of attitudinal, physiological, and behavioral adaptation'.
6. Liver pool **school of tropical medicine** describes health as 'the achievement of a state of harmony between man's internal and external milieu'.
7. **Perkin** viewed health as a state of relative equilibrium of body and function which results from its successful, dynamic adjustment to forces tending to distribute it. It is not passive interplay between body substance and forces impinging upon it, but an active response of the body forces working toward adjustment.

8. ***SC Seal*** defines health as 'a flexible state of body and mind which may be described in terms of range within which a person may stay from the condition wherein he is at the peak of enjoyment of physical, mental and emotional experience, having regard to environment, age, sex, and other biological characteristics due to operations of internal and/or external stimuli and can regain without outside aid'.

9. ***WW Bauer*** defines health as 'a state of feeling well in body, mind and spirit together with a sense of reserve power. It is based on normal functioning of tissues and organs of the body, and harmonious adjustment to the physical and psychological environment together with an attitude which regards health is not an end itself, but a means to a richer life as measured in constructive service of mankind'. Thus good health is based upon the capacity of an individual physical, mental and emotional and takes into what the individual does during his life.

10. ***Planning commission of India*** defined health as "a positive state of wellbeing in which harmonious development of mental and physical capacities of the individuals lead to the enjoyment of a rich and full life. It implies adjustment of the individual to his total environment, physical and social. The commission also states that health is fundamental to the nation progress in any atmosphere-in terms of resources for economic development, nothing can be considered of higher importance than health of the people which is a measure of their energy and capacity as well as of the potential man-hour for productive work in relation to the total number of persons maintained by the nation. For the efficiency of industry or of agriculture, the health of the worker is an essential consideration."

11. ***Dubi*** equates the states of health within an individual ability to control his environment and defines health as 'a state of competence of emotional, mental, and physical strength enabling (a person) to set goals, investigate alternatives, make decision, and take action of control environment'.

12. ***Florence Nightingale*** states than health as "being well and using to the fullest extent every power we have." She shows disease as a reparative process that nature instituted because some want of attention. She also envisioned health as being maintained through prevention of disease via environmental health factors.

13. ***Virginia Henderson*** assumed that 'health is a quality of life, it is basic to human functions. It requires independence and interdependence. The promotion of health is more important than care of sick. Individuals will achieve or maintain health if they have necessary strength will or knowledge'.

14. ***FG Abdellah*** defined health implicitly as 'a state when the individual has no unmet needs and no anticipated or actual impaired function'.

15. ***Patricia Benner*** defined health as what can be assessing where as welling is the human experience of health of wholeness. It is described as not just the absence of disease and illness, also a person may have a disease and not experience themselves as ill because illness as the human experience of loss of dysfunction, whereas disease is what can be assessed at the physical level.

16. ***Dorothy Johnson*** perceives health as an elusive, dynamic state influenced *by* biological, psychological, and social factors.

17. ***Sister Callista Roy*** defines health as a state and process of being and becoming an integrated and the whole person lack of integration represents lack of health. She viewed health along a continuous flowing from death and extreme poor health to high level wellness and peak wellness.

18. ***Betty Neuman*** equates health to wellness and defines health or wellness as the condition in which all parts and subparts (variables) are in harmony with the whole of the client. Disharmony reduces the wellness state.

19. ***Imogene King*** viewed health as a dynamic state in the lifecycle; illness is an interference in the lifecycle. It implies continuous adaptation to stress in the internal and external environment through optimum use of one's resources to achieve maximum potential for daily living. Health is the function of nurse, patient, physician, family, and other interactions.

20. ***Paplau*** defines health as 'a word symbol that implies forward movement of personality and other ongoing human processes in the direction of creative, constructive productive, personal, and community living.'

21. ***World Health Organization*** (WHO) defines health as 'a state of complete physical, mental, social and spiritual wellbeing and not merely absence of disease or infirmity.'

Actually this is a statement included in the preamble of the constitution of WHO, considered as definition of health. Terris a famous epidemiologist, believes that WHO definition should be modified as 'health is a state of physical, mental, social and spiritual wellbeing and ability to function and not merely absence of illness or infirmity'. He thereby replacing 'disease' by 'illness' and excluding 'complete' as health is not an absolute. He added 'and ability to function' which is necessary as definition of health requires both objective and subjective components. Here the objective component being 'the ability to function'. The subjective being 'feeling of well'.

WHO definition is positive and includes more than physical health. It infers that health is an absolute or ultimate state, but all individual cannot achieve the same level of health because of innate differences, some of us are born with some physical and mental differences. Accordingly, the complete wellbeing for all is unattainable goal, with this view the US President Commission states that 'health is an optimal state of physical, mental and social wellbeing'.

R Dubi also believes that WHOs view on health can never be reached because the person never be so projectly adapted to the environment that life will not involve struggle, failure and suffering. Human can adapt environmental conditions, but each new adaptation produces new problem that demands new solution.

Recently the modified definition of health as "a dynamic state of physical, mental, social spiritual wellbeing and not merely absence of disease or infirmity."

However, WHO definition of health connotes a state of dynamic equilibrium among various subsystem of a holistic person, i.e. it concern with the individual as a total system. This definition gives the following characteristics that promote a more positive concept of health:

- A concern for the individual as a total system and touches all aspects or dimensions of health, i.e. physical, mental, social and spiritual.
- A view of health that identifies internal and external environment. Health in its broadest sense is a dynamic state in which the individual adapts to changes in internal and external environment to maintain a state of wellbeing. The internal environment includes many factors that influence on health, including genetic and psychological variables, intellectual and spiritual dimensions and disease processes. The external environment includes factors outside the person that may influence on health, including physical environment, social relationships, and economic variables.
- It is an acknowledgement of the importance of an individual role in life. Health is essential for leading a socioeconomically productive life. The provision of health should be considered a fundamental human right, healthcare is an important mean of protecting that right.

Health is individualized to each person and is affected by so many factors and defining health is very difficult. The most widely accepted definition of health, which includes concepts of wellness, i.e.

"Wellness is more than just good health, it is an active process in which an individual progress toward maximum potential possible, regardless of current status of health. Wellness is influenced by variety of factors including the environment, basic human needs and one's culture."

The primary role of the nurse as a caregiver is to prevent illness, to restore health, and to facilitate coping so as to maximize wellness in clients of all ages, in any setting and in both health and illness. Wellness and health are more than the absence of illness. Health must be defined by each person and must consider the all dimensions of that person, the physical, intellectual, emotional, sociocultural, spiritual, and environmental aspects that compose the whole person. Equal consideration of all these interrelated and interdependent components of the whole person serves as the basic of holistic nursing care.

Holistic Health

Holistic is a term derived from the Greek word *holos*, meaning "whole." Holistic health views the physical, intellectual, sociocultural, psychological, and spiritual aspects of a person's life as an integrated whole. These five aspects cannot be separated or isolated; anything that affects one aspect of a person's life also affects the other aspects. The environment

within which a person lives and the manner whereby the person interacts with that environment are also considerations.

It has been described that health as the maintenance of harmony and balance among body, mind, and spirit. Homeostasis is the balance or stability that the body strives to achieve among these aspects of a person's life by continuous adaptation. Internal physiological homeostasis is a balance of the body's fluids.

Nurses must understand the integration of these aspects of a person's life in order to help clients through healing processes. Figure 1.1 illustrates the holistic perspective.

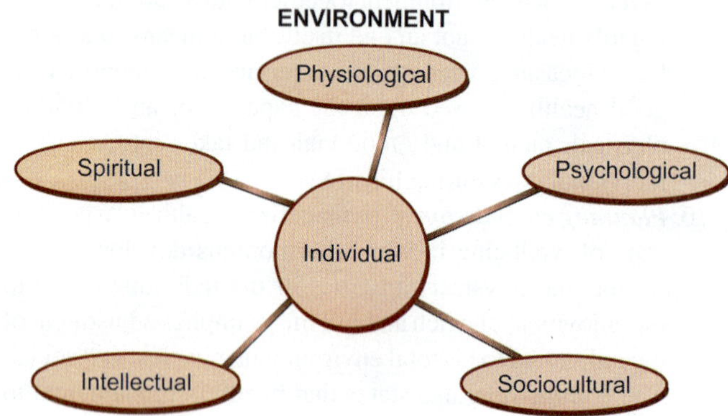

Figure 1.1: Holistic view of an individual

Holistic modalities is gradually becoming integrated into mainstream client care. Holistic care is a care that "considers the whole person, including physical, mental, emotional, and spiritual aspects." The final goal of investigating holistic modalities is to allow the validated therapies to be further integrated into general client care.

Success in using holistic modalities in client care requires an awareness of a fundamental principle of holism: The nurse *facilitates* the client in attaining the best state for healing to occur. Among the holistic modalities most frequently used in nursing are the following:

- Biofeedback
- Exercise and movement
- Goal-setting
- Humor and laughter
- Imagery
- Journaling
- Massage
- Play therapy
- Prayer
- Therapeutic touch.

Nurses must be open to new ideas and must not allow holistic modalities to become just another technology. They must work on developing personal healing qualities and become more aware of healing in their own lives. Among other qualities, a healer:

- Demonstrates awareness that self-healing is a continual process.
- Is familiar with self-development.
- Recognizes personal strengths and weaknesses.

- Models self-care.
- Demonstrates awareness that personal presence is as important as technical skills.
- Respects and loves clients.
- Presumes that clients know the best life choices.
- Guides clients in discovering creative options.
- Listens actively.
- Shares insights without imposing personal values and beliefs.
- Accepts client input without judgment.
- Views time spent with clients as an opportunity to serve and share.

Illness

On examining the definitions of health, it has been defined in terms of individual. Definitions of illness are also individualized to each person, who experiences an alteration in health. Like health, illness is also difficult to define, because the terms disease and illness mean the same process. Disease is a medical term meaning that there is pathological change in the structure or function of the body or mind. It is a condition that has specific symptoms and boundaries where health and illness are individualized perceptions and definitions of oneself. An illness is the response, the person has, to a disease; it is an abnormal process in which the person's level of functioning is changed compared with a previous level. The response is different for each person, and is influenced by self-perceptions; other perceptions, the effects of changes and body, structure and functions; the effects of those changes on roles and relationships; and cultural and spiritual values and beliefs.

- *Culture* – represents nonphysical traits, such as values, belief, attitudes and customs shared by a group of people and passed from one generation to the next. Culture is also the sum of beliefs, practices, habits, likes, dislikes, norms, customs and rituals learned from family during the years of socialization.
- *Ethnicity* – is a sense of identification associated with a cultural groups common social and cultural heritage. The characteristics of an ethnic group includes common language, and dialect, migratory states, race, and religious faith, and practices. People share traditions, values symbols, literature, folklore, music and food preference.
- *Religion* – is a belief in divine or superhuman power (or powers) to be obeyed and worshipped as the creator and ruler of the universe. Religious teachings help formulate a meaningful philosophy and system of practices through the system of beliefs, practices, and social controls having specific values, norms and ethics that vary between religious groups.
- *Illness* – is not merely the presence of disease process. Illness is a state in which a person's physical, emotional, intellectual, social developmental or spiritual functioning is diminished or impaired, compared with that person's experience.

Illness behavior involves the ways persons monitor their bodies, define and interpret their symptoms, take remedial measures/ actions and the use of healthcare systems.

It also can serve as a coping mechanism. It may be a means of obtaining reassurance. Clients may need reassurance that the inability to care for themselves is due to physical disease. Illness behavior can result in clients being released from roles, social expectations or responsibilities.

Determinants of Illness Behavior

- The visibility and recognizability of the illness symptoms.
- The extent to which the person perceives the symptoms as serious (the person's estimate of the present and future roles).
- The person's information, knowledge and cultural assumption and understanding realized to the perceived symptoms.
- The extent to which symptoms disrupt family, work and social activities.
- The frequency of the appearance of the symptoms and their persistence.
- The extent to which others exposed to the persons tolerate the symptoms.
- The extent to which basic needs are denied because of illness.
- The extent to which meeting other competes with illness responses.
- The extent to which the person gives other possible interpretation to the symptoms.
- The availability and physical proximity of treatment resources and psychological and monetary costs of taking action (including costs in time and effort, as well as costs such as stigma, social distance, and feelings of humiliation).

As mentioned earlier that people vary greatly in terms of their response to life situations. Why is this so? Why do some people react to seemingly insurmountable problems with calmness and grace, while others fall apart over seemingly "small" disruptions? The human experience is so complex and interactive that is impossible to make neat little categories that we might add up to determine a score predicting how a person will respond to a given situation. There are several factors, however, that may influence an individual's responses to illness.

Stages of Illness Behavior

Suchman (1972) identified five stages of illness behaviors that people move through as they cope with disruptions to health: experiencing symptoms, sick role behavior, seeking professional care, dependence others, and recovery (Fig. 1.2).

Symptoms Experience

During initial stage, a person is aware that 'something wrong'. A person usually recognizes a physical sensation or limitation in functioning but does not suspect specific diagnosis.

The person's perception of a symptom include awareness of a physical change much as pain, rash or a lump; evaluation of this change and decision that it is a symptom of an illness; and emotional response. For example, a 38 years old women detects a lump during monthly breast examination-due to hormonal changes, not cancer.

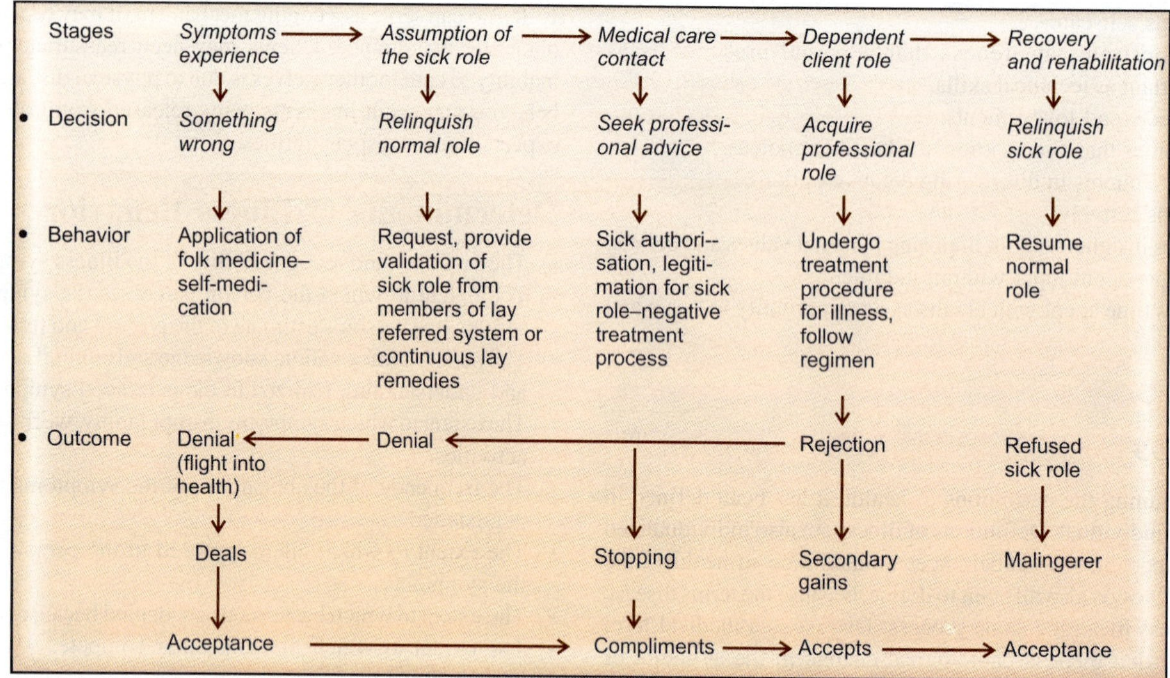

Figure 1.2: Stages of illness behavior

Experiencing symptoms is a signal that illness has begun. If the symptoms are recognizable, such as runny nose, sneezing, and a cough, you may identify the problem as a common cold and turn to previously used remedies. Common problems rarely progress beyond this stage. However, if the symptoms are unusual, severe, or overwhelming, you may progress to the next stage.

Assumption of the Sick Role

If symptoms persists and become severe, client assumes the sick role. At this point the illness become social phenomenon, and sick people seek confirmation from their families and social groups that they are indeed ill and that they should be excused from normal duties and role expectations. The social group recognizes the illness and may also support continued medication.

The assumption of the sick role results in emotional changes such as withdrawal or depression and physical changes. Emotional changes may be simple or complex, depending on the severity of the illness, the degree of disability, and anticipated length of the illness.

Sick role behavior is assumed when you have identified yourself as ill. This role relieves you from normal duties, such as work, school, or tasks at home. The severity of the symptoms and anticipated length of illness determine whether you will progress further along the stages of illness.

Medical Care Contact

If symptoms persist despite the home remedies become severe, or require emergency care, the person is motivated to seek professional health services.

Seeking professional care is the next stage. To reach this stage, you must determine that you are ill and that professional care is required to treat the illness. Persons who seek professional care are asking for validation of their illness, explanations for their symptoms, appropriate treatment, and information about the anticipated length of illness. Health care professionals often bypass this stage, relying on themselves to identify and treat the problem. This is not always the best course of action because it is difficult to the objective when examining yourself.

Dependent Client Role

After accepting the illness and seeking treatment, the client enters this stage. Here the client depends on health care professional, for the relief of symptoms. The client accepts care, sympathy, and protection from the demands and stresses of life. A client adopts the dependent role in a healthcare institution, at home or in a community settings.

The client also adjusts to the disruption of a daily schedule–occupation family, and community.

Dependence on others begins when patient accept the diagnosis and treatment of the health care provider. The severity of the illness and the type of treatment determine the extent of dependence. In some cases this may be limited to listening to the provider's instructions, filling the prescription, and following directions given in the office. However, illness that requires hospitalization is often associated with dependence on nursing staff and hospital personnel for activities of daily living, medications, and treatments. Some people easily make the transition to dependence; others remain as independent as possible even in the face of severe illness. Personal characteristics and values play a large role in determining how each of us will respond to the challenges of being dependent.

Recovery is the final stage of illness. Dependence is given up, and there is a gradual return to normal roles and functioning. In minor illness, this is usually a return to the status quo. Severe illnesses may require a newly defined level of optimum function.

The Nature of the Illness

The nature of the illness affects the way persons react to disruptions. An *acute illness* occurs suddenly and lasts for a limited amount of time. Acute illnesses, such as a cold, flu, or viral infection, may be minor and require no formal health care. Some acute illness, such as strep throat, may require a visit to a health provider for treatment or even hospitalization or surgery, as in cholecystitis (gallbladder inflammation secondary to gallstone formation) or pyelonephritis (infection of the kidney). Although hospitalization and surgery can be quite traumatic, in each case the person is expected to recover. In acute illness a person may experience the disruptions of pain, competing demands, and the unknown. However, an end is in sight. Relief is expected.

In contrast, **chronic illness** lasts for a long period of time, usually 6 months or more, often for a lifetime. Chronic illness requires the person to make life changes. These changes might be regular visits to the clinic or hospital, daily medications, or lifestyle modifications. Examples of chronic illness include AIDS, diabetes mellitus, rheumatoid arthritis, and hypertension. Because of the lengthy period of illness, people with chronic disease often experience periods of remission or exacerbation. A **remission** occurs when symptoms are minimal to none. An **exacerbation** occurs when symptoms intensify. Clients with chronic illness often complain about the unrelenting nature of their health problems. A person with chronic illness may experience virtually all of the disruptions identified earlier.

Why does one client who drinks, smokes, over eats, and avoids exercise live into his 90s, yet another client who "follows all the rules" dies of a sudden heart attack at age 39? Our bodies do not react to the same stressors in the same way. One factor that may contribute to this difference is the person's hardiness.

Hardiness has been described as *developing a very strong positive force to live*–and enjoying the fight! A man with heart problems said, "I guess everybody that's in the situation, who has to fight to live, and has learned the mental wizardry of it, you know, to make yourself want to live on. But if you want to, you develop this–this very, very strong positive force to make it go." It has been reported a study that revealed a 10-year survival rate of 75% "among cancer patients who reacted to the diagnosis with a "fighting spirit," compared with a 22% survival rate "among those who responded with 'stoic acceptance' or feelings of helplessness or hopelessness."

A dramatic example is one woman in an advanced stage of cancer and receiving chemotherapy who got up and went to work every day. Even though it was extremely difficult to drag herself out of bed and get ready for work, she felt much better when she could carry on her normal activities instead of dwelling on her constant pain and the threat of impending death. Carrying on normally is not easy to do, however. It takes a concerted, determined effort to persevere.

Another aspect of hardiness is the willingness to draw on resources within oneself or from others to *break out of old patterns of living* when life situations change. Some people find it too difficult to make life changes, and they just give up. Hardy individuals are willing to seek out information and take initiative in dealing with life situations rather than sitting back and letting someone else control their lives.

Some people don't have many resources to call on. When disruption hits, they lack the cognitive, communicative, creative, and spiritual resources that would support them during difficult times. Ironically, some people blossom during times of adversity. Those who see themselves as hardy tend to approach disruptions with an "I can deal with this" attitude.

Everyone has limits. For health care providers, too many demands over too long a period of time can lead to "burnout," a feeling of being overwhelmed and demoralized. For clients and their families, dealing with the cumulative effect of illness and other life disruptions can break down what might otherwise be excellent coping skills. Therefore, their responses may not be typical of what they usually have demonstrated.

Factors Influencing on Health and Illness

In envisioning health and illness as a continuum, full-spectrum nurses promote wellness regardless of the circumstances that clients face now or in the future. This approach requires the holistic understanding that health is multidimensional. The following are some of the many dimensions of health that persons experience along the health-illness continuum.

Biological Factors: Although biological factors are not entirely within our control, most people consider them when they describe themselves as "well" or "ill." A healthy genetic makeup and freedom from debilitating age-related changes are certainly desired states, and they tip the scale toward the wellness end of the health-illness continuum.

- *Genetic makeup:* For example, the risk of breast cancer increases dramatically in women who have a family history of a mother, sister, or daughter with breast cancer. Recently, a genetic marker for this type of breast cancer has been discovered. Some women with these genetic markers choose to have prophylactic mastectomies to decrease their risk.
- *Gender:* Many diseases occur more commonly in one gender than another. For example, rheumatoid arthritis, osteoporosis, and breast cancer are more common in women, whereas ulcers, color blindness, and bladder cancer are more common in men.

- *Age and developmental stage:* Age and developmental stage influence the likelihood of becoming ill. Certain health problems can be correlated to developmental stage. For example, over 75% of new breast cancer cases are diagnosed in women over age 50. As another example, adolescent boys have much higher rates of head injury and spinal cord injury than the general public because of their tendency toward risk-taking behaviors, which peaks during this stage.

Developmental stage influences a person's ability to cope with stressors that tend to move him toward the illness end of the continuum. Infants or children who are ill, frightened, or hurt have a limited repertoire of experiences, communication ability, and understanding to help them in their responses. As we progress through the stages of development, we develop understanding and skills to help us deal with illness. When disease, loss, or other disruptions occur at a younger age than expected, they change our perception of the event and may present a greater challenge to our coping skills than disruptions that are expected. For example, a child's death may seem more tragic than that of an older adult. It is important, though, not to discount the impact of disruptions that do occur during the period of an individual's life when they might be expected. For example, a client's advanced age does not necessarily make the death of a spouse less traumatic than it would be for a young spouse. Losing someone with whom one has spent most of one's life is an incredible loss, whether or not it is "expected" at that stage of life.

Nutrition: Health requires nourishment, and the most obvious form of nourishment is food. The influence of diet on human health is undeniable: Nutrient-deficiency diseases, such as pellagra and night blindness, are unknown in people who consume a nutritious diet. In addition, many chronic diseases, such as type II diabetes mellitus and heart disease, are known to be influenced by our diets, and nutrition appears to play at least a moderate role in a variety of other diseases, such as osteoporosis and some forms of cancer. As more studies look at the protective properties of some foods (e.g. phytochemicals, antioxidants) and the hazards of others (e.g. simple carbohydrates, trans fatty acids), the phrase "You are what you eat" seems more accurate each day. In Kannada language saying that "Oota Ballavanige Rogavilla" (Those who know proper eating will not get illness).

Physical activity: Healthy people are usually active people. When they are unable to maintain previous levels of activity, they may perceive themselves as less healthy. Studies support the benefit of moderate physical activity in reducing the risk of chronic disease and promoting longevity. As little as 30 minutes of gardening or 15 minutes of jogging on most days of the week can lead to these benefits. In addition, certain types of exercise have been shown to reduce the risk of specific diseases, such as osteoporosis and heart disease. For example, weight training has been shown to increase bone density and reduce the risk of osteoporosis in women over 40, and aerobic activity, such as walking, decreases the risk of heart disease. Some studies even indicate that regular aerobic exercise helps preserve neurological function as we age.

Sleep and Rest: Sleep nourishes health. During sleep, our bodies release the majority of our growth hormone, which assists in tissue regeneration, synthesis of bone, and formation of red blood cells. Sleep is also important to mental health, because it provides time for the mind to slow down and rejuvenate. Perhaps that is why problems often look much smaller in the morning. In controlled studies, people kept awake for 24 hours experienced difficulty concentrating and performing routine tasks. With increasing levels of sleep deprivation, sensory deficits and mood disturbances occurred. Outside the laboratory, mild but chronic sleep deprivation is common, particularly among students, mothers infants and young children, and people in pain.

Meaningful Work: Many people find that work is a healthy way to cope with stressors. It has been observed in *Man's Search for Meaning*, that engaging in meaningful work promotes health and, even in the midst of horrific stressors, can defend against physical and mental breakdown. The definition of meaningful work varies, but many share the view creating something that gives some purpose and meaning. Meaningful work gives some amount of exercises both physical and mental leads to promote health. People also experience meaningful work as a dimension of wellness. For many people, volunteering, pursuing hobbies, and engaging in pleasurable activities can be forms of meaningful work. For example, some find that singing, playing a musical instrument, or listening to music is particularly healing. For others, it may be literature, art, studying the intricacies of the human body, playing basketball, doing counted cross-stitch, gardening, hiking in the wilderness, or even shopping. Remember that being healthy is not all drudgery, such as denying yourself the pleasure of hot fudge sundaes and French fries. By supporting clients' life work, hobbies, and personal interests, you help them nourish their spirit in their unique way.

Lifestyle Choices: People who consider themselves healthy are usually those who make healthy lifestyle choices. They are aware of the threats to health created by cigarette smoking, alcohol consumption, drug abuse, unprotected sex, and other risky behaviors. Consider the following examples:

- A history of smoking increases recovery time from other illnesses, injuries, and surgery. Smoking also increases the risk of infertility, low-birth-weight and preterm babies, and perinatal death.
- Studies have indicated that drinking a glass of red wine each day can reduce the risk of heart disease and slow bone loss. In contrast, excessive alcohol consumption damages the brain, liver, pancreas, and intestines and can lead to malnutrition. It has also been implicated in several forms of cancer and in fetal alcohol syndrome in newborns. Finally, excessive alcohol consumption is implicated in about half of all motor vehicle accidents.
- Drug abuse is a deterioration in health, functioning, social relationships as a result of injection or inhalation of drugs. Even prescription drugs can be abused. Drug abuse is a risk factor in many diseases. For example, people who inject illegal drugs are at increased risk of HIV infection and malnutrition.

Family Relationships: Living in a healthy family is an important dimension of wellness. Moreover, the family influences a person's view of himself as well or ill. For each of the following contrasting pairs of families, which one would help you to experience high-level wellness?

- Some families place a high priority on health promotion, whereas others tend to respond to health issues only in times of serious illness.
- Some encourage adventure and risk-taking, whereas others emphasize caution in new situations.
- Some families are very open about expressing feelings and disagreements, whereas others tend to squelch personal feelings to avoid conflict in the family.
- Some families view themselves as capable and successful, others as powerless victims.
- Some families teach good negotiation skills and build a network of family support and community while encouraging the development of independence. In contrast, some parents do not have a large repertoire of skills to share with their children.

Especially when clients are coping with life threatening disease, family relationships can provide critical sustenance and preserve optimal wellness during the experience.

When illness occurs, some people prefer to be totally independent, priding themselves on never asking for or accepting help. But the reality is that during times of disruption, support from others is crucial. Families, friends, co-workers, healthcare workers, pastors, and counselors may be very effective in helping even rugged individualists deal with difficult life situations. Knowing that support is available, and being willing to accept the support, can greatly affect a person's response to disruptions.

Culture: Culture influences a person's healthcare decisions as well as her view of herself as well or ill. Individual and family health may be influenced by ethnic culture, the culture of a region or a neighborhood, the culture of a school or work environment, the culture of affluence or poverty, or the culture of a religious group. For example, the cultural group may share health-promoting values, such as a nutritious diet or regular physical activity. This is not to say that individuals can be "pegged" by their cultural background. Just as some clients respond in ways unlike their families, some make a conscious decision to break away from culturally conditioned responses.

People response to illness is also partly determined by their culture. For example, people who belong to fundamentalist faiths may interpret illness as a punishment from God for some sort of sin and bear symptoms stoically as retribution for their wrongs. People who identify themselves with the New Age movement may believe that illness is a lesson we give ourselves to teach us something we need to learn for our spiritual evolution. They may therefore try to identify the lesson of their illness–for example, "I need to slow down and be good to myself"–and then attempt to practice it. The culture of health care has traditionally responded to illness with specific therapies aimed at treating a biophysical disorder, whereas nursing, as part of the culture of holism, responds to the physical, emotional, mental, and spiritual dimensions of illness.

Religion and Spirituality: Religion and Spirituality are closely tied to culture, and clients' religious beliefs and practices can influence their healthcare choices. For example, some people believe that spiritual beliefs influence the mind-body connection to promote wellness and healing. When healing is not possible because of terminal illness or external circumstances beyond our control, spiritual reserves can help maintain our view of ourselves as "well."

Environmental Factors: The environment can also nourish wellness. For institutionalized clients, a little corner of the room that is uniquely "theirs," with photos and other mementos, can be healing. Other clients may be soothed by the quietness of a temple, a walk in the country, or even a trip to a shopping mall! Spending time in any place where they feel harmony and peace and draw strength can promote clients' health. On the other hand, environmental pollutants are a common cause of illness.

Finances: It is often said that money doesn't buy happiness. Certainly, this is true. However, money does buy access to health care and healthcare choices and thus nourishes wellness. Health insurance is often tied to employment or income level, and health insurance dictates which providers you have access to and what services are available to you. Even in countries with national health programs, the standard care available may not include the services or medications a person desires. Sometimes healthcare providers wonder why people do not take advantage of services that are available to them. Why do they let things go so long before seeking help–or fail to follow-up with recommended treatment plans? What may seem very reasonable to us as healthcare professionals may seem totally out of reach or unacceptable to those needing the help. A client's apparent lack of concern or lack of compliance to a treatment regimen may be, in reality, a problem regarding access to healthcare resources. Several factors influence access: proximity to the resources; knowledge of available resources; financial ability to access resources; financial ability to make lifestyle adjustments, such as diet or changes in employment; and trust in the resources that are available. Anyone or combination of these factors may keep individuals and families from getting the help that they need.

Factors Disrupt Health

People spend much of their lives trying to maintain good health–eating, sleeping, keeping our bodies at a comfortable temperature–in general, tending to our high-maintenance bodily needs. It's a continual process because of the many disruptions to health we face. Not all of these disruptions are incapacitating, but all challenge our ability to function and enjoy our everyday lives, and they tend to move us toward the illness end of the health-illness continuum.

Physical Disease: Disease disrupts our lives in so many ways. It may reduce individual ability to perform his/her life roles effectively or to engage in activities used to enjoy. The diagnosis of a chronic or life-threatening disease may bring shock, fear, anxiety, anger, or grief: Will I become disabled? How will I support my family? What did I do to deserve this? How can I bear saying good-bye to the people I love? It may also cause clients to question the meaning and purpose of their lives, to become more inwardly focused, or to embrace life even more fully.

Injury: Injury can cause the same symptoms and emotions as disease, but perhaps its most disruptive aspect is its suddenness. For example one patient describes his thoughts in the first days after he recovered consciousness following his cervical spinal cord injury: "The thought that kept going through my mind was: I've ruined my life. I've ruined my life, and you only get one. You can't say, 'I've spoiled this one, so can I have another, please?' There's no counter you can go up to and say, 'I dropped my ice cream cone; could I please have another one?'…. Why isn't there a higher authority you can go to and say, 'Wait a minute, you didn't mean for this to happen to me'".

Mental Illness: Clients with mental illness and their families experience a level of pain, suffering and chronic sorrow that is difficult for healthy people to fully appreciate. In addition, if the illness affects work ability, they experience loss of income and altered role relationships, accompanied by the costs of various therapies. Family members may also live in constant fear of their loved one's committing suicide. Mental illness carried with it a stigma that has been described as the single most debilitating handicap for people with mental illness. This stigmatization can also disrupt the health of family members.

Pain: Whether mild or severe, temporary or long-lasting, pain is a disruption. It's not that we can't live with pain–many people do, every day of their lives. However pain disrupts the smooth operation of our lives. It's hard to concentrate on what we are trying to accomplish when pain is competing for our attention. Pain that is easily remedied with over the counter medications or that is short-lived serves only as a minor disruption in our lives. However, pain that is all-encompassing permeates a person's entire existence. Sometimes that pain is physical, sometimes psychological. One young mother of a profoundly mentally disabled 14-year-old girl spoke of "hurting so bad that my bones hurt."

As discussed earlier, some of our nursing interventions inflict pain. Nurses ask patients to turn, cough, and deep-breathe after surgery, even though it hurts–a *lot*! Nurses put needles in them, catheterize them, and get them out of bed when they would rather sleep. Nurses pull off tape. Nurses invade their physical personal space. Nurses ask them questions about personal things, such as their bowel movements. It is a challenge to be a comforting, healing presence when nurses have to do things that cause discomfort.

Loss: Whether the loss of a job, the end of a romantic relationship, the death of a loved one, or the loss of youth, beauty, functioning, or identity, loss cuts to the core of who we are. Most of us cling to a unique identity, which often does *not* include gaining weight or getting wrinkles and gray hair, let alone being a "patient" or losing major bodily functions. When such losses occur, people typically experience a period of significant disintegration that may continue until they either find a way to cope with the loss or succeed in reinterpreting the loss in a meaningful way.

Impending Death: All people know that they have a 100% chance of dying; however, it is easy for most of them to ignore this finality and live as though death were only a remote possibility. It has been stated that during middle age, even without the presence of life-threatening illness, people tend to become more aware of the compelling reality of death: "One's life is suddenly felt to be limited, finite. It also becomes apparent that one cannot finish everything; there will not be time for all one's projects."

As a nurse, she/he will care for clients who are living in the shadow of death. Some may be aware of their condition; others may choose to deny it, ignore it, or "fight it to the end" by trying a series of conventional and alternative therapies. Caring for dying clients makes us painfully aware of our own frailty and is one of the most difficult experiences you will face as a nurse.

Competing Demands: Even in the normal flow of life, there are many competing demands. Taken independently, they may be easy to handle. Taken together, the cumulative effect wears us down. In times of illness, the other competing demands continue. Children need to be cared for. Aging parents may need care. Bills still need to be paid. Job responsibilities press in. One man with depression reported, "The whole thing bundled together-one caused the other which caused more and it was just a degenerative loop. . . . One thing feeds another which feeds another and so forth until you just constantly go down."

People ignore health issues because the competing demands are too great. Symptoms may even go unnoticed because attention is scattered in so many directions and there is not enough energy to focus on one more issue. Lack of time makes it difficult to research one's symptoms, schedule a doctor's appointment, or follow through with treatments. When a loved one's illness is acute, such as a broken bone, the stress is usually bearable. It is surprising what people can deal with if they can mark off the days on a calendar, knowing how many days are left of a disruption. As nurses, we sometimes find it easy to see how people ought to deal with their situations, even to criticize them. But it is so important to realize that the short amount of time that you spend with someone in a hospital or clinic or in a home visit is only one tiny fragment of the cumulative experience that patients and their families experience, sometimes unrelentingly for years on end.

The Unknown: Even normal life changes present challenges. For example, most new parents bringing their first baby home from the hospital are in for plenty of surprises. Every new squeak, twitch, and rash raises concern. Think of the couple who adds to that equation serious health problems in their infant. They go from anticipating a "bundle of joy" to a new world perhaps involving surgery, breathing treatments, seizures, feeding tubes, clinic visits, and keeping track of numerous medications. With some unknowns, there is time to do research and prepare. For example, if an expectant couple learn via amniocentesis (a prenatal test) that their child has a genetic defect, then during the remaining months of pregnancy they can read about the disorder; and meet with other parents who have had children similarly affected. This can help prepare them to anticipate their child's needs.

Imbalance: Our sense of justice tells us that when we are good, good things should happen. When we are bad, bad things should happen. The Buddhist concept of karma suggests that there is an equitable balance between what one gives to life and what one receives. Thus when we perceive that life has violated this rule, we experience the violation as a disruption. Our sense of balance is perhaps most dramatically disturbed by the death of children. Such deaths are sometimes referred to as "out of order" because children (of any age) "should" not die before their parents. Balance is also disrupted when patients, expecting that their painful and harrowing treatments "should" help them get better, do not get better.

Health Care

Health care is an expression of concern for fellow human beings. It is defined as a "multitude of services rendered to individuals, families and communities by the agents of the health services or professions for the purpose of promoting, maintaining, monitoring or restoring health. Such services might be staffed, organised, administered and financed in every imaginable way, but they all have one thing in common: people are being "served" that is, diagnosed, helped, cured, educated and rehabilitated by health personnel.

Health care is the preventive, curative, restorative and promotive services provided by the official and non-official agencies of a country to its citizens. In many countries, health care is completely or largely a government function. Health care includes 'medical care.' Health care and medical care are not synonymous. Medical care is a subset of a health care system. The term medical care refers chiefly to those personal services that are provided directly by physicians or rendered as a result of the physicians instructions (which range from domiciliary care to resident hospital care).

Health care has many characteristics; they include:

- *Appropriateness (relevance)* refers to whether the services is needed at all in relation to essential human needs, priorities and policies.
- *Comprehensiveness* refers to whether there is an optimum mix of preventive, curative and promotional services.
- *Adequacy* refers to if the service proportionate to requirements.
- *Availability* refers to ratio between the population of an administrative unit and the (e.g. population per center, Doctor-population ratio; Nurse-Patient ratio, etc.
- *Accessibility* refers to this may be geographical accessibility, economic accessibility, or cultural accessibility.
- *Affordability* refers to the cost of health care should be within the means of the individual and the state; and
- *Feasibility* refers to an operational efficiency of certain procedures, logistic support, manpower and material resources.

Health care is the job not of a single person, but of a large number of personnel including medical, nursing, paramedical and allied workers. They work not an isolation but together as a team. Until the British Rule, health care in India was ill-organised and based on Unani/Tibbi, Ayurveda, Siddha, and naturopathy system of medicine. After the advent of British rule and upto 1952, the health care work was predominantly curative care based on allopathy. It was available mainly to the city/town dwellers and the rich. The providers of health care were culturally at a different wavelength than the beneficiaries. The people never participated in the health program.

The 'health system' is intended to deliver health services, in other words it constitutes the management sector and involves organisational matters, e.g. planning, determining priorities, mobilising and allocating resources, translating policies into services, evaluation and health education. The components of the health system includes:

- Concepts (e.g. health and disease).
- Ideas (e.g. equity, coverage, effectiveness, efficiency, impact).
- Objects (e.g. hospitals, health centers, health programs).
- Person (e.g. providers and consumers).

The aim of a health system is health development – a process of continuous and progressive improvement of the health system of a population.

Health Care Delivery System

The health care delivery system is the complete network of agencies, facilities and all providers of health care in a specified geographic area. This system depends on a variety of health care professionals who interact with their external environment. This environment includes the patient, the patients family, the community in which the system is operating, the current technology, government agencies, the medical profession in the community, third party participants (e.g. insurance company), and many other forces that affect the patient care. The major goal of the system is to achieve optimal levels of health care for a defined populations through adequate and appropriate health care services.

A health care delivery system is method for providing health services to meet the health needs of individuals. Health services are usually organised at three levels, each level supported by a higher level to which the patient is referred. These levels are:

1. Primary health care: This is the first level of contact between the individual and the health system where 'essential health care' is provided, which includes:

- Health education of prevailing health problem
- Food supply and nutrition
- Water supply and basic sanitation
- M.C.H. and FP services
- Immunizations
- Prevention and control of locally endemic diseases
- Appropriate treatment for common diseases and injuries
- Provision of essential drugs.

A majority of prevailing health complaints and problems can be satisfactorily dealt with at this level. The level of care is closest to the people. In the Indian context this care is provided by primary health centers and their subcenters, with community participation.

2. Secondary health care: At this level, most complex problems are dealt with. This care comprises essentially curative services and is provided by the district hospitals and community health centers. This level services as the first referral level in the health system.

3. Tertiary health care: This level offers super-speciality care. This care is provided by the regional/central level institutions. These institutions provide not only highly specialized care, but also planning and managerial skills and teaching for specialised staff. In addition, the tertiary level supports and complements the actions carried out at the primary level.

The main purposes of the levels of care are as follows:

1. Primary care: The major purposes of primary care are to promote wellness and prevent illness or disability. Care is coordinated by the office of the primary care providers. Traditionally health care system focused on treating illness rather than promoting wellness. Now however the focus is on health promoting behaviors such as regular exercise, reducing fat in the diet, monitoring cholesterol level and reducing air pollution, wellness promotion activities may be directed toward the individual, the family or the community.

2. Secondary care: Services within the realm of secondary care—diagnosis and treatment—occur after the client exhibits symptoms of illness. Acute treatment centers (hospitals) still constitute the predominant site for the delivering of these health care services, but there is a growing movement to provide diagnostic and therapeutic services in locations that are more easily accessed by the population. These are often satellite care centers of major hospital, where holistic care provided.

3. Tertiary care: The major purpose of tertiary (rehabilitative) care is to restoring an individual to the state of health that existed before the development of an illness. When a person is unable to regain previous functional abilities, the rehabilitation goal is to reach the optimal level of health possible. For example, a client regains partial use of an arm after experiencing stroke. Restorable care is holistic in that the physiological, psychological, social, and spiritual aspects of the person are all addressed in the provision of care.

Today there is more of an emphasis on the holistic promotion of wellness and on the preventive aspects of care. Nurses are the professional care giver, when they got intimate contact with clients allows them the opportunity not only to provide physical and emotional support, but also to teach ways to take an active role in maintaining health. WHO places emphasis on combating communicable diseases educating health workers and improving health of all people in the universe. Many persons believe that health or wellness is only absence of disease. In its truest form health is refers to the wellbeing of whole person.

Health Care Team

Team refer to a group of people with different knowledge levels, abilities, skills, personalities, who complement each other and work together to attain common goals. They cooperate with each other and they follow set of rules and regulations. Health care services are delivered by a multidisciplinary team.

A team means a set of specially prepared persons working together for a common goal. Health team consists of particular group of health care professionals to provide total care for clients. In most practice settings, the nurse works with other members of the team. The involvement of many different persons in the client's health care have the risk of fragmenting care. Nurses have the greatest opportunity to interact with all the other professionals in the health care team. They co-ordinate and integrate various services within the care plan.

In the hospital there is a nursing team for the care of patients. The team leader will be the nursing superintendent. She will delegate her responsibilities to the head nurses who are the team leaders of each ward. She is responsible for assigning duties to the other members of the team in the ward for the care of patients there.

Non-professional workers are also required to be considered such as clerks, attenders cleaners, etc. to perform their particular works to meet the needs of the clients and family in the hospital.

Health team is a team put incharge of health and medical institutions, organisations, projects, campaigns, etc. with the avowed objectives of preventive, promotive, curative, and rehabilitative aspects of diseases and disabilities.

Health team is district hospitals level comprises a medical superintendent, residential medical officer, a nursing superintendent, deputy nursing superintendent, physicians, surgeons, radiologists, ophthalmologists, obstetrician and gynecologists, and other specialists, nursing sisters, staff nurses, laboratory technicians, pharmacists, dieticians, medicosocial workers, record keeper and ward boys/ayahs.

Health team at primary health center consists of medical officers, staff nurses, block extension educators, female health assistants (LHV), female health worker (ANM), male health assistants, male health workers, laboratory technicians, store clerk, officer clerk, ward boys/ayahs, and drivers.

It is important that team should be infused with team spirit. The members of the team should work in a co-ordinated manner. The effort of each member should synchronize with that of others so as to produce a synergistic effort. In a team the action of any one has no value of its own. It is worth only in so far that it harmonises with the acts of others and thus carries the team forward toward its objectives. To put it differently, in a team no member is superior to another, no one's actions are more important than those of others; all actions are equal and complementary.

Models of Health and Illness

A model is defined as a way of presenting a situation in logical term to show the structure of the original idea or object. It is a representation of the original order of object that gives direction in much the same way that a pattern of dress is to guide and provide instruction for making a dress.

A model is a theoretical way of understanding a concept or idea. Because health and illness are complex concepts. Models are used to understand the relationships, between these concepts and the client, attitudes toward health and health practices.

Since the definitions of health and illness are not specific, health models have been developed to help describe the concepts and relationships involved in health and illness. Nurses have developed health models to understand clients health behaviors and beliefs so that effective health care can be provided. Health beliefs are a person's ideas, convictions and attitudes about health and illness. Health beliefs may be based on factual information or misinformation, common sense or myths or reality or false expectations. Health behavior usually results from health beliefs, they can positively or negatively affect health. Positive behaviors are activities related to maintaining, attaining or regaining good health, and preventing illness. Negative behaviors are activities or practices actually or potentially harmful to health.

Nurses have developed health models to understand clients health behaviors and belief so that effective healthcare can be provided. These models allow nurses to understand and predict clients' health behaviors including how they use health services and adhere to recommended therapies.

Purposes of Models of Nursing

A nursing model serves as a unifying framework of three different areas; nursing education, nursing practice, and nursing research. In nursing education, a model provides a means for organizing information into a meaningful whole. It serves to identify the content needed to achieve the goal of nursing care, the learning objectives and criteria for evaluating nursing practice. As nursing education continues to expand, the model provides a way to classify and incorporate relevant data and to delete obsolete material.

In nursing practice, a model gives direction for the assessment process and provides a systematic approach to patient care. It shows the nurse that to look for and how to provide nursing care. A model also stimulates scientific inquiry and research to validate nursing theories and concepts and to improve nursing practice.

Components of a Model

The essential components of model answer the questions, who does what? to whom? where? how? why? In the nursing model, these components are as follows:

- Values on which the model is based
- Client or patient as the recipient of the action
- Goals of the action or intervention
- Intervention or service provided in terms of framework, the procedures, the agent, and the source of energy.

These components identify what the nurse will assess and what is to be done about the health problems presented by the client or patient. Because nursing is a service performed for the people, values are important aspect of the model. The goals established for nursing care must be consistent with cultural values and beliefs of the patient. The manner in which one views the recipient of nursing care is based on one's values about man as 'a biopsychosocial being', one's belief about health and illness, and one's belief about the relationship between the nurse and the recipient of nursing care. A model also prescribes the method and the actions used to achieve the goal setting in which the nursing care takes place, and the source of energy involved.

A model can be defined as a symbolic depiction in logical terms of idealized relatively simple situation showing the structure of the original system. A model, then is conceptual representation of reality.

A theory may be defined as a scientifically acceptable general principle which governs practice or is proposed to explain observed facts. Theory is a different level of reality representation than a model is, and provides the working insides of a model.

Model may represent structure while theory cannote function.

Health-Illness Continuum Model

According to this model, health is a dynamic state that continuously alters, as a person adapts to changes in the internal and external environment to maintain a state of physical, emotional, intellectual, social developmental and spiritual well-being. Illness is a process in which the functioning of a person is diminished or impaired on one or more dimensions, when compared with the persons previous condition. That means health is a constantly changing state, with high level wellness, and death being on opposite ends of a continuous or graduated scale. Because health and illness are relative qualities, existing on varying degrees, it is more accurate to consider health and illness on terms of point on scale given below (Fig. 1.3).

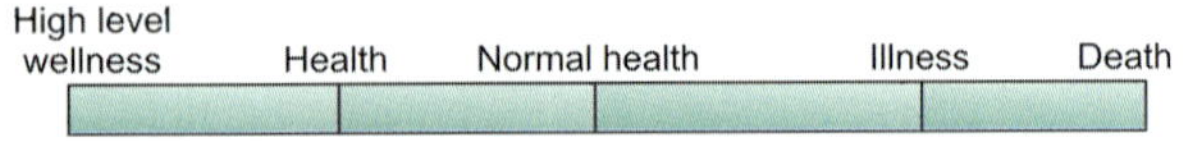

Figure 1.3: Health and illness scale

The nurse must be aware that a client with a chronic illness may place himself or herself at different points on the continuum at any given time, depending on how well the client believes he or she is functioning for the illness. According to Neuman (1990) health on a continuum is the degree of client wellness that exists at any point of time, ranging from an optimal wellness condition, with available energy at its maximum to death, which represents total energy depletion.

High Level Wellness Model

Halber Dunn (1961) described his model of high level wellness as functioning to one's maximum potential while maintaining balance and purposeful direction in the environment. He differentiates, wellness from good health believing that good health is a passive state, wherein the person is not ill. Wellness on the other hand, is a more active state, oriented towards maximizing the potentials of the individual, regardless of the state of health. He also defined processes that help the individual to know who and what he or she is. The processes are:
- Being recognizing self as separate and individual
- Belonging (being part of a whole)
- Becoming (growing and developing)
- Befitting (making personal chances to befit the self for the future).

The model is a holistic in nature, allowing nurses to care for the individual with regard to all dimensional factors affecting the persons state of being as he or she strives to reach maximum potential.

The concept of high level wellness can be applied to the individual, family, community, environment, and society. This model requires the individual to maintain a continuum of balance and purposeful directions within the environments. It involves progress towards a higher level functioning an open ended and ever expanding challenge to live at the fullest potential. Last, there is continued integration of health practices by the individual at increasing higher levels throughout the life. According to this model healthcare directed at helping a client achieve high level wellness emphasizes health promotion and illness prevention activities rather than treatment of illness.

Agent-Host-Environment Model

Agent-host-environment model was originally developed by Leavell and Clark (1965) to describe health in a community, but it is also useful in when examining the cause of the disease in an individual. Accordingly the level of health and illness of an individual or group depends on the dynamic relationship of the agent, host and the environment (Fig. 1.4).

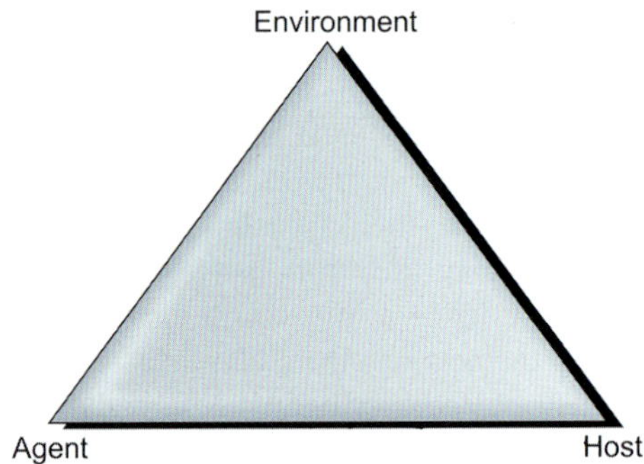

Figure 1.4: Agent-host-environment model

The agent is an internal or external factor that must be present or absent for an illness. Agents can be biological, chemical, physical, mechanical or psychosocial.

The host is the person or persons who may be susceptible to a particular illness or disease, i.e. living being, human or animal capable of being infected or effected by an agent.

Host factors reaction is influenced by family history, age, sex, kind of lifestyles.

The environment is that everything external to the host that makes illness more or less likes. Physical environment includes economic level, climate, living conditions and air, water, food, light, housing ventilation. Social environment consists of factors that are involving individuals and group interaction with others, causing physiopsychosocial illness.

This model is actually more useful in predicting illness than in promoting wellness, although recognition of risk factors resulting from interaction of agent-host-environment is important in the promotion and maintenance of health.

Health Belief Model

Health belief model developed by Rosestoch *et al* (1974) is based on what people perceive, or believe to be true about themselves in relation to health. Health-belief model has three components (Fig. 1.5).
- Perceived susceptibility to a disease, e.g. smokers suspect of cancer.
- Perceived seriousness of a disease and its effect on individual lifestyle, e.g. cancer affects on lifestyle.
- Perceived value of action, e.g. preventive measures or curative measures.

The first component of this model involves the individuals perceptions of susceptibility to an illness. The second component is the individuals perception of the seriousness of illness. This perception is influenced and modified by demographic variables (age, sex, race, ethnicity, etc), socio-psychological variables (personality, social class, peer and reference groups, pressure groups, etc), perceived threats of the illness, and cue for action (advice from others, family friends and medical profession, mass media, etc). The third component, i.e. the likelihood that a person will take preventive action, is the perception of the benefits of taking action. Preventive actions may include lifestyles changes, increased adherence to medical therapies or a search for medical advice and treatment.

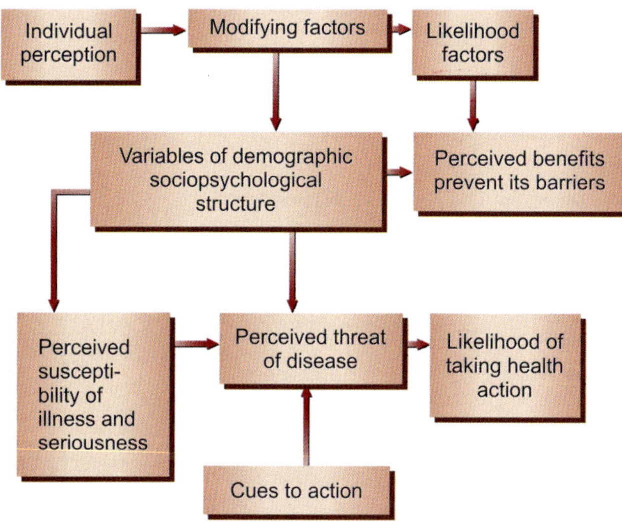

Figure 1.5: Health belief model

This health belief model helps nurses understand factors influencing clients' perceptions, beliefs and behaviors, and plan that will most effectively assist clients in maintaining regarding health and preventing illness. This model is also useful in teaching individuals about their health and illness.

Dimensions of Health and Illness

The factors that influence health and illness related to the person in terms of the human dimensions are as follows:

Each person is a composite of physical dimension, emotional dimension, environmental dimension, intellectual dimensions, social cultural dimensions and spiritual dimension and each dimension influences the behavior of the person receiving care (Fig. 1.6).

Physical dimension: It includes genetic make up, age, developmental level, race, and sex. All are parts of individuals, which strongly influence health status, and health practices.

Emotional dimension: It express that how the mind and body interact to affect body function and to respond to body; emotion also influences health. Long-term stress affects the body system and anxiety affects health habits. Calm acceptance and relaxation can actually change the body responses to illness.

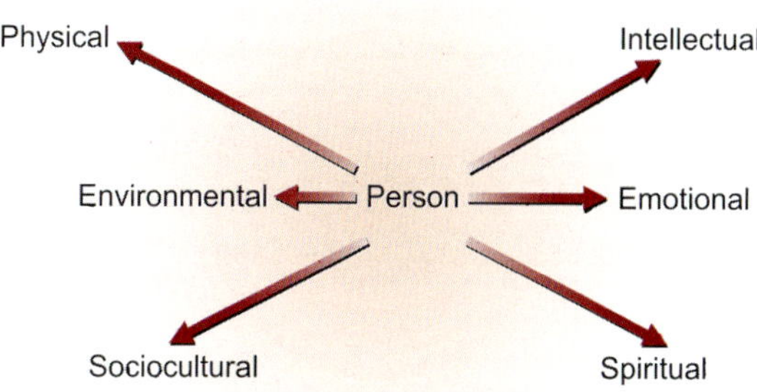

Figure 1.6: Factors affecting health and illness

Intellectual dimension: It encompasses cognitive abilities, educational background and past experiences. These influence a client responses to teaching about health and reactions to nursing care during illness. They also play major role in health behaviors.

Environmental dimension: It has many influences on health and illness. Housing, sanitation, climate and pollution of air, food and water are aspects of the environment, which causes illness.

Socio-cultural dimension: It includes individual's economic level, educational status, lifestyle, family, and culture. These are all with influence on the health and illness of the people.

Spiritual dimension: Spiritual and religious beliefs and values are the important components of how a person behaves in the health and illness. It is important that nurse respects these values and understand their importance to the individual client.

Nursing focus on health: Health is a state of complete physical; social and psychological wellbeing that may coexist and interact with illness. Health and illness are viewed as polar opposites but degrees of health and illness are noted from peak wellness to death (Fig. 1.7).

The Lamberton model of health and illness as separate but coexisting continual development and ecology are viewed as interacting axes which influence the two-continuum (Fig. 1.8).

Health and illness are two separate phenomena. The types of care for each are different (Fig. 1.9).

Health and illness are separate but coexisting and interacting phenomena. On the health continuum the interventions include health promotion for high level wellness, prevention of disruption in health, detection of possible alteration in health, and restoration of actual alteration in health. On the illness continuum the intervention includes prevention of potential disease, detection of possible disease, treatment of common illness, maintenance of stable illness, and treatment of acute illness. All those involved

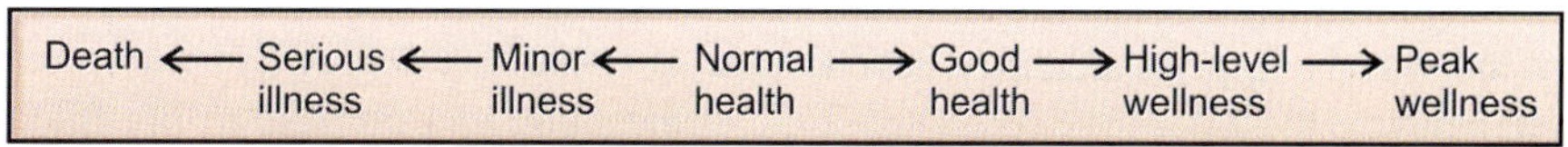

Figure 1.7: Degrees of health and wellness

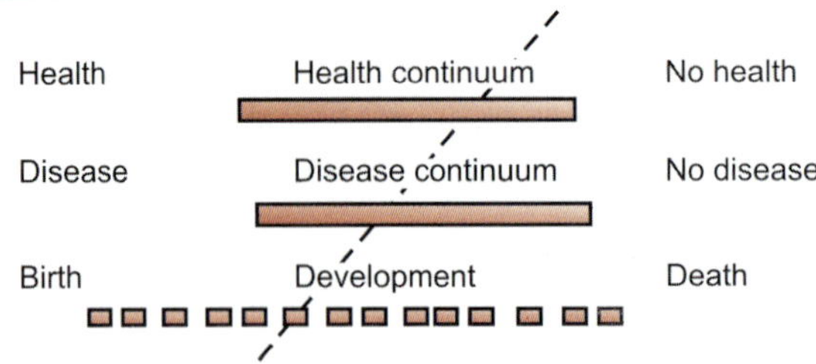

Figure 1.8: Lamberton model of health and illness

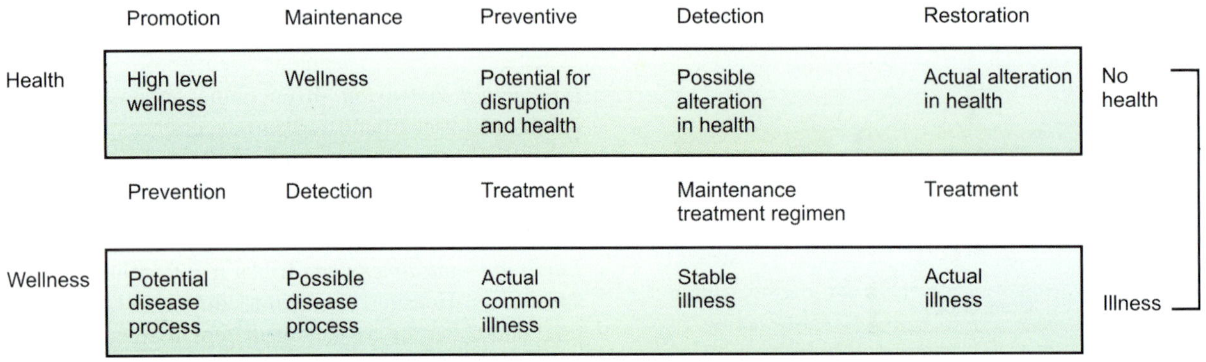

	Promotion	Maintenance	Preventive	Detection	Restoration	
Health	High level wellness	Wellness	Potential for disruption and health	Possible alteration in health	Actual alteration in health	No health
	Prevention	Detection	Treatment	Maintenance treatment regimen	Treatment	
Wellness	Potential disease process	Possible disease process	Actual common illness	Stable illness	Actual illness	Illness

Figure 1.9: Care for health and wellness

in the health and illness care system contribute to one or both types of care at some level of intervention. The nurses' primary focus, however is health and the physician mainly emphasizes on illness. Rehabilitation or assistance to peaceful deaths are interventional that incorporate both health and illness care.

Nursing care however, emphasizes detection of an alteration of those areas of health continuum, that require the most care, for instance, sleep activity, comfort, skin integrity, nutrition, and self care. The recognition of the major role that environment and lifestyles have on both health and illness statures required responsibility of the people for their own health.

Wellness

Health is a complex phenomenon that involves physical, mental, and spiritual aspects. Having good health is an almost universal desire. Wellness is a way of life oriented towards optimal health and wellbeing.

Wellness is a dynamic status of health in which an individual progresses toward a higher level of functioning, achieving an optimal balance between internal and external environment.

Wellness is defined as a state of optimal health wherein an individual maximizes human potential, moves toward integration of human functioning has greater self-awareness and self-satisfaction, and takes responsibility for health and also behaviours exhibited by individuals. Experts identified seven areas of wellness as given below:

- *Emotional wellness*: Emotions bridge the gap between body and mind. The individual who is emotionally well understands his own feelings and knows when to express them appropriately. This person accepts limitations, copes with stress in healthy ways, has the ability to adjust to change, is optimistic and happy, enjoys life, and shows respect and affection to others.
- *Mental wellness*: The person who is mentally well is alert, curious, clear thinking, open-minded, creative, logical and accepting of others. This person also has a good memory, common sense, and a desire for continual learning.
- *Intellectual wellness*: Intellectual wellness is revealed by an ability to think, process information, and solve problems. The intellectually well person questions and evaluates information and situations, is creative, flexible, and open to new ideas, and learns from life experiences.
- *Vocational wellness*: The individual who is satisfied in school or college and/or job and who works in harmony with others enjoys vocational wellness.
- *Social wellness*: The person who shows affection, fairness, concern, and respect for others; communicates effectively; has satisfying relationships; and interacts well with others enjoys social wellness. This person has a network of friends and family, is a member of various organizations and enjoys working together. Other behaviors exhibited are confidence, loyalty, honesty, and tolerance.
- *Spiritual wellness*: Spiritual wellness gives direction, meaning, and purpose to life through values, morals, and ethics. The spirituality healthy person has optimism, faith, and high self-esteem.

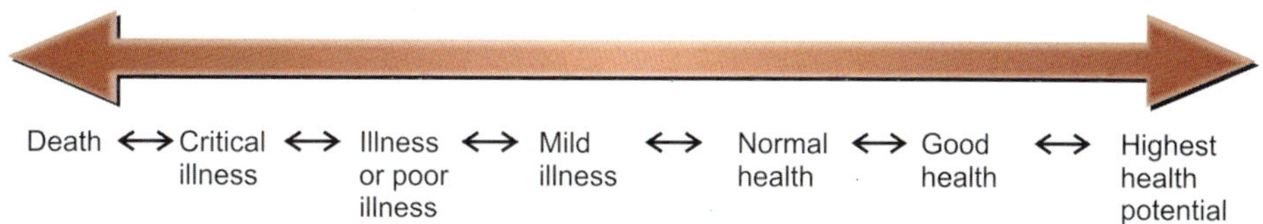

Figure 1.10: Health continuum

- *Physical wellness*: Physical wellness is seen in individuals who exercise regularly, eat a well-balanced diet, and have regular physical examinations. They avoid risky sexual behavior; try to limit exposure to environmental contaminants; and restrict the intake of alcohol, tobacco, caffeine, and drugs.

Nursing the whole person, or holistic health care, is a comprehensive approach to health care. It considers physical, intellectual, sociocultural, psychological, and spiritual aspects, the response to illness, and the effect of illness on a person's ability to meet self-care needs. Also taken into account is the individual's responsibility for personal wellbeing. Teaching preventive care is always a focus. The details of different aspects of wellness discussed in later part of this chapter.

Nurses work with people throughout life to promote wellness and prevent illness. The highest level of wellness should be the goal of each nurse and every client.

Wellness is a responsibility, a choice, a lifestyle design that helps maintain the highest potential for personal health. The health continuum is a way to visualize the range of an individual's health, from highest health potential to death (Fig. 1.10).

An individual's place on the continuum may change daily or even hourly depending on what is happening to that individual. Constant effort is required to balance all aspects of life and to maintain the highest level of health. A person at the highest level of wellness is one who demonstrates good physical self-care, emotional well-being, creative expression, and positive relationships with others.

Wellness incorporates physical, intellectual, sociocultural, psychological, and spiritual wellness. To provide holistic care, all aspects of the individual's wellness must be addressed.

Maslow's Hierarchy of Needs

Abraham Maslow developed a theory of behavioral motivation based on needs. This theory is often referred to as Maslow's Hierarchy of Needs. There are live levels in this hierarchy. The basic physiological needs must be met to maintain life. The rest of the needs are related to quality of life. They are safety and security, love and belonging, self-esteem, and self-actualization. The needs of the lower levels must be met before a person is motivated to meet the needs of the next higher level (Fig. 1.11).

Many nursing programs use Maslow's Hierarchy of Needs as a basis for planning the care of clients. This ensures that basic physiological needs as well as the other needs are assessed and addressed in individualized care plans.

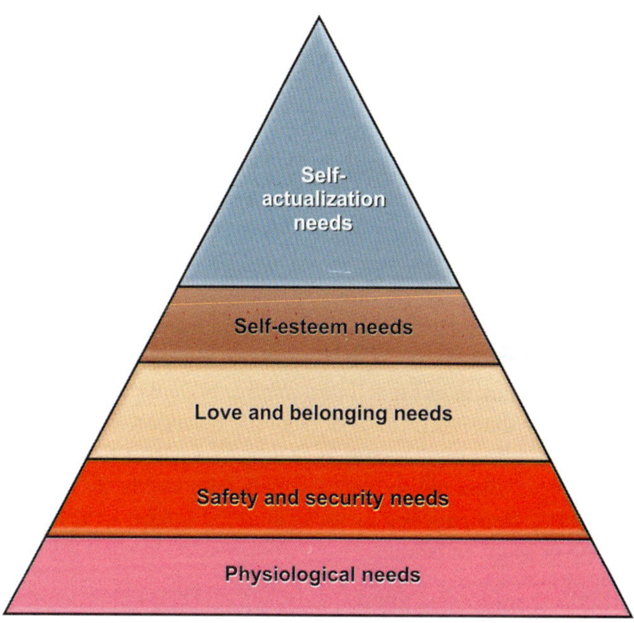

Figure 1.11: Maslow's hierarchy of needs

Physiological needs: Although Maslow (1954) did not specifically identify the physiological needs, they are generally accepted to be the needs of oxygen, water, food, elimination, rest (sleep)/activity (exercise), and sex. With the exception of sex, all of these needs must be met for the life of the individual to be maintained. Satisfying the sexual need, while not necessary for individual survival, is necessary for survival of the human race. The basic physiological needs must be met before higher-level needs become motivators of behavior. For example, a person who is truly hungry is motivated by that need, and behavior is focused on getting food.

Safety and security needs: The next level, safety, encompasses the needs for shelter, stability, security, physical safety, and freedom from undue anxiety. Safety needs include both physical and emotional aspects. Illness is often a threat to safety because the stability of life is disrupted.

Love and belonging needs: The third level of the hierarchy. love and belonging, incorporates not only giving but also receiving affection, Having friends and participating with others in groups and organizations are two ways to meet these needs. Meeting these needs is extremely important fix mental health.

Self-esteem needs: The needs of the self-esteem level are met by achieving success in work and other activities. Recognition from others increases self-esteem and feelings of pride in one's accomplishments.

Self-actualization needs: Self-actualization is the highest level of the Maslow hierarchy. A person who has met these needs is confident, self-fulfilled, and creative; looks for challenges; and sees beauty and order in the world.

Maslow contends that because most people are so busy meeting the physiological and safety and security needs, little time or energy is left to meet the love and belonging, self-esteem, and self-actualization needs: thus, most people are less than satisfied at higher levels of the hierarchy. Even when the lower two levels are met without much trouble, many people have personalities and attitudes that make meeting the needs of the three higher levels difficult, if not impossible.

An individual does not move steadily up the hierarchy. As life situations change, a person's unmet needs change, and behavior is motivated by different levels of the hierarchy. For example, if a person who is working to meet the self-esteem need is suddenly laid off at work, the safety and security need of providing financially for self and family suddenly becomes the unmet need that motivates that person's behavior.

For providing quality care to clients, first nurses to aware of themselves. Then taking care of their own needs (Maslow's Hierarchy). Self-care is a factor in all nurses to be an effective care giver as given below.

- **Self-awareness of Nurses**

Self-awareness is consciously knowing how the self thinks, feels, believes, and behaves at any specific time. Being self-aware is a constant process that is focused on the present. A person's thoughts, feelings, and beliefs are interrelated and greatly influence behavior. Being self-aware influences a person in several ways.

Self-awareness may make a person uncomfortable. Awareness allows the person to either accept or alter feelings, beliefs, and behavior. One can learn to be self-aware.

Self-awareness is extremely important for nurses. Nurses must understand themselves so that their personal feelings, attitudes, and needs do not interfere with providing quality client care. The nurse who is self-aware is more likely to make decisions in response to the client's needs rather than the nurse's own needs. For example, student nurses–and even experienced nurses–are often anxious about caring for a specific client. By taking some time to practice self-awareness, the nurse might discover that the anxiety stems from never having performed the procedure in question. The nurse can then deal directly with the situation by reviewing the procedure and requesting assistance from an instructor or supervisor. All decisions about client care must be made in response to the client's needs, not the nurse's needs.

- **Development of Self-Concept**

Self-concept is how a person thinks or feels about himself. These thoughts and feelings come from the experiences the person has with others and relied how the person thinks others view him.

Self-concept begins forming in infancy. An infant whose needs are met feels satisfied and good. Experiences, both positive and negative, influence a person's self-concept. Interactions with significant others, such as parents, extended family, and friends, have a great impact on self-concept. This is true not only during the developing years, but also throughout life. Because of its influence on client care, it is important for the nurse to be aware of how her own self-concept has developed. Self-concept develops through feedback from others. The nurse is responsible for providing feedback that will not negatively affect the client's self-concept.

An individual who is constantly ignored or who receives messages such as "Don't bother me," "Can't you do anything right?" or "You don't have any sense" may very well begin to view himself in these terms, with the likely result being a negative self-concept. On the other hand, a person who is shown caring and who hears messages such as "Let me help you in a minute." "Let's try it this way." or "Have you thought about. . . ?" will move toward a positive self-concept.

The most effective means to teach wellness is by positive example. By first practicing good health habits as a nursing student, then become, by an example of an important factor in your clients' overall well-being and good health. Reminds that health is a personal choice and that each person has control over his or her own wellness.

Nurses helping clients recognize how their own actions can prevent many of the conditions that cause illness. Choosing to exercise regularly, to eat a balanced diet, to eat breakfast each day, to control fat content, and to select from the basic food groups are good rules for wellness. Choosing to not smoke, to practice moderation in the use of alcohol, to avoid all nontherapeutic drugs, and to practice safe sex can help prevent many of the conditions that cause disease and death.

While emphasizing health promotion and client education, the nurse must also encourage and respect the client's responsibility for wellness. This respect allows the client to become an active partner in, rather than a passive recipient of, health care. It is not enough to tell a client *what* can be done to improve health; the nurse must also be prepared to explain *why*. If a client understands the reason behind an action, the likelihood of compliance increases.

Just as nurses are aware of themselves as a whole person with many components, help their clients see themselves and their health care as more than physical health. Help clients understand how physical, intellectual, sociocultural, psychological, and spiritual health are all related and can lead to an overall sense of well-being. This is the full meaning of holistic care.

(a) Physical Wellness

Physical wellness refers to a healthy body that functions at an optimal level. To achieve physical wellness a person must practice good grooming; use proper body mechanics; have good posture; refrain from smoking and the use of drugs and alcohol; and have adequate nutrition, sleep, rest, relaxation, and exercise.

- **Grooming:** The nurse communicates a message of health and well-being by being clean and neatly dressed. A daily bath or shower and the use of a deodorant form the basis of good grooming. Hair should be clean, combed, and neatly styled, Perfume should not be worn, because it may be offensive to clients. Frequent brushing, regular denial check-ups, and avoiding refined sugars helps control dental caries,

  While important for client safety, good hand hygiene is also crucial to the nurse's wellness. Antiseptic hand lotion can be used to prevent cracked, dry skin. Fingernails should be kept short, because long nails not only harbor dirt and microorganisms but can also scratch clients. Standard precautions have been established. These precautions are designed to protect all health care workers and their clients from the transmission of communicable disease. Good hand hygiene is an integral part of Standard Precautions. As soon as nurses have been taught the skill of hand hygiene practice it. Make it a part of daily life. Encourage your clients to establish good hand hygiene habits. Jewelry, which can harbor bacteria, and excessive make-up are both inappropriate for the Burse in uniform. Clothing should be clean and free of stains and wrinkles. Clients will have confidence in the nurse who maintains a professional appearance and who practices good hygiene.

- **Body Mechanics:** Wellness involves more than just good grooming practices. It also requires proper body mechanics, (i.e. using the body in the safest and most efficient way to move or lift objects). The use of proper body mechanics is very important because many of the skills and tasks that will perform as a nurse involve lifting or moving clients or objects. Bending, lifting, or stooping can cause injury if done incorrectly. One of the first skills you will study involves the practice of proper body mechanics to prevent physical disability, including safe methods for bending, lifting, and moving.

- **Posture:** Good posture is the basis for proper body mechanics. Good posture means the ability to carry oneself well and in correct body alignment. Posture can also send messages about a person. A person who stands with feet, spread apart and with hands on hips, for example, may be perceived as aggressive or authoritative, whereas one who holds the arms tightly folded over the chest may be viewed as closed minded. Observe those around as they communicate with others. Notice the differences in posture. Does the person who stands in good alignment, with shoulders back and head up, convey self-confidence and capability? Does the individual whose shoulders are drooped and head bowed convey depression, sadness, or lack of self-confidence? As continue studies and begin client care, will realize that clients appreciate having nurses who appear confident in their own abilities and decision making. When with clients, nurse must be particularly careful of the way she stand. Remember that nurses posture sends messages about their attitude and feelings. The client should feel that nurses are confident, caring, relaxed, and willing to listen.

- **Smoking:** Smoking contributes to many health hazards and illnesses. It may also be personally offensive to clients. The odor of smoke on clothing or the breath (halitosis) may precipitate allergic reactions or lead to a feeling of nausea in some clients. Most health care facilities have strict rules about smoking. Many facilities are "smoke free." The nurse should never smoke in a client's room. Furthermore, great care should be taken to ensure that no offensive tobacco odors remain if the nurse uses or is in dose proximity to tobacco products. In each situation, every effort should be made to enforce all safety rules for clients and visitors. "No smoking" signs should be posted and strictly enforced when oxygen is in use.

- **Drugs and Alcohol:** A frightening trend is that increasing rate of alcohol and drug abuse. Drug abuse has become so widespread within the health professions that impaired caregiver programs have been implemented. Many states now provide access to treatment for the impaired nurse through the state board of nursing. Drug abuse can begin very insidiously when a nurse says to herself, "I'll borrow a pill just this once for my headache." The second time is easier, and the downward spiral begins. A nurse should never give or make a drug available to anyone without the written order of a physician or other person who can legally prescribe medications, such as a nurse practitioner.

- **Nutrition:** Nursing is emotionally, mentally, and physically demanding. Nurses must be able to think clearly and work efficiently. A balanced diet, including fruits and vegetables, whole grains and cereals, milk and milk products, and meats or other protein foods, is required for optimal body function. Nursing students may be tempted to skip meals, omit breakfast, eat snacks, and follow fad diets. This is never a wise practice. The need for food must be satisfied before you will be motivated to meet the need to learn or to study. Always eat a balanced breakfast. Pastries and coffee, although satisfying in the moment, elevate the blood sugar level only for a short while before the level plummets. This reaction leaves a person drained, irritable, and hungrier than before. Try to avoid snacking on junk foods, which contain empty calories, or those having very little nutritional value. Instead, plan to eat fruit or high-protein snacks. Plan a routine for mealtimes, and stick to it. Doing so helps prevent the urge to binge on unhealthy snacks. Also, drink plenty of water. Water is the body's most important nutrient. A human being can survive for weeks without food but only for a few days without water. By weight, approximately 60% of the adult body is water. In order to maintain proper fluid balance and to facilitate the elimination of body wastes, it is necessary to drink plenty of fluids. Most authorities agree that the average adult needs six to eight (8-ounce) glasses of water each day. It is important to maintain a balance in the diet for optimal wellness.

- **Sleep, Rest, Relaxation, and Exercise:** Wellness implies more than eating balanced meals, avoiding harmful substances, and practicing good grooming. Wellness also means taking time to enjoy yourself. It means making time for sleep, rest, relaxation, and exercise.

Sleep is time for the body to replenish its energy reserves and to heal itself. The amount of time needed may vary with the individual or even with the day. One person may need 8 hours of sleep after a heavy workday but need only 6 hours after a less strenuous day. An infant, of course, needs more sleep than does a young adult. Sleep is necessary to allow the body's organs to function at their most minimal levels. This period of rejuvenation for the body is necessary for total wellness.

Rest, meaning conscious freedom from activity and worry, is just as important as sleep. Rest is a time of inner quiet and physical inactivity. Only when a person is relaxed and at inner peace can that person rest.

Relaxation means doing something for the fun of it. That which is relaxing to one person may not be relaxing to another. Examples or relaxation activities include reading a novel, reading to children, playing cards or other games, fishing, painting, or sewing or other handwork. Many experts agree that the best rest follows planned exercise. During exercise, heart rate and breathing increase, circulation improves, and muscles stretch. Exercise is also a time to free the mind of anxiety producing thoughts. Sometimes after a day's work, a brisk walk frees the mind and allows the body to relax in preparation for rest.

Whichever form of exercise, rest, and relaxation is best for you, make time for it in each day, Rest and relaxation as well as regular sleep and exercise are essential ingredients for wellness and result in reduced fatigue and irritability and possibly increased resistance to colds, flu, and serious infections. Furthermore, the capacity to concentrate increases, which should make a significant difference in your studies.

(b) Intellectual Wellness

Intellectual wellness is the ability to function as an independent person capable of making sound decisions. Such decisions are based on the individual's needs but at the same time take into account the needs of others. Clear thinking, problem-solving skills, good judgment, and the desire to continually learn are all qualities found in the person who is intellectually well.

Nursing requires making many decisions, some of which may mean life or death to the client. The nurse must have intellectual wellness to be able to make the best decisions possible with regard to client care,

(c) Sociocultural Wellness

Sociocultural wellness is the ability to appreciate the needs of others and to care about one's environment and the inhabitants of it. As a nurse, you will care for clients of all ages and races who speak different languages and come from various cultural groups. Each client's culture (behavior, customs, and beliefs of the family, extended family, tribe, nation, and society) influences the way that person views wellness and responds to illness.

It is important that the nurse understand that while everyone's basic needs are the same, the ways that those needs are met may vary based on the client's culture. Today's population is working,

playing, and contributing to society for more years than ever before. People are more health conscious, better educated, and more involved in making health choices than perhaps any previous generation. Nurses should encourage such involvement and work to dispel discrimination by accepting each person as an individual.

(d) Psychological Wellness

Psychological wellness encompasses the enjoyment of creativity, the satisfaction of the basic need to love and be loved, the understanding of emotions, and the ability to maintain control over emotions. Emotions are an integral part of the balance sought in life and are important factors in the way a person relates to others. They are measures of inner thoughts and feelings and are apparent in actions or behaviors.

Wellness requires that individuals recognize emotions and control their reactions in various situations. By controlling their emotions, nurses help create a therapeutic environment within which to help clients. Another aspect of emotional wellness is a positive attitude. An attitude is a feeling about people, places, or things that is evident in the way one behaves. It can be positive or negative. Studies have described the role that a positive attitude plays in helping conquer illness. Many authorities believe having a positive attitude is at least as important as having the best treatment for an illness. Nursing requires that you see the best in people during the worst of times. In order to survive and function well, the nurse needs to see life as a challenge and as a gift to cherish and enjoy.

Positive attitude is so important for nurses when caring for their clients, it is vital that nurse share their with them. An attitude can become a habit. If nurse repeatedly think positively, soon he/she will unconsciously and seeing the positive aspects in any given situation. Whereas having a negative attitude will increase chances of being miserable and unsuccessful, having a positive attitude will help the day go smoother and increase the likelihood of coworkers being cheerful and willing to help. Having a positive attitude will also help in studies. It will help open mind and will spill into daily life, making that life more enjoyable.

(e) Spiritual Wellness

Spiritual wellness manifests as inner strength and peace. Spirituality is a broader concept than religion and involves one's relationship with self, others, the natural order, and a higher power. It manifests as meaningful work, creative expression, familiar rituals, and religious practices. Spirituality involves finding meaning in everything, including life, illness, and death. Spiritual needs include love, meaning in life, forgiveness, and hope. The human spiritual dimension is a major healing force. It can mean the difference between life and death, wellness and illness.

Florence Nightingale spoke boldly about the importance of the spiritual aspect of client care. It has been stated that the richness of a person's interactions with others correlates with positive health outcomes, and that practice of any religion correlates with greater health and increased longevity. Nurses are not asked to take over the role of spiritual counselors. Rather, nurses are encouraged to integrate a holistic approach by extending love, compassion, and empathy; motivating clients to address spiritual issues; and suggesting how they might do so. There has been two suggestions regarding nursing and spiritual wellness: (1) Nurses who have strong religious convictions should not impose those convictions on their clients, and (2) nurses should never assume that clients who have no religious interests have no interest in spiritual values. Clients not interested in religion can be encouraged to become involved in some humanitarian endeavor or to look at life's everyday wonders in a different way.

Nurses play a key role in helping clients find hope and meaning in life, it is important that nurses understand spirituality. For many, religious practices are an expression of their spirituality. An important function for the nurse is to respect the religious beliefs of clients, provide clients with privacy to practice those beliefs, and make spiritual guidance available through the client's minister, priest, rabbi, or other representative, when requested.

Tips for Wellness

Encourage clients to adopt the following tips for wellness:
- Eat healthy meals and healthy snacks.
- Eat breakfast.
- Do not use tobacco products.
- Exercise regularly.
- Do not use drugs.
- Do not drink alcoholic beverages or drink only in moderation.
- Focus on one problem at a time.
- Get enough sleep every night.
- Practice having a positive attitude.
- Think before speaking.
- Make a list of goals for each day.

The worthy and demanding profession of nursing requires unselfish caring for others. Those who select nursing as a career generally want to make a difference in people's lives. The demands of clients, employers, and coworkers can cause stress for the nurse. The nurse's personal life may also be a source of stress. Many caregivers do not know how to care for themselves. Those who do not nurture themselves will suffer stress symptoms and illnesses.

Persons who are well physically, intellectually, socioculturally, psychologically, and spiritually lead productive, creative lives. They are better able to meet life's challenges and to control their stressors. For nurses, wellness means practicing wellness habits daily. As role models for clients, nurses should be examples of the holistically healthy individual.

Hospital

The English word 'hospital' comes from the French word *'hospitale'* as do the words 'hostel' and 'hotel'. The three words, i.e. hospital, hostel, hotel, and are derived from same source, are used in different sense, but basically the meaning of the word will be the same. For example, in hotel, hotel authorities take care of the clients, who wish to stay there and client will receive the hospitality according to their affordability. In hostel also, the hostel authorities are expected to treat their clients by providing basic amenities and other facilities as needed by their clients. In the same way, hospital authorities also receive their clients as their guests and are expected to show more hospitality than those of hotel or hostel. Likewise all these three institutions are meant for treating their clients, but style of treatment is different. Now the term 'hospital' means an establishment where in temporary space be occupied by the sick or injured. In other words the hospital is an institution in which sick or injured persons are treated.

Health care has come a long way since Florence Nightingale tended the wounded soldiers in the Crimean war, it was largely tender loving care. There was not enough of treatment and health care; now in some places, there is too much. Screams of pain used to come from the cut lines of the surgeons scalpel–because there was no anesthesia in those days. In Florence Nightingale times healing the sick was merciful service.

Definitions of Hospital

Hospital is an institution suitably located, constructed, organized, staffed to supply scientifically, economically, efficiently and unhindered, all or any recognized part of the complex requirements for the prevention, diagnosis and treatment of physical, mental and medical aspects of social ills with functioning facilities for training new workers in many special profession, technical and economical fields, essential to the discharge of its proper functions; and with adequate contacts with physicians, other hospitals, medical schools and all accredited health agencies engaged in the better health programs (Dorland's Illustrated Medical Dictionary).

Hospital is an institution for the care, cure, and treatment of the sick and wounded; for the study of diseases; and for the training of doctors and nurses (Steadman's Medical Dictionary).

Hospital is an institution for medical facility primarily intended, appropriately staffed, and equipped to provide diagnostic and therapeutic service in general medicine and surgery or in circumscribed field or fields of restorative medical care, together with bed care, nursing care, and dietetic service to the patients requiring such care and treatment (Blakiston's New Gould Medical Dictionary).

Hospital is an integral part of a social and medical organization, the function of which is to provide for the population complete healthcare, both curative and preventive, and whose outpatient services reach out to the family and its home environment. The hospital is also a center for the training of health worker and for biosocial research (World Health Organization).

A modern hospital is an institution which possesses adequate accommodation and wellqualified and experienced personnel to provide services of curative, restorative and preventive character of the highest quality possible to all people regardless of race, color, creed or economic status, which conducts educational and training programs for the personnel, particularly required for efficacious medical care and hospital services, which conducts research assisting the advancement of medical service and hospital services and which conducts programs in health education.

Thus hospital is an institution for the delivery of the healthcare in the modern world, offers considerable benefits to the individual and society. Individual point of view, the sick and injured person has an accessibility of centralized medical knowledge and technology on as to render treatment much more thorough and efficient, which is meant to say that a large number of professionally and technically skilled people apply their knowledge and skill with the help of sophisticated equipment and appliances to produce/provide qualitative care to the patients. In view of the stand point of society, hospitalization protects the family from many of the disruptive effects of caring for the diseased persons in the home and operates as a means of guiding the sick and injured into medically supervised institutions, where their problems are less disruptive/ complicated for the society.

Philosophy of the Hospital

A philosophy is an abstract system of thought or belief that is concerned with the conduct of man's endeavors. It is good for every individual or group to have philosophy of their own to lead their life and dealing with any such matters concerned to them. Since hospital organization is an essential part of the medical care, it should have its own philosophy. In practice, for many hospitals it is hard to fit into definition of its philosophy. It may be due to changing the needs of the society.

A philosophy is a statement of the values and beliefs that directs individuals or groups in their attempts to achieve a purpose; it explains why things are carried out in the way that they are and it serves as a directive to the way a purpose is achieved. A purpose is a reason for an organizations existence, it is the why of the organizations.

However, every hospital needs to discuss, critique and write down its philosophy in clear terms. No statement of philosophy of an institution is permanent document, it may change according to changing needs and circumstances of the society at large. The philosophy of the hospital is presented in its statement of definition.

Accordingly authorities believe that:

1. Hospital is to maintain the highest quality of services of curative, restorative and preventive services to all persons who seek its services irrespective of race, origin, religion, caste, creed, color or economical status through the excellence of medical practice, nursing practice and nursing service, technical skills and management in an environment that is conducive to the protection and continuous improvement of the total hospital healthcare system.

2. It is expected to render high standard of patient care in all functional areas of the hospital, which include outpatient services, inpatient services, ambulatory care services, emergency services, homecare services, etc.

3. A hospital that believes that high quality of patient care is closely related to a dynamic, stimulating, educational setting will define its role and commitment to educational and training programs, for which/so it conducts educational and training program for the personnel, particularly required for efficacious medical care and hospital service.

4. Hospital may define its commitment to research in patient care, educational training, and management for which it conducts research for assisting the advancement of medical service, nursing services and hospital services as a whole.

5. A hospital that believes it defines its leadership role in the community and possibly the region depending upon its size, type and facilities and in relation to regional area, planning for hospital.

6. A hospital thus believes that it would define its commitments as screening and referral, center for patient suffering from particularly complex health problems, i.e. CCF, head injuries, kidney failure, psychiatric problems, etc.

Objectives of the Hospital

As stated in the definition and philosophy of the hospital, its main objectives are as follows:

- Provide optimum health services to all people, irrespective of race, color, caste, creed and regardless of socioeconomical status.
- Provide care, cure, preventive service to all people, irrespective of race, color, caste, creed economic and social status.
- Protect the human rights of clients who while taking care in its jurisdiction/ in all areas of its services.
- Provide training for professionals, i.e. doctors, nurses, pharmacists, dentists and others technical personnels who are involving in health care services.
- Provide in-service/continuing education in all discipline professional/technical personnels involving in healthcare. For updating their knowledge, skills, etc.
- Participate/conduct research (and investigations in basic and applied biomedical, social and technological sciences) that will benefit patient care, improve the community health status, the management of hospital services and the education of individual who perform the required service.
- Define its leadership role in the community and possibly the region depending upon its size, type and facilities in relation to regional area planning or hospital.

Goals are broadly stated terminal or long-term outcomes of a program/ process. Objective is a short statement of outcomes, objectives are specific, operational terms that signify significant points necessary for eventual goal attainment. They are statements directing activity toward the achievement of the departments purposes.

Scope of Hospital

As stated in the objectives of the hospital, optimum healthcare services have the basis of scientific method, and should be applied in a personalized manner with full recognition and attention to personal dimensions in client needs and is carried out within a framework of social responsibility. It should be available and accessible to everyone who needs it through his own community. The optimum health services consists of following elements:

Team approach: The care of the needy person will be taken by the team of professional members (doctors, nurses, etc.) and para-professionals technicians under the leadership of medically qualified persons with integration and co-ordination.

Contents of service: A spectrum of services that includes diagnosis, specific treatment, nursing rehabilitation, education and prevention.

Co-ordination: Clients' care will cover the co-ordinated efforts of all agencies, which have the required facilities at all levels.

Continuity care: Continuity of client care will be available and rendered by the particular agency with specific services whenever needed.

Integration: Organization of the hospital care of both ambulatory and nonambulatory patients into a continuum with common integrated services.

Evaluation and research: Periodic evaluations, programs and provision of conducting research included in the optimum health services for adequacy in meeting needs of the patients and the community.

Functions of the Hospital

Patient care: Care to the sick and injured and restoration of the health of a diseased person without any discrimination.

Diagnosis and treatment of disease: There are diagnosis and treatment services to in-patients. Within this broad function there are many subdivisions of medical, surgical, obstetrical, gynec, pediatric, psychiatric and other forms of care and rehabilitation. Involved in all of the inpatient services are, various modalities, including nursing, pharmaceutical skills, laboratory and X-ray services and varying refinement of diagnosis and therapy.

Outpatient services: These are services to outpatients with an equally wide range of specialties and technical modalities.

Medical education and training: Hospital provides professional and technical education for many classes of health personnel. They must work in hospital to receive proper training of their choice, i.e. medical, nursing, pharmacy, dental, Lab technicians, X-ray technicians, etc.

Medical and nursing research: Since accumulation of different types of patients, the hospital provides the basis for scientific investigation into causes, diagnosis, treatment and nursing management of diseases, and hospital administration, ward unit administration in hospitals.

Prevention of disease and promotion of health: Hospital provides services to surrounding populations that may be preventive care and promoting their health. There are many ways that hospitals, as centers for technical skills, can offer services to people before they are sick or can project patients from the hazards of disease beyond that for which they have come to the hospital.

Evolution of Hospitals in India

In India, hospitals have existed from ancient times. During the time of Budda (6th century) there were a number of hospitals to look after the crippled and the poor. More such hospitals were started by devotees of Buddha in various parts of India and outside the country. The outstanding hospitals in India at that time were those build by King Ashoka (273-332 BC). The Upakalpaniyam Adyayam of Charaka Samhitha gives specification for hospital buildings, labor rooms and children wards. The qualifications for hospital attendants and nurses as well as specifications for hospital equipment, utensils, instruments and diets have also been given. There is evidence to show that there were many hospitals in South India in olden days, as observed in the Chola and Malakapuram edicts.

During 16th century, the use of allopathic system of medicine started in India particularly by the European missionaries in South India. It was during the British rule that there was some progress in the building of hospital. The first hospital in India was probably built in Goa, as mentioned in foreign traveller. The first hospital in Madras was opened in 1664, the establishment of hospital in Bombay was under discussion in 1670 but apparently it was not actually taken up till 1676 the earliest hospital in Calcutta was built in 1707-1708 and in Delhi in 1874. The Portuguese organized hospitals of the European type at Calicut (Kerala), Goa and Santhome (Madras) through missionary organizations. They set up treatment centers and trained local men and women as dressers, nurses, etc.

As stated earlier in 1664, East India Company established its first hospital in Madras for its soldiers and another in 1688 for the civilians. Complete medical care based on modern medicine spread all over India, mainly through the efforts of the missionaries, lead to built hospitals.

In 19th century, the first medical school for organized medical training was started in Calcutta, i.e. the Native Medical School, followed by one more in Madras. A hospital assistants course of two years duration was started by the army. The medical school in Calcutta was converted into college in 1835. Later on Universities, came into existence and took over all medical schools converted into medical colleges. For which some hospitals at the provincial headquarters were converted into teaching hospitals and attached to medical colleges.

In late 19th century, the status of nursing that had began in Madras around 1870s started with training of women for improving nursing care in military hospitals. In this period nursing services were being established in the hospitals by and large with the assistance of nurses from the western countries. And the nurses training in regional languages also was started in this period.

In the beginning of 20th century, some more nursing training centers were started in India. Most of these were started in Bombay, Calcutta and Madras, the nursing services were concerned with patient care services in the hospitals.

In 1943, Health Survey and Developments Committee had been constituted by the Government of India, under the chairmanship of Sri Joseph Bhore, to work out an integrated health system in India. The Bhore committee submitted its report in 1946; the recommendation of this report, includes the raising of bed population ratio in hospitals (0.24 to 1.03/1000), establishment of dental section and hospitals, provision of housing accommodation for health staff, establishment of primary health centers and staffing patterns of health institution, etc. Later on so many health committees constituted by the Government of India, also made various recommendations for improving and strengthening hospitals and health centers in India.

The last few decades have seen a spectacular development in the health and hospital consciousness of the Indian public. The general public is now more alert to its health and in accepting the role of the hospitals in its daily life. People have gradually rid themselves of their old prejudices. The patients of yesteryear approached the hospital with reluctance, apprehension and fear of death; today they enter it willingly with confidence and with hope of improved health and longer life.

Classification of Hospitals

Hospitals have been classified in many ways. Each hospital is distinct in its characteristics as it differs in structure, functions, performance, and the community it serves. However, we can classify the hospitals into different types depending upon different criteria. The most commonly accepted criteria for classification of the modern hospital are according to:
- Length of stay of patient (long-term and short-term)
- Clinical basis
- Ownership / control basis
- Objectives
- Size
- Management
- System of medicine.

Classification According to Length of Stay of Patient

A patient stays for a short-term in a hospital for treatment of diseases that is acute in nature, such as pneumonia, peptic ulcer, gastroenteritis, etc. A patient may stay for a long-term in a hospital for treatment of diseases that are chronic in nature, such as tuberculosis, leprosy, cancer, psychotics. The hospital according to long-term and short-term also known as chronic care hospital and acute care hospitals, respectively.

Classification According to Clinical Basis

These are hospitals licensed as general hospital, treat all kinds of disease, but major focus on treating speed disease or conditions such as heart disease, or cancer, or ophthalmic, or maternity, etc.

Classification According to Ownership/Control

On the basis of ownership of control, hospitals can be divided into four categories:

Public hospitals: These hospitals are run by the central or state governments or local bodies on noncommercial lines. These may be general hospital or specialized hospitals or both.

Voluntary hospitals: These hospitals are established and incorporated under the societies registration act 1860; or public trust act 1882 or any other appropriate act of central or state governments. They are run with public or private funds on a noncommercial basis.

Private nursing homes/hospitals: These are generally owned by an individual doctor or a group of doctors. They run the hospital or nursing home on a commercial basis. They accept patient suffering from infirmity, advanced age, illness, injury, chronic, disability, etc. But, do not admit patient suffering from communicable disease, alcoholism, drug addiction or mental illness. Usually they prefer patient from wealthy families.

Corporate hospitals: These hospitals are public limited companies formed under the companied act. They are normally run on commercial lines. They can be either general or specialized or both (e.g. Hinduja hospital, Mallya hospital).

Classification According to the Objectives

According to the objectives, hospitals can be classified into the following categories:

Teaching-cum-research hospitals: A hospital to which a college is attached for medical/nursing/ dental/pharmacy education. The main objective of these hospitals is teaching based on research and the provision of health care is secondary. For example, AIIMS, New Delhi; PGIMER, Chandigarh; JIPMER, Pondichery; KR Hospital, Mysore; Victoria hospital, Bangalore belong to this type.

General hospitals: These hospitals provide treatment for common diseases and conditions. All establishment permanently staffed by at least two or more doctors, which can offer in patient accommodation and provide active medical and nursing care for more than one category of medical discipline such as general medicine, general surgery, obstetrics and gynecology, pediatrics, etc. The main objective of these hospitals is to provide medical care to the people. While teaching and research is secondary and incidental. For example, all districts and taluk or PHC or rural hospitals are belonged to this type.

Specialized hospitals: These hospitals are providing medical and nursing care primarily for only one discipline or a specific disease or condition of one system. In other words, these hospitals concentrate on a particular aspect or organ of the body and provide medical and nursing care in that field. For example, tuberculosis, ENT, ophthalmology, leprosy, orthopedics, pediatrics, cardiology, mental health/ psychiatric, oncology, STDs, maternal, etc. The specialized department, administration attended to a general hospital will not be considered as specialized hospital.

Isolation hospital: This is a hospital in which the persons suffering from infections/ communicable diseases requiring isolation of the patients. For example, epidemic diseases hospital, Bangalore.

Classification According to Size

On the basis of health committee report, it is recommended that the following pattern of development of hospitals to be adopted according to size, i.e. bed strength:

(a)	Teaching hospital	500 (bed to be increased according to the number of students).
(b)	District hospital	200 (may be raised up to 300 beds depending upon population).
(c)	Taluk hospital	50 (may be raised depending upon population to be served).
(d)	Community health center	30 beded hospital or more depending upon needs
(d)	Primary health centers	6 (may be increased up to 10 depending upon needs).

Classification According to Management

Union government/government of India: All hospitals administered by the government of India. For example, hospital run by the railways, military/defence, mining/ or public sector undertakings of the central government.

State governments: All hospitals administered by the state/ union territory. Government authorities and public sector undertaking operated by the state/union territories, including the police, prison, irrigation department, etc.

Local bodies: All hospitals administered by local bodies, i.e. municipal corporation, municipality, jilla parishad, panchayat, e.g. corporation maternity homes.

Autonomous bodies: All hospitals established under special act of parliament or state legislation are funded by the central/ state government/ union territory. For example, AIIMS, New Delhi; PGIMER, Chandigarh, NIMHANS, Bangalore; KMIO, Bangalore.

Private: All private hospitals owned by an individual or by a private organization, e.g. MAHE, Manipal; Manipal hospital, Bangalore; Hinduja hospital, Mumbai.

Voluntary agencies: All hospitals operated by a voluntary body/ a trust/charitable society registered or recognized by the appropriate authority under central/state government laws. This includes hospitals run by missionary bodies and cooperatives e.g. CMC hospital, Vellore.

Classification According to System

According to the system of medicine we can classify the hospital as follows:
(a) Allopathic hospitals.
(b) Ayurvedic hospitals.
(c) Homeopathic hospitals.
(d) Unani hospitals.
(e) Hospitals of other systems of medicine.

Hospital Departments

Outpatient Department (OPD)

An outpatient department is a distinct and important part of the hospital. In the past, OPD was frequently housed in a separate building away from the main body and the hospital. Also, the staff was separate, so that there was no community feeling and no unity of efforts. In recent years, the center of gravity of a hospital has been shifting more and more from wards to outpatient department. So in modern planning, these facilities (OPD) are no longer separated. In order to function properly the OPD must take its place with other departments of the hospital in all consideration of the hospital organization, i.e. policy, facilities, financing, patient care, teaching and research, etc.

An outpatient department is the point of contact between hospital and community. Many patients gain their first impression of the hospital from the OPD. The activities of the OPD will influence those of all other departments of the hospital and the activities of all other departments of the hospital will produce the effect on those of OPD. All the patients suffering from diseases of minor, serious, acute, chromic nature are first examined in the OPD.

An OPD should be within the main body of the hospital. The department should be located close to public entrance, particularly where public transportation is provided. The department should also be adjacent to the casualty and emergency service and admitting unit. At the entrance to OPD there should be a reception and enquiry counters, with proper communication facilities like telephone, etc. The OPD space can be utilized for emergency services. It is also effective to have clinics of different speciality, X-ray, laboratory, pharmacy, rehabilitation center, injection room and other facilities depending on the type of hospital.

The number and type of clinics will depend on the needs of the patients served and the interest of medical personnels. In modern days we have number of clinics, conducted in the OPD such as eye, ear, nose, throat, dental, medical, surgical, obstetric and gynecology, and mental health clinics, pediatric, etc. And also we have specialized clinics like orthopedics, genitourinary, neurosurgical, cardiovascular, diabetics, and so on.

In an active OPD there should be a laboratory and other diagnostic facilities to have routine laboratory examinations like urine analysis, common blood examination and others; and also diagnostic facilities like ECG, X-ray; and also there should be pharmacy for distribution of drugs which meets the requirement of outpatient; and also there should be facilities to get them injection, vaccine, proper facility.

An outpatient department should provide an environment which will acquaint the patient with matter of health and hygienic practice. For which suitable posters, can be displayed on the respective units of the OPD.

There are three aspects of outpatient work that need to do considered:

- Emergencies and accidents
- Unreferred patients
- Referred patients.

The provision has to be made for dealing properly and efficiently with medical and surgical emergencies for whatever cause. Every hospital must have provision for receiving and dealing with 'walking casualties' very single fractures, cuts needing suturing, abscess conditions, hard injuries, fractures, burns, poisoning, tetanus, and other conditions.

The casualty department provides round-the clock, immediate diagnosis and treatment for illness of emergent nature and injuries from accident. Simple cases after administering preliminary treatment are dismerged with instructions to attend OPD as a follow-up measure. Cases of serious nature are admitted in casualty wards to provide immediate care, after keeping them in required period, they will be discharged and transferred to respective in-patient wards.

Unreferred patients refer to those who have not been seen by and outside doctor, who present themselves at the hospitals with a wide variety at ailments, and who regard the hospital as a kind of dispensary.

Referred patients refer to those who have been sent by a family doctor or health center to the outpatient department of a hospital for a particular service, i.e. pathological and radiological examination or for consultation for a specialist.

Medical Unit or Department of Medicine

Usually all general hospitals have a medical unit. The surgery unit in teaching hospital will be called as a department of medicine. In general hospital, medical units are usually headed by senior physician with their associates whereas in teaching hospital, there will be a head of the department and professors, asst. professors, lecturers and clinical tutors.

Other medical unit or department in a hospital includes all patients who admitted to the hospital for treatment other than surgery with certain exceptions. The medication services provides for disease entitles that may further divided into subspecialities such as cardiological, neurological, nephrological, thoracic, gastroenterological, dermatological, etc. units. The department also serves in a consulting capacity to the surgical, obstetrical, gynecological, psychiatric and pediatric cases where such patients develop medical complications.

The nurses play vital role in the medical units, that is, they take over all responsibility of the respective wards and manage wards efficiently for the welfare of the patients in all aspects related to nursing profession and also taking main roles and responsibilities in assessing conditions, identifying problems, providing direct care to patients. In addition, they help physician in making proper diagnosis by assisting in performing related medical diagnosis procedures and carrying out medical prescription to treat patients effectively.

Surgical Units/Department of Surgery

Today the surgical services comprise a major sphere of hospital practice, with accompanying problems and personnel, supply and regulation. The surgical unit can be more or less complex depending on the size of the hospital. If we want to have surgical unit, there should be hospital with 100 to 200 bed capacity. Just like medical unit or department there are subspeciality division and surgical side, which includes general surgery, orthopedics, urology, gynecology, eye, ear, nose and throat, neurosurgery, vascular surgery, thoracic surgery can be seen in teaching hospitals.

There are many advantages to the physical separation of surgical and medical beds. The benefits of centralization of equipment, the grouping of nurses skilled mainly in one area, and the facilitation of daily medical and surgical rounds are readily ready apparent.

Depending on the size and location of the institution surgical privileges are granted in accordance with one of the following pattern:

- Every doctor with MBBS degree has privileges to operate or assist in small hospital, in rural area (minor surgeries)
- Only surgeons with PG qualification like MS, D. Orth., DM, DLO, etc. are eligible to perform surgery
- General practitioner without surgical privileges are not eligible to perform surgery
- In our set-up we have, super specialist surgeons, i.e. MCh i.e. MD or MS degree designated as surgeon, deputy surgeon and assistant surgeon. In teaching hospital they can be designated as professor, asst. professor, lecturers of surgery.

Surgical

At present, about half or more of the patients occupying beds in general hospitals are for surgical treatment. In addition to the fact that there is increase in the number of patients needing surgery, new surgical procedure are being developed, some of which require that patient be in the operating room for considerable length of time. Surgical procedure or operation of longer duration, also tend to increase the demand for operating space. It is ideal to have one operating room/theatre for every 50 beds of surgical patients. One of the study (N Wadiya, A Lazaru SF Singh) conducted on some Bombay Hospitals, it was observed that municipal hospital has 12 specialized operation theatre out of 15 operation theatres, for a bed strength of 1,655.

Apart from the surgeons, the role of other personnels in operation theatres, Le. nurses, technicians is very important. To great extent the optimum use of the operation theatre also depends on the coordination and cooperation between specialized staff of the operation theatre like the surgeons, anesthetist, nurses and others who are working in the theatre.

Operation theatre should have the following facilities:

1. *Operating room* – consists of OT tables.
2. *Lay-up room* – which connects directly with operating room, is used to prepare trolleys with all the equipment needful for an operation. Much of the sterilized material come to this room in package for the CSSD. A probable exception in the surgical instruments themselves, which may be sterilized in this room.
3. *Wash-up room* – opening immediately off the operating room, contains sinks and disposal lifts. All used and dirty material go into this room. Some items are sent away immediately by the; disposal lifts; others are rough washed before return to the CSSD.
4. *Anesthesia room* – which is also open directly into the operating room is equipped permanently for the use of anesthetist. Since some anesthetic gases are explosive, proper precautions must be taken to prevent hazards and precautions are also needed against static electricity.
5. *Scrubbing-up room* – in which the surgeons and nurses scrub-up and put on sterilized gowns, gloves and masks. It is ideal to have separate scrubbing-up room for surgeons and nurses.

In addition, the operation theatre should be equipped with necessary equipments, supplies which include linen, surgical instruments, OT tables, Boyer apparatus, O_2, N_2 and other gases. Anesthetic ether and other gases/drugs, etc.

And also it is ideal to have recovery room should be attached to operation theatre for the reception of patients immediately following surgery. Patients remain in the recovery room for varying length of time depending on their condition and on hospital policy.

Maternity Unit/OBG Unit

Maternity unit is very essential in general hospital. The same unit in teaching hospital is referred to as the department of obstetrics and gynecology. This unit or department should serve both in physical set-up and in personnel to provide every care and comfort for the lying-in mother and her newborn. The maternity wards can easily be made attractive, comfortable and restful. The extent of the provision that should be made for institutional confinements is conditioned as:

1. The number of women who should desire a hospital bed, if available.
2. The number of women who ought on medical grounds to have a hospital delivery, and
3. The length of stay in a hospital of normal case.

Antenatal care, the great preventive branch of obstetrics is the systematic medical supervision of women during pregnancy. Its aim is to preserve the physiological aspects of pregnancy and labor and to prevent or detect all the pathological conditions of pregnancy as early as possible. The ideal outcome of childbirth is a healthy mother in possession of a healthy child. The earlier in pregnancy a women comes under medical supervision, the better, and it is ideal that such care be carried into the postpartum period for a reasonable length of time. In order to provide such adequate care of the expectant mother in a hospital, a properly organized department with medical and ancillary services must be available. The antenatal clinic should be situated, where practicable on part of the ground floor off, or adjoining, the maternity wing. The size of the clinic will be governed to some extent by the number of times the obstetrician will wish to see a expectant mother before delivery. The responsibilities of nurses in antenatal clinics include the setting up of examination rooms, preparation for pregnant women for examination and care of supplies and equipments used during the clinic sessions.

All prima gravida and multipara may not need admission in hospitals. The delivery may be conducted at their own houses if they have proper facilities for maintenance of cleanliness and other related aspects. Actual admissions must, of course, be governed by the number of lying-in beds available and if there are insufficient to meet all requests for admission; priority must be given to women having abnormal medical or obstetrical conditions.

The nurses have to play a major role in maternity unit.

Their duties are to correlate all nursing functions in the maternity clinics with those of the inpatient department. Inpatient facility of maternity department will include admitting room, labor and delivery room, equipment for anesthesia, recovery room, postpartum wards, etc. The roles and responsibility of nurses will include: they will be over all manager of the unit, Le. admitting clinic, preparing mother for delivery, conducting delivery, taking care of the mother and newborn, providing postpartum services, and a number of activities related to mother and child.

Pediatric Unit

The pediatric services will constitute a substantial proportions of the whole hospital. In developing countries, the proportion of children to adults in hospital may reach 40 percent. The pediatric services of the hospital should form part of an integrated service to the community. It should contribute to community medium and community health in the area served by the hospital.

The outpatient services for children is an important part of the pediatric service. In pediatric clinics, more space, her to kept open to enable the clinic to accept a patient, without appointments who present themselves with urgent conditions, i.e. many children's diseases are of sudden onset and it is important that the children's OPD should enable children to be seen without delay.

Hospital services for children usually pose many problems, because most hospitals are organized to take care for adults.

However, every hospital must provide some care for children and for newborn delivered in its obstetrical service. The nursing, medical, dietary and other services for children require specialized knowledge and an understanding of children if they are to be effective. The basic needs of children are best met when they are grouped and located in a quiet area of the hospital, removed from the most of the hospitals traffic. The larger the pediatric unit, the better the comprehensive care. If possible, the children section should be the obstetrical service and the newborn nurseries. The grouping of children helps in providing effective isolation of infants and young children and providing suitable recreational facilities.

Generally, children are better grouped by age than by diagnosis, and more attention should be given to the emotional development of the child than to his chronological age. For administrative purpose, most children admitted to pediatric services are between 12 to 15 years or early adolescence.

In designing the pediatric unit, the needs of the two groups must be considered; those of the patient and his parents and those of the hospital staff. The special requirement in planning for children includes the provision of a large proportion of isolation room and facilities for mothers to come into the hospital with their children. There is also a need for large play rooms and for a school room. And also there should be a unit for premature infant should preferably be within the pediatric department. Here a separate, glass walled cubicle is desirable for each infant. Each cubicle should be equipped with devices for controlling temperature and humidity (except in hot, humid climates) and each should be connected to an oxygen supply, although the risks of retrolental fibroplasia in high oxygen tensions must always be born in mind. As premature babies are particularly prove to infection, which may easily prove fatal, facilities should be readily available to enable the staff entering a cubicle to put on sterile gowns and masks, separate gowns and fresh masks being provided for each cubicle.

Nowadays, the hospital authorises proper cubicle partitions for children beds. If cubicle partitions are used they should be made of shatter proof glass (about the height of the bed mattress), 7 feet high and extends 7 feet from the wall. They should also be constructed to allow visibility by nurses and patients in the same room. It is well to have good view of all patients from the nurses station. A proportionately large amount of space may be needed because of the amount of nursing attention is necessary.

The advantages and disadvantages of cubicle are as follows:

Advantages
1. They demarcate areas potential infection and facilities precautionary maintenance.
2. They limit space devoted to a single patient and seem to set a finite value for the hospital bill.
3. They discourage the practice of throwing toys from on area to another, and
4. They encourage visitors to confine their attention to one patient.

Disadvantages
1. They separate children who otherwise would be able to fraternize and have a happier hospital experience.
2. They are relatively expensive to install and keep clean.
3. They diminish air circulation in hot weather and contribute to discomfort, and
4. They reduce the flexibility of the unit.

However, this is up to the discretion of the hospital to adopt cubicle partitions in respect to children wards.

Dental Department/Unit

The dental department in a general hospital should be largely a referred center for cases of diagnosis or operative difficulty sent to the hospital by dental surgeons either in private practice or working in clinics. The services of the hospital dental specialist are also needed for collaboration with the orthopedic or general surgeon in the treatment of fracture of the jaw. In addition to the above functions, the dental specialist should exercise general supervision over peripheral dental clinics dealing with adults (especially expectant mothers) and caring for the dental welfare of healthy children.

Department of Radiology or X-ray Department

Department of radiology deals with radiodiagnosis and radiotherapy. Similarly it will be known as X-ray department. The X-ray department needs to provide services for in-patients, out-patients, casualties and patient referred for X-ray by general practitioners. There are a number of diagnostic procedures performed in the X-ray department, such as barium-meal, intravenous pyelography, myelogram and so on, in addition diagnostic type of practice.

Now radiotherapy is one of the dramatic method of treatment to certain conditions, which carefully administered in sufficient doses. Radiation beams were found to provide an effective method of treatment in many disease (e.g. cancer). The beams were those emitted from X-ray tubes, and those arising from natural or artificial radioactive isotopes and from such devices as betatrons and cyclotrons. Radiation beams include X-rays, alpha, beta and gamma rays, electrons, neutrons, protons and other forms of ionizing energy.

In modern hospital much scientific progress is being made and the uses of diagnostic and therapeutic radiation procedures are increasing.

Department of Pathology/Laboratory

Although the term 'laboratory' has been in popular use, some doctors who specialized in this area prefers to use term "department of pathology." The primary function of pathology services is to give assistance to the attending doctor in the diagnosis and treatment of patients. Investigations made by this service reveals normally other degree of deviation from normal. Tissues, blood, bone marrow, cerebrospinal fluid and other body fluids, excretions (urine, stool, sputum, etc.) and other materials collected from or administered to the patients are examined. Post-mortem examination are conducted to determine the causes of death and to study disease processes.

The medical laboratories may be divided into two groups; i.e. hospital laboratories, which are concerned with tests for the diagnosis, prognosis and response to therapy of disease in individual patients, and public health laboratories which are concerned with the origin, spread and control of disease in the community. Members of the hospital personnel are interested in laboratories as diagnostic tool; public health personnels are interested in them as measuring rods of community health.

The laboratory situated in the hospital also will be concerned with diagnostic laboratory tests, not only for inpatients and outpatients but also for special services clinics, for general practitioners in the area, for public health services and possibly and desirably for certain aspects of industry. Because of these number of responsibilities, the laboratory will have to carry out toxicological studies and physiological function tests as well as hematological, microbiological, biochemical and histopathological investigations.

The pathologist who carries all the activities with the assistance of qualified medical laboratory technicians and also to some extent with nurses.

Department of Psychiatry/Mental Health

Psychiatry as a basic medical science, as a field of therapeutics and as a branch of public health and preventive medicine can also play its role in the general hospital endeavor to improve education, training and research. The general hospital can, by having it own psychiatric facilities, help the community in detecting, diagnosing and treating at an early stage of patients who are then still relatively easy to treat.

Psychiatric services in the general hospital should, if possible, include an outpatient department, liaison services for contact with mental hospitals, long-stay annexas, pre and after care facilities and general and psychiatric community services, day and night treatment facilities and an inpatient unit.

Department of Pharmacy

The pharmacy is the department of the modem hospital which has undergone the greatest recent change and advanced fairly well. The main function of this department will include the stocking of drugs and other medical supplies and equipment, and distribution of drugs and other to different department as and when they required and also manufacturing of medication in hospital pharmacies. Since commercial supplies of materials are relatively less expensive, the manufacturing of certain

medication is disappearing, but preparation of fluid and electrolytes in the hospital in the country.

Now in some hospital purchasing and charging of pharmaceutical are handled by the chief of the pharmacy department in collaboration with the medical superintendents and resident medical officer of the hospital.

The pharmaceutical services in most of the hospitals in India today represent the functions of procurement and distribution of medicaments by medical stores and compounding and dispensing of medicine on doctors prescriptions by persons hitherto known as pharmacists, generally under the control of medical officer.

Laundry

All hospitals are concerned with the dangers of cross-infections and the need for using only sanitary, germ-free linen. So there is a need of an efficient mechanical laundry to ensure the availability of germ-free washed linen. Laundry is closely associated with nursing service. The person who manages laundry must be familiar with problems of nursing service, and nursing personnel should understand the laundry difficulties. Nursing supervisors can be taken on rounds of the laundry periodically to know the problems. Everything that laundry does is of interest to the nursing service. Surgical linens are autoclaved in the surgical area to ensure sterility and further safeguard the patients. When laundry personnel prepare surgical packs, the specification should come from nursing. Isolation techniques established by nursing should be followed by laundry personnel where applicable, and the procedures sometimes may be taught by nursing. All linen levels are established by nursing and the nursing services advises the type of linen required for them to work in wards and other departments.

Dietary Department

The purpose of the dietary service department in every hospital is the preparation of nutritionally adequate, attractive meals. The goals of dietary service to hospital will include the following:
1. Optimum nutrition of the patient.
2. The maintenance of morale.
3. The dietic education of patients, and
4. The achievement of these goals, with maximum effectively and resulting economy.

The functions of the dietary service are determined by these goals. The proper nutrition of patients requires intelligent purchasing of equipment and goods, the professional planning of standard and therapeutic diet, scientific food production and well-planned system of food distribution from "kitchen."

The morale function will apply equally to food prepared for hospital personnel, requires consideration of the esthetics of food service including color, consistency, etc. The way of food distribution also affects the patient reactions to well prepared food.

The educational function are interrelated. Saintly planned, prepared and served meals may, in themselves be an education to some patients, and which discharging the patient, that dischargeship also gives more amount of nutrition education to patient.

The nursing department has a right to expect that the dietary personnel will be trained in correct food handling techniques and will know proper utensils to use for food serving. It is also expected that dietary department will serve correct, complete trays to patients and that the nurse in-charge will be notified where trays are ready to be served. All agreed them, that nurses should be bold when a tray is delivered to a patient who has to be fed.

The dietary service must expect, that the nursing department will notify them promptly about diet changes and that not all of the nursing staff will go to take meals together and leave and patients area without nursing supervision during meals timing. Nurses are expected to discharge doctors from making rounds at meal times so that there will be no dressing done to patients during that time. It is important that the patients room or ward be quite and peaceful at meals time. Food served is an attractive manner provides an incentive for the patient to eat.

Central Sterile Supply Services Department (CSSSD)

The central sterile supply department is supposed to store, sterilize, maintain and issue those instruments, materials and garments which are required to be sterilized. This requirement may steadily decrease as the use of disposable items become more economical. The CSSSD should have direct lines of communication with all wards, operation theatres, outpatient and casualty departments and to a lesser extent with X-ray and pathology department. Air control in this department is essential to check contamination through air. Proper control with indicators for sterilization procedures are essential.

Department of Nursing

Nursing is a major force in the health and medical team which is so essential for providing services to the hospital. Nursing personnels consist of professional nurses, practising nurses and nursing assistant of various types. The position of nurses in India are staff nurses, ward sisters, assistant nursing superintendent, deputy nursing superintendent, nursing superintendent and chief nursing officers, nursing directors, who are used into the hospital nursing services.

Philosophy of Nursing and Modes of Organising Patient Care

Each institution in which nursing is taught or practiced, as well as each individual nurse, has a philosophy of nursing. A philosophy is a statement of beliefs that include one's behavior and, in this case, influence the practice of nursing. An understanding of one's own beliefs, feelings, values, attitudes, and culture precedes the development of a philosophy of nursing. Until the nurse has knowledge of self, it is difficult to state beliefs to guide nursing practice. Several concepts must be discussed in any nursing philosophy. These include human beings, health, illness, and nursing. Writing a personal philosophy of nursing is a task that requires a great deal of though and self-knowledge. Each of the previous self-assessments related to values, attitudes, feelings, and culture provides data that will help the nurse to express personal beliefs. The nurse makes a statement of personal beliefs related to each of the identified concepts. This is a deliberative, rational process that involves a great deal of introspection. For example, the nurse who believes in the Christian religion may express as belief that the human being possesses a life after death and that one function of nursing is to assist the individual to attain this life. These beliefs may influence the care the nurse gives to a dying patient.

Example of a Philosophy of Nursing (Dist McGann Hospital Nursing Service)

The practice of nursing is the care of patients through a professional interpersonal relationship. Nurses apply behavioral scientific principles, biologic scientific principles, and principles of humanism in a skillful, concerted, and compassionate manner to bring patients and their families to optimal health status, personal growth, dignity and peace. Nurses demonstrate the professional use of self and the collaborative involvement of families and related health care provides in bringing about desired change, as established in the patient-nurse contract. Nurses advocate, teach, conduct clinical inquiry, institute planned change, make critical decisions, coordinate and synthesize the efforts of other disciplines, create therapeutic interpersonal contact, perform therapeutic procedures, and establish a therapeutic milieu. The process of nursing causes learning, growth, maturity and acceptance of responsibility by both the patient and nurse.

The primary function of the nursing department is to provide patient services in a manner conducive to the education of health professionals and supportive of appropriate research activities. The department affirms its commitment to optimal patient outcomes and the highest standards of care possible in the face of increasing technical patient care requirements and the need to make intelligent decisions about the use of resources. Given finite resources, nurses exercise conscious decision making the problem solving, managing environmental and support structures for positive patient care outcomes, thereby realizing a satisfying level of nursing practice.

All patients at the McGann Hospital, Shivamogga are entitled to excellence in the nursing care they receive. The quality of care given is irrespective of race, sex, religious or political belief, socioeconomic status, or ethnic background.

Nursing is the primary professional service received during hospitalization. Post-hospitalization, nurses provide continuity of care and contribute to effective interface between hospital and community, emphasizing preventive, health maintenance, and rehabilitative service.

The department commits to the development of professional nursing through modeling the nursing role in caring for patients, developing new healthcare providers and expanding nursing knowledge. Nursing will demonstrate a leadership role in this environment by promoting improved models of organizing and delivering patient care, such as primary nursing, in order to increase and clarify our responsibility and accountability for practice.

Children's Hospital Philosophy of Nursing

We believe that man is holistic (biopsychosocial spiritual) being capable of adapting to many adverse conditions depending upon his stages of developments, family dynamics, environment, and cultural influences. We believe that children are individuals as well as members of a family and that they have a right to:

(a) Be treated as an individual.
(b) Health care to achieve a better quality of life of dignity in death.
(c) Be informed.
(d) Privacy and confidentiality.
(e) Emotional support.
(f) A safe environment.
(g) Maintain family ties in times of disequilibrium.
(h) An environment where the child experiences continued sense of parenting.

We believe that family-centered patient care requires a collaborative interdependence with other disciplines within children's hospitals as well as within the community. This is dependent upon a work environment that promotes critical inquiry, free exchange of ideas, and humanistic treatment of personnel. We further believe that decision making must take place at the most effective level of the organization.

We believe that a professional nurse is a skilled, educated provider of patient care with a clear definition of purpose and standards of practice. The nurse if accountable to the child and his family, him/herself, the institution, and society for integrating quality patient care.

We believe that nurses within the department have the responsibility of developing, implementing, coordinating, and evaluating patient care services to insure that the child receives optimal health care. The professional nurse diagnoses and treats human responses to facilitate effective living by the child and his family as they experience actual or potential health problems.

We believe that the professional nurse:

– Is able to use the process of assessment, planning, implementation, and evaluation as a base for practice.
– Is able to use of organizational skills to efficiently direct and implement the appropriate components of a patient care delivery system.
– Participates in formal and informal learning opportunities to increase skill and knowledge, and communicates new knowledge to other personnel.
– Performs, analyzes, implements, and communicates nursing research to modify nursing practices for more effective patient care.
– Has the responsibility to adhere to policies and procedures and assume initiative for improving personal and institutional practices.
– Fosters open lines of communication with all health team members to assure the best possible care for the client.
– Conducts formal and informal sessions of facilitate the child's and family's knowledge of his condition and environment.
– Provides for continuity of the child's care.

Modes of Organizing Patient

Nursing Care in Hospital

There are five primary means of organizing nursing care for patients are:

Case Method Nursing or Total Patient Care

Case method is an oldest mode of organizing patient care. In this method, nurses assume total responsibility for meeting all the needs of assigned patients during their time on duty. It involves the assignment of one or more clients to a nurse for a specific period of time, such as shift, complete care, including treatments, medication administration and nursing care planning, is the assigned nurses responsibility.

Even though the case method is one of the earliest method of nursing care delivery, it is still widely used in hospitals and in home health agencies. It is developed and communicated through written sources, its usage remains in contemporary practice. Students most frequently learn within this model, private duty nurses practice with this design, and specialty units, such as ICU, ICCU, etc. are most often use this model.

Case method nursing provides for nurses with high autonomy and responsibility. Assigning patient is simple and direct and does not require the planning that other methods of patient care delivery do. The lines of authority and accountability are clear. The patient theoretically receives holistic and unfragmented care during the nurses time on duty. Each nurse caring for the patient can, however modify the care regiment. The merits and demerits of this method as follows:

Merits
The nurse can better see and attend to the total needs of clients due to the time and proximity of intractors. Coordination of all aspects of care is the responsibility of the nurse; physical, emotional, medical regimen, teaching and all other aspects.

- Continuity of care can be facilitated with care.
- Client-nurse interaction/rapport can be developed due to intensity of time and proximity of those involved.
- Client may feel more secure knowing that one person is thoroughly familiar with the needs and the course of treatment.
- Educational needs of the clients can be closely monitored.
- Family and friends may become better known by nurse and more involved in the care of the client.
- Work load for the unit can be equally divided among available staff.
- Nurses accountability for their function built-in.

Demerits
- Many clients do not require the intensity of care inherent in this type of service.
- This method must be modified if nonprofessional health workers are to be used effectively.
- There are not enough nurses to fill the demand of this model; cost-effectiveness must be considered.
- It is difficulty for nurses using this method to become involved in long-term planning and evaluation of care.
- The greatest disadvantage in the case of nursing occurs when the nurse is inadequately trained or prepared to provide total care to the patient.

Functional Method of Nursing

The functional method of delivering nursing care evolved as a result of World War II. Because nurses were in great demand overseas and at home, many ancillary personnels were used to assist in patient care. These relatively unskilled workers were trained to do some simple tasks and gained proficiency by repetition. Personnels were assigned to complete certain tasks rather than care of specific patients, e.g. checking blood pressure, administering medication, changing lines, and bathing patients.

Actually the functional method is a technical approach to nursing care that emphasizes the dependent functions of nursing practice. The available staff on a unit, for a particular period of time, are assigned to selected functions such as vital signs, treatments, medications. All the responsibilities of the unit are assigned to selected people in accordance with their expertize. The only person who has complete responsibility of the client is the head nurse or nurse acting in that role. The following are the merits and demerits of the functional nursing.

Merits
- The person can become particularly skilled in performing assigned tasks; it can be efficient and economical.
- The best utilization may be made of a persons aptitudes, experience and desires.
- Less equipment is needed and what is available is usually better cared for when used only by a few personnels.
- This method saves time because it lends itself to strict organizational protocol.
- The potential for development of technical skills is amplified.

- There is sense of productivity for the task oriented nurse.
- It is easy to organize the work of the unit and staff.

Demerits
- Client care may become impersonal, compartmentalized and fragmented.
- There is a tremendous risk for diminishing continuity of care.
- Staff may become bored and have little motivation to develop self and others, work may become monotonous.
- The staff members are accountable for the task; only the nurse incharge of the unit has accountability for the individual, whole client.
- There is little avenue for staff development, except as it relates to tasks.
- Clients may tend to feel insecure, not knowing who is their own nurse.
- Only parts of the nursing care plan are known to personnel.
- It is difficult to establish client priorities and operationalize the care plan reflecting same.
- It is only safe when the head nurse can coordinate the activities of all members of the staff and make certain that nothing essential in client care in overlooked or forgotten. This is a tremendous responsibility for one person who probably has to think of approximately thirty or more clients, plus the staff.

Majority of them viewed this functional nursing as an economic mean of providing care. Major advantage of this is its efficiency; tasks are completely quickly with little confusion regarding responsibility. For example, in many areas such as operating room, laser room, etc. the functional nursing works well and is still very much in evidence. But functional nursing may lead to fragmented care and the possibility of overlooking priority needs and may lead to low job satisfaction.

Team Nursing/Modular Nursing

Team nursing was developed in 1950s (under grant from the WK Kellogg foundation) directed by Eleanor Lambertson at Teachers College, Columbia University in New York city. It has been developed in an effort to decrease the problems associated with the functional organization of patient care. Majority of people felt that despite a continued shortage of professional nursing staff, a patient care system had to be developed that reduced the fragmented care that accompanied functional nursing.

Team nursing was designed to accommodate several categories of personnels in meeting the comprehensive nursing needs of a group of clients (Donovan 1975). Team nursing is based on philosophy (Kron 1978) in which a group of professional and nonprofessional personnels work together to identify, plan, implement and evaluate comprehensive client-centered care. The key concept is a group that works together toward a common goal, providing qualitative comprehensive nursing care.

In team nursing ancillary personnel collaborate in providing care to a group of patients under the direction of a professional nurse. Actually the team nursing involves decentralization of a nursing unit and professional head nurses authority, in which the unit divided into teams. Each team composed of team leader, team members and patients. Staff and clients are usually divided evenly, often written unit proximity such as a wing of floor. Comprehensive care for the client is the responsibility of the entire team, but is led by the team leader who should be a registered nurse. Assignments are made according to the capabilities of the members and respond to the needs of the group of clients.

In team nursing team leader, the nurse is responsible for knowing the condition and needs of all the patients assigned to the team and planning individual care. The team leader duties vary depending on the patients' needs and workload. These duties may include assisting team members, giving direct personal care to patients, teaching and coordinating patient care activities.

The merits and demerits of team nursing as follows:

Merits
- It includes all healthcare personnel in the groups functioning and goals.
- Feelings of participation and belonging are facilitated with team members.
- Workload can be balanced and shared.
- Division of labor allows members the opportunity to develop leadership skills.
- Every team member has the opportunity to learn from and teach colleagues.
- There is a variety in the daily assignment.
- Interest in client's wellbeing and care shared by several people; reliability of decisions is increased.
- Nursing care hours are usually cost-effective.
- The client is able to identify personnels who are responsible for his care.
- All care is directed by a registered nurse.
- Continuity care is facilitated, especially if team are constant.
- Barriers between professional and nonprofessional workers can be minimized; the group efforts prevail.
- Everyone has the opportunity to contribute to the care plan.

Demerits
- Establishing the team concept taken time, effort and constancy of personnel. Merely assigning people to a group does not make them a 'group' or 'team.'
- Unstable staffing patterns make team nursing difficult.
- All personnels must be client centered.
- The team leader must have complex skills and knowledge, i.e. communication, leadership organization, nursing care, motivation and other skills.
- There is less individual responsibility and independence regarding nursing functions.

Team nursing usually associated with democratic leadership. Group members are given as much autonomy as possible when performing assigned tasks, although responsibility and accountability are shared by the team collectively. The need for excellent communication and coordination skills makes implementing team nursing or organization difficult and requires great self discipline on the part of the team members. Team nursing allows each member to contribute their own special expertise, or skills. Team leader, then, should use their knowledge about each members abilities when making patient assignments. Recognizing the individual worth of all employees and giving team members autonomy result in high job satisfaction.

Progressive Patient/Client Care

Progressive client care is a method in which client-care areas or units provide various levels of care, e.g. (i) intensive care unit for the critically ill, (ii) postintensive care unit, (iii) regular care units, (iv) convalescent unit, (v) self care unit.

Here the clients are evaluated with respect to all level (intensity) of care needed. As they progress towards increased self care (as they become less ethically ill or in need of intensive care or monitoring), they are mared to units/wards staffed to best provide the type of care needed. The merits and demerits of progressive patient care as follows:

Merits
- Efficient use is made of personnel and equipment.
- Clients are in the best place to receive the care they require.
- Use of nursing skills and expertise are maximized due to different staffing patterns of each unit.
- Clients are moved towards self care independence is fostered where indicate.
- Efficient use and placement of equipment is possible.
- Personnels have greater probability to function toward their fullest capacity.

Demerits
- There may be discomfort to clients who are moved often.
- Continuity care is difficult, even though possible.
- Long-term nurse-client relationships are difficult to arrange.
- Heavy emphasis is placed on comprehensive, written care plan.
- There is often times difficulty in meeting administrative need of the organization, staffing evaluation, and accreditation.

Primary Nursing

Primary nursing, developed in the early 1970s, uses some of the concepts of case method. It involves total nursing care, directed by a nurse on a 24-hour basis as long as the client is under care. As originally designed, this method requires a nursing staff comprised totally of registered staff nurses. Here one specific nurse is the client's nurse, at all times directing, planning evaluating and teaching. The primary nurse is essentially, on call all the time and arranged coverage when away.

Actually, the primary nurse assumes 24-hour responsibility for planning the care of one or more patients from admission or the start of treatment to discharge or the treatments end. During work hours the primary nurse provides total direct care for that patient. When the primary nurse is not on duty, care is provided by other junior nurses who follow the care plan established by the primary nurse, that means, eventhough the primary nurse is the director of care for clients, segments of care are often delegated.

As stated earlier, it uses some concepts of case method leads to confusion. The difference exists in the fact that case method involves a specified segment of time, i.e. shift where as the primary nursing is 24-hour responsibility for as long as care needed by the client. Although this method is designed for use in hospitals, this structure lends itself well to home health nursing, hospital nursing and other health care delivery enterprises.

An integral responsibility of the primary nurse is to establish clear communication between the patient, the doctor, the associate nurses and other team members.

Although the primary nurse establishes the nursing care plan, feedback in sought from others in coordinating the patient care. The combination of clear interdisciplinary groups communication and consistent, direct patient care by relatively few nursing staff allows for holistic, high quality patient care. It gives job satisfaction, once nurse develop skill in primary nursing care delivery, they feel challenged and rewarded.

Merits
- There is opportunity for the nurse to see the client and family as one system.
- Nursing accountability, responsibility and independence are increased.
- The nurse is able to use a wide range of skills, knowledge and expertise.
- This method potentiates creativity by the nurse; work satisfaction may increase significantly.
- The scene is set for increased trust and satisfaction by the client and nurse.

Demerits
- The nurse may be isolated from colleagues.
- There is little avenue for group planning of client care.
- Nurses must be mature and independently competent.
- It may be cost effective.
- Staffing patterns may necessitate a heavy client load.
- An inadequate prepared or educated primary nurse may be incapable of coordinating a multidisciplinary team or identifying complex patient needs and condition changes.

The role and functions of the nurse manager in organizing groups for patient care are as follows:

1. Periodically evaluates the effectiveness of the organizational structure for the delivery of patient care.
2. Determines if adequate resources and support exist before making any changes in the organization of patient care.
3. Examines the human element in work redecision and support personnel during adjustment to changes.
4. Uses committees to facilitate group goals, not to delay decision.
5. Teaches group members how to avoid group think.
6. Inspires the work group toward a team effort.
7. Organizes work activities to attain organizational goals.
8. Group activities in a manner that facilitates coordination within and between department.
9. Uses a patient care delivery system that maximizes resources people, material and time.
10. Organizes work in a manner that facilitates communication.
11. Uses committees structure to increase the quality and quantity of work accomplished.
12. Uses knowledge of group dynamics for goal attainment.

2

Concepts of Nursing and its Profession

Introduction

Nursing has been called the oldest of the arts and the youngest of the professions. The term 'nurse' evolved from the Latin word *nutrix* which means 'nourishing'. The roots of medicine and nursing are intertwined and found in mythology, ancient cultures, religion, and reasoned thinking.

Historically the term 'nursing' most often has been used as a verb signifying 'to do'. The word 'nursing' comes from the Latin word *nutrix* meaning to 'nourish or cherish'. The word 'nourish' means to ' supply that which is necessary to life'. Nurse means to foster or cherish, i.e. to nurse one's meager talents; to treat or handle with adroit care, i.e. to nurse one's egg; to bring up, train or nurse; to clasp or handle carefully or fondly, i.e. to nurse a moment to preserve, i.e. to nurse a drink; so the term 'nurse' suggests attendance and service. Its antonym is 'neglect'. When nursing is perceived as a science, the term nursing becomes a noun signifying 'a body of abstract knowledge.'

Today nursing emerged as a learned profession, that is both a science and art. Science is the observation, identification, description, experimental investigations and theoretical explanation of natural phenomena. It is a body of knowledge. Knowledge is an awareness or perception of reality which is acquired through learning or investigation. Science is defined' as both a unified body of knowledge concerned with specific subject matter and the skills and methodology necessary to provide such knowledge. Therefore nursing science is that knowledge of germane to the discipline or nursing plus the processes and methodologies used to gain that knowledge. Goal of science is identification of truths or facts about the subject matter of a discipline ascertaining that–what, where, when, who and how–of phenomena of interest to the discipline.

According to Jean Watson (1979): Nursing is both scientific and artistic. I seek to combine science with humanism… Nursing is a therapeutic interpersonal process… Nursing is a scientific discipline that derives its practical base from scientific research.

Modern nursing involves many activities, concepts and skills related to basic sciences, social sciences, growth and development, contemporary issues; and other areas of nursing. Nursing as profession is unique because it addresses the responses of the individuals and families to actual or potential health problems in a humanistic and holistic manner. Now nurses have many roles, such as care takers, decision makers, advocates and teachers and they often assume several roles at the same time. Because of the diversity of nursing role, nurses need a philosophy of nursing to guide their practice.

Nursing has a fascinating history that parallels the history of humankind. For a long as there has been life so has there been the need to seek care and confort from illness and injury. From the dawn of civilization, evidence prevails to support the premise that nursing has been essential for the preservation of life. Survival of the human race, therefore, is inextricably intertwined with the development of nursing.

Nursing is an art. Art is the application of knowledge and skill to bring about desired results. Art is an individualized action. Nursing art is carried out by the nurse in a one-to-one relationship with the patient, and constitutes the nurse's conscious responses to specific and the patient's immediate situation. The art of clinical nursing is directed toward achievement of the four main goals:

1. Understanding of the patient and his/her condition or situation and need.
2. Enhancement of the patient's capability.
3. Improvement of his/her condition or situation within framework of medical plan for his/her cares, and
4. Prevention of the recurrence of his/her problem or development of a new one which may cause anxiety, disability or distress.

Nursing art involves three initial operations: stimulus, preconception and interpretation. Nurses' action may be rational, reactionary or deliberative.

Nursing is the art and science of assisting individuals in learning to care for themselves whenever possible and of caring for them when they are unable to their own needs. Nursing has developed into a scientific profession from an unorganized way of caring for the ill, resulting in change from mystical beliefs to sophisticated technology and caring. Nursing uses caring behaviors, critical thinking skills and scientific knowledge. Nursing focuses on the client response to illness rather than on the illness. Nursing promotes health and assists client's move to a higher level of wellness, including assistance during a terminal illness with the maintenance of comfort and dignity during the final stage of life.

Florence Nightingale (1876) viewed that nursing has been limited to signify little more than the administration of medicine and the application of poultice. It ought to signify the proper use of fresh air, light, warmth, cleanliness, quiet and the proper choosing and giving of diet – all at the least expense of vital power to the patient. As stated earlier nursing has been called the oldest arts and the youngest of the professions. As such, it has gone through many stages and has been an integral part of societal movements. Nursing has been involved in the existing culture shaped by it and helping development.

Nursing means the care and nurturing of healthy and ill people individually or in groups and communities. Nurses provide care for people in the midst of health, pain, loss, fear, disfigurement, death, grieving, challenge, growth, birth, and transition on intimate front-line basis. Expert nurses call this 'privileged place of nursing'.

Definitions of Nursing

International Council of Nurses (ICN, 1973) defined nursing according to the belief of Virginia Henderson (1966):

"The unique function of the nurse is to assist the individual, sick or well, in the performance of those activities contributing to health or its recovery (or peaceful death) that he would perform unaided if he had the necessary strength, will or knowledge."

Now, nursing throughout the universe has changed. Because advances in health care have altered the type of care required by clients. Nurses have taken on expanded roles, and there is renewed interest in providing care outside the hospital. Keeping in view of these changes the ICN (2003) defines the nursing as follows:

"Nursing encompasses autonomous and collaborative care of individuals of all ages, families, groups and communities, sick or well and in all settings. Nursing includes the promotion of health, prevention of illness, and the care of ill, disabled and dying people. Advocacy, promotion of safe environment, research, participation in shaping health policy and inpatient and health system management, and education are also key nursing roles."

American Nurses Association (1980) defined nursing as "the diagnosis and treatment of human responses to actual and potential health problems." Since nurses are a heterogenous group of people with varying skills.

WHO perform activities designed to provide care ranging from basic to complex in a growing number of settings. It is very difficult to describe the professional boundaries. So, in 2003 ANA acknowledged six essential features of professional nursing i.e.,

- Provision of a caring relationship that facilitates health and healing;
- Attention to the range of human experience and responses to health and illness within the physical and social environments;
- Integration of objective data with knowledge gained from and appreciation of the patient or groups subjective experience;
- Application of scientific knowledge to the processes of diagnosis and treatment through the use of judgment and critical thinking;
- Advancement of professional nursing knowledge through scholarly inquiry; and
- Influence of social and public policy to promote social justice.

Keeping in view of the above essential features, the ANA (2004) redefined professional nursing as:

"The protection, promotion, and optimization of health and abilities, prevention of illness and injury, alleviation of suffering through the diagnosis and treatment of human responses, and advocacy in the care of individuals, families, communities and populations."

"… It will never be possible to define, precisely and in great detail, which activities are inside and which are outside the boundaries of nursing. This is partly because the "state of the art" of health care and nursing are changing so rapidly that such lists become outdated almost before they are completed, and partly because the file has become far too complex to be reduced to lists of tasks and procedures. As the nursing profession matures and the body of nursing knowledge expands, it will become easier to clearly desirable the principles, models, and functions that are the basis of nursing" (CNA, 1993).

Views of Experts on Nursing

As stated earlier, the word 'nurse' originated from Latin word *nutrix* meaning 'to nourish'. Definitions of the nurse and nursing are based on this word origin to describe the nurse as a person who nourishes, fosters, and protects; a person prepared to take care of the sick, injured, and aged people. Defining nursing is a difficult task since nursing in not static but is always responding to new advances, increased knowledge and consumer needs. However, the expanding roles and functions of a nurse in present days have made anyone definition too limited. In the decades since Nightingale thought about, preached, wrote about the transformed nursing, many others have attempted to distill into one definition the essence of nursing. So it is better to review the number of definitions of nursing that evolved over the years, with its themes and goals.

Florence Nightingale (1859) 'Nursing ought to signify the proper use of fresh air, warmth, cleanliness, quiet and the proper selection and administration of diet–all at the least expense of vital power of the patient'.

Nurse means any person incharge of the personal health of another. Nursing means to have charge of the personal health of somebody and what nursing has to do–is put the patient in the least condition of nature to act upon him.

The theme of this definition is that 'the nurses' center of concern is patient'. Nature, a healthful, restful environment are nurses' allies. The goal of nursing is to facilitate body's reparative process by manipulating clients environment, client manipulated environments include appropriate nursing, nutrition, hygiene, light comfort, socialization and hope. In brief, health maintenance and restoration are the nurses' goals.

Shaw (1907) Nursing is an art… it properly includes as well as the execution of specific orders, the administration of food and medicine, the personal care of the patient. To fill such a position requires certain physical and mental attributes as well as special training.

The theme of this definition is that more than knowledge and skills needed by nurse, the attribute of personal caring is also needed.

Harmer (1922) Nursing is rooted in the needs of the humanity. Its object is not only to cure the sick but to bring health and ease, rest and comfort to mind and body. Its object is to prevent disease and to preserve health. The theme here is disease prevention and health promotion.

Harmer and Henderson (1939) Nursing may be defined as 'that service to an individual that helps him to attain or maintain a health state of mind or body'. The definition tells that nursing deals with the health of body psyche (mind and body).

Mother Olivia Gowan (1943) Nursing is both an art and science involving the total patient, as promoting spiritual, mental and physical health, stressing health education and health preservation, ministering to sick, caring for the patients, environment and giving health service to the family, community and to the individual.

Hildagard E Paplau (1952) 'Nursing is a significant, therapeutic, interpersonal process'. It functions co-operatively with other human processes that make health possible for individuals in community. Nursing is an educative instrument that aims to promote forward movement of personality in the direction of creative, constructive, productive, personal and community living.

This definition tells that effective nursing results from a therapeutic relationship between nurse and patient. Accordingly the goal of nursing is to develop interaction between nurse and client. Nurses participate in structuring health care systems to facilitate natural ongoing tendencies of humans to develop interpersonal relationship.

Virginia Henderson (1955) The unique function of the nurse is to assist the individual, sick or well, in the performance of those activities contributing to health (or its recovery or to a peaceful death) that he would perform unaided, if he had the necessary strength, will or knowledge. And to do this in such a way as to help him gain independence as rapidly as possible.

Henderson translates this unique function as (the nurse) in temporarily the conscious or the unconscious; the love of life for the suicidal; the leg for the amputee; the eyes for the newly blind; a means of locomotion for the infant; knowledge and confidence for the young mother; the voice for those who are too weak or withdrawn to speak; and she also argues that in these activities nurse should be an independent practitioner. The main theme of this definition is both well or ill people are the focus of nursing. Responsibility for care is shared by nurse and patient. The goal of nursing to work interdependently with other health care workers assisting client to gain independence as quickly as possible, to help client gain lacking strength.

Faye Glen Abdellah (1960) Nursing is a helping profession. Nursing care is doing something to or for the person or providing information to the person with goal of meeting needs, increasing or restoring self help ability or alleviating an impairment. Abdellah concept of 21 problems are the main focus of nursing. The nurse is a problems-solver and decision maker. The goal of nursing is to provide services to the individuals, families and society. A nurse should not only be kind and caring but also intelligent, competent and technically well prepared to provide this service.

Dorothea E Orem (1960) Nursing is described as the giving of direct assistance to a person, as required, because of the person's specific inabilities in self care resulting from a situation of personal health.

This tells nursing is doing for a person what he cannot do at this time due to health related limitations. The goal of nursing is to care for and help client attain total self care or return to self care is the goal (1971). Nursing care becomes necessary where client is unable to fulfill biological, psychological, developmental or social needs (1985), as nursing is giving assistance to persons who are unable to meet their own needs.

Ida Jean Orlando (1961) The function of professional nursing is conceptionalized as finding out and meeting the patient's immediate need for help.

Orlando viewed three dimensions, i.e. client behavior, nurse's reactions and nurse action, compose nursing situation. The goal of nursing is to respond to client behavior in terms of immediate needs. To interact with client to meet immediate needs by identifying client behavior, reaction of nurse and nursing action to be taken.

Lydia E Hall (1962) Nursing can and should be professional. The professional nurse functions most therapeutically when patients have entered the second stage of their hospital stay (the second stay in the recuperating or nonacute phase of illness).

Hall viewed that client is composed of the overlapping parts, i.e. person pathological stage (core) and treatment (cure) and body (care). Nurse is a caretaker. The goal of nursing is to provide care and comfort to client during disease process.

Ernestine Weidenbach (1964) Nursing is a service, helping art, a goal directed activity. The purpose (goal) of clinical nursing is to facilitate the efforts of the individual to overcome the obstacles which currently interfere with his ability to response capably to demand made of him by his conditions, environment situation and time.

Nursing is a practice which is related to individuals who need help because of behavioral stimulus. Clinical nursing has four interlocking components, i.e. philosophy (way), purpose (why), practice (what), and art (how).

Myra Estrin Levine (1966) Nursing is a human interaction. Nursing intervention is based on four conservation principles of nursing, i.e. conservation of energy, conservation of structural integrity, conservation of personal integrity, and conservation of social integrity.

The goal of nursing is to use conservation activities aimed at optimum use of clients resources.

Dorothy E Johnson (1968) Nursing is an external force acting to preserve the organization of patient behavior while the patient is under stress by means of imposing regularity mechanism or by providing resources.

Nursing is an art and science, it supplies external assistance both before and during system balance disturbances and therefore requires knowledge of order, disorder and control.

The goal of nursing is to reduce stress so that client can move more easily, through recovery process.

Martha E Rogers (1970) Nursing is a humanistic science dedicated to compassionate concern for maintaining and promoting health, preventing illness and caring for and rehabilitating the sick and the disabled.

Her unitary man evolves along life process. Client continuously changes and co-exists with environment. Accordingly each person has a personal maximal health potential. Nursing seeks to strengthen each human being's capacity to achieve that potential. The goal of nursing is to maintain and promote health, prevent illness and care for and rehabilitate ill and disabled through humanistic science of nursing.

Imogene King (1971) Nursing is viewed as an interpersonal process of action, reaction, interaction and transaction, in which perceptions of nurse and client influence the interactional process. Nursing is an observable behavior found in the health care systems in society.

'Nursing is a process of human interactions between nurse and client where each perceives the other and the situation and through communication, they set goals, explore means and agree on means to achieve goal'.

The goal of nursing is to help individuals and group attain, maintain and restore health or die with dignity and to use communication to help client re-establish positive adaptation to environment.

Joyce Travelbee (1971) Nursing is an interpersonal process whereby the professional nurse assists an individual or family to prevent cope with the experience of illness and suffering and if necessary assists the individual or family to find meaning in these experiences.

Travelbee views nurse as a supporter, sustainer, and change agent. The goal of nursing is to assist individual or family to prevent or cope with illness, regain health, find meaning in illness or maintain maximal degree of health.

She also views an interpersonal process as human-to-human relationship formed during illness and experiences of suffering.

Betty Neumen (1972) 'Nursing' is a unique profession in that it is concerned with all of the variables affecting an individual's response to stress and believes that nursing is concerned with the whole person.

The goal of nursing is to assist individuals, families, and groups to attain and maintain maximal level of total wellness by purposeful interventions. The nursing interventions include primary, secondary and tertiary level of preventions.

Sister Callista Roy (1979) Nursing is defined broadly as "a theoretical system of knowledge which prescribes a process of analysis and action related to the care of the ill or potentially ill."

Roy differentiates nursing as a science from nursing as a practice discipline. The goal of nursing is to identify types of demands placed on client, assess adaptation to demands, and help client adapt as nursing is promoting a positive adaptation to changing internal and external environment.

Madeleine Leininger (1978) Nursing is a learned humanistic art and science that focuses upon personalized care behaviors, functions, and process directed toward promoting and maintaining health behaviors or recovery from illness which have physical, psycho-cultural and social significance or meaning for those being assisted generally by a professional nurse or one with similar role competencies.

The goal of nursing is to provide care consistent with nursing's emerging science and knowledge with caring as central focus.

Jean Watson (1979) Nursing is a philosophy and science of caring, and the nursing practice based on 10 creative factors, in which each has a dynamic phenomenological component that is relative to the individuals involved in the relationship as assessed by nursing.

The goal of nursing is to promote health, restore client to health and prevent illness. Watson believes that nurses have the responsibility to go beyond the 10 creative factors (see theory) and to facilitate clients development in the area of health promotion through preventive health actions. This goal is accomplished by teaching clients personal changes to promote health, providing situations support, teaching, problem solving methods and recognizing coping skills and adaptation to loss.

Kathryn E Barnard (1981) Nursing is a process by which the patient is assisted in maintenance and promotion of his independence. This process may be educational, therapeutic or restorative. It involves facilitation of change, most probably change in the environment.

Nursing is the diagnosis and treatment of human responses to health problems (1981).

Deyoung (1981) Nursing is the caring and nurturing of the physical, social, spiritual, cultural, and emotional well-being of an individual, family, or community.

Rosemarie Rizzo Parse (1981) Nursing is a human science. The nursing responsibility to society relative to nursing practice is guiding in choosing of possibilities in the changing health process. The nursing practice is directed towards illuminating and mobilizing family interrelationship in light of the meaning assigned to health and possibilities as languaged in the co-related patterns of relation.

The goal of nursing is to focus on man's qualitative participation with health experiences.

Patricia Benner (1982) Nursing is viewed as caring practice whose science is guided by the moral art and ethics of care and responsibility. Nursing practice is the care and study of the lived experience of health, illness and disease and the relationship between these three.

Helen C Erickson et al Nursing is the holistic helping of persons with their self care activities in relation to their health. This is an interactive, interpersonal process that nurtures strengths to enable development, release, and channeling of resources for coping with one's circumstances and environment.

The goal of nursing is to achieve a state of perceived optimum health and contentment.

Nursing is a helping profession and, as such provides services which contribute to the health and well-being of people.

Nursing is a vital consequence to the individual receiving services. It fills needs that cannot be met by the person, family or other persons in the community.

Three essential components of professional nursing 'are care, cure and coordination. The care aspect is more than to take care of'; it is also 'caring for' and 'caring about'. It is dealing with human beings under stress, frequently over long period of time. It is providing comfort and support in times of anxiety, loneliness, and helpfulness. It is listening, evaluating, and intervening appropriately.

The promotion of health and healing is the cure aspect of professional nursing. It is assisting clients to understand their health problems and helping them to cope with. It is the administration of medication and treatment. It is also the use of clinical nursing judgement in determining on the basis of patient outcomes, whether the plan of care needs to be maintained or changed. It is knowing when and how to use existing and potential resources to help patients toward recovery and adjustment by mobilizing their own resources.

Professional nursing practice is this and even more. It is sharing responsibility for the health and welfare of all people in the community, and it is participating in programs designed to prevent illness and maintain health. It is conditioning and synchronizing medical and other professional and technical services that affect patient care. It is supervising, teaching and directing all those involved in nursing care.

The Congress of Nursing Practice defined nursing as 'the diagnosis and treatment of human responses to actual or potential health problems.' This definition involves the characteristics of nursing, i.e. phenomena, theory application, nursing action, and evaluation of the effects of action.

- *Phenomena:* They are the human responses to actual or potential health problems. The nurse identifies the clients responses by assessing health status and obtaining data.
- *Theory application:* The nurse applies nursing theory to understanding these human responses.
- *Nursing action:* The nurse takes action to resolve actual or potential health problems.
- *Evaluation:* The nurse evaluates the effects of the actions on the clients responses.

These above characteristics are related to the nursing process.

CNA definition of nursing The nursing profession exists in response to a need of society and holds ideals related to man's health throughout his lifespan. Nurses direct their energies toward the promotion, maintenance and restoration of health; the prevention of illness, the alleviation of suffering and the insurance of a peaceful death when life can no longer be sustained. Nurses value a holistic view and regard an individual as a biophysical being who has the capacity to set goals and make decisions and who has the right and responsibility to make informed choices congruent with personal belief and values. Nursing, a dynamic and supportive profession guided by code of ethics, is rooted in caring, a concept evidence through its four fields of activity–practice, education, administration, and research.

In most of the definitions, the central focus is the person receiving care who may be called as the patient or client and includes the physical, emotional, social, and spiritual dimension of that person. Nursing is no longer considered to be primarily concerned with illness care, the concepts and definitions have expanded to include prevention of illness, the promotion of wellness, and the maintenance of health for individual, family and community.

(For more views on nurse experts, please read author's text on "NURSING THEORIES")

Nursing as a Profession

The views and definitions of nurse leaders and educators on nursing have expanded to describe more clearly the roles and actions of nurses; increased attention has focused on the question of nursing as a profession and as a discipline. Nursing is gaining recognition as a profession based on certain basic criteria.

Occupation is often used interchangeably with profession, but their definitions differ. Webster defines occupation as 'what occupies, or engages, one's time, business, and employment'. Profession is defined as 'a vocation requiring advanced training and usually involving mental rather manual work, as teaching, engineering, etc. especially medicine, law or theology'. There is an overall agreement that a profession is different from an occupation in at least two major ways, i.e. preparation and commitment.

Professional preparation usually takes place in a college or university setting. Preparation is prolonged in order to include instruction in the specialized body of knowledge and techniques of the profession. Professional preparation includes more than knowledge and skills, however, it also includes orientation to the beliefs, values and attitudes expected of the members of the profession. Standards of practice and ethical consideration are also included.

Professional commitment to the profession is strong. They derive much of their personal identification from their work and consider it an integral part of their lives.

In occupation, training may occur on the job, and the length of training also varies. The values, beliefs, and ethics are not prominent features of preparation. The commitment and personal identification also vary. In occupation people often change jobs. In these settings, workers are supervised and accountability rests on the employer.

A profession is an occupation with ethical components, i.e. devoted to the promotion of human and social welfare. The services offered by a profession are based on specialized knowledge and skills which have been developed in scientific and learned manner. Whereas occupation is principal areas of work classified according to various features such as preparation, skills and knowledge required; the nature of work itself; supervision; motivation, etc. Professions are those occupations possessing a particular combination of characteristics generally considered to be the expertise, autonomy, commitment, and responsibility.

A profession is an occupation based on specialized intellectual study and training, the purpose of which is to supply skilled services with ethical components and others for a definite fee or salary. The economists view that the profession is a non-cooperating group. The socialists view that professional worker is subject to institutional or normative control.

Criteria of Profession

Many writers have listed the criteria of profession. Some of them are as follows:

Abraham Flexner (1916)

Flexner believed that professional work:
- is basically intellectual (as opposed to physical);
- is based on a body of knowledge that can be learned;
- practical rather than theoretical;
- can be taught through a process of profession education;
- has a strong internal organization of members;
- has practitioners who are motivated by altruism.

On these beliefs Flexner listed following criteria for profession:
1. The profession involves essential intellectual operations accompanied by large undivided responsibilities.
2. They are learned in nature and members are constantly resorting to laboratory and seminar for fresh supply of facts.
3. They are not merely academic and theoretical, but are definitely practical in their aims.
4. They possess a technique capable of communication through a highly specialized educational discipline.
5. They are self organized with activities and duties and responsibilities which completely engage their participants and develop group consciousness.
6. They are likely to be more responsible to public interest than that of unorganized and isolated individuals and they tend to become increasingly concerned with the achievement to social bids.

William Shephard (1948)

William Shephard listed following criteria of profession:
1. A profession must satisfy an indispensable social need and be based upon well established and socially accepted scientific principles.
2. A profession must demand adequate pre-professional and cultural training.
3. A profession must demand the profession of a body of specialized and systematized knowledge.
4. A profession must give evidence of needed skills which the public does not possess, i.e. skills which are partly native and partly acquired.
5. A profession must have developed a scientific technique which is the result of tested experience.
6. A profession must require the exercise of discretion and judgement as to time and manner of the performance of duty. This is in contrast to the work which is subject to immediate direction and supervision.

7. Profession must be a type of beneficial work, the result of which is not subject to standardization in term of unit performance or time element.
8. Profession must have group consciousness designed to extend scientific knowledge in technical language.
9. Profession must have sufficient self impelling power to retain its members throughout life. It must not be used to mere stepping stone to other occupations.
10. A profession must recognize its obligations to society by insisting that its members live up to an established code of ethics.

Bixler and Bixler (1959)

Bixler and Bixler criteria of a profession included the following:
1. A profession utilizes in its practice, as well defined and well organized body of specialized knowledge which is on the intellectual level of the higher learning.
2. A profession constantly enlarges the body of knowledge it uses and improves its techniques of education and service by the use of scientific method.
3. A profession entrusts the education of its practitioners to institutions of higher education.
4. A profession applies its body of knowledge in practical services which are vital to human and social welfare.
5. A profession functions autonomously in the formulation of professional policy and in the control of professional activity thereby.
6. A profession attracts individuals of intellectual and personal qualities who consider service above personal gain and who recognize their chosen occupation as a lifework.
7. A profession strives to compensate its practitioners by providing freedom of action, opportunity for conscious professional growth and economic security.

A comparison of above criteria reveals many similarities. General agreement exists about that constitutes a profession, but not all people agree about which occupations are profession.

Kelly (1981)

Kelly reiterated and expanded Flexner's criteria and listed following characteristics of a profession:
1. The services provided are vital to humanity and welfare of society.
2. There is a special body of knowledge which is continually enlarged through research.
3. The services involve intellectual activities. Individual responsibility (accountability) is a strong feature.
4. Practitioners are educated, in institutions of higher learning.
5. Practitioners are relatively independent and control their own policies and activities (autonomy).
6. Practitioners are motivated by service (altruism) and consider their work as an important component of their lives.
7. There is a code of ethics to guide the decisions and conduct of practitioners.

8. There is an organization (association) which encourages and supports high standards or practice.

Nursing is gaining recognition as a profession based on the criteria that a profession must have:

- a well defined body of knowledge,
- a strong service orientation,
- recognized authority by a professional group,
- a code of ethics,
- a professional organization that sets standards,
- ongoing research,
- autonomy.

In the context of the above criteria formulated by different experts 'nursing' of today has been called as one among the noble professions of the university as it fulfills all the criteria.

Nursing as a Discipline

A discipline has a specific and unique body of knowledge that uses existing and new knowledge to solve problems creatively and meet human needs within everchanging boundaries. To be considered a discipline, certain criteria must be fulfilled:

- An impressive body of lasting works
- Should have suitable techniques
- Should concern with that are relevant to human activities
- Relevant traditions that inspire future knowledge development
- Should have considerable scholarly, recognition and achievement.

Nursing involves specialized skills and application of knowledge based on education that has both theoretical and clinical components. Nurses uphold standards set forth by professional organizations and follow an established code of ethics. The concerns of nursing focus on human responses to actual or potential health problems and are increasingly focused on wellness, an area of caring that encompasses nursing unique knowledge and abilities. Nursing is rich in tradition. Furthermore, nursing is increasingly being recognized as scholarly, with academic qualifications, research and publications specific to nursing becoming more widely accepted and respected as a discipline.

Nursing has evolved through history from a technical service to a client centered process that affects the lives of others to allow maximization of potential in all human dimensions. This has been an active process, as the profession and the discipline of nursing has developed by using lessons from the past to gain knowledge for practice in the present and in the future. Now nursing has emerged as one of the important professions and disciplines that provides sincere service to humanity.

Is Nursing a Profession, Discipline, or Occupation?

One strategy used to describe a field is to categorize it as a profession, discipline, or occupation. Although the term *profession* is freely used, a group must meet the following criteria to be considered a **profession** (Starr, 1982):

- The knowledge of the group must be based on technical and scientific knowledge.
- The knowledge and competence of members of the group must be evaluated by a community of peers.
- The group must have a service orientation and a code of ethics.

Nursing appears to meet all criteria of a profession as defined by Starr. Entry-level nursing education requires coursework in basic and social sciences as well as humanities, arts, and general education. Nursing education and practice are increasingly based on research from nursing and related fields. State or provincial regulatory bodies have defined the criteria that nurses must meet to practice, and they monitor members for adherence to standards. Nursing is clearly focused on providing service to others, and the major professional organizations have developed ethical guidelines to guide the practice of nursing.

Donaldson and Crowley (1978) define a **discipline** as "a unique perspective, a distinct way of viewing all phenomena, which ultimately defines the limits and nature of its inquiry". To be considered a discipline, a profession must have a domain of knowledge that has both theoretical and practical boundaries. The theoretical boundaries of a profession are the questions that arise from clinical practice and are then investigated through research. The practical boundaries are the current state of knowledge and research in the field. This is the known, or the facts that dictate safe practice.

A case can be made that nursing is both a profession and a discipline. It is a scientifically based, self-governed profession that focuses on the ethical care of others. It is also a discipline that is driven by theoretical and practical aspects, demanding thorough knowledge of its scientific basis and clinical skills. Put simply, nursing requires theoretical knowledge and practical skills.

In spite of meeting criteria for both designations (profession and discipline), nursing is often described as an occupation or job. Unlike physicians, most of whom are in control of their practice environment, working conditions, and schedule, most nurses are hourly wage earners. The employer, not the nurse, decides the conditions of practice and the nature of the work. Nurse practice acts do not preclude nurses from functioning more autonomously, however. The following may improve the status of nursing:

- Standardizing the educational requirements for entry into practice
- Enacting uniform continuing education requirements
- Encouraging the participation of more nurses in professional organizations
- Educating the public about the true nature of nursing practice

(For some more details regarding nursing profession please read author's text on "Nursing Administration").

Goals of Nursing

According to views and definition of nursing, it is possible to identify following main areas of nursing, i.e. maintenance of health, promotion of health, restoration of health, prevention of illness, facilitation of coping and the care of the dying. These areas help us to formulate the following goals of nursing:

1. Maintenance of health.
2. Promotion of wellness/health.
3. Restoration of health.
4. Prevention of illness.
5. Facilitate coping.
6. Care of the dying.

To meet these goals of nursing, the nurses use knowledge and skills to give care in a variety of traditional and expanding nursing roles. The primary role of the nurse as caregiver is given shape and substance by the interrelated roles of communicator, teacher, counselor, leader, researcher, and advocate. The brief description of nurse's role in these goals is as follows:

Maintenance of Health

Activities within the roles of nurses are carried out by the nurses in many different settings including hospitals, nursing homes, clinics, offices, mobile units and the home and the community settings. Nurses work in many settings where the goal of health care is the maintenance of health. Residents of nursing homes utilize the skills of nurses to continue maximum functioning. In school campus, nurses provide a variety of educational program focused on the health maintenance as a part of student health service.

Promotion of Health/Wellness

Wellness is a state of human functioning that may be defined as the achievement of one's maximum attainable potential. When promoting health is the goal of nursing, the person is already in an acceptable state of health but is seeking an improved state of health, a higher level on a continuum between illness and health. The objective of health or wellness is to enhance the quality of a person's life through activities that are designed to continually improve the state of his physical, mental, social, emotional, and spiritual well-being.

Promotion of wellness is the framework of the nursing activities. The client's self awareness, health awareness, wellness skills, and use of resource are all considered as the nurse provides care. Through her knowledge and skill, the nurse:

- facilitates decisions about lifestyle that enhance the quality of life and encourages acceptance of responsibility for one's own health,
- increases health awareness by assisting in the understanding that health is more than just not being ill and by teaching certain behaviors and factors that can contribute to or diminish wellness,
- teaches wellness skills by promoting decision making so that self care activities maximize achievement of goals that are realistic and attainable, and by serving as a role of model,
- encourages the use of wellness resources by providing information and referrals.

For example, an individual who wants to improve physical fitness seeks nursing help in determining that it is safe to begin an exercise program after careful examination by the doctor, the nurse may work with person to plan diet and exercise program.

Restoration of Health

Generally, people expect that the nurses have to do with the nurse caring for sick persons, and the majority of nurses do function in these settings. Nurses who work in hospitals and clinics spend most of their time working to restore the health of patients. Activities to restore health include the following:

- Providing direct care of the person who is ill by such measures as providing physical care, administering medications, and carrying out procedures and treatments
- Performing diagnostic measurements and examination that detect an illness
- Referring question and abnormal findings to other health care providers as appropriate
- Planning teaching, and carrying out rehabilitation for illness such as cardiac disease, arthritis, and neurological disorders
- Working in mental illness and chemical depending persons or drug addicts, alcoholics.

Facilitate Coping

In addition to the above the nurses also facilitate client and family coping with altered functions, life crisis and death. Altered functions result in a decrease in an individuals ability to carry out activities of daily living and expected roles. Nurses can facilitate an optional level of function through maximizing strengths and potentials, teaching and knowledge of and referral to community support system. Nurses provide care to both client and families during the terminal illness, and they do so in hospitals, long-term nursing facilities, and homes.

Prevention of Illness

The goals of illness prevention activities are to reduce the risk of illness, to promote good health habits and maintain the individual's optimal function. Nurses primarily promote health by teaching and by giving personal example. Such activities include the following:

- Educational programs in areas such as prenatal care for pregnant women, smoking cessation program, de-addiction program, and stress reduction education
- Community program and resources that encourage health lifestyles including aerobic exercise classes, gymnastics, physical fitness program
- Literature, and television information on diet, exercise and the importance of good health habits
- Health assessments in institutions, clinics, and community settings that identify areas of strength and the potential for illness.

Care of the Dying

Another goal of nursing is to provide care for dying patients, because care and the restoration of health are not always possible. Most of the patients will die in hospitals, but others depending on circumstances, cultural practices, or disease conditions, choose to die at home. Whether patient dies in hospital or home, in such circumstances nurse helps the person to die in dignified and peaceful ways or teach the relatives and friends and family that how best they can help the person to die in dignity and peace.

Although a comprehensive definition of nursing is difficult to formulate, all definitions agree that nursing is about caring.

The recipients of nursing care as "individuals, groups, families, or communities… The recipient(s) of nursing care can be referred to as patient(s), client(s), or person(s)." Nurses may work independently or with other health care providers to care for patients. **Direct care** involves personal interaction between the nurse and clients (e.g., giving medications, dressing a wound, or teaching a client about medicines or care). Nurses deliver **indirect care** when they work on behalf of an individual group, family, or community to improve their health status (e.g., restocking the code blue cart [an emergency cart], ordering unit supplies, or arranging unit staffing). A nurse may use independent judgment to determine the care needed or may work under the direct order of a primary care provider.

Purposes of Nursing Care

Nurses provide care to achieve the goals of health promotion, illness prevention, health restoration, and end-of-life care. Together these aspects of care represent a range of services that cover the spectrum from complete well-being to death.

(i) *Health Promotion*

The World Health Organization defines **health** as "a state of complete physical, mental, and social well-being, and not merely the absence of disease or infirmity". This inclusive definition can be applied to individuals, groups, families, or communities. **Health promotion** activities are any activities that foster the highest state of well-being of the recipient of the activities. For example, you might counsel a pregnant client about the importance of adequate prenatal nutrition to promote health at the individual level. Group and family-level health promotion activities might include teaching about nutrition during pregnancy in prenatal classes and in family education programs. On a community level your nursing activities would be focused on reaching a larger number of people. For example, you could advocate for prominent billboards highlighting the importance of prenatal care and nutrition, post signs in grocery stories recommending food sources for pregnant women, and lobby for labeling of substances that should be avoided in pregnancy.

(ii) *Illness Prevention*

Illness prevention focuses on avoidance of disease. Activities are targeted to decrease the risk of developing an illness or to minimize the risk of exposure to disease. To avoid disease, people must know the causes of disease and the route of disease transmission. For example, pneumonia causes many deaths every year. Those affected are society's most vulnerable: the very young, the very old, and the very ill. Some nursing activities to decrease the risk of pneumonia include:

- Teaching the importance of hand washing to decrease the transmission of infection.
- Advocating for and administering pneumonia immunizations to those at high risk.

(iii) *Health Restoration*

Health restoration encompasses activities that foster a return to health for those already ill. To restore health, the nurse provides direct care to ill individuals, groups, families, or communities. This aspect of care is what most people think of when they envision the nursing role. Recall that health has physical, mental, and social dimensions. When you engage in health restoration activities, your care should address each of these dimensions. Health-restoration activities include the following:

- Providing hygiene and nutrition for someone unable to do so independently.
- Assessing an ill client's health status.
- Performing diagnostic tests on a client.
- Administering medications or treatments.
- Counseling individuals or groups.
- Tracking clients with a communicable disease to ensure that they receive appropriate therapy.
- Lobbying for community changes to decrease the prevalence of disease within a community.

(iv) *End-of-Life* Care

Not all nursing activities can be directed toward promoting or restoring health, or preventing disease. Death is an inevitable consequence of life. Nurses have been active in promoting the respectful care of those who are terminally ill or dying. Nursing activities for the dying are designed to promote comfort, maintain quality of life, provide culturally relevant spiritual care, and ease the emotional burden of death. Nurses work with dying individuals, their family members and support persons, and with organizations that focus on the needs of the terminally ill.

Settings of Nursing Care

As nurses will have the opportunity to work in a variety of settings. During their education, nurses will be placed in many settings and clinical units that will allow them see some of the possible options available upon graduation. Approximately 60% of nurses work in hospitals. The remaining 40% work in extended care facilities, ambulatory care, and community or home health settings.

Hospitals provide services to clients who require round-the-clock nursing care. This type of care is frequently referred to as *acute care*. Length of stay is limited to the amount of time that the client requires 24-hour observation.

Extended care facilities provide care for clients for an extended period of time-usually longer than one month. These facilities include skilled nursing facilities (SNF, also known as convalescent hospitals) and rehabilitation facilities. Clients may begin receiving care at these sites directly or may be transferred there for ongoing care after hospitalization.

Ambulatory care is synonymous with outpatient care. Clients reside at home or in non-hospital settings and come to the site for care. Ambulatory care sites include private health and medical offices, clinics, and outpatient therapy centers.

Home care is provided to clients who are homebound or unable to get themselves to ambulatory care centers for services. Services are usually coordinated by a home health or visiting nurse service and include nursing care as well as various therapies and home assistance programs. Home care services may also be employed when the client or family decides that home is the preferred site of care–particularly when the client is terminally ill. Home care is also appropriate when clients still requiring skilled care are discharged from the hospital because their reimbursable length-of-stay has expired.

Community health deals with provision of care for the community at large. Community health nurses provide services to at-risk populations and devise strategies to improve the health status of the surrounding community. Examples of community health programs include health care for the homeless and school-based programs designed to decrease the incidence of teen pregnancies.

Standards of Nursing Care

The standards of nursing practice in clinical setting are given below (Table 2.1).

Table 2.1: Standards of Clinical Nursing Practice		
Standards of Care		
Standard 1	Assessment	The registered nurse collects comprehensive data pertinent to the patient's health or the situation.
Standard 2	Diagnosis	The registered nurse analyzes the assessment data to determine the diagnoses or issues.
Standard 3	Outcome identification	The registered nurse identifies expected outcomes for a plan individualized to the patient or situation.
Standard 4	Planning	The registered nurse develops a plan that prescribes strategies and to attain expected outcomes.
Standard 5	Implementation	The registered nurse implements the identified plan.
Standard 5A	Coordination of care	The registered nurse coordinates care delivery.
Standard 5B	Health teaching and health promotion	The registered nurse employs strategies to promote health and a safe environment.
Standard 5C	Consultation	The advanced practice registered nurse and the nursing role specialist provide consultation to influence the identified plan, enhance the abilities of others, and effect change.
Standard 5D	Prescriptive authority and treatment	The advanced practice registered nurse uses prescriptive authority, procedures, referrals, treatments, and therapies in accordance with state and federal laws and regulations.
Standard 6	Evaluation	The registered nurse evaluates progress toward attainment of outcomes.
Standards of Professional Performance		
Standard 7	Quality of practice	The registered nurse systematically enhances the quality and effectiveness of nursing practice.
Standard 8	Education	The registered nurse attains knowledge and competency that reflects current nursing practice.
Standard 9	Professional practice evaluation	The registered nurse evaluates one's own nursing practice in relation to professional practice standards and guidelines, relevant statutes, rules, and regulations.
Standard 10	Collegiality	The registered nurse interacts with and contributes to the professional development of peers and colleagues.
Standard 11	Collaboration	The registered nurse collaborates with patient, family, and others in the conduct of nursing practice.
Standard 12	Ethics	The registered nurse integrates ethical provisions in all areas of practice.
Standard 13	Research	The registered nurse integrates research findings into practice.
Standard 14	Resource utilization	The registered nurse considers factors related to safety, effectiveness, cost, and impact on practice in the planning and delivery of nursing services.
Standard 15	Leadership	The registered nurse provides leadership in the professional practice setting and the profession.

Roles and Functions of Nurses

Traditionally, the role of the nurses was to provide care and comfort as they carried out specific nursing function, but changes in nursing of the day have expanded the role to include increased emphasis on health promotion and illness-prevention, as well as concern for the client as a whole. At present nurse functions in the interrelated roles as given below.

Care Giver

Care giving role is a primary role of the nurse. The provision of care to clients that combines both the art and science of nursing in meeting physical, emotional, intellectual, sociocultural, and spiritual needs. As a caregiver, the nurse helps the client regain health through the healing process. The nurse addresses the holistic health care needs of the client, including measures to restore emotional and social well-being. The care giver also helps the client and family set goals with minimum cost of time and energy. As a care giver, the nurse integrates other roles to promote wellness through activities that prevent illness, restore health, and facilitate coping with disability or death.

Communicator

The role of communicator is central to other nursing roles. The quality of communication is a critical factor in meeting the needs of the client, without clear communication effective nursing care is impossible. The use of effective interpersonal and therapeutic communication skills to establish and maintain helping relationships with clients of all ages in a wide variety of health care setting.

Teacher/Client Family Educator

The use of communication skills is to assess, implement and evaluate individualized teaching plans to meet learning needs of clients and their families. As a teacher, the nurse explaining to clients concepts and facts about health, demonstrates procedures such as self care activities, determines that the client fully understands, reinforces learning or client behavior, and evaluates progress in learning. Teaching may be unplanned and formal. (e.g., responding to question while casual conversation) or planned or mere formal (e.g., teaching diet plan for diabetes).

Counselor

The use of therapeutic interpersonal communication skills to provide information, make appropriate referrals, and facilitate the clients problem solving and decision making skills.

Decision Maker

To provide effective care, the nurse uses decision making skills, throughout the nursing process. Before undertaking any nursing intervention, whether it is assessing the client's condition, giving care or evaluating the results of care, the nurse plans the action by deciding the best approach for each client, by using decision making skills.

Leader/Manager

The assertive, self confident practice of nursing, when providing care, effective change and functioning with group. Nurses coordinate the activities of other members of the health care team, such a dietician, and physiotherapists, when managing client needs and nurses also direct their subordinates for quality of nursing care. Nurses must also manage their own time and the resources of the practice setting when concurrently providing care to several clients. As manager/leader, nurses coordinate and delegate care responsibilities and supervise other health care workers.

Comforter

The role of comforter caring for the client as a person, is a traditional and historical one in nursing and has continued to be important as nurses have assumed new roles. Because nursing care must be directed to the whole person rather than simply the body comfort and emotional support often helps give the client strength to recover, while carrying out nursing activities, nurses can provide comfort by demonstrating care of the client as an individual with unique feelings and needs.

Rehabilitator

Rehabilitation is the process by which individuals return to maximal levels of functioning after illness, accidents or other disabling events. Usually the clients experience some improvements and all aspects of health, the nurse helps them to adapt as fully as possible, by using her/ his knowledge and skill of many concepts which she/he learned.

Protector and Advocater/Client Advocate

The protection of human or legal rights and the securing of care for all clients based on the belief that clients have the right to make informed decision about their own health and lives.

As a protector the nurse helps to maintain a safe environment for the client and takes steps to prevent injury and protect the client from possible adverse effect of diagnostic or treatment measures. For example, confirming that a client does not have an allergy to medication.

As an advocate, the nurse protects the client's human and legal rights and provides assistance in asserting those rights if the need arises, e.g., providing additional information to accept treatment.

Career Roles (Expanded Roles)

Clinical Nurse Specialists

A nurse with an advanced degree, education or experience who is considered to be an expert in a specialized area of nursing, carries a direct client care, consultation, teaching clients, families and staff, and conducts research.

Nurse Practitioner

A nurse with an advanced degree certified for a special area or age of client care, works in a variety of health care settings or in independent practice to make health assessment and deliver primary care.

Nurse midwife: A nurse who completes a performance in midwifery, provides prenatal and postnatal care and conducts deliveries to women with uncomplicated pregnancies.

Nurse anesthetist: A nurse who completes a course of study in anestheseology, carries out preoperative visits and assessments, administers and monitor anesthesia during surgery, and evaluates postoperative status of clients.

Nurse educator: A nurse usually with an advanced degree teaches in educational, or clinical setting, teaches theoretical knowledge and clinical skills and conducts research.

Nurse administrator: A nurse who functions at various levels of management in health care setting is responsible for the management and administration of resources and personnel involved in giving client caring.

Nurse researcher: A nurse with an advanced degree conducts research relevant to the definition and improvement of nursing practice, education and administration.

Nurse entrepreneur: A nurse usually with an advanced degree may manage a clinic or health related business, conduct research provide education, or serve as an adviser or consultant to institution, political agencies or business.

The definitions given by nurse leaders are statements of how individuals have viewed nursing. Each definition has been studied, debated, and investigated. Individual school of nursing and health care institution each selects a definition that seems to best reflect the purpose of their unique organization. The ANA defined nursing practice as "a direct service goal oriented, and adaptable to the needs of the individual family and the community during health and illness". The CNA defines, "the nurses direct their energies toward the promotion, maintenance and restoration of health, the prevention of illness, the alleviation of suffering and the ensuring of a peaceful death when life can no longer be sustained."

The ICN adapted following definitions that has been approved by CNR (1987), i.e. nursing as integral part of the health care system, encompasses the promotion of health, prevention of illness and care of physically ill, mentally ill and disabled people of all ages, in all the health care and other community settings. Within this broad spectrum of health care, the phenomenon of particular concern to nurse is individual, family and group response to actual or potential health problems. These human responses range broadly from health restoring reactions to an individual episode of illness to the development of policy in promoting the long-term health of a population.

The unique functions of nurses in caring for individuals, sick or well, is to assess their responses to their health status and to assist them in the performance of those activities contributing to health, recovery or to dignified death, then they would perform unaided, if they had the necessary strength, will or knowledge and to do this in such a way as to help them gain full or partial independence as rapidly as possible, within the total health care environment nurses share with other health professionals and those in other sectors of public service the functions of planning, implementation and evaluation to ensure the adequacy of the health system for promoting health, preventing illness and caring for ill and disabled people. Table 2.2 summarizes the roles and functions of the nurse.

Factors Influence in Nursing Practice

Two types of factors influence contemporary nursing practice: Those in society at large and outside the profession, and those within nursing and health care.

Trends in Society

Historically evolution of nursing influences current nursing practice and will inevitably continue to influence its future development. In addition, nursing is currently influenced by trends in the economy, increased consumer knowledge, legislation, the women's movement, and collective bargaining:

- *The national economy* has a tremendous impact on nursing. In every country, health care is provided as a right of citizenship. In some states, health insurance coverage is linked to full-time employment in large companies with health insurance benefits. Thus, as unemployment figures rise, the number of people without insurance escalates. Fearing the high costs of medicines and health care, many uninsured people delay seeking needed care. The effect is that clients are often sicker when they enter the health care system. This taxes the system's resources and raises the level of nursing care required. Another consideration is that the health care industry—even in a strong economy—is very expensive to operate. Downturns in the economy affect institutional investments and profits, and may limit medications and services available. Similarly, the salaries of health care providers are influenced by national economic trends.
- *The role of the health care consumer* also affects nursing. Historically, patients relied on the knowledge and decision making of the health care team. Now, however, consumers are demanding greater choice in the decisions that affect their health.
- *Patients have access to vast amounts of health and medical information, particularly through the Internet.* Websites such as WebMD and PubMed, and online medical and health journals give consumers accurate and up-to-date health

Table 2.2: Roles and Functions of the Nurse

Role	Function	Examples
Direct care provider	Addressing the physical, emotional, social, and spiritual needs of the client.	Assessing the client Giving medications Patient teaching
Communicator	Using interpersonal and therapeutic communication skills to address the needs of the client, to facilitate communication in the health care team, and to advise the community about health promotion and disease prevention.	Counseling a client Discussing unit staffing needs at a meeting Providing HIV education at a local school
Client/family educator	Assessing and diagnosing the teaching needs of the client, group, family, or community. Once the diagnosis is made, nurses plan how to meet these needs, implement the teaching plan, and evaluate its effectiveness.	Preoperative teaching Prenatal education for siblings Community classes on nutrition
Client advocate	Supporting clients' right to make health care decisions when they are able to voice their opinions and protecting clients from harm when they are unable to make decisions.	Helping a client explain to his family that he does not want to have further chemotherapy
Counselor	Counseling clients on health-related issues through the use of therapeutic communication skills.	Counseling a client on weight-loss strategies
Change agent	Advocating for change that enhances health. The nurse may use counseling, communication, and educator skills to accomplish this change. Change may be advocated on an individual, family, group, community, or societal level.	Working to improve the nutritional quality of the lunch program at a preschool
Leader	Inspiring others by setting an example of positive health, assertive communication, and willingness to improve.	Florence Nightingale Mother Teresa
Manager	Coordinating and managing the activities of all members of the team.	Charge nurse on a hospital unit (e.g., assigns patients and work to staff nurses)
Case manager	Coordinating all care delivered to a client.	Coordinator of services for clients with tuberculosis
Research consumer	Incorporating research into practice to provide the most appropriate care, to identify clinical problems that warrant research, and to protect the rights of research subjects.	Reading journal articles Attending continuing education; seeking additional education

information. This access has allowed consumers to be active participants in discussions about their health problems and therapy options.

- *Direct-to-consumer marketing* is another form of health information, in which companies advertise medicines and therapies directed at the potential user. Advertisements appear in magazines, on television, on billboards, and in the newspaper. Pharmaceutical companies rely heavily on this advertising to generate interest in new therapies. Clients may make direct requests for therapies they have heard about in the media. Nurses need to be prepared to address the truthfulness of the advertisements and to present balanced information to clients.
- *Consumer interest has also generated legislation* that affects nursing care. Legislation directed at patient's rights (Patient's Bill of Rights), the patient's right to know (informed consent), and the patient's right to a dignified death (living will/advanced directives) all govern the care that nurses render to patients.

- *The women's movement* has also influenced the nursing profession and those considering a career in nursing. Historically, women were allowed to practice nursing only while they remained single. As the women's movement gained momentum, women began to enjoy more equitable treatment and were no longer forced out of nursing if they chose to have a family. However, the women's movement also opened up more career choices for women, and nursing has become just one of many options as opposed to a preferred career pathway. Also, as you have seen, societal views of nursing as a women's profession affect men's entry into nursing.
- *Collective bargaining* is a form of negotiating that allows nurses to seek better wages and working conditions as a group rather than individually. A union or organization that represents the nurses usually conducts collective bargaining. Collective bargaining has resulted in major improvements in wages, benefits, and working conditions for nurses. These improvements have made nursing more attractive as a career choice. Not all states have collective bargaining groups for nurses.

Trends in Nursing and Health Care

Many trends in nursing and health care also affect contemporary practice. The most significant of these trends as given below:

Increased Use of Complementary and Alternative Medicine: Health care treatments or services outside the traditional health care system are complementary and alternative medicine. They include medical systems, such as homeopathy, naturopathy, chiropractic, and traditional Chinese medicine, as well as specific treatments, such as herbal medications, dietary changes, massage therapy, yoga, aromatherapy, prayer, and hypnotism. Many of these therapies have evolved alongside traditional health care. For example, many powerful drugs are derived from herbs, and conventional physicians have always prescribed dietary remedies for certain ailments. The following factors have contributed to this interest in the traditional system.

- Rising costs of traditional care, including prohibitive insurance costs.
- Widespread reporting of treatment errors in the media. Some people are now uncertain about the validity of traditional health care.
- Growing distrust of the role of insurance and managed care organizations in determining treatment options.
- Ever-changing health recommendations over the last 20 years. For example, there have been numerous studies to examine the pros and cons of hormone replacement therapy for post-menopausal women.
- Increasing cultural diversity of the population, and the accompanying exchange of information about therapies from different cultural traditions.
- Creation of the National Center for Complementary and Alternative Medicine at the National Institutes of Health.

Expanded Variety of Settings for Care

This trend toward increased diversification in practice sites is expected to continue. As the site of employment shifts away from the hospital, nurses must be prepared to function in these alternative settings. This change requires entry-level education programs to prepare nurses for this type of work. For those already in the field, it may require retooling to deal with this change. In the hospital, nurses have access to support personnel, consultation with other nurses and health care providers, ready access to equipment and diagnostic testing services, and increased access to the patient. As more care is delivered in outpatient, community, or home settings, nurses must be prepared to function more autonomously and creatively. Nurses must adapt care to the equipment available at the site, and they must rely heavily on the skills of patients and family members to detect change and report the need for additional services.

Increased Autonomy and Advanced Practice Roles

The growing role of nursing outside the hospital, the increasing complexity of care, the limited supply of nurses, and the increased use of technology have changed nursing from a largely supportive role to one of increasing responsibility. In addition, the increased use of advanced practice nurses has resulted in greater public exposure for nurses. Professional and public reports demonstrate high patient satisfaction. Studies have also shown comparable, and at times superior, patient outcomes over physician provided care (e.g., better understanding of and compliance with treatment regimen, and fewer hospitalizations). This positive exposure has resulted in increased acceptance and support for all nurses.

Increased Use of Unlicensed Assistive Personnel

Unlicensed assistive personnel (UAP) are health care providers who help nurses and physicians provide patient care. Common UAP roles include nurse aide, assistant, orderly, and technician. UAPs may perform simple nursing tasks (e.g. providing bath, taking temperatures, or making beds) under the direction of the licensed nurse. This redistribution of work load has prompted much controversy.

Although it may seem appropriate to allow the UAP to assume the simple tasks, this change distances the licensed nurse from many aspects of direct patient care. The nurse retains ultimate responsibility for the patient yet may have to base important patient care decisions on information obtained by someone else. Unfortunately many nurses now in practice were never taught in their formal nursing programs about delegation and supervision. This can create problems on nursing units, because some nurses are uncertain about what can safely and legally be delegated and how much responsibility they retain. To remedy this problem, many schools are now adding coursework on delegation to their curricula, and textbooks such as this one are including information about delegation.

As progress through program, person will notice that nurses often gather different information from a client encounter than someone without nursing experience. For example, a nursing aide may provide a bedbath to an elderly client. The aide will be able to tell the RN that there are no open areas on the skin. However, a nurse performing the same task would be able to do an extensive client assessment while giving the bath. The nurse would be able to comment on the client's level of cognition (orientation to surroundings and self), the client's tolerance for activity, breath sounds, heart sounds, bowel sounds, and the condition of the skin. The nurse might use the time during the bath to educate the client about his condition or to gather information about the client's home and support system that can be used for discharge planning.

Influence of Nurses on Health Care Policy

Professional nursing organizations have been actively involved in politics at the local, state, and national levels. Each of the major professional organizations actively lobbies and educates elected and appointed officials about the role nursing plays in health care. Nursing organizations sponsor legislation that promotes the interest of the profession and supports changes that positively influence health outcomes. Nurse-sponsored legislation has addressed safe staffing in hospitals, needle-exchange programs to decrease the transmission of HIV, and funding to increase nursing enrollment during times of nursing shortages.

As individuals, nurses should vote, lobby their elected representatives, and run for political office. Together, nurses represent the largest health professional group; as a voting block, they have strong political power. Many nurses have also promoted nursing by organizing local nursing groups to support candidates or legislation, or by speaking out in the community on health and nursing issues. Nurses are typically trusted and respected political candidates, running successful campaigns at the local, state, and national level. Nurses should consider all of these political activities as they move into the profession.

Recent advances in health care technology have prolonged the lives of patients who are critically ill, such as premature newborns and elderly patients with advanced cardiovascular, pulmonary, or renal disease. The increasing use of this technology has led to numerous legal and ethical dilemmas, particularly about end-of-life care. This trend is in sharp contrast to the concurrent trend toward holism and high-touch therapies, which often avoids technology. One of the biggest challenges in health care is integrating these two divergent trends.

Nursing Theories

As a science, nursing is in its infancy. Professional nurses are aware of this and conscious of the need for both nursing theory development and theory based practice. As nursing comes of age, not only as a practice discipline but also as a scholarly discipline, there will be increasing interest in delineating the theory base of nursing. Some believe that theory development is the most crucial task facing nursing (Chinn and Jacob 1978).

Theories are general explanations which scholars use to explain, control and understand commonly occurring events. Theories are best understood as preliminary explanations that reflect the current understanding of events. "Theory is defined as a set of propositions used to describe, explain, predict and control events." Here set refers to a group of circumstances, situations, and so on, joined and treated as a whole; propositions refer to statements about how two or more concepts are related; concepts refer to an abstract classification of data, temperature; describe means of tell about in details; explain means to offer reasons for; predict means to foretell/forecast; control means to exercise as regulating influence over; and phenomena refer to theory includes the joint functions of theory, i.e. description explanation, prediction and control.

Theory helps in providing knowledge to improve practice by describing, explaining, predicting, and controlling phenomena. Nurse's power is increased through theoretical knowledge

because systematically developed more likely to be successful. In addition, nurses will know why they are doing, what they are doing if challenged. Theory provides professional autonomy by guiding the nursing practice, education and research functions of profession. And also there has been interest in identifying a body of nursing knowledge that is essential to professional nursing practice. Theory development contributes to knowledge building and is seen a means of establishing 'nursing as a profession.'

The commitment to that nursing practice based on sound, reliable knowledge is intrinsically valuable to nursing. That is to say, knowledge is desirable by its very nature. The growth and enrichment of theory and of itself is an important goal for nursing as a scholarly discipline, to pursue. Now nursing practice settings are complex, and the amount of data available to nurses are virtually endless. Nurses must analyze a tremendous amount of information about each patient and decide what to do. If a theory helps practising nurses categorize and understand what is going on in nursing practice, if it helps them predict patients responses to nursing care, and if it is helpful in clinical decision making, it is useful as a guide to nursing practice.

This study of theory helps to develop analytical skills, challenge thinking, clarifies values and assumptions, and determines purposes for nursing practice, education, and research.

The contributions of many theorists outside of nursing profession formed the knowledge based for nursing practice for many years. New disciplines are often slow to develop their own theories and nursing was no exception. Even now, theories from the physical, biological, social, and behavioral sciences in addition to more recent nursing models and theories are used extensively in nursing practice.

The development of nursing science and theory is a scholarly activity. Developing this science involves generating knowledge; although this knowledge can be used with knowledge from other disciplines, it is designed to advance and support nursing practice and health care. As nursing continues to evolve, nurses theorize about the nature of nursing practice, the principles on which practice is based, and the proper goals and functions of nursing in society. Conceptional and theoretical nursing models are used to provide knowledge to improve practice, guide research and curricular and identify domain and goals of nursing practice. Nursing theories provide the nurse with goals of assessment, nursing diagnosis and intervention; common ground for communication; and professional autonomy and accountability. They also guide future directions for nursing research; practice, education, and administration.

Theories of nursing can help the nursing student to understand how the roles and actions of nurses fit together in nursing. The brief descriptions of selected nursing theories are as follows:

(i) Nightingale's Theory (Environment Model) 1860

Florence Nightingale, the matriarch of modern nursing, who is establishing the discipline of nursing, spoke with firm conviction about the 'nature of nursing as a profession that required knowledge distinct from medical knowledge'. The overall goal of this knowledge has explained the practice of nursing as different and distinct from the practice of medicine, psychology, and social work.

Nightingale conceptualized disease as a reparative process and described the nurses' role as manipulating the environment to facilitate this process. Her ideas regarding ventilation, warmth, light, diet, cleanliness, variety and noise are presented in her classic nursing textbook, i.e. *Notes on Nursing* (1859).

Nightingale believed that every woman at one time or another, would be a nurse, in the sense that nursing was to have the responsibility for someone's health. This she proved women with guidelines for nursing care and advice on 'how to think and how to nurse.'

The major concepts as defined by Nightingale are as follows:

- Patient, viewed as individual or person, is responsible, creative in control of his life and health, and desiring good health. However, the patient is regarded as being acted upon by the nurse or affected by the environment.
- Health viewed as a state of being well; using ones power to the fullest.
- Illness defined as the reaction of the nature against the condition in which we have placed ourselves. Disease is a reparative mechanism, an effort of nature to remedy, a process of delay.
- Environment refers to that external to the persons, but affecting the health of both sick and well persons. Environment, one of the chief sources of infection, must include fresh air, fresh water, efficient drainage, cleanliness, and light.
- Nursing, defined as a service to people, is intended to relieve pain and suffering. Goal of nursing is to promote the reparative process by manipulating the environment. Client's environment is manipulated to include appropriate noise, nutrition, hygiene, light, comfort, socialization, and hope.

Nightingale's descriptive theory provides nurses with a way to think about nursing or a frame of reference that focuses on patients and the environment. Her principles encompass the areas of practice, research, and education.

(ii) Paplau's Theory (1952)

Hildagard E Paplau, was born on September 1, 1909, and graduated from Potts town, Pennsylvania Hospital, School of Nursing in 1931. The nature of science and nursing refers to the body of verified knowledge found within the discipline of nursing, i.e. mainly knowledge from the biological and behavioral sciences. The synthesis, recognition, or extension of concepts drawn from the basic and applied sciences, which is their reformation tend to become new concepts have led to the growth of nursing science. Then the evolution of Paplau's theory of interpersonal relations resulted. Paplau's theory focuses on the individual nurse and the interaction process; the result is the nurse-client relationship. The major concepts defined/viewed are as follows:

Psychodynamic Nursing

Psychodynamic nursing is being able to understand one's own behavior to help others identify felt difficulties, and to apply principles of human relations to the problems that arise at all levels of experience. She describes the structural concepts of interpersonal process and both the nurse-patient relationship to be based on psychodynamic nursing.

Nurse-patient Relationship

Nurse-patient relationship described by the Paplau in four phases, i.e. orientation, identification, exploitation, and resolution:

- In orientation phase, the individual has a felt need and seeks professional assistance. The nurse helps the patient recognize and understand his problem and determine his need for help.
- In identification phase the patient identifies with those who can help him (relatedness). The nurse permits exploration feelings to aid the patient in undergoing illness as an experience that reorients feelings and strengthens positive forces in the personality and provides needed satisfaction.
- In exploitation phase the patient attempts to derive full value from what is offered to him through the relationship. Now goals, to be achieved through personal efforts can be projected and power shifted from the nurse to the patient as the patient delays gratification to achieve the newly formed goals.
- In the phase of resolution, old goals are gradually put aside and new goals are adopted. This is a process in which the patient frees himself from identification with the nurse.

Nursing Roles

Paplau describes six different nursing roles that emerge in the various phases of the nurse-patient relationship as given below:

Role of the stranger: In this role both nurse and patient are stranger to each other, the patient should be treated as he is and with ordinary courtesy. This coincides with the identification phase.

Role of resource person: In this role nurse provides specific answers to questions, especially health information, and interprets to the patient the treatment or medical plan of care. Here the nurse also determines, what type of response is appropriate for constructive learning, either straightforward factual answers or providing counseling.

Teaching role: It is a combination of all roles. Paplau separates teaching into two categories, i.e. instructional which consists largely of giving information and is the form explained in educational literature, and practical which is using the experience of the learner as a basis from which learning products are developed.

Leadership role: It involves the democratic process. The nurse helps the patient meet the tasks at hand through a relationship of cooperation and active participation.

Surrogate role: The patient casts the nurse in the surrogate role. The nurse's attitudes and behaviors create 'feeling tones' in the patient that reactivate feelings generate in a prior relationship.

The nurse's function is to assist the patient in recognizing similarities between herself and the person recalled by the patient. She then helps the patient see the differences in her role and that of the recalled person. In this phase, nurse and patient defines areas of dependence, independence and finally interdependence.

Counseling role: Paplau believes the counseling role has the greatest emphasis on psychiatric nursing. Counseling functions in the nurse-patient relationship by the way nurses response to patient demands.

Nursing

Nursing is described by Paplau as a significant, therapeutic, interpersonal process. It functions comparatively with other human processes that make health possible for individuals in communities. When professional health teams offer health services, nurses participate in the organization of conditions that facilitate natural ongoing tendencies in human organism. 'Nursing is an educative instrument, a maturing force that aims to promote forward movement of personality in the direction of creative, constructive, productive, personal, and community living.'

Person

Person refers to man. Man is an organism that lives in an unstable equilibrium.

Health

Health is defined by Paplau as 'a word symbol that implies forward movement of personality and other ongoing human processes in the direction of creative, constructive, productive, personal and community living.'

Environment

Environment is defined in terms of 'existing forces outside the organism and in the context of cultures', from which morals, customs, and beliefs are acquired. However, general conditions that are likely to lead to health always include the interpersonal process.

According to this theory the client is an individual with a felt need, and nursing is an interpersonal and therapeutic process. Nursing's goal is to educate the client and family and to help the client reach mature personality development. Therefore nurse strives to develop a nurse-patient relationship in which the nurse serves as a research person, counselor and surrogate. This theory creates a 'making force' through which interpersonal effectiveness assists in meeting the client needs.

(iii) Henderson's Theory (1955)

Virginia Henderson was born in 1897, a native of Kansas city, Missouri, spent her developmental years in Virginia because her father practised law in Washington DC. During World War I, she developed an interest in nursing. The major concepts defined by Henderson are as follows:

Nursing

Henderson defines nursing in functional terms, i.e. 'the unique function of the nurse is to assist the individual, sick or well, in the performance of those activities contributing to health or its recovery (or to peaceful death) that he would perform unaided if he had the necessary strength, will or knowledge. And to do this is such a way as to help him gain independence as rapidly as possible.'

Health

Henderson did not define health, but looking into several definitions of health, she views health in terms of patient's ability to perform unaided the 14 components of nursing care. She says it is 'the quality or health rather than life itself, that margin of mental, physical vigor that allows a person to work most effectively and to reach his highest potential level of satisfaction of life.'

Environment

By using Webster's definition, Henderson defines 'environment as the aggregate of all the external conditions and influence affecting the life and development of an organism.'

Person (Patient)

Henderson views the patient as an individual who requires assistance to achieve health and independence or peaceful death. The mind and body are inseparable. The patient and his family are viewed as a unit.

Needs

Henderson did not define a need, but she identifies 14 basic needs of the patient, which comprise the components of nursing care. These include the need to:
* Breathe normally,
* Eat and drink adequately,
* Eliminate body wastes by all avenues of elimination,
* Move and maintain a desirable position,
* Sleep and rest,
* Select suitable clothing, i.e. dress and undress,
* Maintain body temperature within the normal range by adjusting clothing and modifying the environment,
* Keep the body clean and well groomed and protect the integument,
* Avoid dangers in the environment and avoid injuring others,
* Communicate with others in expressing emotions, needs, fears or opinions,
* Worship according to one's faith,
* Work in such a way that there is a sense of accomplishments,
* Play or participate in various forms of recreation, and
* Learn, discover or satisfy the curiosity that leads to normal development and health and use the available health facilities.

Henderson viewed nursing as an art and a discipline separate from medicine, and viewed the nurse's role as that of a substitute for the patient, a helper to the patient, and a partner with the patient. The fourteen basic needs compose Henderson's components of nursing care.

(iv) Abdellah's Theory (1960)

Faye Glen Abdellah was born in New York city. A 1942 Magna cum Laude graduate of Fitkin Memorial Hospital, School of

Nursing, she received B.S., M.A. and Ed.D from Teachers College at Columbia University. She completed her doctoral work in 1955.

The nursing theory developed by Faye Abdellah *et al*, emphasized delivering nursing care for the whole person to meet the physical, emotional, intellectual, social, and spiritual needs of the client and family. The major concepts defined by Abdellah are as follows:

Nursing

Abdellah defined nursing as service to individuals and families, therefore to society. It is based upon an art and science which mould the attitudes, intellectual competencies and technical skills of the individual nurse into the desire and ability to help people sick or well to cope with their health needs, and may be carried out under general or specific medical direction.

Abdellah was clearly promoting the image of the nurse who was not only kind and caring, but also intelligent, competent and technically well prepared to provide service to the patient/ mankind.

Nursing Problem

Nursing problem is a problem that is presented by the patient in a condition faced by the patient of family which the nurse can assist him or them to meet through the performance of her professional function. The problem can be either an overt or covert nursing problem:

- An overt nursing problem is an apparent condition faced by the patients or family which the nurse can assist him or them to meet through the performance of her professional functions.
- A covert nursing problem is a concealed or hidden condition faced by the patient or family which then nurse can assist him or them to meet through the performance of her professional functions.

The functions of the nurses are to identify and solve the specific problems of clients. This identification and classification of problems was called the 'typology of 21 nursing problems,' i.e. Abdellah 21 nursing problems were divided into the following three areas:

A. Physical, sociological and emotional needs of the patient.
B. Type of interpersonal relationships between the nurse and patient.
C. Common elements of patient care.

The 21 nursing problems are as follows:

1. To maintain good hygiene and physical comfort.
2. To promote (achieve) optimal activity, exercise, rest, sleep.
3. To promote safety through prevention of accidents, injury or other trauma and through the prevention of the spread of infection.
4. To maintain good body mechanics and prevent and correct deformity.
5. To facilitate the maintenance of supply of oxygen to all body cells.
6. To facilitate the maintenance of nutrition of all body cells.
7. To facilitate the maintenance to elimination.
8. To facilitate the maintenance of fluid and electrolyte balance.
9. To recognize the physiological responses of the body to disease conditions - pathological, physiological and compensatory.
10. To facilitate the maintenance or regulatory mechanisms and functions.
11. To facilitate the maintenance of sensory function.
12. To identify and accept positive and negative expressions, feelings, and reactions.
13. To identify and accept interrelatedness of emotions and organic illness.
14. To facilitate the maintenance of effective verbal and nonverbal communications.
15. To promote the development of productive interpersonal relationships.
16. To facilitate progress toward achievement of personal spiritual goals.
17. To create and/ or maintain a therapeutic environment.
18. To facilitate awareness of self as an individual with varying physical, emotional and developmental needs.
19. To accept the optimal possible goals in the light of limitations, physical and emotional.
20. To use community resources as an aid in resolving problems arising from illness.
21. To understand the role of social problems as influencing factors in the cause of illness.

When using Abdellah's approach, the nurse needs knowledge and skills in interpersonal relations, psychology, growth and development, communication and sociology as well as knowledge of the basic sciences and specific nursing skills.

Problem Solving

Problem solving refers to the process of identifying overt and covert nursing problems and interpreting, analyzing, and selecting appropriate causes of action to solve these problems. This process closely resembles the nursing problems.

The nurse is a problem solver and decision maker. The nurse formulates an individualized view of the client's needs, which may occur in the following areas:

1. Comfort, hygiene, and safety.
2. Physiological balance.
3. Psychological and social factors, and
4. Sociological and community factors.

The specific client's needs, which are often referred to as Abdellah 21 nursing problems, that are useful in identifying the needs and plan and implement the nursing intervention, accordingly.

(v) Orlando's Theory (1961)

Ida Jean Orlando was born in August 12, 1926. In 1947, she received a diploma in nursing later on received BS (PHD) and MA in mental health consultation. From Macheri College, Columbia University, she worked as a staff nurse, nursing supervisor, teacher, research associate.

Orlando describes her model as revolving around five major interrelated concepts:

1. Function of professional nurses.
2. Present behavior of the client.
3. Immediate reaction or internal response to nurse.
4. Nursing process discipline, and
5. Improvement.

Major concepts of her model defined are as follows:

(i) Nurse's responsibility means whatever help the patient may require for his needs to be met.

(ii) Need situationally, defined as requirement of the patient which is supplied, relieves or diminishes his immediate distress or improves his immediate sense of adequacy or well-being.

(iii) Personal behavior means any observable, verbal or nonverbal behavior.

(iv) Immediate reactions include both the nurse and patient's individual perceptional, thoughts and feelings.

(v) Nursing process discipline includes the nurse communicating to the client, his or her own immediate reactions, clearly identifying that the item expressed belongs to the nurse, then asking for validation or correction.

(vi) Improvement means to grow better, to turn, to profit, to use, to advantage.

(vii) Purpose of nursing refers to supply the help a patient requires in order for his needs to be met.

(viii) Automatic action, i.e. those nursing actions decided upon for research other than the patient's immediate need.

(ix) Deliberate action, i.e. those actions decided upon after ascertaining a need and then meeting this need.

(x) Orlando views that nursing should be a distinct profession that functions autonomously. Although nursing has been historically aligned with medicine and continuous to have close relationship with medicine, nursing and practice of medicine are clearly separate profession. She states that function of professional nurse is conceptualized as finding out and meeting the patients immediate need for help. Accordingly the goal of nursing is to respond to client's behavior in terms of immediate needs. To interact with client to meet immediate needs by identifying client behavior, reaction to nurse and nursing action to be taken.

To Orlando, the client is an individual with a need that when met, diminishes distress, increases adequacy or enhances well-being. Her theory focuses on nurse's reactions to client behavior in terms or the client's immediate need. This theory contains those main elements–client's behavior, nurse reaction and nurse action which compose the nursing situation. After nurse thoroughly assesses the client's needs, she recognizes the impact of that need on the client's level of health and then acts automatically or deliberately to meet the need, ultimately reducing client's distress.

(vi) Hall's Theory (1962)

Lydia E Hall began her career in nursing as a graduate of the York Hospital, School of Nursing in York, Pennsylvania. She then earned her BS and MA degrees from Columbia University. Nursing circles of care (body), core (person) and cure (disease) are the central concepts of Hall's theory:

- Care alludes to the 'hands on' intimate bodily care of the patient and implies a comforting, nurturing relationship (the body-natural and biological sciences intimate bodily care-aspects of nursing 'the cure').

- Core involves the therapeutic use of self in communicating with the patient. The nurse reflects questions appropriately and helps the patient clarify motives and goals facilitating the process of increasing patient's self awareness (the person-social science therapeutic use of self aspects of nursing - the core)

- Cure is the aspect of nursing involved with administration of medications and treatment. The nurse's functions in this role are as an 'investigator and potential painer.' (The disease–pathological and therapeutical sciences–seeing the patient and family through medical care–aspects of nursing 'the cure').

According to this theory the goal of nursing is to provide care and comfort to client during disease process. The client is composed of the following overlapping parts, i.e. person (core) pathological state and treatment (cure), and body (care). Nurse is a care giver. The professional nurses function most therapeutically when patients have entered the second stage of their hospital stay. This stage is the recuperating or nonacute phase of illness. The first stage of illness is the time of biological crisis, with nursing being an ancillary to medicine. After the crisis period the patient is more able to benefit and learn from the teaching that nurses can offer.

(vii) Wiedenbach Theory (1964)

Ernestine Wiedenbach's interest in nursing began with her childhood experiences with nurses. She earned masters degree from Columbia University. The major concepts defined by Wiedenbach are as follows:

(i) Patient–she defines patient as an individual who is receiving help of some kind, be it care, instruction or advice, from member of the health profession or from worker in the field of health.

(ii) Need for help–a need is anything that individual may require to maintain or sustain himself comfortably or capably in his situation. A need for help is any measure or action required or desired by the individual, which has potential for restoring or extending his ability to cope with the demands implicit in his situation.

(iii) Nurse is a functioning human being. For the nurse whose action is directed toward achievement of a specific purpose, thoughts and feelings, has a discipline role to play.

(iv) Purpose—that nurse wants to accomplish through what she does–in the overall goal.

(v) Philosophy—an attitude toward life and reality, evolves from each nurse's beliefs and code of conduct, motivates the nurse to act, guides her thinking about what she is to do and influences her decisions. It stems from both her culture and subculture and is integral part of her. It is personal in character, unique to each nurse, and expressed in her way of nursing.

(vi) Practice–overt action, directed by disciplined thoughts and feelings toward meeting the patient's need for help. It constitutes the practice of clinical nursing, it is goal direction deliberately carried out and patient curaterd. Knowledge, judgement skills are necessary for effective practice. Identification, administration, validation are three components of practice directly related to the patient care.

According to Wiedenbach's theory 'nursing is a practice which is related to the individuals who need help because of behavioral stimulus. The goal of nursing is to assist individuals in overcoming obstacles that interfered with the ability to meet demands or needs brought about by condition, environment, situation or time. Clinical nursing has following components, i.e. philosophy, purpose, practice and art.

Wiedenbach identifies five essential attributes to professional person (nurse). These characteristics are as follows:

1. Clarity of purpose.
2. Mastery of skill and knowledge essential for fulfilling purpose.
3. Ability to establish and sustain purposeful working relationship with others, both professional and non-professional.
4. Interest in advancing knowledge in the area of interest and creating new knowledge.
5. Dedication of furthering the goal of mankind rather than to self aggrandizement.

She also stated the following four assumptions related to person:

1. Each human being is endorsed with unique potential to develop within himself–resources which enable him to maintain and sustain himself.
2. The human being basically strives toward self direction and relative independence and desires not only to make best use of his capabilities and potentialities but to fulfill his responsibilities.
3. Self awareness and self acceptance are essential to the individual sense of integrity and self worth.
4. Whatever the individual does represents his best judgement at the amount of his doing it.

(viii) Levine's Theory (1966)

Myra Estrin Levina obtained diploma from Cook Country, School of Nursing in 1944 and M.SN from Wayne State University in 1962. She views the person is who, we know ourself to be or a sense of identity and views the client as an integrated being who instructs with and adapts to the environment.

In her view 'nursing is a human interaction'. The essence of Levine's theory is that when nursing intervention influences adaption favorably or toward renewed social being, then the nurse is acting in a therapeutic sense, when response is unfavorable, the nurse adds supportive care. The goal of nursing is to promote wholeness. Whole, health, hale are all derived from Anglo-Saxon word 'hat'. Wholeness (Holistic) emphasizes

a sound, organic, progressive, mutually between diversified functions and parts with an entirety, the boundaries which are open and fluent. 'Holism' mean that human beings are more than the different from the sum of their parts. Perceiving the 'wholes' depends upon recognizing the organization and interdependence of observable phenomena.

Levine believes that nursing intervention is a conservation activity, with conservation of energy as a primary concern. Health is viewed in terms of the conservation of energy in the following areas, i.e. which Levine calls the 'four conservation principles of nursing':

1. Conservation of client energy.
2. Conservation of structural integrity.
3. Conservation of personal integrity.
4. Conservation of social integrity.

Integrity is from Latin *integer,* meaning 'being control of one's life'. Conservation is also from the Latin word *'conservatio'* meaning to keep together. Conservation describes the way by which complex system are able to continue to function even when severally challenged. The brief description of conservation principle of nursing is as follows:

Conservation of energy: The individual requires a balance of energy and constant renewal of energy to maintain life activities. That energy is challenged by process such as healing and aging. Conservation of energy has long been used in nursing practice even with the most basic procedures.

Conservation of structural integrity: Healing is the process of restoring structural integrity. Nurses should limit the amount of tissue involved in disease by early recognition of functional changes and by nursing interventions.

Conservation of personal integrity: Self worth and a sense of identity are important. Nurses can show patients respect by calling them by name, respecting their wishes, valuing personal possessions, providing privacy during procedures, supporting their defenses, and teaching them. The nurse's goal is always to impart knowledge and strength so that the individual can resume a private life–no longer patient, no longer dependent.

Conservation of social integrity: Life gains meaning through social communities and health is socially determined. Nurses fulfill professional roles, provide family members, assess with religious needs, use interpersonal relation to conserve social integrity.

Adaptation is a process of change whereby the individual retains his integrity within the relation of his environment. In Levine's approach, nursing care involves conservation activities aimed at the optimal use of the client's resources.

(ix) Johnson's Theory (1968)

Dorothy E Johnson was born on August 21, 1919, in Savannah and received BA from Armstrong Junior College and got M.Ph. degree from Harward University in Boston, 1948.

Johnson's perceived nursing is an external force aiming to preserve the organization of the patient behavior, while the patient is under stress by means of imposing regulatory mechanism or by providing resources. As an art and science, it supplies external assistance both before and during system or balance disturbance and therefore requires knowledge of order, disorder, and control.

She views man as a behavioral system with patterned, repetitive and purposeful ways of behaving that link him to the environment. Person is a system of interdependent parts that requires some regularity and adjustment to maintain balance.

She perceives health as an inclusive dynamic state influenced by biological, psychological, and social factors. Health is the desired value by health professionals and focuses on the person rather than illness.

Johnson's theory of nursing focuses on how the client adapts to illness and how actual or potential stress can affect the ability to adapt. The goal of nursing is to reduce stress, so that the client can move more easily through recovery. This theory focuses on basic needs in terms of the following categories of behavior:
1. Security-seeking behavior.
2. Nurturance-seeking behaviors.
3. Master of oneself and ones environment according to internalize standards of excellence.
4. Taking nourishment by socially and culturally acceptable ways.
5. Ridding the body of nurse and socially and cultured acceptable way.
6. Sexual roles identify behavior.
7. Self protected behavior.

According to Johnson, nurses assess the client's needs in these categories of behavior, called behavioral subsystem and plans, and provides nursing care to resolve problems in meeting the client's needs.

(x) Roger's Theory (1970)

Martha E Rogers was born on May 12, 1914 in Dalls, Texas. She began her collegiate education at the University of Jannesse and Knoxville and acquired Doctorate degree (Ed.D) from John Hoplun University, Balmier.

Roger felt that historically the term 'nursing' most often has been used as a verb simplifying 'to do' when nursing is perceived as a science. The term 'nursing' being a noun, signifies body of knowledge. She describes nursing as a learned profession that is both a science and an art. 'Nursing is a humanistic science dedicated to compassionate concern for maintaining and promoting health, preventing illness and caring for and rehabilitating the sick and disabled'. Nursing seeks to promote symphonic interactions between the environment and man, to strengthen the coherence and integrity of the human beings and to direct and redirect patterns of interaction between man and his environment for the realization of maximum health potential.

Roger considers man (unitary fullman being) as an energy field co-existence within the universe. An energy field constitutes the fundamental unit of both the living and nonliving. Field is unifying concept and energy signifies the dynamic nature of the field. Energy fields are infinite, so she identified only two, i.e. the human field and the environment field:

The unitary human being (human field) is defined as an irreducible, indivisible, pandimensional energy field identified by pattern and manifested characteristics that are specific to the whole and which cannot be predicted from knowledge of the parts.

The environment field is defined as an irreducible pandimensional energy field identified by pattern and integral with human field. Each environmental field is specific to its given human field. Both change continuously and creatively. Unitary man evolves along life processes. Client continuously changes and coexists with environment.

Roger viewed the terms health and illness as value leader, arbitrarily defined but as part of the same continuum, i.e. health occurs when patterns of living are in harmony with environmental change and illness occurs when patterns of living conflicts with environmental change and are deemed unacceptable.

The four dimensions used in Roger's theory of energy fields, openness (universe of open system) pattern and organization and to derive principles about how human beings develop. Her views on nursing primarily as a science and are committed to nursing research. Nursing, therefore, corporates knowledge of the basic sciences and physiology, as well as nursing knowledge. The science of nursing aims to provide a body of abstract knowledge growing out of scientific research and logical analysis and capable of being translated into nursing practice. Nursing body of knowledge is a new product specific to nursing.

According to this theory the goal of nursing is to maintain and promote health, prevent illness and care for and rehabilitate ill and disabled client through humanistic science of nursing.

(xi) Orem's Theory

Dorothea Elizabeth Orem, one of the American foremost nursing theorists, was born in Baltimore, Maryland. She began her nursing career at Providence Hospital, School of Nursing, Washington DC, where she received diploma in nursing and she was also recipient of B.SN and M.SN of catholic University America.

Orem's self care deficit' theory of nursing as a general theory consists of three related theories:
1. Theory of self care (describes and explains self care).
2. Theory of self care deficit (describes and explains why people can be helped through nursing).
3. Theory of nursing system (describes and explains relationship that must be brought about and maintained for nursing to be produced).

The major concepts defined by Orems are as follows:

Self care

Self care is a learned good oriented activity of individuals. It is behavior that exists in concrete life situations directed by persons to self or to the environment to regulate factors that affect their own development and functioning in the interests of life, health, or well-being.
- Self care requisites are expression of purposes to be attained, results desired from deliberate engagement in self care. There were three categories of self care requisite as given here:

Universal self care requisites: These are common to all human beings and include the maintenance of air, water, food elimination, activity and rest, and solitude and social interaction, prevention of hazards and promotion of human functioning.

Development self care requisites: These are self care requisites that they promote processes for life and maturation and prevent conditions deleterious to maturation or mitigate those effects.

Health deviation self care requisites: These are defined by Orem that disease or injury affects not only specific structures and physiologic or psychological mechanisms, but also integrated human functioning. When integrated functioning is seriously affected, the individuals' developing or developed powers of agency are seriously inspired either permanently or temporarily–discomfort, frustration resulting from medical care also create a requisites for self care to bring relief.

Self care deficit

Self care deficit refers to a relationship between the human properties therapeutic self care demand and self care agency in which constituent developed self care capabilities within self care agency are nonoperable or not adequate for knowing and meeting some or all components of the existent or projected therapeutic self care demand.

Nursing agency

Nursing agency refers to the complex property or attribute of persons educated and trained as nurses that is enabling when exercised for knowing and helping others, know their therapeutic self care demands, for helping others meet or in meeting their therapeutic self care demands, and in helping other regulate the exercise or development of their self care agency or their dependent care agency.

Therapeutic demand is a humanly constructed entity, with an objective basis in information that describes an individual structurally, functionally, and developmentally.

Nursing System

Nursing system refers to a continuing series of actions produced when nurses link one way or a number of ways in helping to their own actions or the actions of the persons under care that are directed to meet these persons' therapeutic self care demands or to regulate their self care agency.

Self care agency is the complex acquired ability to meet one's continuing requirement for care them regulated life processes, maintains or promotes integrity of human structures and functioning, and human development and promotes well-being.

Three types of nursing system (described by Grem) are as follows:

Wholly compensatory nursing systems: These are needed when the nurse should be compensating for a patient's total inability for (or prescription against) engaging and self care activities that require ambulation and manipulation of movements.

Partially compensatory nursing system: It exists when both nurse and patient perform care measures or other actions involving manipulative tasks or ambulation.

Supportive educative nursing system: These are for situations when the patient is able to perform or can and should learn to perform required measures for externally or internally oriented self care but cannot do so without assistance. The methods of assistance will include acting or doing for guidance, i.e. teaching, supporting, and providing a developmental environment.

In Orem's self care deficit theory, nursing care becomes necessary when client is unable to fulfill biological, psycho-logical, developmental and/or social needs. The goal of nursing is to care for and help client within total self care. She viewed person/patient in an individual unable to continuously maintain self care in sustaining life and health, in recovering from disease or injury or in coping with their effects.

According to Orem, health is an ability to meet self care demands that contribute to the maintenance and promotion of structural integrity, functioning, and development. Illness occurs when a individual is incapable of maintaining self care as a result of health related limitations. She perceived environment that any setting in which a patient has unmet self care needs. And nursing is service of deliberately selected and performed actions to assist individuals to maintain self care, including structural integrity, functioning, and development. Accordingly nursing care is necessary when the client is unable to fulfill biological, psychological, developmental and/or social needs. The nurse determines why a client is unable to meet these needs, what must be done to enable the client to meet them and how much self care the client is able to perform.

Orem describes her philosophy of nursing as follows:

Action and the provision and management of it on continuous basis in order to sustain life and health, recover from disease or injury, and cope with their effects. Self care is a requirement of every person–man, women, and child. When self care is not maintained, illness, disease or death will occur. Nurses, sometimes, manage and maintain required self care continuously for persons who are totally incapable. In other instance, nurses help persons to maintain required self care by performing some but not all care measures, by supervizing others who assist patients and by instructing and guiding individuals as they gradually move toward self care.

Orem suggests that a person needs nursing when the person has a health related self care deficit. The areas of nursing practice are:
1. Entering into and maintaining nurse-client relationships with individuals, families or groups.
2. Determining if and how clients can be helped through nursing.
3. Responding to clients' requirements and needs.
4. Giving direct help to clients and families.
5. Coordinating and integrating nursing with the client's daily living, other health care activities, and social or educational services required.

(xii) King's Theory (1971)

Imogene M King earned her diploma in nursing from St John's Hospital of Nursing in St Louis in 1945 and earned M.SN at St Louis University and Doctor of Education degree from Columbia University, New York.

The major concepts in her theory of goal attainment are interaction, perception, communication, transaction, role stress, growth and development and time and space. The definition, of these concepts by King are as follows:

Interaction
Interaction is defined as a process of perception and communication between person and environment and between person to person, represented by verbal and nonverbal behaviors that are goal directed. Each individual in an interaction (nurse and client) brings different knowledge, needs, goals, postexperiences and perceptions which influence the interactions.

Perception
Perception is defined as 'each person's' representation of reality. This includes import and transformation of energy, and processing, storing, and exporting information. Perceptions are related to postexperiences, concept of self socio-economic group, biological inheritance, and educational background.

Communication
Communication is a process whereby information is given from one person to another either directly or indirectly. It is the information component of the interactions. The exchange or verbal and nonverbal signs and symbols between nurse and client, or between client and environment are communications.

Transaction
Transaction is defined as purposeful interaction that leads to goal attainment. It includes observable behavior of human beings interacting with their environment, the valuation components of human interaction.

Role
Role is defined as a 'set of behaviors' expected to persons occupying a position in a social system; rules that define rights and obligations in a position. If expectations of role differ, then role conflict and role confusion exist.

Stress
Stress is a 'dynamic state' whereby a human being interacts with the environment. It involves an exchange of energy and information between the person and the environment for regulation and control of stressors and energy response of an individual to person, objects, and events. An increase in the stress of the individual leads to narrow perception and decrease rationality, and also affect nursing care.

Growth and Development
Growth and development are defined as a continuous changes in the individuals at the cellular, molecular, and behavioral levels of activities conducive in helping individuals to move toward maturity.

Time
Time is defined as a sequence of events moving onward to the future—time is a duration between one event and another as uniquely experienced by each human being.

Space
Space is defined as existing in all directions and is the same everywhere. It is immediate environment in which nurse and client interact.

King's personal philosophy about human beings and life influenced her assumptions. Her theory of goal attainment based on that assumptions that focus on nursing is human beings interacting with their environment leading to a state of health for individuals, which is an ability to function in social roles. Her assumptions are nursing, person's health and environment as given below:

1. Nursing is an observable behavior found in health care system in society. The goal of nursing is to help individuals maintain their health so that they can function in their roles. Nursing is viewed as an interpersonal process of action, reaction, interaction, and transaction. Perception of nurse and client also influences the interaction process.
2. Persons refers to individuals, that they are social beings, sentient beings, rational beings, perceiving beings, controlling being, purposeful beings, action oriented beings, and time oriented beings.

Health
Health is viewed as a dynamic state in the lifecycle; illness is an interference in the lifecycle. Health implied continuous adaptation to stress in the internal and external environment through optimum use of one's resources to achieve maximum potential for daily living. Health is the function of nurse, patient, physician, family and other interaction.

Environment
King states that an understanding of the ways that human beings interact with their environment to maintain health is essential for nurses. Adjustment to life and health care is influenced by an individual's interaction with environment.

King's theory focuses on the interpersonal relationship between client and the nurse. The nurse-client relationship is vehicle for the nursing process, which is a dynamic interpersonal process in which the nurse and client are affected by each other's behavior, as well as by the health care system. The nurses goal is to use communication to assist the client in re-establishing maintaining positive adaptation to environment.

(xiii) Travelebee's Theory (1972)
Joyce Travelebee was a psychiatric nurse practitioner, educator and writer, born in 1925. She had basic nurse preparation and 1946 at Charity Hospital, School of Nursing and earned B.SN from Lavisinia State University and M.SN from Yale in 1954.

Major concepts defined by Travelebee in her theory are as follows:

1. Nursing is defined as an interpersonal process whereby the professional nurse practitioner assists an individual, family or community to prevent or cope with the experience of illness and suffering and, if necessary, to find meaning in these experiences. Nursing is an interpersonal process because it is an experience that occurs between the nurse and an individual or group of individuals.

2. Person defined as human being, both the nurse and patient are human beings. A human being is unique, irreplaceable individual who is in the continuous process of becoming, evolving, and changing.
3. Health refers to the criteria of subjective and objective health. A person's 'subjective' health states in an individually defined state of well-being in accordance with self appraisal of physical, emotional, spiritual status. Objective health is an absence of discernible disease, disability, or defect as measured by physical examination, laboratory test, assessment by spiritual director, or psychological counselor.

Travelebee viewed interpersonal process as human-to-human relationship formed during illness and 'experience of suffering'. The goal of nursing is to assist individual or family to prevent or cope with illness, regain health, find meaning in illness, or maintain maximum degree of health.

(xiv) Neuman's Theory (1972)

Betty Neuman was born in 1924, completed her initial nursing education at Akron, Ohio in 1947, then earned master degree in mental health in 1966 and received doctorate degree in clinical psychology in 1985. She was a pioneer of nursing involvement in mental health.

The major concepts identified in her model are: holistic client approach, open system, basic structure, environment, created environment, stresses, lines of defence and resistance, degree of reaction, prevention as intervention, and reconstruction. Further included the concepts of scholastic approach, content, process input and output, negontrophy, entropy, stability, wellness and illness.

To Neuman, the persons are dynamic composite of physiological, socio-cultural, and developmental variables that function as an open system. As an open system, the person interacts with adjusts to and it adjusted by the environment, which is viewed as stressor. Stressors disrupt the system. She includes intrapersonal, interpersonal and extra personal stressor. Persons' interpersonal stressors such as role exceptions occur between persons, and extra personal stressor such as financial circumstances occur outside the person.

Neuman believes that nursing is concerned with the whole person. She views nursing as a 'unique profession in that it is concerned with all of the variables affecting an individual response to stress'. Because the nurse's perception influences the care program. Neuman equates health to wellness and defines health and/ or wellness as the condition in which all parts and subparts (variables) are in harmony with the whole of the client. So health is a dynamic equilibrium on the normal line of defence. Illness occurs due to reaction to stressor with lines of resistance, internal and external stressors and restrictive factors are the environment. The reduction of the stressors through prevention acts at three levels of nursing.

The goal of nursing is to assist individual, families, and groups in attaining and maintaining maximal level of total wellness. The nurse assesses managers and evaluates client systems. Nursing focuses on the variables affecting the client response to the stressor. Nursing action are earned out on three levels. When the stressor is identified but no reaction has occurred; interventions can decrease the degree of reaction or increase the line of defence. This is called primary prevention. When the reaction/has already happened, secondary prevention is carried out, with intervention aimed at treating symptoms and reducing reactions. After active treatment, tertiary prevention strengthens the lines of defence through education and uses the systems total resources to prevent further occurrence.

Neuman model is applicable to all phases of the nursing process. It can be applied across all clinical areas and is especially useful for individuals and families. It is a holistic approach because each system or subsystem cannot be isolated; rather, the influence of each system on the whole must be considered. The three levels of prevention are useful guidelines for planning nursing interventions.

(xv) Roy's Theory (1979)

Sister Callista Roy, a member of the Sisters of St Joseph of Carondeler, was born on October 14, 1939 in Los Angles, California. She was the receiver of BA in Nursing, MSc Nursing, MA in Sociology and PhD in Sociology.

The major concepts defined by Roy are as follows:

1. *Person:* According to Roy, a person is a biopsychosocial being in constant interaction with a changing environment. She defined the person, the recipient of nursing care, as a living complex, adaptive system with internal processes (the cognator and regulator) acting to maintain adaptation in the four adaptive modes, i.e. physiological needs, selfconcept, role functions, and interdependence. The person as a living system is 'a whole' made up of parts or subsystems that function as a unity for some purpose... patient is a person or family with unusual stressor or ineffective coping mechanism.
2. *Health:* It is a state and a process of being and becoming an integrated and whole person. Lack of integration represents lack of health.
3. *Environment:* According to Roy environment is all the conditions, circumstances, and influences surrounding and affecting the development and behavior of persons or groups. Factors in the environment that affect the person are categorized as focal, contextual, and residual stimuli.
4. *Nursing:* It is defined broadly as a theoretical system of knowledge which prescribes a process of analysis and action related to the care of the ill or potentially ill person.

Roy differentiates nursing as a science from nursing as a practice discipline. Nursing science is a developing system of knowledge about person that observes, classifies, and relates the processes by which persons positively affect their health status. Nursing as practice discipline is nursing scientific body of knowledge used for the purpose of providing an essential service to people, that is, promoting ability to affect health positively.

Roy's goal of nursing is to help man adapt to change in his physiological needs, his self concept, his role function, and his interdependent relations during health and illness. Nursing fills a unique role as a facilitator of adaptation by assessing behavior in each of these four adaptive modes and intervening by managing the influencing stimulants.

As defined by Roy, response to a decrease in body integrity creates a need state, and the individual responds with an act or behavior. The physiologic mode involves oxygenation, and circulation, fluid and electrolyte balance, nutrition, rest and activity and regulations of temperature, hormones and sensory function. The self concept mode concerned with perceptions of one's physical self and personal self including personality, moral ethical beliefs and values. The interdependent mode involves social relationships, including both the need to be interdependent and the need for support by others. The role function involves the behaviors of a person in each role taken on life.

In this model, all nursing activities are aimed at promoting the individuals adaption to health and illness in all four adaptive modes. The nurse determines what demands are causing problems for a client and assess how well the client is adapting to them. Nursing care is then directed at helping the client to adapt.

(xvi) Leininger's Theory (1978)

Made Leine M Leininger is the founder of transcultural nursing and a leader in transcultural nursing and human cure theory.

The major concepts defined in her theory are as follows:

Care: It refers to phenomenon related to assistive, supportive or enabling behavior toward or for another individual (or group) with evident or anticipated needs to ameliorate or improve a human condition or life way.

Caring: It refers to action directed towards assisting, supporting or enabling another individual (or group) with evident or anticipated needs to ameliorate or improve a human condition or life way.

Culture: It refers to the learned, shared and transmitted values, beliefs, norms and life way practices of a particular group that guides thinking, decisions, actions and patterned ways.

Cultural care: It refers to the cogruitively known values, beliefs, and patterned expressions that assist, support, or enable another individual or group to maintain well-being, improve a human condition or life way, face death and disabilities.

Nursing: It is a learned humanistic art and science that focuses upon personalized (individual group) care behaviors, functions, and processes directed toward promoting and maintaining health behaviors or recovery from illness which have physical, psychocultural and social significance or meaning or those being assisted generally by a professional nurse or one with similar role competencies.

The goal of nursing is to provide care consistent with nursing emerging science and knowledge with caring as a central focus according to his theory carrying is central and unifying domain for nursing knowledge and practice.

(xvii) Watson's Theory (1979) (Margaret)

Jean Harman Watson was born in Southern West Virginia. She earned a BSc in 1964, MS in psychiatric mental health nursing in 1966 and PhD in educational psychology and counseling in 1973.

Watson's philosophy of caring attempts to define outcome of nursing activity in regard to the humanistic aspects of life. Her theory and philosophy of caring is based on the values of kindness, concern, love of self and others and respect for the spiritual dimensions of the person.

Watson defined human caring in nursing as "an art and a science in which caring is a human-to-human process demonstrated through a therapeutic interpersonal interactions". The action of nursing is directed at understanding the inter-relationships, with health, illness, and human behavior. Nursing is concerned with promoting and restoring health and preventing illness.

Watson bases her theory for nursing practice on the following ten creative factors, each has a dynamic phenomenological component that is relative to the individuals involved in the relationship as encompassed by nursing:

Formation of a humanistic altruistic system of values: Humanistic and altruistic values are learned early in life but can be greatly influenced by nurse education. This factor can be defined as satisfaction through giving and extension of the sense of self.

Instillation of faith and hope: This factor incorporating humanistic and altruistic values, facilitates the promotion of holistic nursing care and positive health within the client population. It also describes the nurse's role in developing effective nurse-client interrelation and in promoting wellness by helping the client adopt health seeking behavior.

Cultivation of sensitivity to one's self and to others: The recognition of feelings leads to self acutalization through self acceptance for both the nurse and the client. As nurses acknowledge their sensitivity and feelings, they become more genuine, authentic and sensitive to others.

Development of helping trust and relationship: The development of a helping trust relationships between the nurse and client is crucial for transpersonal caring. A trusting relationship promotes and accepts the expression of both positive and negative feelings. It involves congruence, empathy, nonpossessive warmth, and effective communication.

Promotion and acceptance of the expression of positive and negative feelings: The sharing of feeling is a risk taking experience for both nurse and client. The nurse must be prepared for either positive or negative feelings. The nurse must recognize that intellectual and emotional understandings of a situation differ.

Systematic use of scientific problem solving method of decision making: Use of the nursing process brings a scientific problem solving approach to nursing care.

Promotion of interpersonal teaching learning: It is an important factor in which nurse facilitates the process of teaching—learning techniques that are designed to enable the client to provide self care, determining personal needs, and to provide opportunities for their personal growth.

Provision for supportive, protective and/or corrective mental, physical, sociocultural and spiritual environment: The nurses must recognize the influences that internal and external environment have on the health and illness of individual. Accordingly, they should make arrangement to create such conducive environment for the patient in positive direction.

Assistance with gratification of human needs: The nurse recognizes the biophysical, psychophysical, psychosocial, and interpersonal needs of self and client. Client must satisfy lower order needs before attempting to attain higher order ones, i.e. food elimination, ventilation (biophysical lower needs), activity/ inactivity; sexuality (lower psychological needs) and achievement, affiliation, self actualization (higher ones).

Allowance for existential phenomenological force: Phenomenology describes data of the immediate situation that help people understand the phenomena in question. This analysis of human existence in a situation provides a thought provoking experience leading to better understanding of ourselves and others.

As stated above each factor describes the earning prices of how client attains or maintains health or dies peacefully. Caring represents all of the factors the nurse uses to deliver health care to the client.

(For details of theories on nursing and their applications, please read author's text on "NURSING THEORIES").

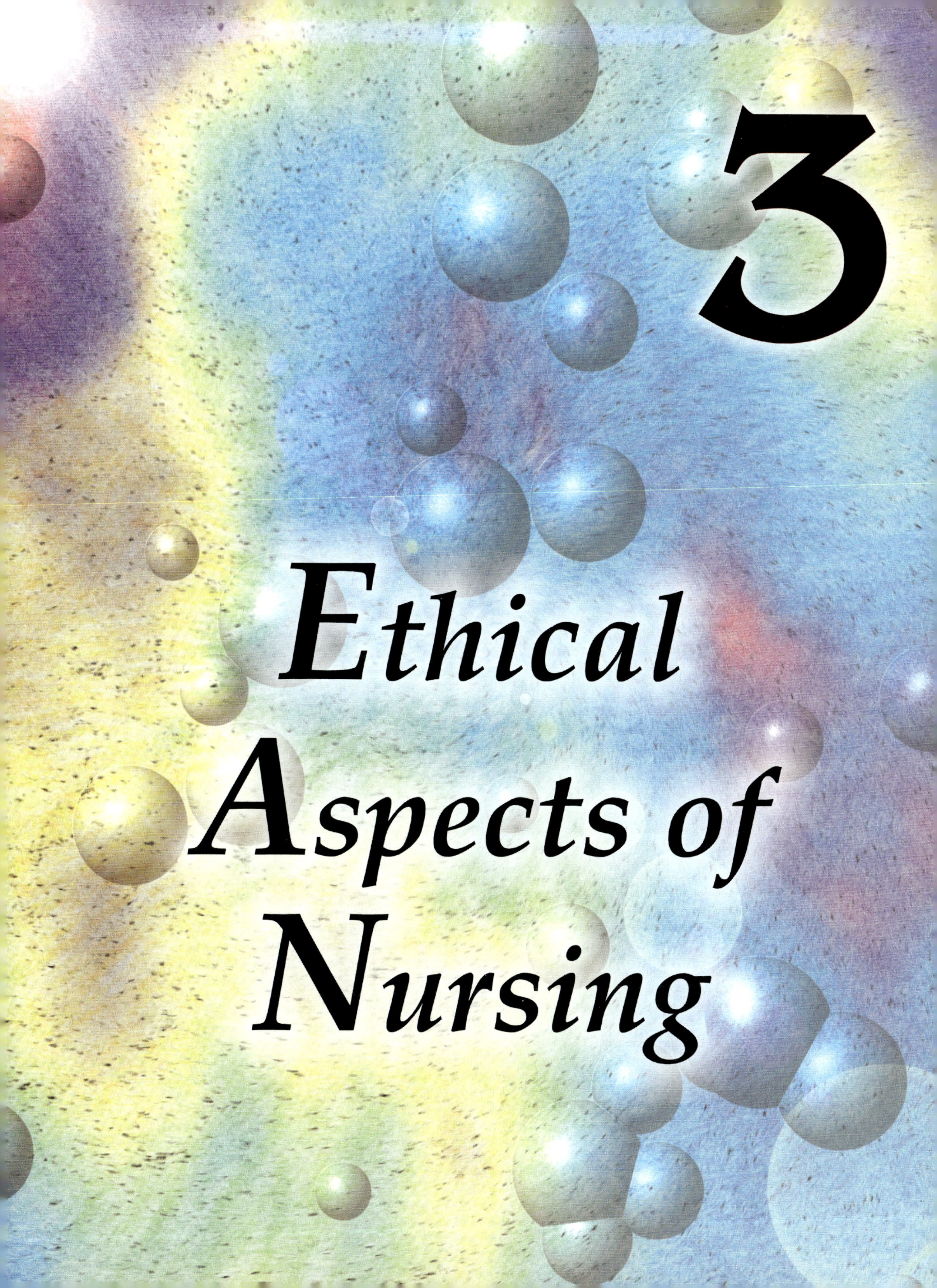

3

Ethical Aspects of Nursing

Introduction

Ethics is the science relating to moral actions and one's value system. Many nurses envision ethics as dealing with principles or morality and what is right or wrong. Ethics is concerned with motives and attitudes and the relationship of these attitudes to the good of the individual. "Ethics has to do with action we wish people would take, not actions they must take". Then, values are interwoven with ethics; values are personal beliefs about the truth and worth of thoughts, objects and behavior.

Ethics may be distinguished from the law as ethics is internal to oneself, looks to the good of an individual rather than society as a whole and concerns the 'why' of one's actions. The law, comprises of rules and regulations pertinent to society as a whole, is external to oneself and concerns one's actions and conduct. What did the person do or fail to do as opposed to why did the person act as he/she did? Ethics concerns the good of an individual within society which law concerns society as a whole as opposed to individual in society. Law can be enforced through the courts and status while ethics are enforced via ethics committees and professional codes.

Ethics are always been an integral part of nursing. Throughout nursing one can find code of ethics, statements of moral principles, treatise on maintaining high ideals, and recorded discussions of moral and ethical issues. Caring for an comforting the sick and protecting the suffering are human activities of nurses. These human activities and how society views directly, affect the morals, customs and beliefs of human kind.

Nursing ethics provides the standards for professional behavior and is the study of principles of right and wrong conduct for nurses. Nursing ethics states the duties and obligation of nurses to their clients, other health professionals, the profession and the community. Ethics promotes the philosophical and theological study of morality, mental judgments and moral problems.

The theoretical knowledge that nurse will need to begin professional practice includes an understanding of the nature of morals and ethics and especially nursing ethics and basic information about factors that affect moral decisions, i.e. values, moral frameworks, professional guidelines, and ethical principle.

Although the terms *ethics* and *morals* are similar in meaning, in modern theory **morals** refers to private, personal, or group standards of right and wrong. **Moral behavior** is behavior that is in accordance with custom or tradition and usually reflects professional or religious beliefs. An example of morality might be a person's opposition to or support of abortion. Another example is the "golden rule," that you should not treat others as you wish to be treated.

Ethics, in contrast, is a systematic study of right and wrong conduct in situations that involve issues of values and morals. Ethics is a formal process for making logical and consistent moral decisions. Morals consider in a broad, general manner what is good or bad, right or wrong (e.g. "In general, it is wrong to steal"). Ethics answers the question "What should I do in a given situation?" (e.g. "Is it wrong to steal if you have to do it to feed your children?"). Ethics uses specific rules, theories, principles, and perspectives to inquire into the justification of an individual's actions in a particular situation.

Ethics is rooted in the legal system and reflects the political values of a society. However, it is important to realize that ethics is not the same as law, religion, institutional practices, or customs. An action that is legal or customary may not be morally right or ethically justifiable. The same holds true of religion. Person cannot assume that an accepted practice of a certain religion is an ethical practice in every situation. For example, there was a time when owning slaves was legal. That did not mean it was morally right. A more current example is that of abortion, which is legal under certain circumstances. However, many people argue that it is morally wrong in all circumstances.

Bioethics refers to the application of ethical principles to health care. Bioethics is concerned with every area of health care, including direct care of patients, allocation of resources, utilization of staff, and medical and nursing research.

The nurse did not need a medical order nor permission from hospital administration to act ethically.

Need for Nurses to Study Ethics

Nurses should study ethics for a variety of reasons as given below:

- *Nurses will encounter ethical problems frequently in their work*: Whether or not you are even aware of it. A consciously made, informed decision must surely be better than one made without awareness of the ethical issues involved. The most difficult question you will face will not be "How do I do this" but "Should I do this?"
- *Ethics is central to nursing:* Commitment to caring for other human beings supports the claim that nursing is a moral art. Traditionally, people have expressed idealism by attending the sick; health and compassion are central values in nursing.
- *Multidisciplinary input is important:* No one profession is responsible for an ethical decision. As situations become more complex, multidisciplinary input becomes increasingly important. For example, physicians are responsible for knowing what surgery to perform and obtaining consent, but the nurse has a part in being sure the patient is adequately informed so that true consent is obtained.
- *Ethical knowledge is necessary for professional acceptance:* Being a professional includes being accountable to others in the profession for the ethical conduct of your work. Professions claim to use professional expertise for social good; therefore, to conduct our work well and have it stand the test of public scrutiny, we need to be clear about the ethics of our work.
- *Ethical reasoning is necessary for nursing to be taken seriously by other disciplines:* Nurses' opinion to be valued by others, you must be able to dearly express your moral position in a logical way. To be a truly accountable practitioner, you must be able *to* (1) understand your own values as they relate *to* basic morality and (2) use ethical reasoning to articulate your moral position.

- *Ethical proficiency is essential for providing holistic care:* Nurses deal with the whole person–that includes providing support for spiritual and moral concerns.
- *Nurses should be advocates for patients*: Advocacy is the communication and defense of the rights and interests of another. Schools have socialized nurses to include patient advocacy in their role conceptions. Currently, Code of Ethics for Nurses, states that the nurse promotes, advocates for and strives to protect the health, safety and rights of the patient. To advocate for patients in ethical situations, nurse must be able to identify the ethical issues and communicate the patient's wishes. Knowledge of ethical principles and decision making can give clarity to the aims of nursing practice and help us keep patients' interests foremost.
- *Studying ethics will help you to make better decisions*: Study of ethics prepares you to analyze moral problems from multiple perspectives rather than relying entirely on your personal values, intuition, and emotions. Practice in analyzing dilemmas will help you to become an informed decision maker, capable of understanding the perspectives of all the people in each situation–to understand.

Most nursing problems have more than one acceptable answer. This is especially true of ethical problems. Each situation is unique in its details. By thinking it through critically from several different angles, you will be assured that yon have done all that you can to provide your client with the highest quality of ethical care.

Moral agency or ethical agency is the ability of nurses to base their practice on professional standards of ethical conduct and to participate in ethical decision making. Simply stated, it means that nurses have choices and are responsible for their actions. An ethical agent must be able to:

- Perceive the difference between good and evil, right and wrong.
- Understand abstract moral principles.
- Reason and apply moral principles to make decisions, weigh alternatives, and plan ways to achieve goals.
- Decide and choose freely.
- Act according to choice (this assumes both the power and the capability to act).

Ethics is a science or study of moral values or principles, including ideals of self-determination, kindness, and justice. To understand ethics and its relationships to health care, the terms morals, ethics, and bioethics must first be clarified.

- *Morals* refer to established rules in situations where a decision about right and wrong must be made. Morals provides standards of behavior. These standards guide the behavior of an individual or social group. Morals reflect the "is" or reality of how individual or groups behave. An example of a moral standard is "good people do not lie."
- If morals reflect the "is" of human behavior, then *ethics* is a term used to reflect the "should" of human behavior. Ethics identify what should be done to live with one another. Ethics are process oriented and involve critical analysis of actions.

If ethicists, people who study ethics, reflected on the moral statement "one should not lie." They would clarify definitions of lying and explore the circumstances under which lying might be acceptable.

- When ethical theories and principles are applied to problems in health care, the field of study is called "bioethics". Bioethics is an area of ethical inquiry came into existence around 1970 when health care began to shift its focus curing disease toward concern for the total patient. A new term, clinical ethics, is increasing being used.

Advances in medicine, science, and technology sometimes create ethical dilemmas. For example, people can now be kept "alive" even when brain dead. But should they be kept alive under these circumstances just because we now have the technology to do to? This kind of issues mandate that nurses must be concerned with what "should" be done for patients they care for. It is that actions be critically analyzed for their appropriateness, since health care professionals possess a good deal of power over those in their care.

Ethics in nursing practice involves many facets of professional conduct. Professional commitment is shown through a desire to help, a sense of obligation, efforts to enhance competence and compliance with professional standards. Professional accountability in one of many important ethical issues. It depends upon an individuals sense of responsibility and personal integrity.

Professional persons are governed by the standards of conduct set forth by their respective professions. Ethics in nursing practice is concerned with the conduct of nurses in performing acts which are deemed ethically right or wrong. Nurses who violate profession ethics may be subject to discipline by nursing associations and may be legally liable for them actions.

It is within the context that nurses need to study code of ethics, ethical theories, and principles, moral developments, ethical dilemmas and ethical decision making models. Such knowledge will increase nurses ability to participate in the resolution of ethical dilemmas.

Today, social values are changing rapidly with the constant advancement of technology and nurses are increasingly confronted by situations that have far-reaching ethical implications. Nurses must know which their legal rights are in such matters as well as those of the patient. It is important for nurses to realize the strength of their personal values in shaping their professional values.

Theories of Ethics

There is no single ethical theory ascribed by all philosophers or ethicists. There are two theories that nurse ethicists have identified as useful. The two basic theories of ethical philosophy that are frequently referenced in literature viz., utilitarianism and deontology.

(i) Utilitarianism

This theory was first described by David Hyme (1771-1776) and was developed further by many notable philosophers including Teremy Bentison and John Stuart Mill. Utilitarianism in sometimes also described on teleology or consequentialism. The primary principle of this philosophy in that actions are "morally right" when the longest number of individuals receive the "best" results (defined as pleasure or happiness) from the action taken. A problem with utilitarianism in the impact of the decision on the minority population.

According to Mill (1863), a "right action" conforms to the "greatest happiness principle." In other words, it is right to maximize the greatest good for the happiness or pleasure of the greatest number of people. Utilitarian ethics calculates the effect of all alternative actions on the general welfare of present and future generations. Thus the position is also referred to as 'calculus mortality.' The utilitarian approach to ethics assumes that it is possible to balance good and bad. The goal in that made people will experience good rather than bad. Benefits are to be maximized for the greatest number of people possible. In this approach, each individual counts as one.

Professional health care employ utilitarian theory in many situations. The concept of triage, where the sick or injured are classified by the severity of their condition to determine priority of treatment, is a example of utilitarianian. In triage, those who are so severely ill or injured, that they cannot possibly recover are not treated at all. Although this seems cruel, when there are many more sick and wounded them available facilities to care for them, triage is accepted worldwide as an ethical basis for determining treatment. Frequently, utilitarianian in the basis for deciding how health care finances will be spent. Money is more likely to be spent on research for diseases that affect large number of people than for research on diseases that affect only a few. A difficulty of this approach that whole the appeal is made to the happiness of the majority, the individual or minority, who also deserves help, may be overlooked.

(ii) Deontology

Deontology as an ethical philosophy describes actions that apply principles and rules. In other words, the rules are to be followed by all individuals at all times. Principles that advocates of the philosophy follow include autonomy, nonmaleficence (not being harmful or evil), beneficence (doing good, acting kindly and charitably), and justice.

The major proponent of deontology was Immanuel Kant (1974-1804). Kant believed that rightness or wrongness of an action depended on the inherent moral significance of the action. He believed that an act was moral if it originated from goodwill. Ethical action consisted in doing one's duty. To do ones duty was right; nor to do ones duty was wrong. Deontology can be further divided into either act or rule deontology. *Act deontologists* determine the right thing to do by gathering all the facts and then making a decision. Much time and energy are needed to carefully judge each situation in and of itself. Once a decision is made, there is commitment to universalizing it. In other words, if one makes a moral judgment in one situation, the same judgment will be made in any similar situation. *Rule deontologists* emphasize that principles guide our actions.

Examples of rules might be "Always keep a promise" or "Never tell a lie." In all situations, the rule is to be followed deontologists are not concerned with the consequences of always following certain rules or actions. If the principles believed is "Always keep promise" the deontologists will keep promises, even if the circumstances have changed.

In nursing, there are many rules and duties that nurses follow. One such rule is "Do no harm" (beneficence). Another justifiable rule is "The patient should be allowed to make his or her own decisions" (autonomy). But consider the situation of a severely depressed young man who wishes to end his life by committing suicide and asks the nurses assistance. Clearly the rule about doing no harm conflicts with allowing young man to make his own decisions. Nurse can see the dilemmas cannot always be resolved using theoretical approaches alone.

Theories of Moral Development

The terms ethics and morality are closely related. Today the terms ethical judgments and ethical principles are used where it once would have been more common to system of moral judgments and moral principles. Moral development describes how a person learns to deal with moral dilemmas from childhood through adulthood. To understand the study of the field of ethics, it is important to review the various theories of ethical or moral development.

John Dewey identified three levels of moral developments:
 (i) The premoral or pre conventional level,
 (ii) The conventional level, and
(iii) The autonomous level.

Using this approach, Dewey stated that an individual would progress through these sequential developmental stages. The lower level – pre moral stage – may be identified by behavior that is motivated by biologic and social impulses. The second level, termed the conventional stage, is exemplified by behavior that is the norm for the group or society. The highest level, that of autonomy, indicates critical thinking and judgment by the individual.

John Piaget used Deweys stages of moral development to identify specific stages in children. Through his study, Piaget identified three similar stages, but linked that with certain ages and developmental levels. Piaget's stages included:
 (i) The premoral stage (0 to 4 years)
 (ii) The heteronomous stage (ages 4 to 8 years)
(iii) The autonomous stage (ages 8 to 12 years).

Lawrence Kohlberg (1976, 1986) proposed three levels of moral development:
 (i) Preconventional
 (ii) Conventional
(iii) Postconventional.

In the preconventional level, the individual is inattentive to the norms of society which responding to moral problems. Instead, the individual perspective in self-centered. At this level what the individual wants or needs takes precedence over right or wrong. Kohlberg saw this level of moral development in most children under nine years of age, as well as in some adolescents and adult, criminal offenders.

The conventional level characterizes by making moral decisions that conform to the expectations of ones family, group or society when confronted with a moral choice, people functioning at the conventional level follow family or cultural group norms. According Kohlberg, most adolescents and adult generally function at this level.

The post conventional level involves more independent modes of thinking than previous stages, so that the individuals is able to define his or her own moral values. People at the post conventional level may ignore both self-interest and group norms in making moral choices. They create their own morality, which may differ from society's norms. Kohlberg believed that only a minority of adults achieve this level.

Each of Kohlberg level, is subdivided into two stages. Progression through the stages occurs over varying lengths of time, but each stage is sequential and is characterized by higher capacity for logical reasoning than the preceding stage.

(i) Preconventional
   – Obedience/punishment orientation
   – Personal interest orientation
(ii) Conventional
   – Good boy/nice girl orientation
   – Law and order orientation
(iii) Postconventional
   – Social contract orientation
   – Conscience orientation.

Kohlberg suggested that certain conditions may stimulate higher level moral development. Intellectual development is one necessary characteristic. Individual higher levels intellectual and generally more advanced in moral development than those operating at lower levels of intelligence. An environment that offers people opportunities for group participation, shared decision-making processes, and responsibility for the consequences of their actions also promotes higher levels of moral reasoning.

Gilligan (1982) was a student of Kohlberg, had recognized that Kohlberg theories had largely been generated from research with men and boys. She believed that Kohlberg's theory was inadequate to explain women's moral development. She suggested that women view moral dilemmas in terms of conflicting responsibilities. The sequence she described included three levels and two transitions, with each level representing a more complex understanding of the relationship of self and others and each transition resulting in a crucial re-evaluation of the conflicts between selfishness and responsibility.

Gilligan's levels of moral development are:
(i) Orientation to individual survival
(ii) A focus on goodness as self sacrifice
(iii) The morality of non-violence.

She believed that the moral person is one who responds to need and demonstrates a consideration of care and responsibility in relationships she described a moral development perspective focused on care. Recent work of Gilligan and her associate has attempted to define the relationship between the two moral orientation of justice and care. They determined that both perspectives were present when people faced real life moral dilemma but people generally tended to focus on one set of concerns and paid only minimal attention to the other perspectives. As expected the care focus was more often exhibited by women, and the justice focus was more often exemplified by men.

The justice and care perspectives in themselves are not competing theories but are two separate moral perspectives that organize thinking in different ways. The justice perspective strives to treat others fairly, whereas the care perspective endeavors not to turn away from someone in need.

Moral Principles

Moral principles are useful in ethical decisions because even if people disagree about which action is right in a situation, they may be able to agree about which principles apply. This agreement may provide common ground for a compromise or other resolution of the problem. Different moral frameworks (to be discussed later) use some of the same principles in ethical reasoning. Autonomy, nonmaleficence, beneficence, fidelity, veracity, and justice as described below:

Autonomy

Autonomy refers to a person's right to choose and his ability to act on that choice. The principle of autonomy rests on the belief that every competent person has the right to determine his own course of action. Maintaining autonomy is one way to show respect for each person's humanity. Individual demonstrate respect for autonomy when treat people with consideration, believe patients' stories about the course and symptoms of their illnesses, and protect patients who are unable to decide for themselves.

The principle of autonomy underlies informed consent–clients' right to decide for themselves whether or not they will agree to a proposed procedure or treatment. Nurse also honor autonomy when she/he respect the patient's or surrogate's right to decide, even when she/he believe those choices are not in the patient's best interest.

Nonmaleficence

The principle of nonmaleficence is the twofold duty to do no harm and to prevent harm. Nonmaleficence refers to both actual harm and risk of harm, as well as to intentional and unintentional harm. In nursing it is rare to find intentional harm, but unintentional harm due to lack of careful planning and consideration does occur.

When using the principle of nonmaleficence to guide treatment regimens, ask the question, "Does this treatment cause more harm or more good to the patient?" Nonmaleficence requires that you think critically about patient care and research situations, weighing the potential risks against the potential benefits. Risk of harm is not always clear. Suppose nurses are about to get a patient out of bed for the first time after surgery. The benefit clearly is that this will prevent postoperative complications such as pneumonia and thrombophlebitis, but the risks, in terms of excessive pain or unintentional damage to the operative site, may be less clear. Weighing risks and benefits is a value laden exercise. Who is to say what amount of pain is excessive–nurse or the patient? To honor the principle of nonmaleficence in this situation, nurse would need to be sure to premedicate the patient and carefully assess his status as you are helping him to ambulate.

Nonmaleficence is a fundamental duty of healthcare professionals. Both the physicians 'Hippocratic Oath and the nurses' Nightingale Pledge state that care providers are to cause no harm to patients. When nurse are careful to prevent medication errors, or provide a walker, or use an ambulation belt for ambulating patients, you are honoring the nonmaleficence principle.

Beneficence

Beneficence is the duty to do or promote good. Nurse can think of this principle as being on a continuum with nonmaleficence. At one end of the continuum is the duty to do no harm; beneficence, at the other end, is the duty to bring about positive good. The following examples illustrate the duties in priority order:

- Do no harm. (Don't push the man into the river.)
- Prevent harm when you can. (If the man is getting dangerously close to the river's edge, warn him that he is about to fall into the river.)
- Remove harm when it is being inflicted. (If you see a struggle and someone is trying to push the man into the river, interfere and try to stop it.)
- Bring about positive good. (If the man has fallen in the river, jump in and try to save him.)

When weighing the risks and benefits of an action, nurses are actually balancing nonmaleficence with beneficence. It is well to remember that patients, family members, and other professionals may identify benefits and harms differently. A benefit to one may represent a burden to another.

In spite of the fact that "doing good" sounds like such a positive goal, beneficence can have negative consequences. One such outcome is **paternalism** (treating others like children). This would occur, for example, if you think you know what is best for a competent client and then coerce the client to act as you wish rather than to act as she wishes. Saying to a patient, for example, "Trust us; we know what is best for you to do in this situation," may seem to be beneficent because you are trying to support the patient. But it is actually paternalistic behavior that inhibits autonomy and lacks respect for the patient.

Fidelity

Fidelity (faithfulness) is the obligation to keep promises. In actual practice individual will often find that competing tasks prevent her/him from being able to deliver something exactly as she/he had promised. Fidelity requires you to make promises in a thoughtful, careful manner to maximize the likelihood that you can keep them. Instead of "I'll be right back with your medication," you might "waffle" a bit and say, "I'll get back with your medication as quickly as I can" or "I must go help another patient for a few minutes, but I'll get here with your medication as quickly as I can."

Being faithful to clients also means meeting their reasonable expectations. For example, clients should expect you to show them basic respect, to be competent, to follow the statements of your professional code of ethics, and to keep their information confidential. They will reasonably expect you to honor commitments you have made to them in terms of informed consent or verbal agreements.

Honoring fidelity is a basic part of every patient care situation. Sometimes the promises are of major significance, such as promising not to share certain information with other members of the healthcare team, and at other times it may be only a promise to come back to check the effectiveness of a pain medication or to bring a requested item back to the client's room. The commitment to fidelity is the same regardless of the level of significance of the promise.

Veracity

Veracity is the duty to tell the truth. This seems very straightforward, and you may wonder why it even needs discussion. However, there are times when veracity may present a challenge. For example, should you tell the truth when you know that it might cause harm to the client? Would it be appropriate to tell a lie in order to relieve extreme patient anxiety? Most nurses would agree that it isn't hard to tell the truth, but at times it may be very hard to determine how much of the truth to tell. For example, healthcare professionals feel uncomfortable giving families "bad news." So instead of saying, ''Your father has a fatal illness and is unlikely to live for more than a month," they may say, ''Your father is very ill, but we will do everything we possibly can for him." In this, as in most situations, the risk of losing patient trust outweighs any benefit of withholding the truth.

Although you always presume the value of telling the truth, there may be times when you are justified to withhold information. In some cultures, for example, families go to great lengths to protect a dying patient from the harsh truth of his prognosis, and the patient himself may not wish to know.

Justice

Justice is the obligation to be fair. It implies equal treatment of all clients. This principle is reflected in the first provision in the Code of Ethics for Nurses (ANA, 2001). Questions of justice will become a part of your everyday experience in patient care, from deciding how to allocate your time among patients to larger decisions, such as how to allocate limited health care resources.

Distributive justice, which is one type of justice that is particularly relevant to health care, requires fair distribution of both benefits and burdens, as in the following issues.

- *Allocating resources:* Distributive justice questions come up when more than one person or group competes for the same resources. One example arises in determining how to spend federal and state tax dollars: Should money he spent to fund AIDS research or to find better treatments for Alzheimer's disease? Other examples surround organ transplantation. Human organs are scarce resources. How do we decide which patient should receive an available organ for transplantation? Is an 18-year-old more deserving of a kidney than a 75-year-old? Is a person with liver disease due to alcoholism less deserving of a liver than someone with liver disease not caused by alcoholism? The decision of who should live and who may die is never an easy decision.

- *Fair access to care:* Access to care is a specific kind of healthcare resource. The principle of distributive justice holds that we should provide equal access to health care for all. The ability to develop sound criteria on which to base the allocation of resources is the challenge of distributive justice.

Compensatory justice focuses on compensation for wrongs that have been done to individuals or groups. This is the type of justice considered when there are malpractice suits, for example, when a patient climbs out of bed and falls and breaks a hip. Groups of citizens may also be harmed, for instance, by a company's unintentional pollution of water in a community. If this pollution were proven to cause cancer in members of the community, a monetary settlement might be made.

Procedural justice is relevant in processes that require ranking or ordering. Often the unwritten rule of "first come, first served" is used as a basis for delivery of services. In many situations, this is considered fair. Institutional policies are written to ensure that the same procedures apply to all clients or employees in the same way (e.g. visiting hours, working on holidays, sick leave).

Moral Frameworks in Nursing

Moral (or philosophical) frameworks are systems of thought (theories) that are the basis for the differing perspectives people have in ethical situations. Such frameworks have existed since ancient times, for example, in the works of the Greek philosophers Plato and Aristotle. No matter how well you know the theories and principles, though, they will not provide answers for specific patient situations. They simply offer a lens through which you can look to examine an ethical problem.

There is no single "best" theory that will give you all the answers or provide the one "true" answer to an ethical problem. Each provides a different perspective. By using more than one framework to analyze a situation, you will perform a more comprehensive analysis of the problem.

Consequentialism

In consequentialist theories, the rightness or wrongness of an action depends on the consequences of the act rather than on the act itself. Theories of this type are also called teleology, from the Greek word *telos,* meaning "end" or the study of ends (also called *final causes).* Utilitarianism, the most familiar consequentialist theory, takes the position that the value of an action is determined by its usefulness. The *principle of utility* states that an act must result in the greatest good for the greatest number of people. When we say "good" here, we mean positive benefit. Any act can then become the ethical choice if it delivers "good" results. In health care, the principle of "most of all, do no harm" is consequentialist in nature. Because of this principle, we are always concerned about weighing the risks and benefits of our care (e.g. a medication may kill cancer cells, but side effects may harm the patient's quality of life).

Using utilitarianism to resolve an ethical problem, you would evaluate every alternative action for its potential outcomes, both positive and negative–similar to a technique you may already use when making a decision, that is, making a list of pros and cons. You would then select the action that results in the most benefits for the greatest number of people involved in the situation. The following is an example of utilitarian reasoning: The practice of triage is used in a disaster when emergency workers have to sort patients to determine who will be treated first or who will receive limited resources (e.g. oxygen or intravenous therapy). If a victim has little potential for survival, he may not be treated at all, or his treatment may be postponed to free the healthcare team to treat those victims (i.e. "the greatest number") with the greatest potential to survive.

Deontology

Deontology is almost the opposite of the utilitarian model in that it considers an action to be right or wrong independent of its consequences, This system of ethical decision making is also called **formalism;** decisions are based on moral rules and unchanging principles, A famous early philosopher, Immanuel Kant (1724-1804), established the principle of the **categorical imperative,** which states that one should only act if the action is based on a principle that is universal (or in other words, if you believe that everyone should act in the same way in a similar situation). Another deontology principle, also formulated by Kant, is to treat people as ends and never as means. Treating people as an *end* means that the person is more important than whatever else you may be trying to accomplish. Can you imagine the ethical concerns of research situations in which the research subjects were exposed to some amount of risk (e.g. a new surgical procedure) to find a drug or treatment that will benefit many other people?

When using a deontological model, nurse would critically examine a situation to determine which actions are right or wrong according to rules and principles such as justice, autonomy, doing good, and doing no harm. These principles are regarded as unchanging and absolute, and they come from the same universal values that underlie all major religions.

Deontological frameworks also emphasize rights (e.g. the right to freedom, the right of self-determination) and obligations (duties). For example, nurse must help someone in need because nurse have a duty to help others, not because helping will produce good consequences. In fact, a duty to help even if helping may produce some bad consequences.

One difficulty with deontology occurs when choosing between conflicting universal principles, it is also important to consider motives.

Feminist Ethics

Feminist ethicists have created a model based on the belief that because traditional deontological models focus on abstract principles such as fairness, justice, and rights, they provide a mostly masculine perspective. In contrast, virtues such as love, relationships, caring, nurturing, and sympathy are more relevant to women but are rarely seen in traditional moral theories. They assert that focusing on deontological principles allows one to be distracted from dealing with larger social issues. Feminist ethics values relationships and stories about relationships over using universal principles. Feminists argue that it is impossible to avoid being influenced by one's relationships. They see that influence as positive and believe it should not be muted by an attempt to be objective–because objectivity is impossible anyway.

Feminist ethics does consider principles and the consequences, but it also asks you to look at social issues surrounding the ethical situation to ensure that social facts are not forgotten. Feminist ethical reasoning addresses issues of gender inequality within each situation. Part of the reasoning would be to ask, "How is this decision affecting the woman?" An example of the feminist ethical approach arises in deciding whether to allocate federal healthcare resources to younger people or to older adults. Feminist reasoning might say that, all other considerations being equalation.

- There are more older women than older men.
- Older women tend to be poorer and are more likely to be alone than are men.
- Therefore, if health care for older adults were to be rationed, it would negatively affect women more than men.
- Therefore, it would be unfair and unethical to allocate more healthcare resources to younger people than to older people.

The **ethics-of-care,** a nursing philosophy, directs intention to the specific situations of individual patient viewed within the context of their life narrative. Can theories are derived directly from the feminist ethic model and especially promote nurturing of patient and caregivers. An ethics-of-care way of thinking emphasizes the role of feelings, not at the expense of some of the principles part of conventional ethics, such as autonomy (self-determination) or beneficence (doing good).

In this model, nurses incorporate a responsibility to care as a part of their professional behavior. Leininger (1988) defines care as "the central unifying domain from the body of knowledge and practices nursing." Some aspects of care include the ability and obligation to appreciate, understand, and even share the patient's pain or condition. Using a caring model, your ethical analysis would focus on relationships and client stories. The following are specific perspectives within the ethics-of-care model:

- Viewing caring as the central force in nursing
- Promoting dignity and respect for patients as people
- Attending to the particulars of each individual patients
- Cultivating responsiveness to others
- Redefining fundamental moral principles to include virtues such as kindness, attentiveness, empathy, compassion, and reliability.

An advantage of including the caring perspective and client stories in ethical dialogue is that it tends focus discussion at the level where the relationship are located, rather than in an intellectual plane. Critics of the ethics-of-care suggest that the term *care* can be misconstrued to become too sentimental at therefore, ineffective. If nursing is sentimentality through overemphasis on caring, nursing will be so as less strong than medicine.

An ethics-of-care model does provide an alternative to the heavily intellectual camps of utilitarianism and ontology. It can give a refreshingly new perspective of moral situations. Some questions that might reflect this model of discourse include the following:

- Should we provide free medical care to the homeless? An ethics-of-care position would say yes, even though it might not, for example, provide the greatest good for the greatest number of people.
- Our healthcare system uses discharge criteria that allow patients to be sent home from hospitals while they are still too ill to care for themselves. What does that say about caring in the health care system?

In addition to moral frameworks, consult professional guidelines when making ethical decisions. One of the characteristics of a profession is that it states publicly the ethical standards for its members. Professionals, especially those who provide health care, have an obligation to society to be competent in their field, to control entry into the profession to those who are qualified, to discipline members of the profession who do not practice at an acceptable level, to do no harm, and to use high moral and ethical standards to resolve dilemmas. One can find ethical standards for nurses in codes of ethics, standards of practice, statements of patients' rights, and in various laws.

Ethical Principles

There are four major principles of ethics which include:
1. The principle of justice
2. The principle of autonomy
3. The principle of beneficence
4. The principle of veracity.

Justice

The principle of justice states that equals should be treated the same and that unequals should be treated differently. In other words, patients with same diagnosis and health care needs should receive the same care. Those with greater or lesser needs should receive different care. In health care, the most common concern about justice relates to allocation of resources and services to clients. Numerous models have been developed for distributing health care resources. These models include:

- To each equally.
- To each according to merit. This may include future contributions to society.
- To each according to what can be acquired in the market place.
- To each according to need.

Justice as a principle often leaves in with questions that answers. It raises our consciousness about making decisions but certainly does not determine what the answer should be.

Autonomy

The principle of autonomy in the claim that individuals are permitted liberty to determine their own actions according to plans they themselves have chosen. Freedom to make one's own decision, is respected under the principle of autonomy. The principle refer to the control individuals have over their own lives. Respect for the individual is the cornerstone of this principle. Autonomy applies to both decisions and actions. Autonomous decisions have several characteristics. They

- are based on individual values
- utilize adequate information
- are free from coercion
- are based on reason and deliberation.

An autonomous action is one that results from an autonomous decision. Health care professionals often take actions that profoundly affect patients lives without adequate consultations with the patients. Incorporating the principle of autonomy in all health care situations is difficult, if not impossible. Patient cannot always make their own choices. Example of those unable to participate in decisions include infants and or small children, mentally incompetent patients, and unconscious patients. Other patients may be unable to participate in decision making because of external constraints such as financial limitations, lack of necessary information, or the norms of their culture.

Beneficence

Beneficence is commonly defined as "the doing good." Frankene (1973), involved several duties with this principles which include:

- Not to inflict harm or evil (nonmaleficence)
- To prevent harm or evil
- To remove harm or evil
- To promote or do good.

The first duty, not to inflict harm, taken priority over through following duties. Even so, all four duties are obligations that must always be taken into account. Additional consideration may take precedence when there is conflict about the appropriate cause of action. For example, a surgical procedure will inflict harm, on the body but potentially has long term benefits. The procedure may be life saving, or it may diminish pain or increase mobility. In this sense, even though it inflicts harm in the short-term it is justified because of the long-term good that will result.

Virtually every one would agree that causing good and avoiding harm are important to all human beings and certainly to health care professionals. It is therefore surprising how often conflicts center around this principles.

Veracity

Veracity is defined as "telling the truth." Truth telling has long been identified as fundamental to the development and continuance of trust among human beings. Telling the truth is expected. It is necessary to basic communication, and societal relationships are built on individuals right to know the truth.

All communications between individuals has the potential to be misleading. It is easy for information to be misunderstood, misinterpreted or not comprehended. Usually these misunderstands are unintentional. Intentional deception, however, is considered morally wrong. Despite that well established fact, much intended deception occurs between health professionals and people seeking health care. Persons seeking health care often are not fruitful when giving their health histories. An example that commonly occurs relates to truthfulness concerning use of drugs and alcohol or HIV related causes.

At the same time, health care professionals are not always truthful in responding to patients questions. The nurse may choose to answer only part of a question, rather than giving all the known facts. A long tradition of a double standard in truth telling exists in health care. Health care professionals are not responsible for false information given to them by their patients. However, they are responsible for information that they give to patients.

Ethical Dilemmas in Nursing

A dilemma is defined as a situations requiring a choice between two equally desirable or undesirable alternatives. In ethical dilemma, each alternative course of action can be justified by two ways in which a person views the course of action based on his or her value system. Issues in healthcare delivery practices present different alternatives based on whether the issue or course of action is viewed by the patient, the healthcare agency, the legal system or the nurse. Increasingly, staff nurses and nurse managers face difficult decisions caused by tensions between technological capabilities, budgetary structures, and quality of life concerns. Nurses in all clinical and functional specialties face the following ethical dilemmas:

- Need to ration patient care to conserve scarce resources.
- Need to make treatment and care decisions for terminally ill patients.

- Need to obtain patients informed consent for care and treatment orders and measures such as:
  - Do not resuscitate order.
  - Withholding/withdrawing nutrition and fluids.
  - Starting/discontinuing life support system.
- Response to patient request for assisted suicide.
- Need to balance the patients need for confidentiality and privacy against society's needs for protection from unreasonable risk.
- Need to protect autonomy rights of children and incompetent adults concerning consent for research participation.
- Need to protect justice rights of patients who participate in random trials of experimental treatment.

Usually the dilemma occurs when opposing views are seen for the solution of an issue and a decision must be made. There is no set of procedures or easy answers for how an ethical dilemma should be resolved. Ethical decision making is needed in all steps of the nursing process and all phases of the nursing management process. Ethical reasoning is similar to the nursing process in that it requires critical thinking skills. A nurse can best resolve ethical dilemma, by systematically considering all options for solving the dilemma. An ethical dilemma occurs as a result of conflict between moral principles that support different courses of action.

Ethical dilemmas occur frequently in nursing practice. This is to be expected since nurses focus on life and death issues involving human beings. Many ethical dilemmas arise in nursing because of conflicts between patients, health care professionals, and/or institutions. In order to understand these conflicts, the following areas will be explored:

- Personal value systems
- Health care team
- Patients rights
- Institutional and societal issues.

i. Personal Value Systems

A value in the perception of words that is placed on an attitude, action, or object. Value system is defined as "an enduring organization of beliefs concerning preferable modes of conduct or end-states of existence along a continuum of relative importance". Value system are learned beliefs that help a person choose between difficult alternatively. Value system has a beginning foundations on beliefs, purposes, attitudes, qualities and objects that are important to ones parents. Value systems vary from individual to individual. Something important to one individual may hold greater or lesser significant to someone else. For example, a clean, neat home means more to some individuals than others.

Value clarification is an approach to "moral education." It is described as a method of self-discovery, allowing individuals to identify their values. It is also allows individuals to act consistently with their values. This then provides a standard of conduct which the individual follows. Values can be obtained from modeling, reward system, punishment, education, and manipulation. Family and peers reinforce values. Professional values are exemplified by various ethical codes and philosophies.

Working on various roles and settings may place nurses in situations that conflict with their moral and ethical value system. An example of this conflict may be seen in the nurse who believes it is her duty to save lives, yet who is caring for a patient who has 'no code' order. This conflict will most likely leave the nurse feeling depressed, guilty or both.

Variations on value system become highly significant when dealing with critical issues such a health and illness or life and death. Value system enable people to resolve conflicts and decide on a course of actions based on a priority of importance. Value systems are not the same as ethical principles. It is not enough to recognize and act on one's values. In addition, one must determine if the value system is ethical. Only after careful reflection concerning how ethical our value systems are can we as nurses take actions based on our personal and professional values.

ii. Dilemmas in Health Care Team

All practicing nurses participates as a members of the health care team. This involves cooperation and collaboration with other professionals. As its true in all situations between human beings, conflicts can easily develop, particularly in stressful circumstances. These conflicts may be between two nurses, the nurse and physician, the nurse and hospital administration, or the nurse and any other health care professional.

Generally, conflicts can evolve because of differing value systems. One nurse may feel that assisting abortions is wrong, whereas institutions performs many abortions daily. Some conflict will develop because of individuals are not respectful of the human rights of other individuals.

Conflicts in human rights often center around one of the ethical principles i.e. justice, autonomy, beneficence, veracity. In some circumstances the ethical dilemma may result from a violation of even more basic human rights, those guaranteed by the constitution.

iii. Conflicts in Patients Rights

In earlier days, health professionals, particularly physicians were considered "all knowing" experts. Very few patients questioned the physician, let alone demanded that basic human rights. Now consumers of health care are increasingly demanding to have a say in matters affecting that health care. As consumers have become more aware of their right, conflicts between health care professionals and institutions have developed. Many of the rights demanded by consumers are their legal as well as moral rights and have been upheld by the judicial system.

Consumer health care is demanding to be allowed to make more decisions about treatment, elective surgery, and medication. They are exercising their rights as outlined in the "Patients Bill of Rights". Especially in the hospital setting, patients are insisting on current information about their condition, prognosis, and treatment; and their right to refuse treatment. Some hospitals are responding to these consumer attitudes by setting up ethics committees to study the type of procedures to be performed or to be discontinued and to determine whether particular patients should or should not receive treatment.

Many of the rights have identified, but some of them were discussed as given below.

Right to Truth

The right of patients to know the truth about their condition, prognosis, and treatment in an issue between the physician and the patient. The current trend is toward more frankness on the part of the physicians. In the past, the moral obligation to disclose the truth – because the patient has the right to know and adjust to it – was often overcome by the professional need to protect the patient from the potential physical or emotional harm that could be caused by knowledge of a critical or terminal condition. In some cases, the professional could not deal with the truths, and therefore, avoided discussion of the situation with the patient.

Because of their extended contact with patients, nurse often find it difficult to accept a physicians decision not to tell a patient the truth about his or her condition. Because of the conflict between physicians decisions and nurses personal feelings it may be advisable for the health care team to meet in order to resolve the problem and to devise a consistent approach to the patient.

Right to Refuse Treatment

For religious reasons or reasons that are sometimes know only to themselves, patient may refuse treatment even though lack of treatment may result in their death. The question of refusal of treatment may have to be decided in court. Many times, the courts rule that patient cannot be forced to accept treatment. On the case of a minor child, however, that courts are likely to rule that parents cannot withhold treatment from a child for any reason. The child is usually made a temporary word of the court and treatment is allowed to begin.

A patient's decision to die rather than to accept treatment may be difficult for a nurse to understand. Nurses must recognize a patient's right to individual and personal attitudes and beliefs, however, and must not allow personal feelings to interfere with patient care. If nurses cannot reconcile that ethical values with those of a patient, they should ask to be taken off the care in the interest of the patient, or they should obtain assistance in coping with the situation.

Informed Consent

The issue of informed consent applies to many health care situations in both legal and ethical ways. Patients have the right to be given accurate and sufficient information about procedure both major and minor, so that their consent undergo those procedures is based on realistic expectations.

Although the responsibility for imparting information about major surgery or complicated medical procedures lies with medical professionals, nurses should inform their patients, in terms of procedures before the procedures are started.

In obtaining legal consent, cairts have generally ruled that consent requires three elements—capacity, information, and voluntariness. Determination of a patients capacity involves consideration of the persons age and his or her competence (the mental ability to understand the effects of his or her choices). The information that is provided to the individual must be understandable by that patient. The information given must include the following elements in order to be considered "informed":

- An explanation of the procedure(s), to be done.
- An explanation of the anticipated results of the procedure(s).
- A description of risks and discomforts.
- An anticipated benefits of the procedure.
- Identification of alternatives.
- An opportunity for questions (and answers).
- The opportunity to withdraw consent at any time.

The patients consent must be given voluntarily, without coercion of prior, written, informed consent to perform a procedure is not obtained, legal action or disciplinary action can involve nurses and other health care professionals. Individuals providing treatment without consent may be liable for assault, battery or negligence.

Since nurses spend considerable periods of time with patients, they are likely to be most aware of their patients questions and concerns. Many times, these concerns should be brought to the attention of attending physicians who, because they see the patients less frequently, may be unaware of the problems. An ethical dilemma occurs when nurses are aware that all aspects of informed consent have not been followed. They are thus faced with the question of what action to take.

Human Experimentation

Research and human experimentation are primarily concerns of the scientific and medical professions. However if nursing care is required for the subjects involved in such experimental project, then nurses become involved. In these cases, nurses responsibilities and ethical decisions are related to making sure that informed consent is given for participation in the research experiments and that the safety of their patients is protected.

Nurses have a responsibility to take action to safeguard patients/clients when care and safety are affected by the incompetent, unethical, or illegal conduct of any person. Further that nurses are to participate in research activities only when they are assured that the rights of the individual subjects are protected. The nurses role, long considered to be that of patient advocate, may, in these situations, place them in direct conflict with research staffs and sponsoring agencies as well as human subject research committees.

Behavior Control

The issue of informed consent is critical question in any form of behavior control, the use of drugs or psychosurgeon further complicate a highly complex topic.

Controversy persists over the right of society to decide what is or is not desirable or acceptable behavior. The issue involves both personal and public behavior. Moreover, it also concerns whether individuals have the right to decide for themselves what is suitable personal behavior, or whether others can decide for them based on some other concept of suitable personal behavior.

In this regard, one of the ethical questions that may be confronted by nurses involves informed consent for treatments that are intended to control behavior. Nurses may question whether individuals who are candidates for drug therapy or psychosurgery are able and competent to give informed consent, and whether these patients, too, have the right to refuse treatments.

Confidentiality

Patients often confide matters of personal concern or highly personal information to nurses, trusting them not to divulge the information carelessly. Nurses must learn to weigh the relevance of such information against the current clinical condition of the patient before revealing any data to physician or co-workers. In order to maintain open communication, nurses may wish to inform patients that confidentiality may not be possible if the information will harm either the patient or other individuals.

The nurses of the specific patient, should never be used when writing nursing care plans or presenting care studies except when these care plans or studies are recorded directly in the patient's chart and are used as a basis for ongoing patient care. Instead, patients should be referred to by their initials to conceal identity in the event that the document is lost and falls into wrong hands. Details of a patients history or status should not be discussed in elevators or cafeterias, or in any other public places. Discussing a patient merely for the sake of gossip is highly unethical and unprofessional. Indiscriminate use of confidential information is also unethical, however, there are times when certain details of patients history may be shared discretely for medical or educational purposes.

Right to Treatment

Health organization identifies the basic rights and responsibilities of patients, in which key patient right to access to care. It is generally held that all patients must be treated with an accepting attitude on the part of the nurses or other health care professionals, regardless of the circumstances causing their health problems. Health professional, must be non-judgmental in their decision making.

In terms of these ethical standards, many health care providers, including nurses find themselves in an ethical dilemma when confronted with the unknown. Recently, this type of ethical conflict has been most prevalent in the care of patient with AIDS. Health care workers providing care to these patients have had to weight that risk of exposure to the disease against that ethical obligation to provide care to their patients. Other ethical conflicts may arise in caring for patients undergoing abortions, providing contraception to teens, participating in organ transplant procedures and a multitude of other situations.

It is important that nurses recognize conflicts between their personal feelings and their professional ethical (and sometime legal) duties. After determining these personal philosophy of nursing, areas of potential ethical conflicts, and the needs of the patient, the nurse must decide what action(s) to take. Sometimes the answers brings the nurse into conflict with other health care professionals. There is not always a correct or best response.

Nurses experience ethical dilemmas when conflicts between policies of their employing institution and themselves controversial health care policies at local, state, or national level can also interfere with the nurses ability to implement care safely and effectively.

In recent years, grave concerns over health care have centered around the cost of care. The rising cost of health care over the past quarter century is a matter that has prompted worry for individuals, groups, and communities as well as government officials. All health care agencies stressing cost containments measures in order to survive. At time, cost containments policies conflict with nurses, value system, whose goal is to provide high-quality, individualized patients care.

Other institutions and societal concerns care result in ethical dilemmas for the nurse whose personal value system does not support the policies set forth by those in authority. Examples include policies concerning access to health care for the elderly, children, and persons with AIDS.

Ethics committees have been/have to be created to deal with the ethical dilemmas in institutional setting.

Bioethical Issues

Bioethics relates specifically to those ethical issues that are raised because of new technologic developments in medicine and biological sciences, applied ethics, or practical ethics, has been an emphasis of bioethical studies since early times, but its importance has increased since the mid-1960s because of the rapid increase in technologic advances.

Nurses and other health care providers seem to be primarily involved with the many ethical issues related to the extremes of the lifespan—birth to death. Other issues that confront nurses are those matters related to life-supporting measures and to the rights of patients. Ethical issues may also be classified according to following categories:

* Inequality
* Environmental
* Obligations to future generations and
* War and peace.

Ethical issues related to birth involve processes that prevent conception or terminate pregnancy prematurely, as well as processes that enable conception and pregnancy to occur through technological intervention rather than through normal developments. Sterilization, contraception, and abortion on the one hand and 'test tube' conception, and artificial insemination on the other, evoke strong feelings from various groups and individuals. Each of these issues has its own ethical ramifications, risks and consequences which must be weighed against the desired outcome. In addition some other bioethical issues are sexually active children (may promote pregnancy or STDs). In

Vitro Fertilization (test-tube conception), surrogate motherhood (due to test-tube conception, artificial insemination and frozen embryos), artificial insemination, genetic research, fetal abuse, fetal surgery, and fetal research.

Ethical issues related to life or death—with the invention of life-saving apparatus, such as the kidney dialysis unit, artificial respirator, heart and lung machine, and fetal monitor, and with the development of new surgical procedures, and new technology, it has become necessary to redefine the terms of life and death, both medically and legally. Many court cases have been generated as a result of decision either to 'pull the plug' of life-sustaining machine or to maintain life support systems in seemingly helpless cases. Likewise, difficult decisions must be made where there are more patients who need kidney dialysis than there are machines to treat them – essentially a decision about who will live and who will die.

Discovery of organ transplantation is another bioethical issues, which conflict of interest between potential donor and recipients.

Other ethical issues, that nurse will come across are euthanasia. Ethical decision involving patients with AIDS. Testing for drug use, drug testing and safety, availability of health care, extra-ordinary care, etc.

As new technology emerges, new issues will arise, and nurses must be prepared to confront them with both changing technical skills and a value system that adapts to the demands of society. Nurses have traditionally met this challenge with renewed dedication to provision of quality of health care.

Sources of Ethical Problems for Nurses

Several factors contribute to the frequency of nurses' ethical problems, including societal factors, the nature of nursing job, and the nature of' the nursing profession itself.

i. Societal Factors

Societal factors that give rise to ethical problems include increased consumer awareness, technological advances, transition from a homogeneous to a multicultural society, and efforts at cost containment in health care.

- *Increased consumer awareness*: Now the health care system operated in a very paternalistic manner. Sick people sought the advice of a physician and then usually followed the physician's orders without question. Partly as a result of increased consumer awareness, professionals now are expected to share knowledge with patients and to obtain truly informed consent for treatments.
- *Technological advances:* With every new technology, new issues arise. For example, techniques of *in vitro* fertilization and embryo transfer have brought about questions of what should be done with embryos that are not implanted into a uterus. Can they be disposed of? What is their status as persons? Other ethical questions surround organ transplants, amniocentesis capable of revealing fetal defects, genetic engineering, cryogenics, and technical advances that allow

loved ones to be maintained on life support beyond what anyone might have imagined earlier.

- *Multicultural population:* In the not too distant past, it was safe to assume that your value and beliefs would be fairly consistent with those of your patients; we had a fairly homogeneous society with a shared value system. We now live in a multi-cultural, multi-faith society, and that assumption is no longer valid. You will work with patients and colleagues from a variety of cultural backgrounds, who probably hold very different sets of values. You will need to respect a variety of belief systems, and you will need to serve as a patient advocate even when the patient's value system is very different from your own.
- *Cost containment:* The emphasis on cutting healthcare costs creates many morally questionable situations. For example, patients are being sent home from the hospital while they are still very ill. On being discharged, they discover that insurance payments are limited for services outside the hospital, including specialists, home care, and medical supplies (e.g. bandages, walkers).

Cost containment efforts and the nursing shortage have led healthcare agencies to increase the number of patients each nurse is expected to care for. As a nurse, you will undoubtedly find yourself in situation where fewer nurses are available than patient acuity requires. You will have to make personal decisions about how far you will stretch your own resources.

ii. The Nature of Nursing Job

The nature of moral problems in nursing is that they are immediate, serious, and frequent. In the classroom, you have the luxury to leave questions unsettled. In the real world, you must always decide: Either you take action, or you do not. But for a nurse, deciding *not* to act is, in effect, an act. For example, suppose the family wishes a patient to have aggressive Code Blue (resuscitation) efforts; however, you know the patient does not wish to be "coded." When the patient dies, whether or not you know the "right" thing to do, you must decide immediately to carry out or not carry out the Code Blue. If you wait too long to ponder the ethical issues, it may be too late to carry it out. If you do not decide, the effect is the same as though you had decided *not* to code.

The nurse's unique position in healthcare organizations also creates problems. Nurses have multiple obligations and relationships, and sometimes conflicting loyalties. Nurses are employees (with a relationship with the agency) as well as professionals (with a special relationship with patients). In addition, they have peer relationships and a unique relationship with physicians. Although nurses are usually not employed by a physician, they are expected to follow physician orders regarding patient care. Additionally, in most organizations, physicians are higher on the power and status hierarchy than are nurses. Ethical questions arise when nurses experience conflicts among their loyalties to patients, families, physicians, employers, and other nurses. Consider the following example: A patient wants to know his test results; the physician is reluctant to tell him. What me the conflicting loyalties? Should the nurse give the patient the information or not?

1. *Tell:* The nurse could honor the principle of personal autonomy and her obligation to the patient by telling him his test results. But this might harm the patient's relationship with the physician, which is important to the patient's wellbeing. Furthermore, if the nurse tells the patient his test results, it may create problems between the physician and the employer (e.g. the hospital). Additionally, this action may in some instances violate hospital policies and therefore harm the nurse's relationship with the hospital. It will certainly affect her relationship with the physician.

2. *Don't tell:* The nurse could preserve the patient-physician relationship by withholding the test results from the patient. This choice does not honor her relationship with the patient. Also, if the nurse does not tell the patient his test results, the patient may find out anyway and be angry with the hospital, the physician, and the nurse.

According to professional ethics, your first allegiance is to the patient. However, the patient's needs often conflict with institutional policies, family desires, or even laws of the state. There may also be conflicts in your relationships with the patient and his family. You can see an example of this in the "Meet Your Patient" scenario, wherein the nurse finds it impossible to honor the parents' autonomy and at the same time advocate for Alan. You may also encounter this type of conflict when a patient does not want any heroic measures and wishes only to die peacefully, but the family has not yet been able to accept the imminent death and are insisting on full resuscitation.

iii. The Nature of the Nursing Profession

Some ethical problems arise because of value conflicts and a lack of clarity within the nursing profession. We have unresolved questions about the nature, scope, and goals of our practice, as well as our professional values. Notice the conflicts of values in the following items:

- Nursing values caring, humanistic care, and nurse-patient relationships–however, nurses now spend less time at the bedside (with patients) than ever before. One reason is the nursing shortage and heavier patient loads, but there are other factors: the use of technology, the need for careful documentation, and the emphasis on leading, managing, and delegation instead of hands-on care.
- On one hand, we believe nurses should have autonomy and equal status with other healthcare professionals–on the other hand, many nurses want to escape hard choices by "letting the doctor decide."
- Most nurses believe we deserve higher pay–yet, claim nurses are cost-effective because we w more cheaply than physicians.
- On one hand, we claim the nurse is a professional, citing critical thinking, knowledge, and management skills—on the other hand, we emphasize caring, with the nurse at the bedside offering comfort and doing hands-on tasks.

In most of those examples, we value both of the opposites. We would not wish to give up either one. But specific situations require us to choose between them, and that is one source of our discomfort.

By now you should have an idea of the nature morals and ethics and of the need to study nursing ethics. We turn our focus now to some basic theoretical knowledge about factors that are involved in making moral decisions: values, ethical principles, moral frameworks, and professional guidelines.

Application of Ethical Principles in Nursing

Ethical principles actually control professionalism nursing practice much more than to ethical theories. Principles encompass basic promises from which rules are developed. Principles are the moral norms that nursing, as a profession, both demands and strives to implement to every day clinical practice. Ethical principle that the nurse should consider when making decisions are as follows:

- Respect for persons
- Respect for autonomy
- Respect for freedom
- Respect for Beneficence (doing good)
- Respect for nonmaleficence (avoiding harm to others)
- Respect for veracity (truth telling)
- Respect for justice (fair and equal treatment)
- Respect for rights
- Respect for fidelity (fulfilling promises)
- Confidentiality (protecting privileged information).

Respect for Persons

Respect for persons not only applies to clinical situations, but also to all life's situations. It directs individuals to treat themselves and other, with a respect inherent to man's humanness. It requires recognition on a sense that all mankind shared a common human destiny. The respect to persons needs to be simplified as it affects nursing practice.

Autonomy

Autonomy that individuals are able to act for themselves to the level of their capacity. It is the right of individual to govern their actions according to their own purpose and reason. Respect for autonomy requires that persons honor another's right to govern himself or herself. The legal doctrine of informed consent is the direct reflection of autonomy. So it requires, that health personnel obtains a patient's informed consent for treatment and for participation in research. The followings are required for a patient to give informed consent for either:

Disclosure: Adequate presentation of relevant information about the proposed treatment or study.

Understanding: Adequate comprehension of the disclosed information.

Voluntary agreement: Free assent, influenced by external controlling factors.

Competence: Adequate decision making capacity. There are three type of autonomy, i.e. freedom of action, freedom of choice and effective deliberation.

Freedom

The principle of individual freedom decrease that patients be exempt from control by others to select and pursue personal health goals. Nurses as a group believe that patient should have greater freedom of choice within the nations healthcare system. This principle should be observed by staff nurses when planning patient care; by nurse manager when leading subordinates.

Beneficence

The beneficence principle states that the actions one takes should promote good. It dictates that a person is obliged to help others to advance their legitimate and important interests. It requires the balancing of harms and benefits. Benefits promotes the clients' welfare and health, whereas harms or risks detract from the clients health and welfare. In other words, providing benefits that enhance the others welfare. Whereas balancing the benefits and harms of intervention made on the others behalf.

Professional education provides an awareness that most nursing interventions are capable of producing undesirable, as well as desirable, patient outcome. Therefore the nurse is obliged to ascertain each care measure, likelihood of success, and balance the measures probable benefits and risks in order to select interventions that maximize patients welfare.

Nonmaleficence

The corollary of beneficence, the principle of nonmaleficence' states that one should do no harm. The nurse should interpret the term 'harm' to mean emotional and social as well as physical injury. Harm is thwarting, defeating, or setting back one person's interest through invasive action by another. Many nurses find it difficult to follow the principle when performing treatment and procedures that bring discomfort and pain to patients. When the principle of sanctity of human life guides healthcare decisions, the principle of nonmaleficence prohibits active and passive enthusive by caregivers of terminally ill patients.

As nurse manager performing performance evaluation of subordinates should emphasize their good qualities and give positive direction for growth. Destroying the employees' self esteem and self worth would be considered doing harm their principles.

Veracity

Veracity concerns truth telling an incorporates the concept that individuals should always tell the truth. It requires professional caregivers to provide with accurate, reality-based information about their health status and care or treatment prospect. Truth telling is an ethical concern for nurse, because truth is the basis for mutual trust between patient and nurse, and trust is the basis for patient's hope of benefit from nursing services. Nurse managers use this principle when they give all the facts of a situation, truthfully and assist their employees to make decisions. However, truth telling may be difficult in a healthcare relationship. Some information that is transmitted from nurse to patient is depressing and/ or frightening, e.g. bad news about personal health status.

Justice

Justice concerns the issue that persons should be treated equally and fairly. This principle of justice requires treating others fairly and giving persons their due. When there are resources to distribute in healthcare, nurses should allocate them in such a way that equal shares go to equal recipients. The following problems complicate the application of justice:

- Not everyone is equal in every way, sometimes there are situations in which it seems that one person should receive a greater or lesser share than another.
- Resources are limited. There is not always enough for each persons to receive an equal share.

Questions of justice relate to the fairness with which benefits and burdens are distributed among people. Experience in turn found various principles have to be proposed to guide fair distribution of society's good are as follows:

- Each person should receive an equal share.
- The amount given to each person should be proportional to his or her need.
- The amount given to each person should be proportional to the amount of his or her work effort.
- The amount given to each person should reflect the value of his or her work product.
- The amount given to each person should reflect his to her value to society.
- The amount given to each person should be determined by free market exchange.

These principles usually arise in times of short supplies or when there is competition for resources of benefits.

Rights

Right is an entitlement to behave in certain way under circumstances, such as nurses entitlement to freely express personal beliefs and preferences by voting in a political election. Another right is the prerogative to define another's behavior in selected situations, such as managers prerogative to give assignments to subordinates. A right is also a claim to a specific good, service or prerequisite such as tea break time. Right is also used to mean agreement with justice, law and morality. So right may be mental rights or legal rights related to respective profession.

- The patient has the right to every consideration of his privacy concerning his own medical care program.

- The patient has the right to expect that all communications and records pertaining to his care should be treated as confidential.
- The patient has the right to expect that within its capacity a hospital must make reasonable response to the request of a patient for services.
- The patient has the right to obtain information as to any relationship of his hospital to other healthcare and educational institutions in so far as his care is concerned and any professional relationships among individuals, by name, who are treating him.
- The patient has the right to be advised if the hospital proposes to engage in or perform human experimentation affecting his care or treatment (and) has the right to refuse to participate.
- The patient has the right to expect reasonable continuity of care.
- The patient has the right to examine and receive an explanation of his bill regardless of source of payment.
- The patient has the right to know what hospital rules and regulations apply to his conduct as a patient.

Fidelity

Fidelity is keeping one's promises or commitments. The principle of fidelity holds that a person should faithfully fulfill his duties and obligations. Fidelity is important in a nurse because a patient's hope for relief and recovery rests on evidence of caregivers conscientiousness. Nurse managers abide by this principle when they follow through on any promise they have previously made to employees, such as promised leave, a certain shift to be worked or a promotion to perception within the unit.

Confidentiality

Confidentiality is the duty to respect privileged information. The principle of confidentiality provides that caregivers should respect a patient need for privacy and use personal information about him or her only to improve care. Nurses should practice confidentiality to decrease patient vulnerability and share from widespread knowledge of personal information divulged during care.

Nursing Codes of Ethics

Professional codes of ethics are formal statements of a group's expectations and standards for professional behavior generally accepted by members of the profession. Codes of ethics set forth ideal behaviors and, of course, are only as effective as the behaviors of the members of the profession who live up to the codes. The purposes of a nursing code of ethics are to:

- Inform the public about the profession's minimum standards
- Demonstrate nursing's commitment to the public it serves
- Outline major ethical considerations of nursing
- Provide general guidelines for professional behavior
- Guide the profession's self-regulating functions

- Remind us of the special responsibility we assume in caring for the sick.

Codes of ethics are open to public scrutiny. Therefore, others may observe and judge your professional behavior. The ethical aspects of your work, just as the technical aspects, are subject to review by professional groups and licensure boards, who may use sanctions to punish code violations. Nursing codes are not legally binding. However, codes often exceed legal obligations. In most states, the state board of nursing uses the nursing code of ethics as the standard against which to evaluate a nurse's ethical behavior. The board has the legal authority to censure or reprimand the nurse who does not practice within the boundaries of ethical practice.

Three nursing organizations have had longstanding codes to guide nurses' ethical decision making. The codes differ in specific details, but they are based on similar principles.

Code of Ethics

International Council of Nurses

The International Council of Nurses (lCN) first adopted its Code of Ethics for Nurses in 1953 as "a guide for action based on social values and needs" (lCN, 2000). It was revised in 2000. The Code has served as the standard for nurses worldwide since it was first adopted. The ICN Code stresses respect for human rights, including the right to life, right to dignity, and right to be treated with respect. The code is designed as a guide for nurses in everyday choices, and it supports their refusal to participate in activities that conflict with caring and healing.

Within any given profession, a code of ethics serves as a means of self-regulation and a source of guidelines for individual behavior and responsibility. Professional codes of ethics are a system of rules and principles by which that profession is expected to regulate its members and demonstrate its responsibility to society. In India, nurses are following the International Council of Nurses Codes for 1993 as given below:

- The fundamental responsibility of the nurse is four-fold, i.e. to promote health, to prevent illness, to restore health, to prevent illness, to restore health, and to alleviate suffering.
- The need for nursing is universal, inherent in nursing is respect for life, dignity and rights of man. It is unrestricted by consideration of nationality, race, creed, color, age, sex, politics or social status.
- Nurses render health services to the individual, the family, and the community and coordinate their services with those of related group.

Nurses and People

- The nurses primary responsibility is to those people who require nursing care.

- The nurse in providing care, promotes an environment in which the values, customs and spiritual beliefs of the individual are respected.
- The nurse holds confidence personal information and uses judgment in sharing their information.

Nurses and Practice

- The nurse carries personal responsibility for nursing practice and for maintaining competence by continual learning. The nurse maintains the higher standards of nursing care possible within the reality of a specific situations.
- The nurse uses judgment in relation to individual competence when accepting and delegating responsibilities.
- The nurse when acting in a professional capacity should at all times maintain standards of personal conduct which reflects credit upon the profession.

Nurses and Society

The nurse shares with other citizens the responsibility for initiating and supporting action to meet the health and social needs of the public.

Nurses and Coworker

- The nurse sustains a cooperative relationship with coworkers in nursing and other fields.
- The nurse takes appropriate action to safeguard the individual when his care endangered by a coworker or any other person.

Nurses and Profession

- The nurse plays the major role in determining and implementing desirable standards of nursing practice and nursing education.
- The nurse is active in developing a care of professional knowledge.
- The nurse acting through the professional organization, participates in establishing and maintaining equitable social and economic working conditions in nursing.

The **Florence Nightingale pledge**, prepared by Gretter included the basic principles governing ethical practices as given below:

I solemnly pledge myself before God and in the presence of assembly; to pass my life in purity and to practices my profession faithfully;

I will abstain from whatever is determines as mischievous and will not take or knowingly administer any harmful drug;

I will do all in my power to maintain and elevate the standard of my profession; and will hold in confidence all personal matters committed to my knowledge in the practice of my calling;

With loyalty I will endeavour to aid physician in the work, and devote myself to the welfare of those committed to my care.

American Nurses Association Code of Ethics for Nurses

1. The nurse, in all professional relationships, practices with compassion and respect for the inherent dignity, worth, and uniqueness of every individual, unrestricted by considerations of social or economic status, personal attributes, or the nature of health problems.
2. The nurse's primary commitment is to the patient, whether an individual, family, group or community.
3. The nurse promotes, advocates for and strives to protect the health, safety and rights of the patient.
4. The nurse is responsible and accountable for individual nursing practice and determines the appropriate delegation of tasks consistent with the nurse's obligation to provide optimum patient care.
5. The nurse owes the same duties to self as to others, including the responsibility to preserve integrity and safety, to maintain competence and to continue personal and professional growth.
6. The nurse participates in establishing, maintaining and improving health care environments and conditions of employment conducive to the provision of quality health care and consistent with the values of the profession through individual and collective action.
7. The nurse participates in the advancement of the profession through contributions to practice, education, administration and knowledge development.
8. The nurse collaborates with other health professionals and the public in promoting community, national and international efforts to meet health needs.
9. The profession of nursing, as represented by associations and their members, is responsible for articulating nursing values for maintaining the integrity of the profession and its practice, and for shaping social policy.

Nursing is a profession, one of the essential characteristic of profession is that they have a code of ethics. A code of ethics is an implied contract through which the profession informs society of the principles and rules by which it functions. Ethical codes help with professional self-regulation. They serve as guidelines to the members of the profession who there can meet the societal need for trustworthy, qualified, and accountable caregivers. It is important to remember that codes are useful only if they are upheld by the members of the profession.

Nurses are frequently caught in situations in which patients or their families no longer want to continue the kind of existence and health care system not developed adequate legal and decision mechanisms to deal with patients desires. For example, new technologies, such as ventilators, now keep people in comas alive even though the quality of life is no longer what they would have desired. Lifetime savings of families may be wiped out by maintaining a family member in an persistent vegetative state.

In response to the need for guidance on ethical issues, a special task force of the ANA (1985) created document entitled the

"Code for Nurses" to help nurses clarify their responsibilities. The code identifies the nurses professional responsibility to the patient. The code will be revised as new issues arise. ANA code of Ethics (1985) as given below:

1. The nurse provides services with respect for human dignity and the uniqueness of the client unrestricted by considerations of social or economic status, personal attributes, or the nature of health problems.
2. The nurse safeguards the clients right to privacy by judiciously protecting information of a confidential nature.
3. The nurse acts to safeguard the client and the public when health care and safety are affected by the incompetent, unethical, or illegal practice of any person.
4. The nurse assures responsibility and accountability for individual nursing judgments and actions.
5. The nurse maintains competence in nursing.
6. The nurse exercises informed judgment and uses individual competence and qualifications as criterion in seeking consultations, accepting responsibilities, and delegating nursing activities to others.
7. The nurse participates in activities that contribute to the ongoing development of the profession's body of knowledge.
8. The nurse participates in the professions efforts to implement and improve standards of nursing.
9. The nurse participates in the professions efforts to establish and maintain conditions of employment conducive to high quality nursing care.
10. The nurse participates in the professions effort to protect the public from misinformation and misrepresentation and to maintain the integrity of nursing.
11. The nurse collaborates with members of the health professions and other citizens in promoting community and national efforts to meet the health needs of the public.

The International Council of Nurses (ICN) (1973) also has a code of ethics for the profession. This document discusses the rights and responsibilities of nurses around the world.

The ICN first adopted a code of ethics in 1953. Its last revision in 1973 represents agreement by 80 national nursing associations (including India) that participate in the international association. The ICN code identifies four major responsibilities for the nurse—promote health, prevent illness, restore health and alleviate suffering. The ICN code for nurses in nursings respect for the life, dignity, and rights of all people unmindful of nationality, race, creed, color, age, sex, policies or social status.

The ICN has written its own "People for Nurses." If all nurses followed the ICN code and pledge in nursing practice, the quality of nursing care would improve vastly. The public image of the nursing profession would also be enhanced. The ICN is continually studying the ever-changing designation of the nurse, based on the increasing responsibilities being placed on the increasing responsibilities being placed on the nursing profession.

The nurses pledge was written by nurse (Marion G. Howell) in support of her ethical convictions as given below:

I solemnly pledge myself before God and in the presence of this assembly, to faithfully practice my profession of nursing.

I will do all in my power to make and maintain the highest standards and practices of my profession.

I will hold in confidence all personal matters committed to my keeping in the practice of my calling.

I will loyally assist the physician in his work and will devote myself to the welfare of my patients, my families, and my community.

I will endeavor to fulfill my rights and privileges as a good citizen and to take my share of responsibility in promoting the health and welfare of my community.

I will constantly endeavor to increase my knowledge and skills in nursing and to use them wisely.

I will zealously seek to nurse those who are ill wherever they may be and whenever they are in need.

I will be active in assisting others in safeguarding and promoting the health and happiness of mankind.

CNA Code of Ethics (Table 3.1)

This code is organized around the above described eight values. In the code, each value is further described by explanatory responsibility statements based on each value.

In addition to its Code of Ethics, the American Nurses Association (ANA) sets standards for all aspects of clinical, practice. In the newly revised *Nursing: Scope and Standards of Practice* (2004), standard 12 focuses on ethical practice. This standard directs nurses to practice within the parameters described in the Code of Ethics for Nurses. Standard 12 speaks to the nurse's responsibilities to patients and directs nurses to manage ethical dilemmas and to report practices that are illegal, incompetent, or impaired.

The registered nurse integrates ethical provisions in all areas of practice.

The registered nurse:

- Uses the Code of Ethics for Nurses with Interpretive Statements to guide practice.
- Delivers care in a manner that preserves and protects patient autonomy, dignity, and rights.
- Maintains patient confidentiality within legal and regulatory parameters.
- Serves as a patient advocate assisting patients in developing skills for self-advocacy.
- Maintains a therapeutic and professional patient-nurse relationship with appropriate professional role boundaries.
- Demonstrates a commitment to practicing self-care, managing stress and connecting with self and others.
- Contributes to resolving ethical issues of patients, colleagues, or systems as evidenced in such activities as participating on ethics committees.
- Reports illegal, incompetent, or impaired practices.

Table 3.1: Canadian Nurses Association Code of Ethics for Registered Nurses

Safe, competent and ethical care	Nurses value the ability to provide safe, competent and ethical care that allows them to fulfill their ethical and professional obligations to the people they serve.
Health and well-being	Nurses value health promotion and well-being and assisting persons to achieve their optimum level of health in situations of normal health, illness, injury, disability or at the end of life.
Choice	Nurses respect and promote the autonomy of persons and help them express their health needs and values and obtain desired information and services so they can make informed decisions.
Dignity	Nurses recognize and respect the inherent worth of each person and advocate for respectful treatment of all persons.
Confidentiality	Nurses safeguard information learned in the context of a professional relationship and ensure it is shared outside the health care team only with the person's informed consent, or as may be legally required, or where the failure to disclose would cause significant harm.
Justice	Nurses uphold principles of equity and fairness to assist persons in receiving a share of health services and resources proportionate to their needs.
Accountability	Nurses are answerable for their practice, and they act in a manner consistent with their professional responsibilities and standards of practice.
Quality practice environments	Nurses value and advocate for practice environments that have the organizational structures and resources necessary to ensure safety, support and respect for all persons in the work setting.

Patients, when hospitalized, should expect the following:

- High-quality care, including the right to know the identity of caregivers.
- A clean, safe environment, including safety, freedom from abuse and neglect, and discussion of any changes in care.
- Respect for healthcare goals, values, and spiritual beliefs.
- To be involved in making decisions about their care and treatment. This includes receiving information about:
  - Health condition and treatments
  - The benefits and risks of treatments, and whether a treatment is experimental or part of a research study
  - What the patient and family will need to do regarding treatment follow-up after leaving the hospital.
- Information about the right to make decisions and to refuse care, including advance directives and counselors or chaplains available to help with decision making.
- Protection of their privacy and confidentiality.
- Help with the bill and filing insurance claims.
- Preparation and information when leaving the hospital, including:
  - Identification of sources for follow-up care and whether the hospital has a financial interest in any of the referrals
  - Coordination of hospital activities with caregivers outside the hospital
  - Information and training about the self-care the person will need at home.

When clients are admitted to hospitals or to extended care facilities, they are entitled to specific rights in terms of their treatment: the right to make their own decisions, to be active partners in the treatment process, and to be treated with dignity and respect. Because rights are rooted in values, and because values are derived from culture, patient rights are different throughout the world. Now *Bill of Rights* replaced with a document called *Patient Care Partnership*. Instead of using "rights" language, this document is written in terms of patient expectations and responsibilities.

The *Patient Care Partnership* encourages healthcare providers to be more aware of the need to treat patients in an ethical manner and to protect client rights.

Nurses are likely to encounter several ethical issues that occur in healthcare. For example, ethical questions arise in the following situations:

- Acquired immune deficiency syndrome (AIDS)
- Abortion
- Allocation of healthcare goods and services
- Confidentiality and privacy (e.g. reporting gunshot wounds and child abuse)
- Honoring advance directives
- Do Not Attempt Resuscitation (DNAR) orders
- Assisted suicide and euthanasia
- Using extraordinary (heroic) measures to prolong life
- Withdrawing or withholding life-sustaining treatments (e.g. ventilators, artificial nutrition and hydration)
- Informed consent
- Organ transplantation
- Reproductive technology (e.g. *in vitro* fertilization, surrogate mothering, sex preselection).

Ethical Decision-making in Nursing

Society is rapidly changing its attitudes about major ethical issues. These changes have a direct effect on nursing practice. Nurses in many instances are faced with providing nursing care in situations which contradict their own personal values.

Changing social values and attitudes impact in various areas of concern to nurses and on the decisions they have to make. New emphasis on equal rights and individual rights brings-up issues such as changes in the role of women, marriage, family and minorities; changes in health care emphasis from episodic to prevent care; and an expanded role for patients/clients in making informed decisions about their own care, treatments, and about their right to die with dignity, changing social attitudes about birth control, sterilization, abortion (MTP), and the possibility of genetic manipulation raise issues concerning the right to life and the value of human life.

Nurses encounter situations daily that require them to make professional judgments and act on those judgments. The judgments or decisions are often made in conjunction with other persons involved in the situations: patients, families and other health care professionals. Whether involved in a collective or individual decision, nurses need to be knowledgeable about the steps in ethical decision making.

Having to make decisions on ethical issues is a contributing factor to stress in nurses work. These ethical decisions are unavoidable in nursing practice. Societal factors that bring about changes in social values which are in conflict with the individual nurses values may cause further stress. This is especially true when these changes cause conflict between nurses and hospital administrators or physicians with regard to ethical decisions. Nurses should be aware of the resources available to assist them in making such decisions.

Decision-making Models

These are various models to assist in ethical decision making have been developed and published in professional publications. The most commonly cited models include those of Rebecca Bergman, Irma Goertzen, and Joyce, Henry Thompson, and Silva.

- **Rebecca Bergman** has developed a complex process of dealing with complex ethical issues. It is a pattern which is closely related to the steps of the nursing process. The steps include:
  - Presentation of the situation.
  - Gathering of facts.
  - Classifications of situation reconstruction, bringing to bear, knowledge and philosophy.
  - Alternative decisions.
  - Actions.
  - Evaluation, and
  - Generalization for future use.
- **Irman Goertzen** also has identified several steps for ethical decisions making.
  - Define the problem.
  - Identify the objective to be achieved.
  - List all alternatives to meet the objectives.
  - Evaluate each alternative.
  - Choose the best alternative and
  - Evaluate the results.

- **Thompson and Thompson (1985)** identified ten steps necessary for making ethical decisions, which include:
  - Review the situation to determine health problems, decision needed, ethical components, and key individuals.
  - Gather additional information.
  - Identify the ethical issues in the situation.
  - Identify personal and professional values.
  - Identify the values of key individuals.
  - Identify any existing value conflicts.
  - Determine who should decide.
  - Identify the range of actions and anticipated outcomes.
  - Decide on a course of action and carry it out.
  - Evaluate the results.
- **Silva (1990)** draw from components of several ethical decision making frameworks to present a five part model.

(i) Data collection and assessment
  - (a) Situational consideration
  - (b) Health team consideration
  - (c) Organizational consideration.

Collection and assessment of data related to an ethical dilemma are integrate to the decision-making process. In regard to steps 'A' situational consideration, one must determine if situation is an ethical dilemma or another type of dilemma considering health team consideration, it is important to determine what persons will be affected by the decision and how they will be affected. Regarding organizational consideration, one must identify how the organizations particularly its procedures and policies may affect the resolution of an ethical dilemma.

(ii) Problem identification
  - (a) Ethical consideration
  - (b) Non-ethical consideration.

A clear understanding of the ethical problem in crucial to resolving a dilemma. Both ethical and non-ethical considerations must be identified. In the nurses professional role, the code for nurses (ANA) clearly outlines the nurses first priority as the patients.

(iii) Consideration of possible actions
  - (a) Utilitarian thinking
  - (b) Deontological thinking.

Once the ethical problem is identified, possible actions must be considered. Serious consideration should only be given to those actions that are reasonable to implement.

(iv) Decision and selection of course of actions
  - (a) Contribution of internal/group factors
  - (b) Contribution of external factors
  - (c) Quality of decision and course of action.

It is not time to make a decision. Both internal (people-related) and external (legal, institutional and social) factors should be considered.

(v) Reflection on decision and course of action
  - (a) Reflection on decision
  - (b) Reflection on course of action.

After a decision is implemented, the result must be evaluated for its effectiveness. If the action accomplished its purposes resolution of the ethical dilemma will presumably have occurred. If the dilemma is not resolved additional problem-solving approaches will need to be implemented.

Decision models used in bioethics do not offer pat, easily arrived at decisions, but they do provide a guiding structure to follow to arrive at the best answer in specific situations. Decision models can help you decide on a course of action even if they do not tell you absolutely that the action is right or wrong.

Nurses decisions are increasingly constrained by ethical issues. Ethical decision making involves reflection on the following:

- Who should make the choice
- Possible options or courses of action
- Available options
- Consequences, both good or bad, of all possible options
- Rules, obligations and values that should direct choices, and
- Desired outcomes.

When making decisions, nurses need to combine all of these elements using an orderly, systematic, and objective method. There are various models for ethical decision making. Perhaps the easiest ethical decision making model to remember and to implement in practice is the" moral model" developed by Thirona and Halloraw as follows:

M – *Massage the dilemma:* Identify and define the issues in the dilemma. Consider the opinions of all major players in the dilemma as well as their value system. This includes patients family members, nurses, doctors, priest and any other interdisciplinary healthcare team member.

O – *Outline the options:* Examine all options including those less realistic and conflicting. This stage is designed only for considering options and not for making final decision.

R – *Resolve the dilemma:* Review the issues and options, applying the basic principles of ethics to each option. Decide the best option based upon the views of all those concerned in the dilemma.

A – *Act by applying chosen action:* This step is usually the most difficult as it requires actual implementation. While the previous steps had only allowed for dialogue or discussion.

L – *Look back and evaluate the entire process including the implementation:* No process is complete without a through evaluation. Ensure that those involved are able to follow through on the final option. If not, a second decision may be required and process must start again at the initial step.

Another exchanges of traditional model of ethical decision making are as follows:

1. Identify the problem.
2. Gather data to analyze the causes and consequence of the problem.
3. Explore the optional solutions to the problem.
4. Evaluate the optional solution.
5. Select the appropriate solution from all the options.
6. Implement the selected solution.
7. Evaluate the result.

Ethical Responsibility in Caring

1. Caring demands the provision of helping services that are appropriate to the needs of the client and significant others.
2. Caring recognizes the client's membership in a family and community and provides for the participation of significant others in his or her care.
3. Caring acknowledges the reality of death in the life of every person, and demands that appropriate support the provided for the dying person and family to enable that to prepare for, and to cope with death when it is inevitable.
4. Caring acknowledges that the human person has the capacity to fact up to health needs and problems in his or her own unique way, and directs nursing action in a manner that will assist the client to develop, maintain or gain personal autonomy, self-respect and self-determination.
5. Caring, as a response to a health need, requires the consent and the participation of the person who is experiencing the need.
6. Caring dictates that the client and significant others have the knowledge and information adequate for free and informed decisions concerning care requirements, alternative and preferences.
7. Caring demands that the needs of the client supersede those of the nurse.
8. Caring acknowledges the vulnerability of a client in certain situations, and dictates restraint in actions which might compromise the client's rights and privileges.
9. Caring involving a relationship which is, in itself, therapeutic, demands mutual respect and trust.
10. Caring acknowledges that information obtained in the course of the nursing relationship is privileged, and that is requires the full protection of confidentiality unless such information provides evidence of serious impending harm to the client or to a third party, or is legally required by the courts.
11. Caring requires that the nurse represents the needs of the client and that the nurse takes appropriate measures when fulfillment of these needs is jeopardized by the actions of other persons.
12. Caring acknowledges the dignity of all persons in the practice of educational setting.
13. Caring acknowledges, respects and draws upon the competencies of others.
14. Caring establishes the conditions for the harmonization of efforts of different helping professionals in providing required services to clients.
15. Caring seeks to establish and maintain a climate of respect for the honest dialogue needed for effective collaboration.
16. Caring establishes the legitimacy of respectful challenge and/ or confrontation when the service required by the client is compromised by incompetency, incapacity or negligence or when the competencies of the nurses are not acknowledged or appropriately utilized.

17. Caring demands the provision of working conditions which enable nurses to carry out their legitimate and responsibilities.
18. Caring demands resourcefulness and restraint-accountability for the use of time, resources, equipment, and funds, and requires accountability to appropriate individuals and/or bodies.
19. Caring requires that the nurse bring to the work situation in education, practice, administration or research, the knowledge, affective and technical skills required, and that competency in these areas be maintained and updated.
20. Caring commands fidelity oneself, and guards the right and privilege of the nurse to act in keeping with an informed moral conscience.

Application of Decision-making Models

It would be easy to decide how to apply moral principles and decide what to do. However, it is common in moral situations for one ethical principle to be at odds with another equally important principle, or for a philosophical framework to produce more than one acceptable option. An **ethical dilemma** is a situation in which a choice must be made between two equally undesirable actions. There is no dearly right or wrong option. Such situations are emotionally painful for everyone in the situation.

However not all moral problems are dilemmas. In fact, you will comfort a true dilemma only occasionally. Not all moral problems are complex and difficult. Some questions are easily answered (e.g. "Should I take the patient's morphine to relieve my back pain?") It is probably more accurate, then, to refer to "moral questions," "moral problems," or "moral situations" and not use the term *dilemma* loosely. Only those problems that pose a question between competing and equally valuable interests are true dilemmas.

Once having identified an ethical problem, a decision model will help to think logically about the best action to take, Nonetheless, in the case of a true ethical dilemma will probably not be comfortable with any course of' action, no matter how logically think it through. It is important to be aware of the ethical issues in patient care situations, but how will you recognize them? The key is that there is usually a conflict. Conflict may occur:

* About the right action to take
* Between the duties and obligations of healthcare professionals (or they are unclear)
* Between the needs and interests of an individual and a group of clients
* Between what the family wants and what the client wants or needs
* Between the family and health professionals
* Between ethical principles or values.

There is no easy way to decide which principle should outrank another principle, or which person's values are best in a given situation. For this reason, healthcare institutions have ethics committees. These typically interdisciplinary committees include nurses, doctors, clergy, ethicists, and lay representatives. Ethics committees write guidelines and policies, provide education and counseling, and, in the case of ethical dilemmas, review the case and provide a forum for the expression of the diverse perspectives of those involved.

Ethics committees usually follow one of three distinct models when discussing a dilemma: the autonomy model, the patient benefit model, and the social justice model.

1. The **autonomy model** is useful when the patient is competent to decide. This model emphasizes patient autonomy and choice as the highest value.
2. The **patient benefit model** assists in decision making for the incompetent patient by using substituted judgment (i.e. what the patient would want for herself if she were capable of making these issues known).
3. The **social justice model** focuses more on broad social issues involving the entire institution, rather than on a single patient issue. Such a committee might consider whether, in general, an institution ought ever to seek a legal order to act against the wishes of the parents. Or they might discuss whether supporting parents' religious belief's in this instance might have implications for supporting other types of religious beliefs in future cases.

The following suggestions will helps to be as well prepared as possible when ethical issues arise.

* *Use theoretical knowledge:* Review nursing and other literature for discussion of cases and experiences of other nurses. This will give you a broader view of the problems you may confront and the strategies for managing them. Become familiar with the various codes of ethics and the *Patient Care Partnership,* as well as the moral frameworks and principles.
* *Use self-knowledge:* Examine your personal value system. Explore the influences of your religion, cultural beliefs, and personal experiences. This will help you to recognize your comfort zone with specific ethical issues.
* *Use practical knowledge:* While still a student, you should ask to attend either ethical rounds or an ethics committee meeting. As a graduate nurse, you could benefit by volunteering to sit on your institution's ethics committee or plan to attend nursing ethics rounds to familiarize yourself with the types of ethical problems that occur at your institution.
* *Consult reliable sources:* Attend ethics education programs, and talk about issues with other healthcare providers. Attorneys, ethicists, and members of the clergy can provide helpful perspectives.
* *Share:* Regularly engage in discussions with the staff on your unit to determine differences in value systems and to collaborate proactively to work out methods that can be used to resolve ethical dilemmas effectively. When you are faced with a difficult moral decision, consult with peers, co-workers, and teachers. Seek guidance and support.

• *Evaluate:* After the situation is resolved, evaluate your decision and the effects of your actions. You should be able to learn from even the worst decision. And when everything goes well, you can file your strategies away to use in similar future situations.

Nurses should play a role of advocates is to safeguard clients against abuse and violation of their rights. Why do nurses think this is so important? Why can't patients do this for themselves? The following are some of the reasons.

1. *Nurses have special knowledge that the patient does not have:* Diseases, treatments, and the healthcare system are so complex that when clients become ill, they may not have the energy to deal with the complexity, even if they do have the necessary knowledge. Nurse may need to help them to "jump through all the necessary hoops" to get what they need. When patients' rights are denied or when patients do not have the ability to exert their rights, nurses have a responsibility to step in. "Without the advocacy and protection of rights there really are no rights."

2. *One aspects of nurses professional role to defend patients' autonomous decisions:* Ethics requires nurses to be a patient advocate. As a nurse, you will he called on to defend your patient's autonomous decisions even if you do not agree with them and even if they conflict with the opinions of others involved in the patient's care. You may find yourself the sole champion of a patient's right to choose for himself the direction of his care.

3. *Nurses have a special relationship with patients:* Nurses may find that they are able to acquire information about a client that is not available to professionals of other disciplines. In general, nurses interact with patients over longer time intervals and are involved in very intimate activities, especially in inpatient settings. They often become the most trusted caregivers. Details about family life, coping styles, personal preferences, fears, and insecurities are all more likely to come out over the time involved in nursing interventions than in the brief minutes of interaction when the physician makes rounds. Additionally, patients may perceive less social distance between themselves and the nurse and, therefore, feel more free to confide in them. The nurses' point of view can be a valuable asset to resolving an ethical problem satisfactorily. Of course, many physicians have long-standing relationships with their patients; however, this does not negate the importance of the nurse's input, which may provide a different perspective.

Nurses role as an advocate is to inform, support, and communicate. Nurse should inform clients of their rights and provide the information they need to make informed decisions, if they are capable of doing so. Then nurse must remain objective and support them in the decisions they make, even when they believe it to be wrong. If others are not respecting client choices, nurse will need to intervene on the client's behalf. This may simply be a matter of conveying information and clarifying the client's wishes to family or healthcare professionals (e.g. "I know how hard it is for you to let him go, but Mr. Sharat says he has made peace and is ready to die. His treatments make him feel even more ill, and he simply does not want to fight anymore.") Advocacy may require you to arrange for the client to consult with clergy or an attorney for advice and support or may require you to consult an institutional ethics committee.

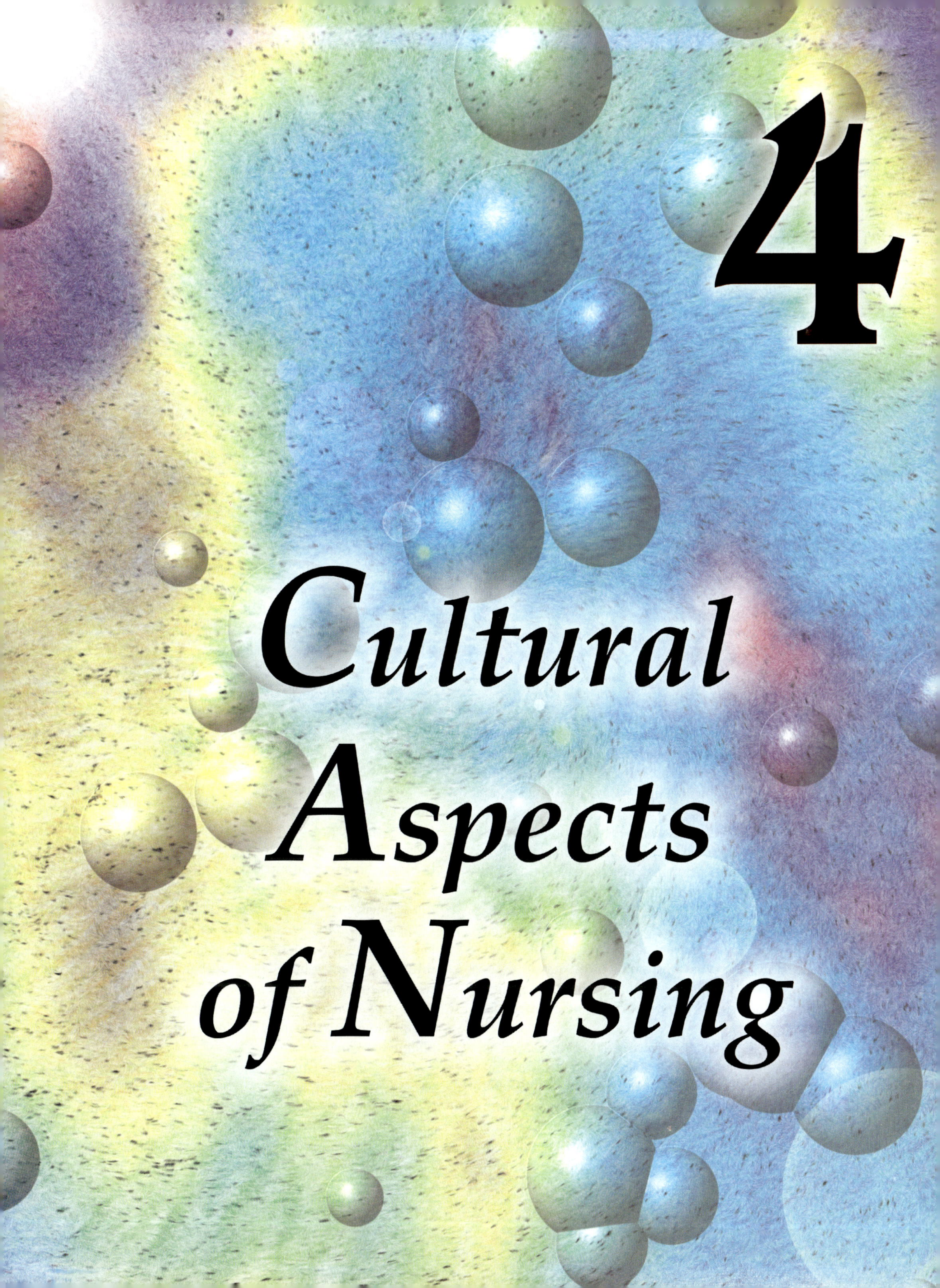

4
Cultural Aspects of Nursing

Culture represents nonphysical fruits, such as values, beliefs, attitudes and customs, shared by a group of people and passed from one generation to the next generation. It is also the some beliefs, practices, habits, likes, dislikes, norms, customs, and rituals learned from the family during the years of socialization. Many people's beliefs, thoughts and actions, both conscious and unconscious, are determined by their cultural background.

Providing care to a culturally diverse population has become a challenge for nurses. Nursing care that is appropriate for the dominant cultural group may be ineffective and inappropriate for people with a different cultural heritage.

Of course it is impossible to know about every culture, but it is important to learn about the ones nurse will encounter most often in their practice. In addition, nurse will need to delegate and supervise others, ensuring that all clients have equal access to culturally appropriate care. Nurse need a good understanding of culture and ethnicity not only for providing direct care, but also for teaching and role-modeling culturally competent care for other care providers.

Meaning of Culture

To provide care in a culturally diverse population, nurse will need to understand concepts related to culture. Start at the beginning by learning what the word *culture* means. Rooted in sociology and more specifically anthropology, we know that culture is both *universal* (everyone has it) and *dynamic* (active). Put simply, **culture** is what people in a group have in common, but it changes over time.

Purnell and *Paulanka* (2003) define culture as "the totality of socially transmitted behavior patterns, arts, beliefs, values, customs, life ways, and all other products of human work and thought characteristic of a population of people that guide their worldview and decision making."

Culture may be defined as 'the learned ways of acting and thinking which are transmitted by group members and which provide for each individual readymade and tested solutions for vital problems.

Culture includes, the areas as diet, language and communication process, religion, art and history, family processes, social groups interactive patterns, value orientations, and healing belief and practices. How persons resolve problems related to basic human needs is strongly influenced by these cultural elements. Because culture is devised by people to solve human problems, it is universal.

Culture is broadly defined, as a view of the world, as well as a set of values, beliefs and traditions that are handed down from generation to generation. As already, stated it includes the beliefs, habits, likes and dislikes, and customs and rituals learned from one's family. The culture also includes all human activities taking material and nonmaterial forms and expressions, the political economic, social, religious, educational, philosophical, technological and environmental contexts in which human beings live and function.

Culture can viewed as learned, shared behavior and understanding that form an interrelated whole. Culture is the social clue that holds relationships together and the mechanism by which we share our values with one another and understand other people. Culture is behavioral map and perceptional filter.

Characteristics of Culture

A culture is learned, a person learns behaviors, values, attitudes and beliefs within his cultural family system. This learning is influenced by the persons social status within a society and adaptation to his environment. Culture is capable of change but remains stable; language, traditions and norms or customs may act as stabilizers for a culture. Components or patterns are present in every culture. These components and patterns include communication system, means of economic and physician survival, transportation systems, family systems, social customs and moves and religious systems. Culture guides behavior into acceptable ways for the people in a specific group. It is shared by and provides for an identity for all members of the same cultural group. Culture is learned by each new generation through both formal and informal life experiences. Language is the primary means of transmitting culture. The practices of particular culture often arise because of the groups' social and physical environment. Cultural practices and beliefs are adapted over time, but they mainly remain constant as long as they satisfy needs. Culture influences, the way of people of a group, have expectations and behaves in response to certain situations. Because a culture is made up of individuals, differences within cultures as well as across cultures are found.

To determine what is meant by culture or cultural, keep in mind the following characteristics:

- *Culture is learned:* Learning occurs through life experiences shared with other members of the culture.
- *Culture is taught:* Cultural values, beliefs, and traditions are passed down from generation to generation, either formally (e.g. in schools) or informally (e.g. ill families).
- *Culture is shared by its members:* Cultural norms are shared through teachings and social interactions.
- *Culture is dynamic and adaptive:* Cultural customs, beliefs, and practices are not static, but change over time and at different rates. Cultural change occurs with adaptation in response to the environment.
- *Culture is complex:* Cultural assumptions and habits are unconscious and thus may be difficult for members of the culture to explain to others.
- *Culture is diverse:* Culture demonstrates the variety that exists among groups and among members of a particular group.
- *Culture exists at many levels:* Culture exists in both the material (art, writings, dress, or artifacts) and the nonmaterial (customs, traditions, language, beliefs and practices).
- *Culture has common beliefs and practices:* Members of the culture share the same beliefs, traditions, customs, and practices as long as they continue to be adaptive and satisfy

the members' needs. Some members of the group may deviate from cultural norms, but for a norm to be considered cultural many members must follow it.

- *Culture is all encompassing:* Culture can influence everything its members think and do.
- *Culture provides identity:* Cultural beliefs provide identity for its members as long as they do not conflict with the dominant culture and continue to gratify its members.

Bicultural is a term that describes a person who identifies with two cultures and maintains some of the values and lifestyles of each. Consider a Hindu man who marries an Italian woman. Their bicultural children may choose to follow Hindu tradition while still holding some of the values and beliefs of their Italian heritage. A bicultural person may experience divorced loyalties. **Multicultural** refers to many cultures and is used to describe groups rather than individuals. Many regions of the country are multicultural, meaning that the region is population by individuals from many different cultural groups. The same can be said about workplace settings. Remember that culture does not always refer to the ethnicity of a group. Think of a hospital: Caregivers may be members of various ethnic and religious groups and the nurses, physicians, physical therapists, and students each comprise a different subculture. A hospital is thus a multicultural setting.

Concepts Related to Culture

There some concepts relevant to culture are as follows:

Holism

The concepts of holism require that human behavior is to be considered within the context in which it occurs. Similarly, culture is best viewed and analyzed as a whole. The various components of culture, such as the political, economic, religious, kinship and health system, perform separate functions but form an operating whole. Thus to understand anyone system, one must view each in relation to the others and the entire culture. A culture is often said to be more than the sum of its parts.

Cultural Change

Any change in one or more systems affects the whole culture. Culture is never static but is constantly adding or deleting elements. This process of cultural change is a result of contact between groups and of forces within a group. Cultural change usually creates new challenges and problems. It involves creative adoption of behavioral precedents that are passed through language, customs, beliefs, attitudes, values, goals, laws traditions, and moral codes. At times precedents become outmoded or maladaptive and thus provide a potential source of conflict. The health status of society is related to its ability to adapt to change. In India western medicine gained status because of political, social and legal changes during British Government.

Enculturation

The process of becoming a member of a cultural group is called 'enculturation.' Cultural behavior or knowing how to act appropriately, is socially acquired, not inherited. Patterns of cultural behavior are learned through the process of enculturation, sometimes called socialization. Enculturation is process of acquiring knowledge and internalizing values. Through this process people achieve competence in their own culture. Children acquire their culture by watching adults and making interferences about the rules of behavior. Cultural patterns provide explanations of life events such as birth, death, puberty, child bearing, rearing of children, illness and disease. It is important for the nurse to understand these explanations, according to their culture and translate these concepts into modern version, as accepted by the universe/society.

Culture-bound

The process of socialization profoundly influences one's world view. A person's whole view is just that the way that individual sees the world. It is the frame of reference out of which all of us function with relation to all aspects of the environment and one another. Each person's world view is learned in the context of specific culture. A person may be blind to his or her own culture, not recognizing that his culture is one of many. Those people who do not know or appreciate differences in world views are 'cultural bound'. This existence of being cultural bound means whenever people learn a culture, they are to some extent imprisoned without knowing it, that is living with a particular reality that is considered as the reality. Everyone has learning and ways to interpret world based on one's enculturation.

Nurses are cultural bound within their own culture and profession. Being cultural bound within nursing, means that nurses are likely to view the modern scientific approach to health and illness on the only possibility. Clients may view this modern scientific approach differently, judging that in some way it meet their needs, and in other ways it does not. Dissatisfaction with medical treatment and doctor, the movement toward self-care, and striving for freedom of choice and individual responsibility have lead to increased interest in alternative health services. Western medicine is often practised in unscientific ways. Desirable outcomes may occur independently of the doctors intervention, or the doctors actions may lead to iatrogenic (treatment related) consequences such as adverse drug reaction.

Ethnocentrism

Ethnocentrism is the belief that one's own cultural view point is the best. It is important for nurses not to consider their own way the best and other people's ideas as ignorant as inferior. The ideas of lay persons may be valid and certainly influence their health care behavior. Culturally appropriate health care begins with the awareness that people may live by different rules and priorities from those of the health care providers. The term cultural relativism denotes that different cultures are neither inferior nor superior to one another. Health professionals must recognize the role of cultural relativism in regard to modern scientific medicine. Nurses must realize that not even their own beliefs and professional practice are immune to scientifically unsound behavior.

Ethnocentrism is the tendency to think that your own group (cultural, professional, ethnic, or social) is superior to others and to view behaviors and beliefs that differ greatly from your own as somehow wrong, strange, or unenlightened. The tendency to ethnocentrism exists in all groups, not just in the dominant culture.

Stereotypes

Stereotypes are exaggerated beliefs and images that are popularly depicted in the mass media and folklore. Usually these images are false; they obscure important differences among members of a group and exaggerate those between groups. The perceived, exaggerated differences between two groups are used to justify negative behavior of people in one group toward the other groups. Although individuals may be found fit the stereotypes, most do not. Stereotypes commonly reflected by false and insensitive statements such as 'Indians are monks; blacks are lazy' nurses are passionate, etc. Stereotyping can lead to inaccurate assessment and interventions based on perceived notions. Health professionals must remain sensitive to individual variations within groups.

Cultural Values

A value is a type of belief about how one should or should not behave. Beliefs are statements which based on empirical evidence. All belief systems are cultural bound because they are based on cultural factors and meaning that individuals ascribe to these factors. Individuals assign meaning to health and illness based on their values and believes. Therefore behavior of clients in regard to health and illness can be more accurately understood by knowing something about their beliefs and values. Cultural values are the prevailing and persistent guidelines influence how people think and act. Beliefs and values influence that kind of health care, a person considers acceptable or desirable. Values provide powerful motivation and standards for behavior. Health care providers need to consider that clients actually believe about their health problems and how should they be treated.

Ethnicity

Ethnicity refers to groups whose members share a common social and cultural heritage that is passed down from generation to generation.

Ethnicity is the sense of identification of a collective cultural group. Largely based on the group's common heritage, one belongs to a specific ethnic group either through birth or through adoption of characteristics of the group. People within an ethnic group share common and unique cultural and social beliefs and behavior patterns, including language and dialect, religious

practices, literature, folklore, music, political interests, food preferences, and employment patterns. Ethnicity largely develops through day to day life with family and friends within the community.

Ethnicity is associated with a cultural group having common social and cultural heritage. Ethnicity is complex, ambivalent, paradoxical and elusive. A person is born into an ethnic group but also may adopt characteristics of another ethnic group. The characteristics of an ethnic group include common language and dialect, migratory status, race, and religious faith and practices. People share traditions, values, symbols, literature, folklore, music, food preferences. Settlement and employment patterns and special political interests are often similar. There are several ethnic group in India.

Religion

Religion refers to an ordered system of beliefs regarding the cause, nature, and purpose of the universe, especially the beliefs related to the worship of a God or Goddess.

Religion is a belief in a divine or superhuman power or powers to be obeyed and worshipped as the creator and ruler of the universe. Ethical values and religious beliefs and practices further clarify ethnicity by providing a frame of reference and a perspective within which to organize information. Religious teachings help formulate a meaningful philosophy and system of practices through a system of beliefs and practices, and social controls having specific values, norms and ethics that vary between religious groups. Some religious practices are health related; for example, some religions teach that adherence to a code or mandate is conducive to harmony and health and that breaking it may cause disharmony or illness, e.g. ekapathni vrata.

Race refers to the grouping of people based on biological similarities. Members of a particular race share distinguishing physical characteristics such as skin color, blood type, or bone structure.

Ethnicity and race are overlapping concepts. Race is usually refers to a group of individuals who share common biological features. Ethnicity sometime has similar meaning but also may refer to a shared culture rather than shared biological characteristics. From this perspective, individuals who share a common culture mayor may not have similar biological characteristics. Ethnicity has been defined as classification of humans based on some commonalty or affiliation. Ethnic group refers to designated or basic division or groups of human king, distinguished by customs, characteristic or language. In short, ethnicity is a difficult concept rooter in the designators own cultural beliefs about what is different or distinguishable. Culture, ethnicity, and religion, race are often used interchangeably, making the concepts difficult to understand.

A person never acquires a culture as a complete and absolute pattern, instead he merely learns the main components of subculture. Subculture is a large group of people who are members of a large cultural group but have certain ethnic, occupational or physical characteristics that are not common to the large

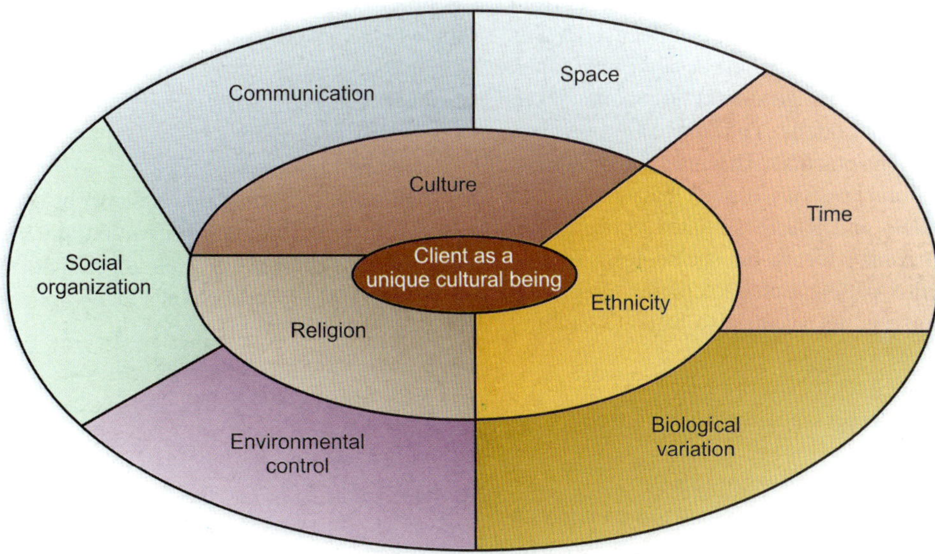

Figure 4.1: Cultural phenomena

culture; for example, nursing is subculture, of health care system. Variations within the cultural groups usually occurs because of individual differences. The factors related to cultural variations among ethnic/minority groups are as follows:

- Age
- Dialect/language spoken
- Gender identity and roles
- Socioeconomic background
- Geographical location in country of origin or current residence
- Amount and type of interaction between younger and older generation
- Degree of adoption of values in current country.

Cultural Phenomena

There are mainly six cultural phenomena having identified as varying between cultural groups, which includes environmental control, biological variations, social organization, communication, space and time (Fig. 4.1).

Environmental Control

It refers to the ability of members of a particular cultural group to plan activities that control nature or direct environmental factors. Included are the complex system of traditional health and illness beliefs, the practice of folk medicine, and the use of traditional healers. This particular cultural phenomenon plays an extremely important role in the ways clients respond to health related experiences, including the ways in which they define health and illness and seek and use health and nursing care resources and social supports.

Biological variations: There are several ways in which people from one cultural group differ, biologically from members of other cultural group:

- Body build and structures
- Skin color
- Enzymatical genetic variations
- Susceptibility of disease
- Nutritional variation.

Social organization: It refers to the family unit (nuclear/single parent or extended family) and the social group organization, i.e. religious or ethnic with which clients and families may identify. Several social barriers, such as unemployment, homelessness, lack of health intimacy and poverty prevent people from entering health care system.

Communication: Its gaps are presented in many ways, including language differences, verbal and nonverbal behaviors, etc. (spoken language, gestures, and even silences).

Space: Personal space involves people's behaviors and attitudes towards the space around themselves. Territoriality is an attitude towards an area people have claimed and defend or reach emotionally about when others encroach on it.

Within all cultural groups personal space varies depending on the relationship between the people speaking: intimate v/s acquaintances people of the same v/s opposite sea; and a people of a different position within the social hierarchy.

Time: Time orientation (past, present and future) varies among different cultural group-waiting or immediate attendance of service.

Culture is an integral components of both health and illness because of genetic characteristics and the values and beliefs we learn from our families and communities. In order to provide holistic care to people from diverse cultural backgrounds, nurses must be sensitive to the cultural needs, characteristics and values of the individuals, families and groups.

Nurses providing care should consider all patients as individuals, because each person is unique. How a person is influenced as well as the extent of the influentiality varies from the individual to individual. How a person is influenced by his culture depends on the unique life experiences of the individual, i.e. family factors, critical events, age and socioeconomic level. Culture influences behavior patterns, communication process, health and illness, beliefs and practices. The nurse and the patient each have their own cultural lifestyles. It is not that nurse should change her beliefs, values and practices related to health and illness to fit those of her/his patients, but she/he needs to gain understanding of her/his patient's characteristics to provide effective care. If a nurse is not aware of a patient's cultural background, she/he may:

- Misjudge the cultural effect on health care.
- Make culturally incorrect and improper nursing care judgment.
- Provide poor and even unsafe interventions.

To provide individualized nursing care, it will be important that for nurses to develop a positive approach in interacting with patients who are culturally or socially different.

Nurses need to be aware of and sensitive to the cultural needs of clients. The body of knowledge relevant to transcultural nursing is rapidly growing, and it is imperative that nurses from all cultural backgrounds be aware of nursing implications in this area. The practice of nursing today demands that the nurse identify and meet the cultural needs of diverse groups; understand the social and cultural reality of the client, family, and community; develop expertise to implement culturally acceptable strategies to provide nursing care; and identify and use resources available and acceptable to the client.

Cultural Values, and Health

Values are important because they help shape health related beliefs and practices. Do you know what value? Think for a minute about what you "value" in life. What are the five ideals, principles, or what are most important to you? Simply put, a personal value is a principle or standard that has meaning with to an individual. For example is cleanliness. In contrast, a belief is something that one accepts as true (e.g. "I believe this germ cause disease"), and a **practice** is a set of behaviors that one follows (e.g. "I always wash my hands before preparing food"). Do you see how values, belief's, and practices are related?

Our values influence much of what we think and do. This is important to know because values are entangled in all ethical situations. If asked, could you say what your values are? Could you explain how they inform your decisions about right and wrong in a given situation? If so, that's a great beginning.

A **value** is a belief that the person have about the worth of something; it serves as a principle or a standard that influences decision making. Values are ideals, beliefs, customs, modes of conduct, qualities, or goals that are highly prized or preferred by individuals, groups, or society. Individual can value an idea, a person, a way of doing things, or even an object (e.g. money).

People express their values through behaviors, feelings, knowledge, and decisions. For example, the nurse who values compassion will interact with patients in a sensitive, caring manner. Some characteristics of values are that they:

- Are freely chosen
- Are often taken for granted
- Are learned in conscious and unconscious ways
- Are learned through observation and experience in social groups (e.g. the family, school, church)
- Become a part of a person's make-up
- Give direction to life
- Can be individual or shared
- Vary from person to person
- Can change over time
- May be expressed overtly or manifested indirectly.

Our **value set** is our "list" of values. It gives direction for our life and forms a basis for behavior. Our value system is our value set with the values ranked on a continuum from most important to least important. The total number of values a person has is rather small. The number of *significant* values is even smaller. It is easy enough to identify values–for example, love, freedom, courage, responsibility–but how many of our values have a consistent and predictable impact on our actions? Those are the significant values.

Attitudes are mental dispositions or feelings toward a person, object, or idea. Attitudes can include cognitive (thinking), affective (feeling), and some behavioral (doing) components. For example, you might have a positive attitude about cleanliness–that is, you may think it is a good thing (e.g. "The floor is clean. That's nice.") But if you *value* cleanliness, you would be willing to scrub the floor. You would also wash your hands at appropriate times, bathe regularly, and teach others about hygiene.

A belief is something that one accepts as true (e.g. "I believe that germs cause disease and that by washing my hands I remove germs"). Beliefs are sometimes based on faith and sometimes on facts. A belief mayor may not be true. Beliefs mayor may not involve values. Consider the following statements of belief. The first does not involve a value; the second one does.

"I believe the earth is round."

"Working hard to achieve goals is important to me; therefore, I believe that I must work during the summer to save money for college."

Professional Versus Personal Values

Our **personal value system** is a set of values that we have reflected on and chosen that will help us to lead a good life. Nurses have internalized some *societal values* and have come to perceive them as their own (e.g. good manners, such as saying "Please" and "Thank you"). In addition, they probably have some personal values (e.g. friendship, fairness, creativity) that are important to them but may or may not be important to society at large.

Table 4.1: Professional Values and Behaviors

Values	Values defined	Professional behaviors
Altruism	A concern for the welfare and well-being of others. Altruism is reflected by the nurse's concern for the welfare of patients, other nurses, and other health care providers.	• Demonstrates understanding of cultures, beliefs, and perspectives of others. • Advocates for patients, particularly the most vulnerable. • Takes risks on behalf of patients and colleagues. • Mentors other professionals.
Autonomy	The right to self-determination. Professional practice reflects autonomy when the nurse respects patients' rights to make decisions about their health care.	• Plans care in partnership with patients. • Honors the right of patients and families to make decisions about health care. • Provides information so that patients can make informed choices.
Human dignity	Respect for the inherent worth and uniqueness of individuals and populations. In professional practice, human dignity is reflected when the nurse values and respects all patients and colleagues.	• Provides culturally competent and sensitive care. • Protects the patient's privacy. • Preserves the confidentiality of patients and health care providers. • Designs care with sensitivity to individual patient needs.
Integrity	Acting in accordance with an appropriate code of ethics and accepted standards of practice. Integrity is reflected in professional practice when the nurse is honest and provides care based on an ethical framework that is accepted within the profession.	• Provides honest information to patients and the public. • Documents care accurately and honestly. • Seeks to remedy errors made by self or others. • Demonstrates accountability for own actions.
Social justice	Upholding moral, legal, and humanistic principles. This value is reflected in professional practice when the nurse works to ensure equal treatment under the law and equal access to quality health care.	• Supports fairness and nondiscrimination in the delivery of care. • Promotes universal access to health care. • Encourages legislation and policy consistent with the advancement of nursing care and health care.

As nurses move forward in their profession, the will assimilate what they have learn and experience and form **professional values** (Table 4.1).

Additional professional values frequently cited for nursing include the following:

- Equality (having the same rights, privileges, or status)
- Esthetics (qualities of objects or people that are pleasing)
- Freedom (capacity to choose)
- Truth (faithfulness to fact or reality)
- Service (commitment to work useful to others)
- Education (basic and lifelong continuing education for nurses)
- Competence (skill, knowledge, performance of nursing work)
- Loyalty (feeling of duty or attachment to other nurses)

Values Transmission

Person acquire values from social interaction. So how does that work? How are values transmitted? Study adds to the information that values transmission between parents and adolescents can be reciprocal and that the presence of a receptive and supportive parent makes value transmission more likely (Table 4.2).

Values Clarification

Values clarification refers to the process of becoming conscious of and naming one's values. If nurses are clear about their values, they will make better decisions and be better able to avoid imposing these values on others. Because each person has his own unique values set, it is important to appreciate others' values and how they influence their decisions. Clarifying values should be a positive process that leads to a human growth experience resulting in more awareness, empathy, and insight. A full value must be:

- Chosen freely from a list of alternatives after thoughtful consideration has been given to the consequences of each alternative (cognitive)
- Cherished and made known to other people (affective)

Table 4.2: Modes of Value Transmission

Mode	Description
Modeling	Children learn values from a variety of role models (parents, peers, rock stars, significant others) by observation. This modeling may lead to socially acceptable or unacceptable behaviors.
Moralizing	"This way is the only way." Children are taught a complete set of values in an authoritarian approach. If the child does not conform, the parent may inflict guilt and fear on him. This approach by parents, teachers, church leaders, and other authorities may make it difficult for young people to make independent choices because they have no experience selecting values that are good for them.
Laissez-faire	"Doing your own thing." Children are allowed to explore differing sets of values on their own with little guidance or discipline. This may lead to conflict and confusion on the part of the child.
Reward and punishment	The child's behavior is controlled by offering rewards for certain valued behaviors and punishing the child who fails to comply. Rewards can strengthen behavior, whereas physical punishment may teach that violence is an acceptable behavior.
Responsible choice	A balance of freedom and restriction allows children to select the values, explore new behaviors, and experience the consequences. This can lead to personal satisfaction and parental support.

Table 4.3: Values Clarification

Step	Description	Questions to ask your patient
Choosing (cognitive)	Beliefs are chosen:	Do (did) you have any choice about what you do?
	Freely (allows you to cherish your choice)	Do you have any control over what happens? What have you decided to do?
	From alternatives	Can you list some alternative actions? What are your options? What could you do instead of…?
	After considering all consequences (ensures that the alternative is right for you)	What do you think will happen if you do that? What will you gain by doing that? What is the disadvantage of doing that?
Prizing (affective)	Beliefs and behaviors that are chosen are prized:	How do you feel about your decision?
	With pride (feeling good about your choice)	People sometimes feel good after making such a decision. Others feel pressured. How is it for you?
	With public affirmation	How do you intend to tell your family (friends) about this decision? What will you say to your wife (friends, family)? When will you announce your decision to...?
Acting (behavioral)	Beliefs are acted on:	Try to determine whether the client will act on the decision:
	By incorporating the choice into one's own behavior	How do you think your wife (significant other) will react when you do that? When will you actually carry out this decision? Try to predict consistent behavior by asking:
	With consistency and repetition	How many times in the past have you...? What kind of schedule have you worked out? How often and when will you...?

- Translated into behaviors that are consistent with the chosen value and integrated into the lifestyle (conative) (Table 4.3)

Neutrality of Value

Nurses need to be nonjudgmental in providing health care to their clients. As a nurse, you have a duty to provide the best care to clients. You should not assume that your personal values are right, and you should not judge the client's values as right or wrong on the basis of whether they agree with your value system. For example Asha, who was seeking an abortion. A nurse who does not believe in abortion could still provide competent nursing care to Asha even though his values regarding abortion are different from Asha. **Value neutrality** means that we attempt to understand our own values regarding an issue and to know when to put them aside, if necessary, to become nonjudgmental when providing care to clients. However, some health care professionals believe that value neutrality is neither possible nor desirable because it imposes an ethical obligation on health care providers to suppress or modify their own deepest moral and religious beliefs.

Values and morals are learned in conscious and unconscious ways and become a part of your make-up. When we evaluate right and wrong, or good and bad, we are using moral judgment. Therefore, our individual preferences (values) of right or wrong become our moral values. Whether or not you are aware of it, your morals and values shape the manner in which you make ethical decisions in your nursing practice.

So, although ethics are based on a structured set of principles and theories, and ethical decisions are publicly stated in terms of possible alternative behaviors, such decisions are always influenced unconsciously by our own personal values and morals. It is important to clarify the influence of your values and morals each time you enter into a situation where you are called on to be objective in your ethical decision making.

Cultural values, beliefs, and practice are the principles, standards, ideas, and behaviors that members of a cultural group share. An example of a cultural value is the European-American obsession with bodily cleanliness. Other values of the **dominant** culture include youth, beauty, success, independence, and material belongings. You should not assume that clients share your values, beliefs, and practices–nor those of the dominant culture. Instead, become familiar with the specific values, beliefs, and practices of clients from the different cultural and ethnic (ethno-cultural) groups in your community. Remember, though, that individuals within an ethnocultural group vary widely and that *learning commonalities is no substitute for careful assessment of each person.*

Culture universals are the values, beliefs, and practices that people from *all* cultures share. In contrast, culture specifics are those values, beliefs, and practices that are special or unique to a culture. Let's look at an example. All cultures celebrate the birth of a new baby in some way (a culture universal), but different cultures celebrate "birth rates" in different ways (a culture specific). In Belize, a baby is christened before visitors are allowed, a practice carried out to prevent the *evil eye* (bad spells cast by others); in Greece, *amulets* (objects or charms worn to protect from evil spirits) may be placed on the baby; and in Israel, Jewish male infants are circumcised on the eighth day of life. Similarly, people from all cultures practice marriage rituals. In India, a groom is prepared for the wedding ceremony in an elaborate ritual that is culture-specific.

Acknowledging that there are commonalities within a group is not the same as saying that *all* people in the group have those characteristics. Bear in mind there is probably more variation among people *within* an ethnic or cultural group than there is *between* the groups and that much variation stems from socioeconomic differences or regional origin. Each person must be seen as unique–as *influenced* by his heritage, but not *defined* by it. "It is important that the nurse consider specific cultural factors impacting on individual clients and recognize that intracultural variation means that each client must be assessed for individual cultural differences."

Culture Specifics Affect Health

Just as they influence our celebrations of births and weddings, culture specifics affect our health beliefs and behaviors. Thus, knowledge of the culture specifics of groups in your community, will enhance your ability.

The following may also be culture specifics. The first two, religion/philosophy and education, vary among subcultures. The other three (technology, politics/law, and the economy) exert broader effects that can be seen among different countries, but less so among subcultures within a country.

- *Religion and philosophy:* A person's religion may determine what health care is acceptable to him. For example, some religions (e.g. Jehovah's Witnesses) do not accept blood transfusions, and many religions' forbid abortion.
- *Education:* Education influences the perception of wellness and illness and the knowledge of options that are available for health care. These, in turn, affect the person's expectations for care.
- *Technology:* The availability of supplies and equipment determines what is used in the health care setting and what comes to be culturally expected, Nurses in most of North America, for example, assume they will have bed linens, water, electricity, necessary medications, and technology such as electrocardiography and X-ray imaging. In many parts of the world, however, these items are not available.
- *Politics and the law:* Governmental policies affect health care. They determine what practitioners will be available and what programs will be funded; for example, the federal government helps fund Medicare, which provides basic medical insurance for people age 65 and above. The legal system defines roles;' functions, and standards of health professionals.
- *Economy:* The condition of the economy directly affects the availability of funds for publicly funded services. It also affects the individual's ability to pay for health care.

Cultural Competent Care in Nursing

i. Concepts

Purnell's model (Purnell and Paulanka, 2003) describes cultural competence as:

- Developing an awareness of one's own existence, sensations, thoughts, and environment without letting it have undue influence on those from other backgrounds
- Demonstrating knowledge and understanding of the client's health-related needs and concepts of health and illness
- Accepting and respecting cultural differences
- Realizing that the values and beliefs of health care providers may be different from the client's
- Resisting judgmental attitudes, such as "different is not as good"
- Being open to cultural encounters
- Adapting care to make it congruent with the client's culture
- Recognizing culture as a conscious and nonlinear process.

Although Madeline Leininger does not use the specific term *cultural competence,* her theory fits with that concept. The goal of her theory is "to use research findings to provide culturally congruent, safe, and meaningful care to clients of diverse or similar cultures." Nurses can obtain this goal by:

1. Discovering cultural care and caring beliefs, values, and practices
2. Analyzing the similarities and differences of these beliefs among the different cultures.

For more information on Leininger's theory of culture care diversity and universality.

The culturally competent model of care (Campinha-Bacote, 2002) views cultural competence as a process, not an end point, The model identifies five components of cultural competence, using the mnemonic ASKED:

Awareness (cultural sensitivity, cultural biases)

Skills (cultural assessment tools)

Knowledge (cultural worldviews, theoretical frameworks)

Encounters (cultural exposure, cultural practice)

Desire (to be culturally competent).

ii. Barriers Nursing

Nurses ability to provide culturally competent nursing may be hampered by the following barriers:

- *Lack of knowledge* about the cultural and ethnic values, beliefs, and behaviors of people within their community is not unusual among health care providers. It can cause them to misinterpret a client's behaviors.
- *Emotional responses* such as fear and distrust–both nurses and the client's–can arise any time members of different cultural groups meet. If nurse aware that this may happen, he/she may be able to avoid this barrier and communicate with their clients effectively.
- *Ethnocentrism* may negatively affect care. People have a tendency to be biased toward their own culture, believing that their own beliefs and values are right and that those of other cultures are wrong (or at least bizarre). If nurse take

this attitude, their patient may feel that you disapprove of him or, at the least, that you don't understand or respect him.

- A **cultural stereotype** is the unsubstantiated belief that all people of a certain racial or ethnic group are alike in certain respects. A stereotype may be positive or negative.
- Similar to a stereotype, **prejudice** refers to negative attitudes toward other people that are based on faulty and rigid stereotypes about race, gender, sexual orientation, and so on.
- Whereas prejudice refers to people's attitudes, the term **discrimination** refers to the behavioral manifestations of that prejudice. For example, prior to the 1960s many hospitals refused treatment to foreigners. Slightly more subtle discrimination against minority groups still exists in housing, banking, and the job market. It is, in some places, more difficult for a woman, someone who is openly homosexual, or such others to obtain a loan or to be hired for certain jobs.
- Racism is a form of prejudice and discrimination based on the belief that race is principal determining factor of human traits and capabilities and that racial difference produce an inherent superiority (or inferiority). The word *race* alone evokes powerful emotional responses for people who feel that they or their ancestors have been oppressed or exploited, and equally for those who deny such a responsibility. The history of discrimination against other country people has created a focus on differences and racial divisiveness. As a nurse, you must recognize that unconscious racism can play a major role in your ability to communicate with people of other races.
- **Sexism,** widespread throughout history, is the assumption that members of one sex are superior to those of the other sex. For example, women have been viewed as more emotional and less rational than men, and assertiveness, considered a positive trait in men, may be seen as "pushiness" or aggressiveness in women. On the other hand, men who art' nurses must combat the kind of sexism that asserts that it is "unnatural" for men to engage in caring behaviors. Some female nurses may not accept their male colleagues, and some patients–both male and female–may object to their care, at least initially.
- **Male chauvinism** (assumption of male superiority) is common in many cultures and in health care settings. It. may be overt or subtle. In the wider society, for example, men may receive higher pay for performing the same work as a woman. In the health care setting, you might, even now, hear a male physician calling female nurses or patients "dear," or using a voice tone more appropriate to addressing a child. When you have the opportunity to do so, observe a conversation between a male nurse and a male physician. You may note that the male nurse communicates more directly and uses more eye contact than female nurses do with this same physician. We are not assuming that all physicians (or nurses) are chauvinistic; we are simply stating that you will probably be able to observe this kind of interchange among some professionals. As in other settings, the assumption of equality–by either party–changes the way people communicate.

- *A language barrier* will obviously affect your ability to communicate with clients. Language barriers can involve foreign languages, dialects, regionalisms (words or pronunciation particular to a specific region), street talk, and jargon (words or expressions used by a subculture, including medicine). In such a case, you would need to explore the resources and policies of your health care facility. If there were no other options for translation help, you would have to resort to nonverbal language and pictures to communicate until further resources could be found. It's not the best option, but it may be the only one, at least temporarily. However, if a consent issue is involved, the hospital will almost certainly have a policy to handle the situation.

- *Street talk, slang, and jargon* can be as challenging as a foreign language. For example, the word *bad* can mean bad or good; the meaning changes, and not everyone has the same interpretations. Ebonics is a type of English that has, in the past, been spoken primarily by African Americans, but many white youth enamored with hip-hop culture now embrace Ebonics as a way to connect with the street culture.

- *Health care jargon* can often be distressing to client. In the health care field, we have our own terminology, including abbreviations, which we use so often we may forget that our clients don't understand them. For example, you may frighten some clients if you say to them, "I'm going to take your vitals" before assessing their blood pressure. You may be surprised to learn that many patients will not know what you mean if you ask, "Have you voided today?" Even worse, patients may hesitate to ask for clarification because they don't like admitting that they don't understand a certain word. What other examples of nursing or medical jargon can you think of that might be confusing to clients?

iii. Nursing Strategies

Nurses should become familiar with the cultural groups. They are most likely to encounter. Choose one of the transcultural models to help you to use critical thinking and the nursing process to provide the holistic care your clients deserve. Leininger's theory describes the following three "modes" of nursing decisions and actions.

1. *Cultural care preservation/maintenance,* which sustains clients' cultural lifestyles in meaningful ways. These are actions that help the client retain or preserve cultural values related to health.

Example: Encouraging the family to bring ethnic foods that are appropriate for the patient's prescribed diet.

2. *Cultural care accommodation/negotiation,* which adapts clients' lifestyles or nurses' actions. The nurse supports and enables the client to adapt to therapies or to negotiate with professionals to achieve satisfying health outcomes. **Negotiation** acknowledges the gap between the nurse's and client's perspectives. You must negotiate when folk or traditional practices might be harmful to the client.

Example: Negotiating with the client to continue seeing the *curandero,* but to come to the clinic every 6 weeks to have his blood pressure checked. If the client refuses all biomedical or nursing interventions, the only avenue still open is to continue monitoring the client to identify changes in his health status. If a health crisis occurs, it may be possible to renegotiate the care.

3. *Cultural care repatterning/restructuring,* which changes nurses' actions or clients' lifestyles into different patterns. The nurse supports and encourages the client to greatly modify his behaviors and to adopt new, different, and beneficial health behaviors, while still respecting the client's cultural values and beliefs.

Example 1: When the client absolutely refuses to take the prescribed pain medication, the nurse uses massage, distraction, and other nonpharmacological techniques to help relieve his pain (change in nurse's actions).

Example 2: A client refuses to see a biomedical doctor for her family's needs. However, when the folk healer is unsuccessful in treating her child's illness and the child becomes critically ill, the nurse convinces the client to bring the child to the emergency department (modification of the client's behaviors).

There are several specific strategies for nurses to consider and many resources to help them develop strategies specific to various cultural groups. Consider the following as they move forward on their journey toward cultural competence (Table 4.4):

- Consider each client as a unique individual, influenced but not defined by his culture.

- Understand your own cultural values and practices and appreciate how they may differ from those held by people of other cultures.

- Recognize your own biases about people and groups, and consider how they may affect the care you provide.

- Learn as much as you can about the cultural groups in your community and work area.

- Make an effort to incorporate beliefs and practices from various cultures into your nursing care and teaching materials.

- Encourage helpful or neutral cultural practices, and discourage those that are dysfunctional (harmful).

- Suggest alternatives to harmful practices.

- Accommodate cultural dietary practices when possible. For inpatients, some dietary departments can make special foods, and you can encourage families to bring food from home. In all situations, help patients and families adapt cultural foods to therapeutic diets.

- Become familiar with appropriate verbal and nonverbal communication patterns within the cultural groups, and use them selectively in your communication approaches.

- Respect your clients regardless of cultural background, and never force, pressure, manipulate, or coerce them to participate in care that conflicts with their values and beliefs.

- Advocate for all of your clients, but especially for those not from the dominant culture.

- Consider the cultural role of the family member who make, the primary decisions. To ignore this person is to doom your interventions to failure.

- Work with the folk medicine practitioner in the interest of the patient.

- Learn from your mistakes, and don't make them again.

Table 4.4: Cultural Phenomena Affecting Cultural Care Etiquette

Cultural phenomenon	Behaviors	Nursing interventions/Etiquette
Time	Visiting	• Inform clients when you are coming.
	Being on time Taboo times	• Avoid surprises. • Explain your expectations about time. • Ask clients from other religions and cultures what they expect. • Be familiar with times and meanings of client's ethnic and religious holidays.
Space	Body language and distancing	• Know cultural and/or religious customs regarding contact and touch with others.
Communication	Greetings	• Know proper forms of addresses for people from a given culture and the ways by which people welcome one another. • Know when touch (e.g. handshake) is expected and when touch is prohibited.
	Gestures	• Be aware that gestures do not have universal meaning–what is accepted in one culture may be taboo in another.
	Smiling	• Be aware smiles may indicate friendliness to some, but to others may be forbidden.
	Eye contact	• Be aware that avoiding eye contact may be a sign of respect.
Social organization	Holidays	• Know what dates are important and why, whether or not to give gifts, what to wear to special events, and what the customs and beliefs are.
	Special events: Births Weddings Funerals	• Know how the event is celebrated, meaning of colors for gifts, and expected rituals at home or at religious services.
Biological variations	Food customs	• Know what can be eaten for certain events, what foods may be eaten together or are forbidden, and what and how utensils are used.
Environmental control	Health practices and remedies	• Know the general health traditions for a given client, and ask questions to verify that your observations are valid.

This is by no means an exhaustive list. Most likely, you can think of other strategies. It may help you to "take a trip to BALI":

Be aware of your own cultural heritage

Appreciate that the client is unique: influenced, but not defined by his culture

Learn about the client's cultural group

Incorporate the client's cultural values/behaviors into the care plan

Major considerations as nurse become more culturally competent is her ability to communicate with clients from different cultures needs encourage the following guidelines:

• Assess personal beliefs of persons from different cultures.
• Assess communication variables from a cultural perspective.
• Consider both verbal and nonverbal communication in the techniques you use you're your clients.

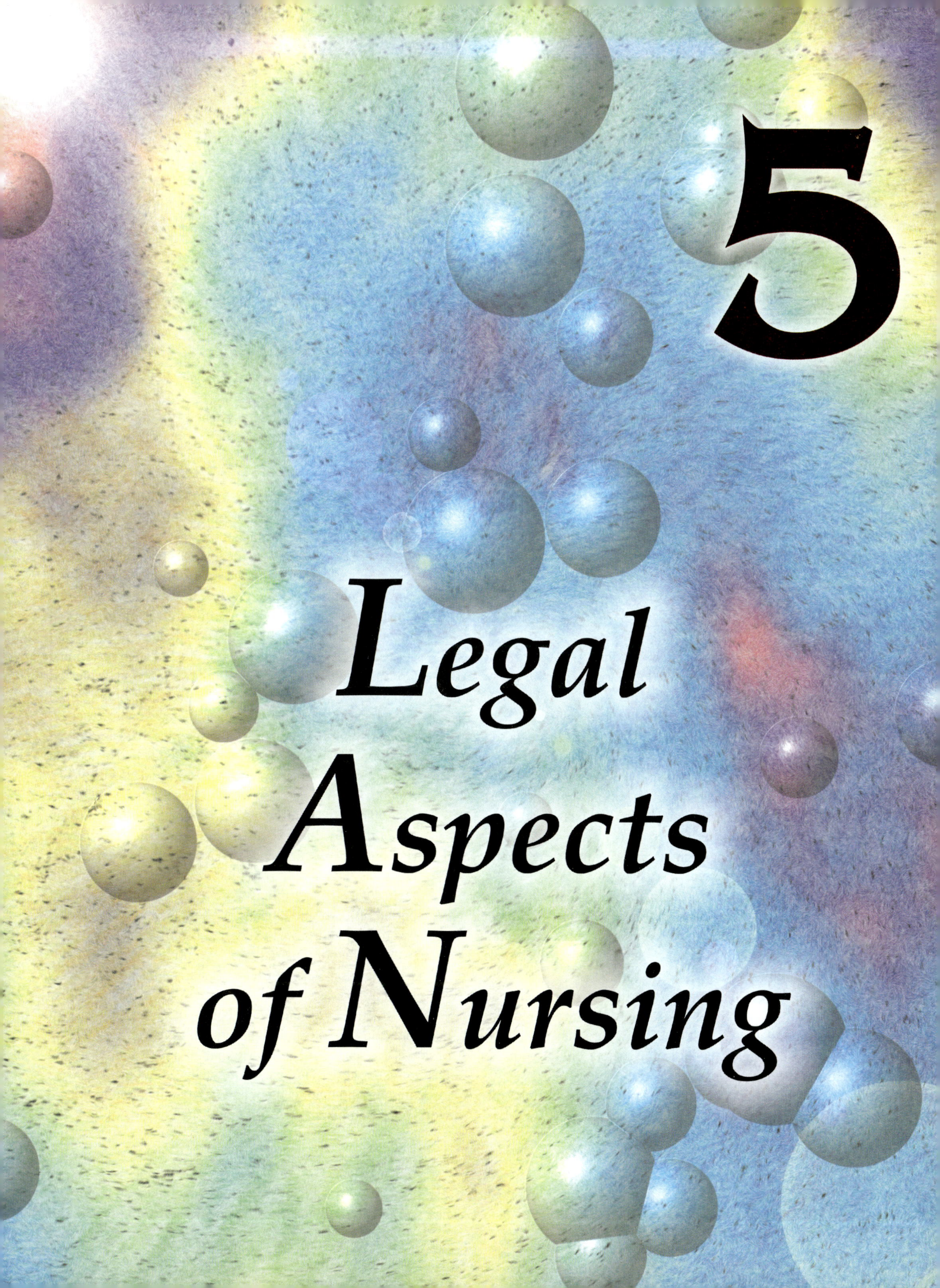
5
Legal
Aspects
of Nursing

The role of nurses and professional nursing has expanded rapidly within the past five years to include expertise specialization, autonomy and accountability, both from legal and ethical perspectives. This expansion has forced new concern among nurses and a heightened awareness of the interaction of legal and ethical principles. Areas of concerns include professional nursing practice, legal issues, ethical principles, labor management and employment.

The term law is derived from its tentoric root 'Lag' which means something which lies fixed on events. In English it means something which is uniform. The word 'Law' is employed in the modern usage in a variety of ways. In physical sciences, like physics and chemistry, it is used to denote the sequence of cause and effect. In social sciences, it refers to the rules which regulate human conduct in various spheres of social life. Laws which govern motives and internal action of humans are known as moral laws and those which regulate external human conduct are known as political laws or positive laws. The former will be enforced by the force of moral sense of the people but the later enjoy the sanctions of the authority of the state.

Laws are sets of enforcible principles and rules established to protect society. Legal principles form a framework within which nurse will practice the art of nursing.

Definition of Law

People ordinarily use the term 'Law' means a body of rules to guide human actions. The various definitions of law given by eminent jurists are as follows:

1. Law is that portion of the established thought and habit which has gained distinct and formal recognition and the shape of uniform rules backed by the authority and power of the government. — Wilson
2. The law constitutes body of principles recognised or enforced by public and regular tribunals has the administration of justice. — Pound
3. The law is a system of rights and obligations which the state enforces. — Green
4. The law is the body of principles recognized and applied by the state and the administration of justice. — Salmaind
5. Law is the command of sovereign continuing a common rule of life for his subjects and obliging them to obedience. —John Ersikene.

Laws may be defined as external rules of human conduct backed by the sovereign political authority. Law and morality are intimately related to each other. Laws are generally based on the moral principles of particular society. Some points of distinction may be brought out as follows:

1. Laws regulate external human conduct whereas morality mainly regulates internal conduct.
2. Laws are universal, morality is variable.
3. Laws are definite and precise whereas morality is variable.
4. Laws are upheld by the coercive power of the state. Morality simply enjoys the support of public opinion and or individual conscience.
5. Laws are studies under jurisprudence but morality is studied under ethics.

Law is system of principles and processes by which members of a society resolve problems and disputes without restoring to physical force. Contemporary law is a composite of all of the rules and regulation by which society governs itself. Without law, society could not deal with disputes and problems in an orderly fashion. The laws of any society are flexible and everchanging through either legislative process or judicial decisions.

Sources of Law

Laws originate from three sources, which includes law, common law, and administration.

1. *Constitutional law* is the judgmental law of the country. It is the law that governs the state. It represents the will of the ultimate and governing–the people. They alone determine how it shall be made, revised or amended. It is the constitutional law that determines the structure of the state. Its power and duties and it also determines the form of government and its relationship with various organs of the government.
2. *Statutory law* is passed by the legislative or parliament of a state in accordance with the constitutional law. In other words, statutory laws are enactments of federal and state legislative bodies. These regularities, relationship between citizens and the state, between individuals and group and between individual and the others, etc. For example, Indian Civil Marriage Act. The statutory law is created by elected legislative bodies of state (Legislative assembly) or the Parliament statutory bodies such as Indian Nursing Council.
3. *Common law* is a body of legal principles that has evolved from court decisions. In other words, it is created by judicial decisions made in courts where cases are decided.
4. *Administrative law* consists of the rules and regulations established by administrative agencies, that have been appointed by the executive branches of Government (President or Governor). It is that part of public law which regulates the conduct of public officials and discharge of their duties. It determines the mutual rights and duties of public officials and citizens. This law is not administered by ordinary courts but by the administrative courts presided over by the administrative or executive officers. It deals with the cases where officials of state violate their powers to all arbitraries.

New structures are continually being enacted, and new court decisions tend to modify older legal principles. Therefore, the body of law is constantly changing. So that all nurses in managerial positions should keep upto date knowledge about legal controls affecting nursing management and practice by attending legal workshops, seminars and readily published reports of law.

Functions of Law in Nursing

The law has many valuable functions which applied to nursing practice. It differentiates nursing practice from the practice of other health care professions. It also describes and protects the rights of clients and nurses. Illness and injury render a person unusually dependent on caregivers. For the most part, institutional caregivers are not personally known to the patients. Of all the health personnels, nursing personnels have most frequent and prolonged contact with the patient and his or her significant others, and as such are most often in a position to intervene protectively on the patient's behalf.

Most of the nursing activities are characterized by intimate touching, critical judgment, skillful manipulation and protective vigilance. Ignorance, carelessness or malice would render a nurses administrations ineffective or harmful. Consequently, nursing practice is regulated by laws that protect patients against deliberate to inadvertent injury by a nurse.

Many nurses view the law with apprehension, because they fear of being nursed in malpractice law-suit. With the increased emphasis on client's rights, nurses today must understand that legal obligations and responsibilities to clients. Nurses who give competent care based on their education will seldom need to worry about malpractice law suit. Now many clients are knowledgeable about their rights related to their health and illness, so nurse should take it as a challenge to become advocates for clients.

Laws governing nursing practice and nursing management can be divided into laws affecting the nurse as an employee, laws then specify the nurse's responsibilities towards patients, laws that regulate a nurse's relationships with doctors, laws that specify the nurse's duty to protect the public, and laws that specify the nurse's duties for record keeping and reporting.

Law can be divided as civil law and criminal law. A brief description of these laws is as follows.

Civil Law

Civil law includes rules and regulations that specify the required course of action to be followed by an individual in business and social relationships with others. It is concerned with relationships among people and the protection of a person's rights. Although violation of civil law might cause harm to an individual or property, no grave threat to society as a whole usually exists. For example, defamatory statements made about a person might lead to personal problems, but they do not threaten society in general.

In a civil case, the courts seek to resolve a dispute between private parties, which may result in payment of money by the defendant to the plaintiff. The **plaintiff** is the person bringing the suit (or making the claim). In a civil case, the plaintiff must prove by a "preponderance of the evidence" that the defendant committed wrong against him. This means that the person must prove to injury that the *allegations* (charges or accusations) made against the **defendant** (the person being sued) are "more likely than not" true. Two types of civil law provide standards for nursing practice: contract law and tort law. We will focus more on tort law, which is seen more commonly in a nursing context.

Contract Law

Contract law controls legally enforceable agreements between individuals, such as employment contracts. A contract may **explicit** (defendant in writing) or **implicit** (defined by behavior and actions). Many nurses do not have explicit employment contracts.

Tort Law

Tort law deals with the duties and rights among individuals that are not covered by contractual agreements. A tort is a civil wrong, such as a claim for malpractice or negligence, usually with claims for damages. **Damage claims** are money demands by the plaintiff for compensation for actual harm or injury inflicted by the defendant. Torts are generally identified under three categories, differing by intent of the defendant: (1) quasi-intentional torts, (2) intentional torts, and (3) negligence and malpractice (unintentional torts).

i. Quasi-intentional Torts

Quasi-Intentional torts all involve speech. There are three torts that fall into this category:

1. **Defamation,** which occurs when a false communication is made to a third person and the communication is harmful; holds the plaintiff up to hatred, contempt, or ridicule; or causes the plaintiff to be shunned or avoided
2. **Slander,** which is a defamatory statement made orally
3. **Libel,** which is a defamatory statement made in writing,

ii. Intentional Torts

"Intentional" conduct is designed to bring about a specific result in the mind of the defendant. Intentional torts include assault, batter, false imprisonment, fraud, and invasion of privacy. Intentional torts may also be prosecuted as misdemeanors or felonies under criminal law. For example, a nurse who has been sued for malpractice may also be charged with a homicide if a patient died as a result of the nurse's act or inaction. So, a patient may sue for damages for assault under civil law, and the government may charge the defendant with assault under criminal law–and the penalties differ.

Assault occurs when a nurse intentionally places a patient in a position of fear that he will suffer harmful or offensive contact (e.g. "Stop that, or I will restrain you"). Battery occurs when intentional, offensive physical contact actually takes place. In the health care context, claims for assault and battery most commonly occur when a nurse or doctor performs a procedure on a patient without informed consent. The physical contact need not result in a physical injury. For example, if you perform a procedure without informed consent, you may be sued for battery even though the patient suffers no physical harm. Keep in mind, however, that to prove a tort case, the plaintiff must make a showing of some kind of damages.

False imprisonment involves an intentional or willful detention of the patient without consent or authority to do so. Claims for false imprisonment most commonly occur in mental health or nursing home settings, when patients claim they were admitted and/or restrained against their will. Competent patients have a right to leave an institution, even if it is harmful to their health. If possible, you should have the person sign a form stating that they are leaving against medical advice (AMA), Restraining a patient without consent is another form of civil false imprisonment.

Fraud is "willfully" or intentionally misleading another person, with the intent to cause legal injury or deprive the person of a right. The nurse may commit fraud when (1) telling a patient a lie; (2) failing to disclose material information, such as during informed consent; or (3) making a statement in reckless disregard of whether it is truthful or accurate. Because actual fraud requires intent, it can never be the result of accident or negligence. In other words, ethics aside, lying to a patient rises to the level of fraud only if it is intended to cause him legal injury or deprive him of a right.

Invasion of privacy violates a person's right to be free from unwanted interference in her private affairs. The law holds that a person has a right to be left alone and not have her personal life held up for public scrutiny. The plaintiff must prove by a preponderance of the evidence that (1) her privacy was violated, (2) public disclosure of private matters occurred, and (3) a reasonable person would object to the intrusion. Examples are a breach of confidentiality, in which the nurse discusses the patient in the lunchroom; filming and making public disclosure of medical treatments without the patient's permission; searching a patient's belongings without permission (and disclosing search results); releasing medical information without the patient's consent; and releasing information to news media.

The right to privacy may conflict with the nurse's duty to report (e.g. reporting a sexually transmitted infection to public health authorities). Or the patient may be a public figure whose medical condition is of importance to the public (e.g. suppose the president has a heart attack). In such cases, you should consult with the agency's legal counsel, public relations department, and the nurse in charge of the unit to be sure that the patient's privacy is not violated.

Invasion of privacy is only one avenue protecting patient privacy. Patient privacy is also upheld by professional codes of ethics, nursing and institutional standards of care, and HIPAA. Note that writing in the patient's chart or discussing pertinent patient data with other involved professionals does not constitute public disclosure. Exceptions to privacy rules are made for mandatory reporting, for example, of suspected child abuse.

Negligence and malpractice actions may be the torts most familiar to health care professionals. Clients and family members who believe that care was unprofessional and did not measure up to standard practice file claims for civil liability. Negligence and malpractice are unintentional torts–nurses can be negligent without intending to do harm. **Negligence** is simply the failure to use ordinary or reasonable care, as dictated by the standards of practice and/or by what a reasonable and prudent nurse would do in the same or similar circumstances. Intent is not an element of negligence. When a nurse or other licensed professional health care provider is negligent and fails to exercise ordinary care, it is called malpractice. In other words, malpractice is simply the professional form of negligence, so it is the form of negligence most relevant to nurses in a professional context.

Elements of Malpractice Liability

To recover damages in a malpractice claim, *all* or the following four elements must be proven by the plaintiff by a "preponderance or the evidence."

1. *Existence of a duty:* The nurse-patient relationship creates a duty by the nurse to the patient. This duty forms when the patient seeks care and treatment from the nurse. Duty also arises when nurse see a patient in need or if nurse observe another provider committing malpractice.
2. *Breach of the duty:* The plaintiff may prove a breach of duty by demonstrating that the nursing actions failed to meet the standards or care. The standard of care will be established by a testifying expert, based on the state nursing practice act and a combination of any of the following sources of' nursing care standards:
    (a) The nurse's job description
    (b) Clinic or hospital policies, procedures, and protocols
    (c) Standards and guidelines adopted by professional organizations to which the nurse may belong, or
    (d) A treatise or textbook that expert witness views as authoritative.
    As a nurses they have a duty to assess, plan, implement, and evaluate care for their patients.
3. *Causation:* Proximate cause must he demonstrated in two distinct steps. Plaintiff' must prove that (1) the nurse's acts (or failure to act) actually *caused* the plaintiff's injury and (2) that the type or injury was foreseeable, or a logical consequence of the breach of the nursing standard.
4. *Damages:* Plaintiff must also prove that there has been an actual injury or damage. For example, even though a nurse administers the wrong medication, if no injury occurred to the patient, then he will not be able to prove a negligence case and recover damages under civil law. The patient may, however, file a complaint before the board of nurse examiners to obtain sanctions against the nurse under administrative law.

The Nurse as a Witness

The nurse also may become a witness in a malpractice action. As a witness, the nurse may testify either for plaintiff or defendant, in the capacity of either a fad witness or an expert witness. For example, nurse may be called as a **fact witness** in a malpractice case if they were an **eyewitness** (present when the act or omission occurred). Nurse could also be called to testify to information found in medical documentation. Nurses can testify to the facts contained in the patient record, even if they do not remember what happened (e.g. "I see from the record that I took the patient's temperature at 8:00 p.m.").

The standard of care in malpractice cases is often brought into evidence by expert testimony. In proving or disproving breach of duty, an **expert witness** has the role of testifying to (1) the actual standard of nursing care in the same or similar circumstances as the incident in question and (2) whether the defendant nurse adhered to the standard or acted as a reasonable and prudent nurse would have in the same or similar circumstances. An expert witness may be asked to summarize volumes of medical records or explain medical terminology to a jury. As a nurse, she/he may be called as an expert based on their specialized knowledge in an area. Experts are allowed to draw conclusions and form opinions regarding the facts in evidence.

Vicarious Liability

Each person is held responsible for his own acts of negligence. In certain circumstances, however, the law imposes vicarious liability. **Vicarious liability** is substitute liability, in which the employer is held responsible for injuries that occur as a result of an employee's negligent acts during the scope of employment. The most common legal theories of vicarious liability under which the nurse-employer relationship may fall include the following:

- *Captain of the ship:* Under this theory of legal liability, the doctor, not the actual employer, may be held liable for the acts of a nurse under the doctor's supervision. Even if the doctor is held liable, the nurse may still be liable for her own actions in the situation; this theory does not protect the nurse.
- *Borrowed servant:* In this instance, the first employer (e.g. an agency) directs the nurse to work for a second employer (e.g. a hospital), which has actual control over the nurse. The second employer then becomes answerable for negligent acts of the nurse. This would apply, for example, to agency nurses.
- *Respondent superior:* This is a Latin term meaning "let the master answer." Under this theory of liability, the health care employer (e.g. a hospital or clinic) becomes liable for the negligent acts of the nurse if the employer knew or should have known of the acts of the nurse. Again, the nurse is still responsible for her own actions and may also be held liable.

Litigation is the formal process that adjudicates legal issues, rights, and duties between the parties. In brief, the litigation process begins when the **plaintiff** (party seeking damages or other relief) files a document called a **complaint,** claiming that a **defendant** (person, persons, or an entity) has violated his rights. If you are the defendant in a civil trial, you will need an attorney. If you have personal liability insurance or can afford to pay an attorney, you can have your own attorney. Alternatively, the employing agency can secure the attorney. You must also notify your employer and your liability insurance carrier if you are served with a complaint.

Criminal Law

Criminal law defines offences that affect public welfare and security and impose penalties. It includes rules forbidding conduct that is injurious to public order and specifying punishments to be administered to individual who exhibits injurious conduct. It is concerned with relationship between individuals and governments and with acts that threaten society and its order. Misuse of controlled substances is an example of criminal conduct for nurses.

A crime is an offense against society that violates a law. Criminal acts are prosecuted in the criminal justice system. There are two classifications of crimes. A felony is a crime of a serious nature that carried a penalty of imprisonment for more than one year or death. A misdemeanor is crime less serious nature, and the penalty is usually a fine or imprisonment for less than a year. In nursing there are few crimes nurses would come out if they practiced within the accepted standards of care.

Two types of common law guiding nursing practice include criminal law and civil law. Although both types fall under both federal and state jurisdictions, there is a distinct difference in the purpose of civil and criminal laws. In a **criminal** case, the federal or state government seeks to penalize the accused for an offense against society. If found guilty under criminal law, a person may be fined, jailed, or even executed. Under civil law, in contrast, a defendant found liable pays money to the plaintiff.

A **crime** is whatever a legislative body has defined it to be. A **misdemeanor** is a minor crime, punishable by a fine and/or imprisonment for less than a year. For example, as a first offense, driving while under the influence of a substance would probably be a misdemeanor traffic violation. A felony is a crime punishable by death or more than one year's imprisonment. State laws may define felonies in other ways, as well. Homicide is a felony and generally leads to severe penalties under criminal law.

So-called mercy killing (active euthanasia) may result in charges of homicide in some states. The same is true of assisted suicide. The American Nurses Association defines **assisted suicide** as providing a patient the means to end his life, with full knowledge of the patient's intentions to do so. Assisted suicide is therefore a form of active euthanasia. It believes that nurses should not participate in active euthanasia (and assisted suicide) because such acts violate the Code of Ethics for Nurses and the ethical traditions of the profession.

Legal Practice of Nursing

To practice nursing legally, a nurse must possess a valid and current license from the appropriate agency in the state where the nurse is employed. Licensure is the process by which a competent authority grants permission for qualified individual to offer her or his skills and knowledge to the public in a particular jurisdiction where such practice would be unlawful without a license.

Licensure may have permissive or mandatory. However, there is a pronounced trend toward, compulsory licensure of professional and practical nurses. Where licensure is mandatory, unlicensed individuals are prohibited from practicing the occupation. When licensure is voluntary, unlicensed individual are denied use of protected title but are not prevented from performing work similar to that of persons licensed to use the protected title. The primary purpose of a licensure law is to protect public from injury by unqualified practitioners through enforcement of minimum practice standards.

The laws governing nursing licensure include the sections that specify licensing board or council, compositions and responsibilities, definition of the professional, personal, educational and evaluation requirements for licensure; testify procedures for determining proficiency; license giving procured for license suspension or revocation and penalties for practicing without license.

Licensing Board/Council

Members of the nursing licensure board appointed by the respective government form a list of candidates submitted by the professional organization. In India, we have Indian Nursing Council and State Nursing Council. It is customary for the councils to include representatives of the medical and educational communities and elected representatives of assembly or Parliament.

Requirements

Most nursing structure specify the following characteristics as requirement for nurse registered/literally:
1. Minimum age
2. Citizenship
3. Demonstration of moral character
4. Educational qualification—general and professional
    In addition to some states conduct tests prior to registration.

Suspension or Revocation

A license or registration can be suspended or revoked by the council of nurses conduct violates provisions containing in the licensory structure. Suspensions is the temporary denial of the right to practice nursing. Revocation is permanent withdrawal of permissions to practice nursing. Revocation may be instituted for those nurses found quality of gross immorality, illegal activity or malpractice. Malpractice is negligence or carelessness by professional personnel. Negligence is a carelessness or failure to act as an ordinarily prudent person would act under the circumstances.

Employee's Rights

Nursing a group are becoming more assertive. Consequently, individual nurses are beginning to assert their rights as plaintiff in employment claim cases. Employment conditions in which nurses are likely to be denied their rights. In such breach of employment contract, nurses can file suit against their employers to obtain their rights:
- Termination of an employee for union organising efforts
- Discrimination in employment on the basis of sex, age, religion and nationality
- Failure makes payment equally
- Failure to provide safe working conditions
- Failure to pay compensation during illness and injury related to work
- Sexual harassment and violating employment right to privacy.

Definition of Professional Nursing

Professional nursing practice encompasses the full scope of nursing practice and includes all its specialties and consists of application of nursing theory to the development, implementation and evaluation of plans of nursing care, for individuals, families and communities.

Professional nursing practice requires substantial knowledge of nursing theory and related scientific behavioral and humanistic disciplines. Professional nursing practice includes the following; but also extended or expanded according to needs:
1. Assessment, diagnosis – planning, intervention, and evaluation of human responses to health and illness.
2. The provision of direct nursing care to individuals to restore optimum functional or to achieve dignified death.
3. The procurement, coordination and management of essential client resources.
4. The provision of health counseling and education.
5. The establishment of standards of practice for nursing care in all settings, induce the development of nursing policies, procedures and protocols for a specific nursing.
6. The direction of nursing practice, including delegation to those practicing technical nursing.
7. The supervision of those who assists, in the practice of nursing.
8. Collaboration with other independently licensed health care professionals, in case finding and clinical management and execution of intervention as identified to be appropriate in a plan of care.
9. The administration of medication and treatments are prescribed by those professional qualified to prescribe under the provision existed acts.

Standards of Practice

Clinical guidelines, standards of professional performance, standards of practice, and *standards of care* are terms that are often used interchangeably. The legal definition of a **standard of care** looks to what a reasonable and prudent nurse would do in the same or similar situation. Standards of practice are developed by various legal and professional groups. Nurses are expected to follow the standards of care that apply to their area of practice, regardless of the source of the standards. In a court ohealthcaref law, various sources may be used to determine what constitutes reasonable care in a particular situation.

Nurse practice acts: Standards of practice may have their basis in the state nurse practice act, which identifies the minimum level of nursing care for a specific patient in specific circumstances. Standards set forth in nurse practice acts are mandatory; that is, they are set forth in statutes and enforced by authority granted by the state. For a summary of minimal acceptable standards of care required in a typical state nursing practice act.

Note: Standards 1 through 6, called Standards of Care, are found in Table 2.1.

Standard 7. Quality of Practice
The registered nurse systematically enhances the quality and effectiveness of nursing practice.

Standard 8. Education
The registered nurse attains knowledge and competency that reflects current nursing practice.

Standard 9. Professional Practice Evaluation
The registered nurse evaluates one's own nursing practice in relation to professional practice standards and guidelines, relevant statutes, rules, and regulations.

Standard 10. Collegiality
The registered nurse interacts with and contributes to the professional development of peers and colleagues.

Standard 11. Collaboration
The registered nurse collaborates with patient, family, and others in the conduct of nursing practice.

Standard 12. Ethics
The registered nurse integrates ethical provisions in all areas of practice.

Standard 13. Research
The registered nurse integrates research findings into practice.

Standard 14. Resource Utilization
The registered nurse considers factors related to safety, effectiveness, cost, and impact on practice in the planning and delivery of nursing services.

Standard 15. Leadership
The registered nurse provides leadership in the professional practice setting and the profession.

State Laws

Some of the state laws affecting nursing practice include mandatory reporting laws, laws regarding patient abandonment, Good Samaritan laws, and nurse practice acts.

Mandatory Reporting Laws

Most states have mandatory reporting laws related to communicable diseases, immunizations, and abuse of children, the elderly, and the mentally disabled. To different degrees, nurses must report to designated authorities (e.g. Child Protective Services) suspected physical, sexual, emotional, or verbal abuse or neglect of patients by health care workers or family members.

Elder abuse laws provide protection to those persons over age 60 "from actions that cause serious physical or emotional injury, caretaker neglect, and financial exploitation." Similar protections are provided to children under the child abuse laws and to the mentally disabled.

Nurse may be wondering how mandatory reporting is affected by privacy laws. To encourage reporting, states provide legal immunity if nurses have made the report in good faith. States vary in their requirements for mandatory reporting of abuse. However, in general, nurses who fail to report suspected abuse or neglect may be held liable under criminal or civil law. In some cases reporting is the responsibility of the employing agency rather than the nurse. Nevertheless, nurses should be familiar with agency policy and state laws for reporting.

Good Samaritan Laws

Good Samaritan laws provide protection for nurses who provide emergency care to people who have been injured (e.g. at the scene of an automobile accident). The specifics of these laws differ among states, so check your state's statutes. A few states may require that citizens stop to render aid, but most do not. For these laws to apply:

1. The assistance provided must have been voluntary (and the person is not paid).
2. The person receiving the help must not object to being helped.
3. Nurses actions must be a good-faith effort to help.

In general, Good Samaritan laws protect nurses from civil liability for damages resulting from their attempt to help people in need. Keep in mind, however, that even ill an emergency situation, negligence and gross misconduct are not defensible. These laws do not apply if the emergency occurs in a hospital. If you do provide emergency care, follow these guidelines to minimize your risk of liability:

- It have someone else call, as soon as you can.
- Do not leave the person unless you transfer care to an equally competent professional. This may mean a trip to the Emergency Department in some cases.
- Place the person under the care of a physician or advanced practice nurse as soon as possible, and follow their instructions.
- Do not accept money or any form of compensation from anyone.

Nurse Practice Acts

Each state legislature has passed a law designed to enact the state nursing practice act. Nursing practice acts are designed to:

- Protect patients or society.
- Define the scope of nursing practice.
- Identify the minimum level of nursing care that must be provided to clients.

A nursing practice act provides for the regulation of nursing practice by an administrative board, such as the board of nurse examiners (or the "state board of nursing"). These boards generally have the authority to regulate nursing practice and education within the particular state.

Licensing

Licensing is meant to ensure that practicing nurses have met the minimum competencies set by the state to protect the public. The licensing procedure varies among states but usually involves some or all of the following steps. The applicant must:

1. Successfully complete an educational program in a state-accredited schools or colleges of nursing.
2. Pass the prescribed RN, a computerized exam developed and administered under the direction of the National Council of Nursing or State Nursing Council.
3. Provide evidence of good mental and physical health.
4. Provide a statement of good moral character.
5. Pay a fee for entrance to the licensing examination.
6. Obtain a temporary license pending outcome of the first attempt at the licensure exam (Note: not all states give a temporary license).
7. Demonstrate competence in English/local language.

All nurses must be licensed by the state in which they practice. Currently certain states, through a **multistate compact** (agreement), allow nurses to be licensed in one state and to practice in all states participating in the compact. Multistate practice often takes place through technology, such as video conferencing and telenursing, where the nurse is licensed in one state, yet gives advice to a patient in another state within the compact.

Credentialing

Credentialing is a voluntary form of self-regulation used by many health care disciplines, including nursing. In the legal sense, credentialing includes accreditation and clarification. Having credentials implies that the person or agency has met higher standards than the minimum (e.g. licensure).

• *Accreditation:* Most nursing councils establish educational requirements for nursing programs and continuing education courses within a given state. The council usually requires that for a nursing program to be **accredited,** it must meet the requirements for accreditation established by the Indian Nursing Council or the respected Universities which runs nursing courses and by the state nurse practice act. This helps ensure that students get a well-rounded education and that patients are cared for by safe practitioners.

Accreditation also applies to noneducational facilities; for example, hospitals seek accreditation by the Accreditation Bodies of Health care Organizations. This is intended to ensure that a minimum standard quality of care is provided.

• *Certification:* Certification is another form of credentialing. Through certification and licensing, the board identifies nurses who are qualified for advanced practice (e.g. clinical nurse specialists, midwives, and nurse practitioners) or for certification in a subspecialty, such as emergency nursing or pediatric nursing. In some states, the board establishes the criteria for certification, including (1) educational preparation, (2) clinical experience, and (3) certification by other professional organizations. In other states, the nurse may obtain an advanced practice license only if she is first certified by a national organization such as a specialty organization. Not all states require certification for advanced practice nurses.

Disciplinary Procedure

Along with specifying the requirements to be able to practice nursing, state boards commonly also enforce the requirements by establishing disciplinary procedure. Generally recommends that the following unprofessional conduct result in disciplinary action: violation of the nursing practice act or rules, fraud, deceit, criminal activity, negligence, risk to clients, physical or mental incapacity, disciplinary action by another jurisdiction, incompetence, and unethical conduct.

The disciplinary procedure conducted by the state board may involve a series of all or some of the following steps:

1. Filing of the sworn complaint with the board by an individual, health care agency, or professional organization
2. Review of the complaint by the board of nursing
3. Hearing and decision by the board determining whether the nurse has acted unprofessionally and violated the state nursing practice act
4. Disciplinary action issued if the board finds that the nurse acted unprofessionally
5. Request by the nurse that a state court review the decision of the nursing board.

Nurse and Law

Legal responsibility in nursing practice means the way in which nurses are obligated to obey the law in professional activities. The law is the final authority for regulating activities of all citizens including professional practitioner. Disobedience of the law results in punishment.

It is always better for all nurses that they should understand their legal responsibility. When assuming a position to take up a client, as a professional nurse needs to update with the fast-changing and advancing professional knowledge to provide safe nursing to their consumer on the basis of their needs. And nursing professional should be aware of their limitations and shall be familiar with the law and nursing practice in their own country. So the nurses should not give any room for any tort, i.e. negligence for malpractice in their practice.

Tort is a civil wrong committed against a person or property. Torts may be subtle. They may be classified as unintentional or international.

1. Unintentional torts include negligence, for example, malpractice.

2. International torts are willfully acts that violate another's right, for example, assault, battery, deformation, invasion of privacy, false imprisonment and fraud.

A brief definition of torts, i.e. uninternational and international are as follows:

Negligence

Negligence is the failure of an individual to do something that a reasonable person would do or the commission of an act that a 'reasonably prudent' person means a person would do in a particular circumstances in standard of care to which a nurse is legally bound, would not do under similar circumstances. It is also defined as exposure of another person's property to unreasonable risk of injury. In other work' negligence' is conduct that falls below the standard of care. It is established by the law for the protection of others against unreasonable risk of harm. It is characterized chiefly by inadvertence, thoughtlessness, or inattention.

If nurses give care that does not meet appropriate standards, they may be held liable for negligence. The problems for which nurses are often found negligence in duties are the following:

1. Failure to use aseptic techniques where required.
2. Leaving a foreign object in a patient's body during surgery, i.e. errors in sponge, instrument or needle count in surgical cases.
3. Failing to respond promptly to patient symptoms impending disaster.
4. Failing to protect an infirm patient from falling, falls resulting injuries to patients.
5. Administering wrong medicine to a patient.
6. Administering a medication inappropriately, i.e. intravenous therapy, errors resulting infiltration or phlebitis.
7. Administering a care in such a manner that a patient suffers injury, e.g. improper handling of hot water bag, burns to clients.

Nurses are responsible for performing all procedures, correctly and exercising professional judgment as they carry out Doctor's orders and duties not ordered by for which they have authority. Any nurse who does not meet accepted standards of practice or care or who performs duties in a careless fashion, runs a risk of being found negligent.

Malpractice

Malpractice is a negligence or carelessness by a professional person. So it concerns professional actions and in the failure of a person, with professional education and skills to act in a reasonable and prudent manner. In other words, it is professional conduct, unreasonable lack of skill of fidelity in professional duties, evil practice or illegal or immoral conduct.

Issues of malpractice have become increasingly more important to the nurse as nursing's authority, accountability and autonomy have increased. There are essentially six elements that must be prevented in a successful malpractice suit as follows:

Nurse (defendant) owned a duty to the client (the plaintiff): There should be an evidence that the nurse owed a duty to the client, e.g. failure to monitor client's response to treatment.

Breach of the duty of care owed the patient: There should be an evidence that nurse failed to meet the prevailing standard of care, e.g. failure to communicate change in status to other care provider.

Forseeability not maintained: Forseeability involves the concept that certain events may reasonably be expected to cause specific results. For example, in children wards, falling of children from bed is common, i.e. there should be an evidence that client suffered due to lack of forseeability by the nurse, e.g. failure to ensure minimum standards are met.

Evidence of causation: It means that the nurse's actions or lack of actions directly caused the patients harm and not merely that patient had some types of harm. So there should be an evidence that nurse's failure to meet that duty likely to cause client injury, e.g. failure to provide patient education.

Evidence: Evidence that nurse's failure was direct cause of client's injury, e.g. patient's falls.

Evidence of damage: There should be an evidence of damage. Damages are valid as malpractice is non-intentional and unintended. Thus, the patient must show financial harm before the courts will allow a finding of liability against the dependent nurse or hospital.

The best way for nurses to avoid being named in law suits is to follow standards of care, give competent health care, and develop empathetic interpersonal relationship with the client. In addition, careful, complete and objective documentation are keys to avoid malpractice. Nurses also must keep current with practice. They should know and follow the policies and procedures of the institutions in which they work. Finally, nurses should be sensitive to the common course of client injury, such as falls. Poor rapport with clients is leading cause of law suits. Clients who believe that nurses performed duties correctly and were concerned with their welfare are unlikely to initiate a law suit.

Nursing managers are charged with maintaining standard of competent nursing care within the institution. Several potential sources, liability for malpractice among nurse managers may be identified-once identified, guideline to prevent or avoid these pitfalls can then be developed. On usual course of malpractice and nursing management are as follows:

Issues of Delegation and Supervision

The failure to delegate and supervise within acceptable standard of professional practice.

Issues Related to Staffing

- Inadequate accreditation standards – adequate number of staff members in a time of advancing patient requirement and limited resources.
- Inadequate staffing, i.e. 'short staffing'.
- Floating staff from unit to unit.

The nurse deals with many people including the client, and family, doctors and other nurses, and other health care personnel as well are employing agency. In nurse-client relationship several legal issues may rise. The brief idea of those issues are as follows:

Assault: It is any wilfull attempt or threat to harm another, coupled with the ability to actually harm the person. The victim believes harm care as a result of the threat. Assault may be subtle. For example, involvement nurse in handling an uncooperative client in the casualty room.

Battery: It is an intentional touching of another body or anything the person is touching or holding without consent. Injury is not a requirement. Informed consent is necessary in such cases. It has been allowed in mental health institutions.

Invasion of privacy: Clients have claims for 'invasion of privacy' which their private affairs, with which the public has no concern, have been publicized. Clients are entitle to confidential health care. All aspects of care should be free from unwanted publicity or exposure to public scrutiny. The precaution should be taken sometimes on individual right to privacy may conflict with public's right to information, e.g. poison case.

Defamation of character: It is the act of holding up of a person to ridicule, scorn, contempt within the community. There are two types of defamation—slander or libel.

- Slander defamation is in the form of spoken words, e.g. if a nurse tells a client that his doctor is incompetent, for which nurse could be held liable for slander.
- Libel defamation is in the form of written words, e.g. the nurse who writes such a comment could be held up for libel.

Informed consent: It is the authorization by the patient or the patient's legal representative to do something to the patient and is based upon legal capacity, voluntary action, and comprehension. It is a person's agreement to allow something to happen based on a full disclosure of facts needed to make an intelligent decision. One who performs a procedure on client without informed consent may be found civilly liable for committing battery. A patient's consent must be obtained before any medical, surgical of nursing treatment is administered. The patient's consent in his or her authorization for another to touch him or her for the purpose of care or treatment. Deliberate touching of another without authorization constitute a tort called battery. Knowingly threatening another will likelihood of immediate harmful or offensive body contact in a tort, called assault.

Assault and battery, which usually occur in conjunction, may be charged against a caregiver who uses undue force to restrain and untruly patient or assists with a diagnostic or treatment procedure for which the patient has not given informed consent. To be legally binding, a patient's consent must be based on full understanding of the proposed treatment. The required information that must be included in the informed consent are as follows:

- An explanation of the treatment-procedure to be performed and the expected results of the treatment/ procedure
- Description of the risk involved

- Benefits that are likely to result because of the treatment/ procedure
- Options to this course of action, including absence of treatment
- Name the persons performing the procedure/treatment, and
- Statement that patient may withdraw his/her consent at any time.

A signed consent form is required for all routine treatment, hazardous procedures such as surgery, some treatment programs such as chemotherapy and research. A client signs general consent form, when admitted. Separate, special consent forms must be signed by the client or a representative before specialized procedures are performed. The following functions must be verified for a consent to be valid:

- The person must be mentally and physically competent and be legally an adult.
- The consent must be given voluntarily. No forceful measures may be sued to obtain it.
- The person giving consent must thoroughly understand the procedure, its risks and benefits and alternative procedures.
- The person giving consent must have the opportunity to have all questions answered satisfactorily.

In many institutions the nurse assumes responsibility for confirming consent. Many nurses serve as witness to the signing the informed consent document and are attesting only to the voluntary nature of the patient's signature. When a nurse takes consent form for patients to sign, the nurse should ask if they understand the procedures which consent is given. If patients deny understanding or the nurse suspects they do not, the nurse is obligated to notify the doctor or nursing supervisor and to make certain that patients are informed before signing.

A patient refusing surgery or other medical procedure/ treatment, must be informed about any harmful consequence. If patient persists in refusing, the rejection should be written, signed and witnessed. In some instances, it is very difficult to obtaining the unforced consent, e.g. children and unconscious patient. In case of pediatric patients, patients are usually the legal guardians. If the patient is unconscious, e.g. consent must be obtained from a person legally authorised to give consent on the patient's behalf.

In emergency situations, if it is impossible to obtain consent from the patients or an authorised or unauthorised person, the procedure required to benefit the client (or perhaps save a life) may be undertaken without liability for failure to obtain consent. In those instances, the law presumes the patient would wish to be treated.

Negligence in Medical Field

The fundamental relationship that exists between a nursing staff and their patient is ordinarily that of an implied contract in which the nurse agrees to provide nursing care to their patient is obliged to pay for services.

1. He/she shall treat the patient with reasonable degrees of skill and nursing care expected of him/her in the circumstances in which he/she is placed.

2. He/she shall exercise due nursing care and diligence in the treatment of his/her patient.

Usually in all cases of alleged negligence against medical practitioner, the following issues require to be clarified: (a) duty, (b) damage, and (c) dereliction on duty.

Duty

As regards to duty, no much controversy is raised. In every case, where treatment has been undertaken by the doctor there is an implied contract in the legal sense.

Damage

As regards to damage, it is an accepted fact that negligence is an object of litigation in tort of which basis is the damage. This damage has been induced in financial loss due to prolonged treatment, complication, mental tort, deformity, disability or death. Each of claims directly or indirectly depends on the treatment given to the patient, the skill utilized and circumstances which will be discussed while discussing the other issues on this point are clarification needs to be made. Apart from culpability what stands on records or brands testified cannot usually is not contradicted even by the doctor. Only the relation of direct causation with dereliction duty is the vital point of evidence in the case.

Dereliction

As regards dereliction of duty, the main point to be established by the claimant, is the deficiency in skill (acquired in training and experience). It is the deficiency in the skill that leads to dereliction of duty that ultimately goes to confirm negligence (e.g. surgical cases – consent before operation, all required investigation before operation, nursing records of all procedures).

Negligence of Assignments of Nurses

A medical practitioner is liable for the negligence of an assignment or a lucum tenens employed by him. But he is not liable for the negligence of nurses at a hospital, when the nurses are not employed by him (Hancke V Hopper 1985) TC.

The institution, however, responsible for the negligence of its employees (e.g. kidney scandal in Bangalore, 1994).

It was held on Marris vs Winsbury while, that the resident medical officer in a hospital and the nursing staff are not the agents of a specialist surgeon who comes and performs an operation.

The Supreme Court on Syad Akbar vs State of Karnataka (1980, ISCC 30/180 Sec (cri) 59) has held that if negligence is an essential ingredient of the offence, the negligence to be established by the prosecution must be culpable or gross and not the negligence merely based on an error of judgment.

A doctor/nurse should not guarantee cure to his patient. All that he/ she can undertake is to make sincere efforts to discharge his/her duties as a medical person and using reasonable skill, care and judgment while treating the patient. He/ she should always bear in mind the importance of preserving a human life from birth till his death.

Common Causes of Nursing Lawsuits

Notice the overlapping in the following categories. For example, "failure to advocate" (by questioning medical orders) could easily lead to a "medication and treatment error." An error usually has many causes which may be:

- Medication and treatment errors
- Failure to follow standards of care (e.g. institutional policies, medical orders)
- Failure to assess and monitor
- Failure to communicate (e.g. failing to report in a timely manner, failing to report significant changes in patient status; poor communication)
- Failure to use equipment in a responsible manner; use of defective technology or equipment
- Failure to act as a patient advocate (e.g. to question incomplete medical orders)
- Infections caused or made worse by poor nursing care
- Failure to document.

Malpractice claims generally result from negligence, a nurse's failure to maintain standards of practice. The most common causes of nursing malpractice claims can be categorized according to where they fall in the nursing process: failure to assess and diagnose, failure to assess plan, failure to implement, and failure to evaluate.

Failure to Assess and Diagnose

The nursing duty to assess assumes four separate requirements. Failure to conduct anyone of these four requirements will result in a breach of the duty to assess.

1. The nurse has the necessary knowledge and skills to observe the patient and interpret the symptoms in the form of a nursing diagnosis.
2. The nurse actually carries out the assessment.
3. When the assessment reveals adverse symptoms, the nurse reports the symptoms to the appropriate provider and carries out the standard nursing care and ordered medical interventions.
4. The nurse continues to assess and monitor until the patient is stable.

One of the most common breaches of the duty to assess is failure to identify and ensure client safety needs, especially involving falls. Others include failure to perform an admission assessment, failure to complete a shift assessment, failure to make ongoing assessments of progress, and failure to listen to and act on a patient's complaints.

Failure to diagnose means not interpreting a patient's signs and symptoms or not recognizing when a patient's condition requires immediate notification of a physician.

Failure to Plan

The Nurses Association standards specifically require nurses to formulate a plan of care. The plan of' care may be written or unwritten, depending on state regulations. Agency policy and procedure may also require that the plan include or be based on protocols, critical pathways, or other tools, such as outcome objectives. Negligence or failure to plan may arise, for example, if you fail to include a turning schedule in the care plan for an immobile, poorly nourished patient who subsequently develops a pressure ulcer.

Failure to Implement a Plan of Care

At the crux of nursing care are the interventions implemented on behalf of the patient. Failure to implement a plan of care may encompass the following:

1. *Failure to respond,* such as not intervening to care for the patient's specific symptoms or expressed request for care.
2. *Failure to educate,* such as not answering questions, not teaching self-care measures, or not explaining procedures or equipment adequately on the patient's discharge.
3. *Failure to follow standards of care and institutional policies and procedures.* This most commonly occurs in the form of medication errors and failure to follow a physician's orders. It also frequently occurs from failure to use equipment responsibly. Among other reasons, a nurse may fail to follow standards of care when the unit is understaffed or the nurse is inexperienced.
4. *Failure to communicate* often comes up when a nurse fails to seek medical authorization for a treatment or fails to notify a physician in a timely manner when a patient's condition warrants action.
5. *Failure to document* the following in the patient's record: assessment data (e.g. drug allergies), patient injuries, medication administration details, patient progress and response to treatment, physicians' orders, and telephone conversations with physicians.
6. *Failure to act as an advocate.* Nurses must frequently intervene to prevent harm to the patient by other health care providers and by relatives and significant others. The following are examples of advocacy errors:
   (a) *Medical and discharge orders:* As an example of failure to advocate, suppose two physicians order the same drug for a patient, but under different brand names. The nurse does not recognize that two drugs are the same, so the patient receives twice the normal amount and has a toxic reaction. Other errors occur when the nurse does not question incomplete or illegible orders or does not question discharge orders when she believes the patient is not well enough to be discharged.
   (b) *Impaired nurses:* You have a duty under most state nursing practice acts to report impaired nursing practice (e.g. as a result of alcoholism or mental illness) to the appropriate licensing agency. Failure to do so is a failure to advocate for patients.
   (c) *Family and significant others:* Advocacy includes reporting neglect and intentional injuries to children, the elderly, and the disabled. Failure to do so may constitute negligence and/or violation of state statutes.

Failure to Evaluate

The duty to evaluate requires an ongoing cycle of the following:

1. Observing for changes after interventions and treatments.
2. Recognizing significance of the change. For example, if Mr. Ashoka's blood pressure (BP) is usually 140/88, a change to 150/90 after exercise would not be significant for him. But for Mrs. Lalitha, whose BP is usually 100/64, a change to 150/90 would be cause for concern.
3. Documenting or reporting symptoms to the appropriate person. If a change is significant, nurse have a legal duty to report the change to the appropriate provider and to document this change in the appropriate medical record.
4. Follow-up: Following up on responses to nursing interventions requires nurses to know the expected outcomes and side effects of medications and treatments, so that nurse can accurately interpret and document anticipated and adverse responses.

Failure to perform any of these aspects of evaluation may rise to the level of negligence.

Tips for Minimizing Malpractice

Most important reference for nurses avoiding malpractice and other legal risks is their states to have nurse practice act. The nurse practice act not only identifies mandatory standards of care, but also provides other legal safeguards for nurses. Be intimately familiar with the tenets of state nurse practice act. For other tips,

i. Observe Mandatory Standards of Care

One way to avoid legal risks is to know and observe mandatory (compulsory) standards of care: those required by law. For the minimum acceptable level of patient care identified in most state nurse practice acts.

Nurse must adhere to these standards to avoid sanctions by the board of nursing examiners and malpractice litigation.

Nurse must be knowledgeable not only about standards of practice identified in their state's nursing practice act, but also about all federal, state, or local laws, rules, and regulations affecting their area of practice as an RN. Ignorance of the law is no excuse for failing to comply with the law, and it is no defense in a malpractice suit.

ii. Use the Nursing Process and Follow Professional Standards of Care

Nurse must use a systematic approach in providing patient care, generally referred to as the nursing process. Use of the nursing process is standard nursing practice and is the legally acceptable model of decision making to be used in nursing practice. It is also a part of the patient care standards of many professional organizations. Nurses documentation should reveal that they have assessed, diagnosed, planned, implemented, and evaluated care. Nurses should also keep current with health care literature, continuing education, agency policy, and so forth, so that they will know what current standards involve.

iii. Avoid Medication and Treatment Errors

Medication errors are among the most common health care errors. Nurse must accurately administer medications and treatments to avoid harm to their patients. Furthermore, as part of their direct duty to the patient, nurses must also know the rationale and side effects of the medications, and should document desired, adverse, or side effects that occur. Nurses can help prevent medication errors by:

- Following the "six rights" of medication administration
- Investigating any patient concerns before giving the medication (e.g. the patient might say, "I didn't get one of those red pills yesterday.")
- Questioning physician orders that are incomplete or that seem inappropriate.

Treatment errors also frequently occur from misuse of equipment. For tips to help nurses to use equipment properly and safely.

iv. Report and Document

For every suggestion for minimizing malpractice risk given in this section, add the reminder: "Document what happened." Remember: "If it isn't documented, it wasn't done." If you are ever required to appear in court, the patient record may be the only proof you have of the care you gave. Do not make false entries or destroy entries in medical records, but do carefully record and detail all care you provide.

Charting

Be sure that nurses to make a record of all interaction with clients, as well as patients' refusal of or noncompliance with treatment. Document telephone conversations with physicians, including time, content of the conversation, and the action they took. Document the facts; do not editorialize (e.g. do not write, "I could not check on the patient as often as ordered because we were understaffed"). Charting should always be:

Factual
Accurate
Complete
Timely

Incident reports

If a standard of care is breached or an unusual incident occurs (e.g. a visitor or patient falls or is somehow injured), nurses should complete an **incident report** (also called *variance report* or *occurrence report*).

These reports are used, in part, for quality improvement in the agency and should not be used to discipline staff members or be placed in employees' files. Do not write "Incident report completed" in the patient record. In some states, an incident report must be made available as a part of discovery in litigation. In other states, however, only the client may be subpoenaed, but if the incident report is mentioned in the chart, the otherwise confidential report may be used as evidence.

When reporting an incident, be sure to identify the patient, date, time, and location dearly. Briefly describe the incident in factual terms. Quote the patient or persons involved if possible. Do not speculate, draw conclusions, or place blame. Identify any witnesses *to* the event or equipment involved.

Example

7:00 PM	Demerol 50 mg given intramuscularly instead of Demerol 15 mg.
7:30 PM	Patient's respirations: 8 per minute; BP 100/60; skin pale.
8:00 PM	Called Dr Krishna. Orders for naloxone (Narcan) 1 mg IV STAT.
8:05 PM	Narcan given as ordered. Resp 12/min, BP 118/70.

v. Obtain Informed Consent

Informed consent is the necessary authorization by the patient for any and all types of care, given with full knowledge *of* the risks, benefits, costs, and alternatives. For hospital admission and for invasive or specialized treatments or diagnostic procedures, the consent must be written and signed by the patient or the person legally responsible for the patient. Written consent is not necessary in an emergency if experts would agree that there was an immediate threat to life or health.

vi. Elements of Consent

To be legally valid, informed consent should include the following elements:

Completeness (disclosure): Health care consumers need a great deal of information to make educated decisions, and they should be told everything they would consider important in making a treatment decision.

Comprehension: The patient (or his surrogate decision maker) must understand the explanation. Ask the patient to describe in his own words the procedure to which he is consenting.

Voluntariness: This means that the patient must be free to accept or reject the treatment. He must not be pressured or coerced to give consent. There must be no actual or implied threat (e.g. "Mom, if you don't let them do this, I am not coming back to see you ever again"). Otherwise, the consent is not valid.

Competence: The person must have the capacity to understand the information and make a choice about *this* situation (e.g. the ability to decide what clothing to wear does not necessarily mean that the person is competent to decide whether to have a risky surgery). The law assumes that minors are not competent in this sense. If it is determined that the person is not a legally competent adult, parents, a legal guardian, next of kin, or a friend can make health care decisions, depending on the state's law.

Generally speaking, a competent adult has the legal right to consent to or refuse any treatment. However, this right does not always extend to situations where an adult is making the decision for a minor. A court sometimes will authorize treatment of a child against parents' wishes. In some states, a minor who is married, serving in the military, or living independently is considered *emancipated* and can consent to or refuse treatment.

Nurse's Role

As a nurse, nurses legal role regarding written consent is to collaborate with the primary provider, usually a physician. Nurse may witness a patient's signature on a consent form, but nurses are not legally responsible for explaining the treatments and options, nor for evaluating whether the physician has adequately explained them. Nurse must, however, determine that the elements of a valid informed consent are in place, communicate the patient's needs for more information to the care provider, and provide feedback if the patient wishes to change her consent.

In addition, nurses should be sure that they have the patient's informal, verbal consent for interventions they perform (e.g. urinary catheterization). The patient's coming to the agency for health care implies that she/he consents to usual treatment, such as injections and catheters. Therefore, nurses do not need to say, "May I catheterize you?" or "May I take your temperature?" for example. But you should always tell the patient what you are preparing to do, the rationale for it, and what she will feel. If the patient objects, discuss it further with him. If the patient questions you or objects, do not proceed until you have the patient's permission.

In addition to state statuts, case law, and agency policy, on Accreditation of Health Care Organizations standards provide valuable guidance regarding informed participation in decision-making.

vii. Attend to Patient Safety

Attend carefully to patient safety. Although institutional policies may address patient safety, following such policy is not an excuse for failing to meet this obligation to the patient. For example, even though you follow the agency's policy and keep the rails raised, nurse may still be found negligent if the patient falls because he called for help and no one came to assist him out of bed. Falls are a common cause of patient injury. Nurse should assess all patients for falls risk on admission to the health care setting and institute falls precautions when needed. Several useful tools have been developed for assessing falls risks.

viii. Maintain Confidentiality and Privacy

Maintain patient confidentiality, unless directed by law to do otherwise (e.g. when a patient is threatening to harm someone). The patient's family and significant others do not have an automatic right to confidential information regarding the patient. For example, parents do not have an automatic right to see the medical records of their child if that child is married and/or declared legally competent to make independent decisions. Of course, nurse need to discuss client's medical conditions with other health team members, but this docs not include chatting about the client's personal life or talking about the patient in the lunchroom. Discuss only health status and discuss it only with those involved ill the patient's care.

ix. Provide Education and Counseling

Nurse educate and counsel their patients. This includes providing information about their illness and medications all other procedures so that the patient can give truly informed consent and perform adequate self-care. It is not adequate just to give information. Nurse must be certain the patient has learned. Ask the patient to repeat instructions to you or to provide a return demonstration of a skill, such as self-injection of insulin.

x. Assign, Delegate, and Supervise According to Guidelines

Nurses should undertake patient care and make assignments in accordance with their education, knowledge, experience, and physical and emotional capability. Nurses must also consider the skill level of the unlicensed assistive personnel to whom they delegate, as well as the condition of the patient. For example, it would be negligent to assign a practical nurse to care for a patient on a ventilator without checking to be certain that the nurse has had training or experience with such patients.

The duty to delegate has a corresponding duty to supervise the care. For example, if nurse assign an aide to take vital signs, and must check periodically to see that the vital signs are taken and reported accurately.

As a rule, nurses will not be held responsible for harm that comes to a patient because of poor staffing, as long as the harm is not due to their own negligence.

xi. Accept Assignments According to Qualification

Nurses can accept an assignment consider whether the assignment is within their level of education, experience, and physical and emotional capability. Refusal to *accept* an assignment does not constitute patient abandonment. Abandonment is a "unilateral severance of the established nurse-patient relationship without giving reasonable notice to the supervisor so that arrangements can be made for continuation of nursing care by others."

Nurse also have a duty to ensure adequate staffing and patient coverage to the extent that they are able to do so. This means that nurse must report to the nurse in charge when leaving the patient care unit. Failure to do this may result in charges of patient abandonment. Never leave a patient, for example, in the preoperative holding area without making certain there is a nurse there to attend to the patient. This does not mean that nurse must work overtime (e.g. a double shift), as long as they give notice and explain their reasoning (e.g. that you are too fatigued to provide safe care).

If nurses do work a double shift, or if a unit is understaffed, they are still liable for any malpractice that they commit. Unfortunately, being "busy" and overwhelmed is not a defense for error, In addition, nurse have the duty to tell supervisors that staffing is inadequate; be sure to do it in writing.

xii. Participate in Continuing Education

Nurse have a duty to participate in ongoing continuing educational training in their area of practice and to keep up with new laws. Be sure to obtain documentation of their attendance. In some states, continuing education is mandatory for relicensure. In states where it is not mandatory, other standards of care still require that you obtain the education and training necessary to implement current nursing procedures and practices. Continuing education is available "for credit" through colleges and universities, hospitals and other health care agencies, in some nursing journals.

xiii. Observe Professional Boundaries

Nurses shall be careful to maintain professional boundaries, not only with the patient but also with other health care providers. Violations of professional boundaries may be physical, sexual, emotional, or financial in nature. Do not accept gifts from vulnerable patients or encourage attempts to have close personal relationships outside the health care setting.

Also be aware of and report the behaviors or staff members who commit sexual harassment. **Sexual harassment** involves the use of power over people lower in the power structure of the organization. It is defined as "unwelcome sexual advances, requests for sexual favors, and other verbal or physical conduct of a sexual nature" if submission to it (1) is a condition of employment, (2) interferes with job performance, (3) is the basis for employment decisions, or (4) creates a hostile and intimidating work environment.

If nurses witness or experience sexual harassment, their first step is to consult the agency's sexual harassment policy. Every agency receiving federal funding must have such a policy in place. It will tells that how to file a grievance, what forms need to use, to whom the incident is reported, and what the procedure is for hearing and resolution.

xiv. Observe Mandatory Reporting Regulations

Most states have laws requiring the nurse to report communicable diseases, known or suspected abuse of patients, and impaired or unsafe professional practice. When you observe violations of' the state's licensing regulations, you have professional and legal responsibility to report them to the appropriate authority. The "authority" varies among states; it may be your immediate supervisor, the board of nurse examiners, or a peer assistance program, often sponsored by the state nurses association. See the section "Mandatory Reporting Laws," earlier in this chapter. Also see the following discussion regarding impaired nurses.

Impaired Nurses

An **impaired nurse** is a nurse whose use of mood-altering substances renders him unable to carry out professional duties or responsibilities in a manner consistent with nursing standards. A recent national survey of 3600 nurses found that 17% reported heavy alcohol use, 6.9% reported inappropriate use of prescription drugs, and 3.9% reported illicit drug use. Most impaired nurses are identified by nonimpaired coworkers, yet in a recent study, only 37% of nurses who worked with impaired co-workers reported them to supervisors. So it is better to avoid unsafe practice is practice by an impaired nurse.

Unauthorized Practice

Nurses must also report the **unauthorized practice** of nursing. This includes reporting persons practicing nursing without a proper license. An example of a practice nurse should report their observation of unlicensed personnel administering medications in an agency.

Nurses have a duty to provide truthful information to the board of nurse examiners. This includes an obligation to correctly answer questions that affect the decision to license, employ, and certify the nurse.

Abuse

State laws also require nurses to report known or suspected abuse, rape, and communicable disease. Laws vary, so she/he will need to know what and to whom to report in their area.

Legal Safeguards for Nurses

In addition to the Good Samaritan laws and the Nurses Association Bill of Rights for Registered Nurses (both previously discussed), safe harbor laws and professional liability insurance offer some legal protection for nurses. The following are some legal safeguards provided to nurses.

Detecting Potential Chemical Dependence in the Workplace

The following may be signs of chemical dependence.

Absenteeism
* Frequent unscheduled absences
* Absences after payday or days off
* Higher than average absence for colds, flu, and minor illnesses.

Absent "On the Job"
* Long coffee breaks
* "Locked door syndrome (excessively long use of restroom)
* Frequent trips to Occupational Health Services for illness on the job.

Difficulty Concentrating
* Medication errors
* Omitted, illogical, incomplete, or illegible charting
* Taking more time to carry out assignments than is expected given the nurse's skill and experience
* Deterioration of handwriting during the shift
* Overlooking the signs of patient's deteriorating condition.

Inconsistent Work Place
- Alternating periods of high and low efficiency
- Minimal or substandard work compared to that of peers
- Frequent requests for help with patient assignments.

Physical or Emotional Problems
- Nervousness, excessive sweating, tremors of the hands
- Physical or emotional condition changes during the shift
- Lack of attention to personal cleanliness or grooming.

Decreasing Efficiency
- Omitting treatments; making bad decisions; showing poor judgment
- Requests to be changed to a less supervised shift.

Poor Relationships on the Job
- Mood swings, from isolation to angry outbursts
- Uncooperativeness
- Avoidance of contact with supervisors
- Patient complaints of irritability, roughness, or verbal abuse.

Medication-centered Problems
- Excessive use of PRN psychoactive medications or narcotics recorded for patients
- Increased waste or breakage of controlled substances
- Missing drugs, unaccounted-for doses
- Omission of dates or times from narcotic sign-out sheets
- Patient complaints about lack of pain relief.

Personal Life Interferes with Job
- Frequent or excessively long phone calls
- Visitors or unexplained errands during work shift.

Safe Harbor Laws

Safe harbor laws, found in the nurse practice act or other state laws, provide for exceptions to certain other laws. For example, they protect nurses from being suspended, terminated, disciplined, or discriminated against for refusing to do (or not do) soliciting nurses believe would be harmful to a patient, for example, refusing to assist with a treatment when a patient has not given truly informed consent. Under these laws, the nurse also has a right to ask for a peer review of either the situation or directives that the nurse believes would violate the nursing practice act. When the situation occurs, nurse must tell their supervisor that you are invoking the safe harbor provision of the nurse practice act. As soon as possible, request and complete the appropriate safe harbor form.

Professional Liability Insurance

Professional liability insurance provides some legal protection from nursing malpractice claims. If nurses are sued, for malpractice, the insurance company pays for the attorney's fees and for any judgment or settlement, up to the limits of the policy. Most insurance policies have **exclusions** (items not covered by the policy). If the patient's claim arises out of excluded activities, the insurance company will not pay for the costs of litigation. The following are common exclusions:
- Transmission of acquired immunodeficiency syndrome (AIDS) from the nurse to a patient
- Sexual abuse of a patient
- Injury caused while under the influence of drugs or alcohol
- Criminal activity
- Punitive damages (damages awarded to punish the defendant for egregious acts or omissions).

There are two types of malpractice coverage. **Occurrence-type** insurance is most often recommended for nurses, because the policy covers malpractice claims for any injury or damage occurring during the time the policy is in force, regardless of when the lawsuit occurs. **Claims made** insurance provides coverage only for malpractice claims made during the term of the policy *and* for injuries that occurred during that period. Nurses should consult an attorney to decide which type of policy is best for them.

As a rule, if nurse work for a hospital or other institution, nurse will be covered by the institution's insurance. However, it covers you only while nurses are working within the scope of their employment. Nurse would not, for example, be covered if he/she volunteer one day a week at a free health clinic. Some legal experts recommend that you purchase individual liability insurance in addition to the coverage provided by the employer. Again, consult a lawyer before making a decision.

Nursing Student Responsibilities

Nursing student nurses are held to the same standards of care as are registered nurses. Nurse must be familiar not only with their state's standards of practice, but also with the policies and procedures in which they have their clinical experiences. Their instructor is responsible for making assignments that are within their competence and for providing clinical supervision. However, this does not excuse from own legal responsibilities. To help protect yourself and your patients:
- Prepare carefully for each clinical experience.
- Never attempt a procedure or make a judgment about which you feel unsure. If you lack the theoretical or practical knowledge for an assignment, notify your clinical instructor immediately.
- Notify your instructor or *a* staff nurse if your patient's condition changes significantly.
- Your nursing school nurse may require you to carry personal professional liability insurance. The school's policy will cover you only for the nursing care you give in your educational experiences. If you work, for example, as an aide, the school's policy will not provide coverage for you at work. Furthermore, you are legally permitted to perform only the procedures contained in your job description. For example, even though you administer injections in your student role, you are not licensed to do so in your role as an aide.

Ethical and legal issues are a major source of conflict for nursing practice. It is important to be clear in you mind that "legal" and "ethical" are not always the same thing. On the one hand, an act may be legal (e.g. abortion), even if you consider it unethical. On the other hand, you may believe that an action (e.g. assisted suicide) is ethically necessary, but the law may forbid it. You should be aware of the legal consequences that your ethical decisions may bring about. For a more detailed discussion of some major legal issues in nursing (organ donation, HIV/AIDS, abortion and other reproductive issues, life-sustaining medical treatment, DNAR orders, and advance directives.

Components and Characteristics of the Legal Process

Judicial or decision law involving the health care delivery system is increasing because issues being litigated between the consumer and health care provider.

Litigation (a law suit) begins when a complaining party (the plaintiff) files a document known as a complaint with the court. This document states the basis for the complaint and outlines the damages (compensation) sought by the plaintiff. The person at whom the complaint is directed is known as the defendant. The filing of a complaint is followed by the issue of summons, which is a court order advising the defendant that a law suit against him is pending. It further notifies the defendant what he must do with respect to the lawsuit and the time constraints involved by the defendant, once served, chooses to do nothing in response to the summons, such as hire an attorney or file a counter-complaint, the court may enter a default judgment against the defendant, which is based on the uncontested testimony of the plaintiff.

A defendant presented with a summons normally retains an attorney, who files a document called an appearance, which prevents the court from entering default judgment. The defendant, through his attorney, then files a response (answer) to the allegations made in the complaint. This response either admits or denies the allegations made. If the response by the defendant includes significant information not referred to in the original complaint, the plaintiff, through his attorney has the option to file a reply.

When all of the allegations by both parties have been addressed, the case is ready to move forward and the parties are said to be 'at issue'. Discovery procedures are then initiated, whereby relevant information is gathered by both sides. Depositions (testimony taken under oath) and interrogatories (written questions) of witnesses are taken from witnesses before the scheduled trail. During this pretrial period, efforts may be made either side to influence the outcome of the lawsuit. Such efforts include, but are not limited, to motions to dismiss the complaint, requisition to change the trail date, and offers to a settlement out of court.

If the motions to dismiss the lawsuit are denied and all other motions have been resolved by the court, the case then goes to trials. The court hears the evidence, comes to certain conclusions, and decides on verdict. Once the judge or jury reaches a decision and a verdict is declared either party may appeal that verdict to an appellate court. If an appeal is granted, the testimony and the procedures of the trail are reviewed by the appellate court. That court may choose to uphold or reverse the decision of the lower court. The right to an appeal is a constitutional right and serves as part of the system of checks and balances on the court system of the country.

Purpose of Legislation

Safeguarding the Public

1. The public safety is guaranteed because the practice of nursing is restricted to those accredited practitioners who would seek to provide the highest possible level of comprehensive care for the individual and the community taking into account the total need.
2. The individual is secured to the event of sickness or disability with no fear of anxiety of being cared for by an competent person.

Legal Safeguard in Nursing Practice

Licensure: All nurses who are in nursing practice has to possess valid licensure, issued by the respective State Nursing Council/ Indian Nursing Council. He/she is being in possession of license to practice which is her/his sole authority. Their practice is confined to that for which they have been prepared by a controlled educational program.

Hence, the purpose of the professional licensure on the one hand to secure to society the benefits which come from the services of a highly skilled groups and on the other hand to protect society from those who are not highly skilled, yet profession to be or from those who being highly skilled are nevertheless to unprinciple as to misuse their superior knowledge to the disadvantage of the people.

Good samaritan laws: In response to health professionals, fear of malpractice claims most states enacted' good samaritan laws' that exempt doctors and nurses from liability when they render first aid during emergency. A nurse who renders assistance at an accident site is held to be same standards of skill, competence, judgment that would be applied to a reasonably prudent person with the same preparation. These laws limit liability and offer legal immunity for people helping in an emergency.

Good rapport: Developing good rapport with the client is very important to prevent malpractice. A lawsuit is often circumvented when the nursing staff treats the client with warrants and caring. So nurses must never underestimate 'rapport' with the client in malpractice prevention. The ability to develop good rapport with clients is dependent on the nurse having good interpersonal communication skills, e.g. listening.

Standards of care: All professionals practicing in the medical field are held certain standards when administering care. Standards of care come from several sources including laws, organizational standards, and institutional policies and procedures. It is always better to follow standards of care to avoid malpractice and do not attempt anything beyond the level of competence.

Standing orders: Although a nurse may not legally diagnose illness or prescribe treatment, she or he may after assessing patient's condition, apply 'standing orders' or treatment guidelines have been established by the physician/ doctor as appropriate for certain problems and conditions. Each nurse supervisor is responsible for persuading the doctor in-charge of the unit to periodically review, sign and date any standing order than nurses are to implement in her or his absence. When a nurse has reason to question a medication order, she or he is expected to promptly notify the patient's physician of the reviewed problem, so that physicians can clarify or modify the order. Nurses do not take chance, if there is any doubt rises in their mind, and seek advise from the service of supervisors of anyone who authorised to do so. And it is always better to follow written orders instead oral orders.

Contracts: A contract is a written or oral agreement between two people in which goods or services are exchanged. Section 13 of the Indian Contract Act defines the word saying that two or more persons are said to consent which they agree upon the same thing in the same sense. Treating a patient without obtaining proper consent can lead to a charge of assault and/or battery. As stated earlier, assault in the threat of an unauthorized touching, battery is unauthorised touching of a patient.

The consent may be expressed or implied, it must be a free consent, i.e. without force, fear or fraud. It must also be a valid, i.e. free consent given by a person legally competent to give consent. Informed consent is a well-recognized doctrine based on the client's rights to autonomy. Section 90 of Indian Penal Code (IPC) excludes consent given under fear of injury under misconception of fact. It also excludes consent of a person of unsound mind, of persons under intoxication, and of a child below 12 years of age.

The other sections of IPC deals with consent are as follows:

Section 87: Act not intended and not known to be likely to cause death or grievous hurt done by consent.

Section 88: Act not intended cause death done by consent in good faith for person's benefit.

Section 89: Act done in good faith for benefit of child or in some person by consent of guardian.

Section 90: Act done in good faith for benefit of a person without consent.

Section 92: Deals with cases when consent cannot be obtained but the acts done by the doctors must be done in good faith and for the benefit of the person concerned. It protects the doctors and nurses from liability.

Professional nurses always seek to ensure informed consent, client's rights and full communication and the consent should be taken in written form specified the respective institution or Government.

Consent for operation and other procedures: A patient coming into hospital still retains his rights as a citizen and his entry only denotes his willingness to undergo an investigation or a course of treatment. Any investigation or treatment of a serious nature, or an operation in which an anesthetic is used, requires the written consent of the patient. A patient may give his own consent if he is of full age, that he has attained the age of 18 years or is a minor who has attained the age of 16 years.

None should be asked to sign an operation consent form before he/ she has full understanding of the procedures involved. The proposed operation is described on the consent form in general terms only. Leaving the exact extent of the surgery to the discretion of the surgeon, but a patient has the right to refuse surgery going 'beyond the extent to which he has agreed to admit. If he does so, or wishes further explanation, the nurse should refer the question to the surgeon before getting the form signed.

If a patient makes any reservation or condition even by word of mouth-when signing, the surgeon must be informed.

For patients under 16 years of age consent of the parent or guardian is normally obtained. In the event of any difficulty, the ward sister should inform the surgeon and the senior and the senior administrative officer. This also applies in those cases where the patient is unfit to give consent and no relative is available.

Correct identity: The nurse or the midwife has the great responsibility to make sure that all babies born in hospital are correctly labeled at birth and to ensure that at no time are they placed in the wrong cot or handled to the wrong mother.

All patients in general hospitals wear to identify bands, in order that mistakes may be avoided. It is very important that the correct band is given to each patient and these are normally checked as part of the admission procedure. With young children or unconscious patients even greater care must be taken to ensure correct identity.

Even patient before being given premedication for an operation should be labeled in the manner approved by the hospital. The label should state the patient's name and hospital number. Moreover, a written request stating the same details should be brought to the ward by the theater porters to ensure that the correct patient is taken to the right theater. In the theater it is the anesthetist's and the surgeon's responsibility to see that they have received the proper patient and that the correct operation is carried out. It is not the nurse's duty to indicate the exact area of operation which digit or whether the left or right side is to be operated upon. But the ward sister or her deputy may be responsible for making sure that before the patient is sent to the theater. The medical staff have indicated clearly the site of the operation and for reporting to the surgeon if this has not been done.

Counting of sponge, instrument and needles: Nurses advocate that sponge, instrument and needle counts be performed for all surgical procedures taking place in operation theater. When an instrument or needle is accidentally left in a patient's body, during surgery, the operating room nurse will probably be liable for any patient injury caused by the presence of foreign body. It is the responsibility of the nurse administrator to establish policies and procedures for sponge, instrument and needle counts in the nursing units, for surgical procedure and also minor diagnostic and treatment procedure involving instruments.

During operation the scrubbed nurse must check the number of all instruments, needles, swabs and packs on her trolley and, as the operation proceeds, check that each item used is returned to her. She will then have to carry out a final check before the body cavity is closed. If any doubt arises she must inform the surgeon, who should delay his final closure until a recount has been taken place. At the conclusion, the theatre nurse in-charge and the surgeon sign the operation register stating that a correct final count was obtained.

Drugs maintenance: The two Acts which control the use of poisons in medicine are as follows:
1. The misuse of Drugs Act, 1971.
2. Dangerous Drug Act, 1965 and 1967.

The Misuse of Drugs Act: It is the aims at checking the unlawful use of the drugs liable to produce dependence or cause harm if misused. Drugs affected by this Act are referred to as controlled drugs and are divided into 4 schedules.

The Dangerous Drug Act: The common drugs controlled under the Dangerous Drug Act include the following:

Cocaine, dimorphine (heroin), levorphanol, methadone, morphine, opium, pethidine and others.

Medical practitioners and registered dentists may prescribe preparations containing these poisons. A prescription must bear the following:
1. Patient's name and address
2. Date
3. Signature of prescriber
4. Total quantity to be supplied, in words or figures.

Every general practitioner is required to keep a record of all purchases of these drugs, and of the amounts issued to individual patients.

In hospitals the use of these drugs is under strict control, although minor variations in details may occur in individual institutions.
1. A special cupboard is used for storing such drugs, and this should be marked 'CD'.
2. The cupboard is kept locked, and the key carried on the person of the state registered nurse in-charge.
3. Renewal of supplies can only be obtained by an order signed by a medical officer; and the drugs can only be given under the written instructions.
4. Each dose of drugs administered must be entered into special registers provided for the purpose, with the date, patient's name and time of giving. The persons giving and

checking the drug must sign this entry. While administering drug, it is always remembered that five 'R's, i.e. right patient, right drug, right dosage, right time and right route.

In most of the hospitals it is a rule that each dose given must be checked by two persons, one of whom should be a state registered nurse. This person should see the bottle from which the drug is taken, and check the dose with the written prescription.

All bottles containing controlled drugs should be marked conspicuously with a special label.

The hospital pharmacial usually checks at intervals the content of the correct drug, cupboard and compares its contents with the records of the register.

Accidents or injury: A patient should sustain injury while in hospital he may bring an action against the hospital authority or against the person to whom he attributes the injury – this may be a member of a medical, nursing or ancillary staff. The hospital has a certain degrees of responsibility for the actions of its staff, but a member of the staff who has been negligent or incompetent and has so caused loss or injury to a patient may be found guilty of culpable negligence and damages will then be awarded against her personally. In the case of a student nurse, it may have to be shown that she has received proper instruction in the procedure undertaken, for example, where a burn has been received from an unprotected hot water bottle.

Accidents can arise to visitors or employees of the hospitals through negligence in such matters as cleaning equipment placed on stairways polish or grease left on the floor, faulty electrical equipment or torn furnishings. Hospital staff should constantly be alerted to the risks entailed and bring them to the notice of the persons concerned or the proper authority. In the case of a pure accident where no negligence or incompetence is involved there is no liability at law.

An action may be brought against the hospital several years after the accident has occurred. It is therefore necessary that at the time of the incident an accurate and full record should be made on the special form provided. This form should contain a complete factual statement of how the accident occurred, of the kind of steps taken, e.g. whether or not X-rays were made, and should list the names of witnesses and of the medical officer called to carry out an examination.

Self discharge of patient: When the patient demands to discharge himself the nurse on duty should try to dissuade him and should inform the medical officer concerned with his care. If the patient is adamant, each hospital will follow its own procedures. It is probable that a senior administrative officer will see the patient and ask him to sign a written statement to the effect that he is discharging himself against medical service. Should he refuse to sign, a note this effect will have to be made and signed by two-witnesses one of whom is usually the administrative officer (by two witnesses, one of whom is usually) concerned and the other the nurse in-charge at the time. The patient must be allowed to leave, except in the case of a mentally disordered patient who is subject to restriction order or where it is felt he may be danger to himself or others, when he may be detained for three days to enable an order to be obtained.

Professional confidence: Guarding the confidence of the patient is an ethical duty of the medical and nursing professions and nurses must take care never to discuss personal informations received by nature of their position, except with senior members of the staff. No confidential information should be divulged to relatives nor friends, or should details of the patient's condition be passed on to his employer as this may cause loss of the patient for which the nurse may be legally liable. This does not mean that near relatives should not be informed of the patient's progress.

Documentation: It is by far the best once a lawsuit is filed. The medical record is a legal document and admissible in court as evidence. It enjoys a privileged status in that it is presumed to be an accurate account of what is transpired. This is because it was written at the time of occurrence, by someone with knowledge of events and before litigation was initiated. From litigation standpoint, the jury often assumes that if something has not charted, it was not done. Nurses should give themselves credit for care they provided thoroughly documenting it in the medical record. While documenting it in the medical record, it is better to use formats of documentation for each activity specified by the respective institutions or Government.

Patient's property: In the department of health, social security requires all hospital under its care to inform patients that the hospital cannot accept responsibility for valuable of money unless they have been handed over for safekeeping money of an unconscious patient admitted as an emergency should be listed, checked by two nurses and put in safe keeping.

While a patient is in hospital, the nurse has no right to go through his locker or personal property without his consent. Searching his possessions may be justified if it is suspected that the patient intends to injure himself or others and has the means to do so. Yet, even in such a case, the nurse will be wise to have a witness.

When a patient dies in hospital his possessions must be recorded in the property book, but money and valuable should be listed and packed separately. The property will then be checked and the book signed by the two persons, usually a nurse and the ward sister or her deputy. Strictly speaking the property should be handed over to the executors to the deceased, but unless property of considerable value is involved, it is usual to hand it over, against a receipt to the next of kin. This may be the responsibility of an administrative officer and in this case the nurse should on no account give property or valuable to relatives or friends of the deceased. Care must be taken in the descriptive terms used; for example, yellow metal is safer term to use the gold and white metal than silver or platinum since the relatives may refuse to accept an article made of base metal that has been incorrectly described.

Making of wills and signing of legal documents: Most hospitals have a rule against or discourage nurses from signing legal documents or witnessing signatures during their professional duties. This is to protect the nurse and should be documented and challenged later, on the ground of the unfitness of the patient. However, the nurse has the duty to pass on immediately any request of this nature on the part of the patient, so that the services of a solicitor may be obtained or those of a hospital administrative officer, who will assist the patient in every way, even in drawing up a simple will, if so required.

Suspicion of theft: The nurse is cautioned not to make accusation of theft against any hospital employee except to a senior trained colleague since without sufficient evidence she may easily lay herself open to an action for slander. The nurse is also cautioned against the all too ready habit of borrowing as this could result in a charge of and conviction for theft.

This refers to hospital property as well as borrowing from a private person. Conviction in turn leads to disciplinary action by the general nursing council, which means that her name may be removed from the nurse's register.

Reporting: In some situations, nurses have obligations or are required to report certain communicable disease or criminal activities such as abuse, gunshot wounds, attempted suicide or rape to the appropriate authority.

Some 'Do's and 'Do not's for the nurses as guidelines for their safe practice are enlisted in Table 5.1.

Legal Responsibilities of Nurse

Responsibility of Appointment and Assignment

Nursing administrators are expected to be aware of legal restrictions affecting personnel appointment and assignment. A manager who departs from agency hiring policies can be held negligent if she or he appoints an employee, without appropriate screening and that employee later injures a patient. The nurse administrator has responsibility for staffing and supervising nursing units to ensure safe, effective patient care. Therefore, they have the authority to temporarily reassign a nursing employee from one unit to another to compensate for emergency staff shortages. In shifting, an employee to compensate for personnel shortage, a supervisor or manager must take into consideration the nurse's capability to discharge duties of the temporary position. In floating nurses to an intensive care unit to compensate for understaffing, the manager should reassign only those nurses whose education and experience have prepared them to perform all of the nursing functions common to an intensive care unit.

Each nurse has legal responsibility to make full disclosure of her or his background knowledge and skills and notify the nurse manager when given an assignment for which she or he is not qualified. The manager is also obliged to adjust the amount and type of supervision to fit the employee's level of maturity and experience. Less-experienced or less-skilled employees need more professional support and advice from the manager.

<table>
<tr><td colspan="2">Table 5.1: Do's and Do Not's Guideline's for Nurses</td></tr>
<tr><td>Do's</td><td>Do not's</td></tr>
<tr><td>

1. Document all unusual incidences.

2. Report all unusual incidents.

3. Follow policies and procedures as established by your employing agency.
4. Keep current year license to practice.

5. Perform procedures that you have been taught and that are within the standard scope of your practice.
6. Protect patient from injuring themselves.

</td><td>

1. Remove side rails on patient's bed, unless there is an order or hospital policy to do so.
2. Allow patients to leave the hospital or nursing home unless there is an order or signed patients to leave the hospital or nursing home unless there is an order or signed release.
3. Accept money or gifts from patients.

4. Give advice that is contrary to doctors' orders or the nursing care plane.
5. Give medical advice to friends and neighbors.

6. Witness a patient's will.
7. Take medications that belong to patients.
8. Work as a nurse in a state in which you are not licensed.

</td></tr>
</table>

Responsibility in Quality Control

The nursing administrators and the authority of the agency at all levels have a legal obligation to ensure nursing care quality. A nurse manager's legal responsibility for quality control of nursing service imposes a duty to observe, report and correct the incompetence of any patient care provider. Usually the head nurse or ward incharge is responsible for quality of patient care given by all personnels including medical in the nursing unit, whether or not these individuals have direct reporting responsibility to the head nurse.

Responsibility for Equipment

To protect patients and employees from injury, a nurse manager must ensure that all patient care equipment is fully functional and that defective equipment is promptly repaired or replaced. He/she must ensure that nursing personnels know how to operate sophisticated equipment, so that he/she is expected to provide instructions in proper care and storage of patient care equipment, even when, there is a service contract providing for maintenance by an outside contractor. Nurses also have duty to refuse to use equipment known to be faulty or that was not designed for use in the situation where it was ordered.

Responsibility for Observation and Reporting

Nursing personnels have more frequent and prolonged patient contact than other caregivers. Nurses are trained to detect significant symptoms and reactions. Consequently nurses have a legal duty to observe patients frequently and report findings that have diagnostic or treatment value of the patient's physician and other members of the patients treatment team. The nurse is expected to observe a patient more closely when his or her condition implies increased health risk. Infants, children, aged, disoriented psychiatric and critically ill patients require more frequent observation than other patients with no evidence of impending respiratory or cardiac emergency.

The nurse has a duty to record and report observations of a patient's condition promptly, so that the physicians can base treatment, decisions upto-date information about the patient's health needs. When the patients condition deteriorates to the point that immediate action is needed to save life, the nurse must report observations of the patient's worsening conditions to the concerned doctor in person or by any mean. The nurse has a duty to report improper medical care through appropriate channels in order to protect patients from doctor's negligence.

Responsibility to Protect Public

The nurse has a legal duty to protect the public from injury by dangerous patients. Each nurse manager or administrator should ensure that the agency in which she or he is employed has a policy describing the procedures to be followed when a patient with violent tendencies who threatens violence to others is discharged or escaped from the health care agency. The manager must ensure that nursing personnel follow the procedures to alert community member to the presence of a potentially dangerous patient in their midst.

Responsibility for Record Keeping and Reporting

Nurses have legal responsibility for accurately reporting and recording patient's conditions, treatments and responses to care. The medical record is a written or computerized account of a patient illness and treatment that includes information submitted by all members of the patient's health care team. The medical record is an information source document that should be used to plan care, evaluate care, allocate costs, educate personnel, research care measure, and substantiate legal claim.

Patient's medical record is essential to proper care, and the medical record is the property of the health care agency. However, patient has a property right to information contained in the report; the patient has right to inspect and copy the record after being discharged. However, it is not advisable to allow a patient to review his or her medical record without medical supervision and explanation, because patient is likely to mis-understand certain record notations.

Failure to record significant patient information in the medical record make a nurse guilty of negligence when the patient is injured because of physician's surgeon's ignorance of significant information, almost medical history, signs and symptoms. The medical record must be accurate to provide a sound basis for care planning. Therefore, errors in nurse's charting must be corrected promptly in a manner that leaves no doubt about the facts.

Every health care agency should have a policy and protocol that direct that an erroneous chart entry be crossed through, labeled or erroneous, signed by the employee who corrects the error and retained in the patient's record. Correct information should then be documented to replace the erroneous data. Pages of the record that contain erroneous and corrected entries should never be destroyed. Nurses who conspire with doctors and others to falsify a patient record for purposes of concealing a criminal violation may be found criminally liable.

All health personnels require to report certain instructions to concerned authorities such as child abuse, ophthalmia neonatarum–infant phenylketonuria, communicable diseases, births out of wedlock, gunshot wounds, suicide, rape and use of unprescribed narcotics. In reporting information about criminal acts obtained during patient care, the nurse must reveal such information only to the police, because it is considered a privileged communication.

Responsibility for Death and Dying

There are many issues surround the events of death. Death occurs when there is an absence of brain function, despite the presence of functions of other body organs. However, nurses must be aware of legal definition of death because they must document all events that, when the patient is in their care. Sometimes there will be issues of euthanasia, either active or passive. Active eutha-nasia is defined as intentional homicide, e.g. intentionally administering a lethal dose of morphine to a patient to cause death. An example of passive euthanasia includes, removing breathing support or with holding blood transfusion from a terminally-ill patient with irreversible brain damage, may raises legal questions.

In addition, documenting all events surrounding death, nurses have other specific legal duties which include, the nurses have the legal obligation to treat a deceased persons with dignity (wrongful handling is a grounds for a law suit) or a close family member (after death). A competent adult can legally give consent to denote specific organs and nurses may serve as a witness to this decision.

Legal Issues in Speciality Practice Areas

Maternal and Infant Nursing

Many legal issues are involved in the care of the mother and her infant. Generally, the causes of lawsuits for malpractice in this area may be divided into two categories who handling the mother and child. Lawsuits brought against physicians/doctors and nurses differ, reflecting the well-recognized differences between these professions and their responsibilities.

A likely, against a doctor who is incharge of looking after mother and infant might be one of the following:

1. Failure to diagnose a high-risk pregnancy.
2. Delay in performing a cesarian section.
3. Improper vaginal delivery of failure to perform a cesarian section.
4. Improper use of forceps.
5. Incidence surrounding inducting labor and the use of oxytocin.
6. Delay in arriving at the hospital.
7. Non-attendance at the delivery.

Common Causes for Lawsuits Against Nurses

Problems of medication: Nurses are authorised to administration of medication. So many allegations against nurses with regard to medication are such as improper client patient identification, wrong medication dosage, route or time, and failure to monitor side effects, e.g. nurses are often involved in the administration of oxytocin for the augmentation of labor.

Failure to adequate client monitoring: Nurses are expected to monitor their clients at appropriate time intervals that depend upon the client's condition. Labor and delivery pose a unique monitoring challenge, in that, there are two clients to monitor– the mother and baby. The delivering mother must be adequately monitored to prevent any maternal complication during prenatal period. Nurses have legal responsibilities regarding fetal monitor during labor, and prompt monitoring will be continued during natal period, postnatal period to prevent complication related to mother and child in respective periods.

Failure to adequately assess the client: Every nurse, regardless of the area of practice, is expected by virtue of his or her licensure to be capable of performing assessment. The nurse is an impor-tant member of the health care team who is with the client constantly, and responsible for the minute by minute evaluation of the client progress. Nurses in all speciality areas must maintain the higher level of assessment skills.

Failure to report changes in the patient: Whenever the nurses assessment indicates that the client's condition has changed, the nurse must notify the concerned physician. For example nurse's failure in reporting changes in the child, denied the physician an opportunity to intervene and possibly save the child's life. When a nurse reports a client's changed condition to the physician, the nurse feels that the physician has not responded in a manner that is in the client's best interest, the nurse must proceed up the chain of command until proper medical care is given to the client. As a patient advocate, nurses must understand that failing to notify a doctor of a problem often leads to a delay in appropriate medical care being implemented. This in turn, can lead to an injury to the client and a lawsuit.

Abortions: It is one of the emotionally-changed issues confronting nurses. Nurses cannot be forced to participate in procedures they find morally offensive. Nurse has right to refuse to assist with abortions. However, nurses cannot attempt to stop an abortion being performed. She can assist with abortion if it is performed under medical treatment of pregnancy Act (MTP Act).

The nurse also has a legal obligation to take care of a patient who has undergone an abortion or who is being treated for complications of an abortion.

Nursing care of newborn: There are certain legal requirement in providing nursing care for newborns, such as properly identifying the infant's mother pair as soon as possible with fingerprints, footprints and wristbands, or blood samples for PKU testing when required by law. Standards of practice include, providing a clear airway, clamping the umbilical cord, applying antibiotics or silver nitrate to the eyes, and minimizing stress of dying and keeping infant warm. Resuscitation equipment must be in the delivery room. When a stillborn is delivered, the nurse must record all events about the delivery. Although the atmosphere in delivery room is disquieting the nurse must complete legal requirements by careful documentation.

Pediatric Nursing

As in all areas of nursing practice, negligence can also involve pediatric clients. Pediatric nurses are responsible for preventing children in their care from accidentally harming themselves. Cribs which sometimes have a restraining device over the top, are designed to keep infants and toddlers from climbing out of bed and injuring themselves. All poisonous substances and share objects should be kept out of the reach of children. Children should be kept under constant surveillance to minimize opportunities for accidental harm.

It is advisable that the health care professional including nurses should report to the concerned authority if they come across the suspected cases of child abuse or neglect. Those who do not report such causes may be liable to civil or criminal legal action.

Medical-Surgical Nursing

As in the case of pediatric clients, disoriented adults may require some form of restraints to prevent accidental self injury. Standard care, laws and regulations about the use of restraints and supervision apply to nursing practice with medical-surgical patient. Siderails are available on most hospital beds for adult patients. Some disoriented older patients may also require belt restraints to prevent them falling out of bed. If patients fall out of bed and injure themselves, they may bring a lawsuit against the nurses and hospital. As in all areas, here also there is a need to avoid malpractice and negligence. Nurses are responsible for performing all procedures correctly and exercising professional judgment. As they carry out doctor's orders and duties not. ordered, but for which they have authority. Any nurse who does not meet the accepted standards of practice or who perform duties in a careless fashion runs a risk of being found negligence. Some common acts of negligence in medical surgical nursing are as follows:

Overlooked sponges, instruments, needles: In the operation theater, it is a responsibility of the nurse to count the sponges, instrument, needles before the closure of the abdomen or any cavity. The nurse may be liable if he/ she makes an error in the count.

Burns: The professional nurses require to know the cause and effect of any heat application so as to avoid burns. Some of the common heat applications are applications of hot water bags, heating pads, double sitz bath, etc. The nurse could be held liable if she/he neglects to take proper safety measures prior to application of such measures.

Falls: The nurse could be held liable if a patient falls from the bed or due to improper securing of patient on examination table or improper application of restraint or provision of a proper bed for an unconscious patient or a child.

Injury: It s due to the use of defective operation or supplies, e.g. defective bed pans injure patients. The nurse could be held liable if she uses equipment or supplies then she/he knows to be faulty, e.g. the use of unsterilized guaze of surgical dressings.

Injury due to administration of wrong medicine, wrong dosage and wrong concentration: Administration of medicine without prescription by the concerned authority, mixing up of poisonous and non-poisonous drug in cupboards leading to errors, and failing to identify right patient for right medication in right dosage at right time, considered as negligent act can be liable to be used.

Loss or damage: The nurse is held liable if a patient's property is lost when it has entrusted to her/ his care.

Assault and battery: Failure to take the informed consent of the patient prior to any procedure, treatment, investigation or operation, the nurse could be held liable.

Failure to report accidents: The nurse has a moral and legal responsibility to report to the concerned authority any accidents, losses or unusual occurrences. Failure to do this is an act of negligence.

Failure of maintain accurate record and reports or removing a position of record: It may also make the nurse liable.

Nurses working in critical care units are also legally accountable for performing their duties. Critical care nurses require additional training and on-going intense education to provide them with information about advances in care methods to handle high tech machines and electric and electronic apparatus in addition to other critical care nursing measures. The possible legal problems for critical care nurses are associated with use of electronic monitoring devices. No monitor can be considered totally reliable and nurse must not completely depend on it. These may be electrical hazards. The equipment should be checked routinely by engineers to ensure that patients will not receive any electrical shock.

Psychiatric Nursing

The practice of psychiatric nursing is influenced by the law, particularly in concern for the right of patients and the quality of care they are receiving. In the past 20 years, civil, criminal and consumers rights have been established and expanded through judicial decision. Previously, powerless and neglected groups such as the mentally ill now using the legal system as both a form for the expression of legitimate grievances and as a vehicle for social change. Many of the laws vary from state to state, and professionals are required to become familiar with the legal provisions of their own state because knowledge of the law enhances the freedom of both the nurse and patient.

A psychiatric nurse should be sufficiently acquired with the legal aspects of psychiatry so that she/he can be aware of the patient's rights and can avoid giving poor advice or innocently involving herself/himself in a legal entanglement.

In psychiatric setting, the process of hospitalization can be traumatic or supportive for the individual depending on the institution, attitude of the family and friends, response of the staff and types of admission. At present three major types are used: informal, voluntary and involuntary.

Informal Admission

Informal type of admission to the psychiatric hospital occurs in the same way as a person is admitted to a general medical hospital. That is, without formal or written application. The individual is then free to leave at any time, as he or she would be in a general medical hospital. The patient is often requested to sign himself out an agreement medical advice, but he or she is not required to do so.

Voluntary Admission

Under this procedure any citizen of lawful age may apply in writing (usually by use of a standard admission form) for admission to a public or private psychiatric hospital. He agrees to receive treatment and abide by the hospital rules. His reason for seeking help may be his own personal decision or may be based on the advice of family or a health professional. If a person is too ill to complete the admission process but voluntarily seeks help, a parent or legal guardian may request admission for his. In most states, child under the age of 16/18 may be admitted if his or her parents sign the required application form.

This is a preferred type of admission because it is similar to that of any medical hospitalization. It indicates that the individual acknowledges problems in living, is seeking help in coping with them and will probably actively participation finding solutions. The majority of patients who enter private psychiatric units of general hospitals are voluntary.

When admitted in this manner, the patient retains all his civil rights. These include such privileges as the rights to vote, possess a driving license, buy and self property, manage personal affairs, hold office, practice a profession, and engage in a business. It is a common misconception of the public that all admissions to a mental hospital involve the loss of civil rights.

If the voluntary patient wishes to be discharged from the hospital, most of states require that he give written notice to the hospital. In some states, he can be released immediately, in others he can be detained from 48 hours to 15 days before being discharged. This allows the hospital staff time to confer with the patient and family member and decide if additional inpatient treatment is necessary. If the patient will not withdraw his request for discharge, the family may initiate involuntary commitment proceedings and thereby change the states of the patient.

Although voluntary admission is most desirable, it is not always possible. Sometimes patients may be actually disturbed, suicidal or dangerous to self or others and yet rejecting of any therapeutic intervention. In these cases involuntary commitments are them initiated.

Involuntary Admission (Commitments)

Involuntary commitments are continuously recognized by the court on the basis of two theories; first, under its 'police power', the state has the authority to protect the community from the dangerous acts of the mentally ill; second, under its 'parens patriae' powers, the state has an interest in providing care for citizen who cannot for themselves, such as some mentally-ill persons.

Involuntary commitments do not always imply compulsion. It means that the request for hospitalization did not originate with the patients and may signify that either it was actively opposed by him or he was indecisive and did not resist. The criteria for commitment vary among states and reflects the confusion present in the medical, social and legal areas of society. Most laws justify commitments of the mentally ill on these grounds:

1. Dangerous to others
2. Dangerous to self
3. Need for treatment.

The impatient element appears to be whether the person can function in a reasonable manner in the outside world without becoming on undue burden on his family or the community. The vagueness of these criteria is reflected in patients committed in psychiatric hospitals. Those suffering from psychosis, account for less than half of all admissions, and the aged, the neurotic and others account for the majority.

State laws on commitment vary, but they attempt to protect the individual who is not mentally ill from being detained in a psychiatric hospital against his will for political, economic, family or other nonmedical reason. Certain procedural elements of the commitment process are common.

Action is begun with a 'sworn petition' by a relative, friend, public official, or any interested citizen starting the person is mentally ill and is in need of treatment. Some states allow only specific individuals to file such a petition. As examination of patient's mental status is then completed by one or two physicians. Some states require at least one of the physicians be a psychiatrist.

The decision as to whether the patient requires hospitalization is then made. Precisely who makes this decision determines the nature of the commitment. Medical certification means a specified number of appointed physicians make the decision. This power to certify is given to all physicians and not limited to psychiatrists. Court or judicial commitment is decided on by a judge or jury in a formal hearing. In this case, the court is required to notify the patient so that he can retain legal counsel to prepare for the hearing if he desires to contest it. A jury trail is not mandatory in most states but can be requested by the patient. Most states recognize the right of the patients if does not have one, administration's commitment is determined by a special tribunal of hearing officers.

If the individual is determined to be in need of treatment, the final step of the commitment process then occurs and he is hospitalized. This may be for varying length of time, depending on the needs of the patients (Fig. 5.1).

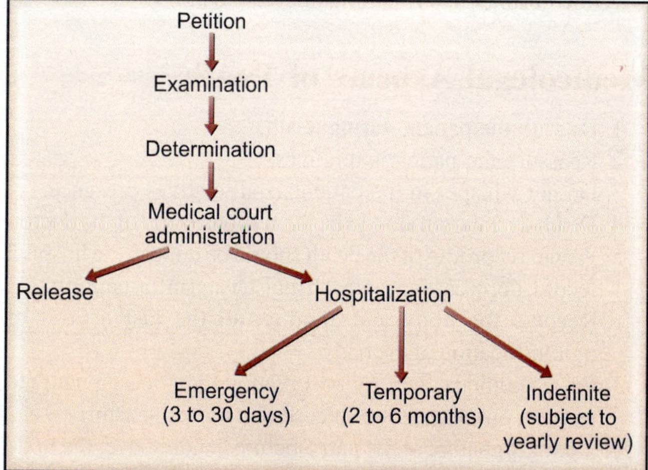

Figure 5.1: Diagrammatic model of involvement-commitment process

The procedures for admission for mentally ill persons in India are as follows:

Immediate restraint of the insane: If an insane person is dangerous to himself or others or if he is likely to injure or squander his property or that to others, he can be lawfully kept under the personal care of attendants or admitted into a mental hospital.

This may be imposed either by the consent of lawful guardian or without his consent if there is no time to obtain it or in an emergency situation. The restraint can last till the danger exists.

Reception direct into a mental hospital voluntary admission: The superintendent of the mental hospital, who are appointed by the state government has the authority to admit any person who is suffering from mental illness and desirous of submitting himself to psychiatric treatment.

Reception order on petition (admission through a magistrate): The family members of the patient have to submit petition for a reception order for admission. The petition must have attained the age of majority and must have seen the patient within 14 days of making the petition. The petition has to be on a special form giving all the particulars of the individual and has to be supported by two medical certificates, written on separate papers one medical certificate has to be obtained from gazetted medical officer or a medical practitioner declared by the government to be a 'medical officer' under Act IV of 1912, the other certificate has to be from any registered medical practitioner. Both the medical men has to examine the alleged lunatic independently, at different times and within seven days of applying for reception order.

The magistrate personally examines and makes the reception order after obtaining consent from the superintendent of mental hospital about his willingness to receive the lunatic and after obtaining in writing from the petitioner that he would been the cost of the maintenance. The only exception to this procedure is a lunatic who is dangerous and unfit to be at large.

Reception order other than on petition (admission through the police): Every officer in-charge of a police station can arrest any person whom he believes to be wandering or a dangerous lunatic, when the magistrate is satisfied about the lunacy of the person, then he is examined by a medical officer like the police surgeon or the civil surgeon. The police officer can adopt the same procedure for obtaining a reception order to a lunatic or a neglected or annually treated by his family or relatives or guardians.

The magistrate has to arrange for a suitable place for detaining the lunatic person till he is transferred to a mental hospital.

Reception after judicial inquisition: If a person is found lunatic after judicial inquisition, the high court or the district court has the authority to issue a reception order for such a person for admission in a mental hospital.

Reception of criminal lunatics: On the order of the presiding officer or a court they have to be admitted in a mental hospital. These criminal lunatics are of three types:

(a) Those who cannot stand the trail by reason of being of unsound mind and incapable of making their defence.
(b) Those who committed the crime, but were acquitted on the ground of being of unsound, mind at the time of committing the crime.
(c) Those who contracted the disease after imprisonment.

Discharge

While discharging psychiatric patient's authority has to follow the procedure laid down in the policies as follows:

- For informal admission and voluntary admissions, the discharge is initiated by the patient and status of civil rights retained in fault by the patient.
- For involuntary admission, the discharge is initiated by hospital or court but not by the patient and here none of the civil rights retained by patients. Sometimes it may depend upon the laws of the nation.

The type of discharge can be observed during discharging a psychiatric patient as follows:

1. *Conditional discharge* — patient may require to attend OPD or other special clinics. But they need no new admission.
2. *Absolute discharge* — a final discharge from the hospital, if he wants, readmission requires new admission procedure.
3. *Judicial discharge — can* be made on appeal by the parents or family need advice from the court for discharge.

The procedure practiced in India for discharging mentally-ill patients who are admitted in the respective mental health institution as follows (This is done under section 31 to 34 of the Indian Lunacy Act, 1912):

1. Any person except a criminal lunatic, can be discharged by an order in writing from the three visitors of the mental hospital, one of the visitors being a medical officer. The notice of discharge has to be communicated to the detaining authority.
2. In case of direct reception, the person can be asked for a discharge by serving a written notice of 24 hours.
3. In case of admissions made on petition, the petitioner has to apply to the superintendent. If the superintendent has opinion that he is not dangerous, and is fit to be at last he is discharged.
4. In cases where the admission is on a magistrate petition order, the person can be discharged after a judicial inquisition has found him to be of sound mind and capable of managing himself.
5. In cases, where the police has admitted the person, he is discharged after:
    (a) The family members or relatives agree in writing to take proper care, and
    (b) The superintendent or the visitor, who is a medical officer opinions that the person is fit to be discharged.
6. In cases of criminal lunatics, the visitors of the hospital have to report every six months about the person's state of mind to the authority which has ordered detention. As soon as they find that the person has become fit to stand the trial, they have to inform about the same to the authority concerned. The person is handed over to the prison officer for further legal action.

Discharge on Parole

Superintendent and the visitors of the mental hospital can discharge any person except a criminal lunatic, on parole and handover to the family members or the relatives. The period of parole ranges from a few days to a few months. This is a temporary discharge and if the person is to be a readmitted to the hospital, he has to be produced before the superintendent before the expiry of the parole period.

Absconding of the Patient

When a patient absconds from the ward, inform immediately to the nursing officer, hospital superintendent, local police station and his relatives. If the patient is a criminal lunatic, then the notice to be brought to the jail superintendent.

Patient's Rights

In 1973, the American Hospital Association issued a patient's bill or rights, which many general hospitals throughout the country have adopted psychiatric hospitals, however, continue to struggle with the issue of the basic civil rights of the individual. In recent years the civil and personal right of the mentally-ill patients have been supported in legislative acts throughout the country in retrospect. The new laws also reflect the registrations and discriminations suffered by the mentally ill in the past. Some plutes are now allowing the committed patient to restless all his civil rights, similar to the voluntary patient except the right to leave the hospital and to terminate treatment.

Medicolegal Aspects of Death

1. Be with the patient during death.
2. Reassure the patient's relatives.
3. Do not whisper in the patients and relatives presence.
4. Death declaration should be the responsibility of the doctor.
5. Proper recording of the death should be done in the hospital record, i.e. in case sheets each register and information book.
6. Respect the body and conduct all the last offices of mummification of the body.
7. Body should be kept for observation for at least 3 hours to prevent misconception in case of cadaver spasm.
8. Taking signature of the party, before handing over the body in death register and case paper.

In case of unknown patient

(a) Intimate the nursing superintendent thereby RMO for further arrangement and body should be sent to mortuary with proper packing and labeling.
(b) In case of MLC, intimate the police through the proper channel and send the body to mortuary for autopsy.

If the individual desired to donate his/her organs, information should be sent to the concerning authority for the removal of organ.

Records and Reports

The medicolegal patient's clinical record is a brief account of the personal and medical history of the patient results of diagnostic tests, findings of medical examination, treatment and nursing care, daily progress notes and advice on discharge.

1. The records are kept under the safe custody of the nurse in each ward of department.
2. No individual sheet is separated from the complete record.
3. Records are kept in a place, not accessible to the patients and visitors.
4. No stranger is ever permitted to read the records.
5. Records are not handed over to the legal advisors without the written permission of the administration.
6. All hospital personnels are legally and ethically obliged to keep in confidence all the informations provided in the records.
7. All records are to be handled carefully, careless handling can destroy the records.
8. All records are filed according to the hospital custom, so that they can be traced easily. Records could be arranged:
   (a) Alphabetically
   (b) Numerically
   (c) With index cards
   (d) Geographically.
9. All records are identified with the biodata of the patients such as name, age, ward, bed No, OP No. diagnosis, etc.
10. Medicolegal records are never sent out of the hospital without the doctor's permission. Reference is made by writing separate sheets and sending to the agency who requests for them, e.g. reference letters, discharge summaries.

Reports

Oral report should be accompanied by written reports.

Nurse is not only meant for providing care to the patient, she should also shoulder some of the responsibilities in respecting the patient's needs, and nurse should know her limitations for this knowledge of laws regarding health is essential. She should adapt some of the legal aspects while discharging her duty in every field.

Community Health Nursing

Community health nursing is the combination of nursing practice and public health practice. The community health nurse is subject to the laws relating to nursing practice and public health practice. The duties of all nurses become legally binding responsibilities for which the nurse is accountable. In addition, the community health nurse has many responsibilities that are unique to public health focused practice. Despite the broad nature and varied roles of community health nursing practice, two legal aspects apply to most practice situations, such as:

1. Professional negligence or malpractice.
2. Scope of practice.

The professional negligence is already discussed in this chapter. The issue of scope of practice involves differentiating between the practices of physicians, nurses and other health care providers. Scope of practice is assessed by the following:

1. Examining the usual and customary practice of profession.
2. Taking into account how legislation defines the practice of profession in a jurisdiction.

The usual and customary practice of community health nursing can be determined through a variety of sources which include the following:

- Contents of community health nursing education profession, general and special
- Experience of other practicing nurses
- Activities and statements, including standards of community health nursing professional organization
- Policies and procedures of agencies employing nurses
- Needs and interest of the community
- Literature, including books, texts and journals.

All these sources can describe and help determine the scope of the usual practice of community health nursing. Legal aspects of the roles and functions of the community health nursing, especially scope of practice and negligence will prove to be useful information for nurses in community health. Every community health nurse must consider legal implication of practice in each clinical encounter, i.e. health education, nutrition education, maintaining sanitation and supply of potable water, maternal and child health including family planning, communicable diseases control, school health, occupational health, mental health and so on. Because the community health nurse may be agent of the Government when implementing a particular health program, consideration must be given to the power of the state or the relationship of this power to individual right. In each clinical encounter, before treating the client, the community health nurse should know what standards of care applies to the situation. Standards of care can be learned from expert nurse witnesses and can be found in agency policies and procedures, nursing and health care literature.

Legal Role of the Nurse

Professional nursing practice is not determined by a simplistic adherence to patient's rights. Rather it emerges from an interplay between the rights of patients and the legal role of the nurse, and her concern for quality psychiatric nursing. There are three roles that the psychiatric nurse moves in and out in the process of completing her/his professional and personal responsibilities. These are the roles of provider of services, employer or contractor of service; and private citizen. These roles are played simultaneously and each role has attendant rights and responsibility.

Nurse as Provider of Care

All psychiatric professionals have legally-defined duties of care and are responsible for their own work. If these duties are violated malpracticed exists. Malpractice involves the failure of a professional person to give the kind of proper and competent care that is given by member of his profession in the community resulting in hard to the patient. Most malpractice claims are filed under the law of negligent tort. A tort is a civil wrong for which the injured party is entitled to compensation. Because under the law, everyone is responsible for his own tort, each nurse can be held responsible in malpractice claims. Under the law of negligent tort the plaintiff must prove the following:

- A legal duty of care existed
- The nurse performed the duty negligently
- Damages were suffered by the plaintiff as a result
- The damages were substantial.

It would be valuable, for the nurse to practice the following preventive measures to avoid possible lawsuits:

1. Implement nursing care that meets the standards of psychiatric-mental health nursing practice (Asst).
2. Know the laws of the state in which one practices, including the rights and duties of the nurse as well as the patients.
3. Keeps accurate and concise nursing records.
4. Maintain the confidentiality of patient information.
5. Consult a lawyer should any question arise.

Nurse as a Employee

As an employee, a nurse has the responsibility to provide adequate supervision and evaluation of those under her/his authority for the quality of care given, to observe her/his employers rights and responsibilities to clients and other employees, to fulfill the obligation of the contracted service adequately, to adequately apprise the employer of circumstances and conditions that impair the quality of care given, and to report observations of negligent care by others when and where appropriate.

Nurse as a Citizen

The role is particularly significant, because all other roles, rights, responsibilities and privileges are awarded because of the inherent rights of citizenship. In our form of democratic government these rights are inherent, civil rights, property rights, right to protection from harm, right to a good name and right to due process. These rights form the foundations for the extension of other legal relationships of the nurse.

6

Communication in Nurse-Patient Relationship

Introduction

Communication is the use of words and behaviors to construct, send, and interpret messages. It conveys varied messages, i.e. information, emotions, human acceptance or rejection. Communication is a dynamic, reciprocal process of sending and receiving messages. These messages may be verbal, non-verbal, or both, and they may involve two or more people. As such, communication forms the basis for sharing meaning and building effective working relationships among individuals, families and the health care team.

Communication is more than the act of talking and listening. Communication is:
- Sharing or transmitting thoughts or feelings.
- A way to meet physical, psychosocial, emotional and spiritual needs.
- A process—the act of sending, receiving, interpreting and reacting to a message.
- Content—the actual subject matter, words, gestures, and substance of the message.

Communication is one of the basic function of human life. The primary purpose of communication is to share information and obtain a response. People use communication to meet their physical, psychosocial, emotional, and spiritual needs.

Communication occurs at any of the three levels as given below:

- **Intrapersonal communication** is conscious internal dialogue, sometimes known as self-talk. Constructional affirmations, or positive self-talk (e.g. this will work) promote success in task. Nurses often engage in intrapersonal communication.
- **Interpersonal communication** is communication between two or more people. Face-to-face conversation between two people in the most frequent form of interpersonal communication. Nurses use this level of communication to gather information during assessment, to teach about health issues, to explain care, and to provide comfort and support. Since professional nurses are accountable for appropriate delegation of activities, they must also communicate effectively with the member of the nursing team and other health care team members.
- **Group communication** is interaction that occurs among several people. Small group communication occurs when engage in an exchange of ideas with two or more individuals at the same time, e.g. staff meetings, committee meetings, educational group and self-help groups. Public speaking is unique of group communication, when the speaker addresses a dozen to hundreds of people. Nurses often engage in public speaking to educate groups of people about health issues and to address professional groups at conferences and conventions.

Communication has two major components, i.e. content and process.

- **The content** of communication describes the actual subject matter, words, gestures, and substance of the message. It is the message everyone may hear or see.
- **Process** refers to the act of sending, receiving interpreting and reacting to a message.

Aspects of Communication

Communication is the process by which information is exchanged between the sender and receiver. The six aspects of communication are sender, message, method, receiver, feedback and influence.

1. **Sender:** The person who has a thought, idea, or emotion to convey to another person called the sender. Messages stem from a persons need to relate to others, to create meanings and to understand various situations.

   The sender initiates the conversations to deliver a message (content) to another individuals. The sender sometimes called the source or the encoder, uses verbal or non-verbal methods to transmit the message. Encoding refers to the process of selecting the words, gestures, tone of voice, signs and symbols used to transmit the message. Encoding is not always consciously intentional, but it is affected by the nature of the message, the relationship between the sender and receiver, and the mood of sender.

2. **Message:** The thought, idea or emotions are person sends to another person is called message. It is a stimulus produced by the sender and responded to by the receiver. The message is the verbal and/or non-verbal information that the sender communicates. It may be a conversation, a speech, a gesture, a letter, and so forth.

   Effective messages are complete, clear, concise, organized, timely, and expressed in a manner that the receiver can understand. The message must be appropriate for the situation and for the developmental level of the person receiving the message.

3. **Method:** The person sending the message must decide how to send the message. The method by which a message may transmitted is verbal or non-verbal. Method may be called as a channel. The channel is the medium used to send the message. Face-to-face communication is commonly used channel. Nurses frequently use touch as a non-verbal way to communicate caring and concern. Other channels include written pamphlets, audiovisual aids, recordings and telephone messages. The type of message, the purposes, and the size of the audience influence the choice of what channel is best suited for communication.

4. **Receiver:** The receiver is the observer, listener, and interpreter of the message. Interpretation, also called *decoding*, refers to relating the message to one's past experiences to determine the senders meaning. The receiver uses visual, auditory, and tactile senses to decode the message. If the decoding meaning matches the intended meaning, then the message was effective. However, messages are sometimes misinterpreted, especially when the receiver is not physically or emotionally ready to receive the message. Here the *physiological* component involves auditory, visual, and kinesthetic processes. The persons

psychological processes may enhance or hinder the receiving message. For example, anxiety may cause an individual to experience an alterations in hearing (act or power of perceiving sound) vision or feeling. The *cognitive* element is the "thinking" parts of the receiving. It involves interpreting stimuli and converting them into meaning, as in listening (interpreting sounds heard and attaching meaning to them).

5. **Feedback:** Once the receiver has received and interpreted the message, he/she may be stimulated to respond by providing feedback to the sender. Feedback is a response from the receiver that enables the sender to verify that the message received was the message sent. When these are nor the same, more messages are sent and received until the receiver understands the message sent by the sender.

   Feedback validates that the receiver received the message and understood it as the sender intended. Feedback may be verbal, non-verbal or both. Verifying the message avoids confusion.

6. **Influences:** Culture, age, emotions, language and attention influences both the sender and receiver as well as the situation within which they find themselves. All of these elements together are called a persons frame of reference. These influences sometimes helps communication, and sometimes they hinder communication.

Methods of Communication

1. Verbal Communication

Verbal communication: It is the use of spoken and written words to send a message. It is influenced by such factors as educational background, culture, language, age, and past experiences. Verbal communication is generally a conscious act in which the sender is able to select the most effective words to communicate a message. When delivering a verbal message, keep the following factors in mind.

Vocabulary: Health care workers have a large vocabulary of technical terms. However, laypersons are often unfamiliar with the language of health care and find its use intimidating or frightening.

Speaking/Listening: Speaking is usually thought of its verbal communication, but the receiver of a spoken message must listen. For communication to take place both speaking and listening must occur. Have you ever spoken to someone in the same room with you and received a nonmeaningful, senseless response from that person or no response al all? The other person probably was only hearing words but not listening to the message.

Communication experts say that people speak at a rate of 125 to 150 words per minute (WPM) but hear at a rate of 400 to 800 WPM. This extra time allows for distractions. Listeners are generally distracted because they are not concentrating on what is being said. Listening is one of the most difficult skills to learn and execute well.

Writing/Reading: The other method of verbal communication is writing. The receiver of the written message reads the words. The reader must understand the words and then attach meaning to them. With a written message there is generally no opportunity for immediate feedback. Therefore, great care should be taken to ensure clarity when composing a written message. A good example is charting. The physician may read the caregivers' notes after they have gone home, allowing no opportunity for immediate feedback. In such an instance, if the notes read that a client was "uncooperative," the physician would have little idea exactly what the caregiver meant. An entry of "refused to eat lunch, refused to get out of bed and sit in chair," however, is far more exact illustrating the clarity in writing that is essential to good communication.

Denotative and Connotative: *Denotation* is the literal (dictionary) meaning of a word. In contrast, *connotation* is the implied or emotional meaning of the word.

Pacing: The pace and rhythm of the delivery can alter the receiver's interpretation of the message. A rapid pace, which does not allow the receiver to track what the speaker is saying, is frustrating and can cause the receiver to lose interest. The pace must be slow enough for the receiver to interpret one thought before the sender moves on to the next thought. By pausing at intervals, the speaker also gives the listener time to interpret the words and respond.

Intonation: Intonation reflects the feeling behind the words. We get a sense of a person's "tone of voice" by noting the pitch (high or low), cadence (rising and falling of the pitch), and volume (soft or loud). These variables help a speaker convey confidence, enthusiasm, sadness, fear, anger, anxiety, or boredom. For example, experiment with the variety of ways you might state, ''Your tests results are in."

Pitch, cadence, and volume can either reinforce or contradict the message. When spoken at a moderate pitch and volume, with a falling cadence, the words, "I understand that I am to report at noon" can be a simple confirmation that the person has received the message. When spoken quietly, hesitantly, and with a rising cadence, it can convey the message that the person actually does not understand at all. Monitor your intonation and that of your clients as you communicate.

People tend to lose interest when someone speaks in a monotone (does not vary the pitch, cadence, and volume). Before presenting lengthy information, whether as individualized teaching or an address to a group, experiment with these variables to ensure that you maintain the listener's engagement with your topic.

Clarity and Brevity: Clarity in communication requires that you select words that convey the intended meaning and that you make sure your spoken words and the non-verbal message are congruent. You can achieve brevity by using the fewest words possible. A conversation that is clear and brief holds the interest of all parties and effectively conveys the message.

Timing and Relevance: Timing is crucial to the communication process. Before starting a conversation, assess your client. A person who is distracted by pain, hunger, or other physiological needs will not receive the message as you intended it. Similarly, a client attempting to cope with stressors, such as limited finances, an upcoming surgery, or a terminal diagnosis, may be unable to listen effectively.

The presence of others is another consideration in timing. For example, asking a client about a personal issue in a public corridor may inhibit his response. You will receive a different response if you ask the same question in a more private setting. In contrast, if you are instructing a client about a recommended diet, be sure that the person who is responsible for shopping and cooking is also present. If your client does neither in his household, he may pay little attention to your instruction.

Timing also involves relevance and response time. Communication is effective when both parties value the interaction and find the discussion relevant. For example, to teach your client about his medicines, choose a time when he is alert, pain-free, and not distracted, and begin by reminding him of the purpose of the discussion: "I'm going to teach you how to take this medication so that it effectively controls your pain." The interaction must also allow time for response. Incessant questions or one-sided conversations inhibit interaction. The conversation must also be relevant.

Credibility: Clients judge the credibility of the message on the credibility of the sender. A pattern of honest and timely response to patient concerns fosters credibility. As a nurse, you will be called on to provide information on a wide variety of topics. Provide information only if you are certain of the facts. A response such as, "I don't know, but I'll find out and let you know" is far more credible than an incorrect answer or guess.

Never lie to the patient; lying destroys trust. Lying can take many forms. If you tell the patient you will be right back with pain medication but do not return until she reminds you an hour later, she may doubt your credibility. If a patient care situation makes you uncomfortable it is best to acknowledge your discomfort rather than risk loss of credibility.

To be credible, your non-verbal communication must match your spoken words. This cannot be overemphasized. For example, if your client asks you if his wound is "ugly," he will pay attention to your facial expressions as well as your spoken response. If you respond that "The wound looks good," but you frown, the client will most likely believe that you are not being completely honest. This may jeopardize future interactions.

Humor: Humor and laughing can have a positive influence on attitude and healing. Laughter can create physiological changes that contribute to well-being and provide an emotional release in a tense situation. However, use humor cautiously. Humor is highly subjective and depends on cultural norms. Never direct humor at the client, disease process, or treatment team. Misused humor can have a negative effect on self-esteem, self-confidence, or the client's confidence in the treatment team. Consider the different affects the following uses of humor might have. Imagine

that your patient has had vomiting and diarrhea for the last 8 hours. When you enter the room you jokingly say, "Oh my! You look like you had too much to drink last night." Although the intent was to lighten the mood, this statement may offend your patient. In contrast, imagine that you notice that an older patient thoroughly enjoys visits from his young grandchildren. You might consider sharing with him an amusing story about your own children.

2. Non-verbal Communication

Non-verbal communication (or body language): It is the exchange of messages without the use of words. Verbal communication is a highly conscious activity in which we choose words to communicate. However, non-verbal communication occurs on a more unconscious level. Because non-verbal language communicates how someone is feeling, it more accurately conveys the true meaning of a message. It may thereby reinforce or contradict the spoken message.

Non-verbal communication, or body language, is a method of sending a message without using speech or writing. Communication without words, is done in many ways including gestures, facial expressions, posture and gait, tone of voice, touch, eye contact, body position, and physical appearance.

Non-verbal communication, which is part learned behavior and part instinct is generally unconscious, Feelings are believed to be most honestly expressed non-verbally because there is little conscious control over non-verbal communication.

Clients are particularly sensitive to non-verbal messages and seem to believe them. Nurses must therefore make every effort to be aware of the non-verbal messages they may be sending to clients, Consider, for example, the nursing skills that are not pleasant yet must be done. How would the client feel if the nurse had a facial expression of disgust or revulsion when emptying a bed pan?

Nurses must also be aware of and sensitive to the client's non-verbal messages. Many clients do not want to bother "busy" nurses, so they say they are fine or do not need anything when in fact they do. The perceptive nurse will observe non-verbal signs such as clenched fists, stiff posture, or a frowning expression and know that something is not right. The nurse would then proceed with further assessment to determine the reason the client is sending those non-verbal clues.

Facial Expression: Expressions of the face and especially the eyes are some of the most demonstrative forms of non-verbal communication. Facial expressions communicate joy, anger, sadness, concern, or fear. Raised eyebrows, staring, squinting, or darting eyes all convey meaning.

Smiling is one expression that is understood universally. In contrast, the interpretation of many other facial expressions is culturally dependent. For example, downcast eyes may indicate sadness, poor self-esteem, a desire to avoid the conversation, respect, powerlessness, or submissive behavior. In Western cultures, eye contact usually indicates an interest in the conversation and a willingness to communicate; however, in Eastern cultures, the amount of eye contact considered acceptable varies.

Although some people have very expressive faces, others do not. A big smile is easily interpreted as indicating happiness. Eyebrows can be very expressive, showing surprise, worry, thoughtfulness, or displeasure. The manner in which the forehead is wrinkled also sends a message.

Nurses must be very aware of their own facial expressions, especially when curing for a client under "unpleasant" conditions, such as when a client is vomiting or suffering from bowel incontinence. An expression of displeasure manifested as a "curled-up" nose or disgust is easily identified by the client. The client, often already embarrassed at requiring such care, will be reassured and comforted by a nurse's facial expression indicating caring, concern, and empathy.

Body Position: Body position is often a good indicator of a person's attitude. For example, crossed arms generally indicate withdrawal, although the person could be cold, open body positions, with the arms held freely at the sides, are usually taken to mean a receptive attitude.

Good posture, with the head held-up, and a purposeful gait are usually interpreted as meaning self-confidence, competence, and a positive self-image. Stooped shoulders, a downward-held head, and a shuffling gait generally convey low self-esteem, depression, lack of confidence, or apathy.

Body position, gait, and posture offer clues to a person's attitudes, emotions, physical well-being, and self-concept. When you see someone with an erect posture, head held high, and a quick gait, what do you think? In Western culture, these are non-verbal indicators of health and a sense of self-assuredness. In contrast, a slow, shuffling gait may signify someone who is ill, is depressed, or has poor self-esteem.

Personal Appearance: Clothing and personal appearance can provide clues to a person's feelings, socioeconomic status, culture, and religion. A person who is ill, tired, or depressed may not have the energy to invest in hygiene and grooming. Lack of attention to personal appearance is especially significant in an individual who typically engages in meticulous grooming. As with all non-verbal data, you need to investigate the meaning of personal appearance to avoid drawing erroneous conclusions.

Dress and adornments are powerful cultural clues. Does the patient dress in a style that differs from local custom? Are pieces of jewelry or religious medallions visible? These are clues to the patient's values, as well as the patient's socioeconomic status. Pay attention to these clues, but do not make assumptions from them. A person who wears an elaborate religious medal may like the ornamentation but not espouse the beliefs that are attached to the symbol.

A person's physical appearance says a great deal about that person. A clean, neat, appropriately dressed individual conveys a positive self-image, knowledge, and competence. A dirty, sloppy, or inappropriately dressed person conveys the message of "I don't care how I look" with the potential implication of

"maybe I am not too knowledgeable or competent," or "I am sloppy in what I do."

It is very important for every nurse to be clean, neat, and professionally dressed. Clients and families understand the non-verbal message that appearance conveys. Appearance does influence communication.

Eye Contact: Eyes it is said, mirror the soul. Have you ever seen joy, sadness, pain, or laughter in someone's eyes? It is very difficult to control these messages of the eyes.

Eye contact is generally interpreted as indicating in interest and attention, whereas lack of eye contact is thought to indicate avoidance, disinterest, or discomfort.

Tone of Voice: Tone of voice has been estimated to convey 23% of the context of a message. When the same words are said in different tones of voice, they can have very different meanings. Tone of voice might be pleasant, sincere, sorrowful, sarcastic, joyful, or angry.

Touch: Touch is a simple yet powerful form of non-verbal communication that even a newborn infant can understand. Touch can communicate caring, understanding, encouragement, warmth, reassurance, or affection. Of course, touch can also communicate anger, displeasure, or a lack or caring and understanding.

Many nursing tasks involve touching the client (i.e. bathing, dressing changes, ambulating). Touch, along with other non-verbal communication such as facial expression, posture, eye contact, and tone of voice, will convey the nurse's caring and acceptance. Most clients accept touch as an integral part of nursing care when it is done appropriately and professionally.

Touch can convey affection, caring, concern, and encouragement. Avoid using touch when dealing with someone who is angry or mentally disturbed, because the touch may be misinterpreted (e.g. as a sign of aggression or sexual attraction). Although touch can be highly effective, use it with conscious awareness of the situation, environment, and receptivity of the patient. For examples of therapeutic non-verbal behaviors and how patients may interpret them,

Gestures: Gestures are often reflected to as "talking with hands." Gestures may be used to help clarify a verbal message, to emphasize an idea, to hold another's attention, or to relieve stress. Finger tapping, fidgeting, or ring twisting generally indicates tension, nervousness, or impatience. Shaking a fist indicates anger, whereas pointing may be used to clarify directions.

Hand and body gestures emphasize and clarify the spoken word. They are good indicators of the feeling tone behind the conversation. Imagine that your client says, "I'm OK." What might it mean if he accompanies his statement with a broad grin and raised arms? What might it mean if, instead, he lowers his head to his hands?

Gestures vary widely among individuals and cultures, so use them with caution. For example, consider the gesture of a "V" made with the second and third fingers of the hand. To some people, this is a peace sign; to others, it is a victory sign; and still others may attach no meaning to it at all. Gestures can help you communicate with individuals with impaired verbal communication. Be careful, however, that you and the patient agree on the meaning of the gestures.

Factors Affect Communication

Environment: Communication is most successful in a favorable environment. A favorable environment is quiet, private, free of noxious smells, and at a comfortable temperature. As a beginning student, you are aware of the noises and distractions in the clinical setting. However, experienced nurses become accustomed to such distractions. Be sensitive to how the environment is affecting your client. Background noise is distracting, impedes hearing, and can create confusion. Lack *of* privacy hinders information sharing. Being around others in pain or distress creates anxiety and fear.

Think creatively to secure the most comfortable environment possible for communicating with patients and families. Hospital chapels, foyers, and activity rooms may be ideal locations for conversation. To discuss private matters, consider talking with the patient in a conference room rather than a shared room.

Developmental Variations: Physical and cognitive development, language skills, level of education, and maturity influence the communication process. Thus, you will need to modify your communication strategies to fit your client's developmental level.

Infants and young toddlers with limited language skills communicate non-verbally. Your response may combine verbal and non-verbal communication. For example, if a hospitalized 1-year-old cries out for his mother, you might cuddle the child with his favorite toy and explain that "Amma will be back very soon." Older toddlers and preschoolers have more verbal ability. Although they may prefer to have a parent present, they are likely to talk with you and answer questions. School-age children are usually quite comfortable interacting verbally. Pay attention to their vocabulary as they speak, and be sure to match it to the extent possible, using words and phrasing the child will understand. *By* the time children reach adolescence, most can process abstract concepts. As a result, they are usually able to understand disease processes, treatments, and other health issues. Bear in mind that children with chronic health problems that have required frequent interventions are often more knowledgeable than would be expected for their age.

Older adults may be affected by sensory alterations, such as hearing loss or vision changes, or any of a variety *of* health care problems that affect cognition.

Factors related to age affect communication. For instance, communicating with a child is different from communicating with an adult and depends on the child's age. Non-verbal communication, particularly touch, and facial expression can be understood by infants. Before learning to understand words, a child can interpret tone of voice and gestures. Preschool children respond well to communication involving toys or play situations.

They should be allowed some choices, but no more than two alternatives should be offered. As the child's vocabulary increases, more verbal communication can take place.

Elderly persons may have some degree of hearing loss or a slowed response time. The nurse should face the elderly client when speaking and allow time for response. The client should be addressed as "Mr." or "Ms." "Shri" or "Smt." Unless she or she asks to be called by his or her first name. These measures reflect respect to the individual from the caregiver.

Gender: Males and females communicate differently and may interpret the same communication differently. It has been stated that women communicate to form connections and establish relationships. In contrast, male communication styles focus on maintaining independence and favorable positions in a hierarchy. In essence, women want to "be connected," whereas men want to "be one up."

The roots of these communication patterns are early socialization differences. Traditionally boys are socialized to participate in hierarchical team sports. Through this play, they learn how to compete, strategize, and win or lose. In contrast, young girls are more likely to engage in one-on-one or fantasy play that requires cooperation and focuses on fairness and negotiation. This early socialization is carried over into communication patterns. Men are more likely to be comfortable in situations that result in a win or loss, whereas women are more likely to attempt to reach consensus.

Gender differences in communication are important to nurses for a number of reasons. Male and female patients may communicate their needs very differently. Similarly, the gender of the nurse may affect the response to the patient's requests. For example, a female patient might state, "I feel so lousy today." A female nurse may interpret this as a desire to talk. In contrast, a male nurse may discuss pain control.

Personal Space: People vary in the amount of physical space they are comfortable with when communicating. The distance that individuals engaged in communication maintain between one another is influenced by the relationship of the individuals, the nature of the conversation, the setting, and cultural influences describes four distinct distances influencing communication: intimate distance, personal distance, social distance, and public distance.

Intimate distance is the area immediately surrounding people that they define as their "private space." It is the distance people prefer to maintain between themselves and others during interactions. In Western cultures, intimate distance is within 18 inches of the other person. Within this distance, people can sense each other's smell and body heat and usually can hear each other speaking at a low volume. It is also at this distance that body contact occurs. As a nurse, you invade a client's intimate distance to perform assessments and procedures. You even breach a client's intimate distance when touching a hand or shoulder to offer support. It is important to recognize that this may make some clients uncomfortable. Before providing nursing interventions in the client's intimate distance, discuss what you are about to do. It is best to ask the client's permission, even for gentle touch, if you are in the slightest doubt about his receptivity.

Personal Distance is from 18 inches to 4 feet. Your interactions with clients and health care team members will commonly occur in this range. This distance facilitates sharing of feelings or personal thoughts and is appropriate to maintain when communicating caring or concern.

Social distance is a distance of 4 to 12 feet. It is used in more formal interaction or when communicating with a group of individuals at the same time. The volume of the spoken words may be loud enough for others to overhear. At this distance, individuals are not within range to be physically touched. Personal feelings and thoughts are shared less often at this distance. If you maintain a social distance from your clients, expect that the clients may be less willing to share personal thoughts. For example, if you stand by the client's door and ask how she is feeling, you will likely receive a more impersonal response than if you were to ask the same question at her bedside.

Public distance is considered to be beyond 12 feet. This distance requires loud and clear enunciation for communication. Public speakers and large educational groups use this form of personal space. This distance is characterized by a lack of individuality and a greater focus on the group or community.

Territoriality: Territoriality refers to the space and things that an individual identifies as belonging to him. Territories may be bounded and visible to others or may be defined by the individual in a way not noticeable to others. In a hospital setting, many clients consider everything within the curtain boundary to be their territory. Clients may be offended if you invade, rearrange, or interfere with this territory by moving furniture, discarding objects, or borrowing items from the client's room, even if they are institutional property. Be aware of this and request permission to rearrange your client's personal territory. Also recognize that hospitalized clients are not in their "home" territory and are therefore likely to be less at ease during interactions.

Sociocultural Factors on Communication: Culture and socioeconomic status strongly influence communication. Facial expressions, non-verbal communication, and even the selection of who to interact with are affected. For example, in some cultures it would be unacceptable for a male nurse to address and provide care to a female patient.

Education is another strong influence on communication. Vocabulary generally increases as well as the ability to discuss and understand concepts and abstract ideas.

Social status also plays a role in communication. Have you ever been present while a physician explained a treatment plan to a patient? Often the patient asks no questions or nods approval, yet barrages you with questions when the physician leaves. One reason for this behavior is that many clients perceive less social distance between themselves and the nurse. Consequently they are more likely to ask you questions or to discuss concerns with you. Social distance can also play a role in how health

professionals view clients. For example, you may see impoverished clients being treated with less respect than wealthy members of the community, although this is certainly not ideal.

Roles and Relationships: The roles of the sender and receiver and the relationship between them affects communication. Relationships affect the choice of vocabulary, tone of voice, use of gestures, and distance associated with the communication. Think of the way you interact with your instructor. Compare your approach with the way you interact with your classmates. What are the differences?

Many patients have preconceived notions about nursing. Some may view you as an authority figure. Others may perceive nursing as a lowly occupation and limit conversation with you to matters of comfort and hygiene. Still other clients become confused by the fact that many health care workers, such as medical assistants and nursing aides, call themselves nurses inspite of the fact that they cannot legally use the title. This makes it unclear whom the patient should speak with about concerns. If you are working with UAPs or other team members, be sure to clarify their roles with the patients.

As a member of the health care team, you will also need to communicate effectively with physicians and health professionals from other disciplines. Each of you shares the common goal *of* providing optimal patient care. This goal should guide the manner in which you communicate, whether at the bedside, at the nurse's station, in care conferences, or via the chart.

A person's emotional state greatly influences how messages are sent or received. Someone who is very anxious or upset, for example, may not hear what is said or may interpret the message differently than the sender intended. This same person typically speaks in an abrupt manner, loudly, and in harsh tones. The depressed person, on the other hand, typically says very little, speaking only one or two words or in very short sentences.

Culture: Each culture has its own standards of communication, especially with regard to non-verbal behavior. In the United States, for example, eye contact is considered a sign of openness and honesty. Those of Spanish heritage, however, believe eye contact to be disrespectful. Similarly, in many parts or Europe, a kiss on the cheek between two men is accepted. People from other parts of the world, however, may look suspiciously on this behavior.

Language: Language certainly influences communication. Speaking the same language assists people in understanding each other, although regional accents or dialects of a language can inhibit communication and understanding. When verbal communication comes to a standstill, non-verbal communication is often employed to assist. Any nurse who works in an area where there is a predominant second language should learn a few words or phrases in that language to help put clients at case and *to* facilitate their understanding.

The amount or attention each individual focuses on a given communication greatly affects the outcome. In selective listening, the receiver hears only what he wants or expects to hear. Pain or discomfort, physical or mental, may result in preoccupation, limiting the attention given to the communication.

Surroundings: Most of people do not want to talk about the intimate details of their health care concerns ill public. Thus, privacy should be provided. If the client occupies a room alone, the nurse should close the door; if the client shares a room, the nurse should take the client to a conference room or *to* another private place, if possible, to discuss personal information.

Therapeutic Communication

Therapeutic communication, sometimes called effective communication, is purposeful and goal directed, creating a beneficial outcome for the client. The locus of the conversation is the client, the client's problems, or the client's needs, not the problems or needs of the nurse.

Goals of Therapeutic Communication

Therapeutic communication has several goals or purposes. One or more of these goals guides each therapeutic communication between the nurse and client. The goals are to develop trust, obtain or provide information, show caring, and explore feelings.

Develop Trust: Clients and nurses are generally strangers when they first meet. The nurse then works to establish trust with each client. Examples of ways to build trust include answering questions honestly, responding to call lights promptly, and following through. When caring is shown, trust develops faster. Mutual trust established between client and nurse is termed rapport.

Obtain or Provide Information: The nurse obtains information from the client about general health and specific health problems. With this information the nurse can make an accurate assessment and plan of care.

The nurse provides information to the client from admission to discharge, beginning with the orientation of a new client to the hospital policies and routines. Sharing of information continues throughout the hospital stay as the nurse explains procedures, treatments, and tests; teaches the client self-care; clarifies instruction from other health care workers; and answers client questions. The discharge instructions constitute the final stage of information provision.

Show Caring: Two ways to show caring are offering a drink of water without being asked or fluffing a pillow. Knocking on the room door before entering and taking time to always greet the client by name are additional ways to show caring.

Explore Feelings: After rapport is established, the nurse can encourage the client to explore feelings. Many clients are anxious about their illness. Some have anxiety about being in the hospital and some fear the results of diagnostic tests. Some individuals will not admit they are anxious or fearful. The nurse is often able to help the client talk about feelings and reduce anxiety by

Activity	Statements to use with activity
Cover the client with a blanket.	"It feels chilly in here. Perhaps this blanket will help."
Assist the client to dress.	"I noticed you're having a little trouble getting your robe on. Perhaps I can help."
Serve a tray to the client.	"It's time to eat. I hope you're hungry because it really looks good."
Offer assistance.	"Here, let me help you. Perhaps together we can arrange these flowers."
Ask when leaving the room.	"Is there anything more I can do for you before I go?" or "I'm leaving now, but I'll be back in 20 minutes."
Move the client up in bed.	"You look so uncomfortable. Let me move you up in bed."
Make the client's bed.	"Now you have a nice fresh bed."
Regulate environmental temperature.	"It seems very warm in here. Perhaps if I turn the air conditioner up, it will help."
Turn the client in bed.	"Changing position really makes a difference, doesn't it?"
Straighten a pillow.	"Let me straighten your pillow for you."

using therapeutic communication techniques. Sometimes, only a clarifying statement is needed to alleviate fear or anxiety. Other limes, fear and anxiety are reduced by allowing the client to talk.

Therapeutic Relationship

The therapeutic relationship focuses on improving the health of the client, whether an individual or community. The client gains information and knowledge and works through issues, concerns, and problems related to health status, treatments, and nursing care.

Therapeutic communication promotes this helping relationship. It is client-centered communication directed at achieving client goals. It is used to establish the therapeutic relationship, provide and obtain health care information, and express interest and concern for the client and family.

The *therapeutic relationship* consists of four phases. As nurse you read about each phase, notice the fundamental role of client-focused communication.

The *pre-interaction phase* occurs before you meet the client. In this phase you will gather information about the client. As a student, you initiate this phase as you prepare for clinical days. The client also experiences a pre-interaction phase, which begins when she identifies the need for health care. This can be an anxious time for the client. In this phase, the nurse and client do not have direct communication.

The *orientation phase* begins when you meet the client. The goal in this phase is to establish rapport and trust. This phase begins with introductions, followed by an initial exchange of information. Information may include the client's purpose for the visit or chief concerns. Ideally there is time to exchange pleasantries and begin to develop a level of comfort. In some clinical situations, such as during an emergency, this phase is extremely brief. This phase ends when the relationship has been defined. During this phase, verbal and non-verbal communication occurs. All of the factors that affect communication (discussed above) influence the interaction.

The bulk of therapeutic communication occurs in the *working phase*, the active part of the relationship. During this phase, caring is communicated, thoughts and feelings are expressed, mutual respect is maintained, and honest verbal and non-verbal expression occurs. Key communication goals are to assist the client to clarify feelings and concerns. A professional relationship is courteous, trustworthy, and confidential, and accomplished by active listening and other techniques of therapeutic communication presented later in this chapter.

The termination phase is the conclusion of the relationship, whether at the end of the nurse's shift or on the client's discharge from the unit, facility, or service. Reviewing and summarizing help to bring the relationship to a comfortable conclusion. If communication has been effective, the termination phase prepares the nurse and client for future interactions. Unsuccessful communication may affect the client's health outcomes or understanding of his disease process, as well as affect the nurse's job satisfaction.

Behaviors and attitudes that enhance therapeutic communication include warmth, active listening, caring, genuineness, empathy, acceptance and respect, and self-disclosure.

Caring: Caring is an attitude that enhances communication as well as a goal of therapeutic communication. Caring is the basis of a nurse-client relationship and makes the client feel important. The client can easily identify a caring attitude.

Keller and Baker (2000) identify four steps to help communicate a caring attitude to clients:

1. *Connect with the client:* Make eye contact; be at eye level when speaking to client; address client formally by the last name.
2. *Appreciate the client's situation:* Listen carefully; focus on what client is saying; acknowledge client's point of view; express concern.
3. *Respond to client needs:* Clarify what is being asked; respond in ordinary language; let client know what to expect.
4. *Empower the client:* Find out what client knows about condition and acknowledge opinions: work as partner to develop plan of care: allow choices as appropriate; encourage questions.

Warmth: Warmth, expressed predominantly by non-verbal communication, makes the client feel relaxed, welcomed and unjudged.

While touch is an important method to show warmth, it must be used appropriately, Society dictates the touching that is appropriate in various situations. Communication may be greatly enhanced by holding a client's hand or pulling a hand on the shoulder. This touching provides a connection between the nurse and the client. Remember touch may not always be welcomed by the client.

Active Listening: As implied, listening is an active process requiring energy and concentration. It involves listening to the spoken words as well as being attentive to the non-verbal messages.

Responses from the nurses indicate that the nurse is really listening to the client. It is important that the nurse concentrate on the interaction at hand and not become distracted by other thoughts.

Genuineness: Effective communication is genuine. The nurse must be honest about personal feelings. Sometimes it is appropriate to cry with a client.

Genuineness means being truthful and not attempting to answer a question when the answer is not known. After admitting not knowing the nurse should after to find the answer and then do so. Knowing that being genuine builds trust, the nurse must use good judgment about confronting a family member, client, another health care worker, or expressing negative thoughts.

Empathy: Empathy, the capacity to understand another person's feelings or perception of a situation, is an objective awareness of, or a sensitivity to another person's feelings and thoughts. Although the nurse is not involved in the thoughts and feelings of the client, through empathy the nurse is able to understand and accept the feelings and thoughts of the client. Sympathy is different from empathy. In sympathy, the nurse shares in the feelings and thoughts of the client. These feelings and thoughts are generally related to a loss.

Acceptance and Respect: Acceptance of clients as individuals with values and beliefs of their own is an attitude that enhances communication. Nurses must accept the fact that clients may have different values and beliefs. It is called being non-judgmental when a client is accepted at face value.

Acceptance is shown by not expressing differing beliefs or values and by simply accepting the statements or complaints of clients. Clients then fed free to communicate and corporate in their care.

After acceptance comes respect. In order to understand clients as unique individuals, they must be accepted in a non-judgmental way, Acceptance and respect by the nurse lets clients know they can be themselves and they will still receive quality nursing care, even though they have different values and beliefs' than the nurse, Respect is shown when the nurse introduces herself and also addresses the client by name (preceded by "Mr.," "Mrs.," or "Ms.").

Self-disclosure: Sharing something about yourself such as thoughts, expectations, feelings, or ideas is termed self-disclosure. It does not mean sharing personal problems, a nurse who shares something, such as personal future goals in nursing, is trusting the client with that knowledge, The client who feels trusted will trust the nurse, and therapeutic communication is augmented.

Techniques of Therapeutic Communication

Certain techniques promote therapeutic communication. These techniques should be learned and incorporated into the nurse's manner of communicating.

Clarifying/Validating: Clarifying or validating are used when the nurse is not sure of the meaning of a message. Clarifying is the technique used to understand verbal messages. For example:

"Do you mean…?"

Validating is used to establish truth or accuracy. It is used for non-verbal as well as verbal messages. Examples are as follows:

"Are you saying that you did not get your medication today?"

"You are holding your side. Are you having pain there?"

Open Questions: Open questions encourage clients to express their own thoughts and feelings. *How, when, where,* and *what* are words with which to begin an open question. Open questions cannot typically be answered with "yes" or "no" or with just one or two words. For example:

"How has this medication affected your vision?"

"What did the doctor tell you about going home?"

Indirect Statements: An indirect statement calls for a response from the client. Because it is a statement and not a question, the client does not feel quizzed. Indirect statements allow the client to determine the direction of the conversation, thus helping the client maintain a feeling of independence. Examples of indirect statements are as follows:

"Tell me about your physical therapy today."

"You were telling me about. . ."

Reflecting: Reflecting is repeating all or part of a message back to the sender. Often, reflecting focuses on feelings and helps the sender "hear" the message from the receiver. This allows the sender a chance to clarify the message and shows that the listener is trying to understand the message. Reflecting can be a very useful technique if not overused. Examples include the following:

Patient: "I'm really nervous about my surgery tomorrow. My friend got an infection after her surgery, I'm very frightened,"

Nurse: "You are anxious about your surgery and afraid of getting an infection?"

Paraphrasing: Paraphrasing is restating the message in the receiver's own words, This lies the sender know how the receiver interpreted the message, Clarification can then be done if necessary. The sender is aware that the receiver is listening and trying to understand the message. For example:

Nurse: "You are afraid that you might have complications from your surgery?"

Summarizing: Summarizing is stating in a sentence or two the major points of a conversation to let the sender know what was heard. The sender can then add more information or clarify what was originally heard. An example might be as follows:

"Let me see, we have discussed…"

Focusing: Keeping communication focused on the topic being discussed can sometimes be difficult. Clients may wander off to other topics, or the topic may shift to the nurse. It is important to keep the focus on the client and not the nurse, For example the nurse could say:

"We can discuss that in a minute, right now I'd like to discuss…."

"A minute ago you mentioned that you'd had an upset stomach after taking your medication. Tell me more about that."

Silence: Silence is one of the most difficult but effective techniques to use. In the dominant culture, most people are uncomfortable with silence and feel the need to fill the gap by saying something. Silence can be a valuable therapeutic technique, allowing the client time to gather thoughts or check emotions. Silence also gives the nurse a chance to decide how best to continue the interaction. If the nurse employs behaviors to enhance communication during the silence, the client will often verbalize thoughts or feelings.

Communication skills can be improved by:

- Minimizing distractions
- Making eye contact
- Listening
- Checking congruency of words spoken with non-verbal cues
- Using clear, easy-to-understand, terminology and explaining medical terms when used
- Asking client to paraphrase important information.

Please see Table 6.1 for verbal therapeutic communication techniques.

Barriers to Communication

Employing behaviors and attitudes to enhance communication will be of little use if the nurse also employs barriers to communication. Although the communication process is intense, it should not be threatening. The purpose in learning about things that block communication is to enable the nurse to identify them and avoid using them. Many mistakes can be corrected when identified. A simple "I'm sorry, I shouldn't have said that" will often take care of the situation. Practice helps sharpen communication skills. The most common barriers are discussed following.

Closed Questions

Questions that can be answered with "yes" or "no" or with only one or two words are considered closed. After the one- or two-word answer, communication is usually ended: there is no other avenue for the communication to follow. This type of question is appropriate in certain circumstances, however, such as when taking a health history or in an emergency. Examples of closed questions are as follows:

"Is the pain gone?"

"Did you sleep well?"

Cliches: Cliches are overused, trite phrases that are almost meaningless. They are impersonal and often used when

Table 6.1: Therapeutic Communication Techniques: Verbal

Verbal techniques	Benefits	Examples
Closed Questioning Focused and seeks a particular answer; usually requires and elicits only a "yes" or "no" or one- to two-word answer	Provides a very specific answer to a very specific question	"How old are you?" "How many children do you have?" "Have you had a tetanus shot in the past 5 years?"
Open-ended Questioning Does not require a specific answer and cannot be answered by "yes," "no," or a one-word response; usually begin with words like "how," "what," "can you tell me about," "in what way"	Allows the patient to elaborate freely; useful in assessing feelings; elicits the patient's thoughts without influencing the response	"How do you feel about having surgery tomorrow?" "What concerns do you have about going home?" "How are these symptoms different from the last time you were ill?"
Restating Repeating to the patient what the nurse believes to be the main point that the patient is trying to communicate; tone of voice rises slightly at the end of the phrase as if asking a question	Lets the patient know if the nurse heard what was said; encourages the patient to offer additional information	Patient: "I'm not sure how I will manage the housework when I get home. My husband will expect me to do the cooking and cleaning just like always, and I don't think I'll be able to do it so soon after my surgery." Nurse: "Your husband will expect you to do the cooking and cleaning when you get home?" Patient: "Yes. I don't think he understands how difficult this surgery has been for me, and how weak and tired I feel."
Paraphrasing Restatement of the patient's message in the nurse's own words	Verifies that the nurse's interpretation of the message is correct	Patient: "I wish I was having a general anesthetic instead of a spinal. My neighbor had a relative who had a spinal anesthetic and never walked again." Nurse: "You are concerned that you might have complications from the spinal anesthetic?" Patient: "I am sure." Nurse: "I can have the anesthesiologist come talk to you some more about the risks and benefits of a spinal anesthetic. Would that be helpful?" Patient: "Oh, yes. Would you do that, please?"
Clarifying Seeks to understand the patient's message by asking for more information or for elaboration on a point; expressed as a question or statement followed by a restatement or paraphrasing of part of the patient's message	Allows the patient to verify that the message received is accurate; particularly useful when the message is ambiguous or not easily understood	Nurse: "How are you getting along with the new blood pressure medication?" Patient: "Well, the doctor told me to take one every day, but they are so darned expensive, I've only been taking them every other day. It seems to be working out okay." Nurse: "Let me make sure I understand this correctly. The cost of the medication is keeping you from being able to take it each day?" Patient: "Yes, I just can't afford it on my fixed income."
Focusing The nurse encourages the patient to select one topic over another as the primary focus of discussion	Allows the nurse to gather more specific information when the patient's message is too vague; focuses on specific data	Patient: "Don't let them give me any morphine. The last time they gave me that I almost died!" Nurse: "Will you please tell me as accurately as you can, what you experienced the last time you were given morphine?"
Reflecting Assists the patient to reflect on inner feelings and thoughts rather than seeking answers and advice from another	Promotes independent decision making; allows patient to see that his ideas and thoughts are important	Patient: "Sometimes I think my family is falling apart. All we ever do is fight and argue. My kids don't take responsibility for themselves, much less help out around the house. This makes my husband furious, and we all end up in a shouting match with everyone feeling miserable. What should I do? Sometimes I just feel like walking out" Nurse "What do you think you should do?" Patient: "I don't know. I would like for us to go to counseling, but I'm afraid my husband won't hear of it" Nurse: "Have you discussed this with him?" Patient: "No. I suppose that is where I need to start"

Contd...

Table 6.1: *Contd...*

Verbal techniques	Benefits	Examples
Stating Observations The nurse makes observations of the patient during an interaction and communicates these observations back to the patient	Allows for clarification of the intended message when verbal cues do not match non-verbal cues; allows for more accurate interpretation of patient concerns	(Mrs. Parvathi denies having any concerns about her upcoming hysterectomy. However, the nurse notes that Mrs. Parvathi's posture and facial expression are tense, her eye contact is brief and darting, and she is fidgeting about in bed. The nurse shares these observations with Mrs. Parvathi.) Nurse: "Mrs. Parvathi, you seem to understand the information about your surgery that we have discussed, but you still seem to be quite tense and anxious. Can you tell me what is bothering you?" Mrs. Parvathi.: "Well, it's just that my husband and I always wanted to have one more child and now that will never happen. It all seems so final."
Offering Information Nurse provides the patient with relevant data and asks for feedback to determining the patient's level of understanding	Useful for patient teaching; promotes informed decision making	Preoperative teaching Diabetes education Discharge instruction
Summarizing Concise review of main ideas from a discussion	Focuses on key issues and allows for additional information which may have been omitted; particularly useful when interaction has been lengthy or has covered several topics	"We've covered a lot of information in the past few minutes. The main things to keep in mind are _____"

individuals are at a loss for anything better to say, They are used without thinking of the impact on the other person and often seem disrespectful of the client's individual circumstances. Examples include the following:

"Hang in there, tomorrow is another day."

"It could be worse."

False Reassurance: False reassurance about the outcome of a situation is often used in an effort to cheer up the client regardless of the facts. False reassurance can be especially traumatic to a terminally ill client who may be desperate to believe assurances even if they are not founded in reality. An example of false reassurance is as follows:

"Don't worry, I'm sure everything will be fine."

Judgmental Responses: Judgmental responses are based on the nurse's personal value system and imply right or wrong. Such responses allow no room for further discussion. For example:

"You shouldn't feel that way."

"You ought to do…"

Agreeing/Disagreeing or Approving/Disapproving: Whether the nurse is agreeing/approving or disagreeing/disapproving, offering an opinion implies that one belief is right and the other wrong. Clients are thus prevented from sharing their feelings and may feel pressured to express the same values and opinions as the nurse. One example is as follows:

"I wouldn't do it that way."

Giving Advice: Giving advice involves offering personal rather than professional opinion. When the nurse does this, the client's responsibility for making decisions is diminished. Furthermore, some clients may end up feeling unable to make their own choices and may therefore become more dependent on the nurse. One example might be:

"I think you should…."

Stereotyping: Stereotyping occurs when individual differences are ignored and a person is automatically put into a specific category because they have certain characteristics. For example:

"Someone your age shouldn't worry about that."

"Boys aren't supposed to cry."

Belittling: Belittling conveys to a person that his thoughts or feelings really have no value, that it is silly to think or feel a certain way, or that he is no different from other individuals in similar circumstances, Examples include the following:

"Many people have it much worse."

"Yes, everyone feels like that."

Defending: Defending is a response to a feeling of being directly or indirectly threatened. The nurse may make statements in defense of self, another nurse, a doctor, or the health care facility. Defending implies that the client is not permitted to criticize or express feelings. This may be one of the most difficult communication barriers to overcome, No one likes to be

Table 6.2: Responses that Block Communication

Category of response	Explanation of categories	Examples	Outcome
False reassurance	Using falsely comforting phrases in an attempt to offer reassurance	"It will be okay." "Don't worry. Everything will be just fine." "You'll be fine."	Nurse may promise something that will not occur or is unrealistic
Giving advice	Making a decision for a client; offering personal opinions; telling a patient what to do with phrases such as "should do," "ought to"	"If I were you I would." "I think you should." "Why don't you."	Takes decision making away from the patient; inhibits spontaneity; impairs decision making; creates doubt
False assumptions	Making an assumption without validation; jumping to conclusions	"You're just afraid to give your own injection." "Your husband isn't very supportive." "You aren't really trying."	Can easily lead to the wrong conclusion; may be viewed as accusatory or argumentative
Value judgments	Trying to impose the nurse's own attitudes, values, beliefs, and moral standards on a patient about what is right and wrong	"Abortion is wrong!" "Having cosmetic surgery is frivolous." "You shouldn't even think that." "He really is a good doctor."	Can lead the patient to doubt his own values; may create feelings of guilt and resentment; may cause friction between the patient and the nurse
Cliche	Stereotyped or superficial comments that do not focus on what the client is feeling or trying to say	"You can't win them all." "Isn't that nice?" "I don't make the rules, I just follow them." "The doctor knows best."	Tends to belittle the individual's feelings and minimize the importance of the message; communicates the message that the nurse is not taking the patient's concerns seriously
Defensiveness	Responding negatively to criticism; often in response to feelings of anger or hurt on the part of the nurse; usually involves making excuses	"I'm doing the best I can." "Oh, I'm sure the night nurse wouldn't have done that." "You must not have heard me right."	Implies that the patient has no right to an opinion; patient's concerns are often ignored or minimized because nurse is focusing on defense of self or others
Arguing	Challenging or arguing against statements or perceptions of the patient	"How can you say you didn't sleep a wink, when I heard you snoring all night long?" "How could your pain level be so high? You were just talking and laughing with your visitor."	Denies that the patient's perceptions are real and valid; implies that the patient is lying, misinformed, or uneducated
Asking for explanations	Asks patient to explain their actions, beliefs, or feelings with "why" questions	"Why aren't you taking your medicine the way the doctor prescribed it?" "Why do you feel that way?" "Why didn't you go to the doctor sooner?"	Frequently viewed by the patient as accusatory; patient may think the nurse knows the answer and is testing them; can cause resentment, insecurity and mistrust
Changing the subject	Inappropriately focusing the discussion on something other than the patient's concern	"We'll worry about that later. It's time for your bath now." "Let's talk about something else. Talking about having cancer is making you too sad."	Rude and shows lack of empathy; blocks further communication and patient may not feel comfortable expressing feelings; thoughts are interrupted and important information may not be shared

criticized or to hear coworkers criticized. A natural first response is to defend why something was said, done, or not done. An example or defending is as follows:

"No one on this unit would say that."

Requesting an Explanation: It can be very intermidating for a client when a nurse asks for an explanation of behaviors, feelings, or thoughts. Often, the client does not know the "why." The usual results are increased anxiety, becoming defensive, and an end to communication, Examples are as follows:

"Why did you do that?"

"Why do you feel that way?"

Changing the Subject: An abrupt change of subject by the nurse generally indicates to the client that the nurse is uncomfortable or anxious about the topic under discussion. It often is used to avoid listening to a client's fear, distress, or problems and is interpreted by the client as a lack of interest.

Patient: "I don't think I'll ever get well."

Nurse: "Isn't it a beautiful day?"

Please refer Table 6.2 for responses that blocks communication.

Nurse-Patient Communication

All communication with clients must take place within the limits of the professional relationship that allow for a safe, therapeutic connection between the professional and the client. The nurse must abstain from obtaining personal gain at the expense of the client and refrain from inappropriate involvement in the client's personal relationships.

One of the most important aspects of nursing care is communication. Good communication skills are essential whether the nurse is gathering admission information, taking a health history, teaching, or implementing care.

Nurses have both an ethical and moral responsibility to use any information gathered from the client in the client's best interest. Information that affects the health status or care of the client should be shared with other members of the health care team. All information concerning a client is confidential and should never be discussed in elevators, the cafeteria, the hallways, or other public places outside the health care facility.

Nurses' competence is often judged by their communication skills. Client satisfaction is increased by good communication, and increased client satisfaction leads to better compliance with the therapeutic regimen.

A key factor in the client's perception and evaluation of the health care services provided is communication.

Formal communication is purposeful and is employed in a structured situation such as information gathering on admission or scheduled teaching sessions. Specific items covered in a planned sequence provide more information in the shortest amount of time.

Informal communication does not follow a structured approach, although it often reveals information that is pertinent to the client's care. For instance, a client may comment that the tape holding her bandage in place is irritating to her skin. This would lead the nurse to assess the wound area and take action to correct the problem. This interaction, although not planned or structured, was nonetheless helpful in ensuring quality nursing care.

Every day conversations with friends, family, and acquaintances are called social communication. Topics usually are those of interest to both parties and reflect the social relationship of the persons involved. Both people share information, feelings, and thoughts, Social communication provides a way to get acquainted with clients to learn about each other, and to begin a nurse-client relationship.

Although social communication is not considered therapeutic communication, it is used in the nurse-client relationship. It is nonthreatening and puts the client at ease, allowing the nurse to get to know the client and what is important to the client. Social communication is often interpreted by clients as expressions of caring on the part of the nurse that is, the nurse cares enough about the client to spend time communicating as a person rather than as a nurse.

Interactions with Client

Nurse-client interactions and relationships progress through three phases. The purpose of the interaction dictates the amount of time spent on each phase.

Introduction Phase: The introduction phase of any interaction is usually fairly short. After greeting the client by name, the nurse should introduce himself and define his role. Then expectations of the interaction are clarified, and mutual goals are set. A good format might be:

"Good morning, Mrs. Asha. My name is Basanthi. I am a student nurse. I will be caring for you today and tomorrow, During this time, I will be teaching you some leg exercises that you will have to do after your surgery tomorrow."

Working Phase: The working phase generally constitutes the major portion of any interaction and is used to accomplish the goal or objective defined in the introduction. Feedback should always be asked for to ensure understanding on the part of the client. In the previously presented scenario, the client's demonstrating the leg exercises and verbalizing why the exercises are necessary would indicate understanding.

Termination Phase: The termination phase is the final phase of any interaction. Seldom do nurses have unlimited time to spend with one client, and there are several ways for the nurse to indicate the end of an interaction. The nurse may ask whether the client has any questions about the topic discussed. Summarizing the topic is another good way for the nurse to indicate closure.

Factors Affecting Nurse-Patient Relationship and Communication

As mentioned previously, factors such as age, education, emotions, culture, language, attention, and surroundings affect both parties in a communication. In nurse-client communications, additional factors relating to both the nurse and client also come into play. The nurse must be sensitive to these factors and avoid personal biases in order to provide appropriate nursing care.

Nurse: Many factors pertaining to the nurse influence nurse-client communication. The nurse's state of health, home situation, workload, staff relations, and past experiences as a nurse, can all impact the attitude, thinking, concentration and emotions of the nurse. These all influence the way a nurse sends and receives messages. Self-awareness (an awareness of all these factors) is very important for the nurse when communicating.

Client: Factors related to the client that must be considered include social factors, religion, family situation, visual ability, hearing ability, speech ability, level of consciousness, language proficiency, and state of illness.

Hearing Ability: If a hearing-impaired person is able to read, writing may be the easiest method of communication; however, many hearing-impaired persons have learned to speech read at least to some degree. This was formerly known as lip read. Communicating with a client who is hearing impaired requires time and patience.

The client may experience frustration when communicating. Such frustration generally stems more from trying to understand others rather than from trying to be understood. Face the client and speak slowly and deliberately using slightly exaggerated word formation. Gesturing can also be very effective. Check to see whether the client has a hearing aid and, if so, encourage its use during the communication.

When taking care of client who has hearing impairments, Nurse should:
- Check to see whether the client wears a hearing aid. Be sure it is in working order and turned on.
- Make every effort to move the client to a setting with minimal background noise.
- Always face the client.
- Speak in a normal tone and at a normal pace.
- Determine whether the client uses sign language. If signing is used, enlist the assistance of an interpreter.
- Pay particular attention to non-verbal cues of the client and to your own non-verbal behavior.
- Provide a pen and a paper to facilitate communication, if necessary.

Speech Ability Dysphasia: The impairment of speech, and **aphasia,** the absence of speech, are most commonly seen as the result of a stroke, although both can result from a brain lesion. Other neurological diseases such as Parkinson's disease may also cause dysphasia. A dysfunction of the muscles used for speech is termed **dysarthria,** which makes a person's speech difficult, slow, and hard to understand. Dysphasia, aphasia, and dysarthria create communication problems.

The person with dysphasia has difficulty putting thoughts and feelings into words and sending messages. It should be noted, however, that seldom does the person with dysphasia have difficulty receiving and interpreting messages: thus, explanations should be given before doing anything. If the client can write, paper and pencil can be used for communication. A picture board, word board, letter board, or computer may also be employed. A person with speech impairments may feel frustrated and helpless. Establishing some method of communication for the client provides hope and maintains self-esteem while minimizing or preventing feelings of depression, anger, and hostility.

Level of Consciousness: True communication cannot be accomplished with unconscious or comatose clients. It should be remembered, however, that unconscious or comatose clients may be able to hear even though they cannot respond. Caregivers should speak to these clients just as they would to alert clients. Always greet the client by name, identify yourself, and explain why you are in the room (i.e. what you are going to do). Then let the client know when you are leaving and, if possible, when you will return. Although one-sided, this interaction is critical to the client's care.

Language Proficiency: The client's ability to communicate effectively through spoken language also influences the nurse-client interaction. Clients who do not speak English generally come from another culture. Learning about the other culture, especially about the values and beliefs, will help prevent the nurse from violating those values and beliefs.

A family member who speaks English could be used as an interpreter. When another health care worker on the nursing unit speaks the same language as does the client, that person could also be used as an interpreter as long as it does not interfere with his or her work. Speak directly to the client whether an interpreter is present or not. Make eye contact with the client and speak slowly and clearly. Use simple words and avoid slang and medical jargon.

Pictures or a two-language dictionary are often helpful. When another language is prevalent in the community, nurse's should learn some phrases in that language to use in client assessment and care. *Remember, gestures, facial expressions, and other non-verbal communication send messages without the use of language.*

Social Factors: Socially acceptable health concerns, such as having the gallbladder or appendix removed or having the flu, are easy to discuss. It may be more difficult to communicate with a woman who is having a breast removed. The symbolic meaning of the breast may make it difficult for the client to accept its removal and may influence how she relates to others. A person who is HIV positive or has another sexually transmitted disease may be very reluctant to discuss the illness.

Stage of Illness: The stage of a client's illness may influence the client's desire to communicate with the nurse. Clients in the early stages of illness may be eager to learn all they can about the illness or may express anger and resentment at their current state of health.

Terminally ill clients may pose special challenges for the nurse. Most terminally ill clients know they are dying and are concerned about those whom they love. It is thus important for the nurse to have the client identify those persons the client considers to be "family." Family and nurses often struggle with effective communication techniques when speaking with one who is dying. Death is not a prime subject for discussion as it is often considered a defeat by health care workers. *Remember that silence and listening are both part of communication and can relay caring, compassion, and acceptance.*

Whenever a client begins talking about death the nurse must be willing to listen and take part in the conversation. Many times nurses hesitate to communicate with the terminally ill for fear they will say the wrong thing. The client who wishes to talk needs a good listener. Allow the client to guide the conversation. Listen and accept what the client says. Trying not to give advice may be very difficult to do.

The nurse and the family must work together to understand the ways that the terminally ill client communicates. It can take persistence and insight to identify and decipher some messages. "Listening" to the client's gestures and facial expressions helps facilitate understanding or messages.

Religion: Communication can be difficult when religious beliefs conflict with those of the health care team. Members of some religions seek healing only through faith and not through conventional medical services, including not receiving blood transfusions.

When a client has a minister, priest, or rabbi visit, privacy should be provided if at all possible.

Family Situation: Illness often unites family members around the client, but communication between the family and client may be strained if the family has not been close to or supportive of the client before the illness. The nurse must be careful not to discuss aspects of the client's condition or treatment in front of family members. It is usually best to ask family members to step out or the room when any nursing care is being given. This maintains the client's right to privacy and confidentiality.

If the client asks for a specific person to remain in the room. it is usually allowed unless specifically contraindicated.

Visual Ability: Communicating with clients who are visually impaired may not seem to be a challenge at first; however, because the non-verbal part of any message, such as facial expressions, gestures, and other body language, is not able to be observed, an important part of every message is lost to the client.

When taking care of client who visually impaired, nurse should:
- Look directly at the client when speaking.
- Use a normal tone and volume of voice.

- Advice the client when you are entering or leaving the room.
- Orient the person to the immediate environment; use clock hours to indicate positions of items in relation to the client.
- Ask for permission before touching the client.

Generally, persons who are visually impaired speak only when spoken to. Their speech is often loud when they are not sure where the other person is. Silence makes them uncomfortable.

When orienting a new client who cannot see, the nurse must include an explanation of "hospital sounds." Describe the room in detail and guide the client around the room if possible. Always speak and identify yourself when entering the room. Each step of a procedure as well as any touching should be described before it is initiated. To prevent startling a client, always inform the visually impaired client before touching.

Communicating with the Health Care Team

Nurses providing care to clients is a team effort, effective communication is necessary. This communication between team members may be oral or written, individual, group, or on computer.

Oral Communication

Oral communication takes place among all health care team members. To provide continuity of care to the client, all persons who provide that care communicate orally concerning that care.

Nurse-Student Nurse: Student nurses communicate not only with their clinical instructor but with the staff nurses too. How well staff nurses interact with student nurses depends on the experiences the staff nurses have had with other student nurses and also on bow the staff nurses were treated as students. Student nurses are present in the clinical facility for very specific learning experiences, which are selected by the instructor and relate to classroom discussion. They will review client records, communicate with and care for their clients, and when possible observe others performing procedures. Depending on how far they have progressed through the nursing curriculum, students may be limited in their nursing activities. Communication between student nurses and staff nurses is essential because staff nurses are responsible for the care of clients even though clients are assigned to students. Usually a helping relationship develops between staff nurses and nursing students.

Nurse-Nursing Assistant: The nurse is responsible for assigning duties to the nursing assistants. A relationship of trust and mutual respect is established by answering questions and providing reasons for specific activities requested.

Nursing assistants are often much more comfortable and confident in providing bedside care. Therefore, they can be of considerable assistance to the new graduate (whether an LP/VN or RN). They often have creative solutions to problems and should be included in planning care.

Nurse-Nurse: Nurse-nurse communications can be either peer-peer or superior-subordinate communication. Peer-peer communication takes place many times every day. When each nurse uses effective communication with peers as well as clients, the unit runs more efficiently, and client care will be more effective. Superior-subordinate communication of tell occurs when the superior discusses client care to be performed by the subordinate. The way this communication is handled affects both the attitude of the subordinate and the client care given.

Nurse-Physician: Nursing education and expertise have evolved over the years to a professional level. Nurses are responsible for their own actions even when under the direction of a physician. Nurses have a duty to secure physician clarification of any order that is illegible or unclear, that violates hospital policy or procedure, or that is below the acceptable standard of care.

Nurses must communicate openly and honestly with physicians, demonstrating competence in assessments, nursing skills, provision of quality care, reporting change in client status, and accurate documentation.

Nurse-Other Health Professionals: Communicate with professionals in other departments on a peer-to-peer basis. The focus of communication should be clarification of goals for each client and ways to meet those goals. Top-quality care is provided to clients by listening to those in other departments and establishing mutual respect for each other's area of expertise.

Group Communication: Client care conferences may be scheduled whenever the need arises or on a regular basis. Some conferences may be only for the staff of a specific nursing unit; others may include some members of other departments. Only persons directly involved with client care should be invited.

The objectives of the conference are established by the conference leader, who makes all necessary arrangements. The meeting site should be a conference room or other private place. One person should record the discussion. When the conference is about a particular client, only facts are to be documented on the client's chart. When the topic is general and not related to anyone client, only a record of the discussion is needed.

Telephone: When a student nurse takes a telephone call, the call should he answered with the name of the department or floor and the student's full name and position (i.e. student nurse). If a message is taken, the student nurse should write it down and read it back to the caller, asking for the caller's name and for the caller to spell out his or her name. The student nurse must never give out any information about clients.

Shift Report: Vital to continuity of client care is the **shift report** (report about each client between shifts). An oral report is the most common. The charge nurse of the outgoing shift may report to all members of the incoming shift or only to the incoming charge nurse who, in turn, shares the information with the appropriate caregivers on the incoming shift.

Sometimes, the report is put on a tape recorder for the next shift. This allows no chance for feedback, which can be a disadvantage.

Another method is it "walking report." The outgoing nurse reports to the oncoming nurse on each client as they walk from bed to bed. This way the client is included and aware of the information provided to the next shift.

The shift report about each client should be complete and concise no matter which method is used. The report should be focused on the clients and given in an orderly, manner. This is not the time for social conversation.

The shift report should contain following informations:
- Name, room and bed, age, sex
- Physician, diagnosis, admission date, any surgery
- Diagnostic tests (results if available) or treatments in past 24 hours
- General status, significant changes in condition
- Changed or new physician's orders
- Nursing diagnoses with nursing order
- Evaluation of nursing interventions
- Last PRN medication given, IV fluids left hanging and amount given
- Any concerns about the client or family.

Written Communication

Most written communication relates to the client's chart. All aspects of a client's care are recorded on that client's chart.

Requisitions to X-ray or to physical or respiratory therapy and requests for laboratory services for a client are all forms of written communication. The reports resulting from these requests become part of the client's chart.

One type of written communication not pertaining to a specific client is the interdepartmental memo requesting equipment, supplies, maintenance, or housekeeping. Such documents are necessary to keep the nursing unit functioning efficiently and effectively.

Electronic Communication

Computers are being used extensively in the business offices of health care agencies and have been so for years. The introduction of computers into the departments of direct client care has been slower, however. Nonetheless, in many places, computers are used by client care departments to send requisitions to other departments and to receive test results. Some hospital pharmacies use computer programs that show safe dosages and drug interactions. There are also programs to aid physicians in diagnosing and treating some conditions. With the expanding use of computers in health care and the corresponding potential for increased use, it is important for all health care workers to have some knowledge about computers.

The Institute of Medicine defines the computerized patient record as an "electronic record that resides in a system specifically designed to support users through availability of complete and accurate data, practitioner reminders and alerts, clinical decision support systems, links to bodies of medical knowledge and other aids." This moves the client record from simply tracking client care to serving as a resource for health care delivery.

As widespread use of the computerised patient record is implemented many questions are being considered, including: How can changes to the data entered be prevented? How will charting errors be corrected? What happens when the computers are down? How will security be maintained? What are the legal implications of electronic or digital signatures? All client records must be confidential, accurate, secure, and protected from unauthorized access and disclosure, regardless of the form.

Telehealth

Telehealth is using telecommunication equipment and communication networks to transfer health care information between participants at different locations. It can be used in almost every area of health care.

Telenursing, an element of telehealth, permits nurses to provide care through a telecommunication system. The simplest form has been used for years-the telephone. Telelmedicine, another element of telehealth, permits physicians to provide care through a telecommunication system. Recognized subspecialties include teledermatology, teleoncology, telepathology, and teleradiology.

The use of two-way video allows the client and health care provider to see, hear, and talk to each other. A stethoscope or otoscope (called peripherals) can be included in the hook-up so that the sounds and visual images can be transmitted . This allows physician specialists in large medical centers to examine a client many miles away. Following points to be kept in mind while maintain telehealth confidentiality:

- Avoid sending or receiving client data by e-mail unless the computer has encryption capabilities.
- During a two-way video consultation, inform the client of any other people who are present in the room, but off camera. Try to ensure that only those persons who must know about the client's condition are present.
- From the office, a home health nurse can watch a client at home change a dressing or self-administer insulin.
- During a video consult, a home health nurse might assist by manipulating the peripherals or actually performing a physical assessment.

Nurses should document all activities, assessment findings, information provided by the client, and any instructions given *to* the client. All data transmissions (e.g. telemetry printouts or videotapes) should be stored in the client's record. Most telemedicine laws require that existing confidentiality rules be maintained.

Guidelines for Communicating with Different Situation

Self-Talk: People talk to themselves every day whether they admit it *or* not. Often, such communication takes the form of thoughts rather than spoken words. What people say to themselves influences their personalities and, therefore, how they interact with others. This self-talk may be positive *or* negative.

i.   Positive Self-Talk: The practice of positive self-talk is key to positive self-esteem. You can send positive thoughts to yourself about yourself, but better yet, say the thoughts out loud. Thinking, saying, and hearing positive statements about oneself reinforces positive self-esteem. When you have had a clinical day, whether in the classroom or clinical area, remind yourself of your good attributes and accomplishments. Every day tell yourself out loud what you learned or what good care you gave to your client(s).

The desire to succeed is reinforced by positive self-talk. When things are not going well and frustration sets in, memories *of* success can serve as positive influences.

Positive affirmation is a positive thought or idea on which a person consciously focuses to produce a desired result. Positive affirmation can be used to change negative inner messages to positive messages. For instance, say, "I know I can pass this test" instead of saying, "I don't know if I can pass this test." Of course, positive affirmation cannot be a substitute for studying and preparing for the test. Positive affirmation merely serves to modify your attitude about the test-or about any other situation.

ii. Negative Self-Talk: Whenever you say to yourself, "If can't do . . ." you are decreasing your self-esteem with the negative self-talk may originate within you or may be a replay of things that others have said about you. Negative self-talk is self-destructive. Your self-image is lowered by your own criticism, and you begin to see yourself as a failure. The following guidelines are helpful in communicating with different situations:

(i) Communicating with patients who are partially known to language

- Assess the patient's non-verbal as well as verbal communication.
- Keep your eyes at approximately the same level as the patient's. This will probably mean you will sit. Assess if the patient is comfortable with eye contact.
- Speak slowly, and never loudly (unless the patient has a hearing impairment).
- Use pictures when possible (Remember: A picture is worth a thousand words).
- Avoid using technical terms.
- Ask for feedback. Provide the patient with paper and pencil.
- Remember that patients understand more than they can express–they need time to think in their own language.

- Remember that stress interferes with the patient's ability to think and speak in English.

(ii) Communication with English speaking patients

If there is an interpreter available:

- Use dialect-specific interpreters, not translators.
- Give the patient and interpreter time alone together.
- Build in time for translation and Interpretation.
- Avoid using children and relatives as interpreters.
- Select same-age and same-gender interpreters.
- Address your questions to the patient, not the interpreter. If there is not an interpreter available:
- Use a translator.
- Determine if there is a third language that is common to you and the patient. It is common for patients from diverse cultures to know several languages.
- Remember that non-verbal communication is more important than verbal.
- Be attentive to both your own and the patient's non-verbal messages.
- Pantomime simple words and actions.
- Remember: "A picture is worth a thousand words." Use paper and pencil.
- Talk with administration about the importance of using trained medical interpreters when caring for the non-English-speaking patient.
- Until medical interpreters are available, use both formal and informal networking to locate a suitable interpreter. If all else fails, owners of ethnic restaurants and grocery stores may be sources for locating interpreters or translators.

(iii) Communicating with patients of different cultures

Dominant language and dialects

- Identify the dominant language of the group.
- Identify dialects that may interfere with communication.
- Explore contextual speech patterns of the group. What is the usual volume and tone of speech?

Cultural communication patterns

- Explore the willingness of individuals to share thoughts, feelings, and ideas.
- Explore the practice and meaning of touch in the given society; within the family, among friends, with strangers, with members of the same sex, with members of the opposite sex, and with health care providers.
- Identify personal spatial and distancing characteristics. Explore how distancing changes with friends compared to strangers.
- Explore the use of eye contact within the group. Does avoidance of eye contact have special meanings? How does eye contact vary among family, friends, and strangers? Does eye contact change among socioeconomic groups?
- Explore the meaning of various facial expressions. Do specific facial expressions have special meanings? Do people tend to smile a lot? How are emotions displayed or not displayed in facial expressions?
- Are there acceptable ways of standing and greeting outsiders?

Temporal relationships

- Explore temporal relationships in the group. Are individuals primarily oriented to the past, present, or future? How do individuals see the context of past, present, and future?
- Identify differences in the interpretation of social time versus clock time.
- Explore how time factors are interpreted by the group. Are individuals expected to be punctual in arrival to jobs, appointments, and social engagements?

Format for names

- Explore the format for personal names.
- How does the individual expect to be greeted by strangers and health care practitioners?

(iv) Communicating with the older adult

- Encourage the patient to wear prescribed glasses and hearing aids. About 40% of adults age 65 years and older have hearing loss sufficient to interfere with daily conversation. About 20% have enough vision loss to prevent clear perception of a communication partner at a conversational distance.
- Face the patient's unaffected side or "better" ear. This positioning increases the patient's awareness of the interaction and enhances the patient's ability to interact.
- Provide sufficient light and remove distractions and background noise. Background noise further impairs the older adult's hearing.
- Use low voice tones and recognize that perception of the sounds *f*, s, *th, ch, sh, b, t, p, k,* and *d* is impaired with age-related hearing loss.
- Allow time for thought comprehension when communicating with the patient. Older adults do not like to be rushed. When they are allowed to function at a moderately slow pace, their comprehension is enhanced.
- Schedule time to listen to the patient's life stories. This helps the nurse learn what is important to the patient.
- Use touch as culturally appropriate.

(v) Communicating with patients who are cognitively impaired

- Reduce environmental distractions while conversing.
- Get patient's attention prior to speaking. Use simple sentences and avoid long explanations.
- Ask one question at a time.
- Allow time for patient to respond.
- Be an attentive listener.
- Include family and friends in conversations, especially in subjects known to patient.

(vi) Communication methods for patients with hearing impairment

- Get the patient's attention. Do not startle the patient when entering the room. Do not approach a patient from behind. Be sure the patient knows you wish to speak.
- Face the patient and stand or sit on the same level. Be sure your face and lips are illuminated to promote lip reading. Keep hands away from mouth.

- If the patient wears glasses, be sure they are clean so that your gestures and face can be seen. If the patient wears a hearing aid, make sure it is in place and working.
- Speak slowly and articulate clearly. Older adults may take longer to process verbal messages. Use a normal tone of voice and inflections of speech. Refrain from speaking with something in your mouth.
- When you are not understood, rephrase rather than repeat the statement.
- Use visible expressions. Speak with your hands, your face, and your eyes.
- Do not shout. Loud sounds are usually pitched higher and may impede hearing by accentuating vowel sounds and concealing consonants. If it is necessary to raise your voice, speak in lower tones.
- Talk toward the patient's best or normal ear.
- Use written information to enhance the spoken word.
- Do not restrict a deaf patient's hands. Never have intravenous lines in both of the patient's hands if the preferred method of communication is sign language.
- Avoid eating, chewing, or smoking while speaking.
- Avoid speaking from another room or while walking away.

(vii) Communication with patients of impaired verbal communication

- Determine language spoken; obtain language dictionary or interpreter if possible and accepted by the patient.
- Listen carefully. Validate verbal and non-verbal expression.
- Anticipate patient's needs until effective communication is possible.
- Use simple communication, speak in a well modulated voice, and smile and show concern for the patient.
- Maintain eye contact at patient's level and read patient's eyes as able.
- Use touch as appropriate. Holding a patient's hand or stroking the arm is a simple, unintrusive way of showing empathy and concern.
- Spend time with the patient, allow time for responses, and make the call light readily available.
- Explain all health care procedures.
- Determine the patient's literacy status.
- Obtain communication equipment such as electronic devices, letter boards, picture boards, and magic slates as indicated.
- Establish an alternative method of communication such as writing or pointing to letters, words, phrases, picture cards, or simple drawings of basic needs.
- If there is a comprehension deficit, keep environment quiet when communicating and get the patient's attention before attempting to communicate (e.g. touch patient's shoulder, call patient's name).
- Give praise for progress noted. Ignore mistakes and watch for frustration or fatigue.
- Never raise your voice or shout at a patient.

The communication techniques discussed thus far are generally applicable to any type of nurse-patient interaction.

Some patients have unique communication needs. Following are examples of three such situations.

(viii) Communicating with ventilator-dependent patients

Patients who are placed on mechanical ventilation via endotracheal tube or tracheostomy will experience an inability to speak because of obstruction of the trachea caused by the tube. This inability to speak can be devastating to patients and can have a negative effect on their sense of well-being and control. In situations such as this, when the patient is unable to produce sound, alternative methods of communication must be identified and implemented.

To determine the most appropriate method the nurse must carefully assess the patient's ability to use a particular alternative method of communication (e.g. cognitive level, literacy, visual acuity, consciousness level, primary language, gross motor skills, and fine motor skills). One method that may be useful is a communication board. Depending on the patient's literacy, a communication board may include the alphabet, commonly used phrases, pictures, or a combination of all three. If able to point, the patient can point to pictures or phrases on the board to communicate a need or thought. If the desired picture or phrase is not on the board, the patient can point to the letters that spell out the message. This is not feasible, however, for the patient who does not read or cannot see well enough to select from the board. If unable to move the arms to point, alternative selection methods will be necessary. This might include setting up a "signal" system, such as one eye blink for "yes" and two blinks for "no." The receiver (e.g. the nurse or a family member) systematically points to items or letters on the board, and the patient "signals" when the correct item is selected. This is a slow and rather cumbersome process for communicating and requires patience on the part of both the patient and the receiver of the message. It can also be very tiring for the patient. However, it can be a helpful tool when no other means of communicating is available or feasible.

(ix) Aphasic patients

Aphasia is a deficient or absent language function resulting from ischemic insult to the brain, such as stroke (brain attack), brain trauma, or anoxia. The patient may experience expressive aphasia, in which the patient cannot send the desired message, or receptive aphasia, in which the patient cannot recognize or interpret the message being received.

Communication methods for patients with aphasia
- Listen attentively, be patient, and do not interrupt.
- Ask simple questions that require yes or no answers. Allow time for understanding and response.
- Use visual cues (e.g. words, pictures, and objects) when possible.
- Allow only one person to speak at a time.
- Do not shout or speak too loudly.
- Encourage the patient to converse.
- Let the patient know if you have not understood him or her.
- Collaborate with a speech therapist as needed. Use communication aids.

Alternative methods of communication for patients who are unable to speak

- Lip reading: patient mouths words to be interpreted by the receiver
- Sign language: hand and finger signals used to indicate letters; used throughout the world for hearing-impaired patients
- Paper and pencil/magic slate: patient writes messages to communicate needs
- Picture board: patient points to pictures on a board or poster of typical patient needs
- Word or picture cards: 3×5 cards with words or pictures on them; patient picks appropriate card or sorts cards into short phrases or sentences
- Magnetic boards with plastic letters: patient moves letters around on board to spell words or phrases
- Eye blinks: predetermined system in which the number of times a patient blinks in response to a question indicates yes or no answer
- Computer-assisted communication: patient uses keyboard to type out messages
- Clock face communicator: messages placed at intervals around the clock face; clock hand scans the messages, and the patient presses a button to stop the hand on the desired message.

(x) Unresponsive patients

It is not certain if, or how much, the unresponsive patient is able to hear or interpret verbal stimuli. Some patients, after regaining consciousness, have reported hearing actual statements that were made in the room while the patient was still in an unconscious state. Because of this, anyone interacting with the unresponsive patient should assume that all sound and verbal stimuli have the potential of being heard by the patient. People in the environment must be cautioned about making negative or anxiety-producing statements in the presence of the patient. Health care providers, as well as family and friends, should be encouraged to speak to the unresponsive individual as if he or she were awake. This may feel awkward, and family members and friends in particular may need support and encouragement to talk with the patient as they would have before the illness or accident. Talking about daily activities and reading books, cards, and newspapers is suggested. Also, the nurse should always explain to the patient any procedure or activity that is to take place involving the patient. Health care providers should never converse about topics that do not place the patient at the center of the discussion or that might cause stress or anxiety if the patient were to hear it.

Interaction cannot take place without something being communicated. Every time a nurse interacts with a patient there is opportunity for a positive or negative outcome. By becoming familiar with therapeutic communication techniques and practicing them to become proficient in their use, the nurse can promote a helping relationship with the patient. By also being aware of factors that affect communication and of blocks to communication, the nurse can prevent interactions that

might negatively affect the patient's self-esteem and sense of worth.

Responses from the nurse such as "go on," "yes," "tell me more," "mmhm," or "what else?" communicate that the nurse is really listening and encourage the client to continue.

Psychosocial Aspects of Communication in Nursing

The psychosocial aspects of communication are important for nurses to understand and then apply when caring for individual clients. Consideration of these aspects makes communication more effective.

The psychosocial aspects of communication include gestures, style, meaning of space, meaning of time, cultural values, and political correctness. These aspects are based on individuality and culture and influence the nurse-client relationship.

Gestures

Gestures are movements of the body to reflect a thought, feeling, or attitude. Some gestures are known globally, such as applause to indicate approval. Some gestures, however, have entirely different meanings in various countries. The nurse must be sensitive to cultural variances and exercise good judgment when caring for clients of different backgrounds and heritages.

The meaning of gestures is not universal. For instance, in many places, a small circle made with the thumb and forefinger means "okay," This is not true in Japan and France, however, where this gesture means "money" and "zero," respectively, And in Brazil and Turkey, this gesture is a symbol for female genitalia and is considered an insult.

Style

Each person has a style of communication reflecting the personality and self-concept of that person. According to Jack (2000), there are three common types of style: passive, aggressive, and assertive. Remember that a person's style of communication is learned and has been reinforced over the years. Because communication style is learned, it can be changed.

The stress, fear, and anxiety associated with being a client in the health care system may change a client's style to passive or aggressive or assertive.

i. Passive

The person using the passive style of communication is not able to share feelings or needs with others, has difficulty asking for help, does not stand up for himself, and is hurt and angry when others take advantage of him, This person has a weak, soft voice: uses apologetic words; makes little eye contact and is often fidgety. The person with a passive style of communication will often go along with others without expressing a personal desire for an alternate plan of action. The client who is generally very compliant, asks for nothing, and gets little attention has a passive style of communication.

In instances when clients block communication, keep the following things in mind:

- The client may not wish to discuss the topic introduced by the nurse or may not wish to talk at all. Everyone needs time alone to think.
- Accept and respect the client's desires to not communicate a particular time.
- Let the client know that you are ready to listen whenever the client is ready to talk.

ii. Aggressive

The person using the aggressive style of communication puts his own needs and feelings first. Communication is done in a haughty or angry manner. The voice is often demanding. This person works to control or manipulate others, shows no concern for anyone else's feelings, and has an attitude of superiority.

iii. Assertive

The assertive person stands up for himself without violating the basic rights of others. True feelings are expressed in an honest, direct manner and others are not allowed to take advantage of him. The voice is firm and confident, and appropriate eye contact is made. Such a person also respects the rights, needs, and feelings of others: takes responsibility for the consequences of his actions; and behaves in a manner that enhances self-respect. A person using the assertive style of communication effectively lets others know his thoughts, feelings, and needs. He also listens to and acknowledges the other person's thoughts, feelings, and needs. If the thoughts, feelings, or needs of the persons communicating are in conflict, a compromise acceptable to both can usually be worked out.

Meaning of Space

For many years Edward T. Hall (1959) studied **proxemics**, the study of space between people and its effect on interpersonal behavior. Hall says that like other animals, humans are territorial. Consider the following examples of human territoriality: People on a beach, mark territory with a towel or blanket; space is marked in waiting rooms, with a hat, jacket, luggage, or newspaper: students in a classroom generally sit in the same place and expect others to respect that space.

How much space do you prefer between yourself and another person? This distance usually varies with the person and the situation. The distance at which one person is comfortable with another person is influenced by age, gender of those interacting, and cultural values. Hall (1959) categorizes these comfort zones as intimate, personal, social, and public space, defined as follows:

Intimate – touch to 18 inches; usually limited to family and close friends; necessary when performing most nursing procedures.

Personal – 18 inches to 4 feet; used with friends and coworkers: effective for many nurse-client interactions involving interviewing or data gathering.

Social – 4 to 12 feet; preferred distance with casual acquaintances.

Public – 12 feet or more; generally used with strangers in public places.

Comfort zone distances vary from person to person. While some people are comfortable being very close to the person with whom they are interacting, others prefer a greater distance. Nurses should always be aware of the client's spatial comfort level.

Much of nursing care involves touching the client, yet on admission, the nurse and client generally do not know each other. The nurse must move from the client's public space to the client's intimate space in a very short span of time to provide care. When care is given competently and professionally it helps the client feel more comfortable as the nurse occupies the client's intimate space.

Meaning of Time

In the United States, great emphasis is placed on schedules and being on time. Time is money. The clock is watched so individuals know where they are to be every hour of the day and night. When scheduled appointments are kept, the person is considered to be dependable.

Some cultures do not have an instrument for telling time. They have other ways of perceiving and dividing time. Some cultures know a day has passed because the sun has risen, set, and is rising again. Scheduling in these cultures often means "when we get around to it."

Cultural Values

It is important that the nurse be familiar with the cultural values of the people in the nurse's region of employment, especially when those values differ from the values of the dominant culture. For example, optimal health for all is the focus of the dominant culture. In some cultures, however, health is not a major concern, and little financial or political effort is dedicated to health. Likewise, individualism is stressed in our culture. In many other cultures, however, the social group, not the individual, is the primary focus.

As another example, consider that a number of cultural groups have learned to enjoy what they have and do not feel the need to keep working for some goal or material object. This contrasts with the dominant culture, where persons must work hard, achieve, and keep busy in order to be considered successful. Finally, in the dominant culture, cleanliness is closely related to optimal health and is a dominant value. Few cultural groups emphasize cleanliness in the way the culture does.

Political Correctness

Politically correct communication uses language that shows sensitivity to those who are different from oneself. It is intended to avoid the use of language that offends and to help eliminate prejudice. Terms that suggest inferior status for members of minority groups and terms that exclude older people, women, and those with handicaps are replaced by politically correct language. Prejudice and false ideas, which often lead to violence, are perpetuated by racist and bigoted language.

The nurse should respect the client's current "home" (e.g. the hospital room) as she would any person's home, knocking on the door before entering the room, not sitting on the bed without permission, and asking before moving any personal articles. These simple courtesies show respect for the client as a person. When the client feels respected, communication is enhanced.

Congruency of Messages

It is important that verbal and non-verbal communications are in agreement, or **congruent.** Saying, "I really appreciate what you just did," in a pleasant tone of voice while smiling is congruent and clear: saying the same words in a disgusted tone of voice while frowning is incongruent and, thus, potentially unclear. The receiver may not know whether the sender is genuinely pleased with what was done or is displeased and being sarcastic. Messages such as these can confuse the receiver, who then may require feedback in order to correctly interpret the message.

It is important for the nurse to watch for congruency between verbal and non-verbal messages and to ask for clarification when incongruity exists.

Listening/Observing

Listening and observing are two of the most valuable skills a nurse can have. These two skills are used to gather the subjective and objective data for the nursing assessment. Because the nursing diagnoses and nursing interventions are based on the assessment, it is imperative that the assessment be accurate.

The term **active listening** has been used to describe the behavior of listening and observing: it reflects the process or hearing spoken words and noting non-verbal behavior. It is listening for the meaning behind the words. This takes energy and concentration. To show undivided attention to the client, the nurse should be at eye level with the client, lean slightly forward toward the client, and make eye contact. In this position the nurse will be able to listen and observe more accurately.

Assessing Communication

When nurses assess the communication of clients, they need to include language development, non-verbal behavior, and communication style.

Language Development

The nurse assesses the following aspects of language development:

- The language skills presented by the client, compared to the language skills normally expected
- Adequacy of the language skills in relation to the individual's need
- The chief method of communicating, e.g. words or gestures
- Obstacles to language development, such as deafness or absence of environmental stimuli
- Specific forms of language impairment, e.g. a school-age child's inability to write or lack of abstractions in the language of an adult
- Cultural influences on language development, e.g. the language used in the home or customs about when and how to speak.

Non-verbal Behavior

In assessing non-verbal communication, the nurse considers the following:

- Gestures used by the individual.
- Posture and facial expressions employed.
- Use of touch as a means of communication.
- The interpersonal distance with which the person feels comfortable, e.g. whether the person assumes an intimate distance for most discussions.
- The grooming and appearance of the individual. These may affect the communication process, e.g. when dress is inconsistent with a setting or presents a stereotype that may evoke biases.

Style of Communication

A person's style of communication is often affected by such factors as health, culture, education, stress level, fatigue, and cognitive ability. In assessing communication style, the nurse considers the following:

- The vocabulary of the individual, particularly any changes from the vocabulary normally used. For example, a person who normally never swears may indicate increased stress or illness by an uncharacteristic use of profanity.
- The use of symbols and gestures to communicate. Some uses of symbols and gestures are culturally determined; for example, a Puerto Rican girl may be taught not to look an adult in the eyes, as a sign of respect and obedience; the gesture should not be interpreted as a sign of guilt.
- The presence of hostility, aggression, assertiveness, reticence, hesitance, anxiety, or loquaciousness (incessant verbalization) in the communication.
- Difficulties with verbal communication, such as slurring, stuttering, inability to pronounce a particular sound, lack of clarity in enunciation, inability to speak in sentences, loose association of ideas, flight of ideas, or the inability to find or name words or identify objects.
- Refusal or inability to speak.

Diagnosing Communication Problems

Impaired verbal communication is the nursing diagnosis given to clients with verbal communication problems. Impaired verbal communication is the "state in which an individual experiences, or could experience, a decreased ability to send or receive messages, i.e. has difficulty exchanging thoughts, ideas, or desires". Contributing factors for impaired verbal communication follow.

Impaired verbal communication related to:
- Development or age-related stage(s)
- Anatomic deficit, such as cleft palate
- Cultural difference or inability to speak dominant language
- Physical conditions such as cerebrovascular accident or brain tumor, or surgery such as laryngectomy or tracheostomy
- Psychologic conditions, such as extreme anger, severe anxiety or panic, moderate and severe depression, fear, shyness, loneliness, and unrealistic or inadequate self-concept
- Pharmacologic therapy, such as central nervous system depressant.

Ineffective individual coping, Ineffective family coping, Anxiety, and Fear may be appropriate diagnoses for some clients.

Assessment

Assessment is essential to effective communication. Your assessment should look for factors that alter a client's ability to receive, process, or transmit information, such as the following:
- *Language barrier*: Clients with limited knowledge of the dominant language often find it difficult to communicate their needs or respond to communication from health care providers. Imagine how difficult it would be if you became seriously ill while traveling in a country where you were unable to speak or read the language. How would you communicate that you were nauseated or in pain; how would you tell them when the symptom started or what makes it worse?
- *Cognitive skills*: Difficulty understanding or engaging in communication may signal cognitive impairment. Developmental delays and physiological conditions involving the central nervous system affect language skills. Gather data about the client's abilities. Does the client have problems with short-term memory, long-term memory, or both? Does the client function at, below, or above expectations for her age?
- *Sensory perceptual alterations*: Assess for hearing deficits, use of hearing aids, or visual problems. Aphasia is a problem that may develop after cerebrovascular accident (stroke) or neurological disease. Receptive aphasia is the inability to receive or interpret verbal or non-verbal messages. Expressive aphasia is the inability to express verbal or non-verbal messages. It is important to distinguish the type of aphasia your client is experiencing. The type dictates the solutions that are effective.

- *Physiological barriers*: Difficulty speaking may be due to respiratory problems, such as dyspnea or the use of artificial airways, or oral problems, such as loose-fitting dentures or cleft palate.

Nursing Diagnosis

Several NANDA diagnoses directly pertain to communication. Note that communication problems may involve the inability to receive, interpret, or express spoken, written, and non-verbal messages.
- *Readiness for Enhanced Communication* is appropriate when the client expresses willingness to enhance communication.
- *Impaired Verbal Communication* is an appropriate diagnosis if the client has (1) expressive aphasia or a physiological problem (e.g. dyspnea, stuttering, or laryngeal cancer) that impairs the ability to speak; or (2) receptive aphasia or sensory deficits (e.g. vision or hearing loss) that impair the ability to receive messages.
- *Impaired Communication* is the preferred nursing diagnosis if the client is unfamiliar with the dominant language or has some other difficulty receiving and sending messages.

Other nursing diagnoses may be the cause of communication problems. For example, clients with acute or chronic confusion often have difficulty expressing or receiving verbal and non-verbal messages. Confusion may be related to physical health problems or mental health problems or be a side effect of medications or sleep deprivation. Mental health problems can also lead to communication difficulties. For example, anxiety impairs the ability to deliver and receive messages, and chronic or situational low self-esteem often results in limited interaction with others. Your assessment data will help you determine whether communication impairment is the primary problem or whether it is a result of other health problems.

Impaired Verbal Communication may be the etiology of other nursing diagnoses, for example:
- Anxiety related to inability to communicate needs.
- Social isolation related to difficulty maintaining relationships secondary to impaired verbal communication.
- Impaired social interaction related to inability to carry on conversation.
- Chronic low self-esteem related to fear of conversing with others secondary to stuttering.

Planning

When problems in communication have been identified, the nurse and client set goals and begin planning ways to promote effective communication. The overall client goal for persons with impaired verbal communication is to reduce or resolve the impaired communication. Specific nursing interventions are planned from the stated etiology. Among these interventions are (a) developing listening skills, (b) becoming aware of how people respond and

(c) developing a helping relationship. More specific interventions may include the following:

- Anticipate needs until effective communication is established.
- Discuss individual methods of dealing with the impairment.
- Keep communication simple, using visual, auditory, and kinesthetic modes for conveying information.
- Plan for alternate methods of communication, such as a typewriter, slate, or letter/picture board.
- Respond with simple, straightforward, honest statements to provide reality orientation and correct faulty perception.
- Use and assist clients to learn facilitative communication techniques, e.g. active listening skills. See the discussion of therapeutic and nontherapeutic communication skills later in this chapter.
- Help the client look at the effects of nonfacilitative communication techniques.
- Teach and encourage expression of feelings.
- Point out discrepancies in verbal and non-verbal behavior.
- Encourage the client to ask for feedback when communicating with others.
- Refer the client to appropriate resources such as speech therapy, group therapy, or individual or family counseling.

Examples of outcome criteria to evaluate the achievement of client goals and the effectiveness of nursing interventions follow.

The client:
- Attends to appropriate communication input.
- Perceives input accurately.
- Gives clear, concise, understandable messages.
- Uses effective communication techniques, e.g. active listening, silence, reflecting, restating.
- Avoids the use of nonfacilitative techniques such as offering advice.
- Expresses congruent verbal and non-verbal behavior.
- Expresses feelings appropriately.
- Uses resources appropriately.
- Establishes a method of communication in which needs can be expressed.

With selected indicators, nurse can use these to write goals for clients' communication problems.

Individualized client outcomes and goals depend on the nursing diagnosis you identify. For example, for Impaired Verbal Communication, you might write the following desired outcomes. The client:
- Uses alternative methods of communication (e.g. writing, picture board, gestures) effectively (specify time frame).
- Demonstrates minimal frustration with communication difficulties (specify time frame).
- Communicates effectively using a translator or interpreter.
- Interprets messages accurately, as evidenced by appropriate verbal or non-verbal feedback.

Implementation

Specific nursing activities for communication problems depend on the etiology of the problem and on the goals selected.

Characteristics of Therapeutic Communication

The therapeutic relationship requires conscious use of your knowledge and skills to effect change in the client. This is often called the *therapeutic use of self*. Five qualities characterize communication in the therapeutic relationship: empathy, respect, genuineness, concreteness, and confrontation.

Empathy

Empathy is the desire to understand and be sensitive to the feelings, beliefs, and situation of another person. To empathize with a client, you must look beyond outward appearance or behavior. Empathy is more than sharing of information. Instead, it involves putting yourself, mentally and emotionally, in the client's place so that you acknowledge the uniqueness of the client. Empathy requires you to be willing to adapt your style, tone, vocabulary, and behavior to create the best approach for each client situation.

Respect

In the therapeutic relationship, you communicate respect by valuing the client and being flexible to meet the needs of your client. As a nurse, you must be willing to adjust to your client rather than expecting the client to adjust to you, the health care environment, or hospital routines. Most health care experiences strip the client of power-clothes are removed, roles are discontinued, clients are separated from loved ones and familiar surroundings, and schedules are altered. When a relationship is grounded in respect, both parties maintain power and self-esteem. You show your respect for clients in the way you address them, the words and intonation you choose, and in your acknowledgment of their strengths and needs. Making even minor adjustments, such as putting off breakfast for an hour to allow the client to sleep, communicates that you respect the client's wishes.

Genuineness

When interviewing clients, we expect them to respond truthfully. After all, many health care decisions are based on the client's responses. Similarly, clients have a right to expect truthful responses from health care providers as well. Genuineness is the ability to respond honestly. If you are unable to answer a client's question, do not offer guesses. Be honest. Tell the client you need assistance before you can answer the question. Genuineness also involves willingness to self-evaluate. How well did I communicate? Did I handle that situation appropriately? How could I improve my communication?

Concreteness and Confrontation

In a therapeutic relationship, you must offer understandable responses to a client's questions or concerns. To do so requires you to express in concrete terms what you mean. The message must be constructed and delivered in a manner that is suitable for the client. Communication is a reciprocal process. If your client is unable to express his thoughts clearly, you must be willing to confront her to request clarification. Similarly, you must be willing to be confronted if you are unclear.

Therapeutic communication requires practice. A strategy commonly used to improve communication skills is called *process recording*. In process recording, two people converse while a third transcribes the conversation. Afterward, the participants analyze the interaction. A tape recorder can facilitate process recording. It effectively captures the words and intonation of the conversation, but it must be supplemented by notes on non-verbal communication. Videotaping allows participants to examine both verbal and non-verbal communication. As you examine an interaction, look for the five qualities just discussed.

Experts identified following skills associated with above said give qualities of therapeutic communications which includes the ability to:
- Appreciate experiences and beliefs that differ from your own.
- Recognize and interpret verbal and non-verbal messages.
- Guide the interaction to accomplish goals.
- Determine whether communication is taking place.
- Speak when appropriate and remain silent when appropriate.
- Adapt to the pace, tone, and remain silent when appropriate.
- Evaluate your own participation in an interaction.

Helping Groups and Communication

Nurses frequently communicate with groups. Group communication occurs when you interact with a family, a community, or a committee. Groups can enhance problem solving and creativity, generate understanding and support, enhance morale, and provide affiliation.

Task groups are developed to address a task or need. Members are chosen based on ability to complete the task. **Short-term groups** dissolve once the task is completed. Short-term groups might include a task force to address holiday scheduling or a panel to critique response to a disaster drill. Because the time together is limited, the focus of communication is on the task at hand. Often time to develop rapport or relationships is limited. Direct verbal communication with congruent non-verbal communication allows the group to function most effectively.

Ongoing groups address issues that are recurrent. Committees are a form of a task group. Common ongoing committees in health care organizations include quality assurance, infection control, and discharge planning. A committee has a chairperson that may be elected from within or appointed. Members have designated roles within the groups (e.g. recorder, time keeper). The size of the group strongly affects communication. In small groups, all members have an opportunity to communicate their opinions. In larger groups,

patterns of communication form; some members voice their opinion regularly, whereas others are often silent. When not all members speak, it is essential to examine non-verbal behavior to determine whether the nonspeaking members are in agreement.

Self-help groups are voluntary organizations composed of individuals with a common need. Members who have met the goals of the group often run meetings. Alcoholics anonymous is the most widely recognized self-help group. Other well-known self-help groups include Weight Watchers, Narcotics Anonymous, and Reach for Recovery (for women with breast cancer). Nurses may be members, facilitators, or consultants for self-help groups. Members are encouraged to share experiences and seek help from other members of the group. The facilitator may serve as a leader of the group or may coordinate room arrangements and schedules but acts as a member during sessions. The facilitator is usually chosen by the members. Consultants may be health professionals or experts in the field who offer advice or education to the group.

Several channels are available to self-help groups. They may have face-to-face meetings, participate in Internet chat groups, or communicate via newsletters. Communication of shared interests is the link that holds these groups together.

Therapy groups are formed to help individual members cope with issues, improve relationships, or address stress. They may be ongoing or have a designated length of operation. Community, public health, and psychiatric nurses sometimes facilitate therapy groups. Group facilitators arrange the time and place of the group and often introduce topics for discussion. Many groups are organized around themes, such as coping with divorce, loss of a spouse, or motherhood. These groups are also called self-awareness or growth groups.

Work-related social support groups help members of a profession cope with the stress associated with their work. The helping professions can be quite emotionally draining. These social support groups provide an opportunity to share concerns and offer mutual support through formal meetings with a facilitator or informal drop-in events.

The formation of a group does not guarantee its success. To be successful, a group must have characteristics that allow the group to function and achieve its goals. A successful group has:
- A clearly defined purpose.
- A set of guidelines apparent to all members under which the group functions.
- A sense of shared responsibility.
- Shared leadership.
- Mutual trust.
- Comfort among members.
- A climate that is cohesive but does not stifle individuality.
- Members who are willing to share feelings, concerns, or beliefs.
- Flexibility to change what is not working.

Therapeutic communication is used throughout the nursing process. In the next few sections we will explore communication problems as well as therapeutic interventions.

Enhancing Therapeutic Communication

The following are activities of nurse can implement immediately to improve their communication with patients and others.

Active Listening

At first glance, the term *active listening* appears to be an oxymoron. People often think of listening as a passive activity. If you have ever been in a one-sided conversation, you are very aware that listening can be passive. In contrast, an active listener focuses on the sender's message with all senses.

An active listener gives undivided attention and allows the sender the opportunity to complete comments without interruption. Active listening requires paying attention to verbal and non-verbal communication and looking for congruence. If a message is unclear, seek clarification through use of probing questions or reflective comments, such as, "Tell me more," or "When you say... what do you mean?"

As a nurse, you can demonstrate active listening by facing your client, making eye contact, and focusing the conversation on issues of importance to the client. If you must take notes during the conversation, record only key words to stimulate your memory at another time, because taking copious notes distracts you from active listening. Active listening behaviors signal a willingness to listen, convey caring, and provide a comfortable environment for the client to share his concerns.

Establishing Trust

Mutual trust is an essential component of therapeutic communication because it facilitates disclosure and honesty. As you and the client establish trust, the client can more easily relay information and share feelings. To establish trust, always greet the client by name, listen actively, respond honestly to the client's concerns, and provide care competently and consistently.

Being Assertive

There are many communication styles. In fact, it may be best to think of these styles as a continuum from passive, through assertive, to aggressive. A passive approach avoids conflict and allows others to take the lead. "Whatever you want. I don't want you to change anything for me," is an example of a passive approach. In contrast, an aggressive approach forces others to lose. The goal is to win and be in control. "My way is the correct way. You don't know what you're talking about," typifies an aggressive approach.

Assertiveness is the ability to express your beliefs or feelings without infringing on another's rights. Assertive communication conveys respect for others, encourages honest feedback, and aims to establish balance and fairness without blame. Assertive communication techniques include the following:

- *Make "I" statements:* "I think this approach might be the best, but I'd like to hear your thoughts." This approach focuses on the issue, not the participants.
- *State facts, avoid judgments:* "The patient is in pain and needs medication," instead of, "Why haven't you given the patient his medications yet?"
- *Don't invite negative responses:* "I would really appreciate it if you could help me weigh Mr. Max on the bed scale," rather than, "Can you help me weigh him?"
- *Use assertive body language:* Face the client, stay calm, make eye contact, and speak clearly.

An assertive individual is one who is confident and comfortable and remains in charge of where the conversation is going. Assertive communication enables you to deal directly with stressful interpersonal communication. An assertive nurse also serves as a role model for the client. The therapeutic relationship is a safe place for clients to practice being assertive and receive feedback about their communication. The characteristics of an assertive nurse includes:

- Maintains eye contact, as culturally appropriate.
- Speaks clearly and firmly.
- Projects a clear tone of voice.
- Is self-confident.
- Maintains professional composure.
- Communicates in a positive manner.
- Refrains from sarcasm.
- Provides congruence between verbal and non-verbal messages.
- Guides the direction of the discussion.

Restating, Clarifying, and Validating Messages

Restating means using your own words to summarize the message you received from the client. This demonstrates concern and active listening. Below is an example:

Client: I'm so worried about this diabetes. I have young kids. I want to see them grow-up. Every diabetic I've known has died young.

Nurse: Diabetes is a serious disease. I understand why you would worry about its effects on you. However, we want to focus on becoming well controlled so that you can avoid complications.

Clarify messages to ensure that you have accurately interpreted the information. For instance, you might state, "I'm not sure what you mean when you say you're so worried about your diabetes." Or, "When you say you're worried, what do you mean?"

To validate the message, ask the client whether you are making a correct interpretation: "When you say you're worried about your diabetes, do you mean you are afraid you will die soon?" These techniques help to identify client concerns and focus communication. They are especially helpful if the client is unclear or vague with his message.

Interpreting Body Language and Sharing Observations

Be attentive to what the patient says and how she says it. Note the tone of voice, rate of speech, distance, eye movement, facial expressions, and gestures. Look for congruence between the spoken message and the non-verbal message. If there is a disparity, share your observations with the patient. You can share your observations by describing the patient's body language or tone or voice. For example, you might state, "I know you said you feel well, but your voice and hands are trembling. How can I help you?" Or more simply, "You're frowning. Has something upset you?"

Exploring Issues

Ask open-ended questions to obtain a clear understanding of an issue and follow your client's thoughts. Probing comments such as "Tell me more" encourage your client to share information.

Using Silence

Learn to be comfortable with silence. When you remain silent but attentive, clients are unlikely to interpret your silence as a gap in rapport. Silence demonstrates acceptance and allows clients to compose their thoughts and provide further information. It is especially effective if your client is emotionally upset.

Summarizing the Conversation

At the end of the conversation, summarize what you have heard. For example, you might say, "Today we talked about diet, exercise, and medications for high blood pressure. Your job is to review the handouts and start taking your medication every morning. I will see you in 2 weeks when you return for your follow-up visit." Summarizing demonstrates active listening and allows the client to clarify any misunderstandings.

Barriers to Therapeutic Communication

As a nurse, you learn to communicate therapeutically, you may find yourself thinking, doing, or saying things that seem to close down your conversation. If so, acknowledge your error and return to therapeutic patterns. The following sections describe the most common barriers to therapeutic communication.

Asking Too Many Questions

Asking questions at the appropriate time is important. However, asking too many questions, especially closed questions (requiring only a yes or no answer) can make clients feel they are being interrogated. Excessive questioning may suggest lack of respect or sensitivity to the client's issues, as in the following dialogue:
Patient: I feel lousy today.
Nurse: Didn't you sleep well?
Patient: No, hardly at all.
Nurse: Did you take anything to help you sleep?
Patient: No.
Nurse: Don't you think you should have taken something?
Patient: I guess.
Nurse: Why didn't you tell the night nurse you needed something?
Patient: I don't know.

As a nurse, you can see, this approach controls the range and nature of responses that the client provides. In contrast, open-ended questions stimulate conversation and exploration. Contrast the preceding conversation with the conversation below.
Patient: I feel lousy today.
Nurse: Lousy? Tell me more.
Patient: Well, my back and neck hurts, and I hardly slept at all. I thought it would go away, but I just lay in bed last night worrying.
Nurse: What kind of things are you worrying about?
Patient: I'm worried about...
In the second conversation, the nurse asked open-ended questions. These prompts encouraged the patient to discuss his concerns.

Asking Why

In many health situations, we want to learn why a patient acted or responded as he did. However, asking why suggests criticism to some people. If you ask, "Why did you stop taking your medication?" the patient may become defensive and halt further communication. A more subtle approach is usually more comfortable for the patient. You might ask, "What concerns do you have about your medicines?" or "Tell me more about your experience with the medicines." Both of these approaches will help you gather more information about the client's concerns, without suggesting criticism.

Review the first dialogue in the previous section, "Asking Too Many Questions," for another example of the effect of "why" questions. How do you think this patient felt?

Changing the Subject Inappropriately

Abruptly changing the topic of discussion makes you appear uninterested. This often occurs when the nurse is intent on one issue and the client is focused on another. For example, imagine that you want to tell the patient about a change in the scheduling for a diagnostic test before you forget. As you enter the room, your patient says, "I am having a lot of pain in my knee today." This situation requires you to address the patient's concern first and postpone discussing the schedule change until the patient can be receptive to the information.

In an ongoing dialogue, changing the subject can stop the flow of conversation cold. Both patients and nurses sometime use this tactic to avoid discussing sensitive topics. The following is an example:
Nurse: This must be a tough time for you. Your wife is very sick. How are you handling this?
Patient's husband: Yes, it's tough, but I went out to a movie last night. Have you seen that new Spielberg movie? It's all about...
Your relationship with the patient's husband and the facts of the patient situation would determine whether you would redirect this conversation back to the original subject or allow him to wander. You may choose to give the husband more time to be comfortable with you prior to approaching this topic again.

Failing to Listen

Failure to listen to your client will result in missed messages or misinterpretation. Consider this example:

Patient: I guess I'm going to surgery tomorrow.

Nurse: (Checking the IV fluids and hanging a medication) Uh-huh.

Patient: The surgeon says I'll be in intensive care for a few days.

Nurse: (Looking at the drainage in the urine collection bag) OK. Your urine looks good.

Patient: I guess this is pretty risky surgery.

Nurse: (Recording on the flow sheet) Yes.

How do you think the patient must feel in this situation? The patient is clearly expressing concern about his upcoming surgery. However, the nurse is busy with a variety of tasks and is not paying attention to the conversation. Undoubtedly the patient will continue to feel anxiety. In fact, his unsuccessful attempts to communicate may even increase his anxiety. If the nurse were listening, this would be an excellent opportunity to discuss the patient's concerns, provide preoperative teaching, and help the patient ease his anxiety.

Failing to Probe

The quality of your care is affected by the interchange between you and your client. A thorough assessment requires you to explore issues in detail. Failing to probe results in incomplete assessment. Review the following conversation.

Patient: I'm having a lot of discomfort in my back.

Nurse: How much does it hurt?

Patient: Quite a bit. I had trouble sleeping last night.

Nurse: I'll get you something for pain.

Compare this conversation with the next example, in which the nurse gathers additional data.

Patient: I'm having a lot of discomfort in my back.

Nurse: Tell me about the discomfort.

Patient: It hurts a lot. I had trouble sleeping last night.

Nurse: When did you first notice this pain?

Patient: It started in the middle of the night.

Nurse: What does it feel like?

Patient: I feel sore. I'd like to turn over to my side, but I can't because of this heavy cast.

Nurse: Let me help you turn (Assists patient to turn and uses pillows to hold the patient on her side).

Patient: Oh, that feels better!

Nurse: How is the discomfort now?

Patient: It's pretty much gone.

Nurse: I'm glad you're feeling better. Would you like something for pain as well?

Patient: I think I'm OK now.

In the second example, the nurse followed her original question with additional probing questions. A few additional questions helped clarify what the patient needed and led to immediate comfort.

Expressing Approval or Disapproval

We offer our friends and family members approval when they do something well or disapproval for doing something wrong. But you should exercise caution when providing approval or disapproval in the nurse-client relationship. Even approval can inhibit further sharing—it puts you in the position of being the judge of what is "right." This often prompts the patient to continue to seek approval. He thinks, "I'd better be careful; she may not approve of the next thing I was going to tell her. She expects me to be *this* way." Consider instead offering recommendations and allowing the client to choose. Read the following exchange.

Patient: I've decided I'm going to have the surgery.

Nurse: That's great. I think you made the right choice.

Compare this conversation with the following example.

Patient: I've decided I'm going to have the surgery.

Nurse: Tell me about your decision.

Patient: Well, my shoulder has been bothering me for several months now. I know I said I wanted to put off surgery, but I think I'll have a faster recovery if I just get the surgery done now.

Nurse: So your choices are to do a trial of physical therapy and anti-inflammatory medicines, to try a steroid injection, or to have surgery.

Patient: Right. But there's a good chance I'll still need surgery even if I try the therapy or medicines. The only thing that will actually fix the problem is surgery. The others don't guarantee improvement.

Can you see how different the conversation becomes if the nurse does not express approval? By allowing the patient to discuss the choices, the nurse has empowered the patient to make his own health care decisions.

Offering Advice

Offering an opinion is rarely helpful. Avoid statements such as, "If I were you..." or, "You should..." These statements impose your opinion on your clients. In effect, your statements function as approval if they agree with the client's thoughts or disapproval if they do not. As with other forms of approval or disapproval, conversation halts. If the client asks, "What should I do?" help her clarify her options, and provide her with information about the choices. Telling the client what you think negates the client's opportunity to participate as a mutual partner in the decision-making process.

Providing False Reassurance

Providing reassurance helps to ease concern, offers comfort, and communicates empathy. Thus, it is an appropriate and therapeutic action—if the reassurance is warranted. For example, consider the client who presents to the emergency department (ED) for treatment of an acute episode of asthma. Because anxiety exacerbates asthma, reassuring the client that he will be cared for promptly and effectively is certainly therapeutic. In contrast, false reassurance is a barrier to therapeutic communication. When patients or family members ask for information or tell you that they are worried, it is easy to reassure them that everything will be okay. However, such responses are uninformed, inaccurate, and may feel dismissive–even condescending-to the receiver. Examine the following scenario:

You are a nurse working at the triage station in the local ED. Your role is to evaluate the condition and prioritize the care of all clients presenting for treatment. An ambulance arrives with a man complaining of severe chest pain. He is ashen and short of breath. He tells you his pain is "crushing." Suspecting a heart attack, you immediately move him to the critical care bay of the ED and request urgent evaluation. Several minutes later his wife arrives by private car and approaches the triage station. She anxiously asks, "How is my husband?" How would you respond?

It may be tempting to offer a response such as, "Don't worry, everything will be all right." But do you really know that will be the case? A better approach is to provide accurate information: "I had him immediately taken in for treatment. I'll get you into see him as soon as I can. Please have a seat, and I'll check on him." This comment is accurate, calming, and avoids misstatements.

Stereotyping

The racial, cultural, religious, age-related, or gender stereotypes distort assessment and prevent you from recognizing the uniqueness of the patient. Examples of statements reflecting a stereotype include, "He's old, he won't remember anything you tell him," or "Men are always the biggest crybabies about pain." Such comments may shut down communication and escalate tension. Avoid their use with patients and colleagues.

Stereotypes may be blatant or subtle. Blatant examples, such as those above, are easily recognized and may create an intense reaction. Subtle stereotypes, however, may be equally disruptive to care. Subtle stereotypes common in health care include the following:

- Believing a patient will be calm and know what to expect because he has had previous hospitalizations for the same diagnosis or has had previous surgeries or other procedures.
- Assuming that patients will understand their health care because of their educational level or work experience, for example, expecting that a physician who has suffered a heart attack needs no explanation of her care.
- Expecting all patients with the same surgery or diagnosis to experience similar responses.

Using Patronizing Language

Patronizing language communicates superiority or disapproval. Statements such as, "You know better than that," are patronizing and offensive to the client.

Condescending approaches, such as, "You should have used the call button before you got up. You're lucky you didn't hurt yourself," do not communicate respect for the client.

Patronizing language may seem innocent. Have you heard staff call patients "Sweetie," "Dearie," or "Mama"? Although the intent is to be endearing, many patients are offended. When you first meet your client, use a formal title–Mr., Ms, and so on. In the orientation phase of the relationship, ask your patient how he would prefer to be addressed. If the patient is unable to respond, ask family members how to address the patient.

Conveying Acceptance

Many issues in the nurse-patient relationship are of a highly personal nature. A patient may be afraid to give the nurse complete information, particularly as it relates to values, beliefs, lifestyles, and practices. This may stem from a fear that the nurse will disapprove of the patient's values, beliefs, or practices, or even fear of being rejected as an individual.

Acceptance is the willingness to listen and respond to what a patient is saying without passing judgment on the patient. It is likely that a patient's values, beliefs, and practices will differ from those of the individual nurse related to variances in sociocultural influences (e.g. economic status, religion, upbringing, cultural background, and age, to mention only a few). The nurse must be careful not to non-verbally communicate disapproval through gestures or facial expressions.

Acceptance and agreement are not synonymous. The nurse is often confronted with a patient whose practices may be detrimental to a healthy lifestyle. The nurse's challenge is to facilitate changes in the patient's health behaviors while maintaining the personal integrity of the patient. This can be approached by demonstrating acceptance of patients' rights to their present beliefs and practices without condoning them. The next step is to communicate a healthier alternative to the present behavior and assist the patient in initiating the new behavior.

Minimal encouragement is a subtle therapeutic technique that communicates to the patient that the nurse is interested and wants to hear more. It usually involves non-verbal, such as maintaining appropriate eye contact and nodding occasionally, and verbal comments, such as "Yes, go on," to encourage the patient to continue.

(For some more details on Nurse-Patient Relationship, please refer Chapter 11 under Helping Relationship).

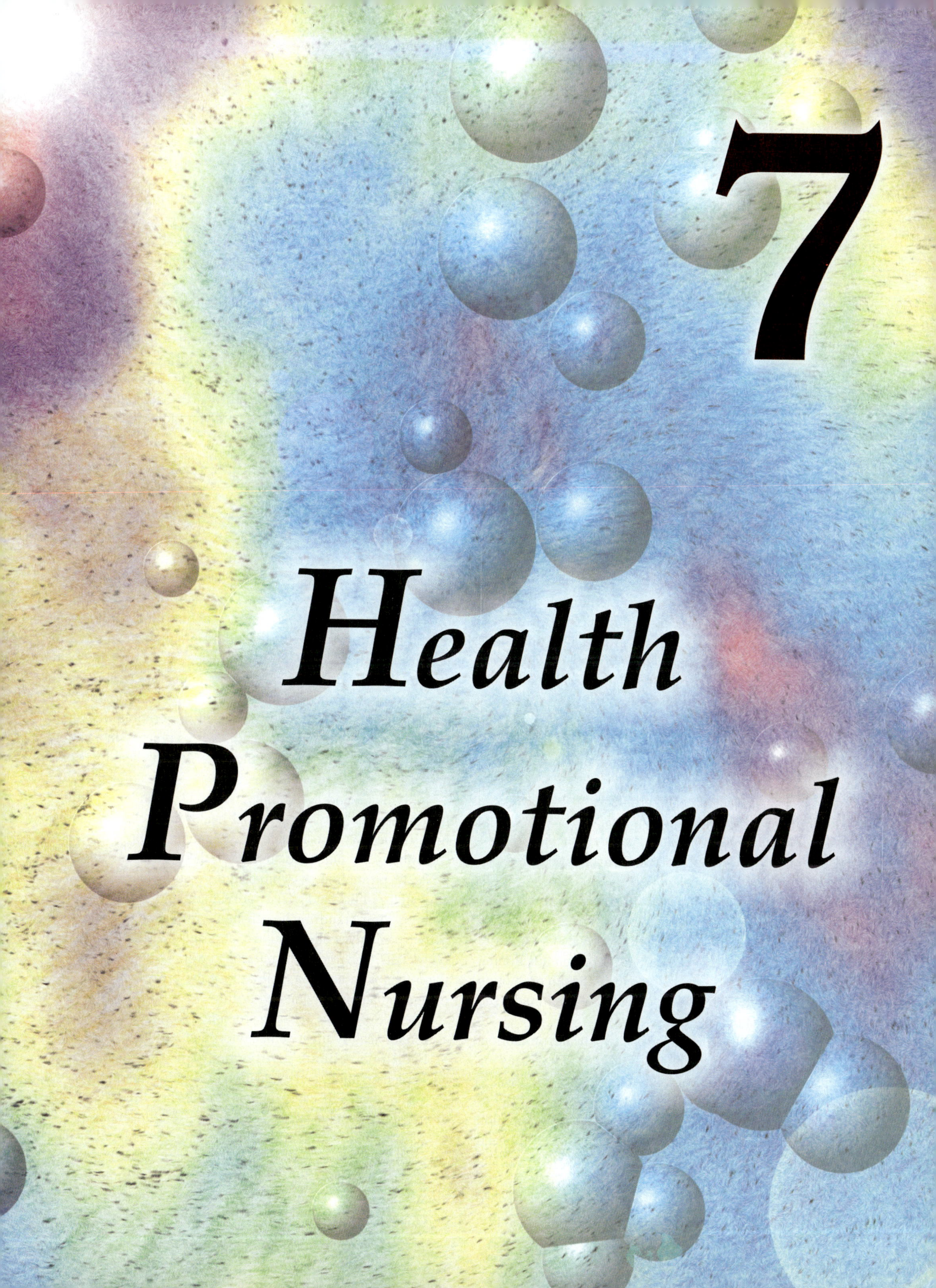

7

Health
Promotional
Nursing

Introduction

Health promotion is an important components of nursing practice. It is a way of thinking than revolves around philosophy of wholeness, wellness and well-being. Now-a-days people are has become increasingly aware of and interested in health promotion. Many of them are aware of relationship between lifestyle and illness and are developing health-promoting basis such as getting adequate exercise, rest and relaxation, maintaining good nutrition and controlling the use of tobacco, alcohol, drugs and other substances that may be harmful to the body.

Health promotion is more than preventing illness. It means assisting individuals to better health, functioning, and well being and to maximizing their potential. Health promotion focuses on choosing healthy behavior rather than eluding illness. The goal is for individuals to control and improve their health. Health promotion is appropriate for the individual and the entire population.

Concept of Health Promotion

Health promotion is defined as "any endeavor directed at enhancing the quality of health and well being of individuals, families, groups, communities, and for nations through strategies, involving supportive environment, coordination of resources, and respect for personal choice and values." Leavell and Clark (1965) defined three levels of preventions; primary, secondary and tertiary, in which there are five steps that describe thee levels as given below:

- *Primary Prevention Focus on*
  1. Health Promotion
  2. Protection against specific health problems
- *Secondary Prevention Focus on*
  3. Early identification of health problems
  4. Prompt prevention to alleviate
- *Tertiary Prevention Focus on*
  5. Restorations and rehabilitation to an optional level of functioning

These three levels of preventions describe as "Health Protection" by Pender, Murdaugh & Parsons (2002). According to them "Health Protection" is behavior motivated by a desire to actively avoid illness, detect it early or maintain functioning within the constraints of illness". In contrast, health promotion is behavior motivated by a desire to increase well-being and actualize human health potential.

It is very difficulty to differentiate behavior health promotion, health protection and prevention of illness. They may be understand well on the basis of following specific activities.

- **Health Promotion:** Individual and community activities to promote healthful lifestyle. Examples of health promotion activities such as improving Nutrition, preventing alcohol and drug misuse, restricting smoking, maintaining fitness, and exercising.
- **Health Protection:** Action by government and industry to minimize environmental health threats. Health protection relates to activities such as maintaining occupational safety, controlling radiation and tonic agents and preventing infection diseases and accidents.
- **Preventive Illness Services:** Actions than health care providers take to prevent health problems. These services include control of high blood pressure, control of HIV/AIDS, STD's, immunizations, family planning and health care during pregnancy and infancy.

Thus, health promotion facilitates an individual or community in a process of self-determining a present health status in order to actively choose ways of altering personal or communal health habits for improvement, and to develop resources and skills to alter the environment so that health is being maintained or self-determined higher level of health can be achieved. So the concepts of health promotions will includes the following (Schultz 1995):

- Health promotion maintains and enhances health
- Health promotion develops the resources and skills of the person or community
- Health promotion alters personnel or communal habits and the environment
- Health promotion defines health as a continuum
- Health promotion is self-directed.

Health care and nursing have traditionally been more oriented toward curing and treating than preventing illness, injury and disability, shifting the focus toward maintaining and promoting health and well-ness is a current challenge. The role of the health promoter provides the nurse with many opportunities to contribute to improved health. The nurse with many opportunity to educate individuals and groups in the community about prevention and maintaining health. Nurses practice in a variety of community settings, where they interact with healthy people and can provide guidance.

Individuals and community who seek to increase require health responsibility for personal health and self-care require health education. The trend toward health promotion has created opportunity for nurses to strengthen the professions influence on health promotion, disseminate information than promotes on educated public, and assist individuals and communities to change long-standing health-behavior. Health promotion activities involve collaborative relationships with both client and physicians. The role of the nurse is to work with people, not for them-than is to act as a facilitator of the process of assessing, evaluating and understanding health.

The role of nurses in health promotion includes the following:

- Model healthy lifestyle behaviors and attitudes
- Facilitate client involvement in the assessment, implementation, and evaluation of health goals
- Teach client self-care strategies to enhance fitness, improve nutrition, manage stress, and enhance relationships
- Assist individuals, families and communities to increase their levels of health
- Educate clients to be effective health care consumers
- Assist clients, families and communities to develop and choose health promoting options

- Guide clients development in effective problem-solving and decision-making
- Advocate in the community for changes that promote a healthy environment.

Health care professionals and consumers are emphasizing on health promotion and illness prevention activities which are designed to help clients to reduce the risks of illness and maintain maximal health. Nurses are major force in the health care delivery system, who emphasizes health promotion and illness prevention activities as important forms of health care.

Promotive nursing refers to the activities involving health promotion and illness prevention. Nurses assist in maintaining good health and improving their levels of health instead of merely providing care after illness occurs. Activities involving health promotion help clients to maintain or enhance their present level of health, whereas the activities of illness prevention protect clients from actual or potential threats to health. Health promotion activities motivate people to act positively to reach the goals of more stable level of health, illness prevention activities motivate people to avoid declines in health of functional levels.

Health promotion services have developed rapidly within the health care delivery system. By keeping people healthy, the overall costs of health care decline. The activities of health promotion will include specific health education programs which are designed to help clients in reducing the risk of illness, maintain maximal function, and promote habits related to good health.

As caregivers, nurses promote health and wellness for people from birth to death. All people, regardless of age, have unique health care needs that result from the physical, emotional, intellectual, social, spiritual, and cultural aspects of their developmental level. To plan and provide holistic and individualized care, the nurse must understand typical growth and developmental characteristics, tasks, and needs for the clients of all ages.

Further details of concepts of health promotion. Please read authors texts on "Community Health Nursing" in "Nursing Theories".

Basic Human Needs

Need is something that is essential to the emotional and physiological health and for survival of humans. All people strive to meet their basic needs. At any given time, an individual need may be met, partially met, or unmet. A person whose needs are met may be considered to be healthy, and a person with one or more unmet needs is at increased risk for illness or health alterations, in one or more of the human dimensions. Needs, i.e. integral parts of each person's human dimension are as follows:

- *Physical needs*—involve all of the body's physiologic processes including breathing, intake and output of fluids and food, temperature, circulation and movement.
- *Emotional needs*—are concerned with the feelings of a person such as fear, happiness, sadness and loneliness.
- *Intellectual needs* – are focused on process such as thinking, learning, problem solving and decision-making.

- *Environmental needs* – deal with physical surroundings as they affect safety and security and include housing, neighborhood, climate, and atmosphere.
- *Sociocultural needs* – relate to relationships and communications a person has with others such as friends, and a sense of belonging to a group community and being loved by others.
- *Spiritual needs* – concern with persons' values and beliefs as they relate to a higher being and to the performance of activities to help others.

Basic human needs are common to all people and are essential to health and survival. They are matters such as food, water, safety and love that are necessary for survival and health. People set their behavior, feeling about their self and other, results of physiological and psychological needs. Although each person has additional unique needs, everyone has the same basic need. The extent to which basic needs are met determine a person's level of health and position on the health—illness continuum. Basic human needs are met or unmet in a variety of ways. Need satisfaction largely depends on an individual, or social environment particularly his/her and community.

While providing nursing care nurses should consider all of the dimensions that affecting basic human needs in health and illness, that allows the nurse to provide proper nursing care, with ensuring to meet basic human needs.

Maslow's Hierarchy of Human Needs

Abraham Maslow (1868-1954) developed a hierarchy of human needs. This hierarchy of human needs arranged the basic human needs in level of priority as follows (Fig 7.1).

1. Physiological needs
2. Safety and security needs
3. Love and belonging needs (social affiliation)
4. Self esteem needs
5. Self-actualization needs.

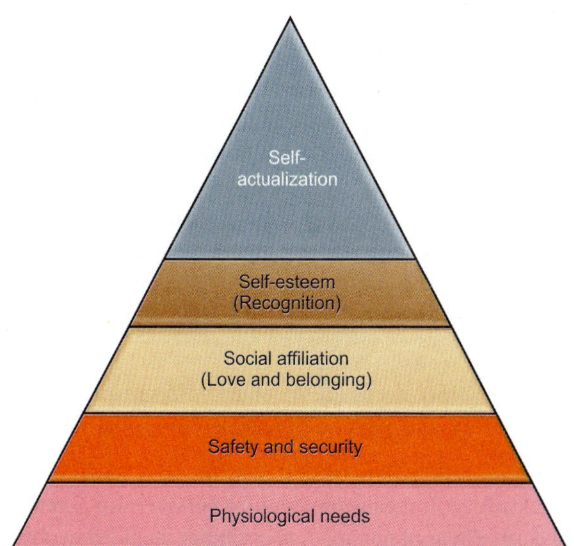

Figure 7.1: Maslow's hierarchy of human needs

Nursing care is often directed towards meeting unmet needs. Usually in nursing, nurses are concerned with physical and psychological needs of each individual. When providing nursing care nurses can use the theory of hierarchy of human needs of Maslow to determine the needs of the client that are the most important at any given time. This theory provides a framework for nursing assessment and for understanding the needs of clients at all levels so that the nursing interventions to meet needs can be planned. To quote an example that when patient comes to casualty department, first nurse immediately concern with physiological need that administers oxygen, if any wound, takes pain relief measure, while administered of O_2 and any pain relief measure, nurse takes safety measures (i.e. precaution of O_2 administration) and put him on comfortable asks the family members to be there for sometimes to meet that need.

Let us examine these needs briefly as follows:

1. *Physiological Needs*
According to Maslow, these needs are located at the base of the hierarchy of needs, that are very essential to life; therefore, they are placed in top priority when unsatisfied and remain as having highest priority until satisfied. They are basic needs which include air (oxygen), water (fluid), food (nutrition), clothing (to maintain temperature), shelter (comfortable room), elimination, sexuality, physical activity and rest. These needs fall under lifesaving (prevention of imminent death) and life sustaining (health maintenance and prevention of complications following bodily insult) dimensions. Physiological needs for survival, i.e. oxygen, fluid, nutrition, temperature, elimination, shelter, rest, and sex. They are actually physical needs, which involve physiological and homeostatic process in the body (Physiological process includes personal hygiene, activity, and sexuality; and homeostatis includes eating, drinking, vital functions, oxygenation, sleep, rest and elimination).

Oxygen: It is the most essential of all the needs; all body cells require oxygen for survival. Nurses evaluate oxygen need by assessing skin color, vital signs, and mental responsiveness of clients. Accordingly, she/he plans to meet that need.

Physical activity: These are also basic physiologic needs. These activities are accomplished by intact functioning of non-muscular and body systems. Like these all physiologic needs are very essential to plan nursing care. The areas of nursing responsibilities in these needs, are to maintain nutrition, providing sleep and rest, support elimination process, prevention of complication, assurance of physiological status and health maintenance, etc.

2. *Safety and Security Needs*
Safety and security needs are involved with self-preservation ; physical safety and psychological or emotional safety and security.

Physical safety: It means protecting a person from potential or actual harm. Areas of nursing responsibility included in physical safety are providing comfort, insisting physical exercises, i.e.

precautions, maintaining personal hygiene. Providing or creating safety environment, etc. Nurses carry out a variety of activities to meet clients physical safety. These activities are as follows:
- Hand washing and using sterile technique to prevent infection
- Using electrical equipment properly with precautions
- Administering medications knowledgeably
- Using skill moving and ambulating patients
- Teaching parents about household chemicals that are dangerous to children and others.

Emotional safety: It involves trusting others and being free from fear, anxiety, and apprehension. An area of nursing responsibility to meet these needs will include encouraging religious practices that are source of strength and support, by providing spiritual comfort and assistance, by providing emotional support, counseling and teaching.

3. *Love and Belonging Needs*
Love and belonging are the needs or social affiliation, in which person expects meaningful interpersonal relationship, group acceptance, and love and belonging. All human have their basic needs which include the understanding and acceptance of others in both giving and receiving love and the feeling of belonging to others. Love and belonging needs are life enhancing needs that one's relationship with the universe, which requires communication identity, affection, modesty, companionship and dependence.

Individuals who perceive that their love and belonging needs are unmet often have a sense of loneliness and isolation, which may lead to withdrawal, and other unexpected experience with the client. When these social affiliation needs are unsatisfied, the nurse may observe boredom in clients, apathy, desire to have friends and family visits and other signs. Accordingly to fulfill these needs nurse can include the family and friends in the care of clients and establishing good rapport based on mutual understanding and trust by demonstrating caring, encouraging communication, respecting privacy and also insisting or encouraging diversional activities, socializing process with privacy.

4. *Self-esteem Needs*
Self-esteem need is the need for a person to feel good about himself or herself, to feel pride and a sense of accomplishment and to believe that others also hold one in high regard. It gives the individual confidence and independence.

When a client first seeks to belong, the positive values of belonging emerge as priorities and should be satisfied if a nurse desires the client to reach fullest potential. Instead of just feeling like a part of systems or group, the person who has esteem needs in focus others, prestige and power, the client may want to be useful in some way, either being personally involved in or by helping in others' care. So the esteem needs which involve self-confidence, usefulness, activeness and self-worth.

Sometime disease process, treatment measures, nurses' actions and others may lower the self-esteem. Nurses can meet clients self-esteem needs by accepting values and beliefs, encouraging clients to set attainable goals, and facilitating support by family or significant others. These actions will promote a sense of worth and self-acceptance. The areas of nursing responsibilities will include and amplification of what has emerged before, but considering the client need for achievement.

5. *Self-actualization Needs*

Self-actualization is the need for an individual to reach his or her potential through full development of the individual's unique capabilities. Self-actualization is the state of having reached one's fullest potential and being able to cope with problems. In other words, it is the state of fully achieving potential and having ability to solve problems and cope realistically with life situations. The process of self-actualization is one that continues throughout life.

The characteristics of self-actualization include the following:

- Solves his own problem
- Assists others in problem solving
- Accepts suggestion from others
- Has broad interest work and social topic
- Possesses good communication skills as Listener and communicator
- Manages stress and assists others
- Enjoys privacy
- Seeks new experience and knowledge
- Shows confidence in abilities and decision
- Anticipates problems and successes
- Likes self.

Since it is a need for reaching individual's full potentials, Maslow enlists the following qualities that indicate achievement of one's potential:

- Acceptance of self and others as they are
- Focus of interest on problems outside self
- Ability to be objective
- Feelings of happiness and affection for others
- Respect for all people
- Ability to discriminate between good and evil
- Creativity as a guidelines for solving problems and pursuing interests.

To meet clients self-actualization needs, the nurse must focus on strengths and possibilities of clients, and to use holistic approach in providing nursing care, which provides a sense and direction, and hope, and engaging in teaching that aimed at maximizing potentials.

Nurses must constantly strive to satisfy the needs of clients at the level of implicitly and explicitly expressed by the person. Maslow's structural framework provides a useful basis by which nurses can determine priorities of clients' needs and accordingly, they can plan the nursing care.

Basic Concepts of Development

Development is a very broad term which, first of all, refers to the process by which individuals' potentialities unfold and appear as new abilities, qualities, and characteristics. It includes the relatively permanent changes resulting from growth, maturation, learning, and achievement. The qualitative or behavioral aspects of progressive adaptation to the environment are called 'development'. An example of these qualitative changes is increased functioning capacity resulting from mastery of several smaller skills. For instance, a significant qualitative and observable change for preschoolers is participating in telephone conversation with their parents. Before developing this capacity, they must develop a small vocabulary, learn to put words together in phrases and sentences, and develop a cognitive understanding of object permanence (that a person or object out of sight still exists). This development, refers to an increase in functional capacity and results from two basic factors, maturation and learning.

'Growth' refers to the increment of bodily tissues, organs, structures and systems or an increase in body size. Physical growth is the qualitative or measurable, aspect of an individual's increase in physical measurement. Measurable growth indicators include height, weight and dental, skeletal, and sexual age. Increase in these indicators demonstrate growth. For example, children generally double birth weight by 6 months of age and double height by 36 months. Also children usually have their primary teeth before 3 years of age and begin to loose them at the end of the preschool period.

'Maturation' refers to the inborn, genetically transmitted capacity for development in all areas. It means their emergence and attainment of maturity of bodily structures and functional powers mainly as a result of periodic genetic stimulation. Thus maturation may be defined as the progressive differentiation of structure and function. Hence, maturation is the process of becoming fully developed and growth. It involves an individual's biological ability, physiological condition, and desire to learn more mature behaviors. To mature, the individual may have to relinquish previous behaviors and learning, integrate new pattern into existing behaviors or both. Maturation influences sequence and timing of the changes associated with growth and development. For example, the infant relinquishes crawling for walking, because it permits more extensive investigation of the environment and more learning. However infant cannot walk until the biological ability and structure to perform the action (that is increased muscles calls and tone) have developed.

'Learning' is the process by which one gains specific knowledge of skill and acquires a habit or attitude. It is the result of experience, experimentation, training and the resultant changes in behavior.

The 'developmental sequence' means that changes are specific, progressive and orderly, and lead eventually to maturity. All children progress through similar stages, but the age for achievement varies, since achievement depends upon the child's inherent maturation capacity, interacting with his physical and social environment. The different areas of growth and development, i.e. physical, mental, emotional, social and spiritual are interrelated, proceed together, and affect each others in various ways.

Principles of Growth and Development

Some principles of growth and development are true for all people. These commonalties are expressed by the following concepts:

1. Individual have adaptive potential for qualitative and quantitative changes by receiving stimuli from and giving stimuli to the environment.
2. Individuals derive uniqueness from the interaction of heredity and environment.
3. The primary goal of development is achievement of potential (Self-realization or self-actualization).

Basic Principles

A. Development follows a set of sequence. The physiological development of the human shows an orderly process of structural changes marked by two interrelated types of sequence: (i) cephalocaudal and (ii) proximodistal, which meant development is directional and proceed along the body axis.

   (i) *Cephalocaudal:* In this sequence growth proceeds from the head to the lower parts of the body. The etymology of the word indicates the direction of early structural growth from the head, through the trunk, to the extremities. This means that the infants' head and brain grow faster and reach each level of maturity earlier than the heart, lungs, or other visceral organs.

   (ii) *Proximodistal:* In this sequence development proceeds from the (proxima, i.e. central areas of the body of outer (peripheral). The proximodistal sequence of maturation merely parallels the caphalocaudal direction in terms of movement and control. Movements close to the body axis mature faster than that of body parts located on its periphery. Head and eye control appear very early in postnatal life. Whole arm and leg movements are seen long before elbow and knee. Joint control in exercise, the coordinate use of the knee and toes for climbing or jumping follow knee-joints control.

B. The functional aspect of behavior follows the sequence from general to specific. This sequence is inherent in all aspects of early development. In emotional development, general excitement proceeds the appearance of specific emotional responses, such as fear, anger or delights fear in turn, differentiates into fear of specific objects animals or situations. In acquiring speech, the child first learns a number of general nouns before he assimilates any specific word. This behavior sequence from general to specific may be further exemplified by such generalization as from simple to complex, from unselective to highly selective, from unselective to highly selective, from concrete to abstract, from tangible to intangible, and from known to unknown.

C. Development is complex, yet predictable, occurring with consistent pattern and chronology. Since development is an orderly sequence in growth, motivation, behavior and possible in personality organizations, it seems logical that, if someone, is an expert in developmental process and behavior and is capable of diagnostic assessment, he can predict or atleast estimate likely growth patterns of motivational structure, achievement, and probable tendencies of self-expression in a particular individual.

D. Human growth is phasic. The course of human growth and decline is marked by both continued slow modifications and rapid transformation, e.g. teach-first set-next set.

E. Development is unique to individuals and their genetic potential, and each individual tends to seek a maximal potential for development.

F. Development occurs through conflict and adaption, and different aspects develop at different rates, creating period of equilibrium and disequilibrium.

G. Development involves challenges for individuals in the forms of certain tasks specific to age and ability.

H. Developmental tasks require practice and energy the focus of which varies with each developmental stage and tasks accomplished.

Elizabeth Hurlock's Principles of Development

1. Development involves changes, the goal of which is self-realization or the achievement of the hereditary potentials.
2. Early development is more critical than later development. Because early foundations are greatly influenced by learning and experience if they are harmful to a child's personal and social adjustment, they can be changed before they settle into habitual patterns.
3. Development comes from the interaction of maturation and learning, with maturation setting limits to the development.
4. The pattern of development is predictable, through this predictable pattern can be delayed or accelerates by conditions within the prenatal or postnatal environment.
5. The developmental pattern has certain predictable characteristics, the most important of which are that there is similarity in the developmental pattern of all children, the development proceeds from general to specific, responses, development in continuous, different areas develop at different rates, and there is correlation in development.
6. There are individual difference in development due partly to hereditary influences and partly to environmental conditions. This is true both for physical and psychological development.
7. There are periods in the developmental pattern, which labeled the prenatal period, infancy to later adulthood.
8. There are social expectation for every developmental period. The social expectations are in the forms of developmental tasks which enable parents, teachers and other interested ones to know these different patterns of behavior and adjustment.

9. Every area of development has potential hazards – physical – psychological – which alter the pattern of development.
10. Happiness varies at different periods in the developmental pattern. The first year of life is usually the happiest and puberty is usually most unhappy.

Although growth and development in each of the dimension are individualized, certain generalization can be made about the nature of human development. These form the principles of that which serve as guidelines for understanding growth and development.

1. Growth and development are orderly and sequential as well as continuous and complex. Every human being experiences the same growth patterns and developmental level. As these patterns and levels are individualized, wide variation in biological and behavioral changes is considered normal. Within each developmental level, certain milestones are identified.
2. Growth and developments follow regular and predictable trends. Cephalocaudal development is the first trend, i.e. head and brain develop first, followed by trunk, legs and feet. The second trend is proximodistal development which means that growth progress from gross motor movements (i.e. learning to lift ones head) to fine motor movements (i.e. learning to pick up a toy with fingers). The last trend is symmetrical development of the body with both sides of body developing equally.
3. Growth and development are both differentiated and integrated. As nerve pathways develop, they become more specialized, allowing to growing child to respond to different stimuli, throughout the life span. Each new learned activity builds on previous learning and abilities, so that increasingly complex tasks can be accomplished.
4. Different aspects of growth and development occur at different stages and at different rates, and can be modified.
5. The pace of growth and development is specific for each person.

Factors Influencing Growth and Development

The human being is a complex, open system influenced by natural forces from within and from the environment. Interaction between these forces affects development. In general, natural factors set the limits for development, whereas external forces/factors present opportunities for achieving that potential. The brief description of relevant influence of factors on growth and development is as follows.

Natural Factors

1. Heredity is a natural force in which genetic endowments – sex, race, hair and eye color, physical growth, and stature, etc. – influence the growth and development.
2. Temperament is also natural force, which is a characteristic psychological mood in which child is born and includes behavioral styles of easy, slow to warn, and difficult.

External Factors

Family: The role of family is to protect its members. Its functions include means for survival, security, assistance with emotional and social development, assistance with maintenance of relationships, instruction about speciality and world and assistance in learning roles and behaviors. Family influences through its values, beliefs, customs, and specific patterns of interaction and communication. Ordinal position and sex influence individual's interaction and communication in family.

Peer group: It provides new and different learning environment. It provides different pattern and structures of interaction and communication necessitating different styles of behavior. Functions of peer group includes the following:

(i) Allowing the individual to learn about success and failure
(ii) To validate the challenge thoughts, feelings and concepts.
(iii) To receive acceptance, support and rejection as unique person apart from family.
(iv) To achieve group purposes by meeting demands, pressures and expectations.

Life experience: Life experience and learning process allow individuals to develop by applying what has been learned to what needs to be learned. Leaning process involves a series of steps which includes the following:

- Recognition of need to know tasks
- Mastery of skills to perform task
- Mastery of task
- Expertise in performing task, which expands capabilities
- Integration into whole functioning
- Use of accumulated skills and experience to develop repertoire of effective behavior.

Health environment: Level of health affects persons' responsiveness to environment, particularly the following:

(i) Prenatal health preconception (i.e. genetic and chromosomal factors, maternal age, health) and post conception (i.e. nutrition, weight gain, use of tobacco and alcohol, medical problems, use of prenatal services) factors affect fetal growth and development.
(ii) Nutrition growth is regulated by dietary factors. Adequacy of nutrients influences whether and how physiological needs as well as subsequent growth and developmental needs, are met.
(iii) Rest, sleep, and exercise balance between rest or sleep and exercises is essential to rejuvenating body. Imbalances diminishes growth, whereas equilibrium reinforces physiological and psychological health.
(iv) Health status, illness or injury potentially hampers growth and development. Nature and duration of health problem influences its impact. Prolonged injury or illness leaves person less able to cope with and respond to demands and tasks of developmental stage.
(v) Living environment factors affecting growth and development include season, climate, housing, and socioeconomic status.

Growth and development in the family: Family is considered responsible for the child's growth and development and behavioral outcome and for the welfare of its members. Family is strongly influenced by its environment as is the child himself, and should bear full responsibility for what the child is or becomes. Family is expected to per child is or becomes. Family is expected to perform the following developmental tasks.

(i) It provides for physical safety, daily routines and economic needs of its members and obtains enough resources to survive.

(ii) It creates a sense of family loyalty and security and a mentally healthy environment for the family's well-being.

(iii) It reproduces and socializes the child or children, teaching values and appropriate behaviors.

(iv) It teaches members to effectively communicate their needs, ideas, feelings, and respect for each other.

(v) It provides social togetherness simultaneously with division of labor, patterning of sexual roles, and performance of family roles with flexibility and cooperation.

(vi) It helps members to develop physically, emotionally, intellectually and spiritually and to develop a personal and family identity, while adjusting to the demands of family life.

(vii) It releases family members into large society–school, religious instruction, organization employment, and eventually another family unit.

The health status of the family members influences family functioning and family functioning, in turn influences its own and society's perceptions of its health. When the family satisfactorily meets its goals through adequate functioning, its members tends to feel positive about themselves and their family. Conversely, they do not meet goals, families view themselves as ineffective. When the family faces health problems, the nurses view the family as context and as client.

When nurses view the family as context, their primary focus is the health and development of an individual member existing within a specific environment, i.e. clients family. And when the family is viewed as a client it is more than sum of its individual members. The family unit is the primary focus of nursing care because any nursing intervention with one member ultimately influences all members. Then nurses assess the family structure, and function and applies the nursing process, whether family is viewed as client itself. The nurse maximizes therapeutic effectiveness by recognizing family influence and using its research to promote individual and family health.

While making family assessment certain behaviors of family to be noted which may be signs of structured or unhealthy family relationships are as follows for proper guidance and counseling family:

1. Lack of communication between spouses or others family members

2. Disregard shown by family members to each other alternating with harshment through arguments or harshness with each other.

3. Lack of decision making or inability to cooperate with care givers.

4. Over possessiveness of children, mates or other family members, extreme behavior or incest.

5. Derogatory remarks by children to parents or *vice versa.*

6. Blame placed among family members for difficulties.

7. High level of anxiety, tension or insecurity present in the interaction between family members.

8. Pattern of immature or regressive behavior in family members.

In addition, nurses who are taking care of the family, also should insist small family norm, health habits and styles in all respects and also identify abuse in the family (abused women, sexual abuses and child abuses, etc) accordingly, educate the family to correct those deficiencies and also can refer certain available community resource to help them to overcome those problems.

Growth and Development Inside the Womb

Human growth and development begin at the moment when the ovum is fertilized by the sperm. Human life begins at conception when the male sperm unites with the female ovum during its journey down the fallopian tube. 'Gestation' is the term used to describe the development of new life that takes place in the womb between conception and birth. This development normally takes about 9 months.

The fertilized ovum or zygote, contains the full complement of genetic information provided by each parent that determines gender and influences personality, intellect and physical and psychological traits. The growth and development of the fetus are orderly and continuous and proceed in the following three stages.

Pre-embryonic Stage or Germinal Stage (Fertilization to 3 Weeks)

The organism life begins after sexual intercourse has occurred, when the ovum is penetrated by the sperm. Fertilization often takes place in the fallopian tube, usually within 12 to 24 hours after the ovum are released from the ovary. The ovum and sperm fuse and the material from both cell nuclei units. The organism has its full genetic complement in one pair of sex chromosomes and 22 pairs of autosomal chromosomes.

During this stage, the cells of the fertilized ovum, now called zygote, multiply rapidly and the new cell mass moves down from fallopian tube to the uterus. The zygote implants on the uterine wall, and has distinct three layers:

- The ectoderm, the outer cell layer, which forms the brain, spinal cord, nervous system, and outer body parts (skin, hair and nails).

- The endoderm, the inner cell layer, which forms the respiratory system, the digestive system, the liver and the pancreas.

- The mesoderm, which forms the skeleton, connective tissue, cartilage and muscles, and the circulatory, lymphoid, reproductive and urinary system.

The fertilized ovum or zygote passes through the fallopian tube to uterus within 4 days. This time zygote continues to divide. By third day, a solid ball of cells, called morula is formed. Morula soon develops a central cavity or blastocyst. Even at this early stage, cells begin to differentiate in structure and function. Cells at one end of blastocyst develop into the embryo, and those at the opposite end from the placenta.

Embryonic Stage (4 to 8th Week)

The embryonic stage occurs from the 4th through the 8th week. Rapid growth and differentiation of the germ cell layers take place, and by the end of this period, all basic organs have been established, the bones have begun to ossify, and some human features are recognizable.

During this stage, the amniotic sac and the placenta are formed. The amniotic sac, is a protective membrane filled with fluid that surrounds the developing embryo, providing warmth, moisture and relative freedom of movement. The placenta is an organ that attaches to the uterine wall and to the fetus by means of umbilical cord. Through the umbilical cord the unborn child receives nourishment and oxygenated blood and disposes wastes. The placenta also serves as a carrier protecting the developing child from potentially harmful agents. Before implantation the embryo is relatively protected from the environment, but with implantation, it becomes more vulnerable to the lazar maternal environment via exchange of materials through placenta. Placenta produces essential hormones that help maintain pregnancy and that permit transfer of materials between the embryo and mother including oxygen, carbon dioxide, nutrients, and waste products. Because the placenta extremely porous, noxious materials such as viruses and drugs can also pass from mother to fetus which leads to harmful effect on fetal growth and development. Thus this period is such period of rapid growth and change, the fetus is especially vulnerable to any factor that might cause congenital anomalies such as maternal use of alcohol, nicotine or drugs of any kind.

Fetal Stage (9 Weeks to Birth)

By 9 weeks gestation, the embryo is recognizably human, with distinct arms, legs, fingers and toes, although head comprises about half its length. It is only about an inch long but already its systems are beginning to function.

The most striking change that occurs during the fetal stage is the dramatic increase in size from approximately 1 to 1.5 inches to an average length of 18 to 20 inches at birth. The systems that began to form in the embryonic stage increases in complexity and maturity. The fetus begins to move by the third months, although this is not usually felt by the mother until the fourth or fifth month, when its actions become more vigorous. By the sixth month, the eyelids open and the fetus begins to take amniotic fluid into its lungs as a rudimentary form of breathing.

The greatest brain development occurs during the last few months of the fetal stage. Until the seventh month, the fetus is virtually incapable of living outside the womb, owing to the immaturity of its nervous system. The seven months fetus is neurologically mature enough to survive in the extrauterine world in a controlled environment. It can breathe, although the lungs are not fully developed until approximately 36 weeks gestation, or just before birth in a full term infant. Also fetus at 7 months, has not accumulated the layers of fat so noticeable is a full term baby, which protect him from temperature changes and enable him to go without nourishment for the first day or two after birth.

The eight and ninth month of fetal development are devoted primarily to maturation of the lungs and nervous system and to the accumulation of fat. Towards the end of ninth months, activity often diminishes as the fetus because cramped for space. Shortly before the onset of labor the fetus becomes 'engaged' in the pelvic cavity, normally with its head down in preparation of birth.

During its period of development inside the womb the fetus is totally dependent on the mother to satisfy its basic needs. She provides nutrients, oxygen, warmth and protection and disposes fetal wastes. Although the placenta provides some protection from harmful agents, others pass through the placental barrier to the fetus. As the fetus is very vulnerable to infection and the effects of noxious stimuli particularly in its early developmental stage, the mother must take care to protect her unborn child from such dangers. And also that maternal emotions affect the developing fetus, so such psychological aspects of the expectant mother also dealt accordingly to have a healthy child.

The following are the needs of the expectant mothers which require particular attention during pregnancy to meet these to get healthy child accordingly (Table 7.1).

Care during Pregnancy

Pregnancy is a chronological event, that occurs traditionally during the stage of early adulthood. We feel that it belongs more logically in a discussion on fetal development. While the unborn child grows and develops inside the womb of the mother, many other changes are occurring that affect the pregnant women herself. The duration of an average pregnancy is 38 weeks from conception or 40 weeks from the last menstrual period which is divided into 3 trimesters of 3 months each.

First Trimester

A woman's first indication that she is pregnant may be the cessation of menses, swollen and tender breasts or she may feel generally out of sorts. During the first trimester of pregnancy there is a marked increase in the production of hormones, particularly estrogen and progesterone. These hormonal changes account for many of the early signs of pregnancy. She may feel tired and her breasts may swell, tingle and feel tender as the milk glands get prepared to produce milk. She may experiences nausea and vomiting especially in morning.

The pelvic structure begins to widen to accommodate the growing uterus. During pregnancy the uterus will increase its weight from approximately 60 gm (prepregnancy weight) to approximately 1100 gm at full term. Many women feel the need to urinate more frequently owing to the pressure of the uterus on

Table 7.1: Needs of Expectant Mothers

	Needs	*Rationales*
1.	Nutrition	Growth and development of new tissues requiring additional nourishment. Fetus is nourished at expense of mother
2.	Elimination	Hormonal changes affecting kidney function and digestion. Expansion of uterus in pelvis and into abdominal cavity
3.	Circulation	Increased in total fluid volume Increased body mass
4.	Comfort, rest, sleep	Weight gain, increasingly body bulk Altered body proportions, making some resting positions difficult
5.	Pain avoidance	Medications may cross placenta and have effects on the fetus
6.	Movement and exercise	Awkwardness due to (i) Weight gain (ii) Increase in fluid volume (iii) Shift to center of gravity (iv) Relaxing ligaments (v) Slowing down of body process
7.	Protection and safety	Dependence of fetus well-being on mother Shift in sense of gravity, affecting balance
8.	Hygiene	Hormonal changes affecting skin texture and secretions
9.	Infection control	Placenta only a partial barrier to harmful agents
10.	Love, security, self-esteem	Possibility that strong emotions may affect fetus
11.	Sexuality	Note: There are conflicting beliefs regarding possible harm to the fetus from intercourse • Altered body proportions • New role of mother

the bladder as well as to hormonal changes. The increase in progesterone has a relaxing effect on smooth muscle, which causes bowel irregularity and in many cases constipation.

The degree to which these changes are felt depends on her physiological make-up and on her emotional response to her pregnancy.

During this trimester fetal cells continue to differentiate and develop into essential organs systems. These processes of cellular change (differentiation) and staged organ change (development) occur at different rates and time, and each organ extremely vulnerable to environmental insult. Interference with growth can cause the congenital absence of an organ system or extensive structural and functional alteration. Agents capable of producing adverse effect on the fetus are called teratogens. Some teratogens produce defect only if the fetus is exposed to the agent when the vulnerable organ is developing. One such teratogen is rubella virus, which can cause abortion, stillbirth or defects of the eyes, ears, and heart, primarily when exposure in first trimester. Many drugs are teratogenic during rapid organ growth (organogenesis) in the first trimester, which include barbiturate, alcohol, hydantoins, anticonvulsants and anticoagulants, etc. smoking and abuse of drugs such as cocaine results low birth weight and congenital abnormalities.

To avoid such hazards in fetal development nurses should assess all those concern for defects, and explore lifestyles changes that can help the women abstinence from tobacco, alcohol, medications, and suggest measures to minimize or prevent infections during pregnancy.

The nurse should focus on these two events during prenatal care. Changes in maternal behavior during this period include planning for the birth, concern for personal safety, and preoccupation with health and appearance. The nurse can help the woman adapt to these changes and plan for the impending birth. This is often a good time for education about gestational events and appropriate maternal rest and nutrition.

Second Trimester

During the fourth to the sixth month of pregnancy the expectant mother usually experiences a feeling of overall well being. Her body has adjusted to the hormonal changes and she has more energy. She can feel the fetus more which usually has a positive effect, many women take on a radiant glow at this time.

By the fourth month weight gain is usually evident. There is a thickening of waist as the uterus expands and rises out of the pelvis. The amount of body fluid increases by approximately 7 liters, about 3 liters of which is increased blood volume. The cervix softens and is closed by a much plug. The breasts including nipples enlarge and may begin to produce colostrums. The nipples may become darker, and a vertical line of dark pigment called 'linea nigra' appears between the public area and the navel. Some women develop stretch marks (reddish streaks) on their breasts and abdomen.

During this trimester some organ systems of fetus continue basic development and the functional capabilities of others are refined. The fetus is considered viable or capable of life outside the uterus, if given intensive environmental support. The fetus weight about 0.7 kg (1.5 lb) and is approximately 30 cm (12") long. Fingers and toes are differentiated, a rudimentary kidney functions, and sex of fetus can be determined. The fetus is covered with vernia caseosa a cheese like substance coating the skin. Lunago or fine hairs, covers most of the body. In this trimester fetal heartbeats become audible and the mother becomes aware of fetal movements.

During pregnancy and labor many women sense a diminution of their self image, a loss of respect on the part of others for their needs and wishes. All too often especially during labor, the pregnant women wishes to have been overruled or ignored in favor of the conveniences of hospital personnel. It should be remembered that while the healthy and safe delivery of the infant are important, so are the needs and wishes of the parents.

(For details read the authors texts on *Community Health Nursing* – Chapter on MCH and also "Midwifery and Reproductive Health Nursing").

Third Trimester

During third trimester, the expectant mother again often experiences fatigue and new feelings of heaviness. A general relaxation of all body ligament occurs in late pregnancy and continuously enlarge in uterus pushed her center of gravity backward. The enlarged uterus is responsible for much of the discomfort and woman feels at this time. It may press on the lungs or the diaphragm or both, causing shortness of breaths; on the bladder, causing urinary frequency; or on the stomach, causing indigestion.

Approximately one month before the birth of the baby 'drop' as its head settles into pelvic cavity. This makes mother centrally more comfortable, although the uterus may now be pressing on the bowel, causing constipation. During this stage, Braxton Hicks contractions, that is, tightening of the uterus muscles in preparation for labor which often occurs.

During this trimester, the fetus skin thickens, lunago being to disappear, and fetal body becomes rounder and fuller. A tremendous spurt in growth of brain begins during this trimester and lasts well into the first few years of life. The central nervous system has established its total number of neurons and connections between neuron, and myelination of nerve fibers progresses at a rapid rate. Exposure to noxious agents and the absence of essential nutrients are the most common causes of damage to the central nervous system during this trimester. The nurse can teach the women about these factors, particularly by nutritional counseling.

At end of third trimester, the normal fetus is physically able to make the transition from intrauterine to extrauterine life. The cardiac system can change its circulation to the end by passing of the lungs. The lungs are capable of maintaining the inflated state for gas exchange. The primitive temperature mountains, system reflexes, and sensory organs are ready for use.

At the end of this trimester, in expectant mother the loss of the mucus plug (show) and the appearance of amniotic fluid are generally good indications that labor is imminent. Labor is the process by which the baby is expelled out from the uterus. It consists of a series of strong contractions, and can be divided into three stages:

- In the first stage labor the cervix shortens and becomes thinner (effacement) and opens (dilation) to allow the baby to pass through
- The second stage labor begins as the baby's head crowns or becoming visible and ends with birth of the infant
- In third stage labor the placenta is expelled out.

Neonate Care

The neonatal period is the first month of life. A birth, neonate must adapt to extrauterine life, and must make several significant physiologic adjustment to do so. Although these adjustments occur in all body systems, the most important ones occur in the respiratory and circulatory systems.

During this stage, the newborn's physical functioning system is mostly reflexive and stabilization of the major organ systems. The physical characteristics of the neonates include the following:

- They reflex that allow sucking, swallowing, blinking, sneezing and yawning
- They labile temperature control that responds quickly to environmental temperature
- They are alert to the environment, see color and form, hear and turn toward sound, and smell and taste and are sensitive to touch and pain
- They can eliminate both stool and urine
- They will drink breast milk, glucose water and plain water.

The impact of these reflexive behaviors is generally a surge of maternal feelings of love that prompt the mother to cuddle the baby.

The neonate also inherits a transient immunity from infection as a result of immunoglobulins that cross the placenta. Breastfeeding provides further protection against bacterial and viral infections through immunoglobulins and leukocytes. The high lactose content of breast milk, combined with limited proteins, promotes and acid environment that is unsuitable for bacterial growth. Antibodies secreted in breast milk help to control some viral infections.

The common health problems which occur in neonates are particular difficulties related to the birth process, the transition to extrauterine life or congenital anomalies. The selected drugs given to mother lead to breathing difficulties; premature neonate experience respiratory distress syndrome. Congenital malformation will include cleft palate, cleft lip, spina bifida. Down syndrome or birth trauma, may be noticed neonate. Physiological jaundice commonly presents in neonates.

Nurses can apply their knowledge of this stage of growth and development to promote newborn and parental health. For example, assessment of the newborn is done immediately after birth. There are several measurement scales, but the Apgar one is commonly used. The Apgar rating scale is applied to neonates at 1 to 15 minutes after birth (Table 7.2).

Normal neonates score between 7 and 10. neonates who score between 4 and 6 require special assistance; those who score below 4 are in need of immediate life saving support.

Table 7.2: Apgar Score

	Scores		
Signs	*0*	*1*	*2*
Heart rate	Absent	Slow (< 100 beats p.m)	100 beat p.m
Respiration rate	Absent	Slow, irregular	Good crying
Muscle tone	Flaccid	Some flexion of extremities	Active motion
Reflex irritability	No response	Weak cry and grimace	Vigorous cry
Color	Blue, pale	Body pink, extreme blue	Completely pink

Nurses must understand all aspects of neonate and identify problems and assist parents to fulfill the demands of the neonates and give education regarding breastfeeding and avoiding mothers' lifestyles such as smoking, consuming alcohol, drugs.

Infant Care

Infancy is the period from one month to one year of age. Rapid physical growth and change characterize this stage. The physical characteristics of the infant includes:

- Brain grows about half the adult size
- Body temperature stabilizes
- Motor abilities develop to allow using building block, trying the feed self, crawling, walking
- Eyes begin to focus and fixate
- Heart doubles in weight, the heart rate slows and blood pressure rises
- Decidual teeth begin to erupt at 4 to 6 months
- Birth weight usually triples by one year.

In addition one can observe cognitive development in the prelinguistic phase. Here babies begin to speak and make pleasurable sounds soon after birth, and by 12 months, they can convey wishes through a few keywords. Language age development has several consistent characteristic regardless of the specific language being learned such as use of syllable repetition (mama, dada, by-bye), identical early phonetic expressions (bubbling sounds), imitation of sounds, and intonations spoken by caregivers.

An infant also shows some psychosocial development advances, aided by the progression from reflexive to more purposeful behavior. He/she is in the oral stage striving for immediate gratification of needs and having a strong suckling need. Then develops trust when the caregiver can be counted on to provide food when infant is hungry; trust also is facilitated by diaper changing, warmth and comforting and meets the developmental tasks by learning to take solid food, walk and talk.

According to Erickson, the infant should learn to trust. Basic trust involves confidence, optimism, acceptance of and reliance on self and others and a sense of hope. A sense of trust forms the basis for later identity formation, social responsiveness, to others, and ability to care about and love others, because of trust may be demonstrated in the infant by the case for feeding, the depth of sleep and overall appearance of contentment. If trust is not developed, mistrust develops. Mistrust, is a sense of feeling dissatisfied emotionally or physically; an inability to believe in or rely on others or self. It is characterized by lethargy, loss of weight, poor eating, excessive cold, lack of sleep and failure thrive. Later they may develop pessimism, suspicious, bitterness toward others and antagonism or may withdrawn.

The nurses have responsibility to educate parents and other caregivers about health promotion behaviors that will positively affect perception of health and self. During the phase of growth and development the nurse can observe the children adaptive potential, because qualitative and quantitative changes occur rapidly.

And the nurses also should aware the expected developmental tasks and she/he can assess the child, that whether the child is showing or performing those tasks accordingly or not. The developmental tasks of infant are as follows.

Developmental Tasks of Infant

Infancy if far from what some have assured – a rigidity and mechanical handling the baby because he seems to have so little capability as an adapting human being. The following developmental tasks are to be accomplished in infancy:

1. Achieve overall physiological equilibrium after birth of oral system
2. Establish perceive self as a dependent person but separate human being from others
3. Become aware of the alive versus inanimate and familiar versus unfamiliar, and develop rudimentary social interaction
4. Develop a feeling of and desire for affection and response from others
5. Adjust somewhat to the expectation of others
6. Manage the changing body and learn new motor skills, develop equilibrium, begin eye-hand coordination, and establish rest activity rhythm

7. Learn to understand and control the physical world through exploration
8. Develop a beginning symbol system, conceptual ability and preverbal communication
9. Direct emotional expression to indicate need and wishes.

In addition the nurses should be aware about the needs of an infant and plan the care for promotion of health or wellness (Table 7.3).

For promoting optimum health of an infant the nurses must emphasize on the following:

Nutrition: Feeding time is crucial for both mother and child. It is the time that strengthen attachment so that child feels love and security and it is time for the child to learn about the environment. So the nurses should encourage the mother to enrich breastfeeding to the child, because the human milk is sterile, digestible, available, inexpensive and contains necessary nutrients except vitamins C and D, and iron. Breast milk is all that baby needs the first month of life as it contains antibodies (immunoglobulin). In addition 4 months onward, the nurse should advise the mother to start weaning, for infant.

Sleep, rest and exercise: The nurse in a key position to teach parents about the child sleep patterns and to promote sleeping in the child. Every child has a unique sleep pattern.

Immunization: The nurses should encourage the parents to get that child immunized according to National Immunization Schedule.

Injury prevention: The nurse is responsible for giving safe care and can teach parents and others about safety measure to the child, for prevention of injuries due to falls, suffocation and burns, etc.

In general the most essential role of the nurse in meeting health care needs of the infant is the prevention of illness (ARI and other) and promotion of wellness through teaching family members. The aspects of concern related to preventive teaching in infancy are as follow.

1. *Accident prevention*
- Associate common accidents to developmental abilities of the infant
- Encourage relaxes, slow feeding and regular bubbling (burping) to prevent aspiration
- Emphasize that bottles should not be propped and left with an unattended infant
- Emphasize the use of Dumper pads and keeping crib sides up at all times to prevent injury related to jumping or falling
- Teach the correct usage of infant care seats
- Emphasize never leaving an infant unattended on table chair or regular bed
- Teach proper positioning of infant for sleeping and discourage the use of pillows to prevent suffocation.

2. *Nutrition and feeding methods*
- Assist the mother with initiation and maintenance of breastfeeding

	Table 7.3: Needs of an Infant	
	Needs	*Rationales*
1.	Nutrition	Immaturity of gastrointestinal system: • Rapid growth of all body tissues, requiring increased nutrition • Appearance of teeth
2.	Elimination	Immaturity of GI system: • Immaturity of neuromuscular structure necessary for the control
3.	Temperature regulation	Immaturity of temperature regularity system
4.	Comfort, rest, sleep	Rapid growth requiring increase rest and sleep
5.	Sensory stimulation	Quality of environment: • Mobility status
6.	Movement and exercise	Neuromuscular development: • Opportunity for exploration of environment
7.	Protection and safety	Lack of experience to perceive danger: • Inability to protect self
8.	Hygiene	Vulnerability to infection: • Sensitivity of skin
9.	Infection control	Maternal antibodies to young infants prolonged by breastfeeding: • Immunization schedule
10.	Security and self-esteem	Mother-infant adjustment is prime importance
11.	Love and belongingness	Mother, infant 'bonding' important: • Quality care, extent of cuddling, affection important.

- If the baby is bottle-fed, provide information on the preparation of formula milk for feeding, expulsion of air from the bottle, nipple types and hole size, and position of the baby while feeding
- Discuss the age at which seem solid and solid foods are needed (i.e. 4 to 6 months)
- Discuss the sequence of solid foods, i.e. cereals, vegetables, fruits, meat and protein products.

3. *Infections*
- Encourage prompt attention of infections, i.e. ARI, diarrhea, etc.
- Encourage completion of required immunization of infancy.

4. *Hygiene and skin care*
- Teach proper infant bathing techniques, i.e. washing eye from inner to outer canthus, washing genitals, umbilical cord care
- Discuss the proper use of creams, oils and powders
- Describe the nature of infant skin and its susceptibility to disturbance
- Teach diapering and hygienic practices related to the disposal of products of elimination
- Teach care related to hairs, nails and genitals.

5. *Developmental performance*
- Provide accurate information about developmental norms. This can prevent unrealistic expectations in caregivers and assist in isolating and treating developmental delays earlier.

6. *Emotional attachments*
- Encourage intimate child caregiver contact in the crucial period, i.e. immediately after birth
- Provide information about the sequence of normal attachment behaviors in infant
- Reassure concerned caregivers that attachment feelings occur at different rates for different caregivers and infants.

Toddler (One to Three Years) Care

Usually one to three years of the child is considered as toddler. Toddler hood ranges from the time when the children begin to walk independently until they walk and run with ease, which approximately from 12 to 36 months. Toddler hood is characterized by increasing independence bolstered by greater physical mobility and cognitive abilities. Toddlers are increasingly aware of their abilities of control and are pleased with successful efforts with this new skill. This success leads them to repeated attempts may lead to negative behaviors and temperature.

During this stage the child continues to grow, although not so quite and so rapidly as during infancy. The proportions of his body begin to change – his head does not appear quite so large, and his limbs begin to lengthen in relation to his trunk. The body systems continue to mature and mental functions increase in complexity. For example, between 18 to 24 months, most children have the neuromuscular capacity for spincter control,

i.e. the capable of controlling eliminations. This is the time most children initiate toilet training. In this stage, raid brain growth; increase in length of long bones of arms and legs; growth of muscles are taking place. Child can use fingers to pick up small objects; child can walk forward and backward, run, kick, climb stairs and ride a tricycle. He can drink from a cup and uses a spoon and also can turn out pages in a book. At age 2, the birth weight can increase to four times. Now child will show normal vital sign such a temperature, pulse and respiration.

Language plays an important role for children at this stage, they are learning to make their wants and needs understood by others. By two years, the average child has a vocabulary of 50 to 100 words; by the age of 3 years, they are capable of forming complex sentences to express their ideas.

By the end of the toddler period, the child should have achieved the following developmental tasks:
- Settled into a daily routine
- Mastering eating habits
- Mastered the basis of toilet training
- Developed physical skills appropriate to the stage of motor development
- Achieved feeling like a family member
- Learned to communicate more effectively

It is the stage that child enters the Erickson stage of autonomy versus shame and doubt. Toddler should develop autonomy instead shame and doubt. Autonomy is shown in the ability to gain self-control; to feel able to cope adequately with problems or get necessary help; to give generously or to hold on; to distinguish between himself, his possession or wishes and other and their possessions; and to have a feeling of good will and pride. Independence in feeling, walking, dressing and toileting as well as the ability to verbally express wishes, facilitate autonomy.

Shame and doubt are felt if autonomy and a positive self-concept are not achieved. Shame is the feeling of being fooled, embarrassed, exposed or small; impotent dirty of wanting to hide, and range against self. Doubt is a fear, uncertainty, mistrust, lack of self-confidence and feeling that nothing done, in any good and that one is controlled by others rather then being in control of self. Toddler may exhibit separation anxiety, negativism and regression. Separation anxiety occurs when a child is afraid of being sent away from those people who loved and serve as security. Negativism is the result of the toddlers effort to have some measure of control over the environment. Regression or behavior that is most characteristic of a younger age, can occur at any time and response to stressful circumstances, e.g. loss of control over elimination.

The family with toddler faces many new tasks, such as:
- Meeting the aspiration costs of family living
- Providing home which is safe, comfortable and had adequate space
- Maintaining sexual involvement which meets both partners need
- Developing a satisfactory division of labor
- Promoting understanding between toddler and his family

- Determining whether they will have any more children
- Rededicating themselves, among many dilemmas, to their decision to be a childbearing family.

Roles of Nurses in Toddler Care

The roles of the nurse in promoting optimum health of the children is very essential. A significant part of teaching in helping caregivers find the means of helping their toddler through encouraging health independence while setting firm limits. Parents sometimes confused about handling the toddler behaviors. Nurses can assist this by outlining some simple rules:

1. Consider limits as more than restriction but rather as a distraction from one prohibited activity to another in which the child can freely participate. For example, if the toddler is not allowed to pull the dogs tail, give him a toy animal. Distraction is very effective with the toddler because of his short attention span.
2. Reinforce appropriate behavior through approval and attention. The child will continue behavior which gains attention, even if the attention is punitive, because negative attention is better than none to the child.
3. Set limits consistently so that the child can rely on the parents judgment rather than testing the adults endurance in each situation.
4. State limits clearly, concisely, simply, positively and in a clam voice.
5. Set limits only when necessary, come rules promote a sense of security, but too many confuse him.
6. Provide an area where the child is free to do whenever they wants to do.
7. Do not overprotect the child; he should learn somethings have a price, such as bruise on scratch.
8. Do not terminate the child's activity too quickly without feeling him the activity in ending.

In addition to the above, nurse can identify the required needs of the toddler, and accordingly teach the parents or caregiver to meet the needs of the toddler. The common needs of toddlers are given in Table 7.4.

The common health problems of the toddler will include accidents, i.e. motor vehicle, poisonings, burning, drowning, aspiration and falls, e.g. dental health problems and other infections, particularly respiratory infection are common. The aspects of health related to preventive teaching for promoting health of the toddler are as follows.

Accident Prevention

- Explain how the autonomy needs of the toddler are to be met with an eye to safety need
- Suggest locking poisons, out of child's reach
- Advices to block stairs with gate and then help the child learn how to maneuver stairs
- Advise not allowing toddler to have small, hard food items, such as popcorn, peanuts, raw carrots or hard candy or ballon which may cause aspiration

- Discourage the toddler from running with food in his or her mouth
- Encourage the proper use of car seats
- Advised never to leave the child unattended near water
- Suggest teaching toddler to danger in clear, simple terms
- Advise against tossing child into the air or swinging the child by the arms.

Table 7.4: Needs of Toddlers	
Needs	*Rationales*
1. Nutrition	• Continued growth and maturation of system
2. Elimination	• Proportional fluid consistency of body in great compared with that in adult • Achievement of control of elimination
3. Sensory stimulation	• Increased mobility and improved motor control, making • Developing sense of autonomy
4. Movement and exercise	• Independence of movement • Improved motor control • Development of motor skills
5. Protection and safety	• Development of independence • Instable curiosity • Improved motor control • Inability to understand danger
6. Hygiene	• Parental teaching • Toilet training
7. Infection control	• Increased contact with other children/ immunization schedule
8. Security	• Developing sense of autonomy • Home atmosphere
9. Love and belonging	• Quality of parent-child interactions • Stability of relationships with parents, siblings • Developing of trust
10. Sexuality	• Gender identification • Relationship with parents and siblings is important

Toilet Training

- Explain developmental tasks necessary for toilet training
- Correct misconceptions about mastery of this task
- Suggest some helpful literature for parents / caregiver.

Negativism

- Held caregivers understand the normality of negativism in toddler-hood and its meaning from child point of view.

Feeding and Nutrition

- Suggest that food can be provided in the forms that toddler can manipulate independently
- Advise caregivers not to be concerned about the merciness of toddler eating habits because the independence gained by the child is more important
- Provide soft finger foods that the child can eat while playing
- Reassure caregivers that short anorexic periods are common in toddler hood.

Hygiene and Dental Care

- Emphasize the teaching of good hygiene habits
- Suggest teaching the toddler how to brush teeth (with assistance)
- Encourage caregivers to take the toddler with them for dentists (if needed).

Infections

- Encourage caregivers to attend to respiratory tract infections promptly because of the high correlation between such infections and media
- Encourage complete immunization as per schedule.

Play Habits

- Encourage the selection of toys that emphasize gross motor skills and creativity
- Advise parents that sharing is not likely to occur and that parallel play is an important precursor to interactive play.

The natural mode of expression for the child is playing, the purposes of playing include the following:

- Develop and improve muscular strength, coordination and balance
- Develop spatial and sensory perception
- Work off excess physical energy
- Communicate with others, establish friendships and develop concern for others
- Learn cooperation and sharing
- Express imagination, creativity and initiative
- Translate feelings, drives and fantasies into action
- Imitate the learn about social activity and adult roles
- Test and deal with reality
- Explore, investigate and manipulate futures of the adult world
- Build self-esteem
- Feel a sense of power, make things happen, explore and experiment
- Provide for intellectual, sensory and language development and deal with concrete experience in symbolic terms
- Assemble novel aspects of environment
- Learn about self and how others see him
- Practice leader and followers role
- Have fun, express joy, feel the pleasure of mastery

- Work through a painful physical or emotional state by repetition and play so that it is more bearable and assimilated into the child's self concept.

Preschoolers (3 to 6 Years) Care

The preschool years are a transition between toddler-hood and the schoolage years. Between 3 to 6 years are considered as preschool years. During this period, the rate of growth is stable and relatively slow down. The physical characteristic of the preschool head is close to adult size by age 6. Motor abilities include skipping, the rowing and catching a ball, copying figures and printing letters and numbers. The full set of 20 decidual teeth and, etc. like this several aspects of physical development continue to stabilize in the preschool years. In short in this period, the preschooler body systems have reached functional maturity. For example, they can handle adult foods and they are capable of controlling their elimination and taking care of their various toilet needs. Although infants are capable of seeking at birth, full visual maturity does not occur until the about age of 5 years. Children develop active immunity through exposure to disease.

Preschoolers continue to master the preoperational stage of cognition. Their vocabularies continue to increase rapidly and by the age of 5, children have more than 200 words that they can use to define, familiarize objects, identify, colors and express their desires and frustrations.

According to Erickson, the principal conflict of this stage is 'initiative vs. guilt'. Initiating is enjoyment of energy displayed in action, assertiveness, learning, increasing dependability and ability to plan. He is expected to learn a sense of initiation rather than guilt. If the child does not achieve initiative, there is an overriding sense of guilt from the tension between the demands of super ego, or others expectations and actual performance. Guilt is a sense of defeatism, anger, feeling responsible for things which he is not responsible for, feeling bad, shameful and deserving for punishment.

An expected developmental tasks of the preschoolers are as follows:

1. Settle into a healthful daily routine of adequately eating, exercising and resting.
2. Master physical skills of large and small muscle coordination and movement.
3. Become a participating member in the family.
4. Confirm to others expectations.
5. Express emotions healthfully and for a wide variety of experiences.
6. Learn to communicate affectively with an increasing number of others.
7. Learn to use initiative tempered by a conscience.
8. Develop ability to handle potentially dangerous situations.
9. Lay foundation for understanding the meaning of life, self, the world, and ethical, religious and philosophical ideas.

Accordingly the development tasks of the family to preschoolers are as follows:

1. Encourage and accept his evolving skills rather than elevating self-esteem by pushing the child beyond his capacity. Satisfaction if found through reducing assistance with physical care and giving more guidance in other respects.
2. Supply adequate housing facilities, space, equipment and other materials needed for life, comfort, health and recreation.
3. Plan for predicted and unexpected costs of family life such as medical care, insurance, education, babysitter fees, food, clothing and recreation.
4. Maintain some privacy and provide an outlet for tension of family members while including the child as a participant in the family.
5. Share household and childcare responsibility with other family members, including the child.
6. Strengthen the partnership with the mate and express affection in ways that keep the relationship from becoming humdrum.
7. Learn to accept failures, mistakes and blunders without piling up feelings of guilt, blame and discrimination.
8. Nourish common interests and friendships to strengthen self-respect and self-confidence and to remain interesting to each other.
9. Create and maintain effective communication within the family.
10. Cultivate relationships with the extended family.
11. Tap resources and serve others outside the family to prevent preoccupation with self and family.
12. Face life lammas and rework moral codes, spiritual values and a philosophy of life.

For achieving the above tasks, the needs of the preschoolers to be taken care of for their promotion of health are discussed in Table 7.5.

Role of the Nurses in Health Care of Preschoolers

Preschoolers continue to have health problems that are common in toddler-hood. Communicable diseases and respiratory tract infections are frequent and also they prone to accidents. The following are the concern and preventive teaching in promoting health in preschoolers.

Accident Prevention and Safety

- Advise the clear boundaries regarding where tricycles or bicycles can be ridden need to be given
- Teach simple road safety (e.g. looking both ways before crossing the street)
- Encourage education of children regarding strangers
- Encourage education about sexual abuse (e.g. avoid inappropriate touch)
- Swimming lessons can begin and basic water safety taught

Table 7.5: Needs of a Preschool Child

Needs	Rationales
1. Nutrition	• Continued growth and maturation of system
2. Elimination	• Functional maturity of systems
3. Sensory stimulation	• Maturation of vision - Improve muscle control making exploration easier
4. Movement and exercise	• Improved neuromuscular control • Development of motor skills
5. Protection and safety	• Lack of awareness of danger • Expanding horizons
6. Infection control	• Increased contact with others • Development of active immunity to infection • Immunization schedule for communicable disease • Nutritional status effects vulnerability to infections
7. Sexuality	• Gender identification with parent of same sex
8. Love and belonging	• Home environment • Development of initiative • Parents and siblings attitude toward child
9. Security	• Development of initiative • Support and guidance from parents • Stability of home • Accustomed routines
10. Self-esteem	• Interaction with peers • Family atmosphere

- Teach the dangers of matches and practice of homefire safety drills.

Infections

- Advise that these are an inevitable result of increased socialization
- Advise teaching children sound hygienic practices (hand wash, disposal of wastes)
- Keep immunizations current.

Sleep Disorders

- Explain to caregiver the commonalty of this problem among preschooler
- Suggest that relaxed bedtime rituals and a night light can help
- Advise that comforting and warm, reassurance and needed which a child is awakened by nightmare—telling stories.

Dental Hygiene

- Teach the preschoolers should be brushing their teeth and flossing with caregiver assistance
- Advise dental visit of needed.

Play Habits

- Advise caregivers that make believe plays and imaginary friends are common and normal in the preschool years
- Encourage caregivers to promote socialization through neighborhood play groups and nursery schools.

Self-esteem

- Encourage caregivers to provide opportunities to make new discoveries and gain a sense of autonomy by experiencing neighborhood and preschool activities
- Advise to avoid frequent criticism and over-protectiveness
- Teach caregivers importance of providing opportunities for the child to plan and carry out activities and giving appropriate praise for accomplishments

School Age Child (Six to Eleven Years) Care

School age of child is otherwise known as middle childhood. During these middle years of childhood the foundation of adult roles in work, recreation and social interaction is laid. The child growth continue at a slow and steady rate. The child's body proportions now resembles those of an adult. There is a further maturation of the body's systems and brain development is virtually complete by puberty. The neuromuscular coordination is further refined. Motor abilities progress from the ability to hold a pencil and print words at the age 6 to the ability to write in script and in sentences at age 12.

Sexual organs grow but are dormant until late this period, when hormonal changes begin. The physical or secondary sex changes that occur in the female, in sequence, during prepuberty or preadolescence are as follows:

- Increase in transverse diameter of the pelvis
- Broadening of hips
- Tenderness in developing breast tissue and enlargement of areola diameter
- Axillary perspiring
- Change in vaginal secretions from alkaline to acid pH
- Change in vaginal layer to thick, gray, mucoid linking
- Change in vaginal flora from mixed to doederlins lactic acid-producing bacilli
- Appearance of public hair from 8 to 14 years; hair first appear in labia and then spreads to mons.

The physical or secondary sex changes that occur in the male, in sequence during this period are as follows:

- Growth spurt at 12 to 16 years (average 14 years); average 4" for 2 ½ years

- Auxiliary perspiring
- Increased testicular sensitivity to persue
- Increase in testes size
- Changes in scrotum color
- Temporary enlargement of breasts
- Increase in height and shoulder breadth
- Appearance of pigmented hair at base of penis
- Increase in length and width of penis.

With regard to cognitive development, the schoolage childhood usually has following characteristics:

- Thinks logically and develops concept of mass volume, weight and measurements
- Deals best with actual objects and people, but relates, concepts and compares events
- Uses inductive reasoning to solve new problems
- Generalizes about the people, places and things
- Develops an awareness and understanding of other people feelings and points of view
- Understands reversal of events.

They will also have well developed language skills, ability to store information, memory, recall whenever needed. Body images, self-concepts and sexuality are interrelated. Sexual development results in a strong need to understand body function clearly and to have accurate information about sexuality.

The period of middle childhood is a critical one in term of psychosocial development. This is a period when the child firmly establishes his sense of independence and defines his social role. According to Erickson, the principal conflict of this period is "industry vs. inferiority". Industry is an interest in doing the work of the world, the child feeling that he can learn and solve problems, the formation of responsible work habits and attitudes and the mastery of age appropriate tasks. A sense of industry involves self-confidence, perseverance, diligence, self-control, cooperation and compromise rather than competition. The danger of this period is that children may develop a sense of inferiority. Inferiority involves a feeling of inadequate, defeated, unable to learn or do task, lazy unable to complete, compromise and cooperate. Children later adult who feel inferior will not like to work or try new tasks. They will be moody, anxious, oversensitive to and isolated from others, excessively meek and lacking in perservance. Regressive or withdrawn behavior, excess fear of bodily injury or / or illness speech disorders or psychomotor disorders may be observed. They may show acting out behaviors, i.e. stealing and others distinctiveness, lack of interest in all activities.

The expected developmental tasks of the school age children are as follows:

Developmental Tasks

1. Decreasing dependence upon family and gaining some satisfaction from peers and other adults
2. Increasing neuromuscular skills so that he can participate in games and work with other

3. Learning basic adult concepts and knowledge to be able to reason and engage in tasks of everyday living
4. Learning ways of communicate with others realistically
5. Becoming a more active and cooperative family participant
6. Giving and receiving affection to family and friends without immediately seeking or giving a gift in return
7. Learning socially acceptable ways of getting money and saving it for later satisfaction.
8. Learning how to handle strong feeling and impulses appropriately
9. Adjusting his changing body image and self-concept to come to terms with the masculine or feminine social role
10. Discovering healthy ways of becoming acceptable as a person
11. Developing a positive attitude toward his own and others social, racial, economic and religious groups.

Accordingly to help the schoolage children, the developmental tasks of the family are as follows:

1. Keeping lines and communication, open among family members
2. Working together to achieve common goals
3. Planning a life style within economic means
4. Finding creative ways to continue mutually satisfactory married life
5. Providing for parental privacy and space for children's play
6. Maintaining close ties with relatives
7. Expanding family life into the community through various activities
8. Validating the family philosophy of life.

Accordingly the needs of schoolage child to be met on priority basis which are given in Table 7.6.

Nurse's Role in Promoting Health of School Age Child

School age child is on a quest of discovery throughout her / his inner-outer selves. He/she asks many questions, seeking to understand every aspect of the world. He/she may want to know where he came from, e.g. or who made this world. He might enjoy taking things apart to see that makes them work. He always too busy with his activities. Parents, teachers, nurses may see this industry at times as restlessness, irritability, rebellion toward authority, and lack of obedience. Accordingly assist him/her to do so without harm/hurting to them.

Sex education began earlier, the parent, teachers and nurses should identify the need and know the facts and explain them at the child's level. Try to make conversation as relaxed as possible and answer all questions as honestly as possible.

The school experience has considerable influence on children, because they are in formative years and spend much time in school. School should help children to learn to do the followings:
- Thinking critically
- Make judgment based on reason
- Develop social skills

Table 7.6: Needs of School Child

Needs	Rationales
1. Nutrition	• Continued growth and maturation of system
2. Movement and exercise	• Further refinement of neuromuscular control
3. Protection and safety	• Understanding relationship of cause and effect
4. Infection control	• Increased contact with other (School and extracurricular) • Development of active immunity • Immunization schedule • Nutritional status
5. Sexuality	• Adoption of social role based on sex
6. Self-esteem	• Establishment of independence • Home atmosphere and school atmosphere • Relationship with peers, adults outside home • Success in endeavor • Parental support
7. Security	• Teacher support
8. Love and belonging	• Stability of home environment • Continuity of school environments • Routines and schedules • Development of social role based on gender
9. Sexuality	• Role model (Parent or parent substitute of same sex)

- Cooperate with others
- Accept other adult authority
- Be leaders and followers.

In addition, the home and other groups, peer or organized clubs are important for intellectual and social development and for promoting sense and social development and for promoting sense of achievement and industry.

The nurses role in promoting health for the school age child involves intellectual and family teaching. The following are the areas of nursing activities related to this school age children.

Accident Prevention

- Emphasize traffic safety
- Encourage the use of seatbelts (if)
- Emphasize bicycle, skateboard, and scooter safety
- Teach children to take water safety program.

Communicable Diseases

- Encourage proper hygienic habits, including not sharing personal items like comb (to avoid pediculosis, etc.)

- Home visits may be acquired to discuss home health practices if child has scabies, or pediculosis
- Advise common treatment methods for conditions like scabies, impetigo and pediculosis
- Teach about STDs including AIDS.

Substance Abuse

- Early preventive teaching about alcohol, nicotine and street drugs that includes guidance for families is essential
- Sex education needs to begin as early as are 7 or 8
- Families need encouragement to talk about sex at home
- Caregivers need encouragement to answer questions honestly and correctly
- Menstruation needs to be discussed by atleast age of 7 because some girls attain menarche at 8 or 9.

Mental Health (Concerns Phobia, Suicide)

- Nurse needs to work with teachers and family so that they learn to recognize behavior that indicates mental health difficulties, e.g. phobias, depression and suicide.

Physical Fitness

- Teach good food choices that are lower in fat, salt and sugar but avoid sternous dieting if child is over height
- Emphasize the importance of physical activity, exercise.

Self-esteem

- Teach caregivers to encourage independent activities and to be sure that success are greater in number than failures
- Provide the child with positive statements that demonstrate being valued, important and loved.

Adolescent Care

Adolescence has been defines as 'the period of psychobiological maturation during which the secondary physical growth spurt is completed and sexual maturity and the ability to reproduce are achieved'. The term adolescent refers to psychological maturation of the individual whereas puberty refers to the point at which reproduction becomes possible.

Adolescence is the period of development during which the individual makes the transition from childhood to adulthood, usually between 13 and 21 years. It is the period in which puberty begins and extends for 8 to 10 years until the person is physically and psychologically mature, ready to assume adult responsibilities and be self sufficient because of changes in intellect, attitude and interests.

The physiological changes in adolescence will include the following;
- Beginning of skeletal growth spurt (at 12 in girls, 14 in boys)
- Beginning of breast development in girls
- Enlargement of testes and scrotal sac in boys

- Appearance of straight, pigmented pubic hair which gradually becomes curly
- Early voice changes (cracks)
- Enlargement of penis and prostate glands (boys)
- Menarche in girls, vulva and clitoris enlarges uterus in girls
- Spermatogenesis (circulation of sperm in boys)
- Progressive enlargement of the ovaries, ripening of graafian follicles in females
- Ovulation and completion of breast development in girls
- Appearance of axillary hair and increased output of oil an seat producing glands which may lead to acne
- Widening and deepening of female pelvis, with deposition of subcutaneous fat that gives rounded appearance to body
- Increase in shoulder width
- Deepening of void, appearance of coarse and pigmented facial hair, and appearance of chest hairs.

In brief, four main physical changes during this period are as follows:
- Increased growth rate of skeleton, muscle and viscera
- Sex specific changes, such as changes in shoulders and hip width
- Alteration in distribution of muscle and fat
- Development of the reproductive system and secondary sex characters.

A wide variation exists in the timing of physical changes associated with puberty and girls tend to begin their physical changes earlier than boys.

In the area of cognitive development, the adolescent differs from younger children in his ability to think and reason in the logical manner. Deductive, reflective, and hypothetical reasoning are possible; and abstract concepts can be handled; long-term goals can be set as the concept of time, its passage and the future become real. These abilities can make problem-solving difficult for the adolescent and challenging the decision-making of adults is common. Egocentrism returns and imaginary audiences and daydreaming are used. The adolescent is often critical of the stage of the world in general and actively seeks to change it. He strives for perfection, yet often gets carried away by his emotions.

Adolescence is characterized by experimentation as the individual seeks to again knowledge about himself and the world around him. During this stage, many adolescents engage in risk taking behavior, often pushing themselves and each other to test their limits. For example, they may drive at high speed, experiments with drugs, alcohol, smoking or engage in sex without precautions against pregnancy. And also experiment with their own self-image, trying on various roles in an effort to establish in true sense of self.

According to Erickson, it is a stage of *identity formation vs. identity diffusion*. Identity means that an individual feels he is a specific unique person, he has emerged as an adult. Identify formation results through synthesis of biopsychosocial characteristics from a number of sources. For example, earlier gender identity, i.e. sexual identity, group identity, family identity, a vocational identity, health identity, moral identity, psychosocial moratorium. Identity formation implies emerging from the era with a sense of wholeness, knowing the self as unique person, feeling responsibility loyalty and commitment to value system. Identity formation implies an internal stability, sameness or continuity which resists extreme change and preserve itself from obvious in the face to stress or contractions. There are types of identity.

- Personal or real identity – what the person beliefs himself to be
- Ideal identity – what he would like to be
- Claimed identity – what he wants others to think he is.

Identity diffusion results if the adolescent fails to achieve a sense of identity; with identity diffusion, he or she feels impotent, insecure and disillusioned.

Developmental Tasks

An expected development tasks of an adolescent are as follows:

1. Accepting the changing body size, shape and understand the meaning of physical maturity.
2. Learning to handle the body in variety of physical skills and to maintain good health.
3. Achieving a satisfying and socially accepted feminine or masculine role, recognizing how these roles have similarities and distinctions.
4. Finding the self as a member of one or more peer groups and developing skills in relating to a variety of people, including those of the opposite sex.
5. Achieving independence from parents and other adults while maintaining a mature affection and interdependence with them.
6. Selecting a satisfying occupation in line with interests and abilities and preparing for economic independence.
7. Preparing to settle down, frequently for marriage and family life, or for a close relationship with another, by developing a responsible attitude, acquiring needed knowledge, making appropriate decisions and forming a relationship based on love rather than infatuation.
8. Developing intellectuality and work skills, and social sensitivities as competent citizen.
9. Developing a workable philosophy, a mature set of values and worthy ideals
10. Achieving new and matured relationships with both males of the same age.
11. Achieving a masculine or famine social role.
12. Accepting one's personal appearance.
13. Acquiring a set of values and an ethical system as guide to behavior.
14. Achieving emotional independence from significant adult.
15. Preparing for a career.

Accordingly developmental tasks of the family in relation to individual are as follows:

1. Provide facilities for individual differences and needs of family members
2. Work out a system of financial responsibility within the family

3. Establish a sharing of responsibility
4. Re-establish a naturally satisfying marriage relationships
5. Strengthen the communication within the family
6. Rework relationships with relatives, friends and associates
7. Broadens horizons of the adolescent and parents
8. Formulate workable philosophy of life as a family.

Accordingly the needs to be met on priority for smooth performing of the above said developmental tasks are discussed in Table 7.7.

Table 7.7: Needs of an Adolescent

Needs	Rationales
1. Nutrition	• Growth spurt – maturation of systems,
2. Oxygen	• Rapid increase in vital capacity of lungs
3. Movement and exercise	• Change in body proportions
4. Protection and safety	• Risk taking behavior
5. Hygiene	• Excessive serum production • Attainment of puberty
6. Infection control	• Sexual experimentation
7. Sexuality	• Establishment of social role • Physical appearance
8. Self-esteem	• Peer relations • Attainment of independence • Establishment of identity

Role of Nurse in Adolescent Health Promotion

The common health problems usually associated with an adolescent period are accidents, substance abuse, suicide, pregnancy (female), nutritional difficulties, sexually transmitted diseases.

The nurses understanding of development provides a unique perspective for helping teenagers and parents anticipate and cope with the stresses of adolescence. Nursing activities, particularly education, can promote healthy development. The nurse can foster identity formation by reinforcement of positive behavior, listening, providing support during trying times; and being a role model identity nurse can teach encouragement about good nutrition, exercise, rest, sleep and proper use of leisure.

The most significant activity of the nurse during this period is that facilitating healthy family relationships, mutual respect, open communications and accurate information exchange among family members pave the way for a health transition from adolescent to adulthood. The aspects concern need to be emphasized during health teaching are as follows:

Substance Abuse

- Advise adolescents of statistics about substance abuse (alcohol, drugs, etc)

- Discuss the risks of substance abuse
- Discuss the physical consequences of substance abuse
- Discuss the psychosocial consequences of substance abuse
- Assist in preparing strategies for saying no to substance abuse.

Motor Vehicle

- Encourage driving education classes for adolescents
- Discuss the relation of alcohol consumption area vs. motor-vehicle accidents.

Suicide

- Assist teachers and caregivers to identify risk factors and data indicative of suicide (e.g. school performance, social withstand)
- Advise adolescents with depression where to seek help (e.g. psychiatrist).

Nutrition

- Discuss healthy eating habits
- Discuss dangers of excessive or nutritionally unsound dieting
- Help caregivers and teachers recognize 'risk' students
- Advise adolescents who legitimately need to lose weight to consult a physician.

Sex Education

- Provide factual informations about physical and psychosexual development
- Discuss the nature and prevention of STDs
- Discuss safe sex practices in relation to STDs and AIDS
- Assist with developing strategies for saying no to sexual activity for those who wish
- If adolescent is or intends to become sexually behavior or birth control
- Provide assistance to pregnant adolescent by discussing options, encouraging medical care/MTP, encouraging psychosocial counseling.

Self-esteem

- Teach caregivers that normal behavior includes belonging to a peer group, the desire to be like everyone else and trying on different roles (which may include hairstyle, clothing, and jewellery)
- Keep lines of communication open
- Encourage caregivers to facilitate independence while providing love and consistent rules.

Brief description of the health promotional aspect like marriage counseling and sex education as follows:

Marriage Counseling

Marriage is a religious and sacred union of two souls in conformity to natures law and custom. Proper and suitable education in the general biology should therefore be given to every child so that he or she can understand the significance of marriage, reproductive, heredity and evolution. Guidance on question of conduct should be given to adolescent boys and girls before they leave the school.

The policy of maintaining silence about sex matters to which young boys and girls have been so much subjected generally leads to crude and loutish notion or strange or fearsome concepts of sexual organs and sex life. The hygiene of the sexual organs and the sex problems should be grasped with frankness by the young persons. Before the onset of puberty, the bodily changes which gradually occur should be explained. The first menstruation in a girl or the first nocturnal emission in a boy, if they happen without warning, may inflict lasting mental torture or injury. The number of nocturnal emissions varies greatly, but up to 2-3 times a month need not to be considered abnormal. At later stage, the question of sexual intercourse must be death with. Marriage is solution which is inevitable.

Every couple relationship is unique. Although no rules guarantee a successful marriage. Some guidelines are useful for building a happy marriage. Before marriage the couple ideally should complete five tasks:

1. They should make certain that their emotions are based on love rather than physical or sexual attraction.
2. Both partners should explore their motivation for wanting to marry
3. They should focus on developing clear communication
4. They should understand that any annoying behavior patterns and habits are unlikely to change after marriage
5. They should determine their compatibility in important beliefs and values.

When establishing a household and family the married couple must begin to work as a team. They have the following tasks:

1. Establishing an intimate relationship
2. Establishing guidelines for power and decision-making issues
3. Deciding on the working toward mutual goals
4. Setting standards for extra family interactions
5. Finding companionship with other people for social life
6. Choosing morals, values, and ideologies acceptable to both.

These major tasks of adults require considerable maturity and self-esteem. When accomplished, however they provide the foundation for a stable relationship. Growth in marriage extend over many years. Success in solving the formidable problems that occur in any marriage officers marital partners insight into each other.

There are some problems which arise after marriage. A few words or timely advice by the parents or family doctor or friends to a prospective bride or bridegroom can do much to save marriage from ship work, for it is absolutely trust that a marriage may be ruined and the couple made unhappy and miserable for years or for whole life on the first night of the honeymoon. The bridge goes to her marriage bed ignorant of the nature of the sexual act, the first intercourse is little more than a rape. The bridegroom should be informed about the difficulties of a bride's first intercourse, and if he loves her, he will be prepare to overcome her desire to woo her afresh with gentleness and not seize her as a matter of right.

A marital relationship generally passes through three developmental stages. The establishment stage begins at wedding and continues as the couple attempts to function as a dyad (pair). They learn patterns of sexual expression and ways to live intimately with each other. The must learn styles of conflict resolution, decision making and role patterns. Next the family orientation stage, that is directed at child bearing and child rearing activities. Parenting roles must be defined and practiced. Nurturing and socialization needs of the children can put pressure on the couples intimate relationship. Last stage will be 'post parental family stage' when the children depart from the household.

Sex Education

Sex plays an important role in influencing our lives. It is an urge which attracts man and woman to each other. When men and women understand their roles, they can better appreciate one another and work together more happily. Marriage is the physical relationship but it becomes an emotional relationship, through which a husband and wife are to express their affection for each other. Sex is the foundation for the development of family life. That is why, proper understanding toward sex is necessary for a richer and happier living. Proper sex education is of paramount importance for a happy life in order to understand, accept, and deal adequately with the changes occurring in the youth and to control and direct the sex drives is socially acceptable ways. Industrialization and urbanization have brought about vast changes in family life. One normal family life is being threatened to change in culture. The families are being uprooted and moved from rural areas to mostly overcrowded and unstable conditions with usually lower standard of life and conduct. There is more individual freedom and less supervision over young people who are confused with the changing standard of conduct. The high divorce rate, unhappy marriage, illegitimate births, criminal abortion, sexual mal-adjustment, sexually transmitted disease / AIDS, prostitution and sex crimes are unwholesome conditions in society which testify to the failure of home, school and community in meeting the needs of youth. Sex education can help to prevent some of these conditions.

Sexuality and sex are two different things. Sexuality is the degree to which a person exhibits and experiences maleness or femaleness physically, emotionally and mentally. It is often described as the sense of being female or male as it has biological, psychological, social and ethical components. Sexuality influences and is influence by life experiences. Sexuality is defined not only by a person's genital but also by attitudes and feelings. It can also defined as learned behaviors as how one behaves in relationships with others. Culture profoundly influence is an integral part of a persons identity and is present in one's demeanor through actions, communication and physical appearance.

The word sex, has a more limited meaning. It usually describes the biological aspect of sexuality such as genital, sexual, activity. Sex may be used for pleasure and reproduction. As a result life changes or a choice, sexual activity may be absents from a persons life for brief or prolonged periods.

The process by which people come to know themselves as females or males not clearly understood. Being born with female or male genitalias and subsequently learning female or male social roles seem to key ingredients; yet this does not explain all variations of sexuality and sexual behavior.

Sources of Sex Education

Home: Children begin to receive sex education, good or bad, at home even before the child goes to the school from servants and animals. The grown-up children receive sex education from radio, TV, motion pictures, magazines and newspapers, etc. Youth from varied background with different attitude towards sex have misconceptions and misinformation due to different backgrounds of their parents. Some parents have had no opportunity to acquire the scientific informations about sex. Some of them cannot express themselves to their children as they do not know what to tell them. Some parents suffer for sexual repressions and taboos carried over their own childhood. Few parents may have had unfortunate experiences and are themselves emotionally maladjusted and unstable. Children from such families are likely to be biased and unsound. In some families there is a disturbed relationship between parents with confusion, unrest, and broken homes. It is always good to set good examples of standard sex codes to children by the parents. In youth the temptation to illicit sexual intercourse is strong. Hard and strenuous work, exercise, pride in a healthy body and avoidance of evil companions, sexy literature, use of alcohol, all help in the fight to the mind and body against sexual instinct.

School: It should play a positive role in sex education to help the students through sound education and wholesome recreation. Teachers should be trained in the scientific knowledge of conception, birth, menses, night pollution, etc. teacher should be emotionally well adjusted. He should be aware of the standard of sex conduct in the community. Sex education in school should be integrated with the total health education program and undue emphases should not be forced upon uninterested student. It should be presented in a dignified way, using dignified vocabulary.

Biological difference between men and women are determined at conception. Female fetuses receive tow 'X' chromosomes, and from each parent and male fetuses receive an 'X' chromosome from the mother and a "Y" chromosomes from the father. Biologic gender in the term used to denote chromosomal development, male (XY), or female (XX). Gender or sexual identity is the inner sense of a person has being male or female which may be the same or different from biologic gender. Gender role is the behavior a person conveys about being male or female which again, may or may not be the same as biologic gender or gender identity. Gender role behavior is encouraged by parents, peers, and the media, differences among individual sexual behavior develop and the cultural factors also the key elements in defining sex roles.

Sexual orientation is the clear, persistent, erotic preference of a person for one sex or the other. The origins of sexual orientation are still not understood. People experience sexual gratification in many ways, and what is considered 'normal' differs from one individual to another and among cultures. Sexual orientation refers to the preferred gender of the partner of an individual. A heterosexual is one who experiences sexual fulfilment with a person of the opposite gender. A homosexual is one who experiences sexual fulfilment with a person of the same gender. Homosexual in male termed as 'gay' and in female it is termed a 'lesbian'. Bisexuality refers to a person who finds pleasure with both opposite sex and same sex partners. A transsexual is a person of a certain biologic gender with the feelings of opposite sex, e.g. taking role of opposite sex, or wearing cloths of opposite sex.

Sexual expressions are the methods by which people gain satisfaction though sexual stimulations are varied. Touch, smell, sight, sounds, feelings, thoughts, and fantasy can all contribute to sexual fulfilment in any forms of expression chosen by individuals. Feeling of love for another person is closely associated with desire. Forms of sexual stimulation include, kissing, hugging, stroking, squeezing, breast stimulation, manual stimulation of genitals, oral genital stimulation and anal stimulation. Sexual stimulation may be physical or psychologic. Erotic stimulation through the use of films, magazines, and photographs is common. Fetishism usually practiced by a male, is sexual arousal with the help of an inanimate object, e.g. shoes, leather, women undergarments. Transsexual express that if a man may think himself as women in a man's body or women may think herself as man in a women body. Transverse bite usually is a heterosexual man who periodically dresses like women for psychological and sexual relied. Masturbation is a technique of sexual expression in which an individual practices self stimulation (penis and clitoris).

Young Adult Care

Childhood and adolescence are the periods of growing up, adulthood is the time for setting down. The changes in young adulthood are related more to sociocultural forces and expectations and to value and cognitive changes than physical development. The young adult is considered to have reached maturity to have completed growth and to have completed growth and to have developed internal and external controls and values acceptable to society.

The young adults have well developed and coordinated organ systems, functioning at peak efficiency. Although some normal changes begin to take place during the later part of the period, for the most part, physical changes are minimal.

The young adult in the 20s, is expected to enter new roles of finding an occupation, establishing a family and demonstrating

responsibility at work at home, and in society and to develop values, attitudes and interest in keeping with these roles. Young adults may have difficulty in their 30s, and 40s if they work at primarily one of these roles at a time and neglect the others, which can create problems for persons in any of these areas.

According to Erickson, the psychosexual crisis is *intimacy versus self isolation*. Intimacy is a reaching out and using the self to form a commitment to and intense, lasting relationship with another person, or even a cause, an institution or a creative effort. Intimacy involves mutual love and trust, sharing of feelings and responsibility to and cooperation with each other. Intimacy includes intercourse, but it means more than physical or genital contact. The person is involved with people, work, hobbies and community issue. Intimacy is when two people (in marriage or in a close relationship) accept all aspects of the other and adjust their behavior to each others behavior and need for mutual satisfaction.

Isolation or self absorption, is the inability to intimate, spontaneous or close with another thus becoming withdrawn, lonely, conceited and behaving in a stereotyped manner. The isolated person often experiences a long succession of unsuccessful relationship, over extends self with out any real interest or feeling and that cannot sustain close relationship. No real exchange of fellowship occurs.

Developmental Tasks of Young Adults

1. Accepting himself and stabilizing self concept and body image.
2. Establishing independence from parental home and financial aid.
3. Becoming established in a vocation or profession that provides personal satisfaction economic independence and a feeling of making a worthwhile contribution to society.
4. Learning to appraise and express love responsibility through more than sexual contact.
5. Establishing an intimate bond with another, either through marriage or with a close friend.
6. Establishing and managing a residence, a home.
7. Finding a congenial social group.
8. Deciding whether or not to have a family.
9. Formulating a meaningful philosophy of life.
10. Becoming involved as a citizen in the community.

According the development tasks of the family for an young adult are:

1. Rearranging the home physically and reallocating resources (space, material, objects) to meet the needs of remaining members.
2. Meeting the expenses of releasing the offspring and redistributing the budget
3. Redistributing the responsibilities among grown and growing children and finally between the husband and wife on the basis of interests, ability, and availability.
4. Maintaining communication within the family to contribute to marital happiness, while remaining available to young adult and other offspring.

5. Enjoying mutual companionship as a husband-wife team while incorporating changes.

6. Widening the family circle to include the lose friends or spouses of the offspring as well as the entire family of in-laws.

7. Reconciling conflicting loyalties and philosophy of life.

Accordingly the needs of an early / young adult to be met for proper performance of development tasks are given in Table 7.8.

Table 7.8: Needs of an Early Adult	
Needs	*Rationales*
1. Nutrition	• Continued growth and development in early adult years • Establishment of own dietary habits • Time and work pressure
2. Movement and exercise	• More sedentary lifestyle • Development of own lifestyle • Gradual decline in physical performance from peak fitness • Feeling of indestructibility
3. Protection and safety	• Risk taking behavior • Strength of sexual drive
4. Infection control	• Choice of sexual partner • Self image
5. Sexuality	• Ability to establish close relationships with opposite sex • Choosing a marriage partner
6. Security and self-esteem	• Decline in physical performance • Relationship with others • Ability to make major decisions
7. Love and belonging	• Ability to form close ties with others

Roles of Nurses in Promoting Health of Young Adult

Usually young adulthood is a time for good health, but physical and emotional problems can result from lifestyle, developmental or situational crises, family history, and the environment.

1. *Lifestyle:* Some actual and potential risks of lifestyles are as follows:
• Violent deaths due to accidents, suicide, and alcohol.
• Sexual relationships lead to STDs and AIDS
• Drug abuse leads to many problem
• Diet and exercises needs leads to health problems, e.g. obesity, anemia, etc.

2. *Situational crime:* Sometimes the lifestyle, occupation and relationship leads to stressors, family centered stressors may be related to both positive and negative factors, marriages, divorce, parenthood, death of a parent, etc. The increased stress may precipitate mental or physical health problems, aggravated by the ineffective coping mechanisms, such as substance abuse, child abuse, spouse abuse, decreased nutrition and rest, and risk taking behavior.

3. *Family history of chronic disease:* Such as hypertension cardiac disease and diabetics increase a risk in an individual.

4. *Environment pollution*: It also leads to many problems
Nursing considerations specific to the young adults are as follows:
• Teaching the need for regular physical examination and dental care, including screening for disease are most common at this age.
• Teaching preventive health practices, related to nutrition, rest, substance abuse, and stress related illness.
• Providing information about sexuality, pregnancy and health of the reproductive system through self breast and self testicular examination, birth control and prevention of STDs.
• Providing and supporting safety, education in the work place and in activities of daily living.

Care of Middle Age/Middle Adulthood

Chronological age of 45 to 65 years is only one definition of middle age. The person will also consider the physiopsychological age conditions of the body; how old she or he acts and feels. The middle adult years are time for change in both physical and psychological dimensions. The changes are gradual and individualized.

Middle age is attributed to improved nutrition, control of communicable diseases, discovery and control of familial disease and other medical advances. It is a time if relatively good health, new personal freedom, maximum command of self, and influence over social life.

The early years of this period of life are marked by maximum physical development and functioning. As time passes, gradual physiologic changes – both internal and external – occur. These are not pathologic changes, but rather normal changes that result from again, self image and self concept must be altered to adapt successfully these changes, which include the following:
• Fatty tissue redistributed; men tend to develop abdominal fat, women thicken through the middle
• Weight gain
• Dry skin
• Wrinkle lines appear on the face
• Grey hair appears
• Man may begin to loss hair on the head
• Cardiac output starts to decrease
• Increased fatigue
• Gradual decrease in muscle mass, strength and agility
• Loss of calcium from bones, especially in postmenopausal women
• Changes in visual acuity, especially for near vision (presbyopia)

- Diminished hearing acuity, especially for high pitched sounds
- Decreasing hormone production results in menopause or andropause.

The middle adult year is a time of increased personal freedom, economic stability and social relationships. It also is a time of increased responsibility and an awareness of one's own mortality. One is faced with the realization that half of one's life is over and many things are still undone. This realization can lead to developmental crisis and situational stressors.

According to Erickson the developmental crisis of middle age is *generativity versus self absorption/or stagnation*. Generativity is concerned about providing for others, that in equal to the concern of providing for the self. The generative person has a sense of parenthood and creativity of being vital in establishing and guiding the next generation, the arts or a profession and if feeling needed and being important to welfare of human kind. The middle ager who is generative takes on the major work of providing for other, directly or indirectly. There is a sense of productivity, mastery, charity, altruism and perseverance, these concepts to motivate actions.

If generativity is not achieved, stagnation or self absorption results. The person hates the aging process and feels neither secure not adept in handling self, physically or interpersonally. The person is withdrawn, resigned, isolated and introspective. Fear of old age may cause regressive to inappropriate youthfulness in behavior or dress or unfaithfulness in marriage.

Middle Aged Developmental Tasks

1. Discover and develop new satisfactions as a mate (if married) and develop a since of unity and intimacy.
2. Helping growing and grown children to become happy and responsible adults.
3. Creating a pleasant, comfortable home, appropriate to his values, interest, time, energy and resources; giving and receiving, and exchanging hospitality and taking pride in accomplishment of self and spouse are on going tasks.
4. Finding pleasure in generativity and recognition in work.
5. Role reversal with aging parents and parents in law.
6. Achieving mature social and civil responsibility being informed as a citizen.
7. Develop or maintain an active organizational membership, deriving from it pleasure and sense of belonging.
8. Accept and adjust to the physical changes of middle age; maintain healthful ways of living.
9. Making as art of friendship; cherishing old friends and choosing new, enjoying active social life with friends of both sex.
10. Using leisure creatively and with satisfaction without yielding too much to social pressures and styles.
11. Continue to formulate philosophy of life.
12. Prepare for retirement with financial arrangement.
13. Recognize the finiteness of life and prepare for eventual personal death.

Accordingly the developmental tasks of the family in relation to middle age are as follows.

Developmental Tasks of the Family

1. Maintain pleasant and comfortable home
2. Assure security for later years, financially and emotionally
3. Share household responsibilities
4. Draw emotionally closer as a couple
5. Maintain contact with grown children and their family
6. Keep in touch with aging parents, siblings their families and other relatives and friends
7. Participate on community life beyond the family
8. Reaffirm the values of life that have real meanings, i.e. philosophic, religious and social.

Accordingly the needs to be met on priority basis for smooth performance of the developmental tasks of the middle age are given in Table 7.9.

Table 7.9: Needs of Middle Age	
Needs	*Rationales*
1. Nutrition	• More sedentary lifestyle
2. Sensory stimulation	• Greater intensity of stimulation required
3. Movement and exercise	• Decline of physical performance • Awareness of preventive value of regular exercise • Availability of the program
4. Hygiene	• Decreased skin integrity
5. Sexuality	• Elimination of fear of pregnancy for women • Decrease in fertility • Self image • Attainment of career and social goals
6. Self-esteem	• Attainment of career and social goals • Decline of fertility and sexual functions
7. Security	• Visual signs of aging process • Mid-life crisis
8. Love and belonging	• Decline of sexual functions • Teen aged children • Aging parents

Role of Nurses in Promoting Health of Middle Aged

Like young adult, the middle adult is also subject to physical and emotional problems from lifestyle, developmental or situational crisis, family history and environment. The leading causes of death in middle years are motor vehicle accidents, occupational accidents, suicide and chronic disease, e.g. cancer in women, heart disease in men.

Middle age does not automatically results in physical and emotional health problems. Many men and women remain healthy throughout their lives, but knowledge of preventive health care and the special needs of these age groups can lead to improved quality and quantity of life.

The nurse plays a major role in promoting health in the middle adult by teaching, serving as a role model and encouraging self care responsibilities. The following health promotion activities are recommended:

Adults Aged 20 to 40 (Female)

- Breast self examinations every month
- Breast examination by a health care provider every 3 years.

Adults Aged 40 or Older

- Breast examination by health care provider yearly
- Self breast examination every month
- Mannorogram as baseline.

All Women

- If age 18 or older and for sexually active people, pelvic examination and Papanicolaou test yearly
- After three or more consecutive normal annual tests, Pap tests may be done less frequently at the health care providers discretion.

All Middle Adults

All middle adults should undergo the following examinations:
- Complete physical examination every 2 years
- Annual dental examination
- Eye examination ever 1 to 2 years
- Maintenance of current immunization
- Annual examination of fecal material for the presence of blood
- Digital rectal examination every year
- Regular self testicular examination and regular prostate examinations
- Cancer screening.

In addition the middle adult should be taught importance of proper nutrition, rest, exercises as well as the dangers of substance abuse. Referrals to support groups and individual counseling may be necessary to strengthening the coping mechanisms and allow acceptance of personal and family changes.

Care of Older Adulthood / Elderly

The beginning age for the elderly actually depends upon many factors. Our society has arbitrarily labeled the older adult to one over the age of 65. It is the final stage of an individual's development that has been called the 'golden age'. It is a time when the individual no longer has to strive to achieve something but he can relax and enjoy the fruits of his labor.

Senescence, the condition of aging or growing old, a label for the years of later maturity, which unfortunately carried a connotations of weakness or infirmity. Senility, the state of oldage, with the weakness, deterioration or infirmity accompanying oldage.

The general appearance of the older adult is determined in part by the changes that occur in the skin, face, hair and posture. The skin develops creases and furrows and begins to sag. Lentigines senilis appears, particularly the dorsum of the hands, arms, and face. There is decrease in skin turgor. The posture of the older adult is one of general flexion. The head is tilted forward; hips and knees are slightly flexed. There are certain changes in bodily system. The normal physiologic changes of older adulthood are as follows:

General Status

- Progressively decreasing efficiency or physiologic processes results in a fragile balance and hinders the body's ability to maintain homeostasis
- Physical or emotional stressors cause an older adult to be more valuable because of decreased physiologic reserves
- The older may continue to engage in all activities of middle age but intuitively adjusts to a modified pace and more frequent rest period.

Integumentary

- Wrinkling and sagging of skin occur with decreased skin elasticity, dryness and sealing are common
- Balding becomes common in men; and women experience thinning of hairs also; hair looses pigmentation
- Skin pigmentation and moles are common, although the skin may become plane because of loss of melanocytes
- Nails typically thicken and brittle and yellowish.

Musculoskeletal

- Decrease in subcutaneous tissue and weight commonly and found in the old age
- Muscle mass and strength decrease
- Bone demineralization occurs and bone becomes porous and brittle
- Joint tends to stiffen and loss flexibility and range of motion may decrease
- Overall mobility commonly slows and posture tends to stop, height decreases slightly.

Neurologic

- The central nervous system responds more slowly to multiple stimuli. Hence, the cognitive and behavioral response of the older adult may be delayed
- Rate of reflex respond decreases

- Temperature regulation and pain perception become less efficient
- The sense of balance declines, and fine movements may become more difficult
- Sleep at night typically shortens and the older adult may awaken more easily.

Special Senses

- Diminished visual acuity (presbyopia) occurs, with increased sensitivities to glare and decreased ability to adjust to darkness, cataracts may further obsecure vision
- Diminished hearing acuity (presbycusis) occur, particularly diminished pitch discrimination in the presence of environmental noises
- The sense of taste and smell are decreased.

Cardiopulmonary

- Blood vessels become less elastic and often rigid and tortous. Venous return becomes less efficient. Fatty plaque deposits continue to occur in the linings of the blood vessels. Lower exterminity edema and cooling may occur; particularly with decrease mobility
- The body is less able to increase heart rate and cardiac output with activity
- Pulmonary elasticity and ciliary action decrease to cleaning of the lungs becomes less efficient. Respiratory rate may increase, accompanied by diminished depty.

Gastrointestinal

- Digestive juices, continue to diminish and nutrient absorption decreases
- Malnutrition and anemia become more common
- With reduced muscle tone and decrease peristalsis, constipation and indigestion and common complaints.

Dentition

- Tooth decay and loss continue for most older adults
- Eating habits may change, particularly if the older adults lacks teeth or has ill fitting dentures.

Genitourinary

- Blood flow to the kidney decreases with diminished cardiac output
- The number of functioning nephron units decreases by 50 percent, waste products may be filtered and excreted more slowly
- Fluids and electrolyte remain within normal ranges but the balance if fragile
- Bladder capacity decreases by 50 percent, voiding becomes more frequent; two or three times a night is usual. A decrease in bladder and sphincter muscle control may result in stress incontinence or incomplete bladder emptying

- About 75 percent men over 65, experience hypertrophy of the prostate gland (may require surgery)
- There is atrophy, decrease secretion and thinning of the older women's genital tract.

Reproductive

- Changes in the sexual function; concentration of testosterone diminished with aging, producing a gradual decline in sexual vigor, muscle strength and active sperm.

As sexual partner, the older man experiences reduction in the frequency of intercourse, i.e. the intensity of sensation, the speak of attaining erection, and the force of ejaculation.

The older women encounters little sexual difficulty if she is in good health, has an open and positive attitude toward sex relations, and has an available and effective sexual partner. Effective sexual capacity and performance among women remains until late 70s or even older.

The psychosexual crisis in old age is an ego integrity versus self-despair. Ego integrity is the coming together of all previous of the lifecycle. Having accomplished the earlier tasks, the persons accept life as it has been. The person demonstrates the characteristics of maturity, achieving both wisdom and an enriched perspective about life and people. Without sense of ego integrity a sense of self-despair and self disgust results. The person becomes hypercritical of others and projects personal self disgust, inadequacy and anger on to other. These fellings are being burden, too slow and worthless.

As expected development tasks of the elderly are as follows:
- Recognize the aging process and resulting limitations
- Adjust to decreasing physical strength and health changes
- Continue a supportive, close, warmth relationship with the spouse or significant other, including a satisfying sexual relationship
- Find a satisfactory home or living arrangements and establish a safe, comfortable household routine to fit health and economic status
- Adjust living standard of retirement income; supplement retirement income if possible with remunerative activity
- Maintain maximum level of health care for self; physically and emotionally by getting health examination and needed medical or dental care, eating an adequate diet, and maintaining personal hygiene
- Maximum contact with children, grand children and other living relatives, finding emotional satisfaction with them
- Establish and maintain affiliation with members of own age group
- Maintain interest in people outside the family and in social, civil, and political responsibility
- Pursue alternate sources of need satisfaction and new interest and maintain former activities to gain status, recognition and a feeling of being needed
- Find meaning in life after retirement and in facing inevitable illness and death of oneself and spouse as well as others.

Table 7.10: Needs of the Later Years	
Needs	*Rationales*
1. Nutrition	• Fixed or diminished income • Reduced caloric intake • Oral problems • Loneliness, depression
2. Elimination	• More sedentary lifestyle • Loss of muscle tone • Poor eating habits
3. Circulation	• Slower heart rate • Fatty deposits around heart • Chronic conditions
4. Oxygen	• Decreased in vital capacity of lungs • Chronic condition
5. Temperature regulation	• Diminished adaptation to extremes of heat and cold
6. Comfort, rest and sleep	• Loss of skin integrity
7. Pain avoidance	• Reduced sensitivity to pain
8. Sensory stimulation	• Diminished perception in all areas
9. Movement and exercise	• Loss of muscle tone, mass • Loss of cartilage • Limited range of motions • Slower coordination
10. Protection and safety	• Loss of cartilage • Bones more fragile • Presence of osteoporosis • Slower reflexes • Diminished sensory perceptions
11. Hygiene	• Loss of skin integrity • Loss to teeth • Dentures, gum disease
12. Infection control	• Loss of skin integrity • Decreased isoimmunity • Immunosuppressive drugs • Chronic conditions
13. Sexuality	• Privacy sexual partner, psychosexual crisis
14. Self-esteem	• Financial status • Leisure, social activities • Dependency status • Attitudes of family, and others
15. Security	• Financial social status • Dependence status • Death of spouse, friends • Attitude of family and others
16. Needs related to terminal illness	• Death of spouse, friends inevitability of own death

Accordingly the needs to be met promoting the health of the elderly are given in Table 7.10.

Nurses Role in Health Care of the Elderly

The nurse must recognize, physiological and psychosocial interrelationships and view the older client holistically. The major goal of nursing care of the elderly is to assist the older client to function as independently as possible and to continue to develop individual potentials. The nurse collaborates with the family and other disciples to prevent complication of illness, to secure a safe and comfortable environment and to promote the clients return to normal health. The general guidelines for nursing care for the elderly are as follows:

- Maintain the client physiologic reserves, carefully assess the client to so that complications are discovered early.
- Prevent multisystem complication. Include nursing care that maintains physical integrity and function, such as skin care and planned rest and activity times. Teach the client and family members what symptoms to report to the health care provider.

- Provide safe and encultured environment with comfortable temperature and good lighting. If the environment is unfamiliar, orient the client to routine and equipment. Teach safety measures in the home, such as using a night light, avoiding throw rugs and having safety bars around the tub and commode.
- Slow your pace of care. Allow the client extra time to carry out activities, particularly those that require physical coordination such as eating.
- Encourage independence, teach the family to allow the client to provide selfcare independently as much as possible.
- Beware of the stereotype of aging. Treat each client as a unique person. Although many older client have similar needs, factors such as background, interests, capabilities, values, culture, and life styles may differ greatly.
- Promote continued development. Assist the client and family to accept physical limitations. Work with them to adapt the environment so that functional health is maintained.
- Be familiar with the resources available in the community, collaborate with the health care team to provide information and referrals for resource for the client and family.

8

Hospital Admission, Transfer, Discharge and Documentation

Admitting a Patient

Admission refers to an entry of a patient into the health care facility that may be hospital or any other health care facility that may be any agency that provides health care.

Admission is an anxious time for patient and their families. The patient usually very concerned about health problems or potential health problems and the potential outcome of treatment. Often the patient is having pain or other discomforts. The first contact with nurses and health care workers is important, anxiety and fear can be reduced and a positive attitude regarding the care to be received can be initiated. Admission routines that are efficient and show appropriate concerns for the patient can ease his or her anxiety. Admission routines that the patient perceives as careless or excessively impersonal can heighten anxiety, reduce cooperation, impair response to treatment, and perhaps aggravate symptoms.

The environment of hospital differs from patient's home in all aspects in relation to new sights, sounds and smell. These may interfere with the patient comforts. It is the responsibility of nurses to assist the patient in maintaining dignity and sense of control and in becoming comfortable in the hospital. Each persons reaction to the hospital is unique that nurse can anticipate some common reactions, such as fear of unknown, loss of identity, disorientation, separation, anxiety and loneliness.

Fear of unknown, which causes insecurity, loss of identity reflects a need for esteem, love and belonging which includes recognition. The reactions of separation, anxiety and loneliness reflect a need for belongingness and love.

Admission into a hospital is an extremely stressful situation or an event. It is an anxious time for patients and their families. The patients often experiences pain and/or some other discomfort. The surrounding of the hospital is different from the patient's home. Sometimes the new surroundings of the hospital such as new sights, sounds and smell that may interfere with patients comfort. Each persons reaction to the hospitalization is unique; however, there are some common reaction's, which the nurse can expect are fear of the unknown, loss of identity, disorientation, separation, anxiety, and loneliness. The fear of the unknown cause insecurity, and the anxiety and loneliness reflect a need for belongingness and love. The loss of identity may reflex a need for self-esteem including recognition.

The nurse may help to reduce the severity of these common reactions to hospitalization with a warm, caring attitude and with courtesy and empathy. Treating each patient with respect, maintaining his dignity, involving him in the plan of care, and whenever possible, adjusting hospital routine to meet his desires will help the patient adaptation to hospital surroundings.

Admission procedure usually begins in the admitting department. Here the admission staff gather information to start the patient's record. This information usually includes name, address and other necessary details related to office for various purposes. When admitting a person to hospital or health care facility the nurses have many responsibilities which include the following:

1. Meeting immediate needs of the person, i.e. physical, emotional.
2. Introduction and orientation.
3. Baseline assessment by observation, physical examination, inspecting and history taking.
4. Care of belongings.
5. Record keeping.

Immediate needs: A brief general assessment of a new patient to ascertain his or her immediate needs is essential. Immediate needs may be either physical or emotional. If a patient is in acute pain, contact the physician immediately regarding orders for medication and care, meanwhile institute nursing measures to relieve pain or follow standing orders to relieve pain. If a patient is upset or distraught, spend a short time listening and talking to the patient; this can facilitate his or her transition to the hospital environment. If a patient feels that those around are concerned about his or her immediate needs and are taking action to meet their relationship or trust may well have begun.

Introduction and orientation: After meeting immediate needs, the nurse can use her/his judgment when to have introduction and orientation according to the condition of the patient. The nursing actions will includes starting with greeting the patient by name and making him feel welcome. The way of greeting should convey interest in and concern for the patient. A person just entering a hospital is really not concerned about nurses problems of staffing or time expect as they directly affect his or her own care. If it is necessary for a patients to wait and explanation is appreciated. Then introducing nurses themselves to patients and others by both name and positions, help the patients to orient himself or herself to what is happening. Other patients who are in the same ward should also be introduced.

The new patient should be given an orientation to the unit and the room/ward. The orientation should include the following:

- The relationships of the room to the nurses station
- The location of lounge areas
- The location of shower and bathroom facilities
- How to call the nurse from the bed and the bathroom
- How to use intercom system
- How to adjust the bed and lights
- How to operate TV/radio/telephone, etc.
- Explanation of policies that are applicable to patients
- Explanation of hospital routines.

Baseline assessment: The information to be gathered in base lines assessment varies from one hospital to another hospital or facility. It almost always includes temperature, pulse, respiration, blood pressure, height and weight. In some facilities a complete physical examination is done by the nurses. In others, the nurse may do a thorough assessment that does not encompass the traditional physical examination. A nursing history is usually taken. Even if a formalized nursing history not used, information in relation to allergies, current medications and patients perception of his/her entering problem, i.e. chief complaints are gathered. An interview is used to gather subjective information regarding the patient. These baseline informations are necessary in order to evaluate future observations and data gathered.

Care of belongings: Usually, jewellary, money and medication should be given to the family to take home. If no family member is present, the valuables may be put in the hospital safe. This is one of the most difficult problems in a hospital, i.e. keeping track of a patient's personal property. The loss of valued items is unsetting to the patients and can be costly to a hospital or health care institution.

The nurses must carefully follow the hospital policy for the patient valuables. Losing the patient valuables can have serious legal implications for both the hospital and the nurse. Most facilities have a routine for checking and noting all personal items brought to worn by a patient. Those items that are not needed can be sent home with family members. This is perhaps the best safeguard. Large sums of money and valuable items are usually kept in safe in the hospital administrative office with proper document attesting to their location and values. Disposition of valuables must be documented on the medical record.

Record keeping: Recording of all parts of the admission process is essential for legal purpose. The baseline assessment swerves as the reference thorough out the period of care; and frequently the record of care of personal effects must be considered. Nurses are responsible for keeping all the records pertaining to the patient *(Admitting mentally ill patient please refer to legal responsibility of nurse in admitting psychiatric patients Chapter 5).*

Procedure for Admitting a Client

When admitting a patient to the nursing division or ward, the nurse completes a number of procedures during the admission process including orientation of the patient to ward and unit procedures, collection of a nursing history and physical assessment, collection of specimen and clarification of patients questions and expectations. The nurse have to perform the accepted procedures for admitting a patient for the following reasons:

- To assist the patient to become comfortable in the hospital environment
- To obtain information about the patient that will serve as a basis for cure
- To begin to establish a nurse-patient relationship.

Before admitting a patient, the nurse should understand the following:

- Principles of communication
- Accurate documentation
- Growth and development
- Physical assessment
- Vital signs assessment

The procedure for admitting a client to a health care facility is extremely important. First impressions of the facility and care-givers are lasting ones. A calm, caring approach instills confidence in the client and the belief that the client's needs are important. Orienting the client to the room, nursing unit, and

facility will help the client to be comfortable in the health care environment.

While admitting a client, nurse should:
1. Assess the client's comfort level about being in a health care facility. Identifies needed nurse-client interactions.
2. Assess client's physical and mental state. Provides basis for nursing care. Shows caring and concern for the client.
3. Assess client's knowledge of reason for admission. Provides basis for nurse-client interaction and client teaching.

Please see Table 8.1 for admitting procedures of patient.

Equipment Needed

- Admission kit: wash basin, emesis basin, pitcher, glass, etc.
- Client orientation materials
- Valuables envelope (if needed)
- Belongings checklist
- Admission Nursing Assessment form
- Sphygmomanometer, stethoscope, thermometer.

After procedure the nurse should see that:
- The client is comfortable in the health care facility.
- The client uses call bell system, bed controls, television, and telephone.
- The client has adjusted to facility routing.

And document the following:
- Complete admitting nursing assessment record
- Time and condition of client on admission
- All valuables sent to the safe
- Client's belongings
- Client's comfort level.

Transferring a Patient

Transferring a patient refers to that, patient may require transfer either from the unit to another or to another health care institution according to the condition of the patient. A patient may be moved to general care unit to special care unit or special care unit to general care unit. Transfer also may be done at the patient request. This transfer combined admission and discharge. The nurse performs the accepted procedure for transferring a patient for the following purposes.
- To match the type of identify of nursing care to patient needs
- To locate the patient in the facility best able to provide care needed
- To accommodate the patient request for a specific type of room.

Discharging a Patient

Discharge a patient refers to releasing a patient from hospital or health care facility to home. The nurse performs the accepted procedure for discharging a patient for the following purposes:

Table 8.1: Admitting a Patient

	Nursing action		Rationale
1.	Welcome client to unit. Introduce yourself by name and title. Ask client to state his or her name.	1.	Verifies identification.
2.	Orient client to room and nursing unit. Describe items such as nurse call bell system, location of bathroom, place for clothing, bed controls, television, telephone, visiting hours, meal times, Standard Precautions, and review items in client education materials such as client rights and other written information about the facility.	2.	Reduces client anxiety: allows fuller participation in care.
3.	Provide privacy for client to change into pajamas or hospital gown, if not already done.	3.	Respects client privacy.
4.	Show client ill bracelet to double-check proper identification. Attach bracelet to wrist. (This may have been done in Admitting Department.) Review drug allergies and attach allergy bracelet to same wrist, according to agency policy.	4.	Confirms client identification; promotes client safety.
5.	Document and store client's belongings and valuables according to agency policy.	5.	Reduces the risk of loss.
6.	Begin nursing assessment, according to agency policy.	6.	Starts development of client database.
7.	Perform any other actions, as directed by agency policy.	7.	Different facilities have different needs, regulations, and guidelines for client admission.

- To assist the patient in making the change from the hospital environment to the home environment
- To provide continuity of care at home so that the patient care returns to the best state of wellness possible

When planning for a patient discharge to home, or to another unit, the nurse responsibilities are similar which includes the following:

- Planning for continuity of care
- Patient teaching
- Final assessment
- Care of personal property
- Business function
- Record keeping.

Planning for discharge must be individualized to the patient's specific needs. Through out the hospital stay the patient should be taught about medication, diet activity treatments and any signs and symptoms to be repeated to the physician general health teaching also to be performed. Discharge orders should be obtained from the physician. No official documentation or process should be initiated until the instruction is written. Afterwards plans are made for continuing care as method. If the patient is going home, this planning can be done with the patient and the family.

As stated earlier, patient teaching should be continued; wherever the patient is going, explain what will happen, where he or she is going and when this will happen. The patient may need information about his or her medication, treatments, activity, diet, and continued health supervision. Before the patient leave from the ward or unit, nurses must prepare a final assessment of his or her total status and the patient ability to continue to participate in his or her own care. Be sure that all personal belongings accompany the patient especially critical dentures, glasses and special appliances, such as crutches. And it is customary for either the patient or the family to consult with the administration office regarding settlement of financial matters, if any. Record keeping must be maintained according to hospital policy.

Sometimes patient will insist on leaving the hospital without physician consent, that is against medical advice. In such events a special form must be signed by the patient in the patient acknowledged leaving without the physician discharge order and that the physician, hospital and hospital personnel will not be responsible for any problem that might occur because of this action.

Procedure for Transferring a Client

Transferring a client to a different unit in a health care facility can be very stressful to the client. It may mean that the client's condition has deteriorated (transferring to ICU) or improved (transferring to a rehabilitation unit after a hip replacement), thus requiring different treatments.

However short the stay before a transfer, the client has a sense of knowing the environment and the health care personnel on that unit. Explaining the reason for transfer to the client and family as well as gathering all equipment, medications, and client's personal belongings, help ease the stress of a transfer,

Introducing the client and family to health care personnel working on the new unit and sharing some of the client's personal preferences in the client's presence (i.e. prefers one pillow and an extra blanket) shows caring and concern for the client and helps ensure continuity of care.

- Assess client's knowledge and feelings about the transfer. Allows for explanations and discussion about the situation.
- Assess which equipment is to be transferred with the client and that those medications and client's personal belongings

Table 8.2: Transferring a Patient

	Nursing action		*Rationale*
1.	Check to see if order is needed to initiate transfer according to agency policy.	1.	Policies differ among facilities.
2.	Call nursing unit of new location to see if bed is ready and to give report.	2.	Provides continuity of care.
3.	Explain the transfer to the client (and family, if appropriate). Answer any questions. Allay anxieties about moving.	3.	Keeps client informed and promotes cooperation.
4.	Review the valuables and belongings checklist completed on admission. Compare with belongings.	4.	Ensures all of client's belongings are transferred with the client. Prevents loss.
5.	Gather records and any other equipment that will be transferred with the client, according to agency policy, such as eye drops, other medications, IV pump, respiratory therapy equipment, and so on.	5.	Helps make transfer more efficient and reduces multiple trips to new area.
6.	Transfer client by appropriate vehicle (wheelchair, stretcher), Accompany client to new unit. Transfer care to another staff member in person. Ensure that call bell is within reach or staff member is in room before leaving client.	6.	Enhances continuity of care. Promotes safety.
7.	Document time of transfer and any other information required by agency policy.	7.	Promotes communication among members of the health care team.
8.	Upon return to unit, notify appropriate personnel according to agency policy that client has left the unit. Arrange for personnel to clean the bed and surroundings the client has left.	8.	Prepares bed for new admission. Reduces transfer of microorganisms.

are ready to move. Provides organization to the transfer and encourages completeness.

- Assess readiness of new unit to accept client. Allows transfer to proceed smoothly with no waiting.

For procedures of transferring patient, please see Table 8.2.

Equipment Needed

- Client's medical record (if not electronic)
- Client's imprint card
- Client's medications
- Stretcher or wheelchair
- Cart to carry client's belongings.

Transferring a client is a skill that ancillary personnel may assist with. The nurse is responsible for transferring the client's medical record and medications and for giving a thorough report to the accepting nurse on the new unit.

After procedure nurse should see that:

- The client understands the reason for transferring to a new unit.
- The client is safely moved with needed equipment and medications and all personal belongings.
- The client's move was communicated to appropriate departments for continuity or care.

And document the following:

- Client's condition when leaving unit.
- Equipment and medications transferred with the client.
- Personal belongings sent with client.
- Report on client given to receiving nurse.
- Departments notified of client's transfer.

Procedure for Discharging a Client

A client may be discharged from a health care facility to another facility or to home. This can be a frightening experience depending on the level of recuperation the client has achieved. The amount and type of medications prescribed, dietary needs or restrictions, and other treatments to be conducted. Being transferred from one facility to another may be seen either as improvement or as a lack of progress in recovery.

Discuss with the client and family the discharge process. Complete all paper work and all discharge teaching. Collect the client's belongings and valuables (as documented on admission) so they can accompany the client. These things will help make the discharge process pleasant and effective. For procedure of discharging of a patient please see Tables 8.3 and 8.4.

Before discharging a client nurse should:

- Assess client's feelings about being discharged. Opens communication about the discharge.
- Assess that family and home or the other facility is prepared to receive the client. Provides a smooth process with less stress for the client.
- Assess client's or family's knowledge of care at home. Ensures continuity of care.

Equipment needed:

- Required facility paperwork
- Stretcher or wheelchair
- Cart for client's belongings.

For discharge to home:

- Prescriptions
- Instructions–care, diet, medications, follow-up appointment.

Table 8.3: Discharging a Patient (Procedure 1)

Nursing action		*Rationale*	
1.	Check order for discharge.	1.	Most agency policies require order for discharge.
Discharge to Another Facility			
2.	Explain discharge to client, and family, if appropriate.	2.	Includes client in care. Promotes cooperation.
3.	Complete intra-agency transfer form, according to policy. Be sure to note last time of medication doses. Complete nursing discharge summary. Prepare transfer paperwork, according to policy.	3.	Facilitates continuity of care. Promotes client safety
4.	Notify receiving agency of impending transfer. Provide report and confirm ability to receive client.	4.	Facilitates continuity of care. Ensures that new facility will accept client before client leaves current facility.
5.	Arrange for transportation to new facility. Call transportation company according to agency policy.	5.	Reduces waiting time; facilitates continuity of care.
6.	Review the valuables and belongings checklist completed on admission. Compare with belongings.	6.	Ensures all of client's belongings leave with the client. Prevents loss.
7.	When personnel from transportation company arrive, assist client transfer to stretcher or wheelchair. Provide transportation personnel with required information, such as client's DNA status, for transfer. See that client's belongings accompany client, along with any required paperwork or equipment.	7.	Provides continuity of care.
Discharge to Home			
8.	Discuss discharge with client, and family, if appropriate. Confirm that discharge teaching has been done. Ask client if there are any questions about self-care at home. If so, follow-up with appropriate personnel (typically, RN).	8.	Promotes client cooperation. Allays anxiety.
9.	Nurse (according to agency policy) reviews with client; prescriptions to be filled, including telling client when next dose is due based on medications administered in the facility; food and drug interactions and any other essential medication information; care of incision or dressings, if indicated; dietary needs or restrictions or other pertinent information; and when client should make appointment for follow-up with private physician.	9.	Promotes continuity of care.
10.	Have client/family provide return demonstration of skills required for self-care at home.	10.	Demonstrates that learning has occurred.
11.	Check that transportation to home is available. Check client room area for any personal belongings.	11.	Reduces waiting time.
12.	Complete any paperwork with client, as required by agency policy.	12.	Meets regulatory requirements.
13.	Escort client to transportation vehicle.	13.	Promotes client safety.
For any Discharge			
14.	Notify appropriate personnel according to agency policy that client has left the unit. Arrange for personnel to clean the bed and surroundings the client has left.	14.	Prepares bed for new admission. Reduces transfer of microorganisms.

After discharge a client nurse should see that:
- The client encountered no problems in discharge to another facility
- The client, with the assistance of family, is confident about care at home.

And document the following:
- Date and time of discharge
- Belongings and valuables with client.

If discharge to another facility:
- Person receiving report on client
- Company transporting client.

If discharge to home
- Mode of taking client to transportation vehicle
- Person taking client home
- Prescriptions and instructions given to client.

	Table 8.4: Discharging a Patient (Procedure 2)			
	Nursing action			*Rationale*
1.	Wash hands thoroughly.		1.	Prevents spread of microorganism.
2.	Make certain there is written discharge order.		2.	Verifies physician's decision regarding time for the patient to be discharged.
3.	If no discharge order has been written, have LAMA form signed by patient.		3.	Generally patients cannot be held against their wishes. The patients signature acknowledge full responsibility for what happens after leaving.
4.	Notify the family or person who will be transferring the patient home.		4.	Avoids delay in discharge.
5.	Verify that the patient and family understand the instructions for care, medication, special diet, exercise.		5.	Helps ensure appropriate home care.
6.	Gather equipment, supplies and prescriptions that the patient is to take here.		6.	Provides service, patient is unable to do.
7.	Check to see that business office has given a release.		7.	Prevents undue wasting for the patient when leaving.
8.	Assist the patient to dress and pack items to go home.		8.	Conserves patients strength.
9.	Check clothing and valuables list made on admission according to policy.		9.	Avoids patient leaving personal items at facility.
10.	Transfer the patient and belongings via wheelchair to the vehicle. Assist patient into the vehicle, if needed.		10.	Provides patient safety and complies with policy of most hospital.
11.	Wash hands thoroughly.		11.	Prevent spread of microorganism.
12.	Record entire discharge procedure.		12.	Documentation of teaching, patient condition and method of discharge complete record. Legally this is important and prevent problems in the future.

Discharge: Leaving Against Medical Advice (LAMA)

Occasionally, the patient or the patient's family may demand discharge against medical advice (AMA) (when a patient leaves a health care facility without a physician's order for discharge). If this occurs, notify the physician immediately. If the physician fails to convince the patient to remain in the facility, the physician will ask the patient to sign an AMA form releasing the facility from legal responsibility for any medical problems the patient may experience after discharge.

If the physician is not available, discuss the discharge form with the patient and obtain the patient's signature. If the patient refuses to sign the AMA form, do not detain the patient. This violates his or her legal rights.* After the patient leaves, document the incident thoroughly in your notes and notify the physician.

STATEMENT OF PATIENT LEAVING HOSPITAL AGAINST ADVICE

This is to certify that I am leaving _________________ Hospital at my own insistence and against the advice of the hospital authorities and my attending physician. I have been informed by them of the dangers of my leaving the hospital at this time. I release the hospital, its employees and officers, and my attending physician from all liability for any adverse results caused by my leaving the hospital prematurely.

Signature of patient _______________________________

I agree to hold harmless the _______________________________ Hospital, its employees and officers, and the attending physician from all liability, with reference to the discharge of the patient named above.

____

(Husband, wife, parent, etc.)

Date _______________________________

Witness _______________________________

* A rational adult patient who will not sign the form cannot be forcibly detained. Only if a court order was issued for the admission, as in some cases of mental illness, can a patient be forcibly detained. A lawsuit for false imprisonment could be filed against the hospital and/or personnel for keeping patients against personal wishes, Documentation of the refusal to sign the form and the information given about the risks of leaving should be made in the patient's chart.

Nursing Process for Patient Discharge

Assessment

Every patient in a hospital requires discharge planning, which is initiated on admission. There are conditions, however, that place a patient at greater risk for being unable to meet continuing health care needs after discharge. The following risk factors should be identified:

- Older adult age group
- Multisystem disease process
- Major surgical procedure
- Chronic or terminal illness
- Emotional or mental instability.

The nurse assesses the patient's and family's needs for health teaching and collaborates with physicians and staff in other disciplines in assessing need for referral.

Nursing Diagnosis

Clustering of defining characteristics from assessment data may reveal the following nursing diagnoses for the patient needing discharge:

- Impaired home maintenance
- Self-care deficit.

Expected Outcomes/Planning

Planning involves the development of individualized goals for the patient based on nursing diagnoses.

- Patient or family member will be able to care for individual needs.
- Health care resources at home will be available.

Implementation

On the day of discharge:

- All equipment, supplies, and prescriptions that the patient is to take home are gathered.
- The nurse verifies that the patient and caregiver understand the instructions for care.
- Have patient or family member perform any treatments to be continued in the home.
- Home health nurse will inspect home environment to assess for obstacles or risks.

Evaluation

- Home health agency has been notified of patient's needs on arrival at home.
- Home health agency's initial visit completed before discharge or soon thereafter.

Documentation

Documentation is the act of recording client status and care in written form. The methods of recording and reporting information – relevant to client care have developed as a response to standards of practice, legal and regulatory standards, institutional standards and policies and society's norms, oral communication about a client's status is called reporting.

Documentation is any printed or written record of activities. In health care it should include the following:

- Changes in the client's condition.
- The administration of tests, treatments, procedures, and client education with the results of, or client responses to them.
- The clients response to an intervention.
- The evaluation of expected outcome.
- Complaints from client or family.

Purposes of Documentation

The client record is a collection of materials that serves as a legal record of the clients health care experience. The two primary purposes for documentation are professional responsibility and accountability. The profession responsibility of all health care practitioners. Documentation provides evidence of the practitioners accountability to the client, institution, the profession and society.

The written records serves the following purposes.

(i) Communication: Documentation is a communication method that confirms the care provided to the client and clearly outlines all important information reporting clients. Health care professionals use the client record to communicate about the client status and care. The record serves as the vehicle by which different health professionals who interact with a client communicate with each other. This prevent fragmentation, repetition and delays in client care.

(ii) Education: Students of medical, nursing and others use the medical record as a tool to learn about disease processes, medical and nursing diagnoses, complications, and interventions. Nursing students can enhance their critical thinking skills by examining the records following in chronological order, health care teams plan of care, including the way it was developed, implanted and evaluated, analyzing the results. A record can frequently provide a comprehensive view of client, the illness, effective treatment, strategies and factors that affect the outcome of illness.

(iii) Legal document: The medical record is a legal document, and in a law suit, it is the record that serves as the description of exactly what happened to a client. The client record is scrutinized by attorneys whenever dispute about a patient care arises. In court, the record is legal evidence of the quality of care given to a client. The legal aspects of documentation require:

- Writing, legible and neat.
- Spelling and grammar, properly used.
- Authorised abbreviations.
- Time-sequenced, and factual descriptive entries.

(iv) Quality assurance: Health care agencies perform chart audits (reviews of client records) to identify ways to improve patient care, decrease lengths of stay, control costs, and design inservice education programs. According agencies review records to ensure delivery of quality care and public safety.

(v) Reimbursement: Insurance companies, budget managers, and facility billing staff use client records to determine the cost of care. From the agency's perspective, when information in the medical record shows compliance with Medicare and Medicaid standards, reimbursement is maximized. Failure to document equipment or procedure used daily (e.g. feeding pump, daily weight, intake and output, IV therapy, drug additives) can result in reimbursement being denied.

(vi) Research: The client record is used to gather data for clinical research. The clients medical record is used by researcher, to determine whether a clients meets the research criteria for a study. Documentation can also indicate a need for research. The treatment plans for number of clients with the same health problems can yield information helpful in treating other clients.

(vii) Nursing audit: Nursing audit is a method of evaluating the quality of care provided to clients. A nursing audit can focus on the implementation of the nursing process in order to evaluate quality care provided. Nursing audit committee examine the data related to:

- Safety measures
- Treatment interventions and client responses to them
- Expected outcomes as basis for interventions
- Client teaching
- Discharge planning
- Adequate staffing.

(viii) Health care analysis: Information from record may assist health care planners to identify agency needs such as over utilized and underutilized hospital services. Records can be used to establish the cost, of various services and to identify those services that cost the agency money and those that generative revenue.

Documentation Systems

Currently there are number of documentation systems are in use which includes source-oriented record, problem-oriented medical record (POMR), Problem Intervention Evaluation (PIE), mould, focus charting, charting by exception (CBE) and computerized documentation and care management.

1. Source-Oriented Record

In hospitals patients receive care from variety of disciplines. Such hospitals use source-oriented records. In this members of each disciplines record their findings in a separately labeled section of the chart. Sections of the source oriented record induces the following.

- Admission data – demographic information, insurance data, contact information
- History and physical examination – summary of the current problem
- Physicians orders – medication, treatments and activities
- Diagnostic reports – findings of texts, X-rays, ultrasound, MRI, etc.
- Laboratory data – compilation of results from laboratory studies
- Nurses notes – chronological charting by nurses on patients responses to care
- Graphic sheets – vital signs flow sheets, intake and output chart, checklists regarding patient activity include dietary intake
- Rehabilitation and therapy notes
- Discharge planning.

Source oriented recording in a narrative recording by each member (source) of the health care team on separate documents. Each discipline uses a separate records often resulting in fragments care and time-consuming communication between disciplines. Narrative charting is a traditional part of the source oriented record which consists of written notes that include routine care, normal findings, and client problems, new narrative recording is being replaced by other systems such as charting by exception and focus.

Still the source oriented records are convenient because care provider from each discipline can easily locate the forms on which to record data and it is easy to trace the information specific to one discipline. The disadvantage is that information about a particular client problems is scattered throughout the chart, so it is difficult to find chronological information on a clients problems and progress.

2. Problem-Oriented Medical Records (POMR)

Problem-oriented records are organized around the clients problem. POMR employs a structured, logical format focuses on the clients problem. There are four critical components in POMR, which includes the following:

- **Data base:** Data base is assessment data, which consists of many parts: demographic data, the history, physical, nursing assessment data and data pertinent to family and social history and baseline diagnostic tests. The data base should be updated when the client condition changes to reflect the clients current status.

- **Problem list:** It is a concise listing of problems that have been identified from the data base, when once problem is resolved it is noted on the problem list. Clients problem numbered according to which identified. If a problem changes or is redefined, the problem list is updated to reflect changes. Here all caregiver may contribute to the problem list, which includes all the needs of client which may be physiologic, psychologic, social cultural, spiritual, developmental and environmental. Physicians write problems as medical diagnoses, surgical procedures or symptoms, nurses write problems as nursing diagnoses.

- **Plan of care:** An initial plan includes outline of goals, expected outcomes and learning needs and further data of needed. The initial list of orders or plan of care is made with reference to the actual problems, which includes physicians orders and nursing care plan for addressing the identified problems. Care plans are generated by the person who lists the problems. Physician writes physician orders or medical care plan; nurses write nursing orders or nursing care plan. Other disciplines may also contribute to the plan.

- **Progress note:** Progress note in the POMR is a chart entry made by all health professional involved in a client care, they all use the same type of sheet for notes. Progress notes are organized according to problem list. Each discipline charts on shared notes. Charting is labeled according to problem number. Progress notes are numbered to correspond to the problems on the problem list and may be lettered for the type of data.

The format in which progress notes are to be written include SOAP, SOAPIE or SOAPIER which are acronym for:

- **S:** Subjective data consists of information obtained from what the client or family states that when it is important and relevant to the problem.
- **O:** Objective data consists of information that is measured or observed by the use of senses (what is observed or inspected) e.g. vital signs.
- **A:** Assessment is the interpretation or conclusions drawn about the subjective and objective data. In other words it is a conclusion reached on the basis of data formulated as client problem or nursing diagnosis.
- **P:** The plan is the plan of care designed to resolve the stated problem includes an expected outcomes and actions to be taken. The initial plan is written by a person who enters the problem into the record. All the subsequent plans including revisions, are entered into the progress notes.
- **I:** Interventions refer to the specific interventions that have actually been performed by the caregiver.
- **E:** Evaluation includes client responses to nursing interventions and medical treatments. This is primarily reassessment data.
- **R:** Revision reflects care plan modifications suggested by evaluation changes may be made in desired outcomes, interventions or target data.

Recent version of this format removes the subjective and objective data and starts with assessment, which combines the both data. The acronym become APIE or APIER. Author kept the subjective and objective data in his PRONE format of Nursing Care Plan, where 'R' is an acronym for "Reason" for the Problem (P) identified.

The advantage of POMR documentation includes:

- There is a common problem list that includes input from all disciplines.
- It is easy to monitor the patients progress because each problem is readily identified in the notes.
- Each discipline has ready access to the findings of the other members of the health teach which may encourage greater collaboration.
- It require cooperative spirit among health care provider.

PIE Documentation Model

PIE is an acronym for problems, interventions, and evaluation of nursing care. This system was to develop streamline documentation. The main parts of this system are an integrated plan of care, assessment flow sheets, and nurses progress notes.

Date	Hour	Progress notes
14-02-2007	08.30	**P:** Disturbed body image r/t bilateral mas **I:** Encourage verbalization of feelings and concerns and remain alert for clients comments about body image **E:** Glanced at chest during dressing change. Continue encouraging.

As stated above after the assessment, this nurse establishes and records specific problems on the progress notes often using NANDA diagnosis to word the problems. The problem statement is labeled "P" and referred to by number. The interventions employed to manage the problem as labeled "I" and numbered according to problem. The evaluation of the effectiveness of the interventions is also labeled and numbered according to the problem.

This system eliminates the traditional care plan and incorporates an ongoing care plan into the progress notes. There is no need to create and update separate plan. But the nurse must review all the nursing notes before giving care to determine which problems are current and which intervention are effective in taking care of clients.

Focus Charting

Focus charting highlights the client concerns, problems or strengths. Focus charting is a documentation system using a column format to Data, Action, and Response. Usually the focus is a nursing diagnosis but it may also be:

- A sign or symptom (e.g. abnormal vaginal bleeding)
- An acute change in the client condition (e.g. sudden increased in BP)
- A special need (e.g. a discharge referral)

Data reflect the assessment phase of nursing process and consists of observation of client status and behaviors including data from flow sheets (vital signs, papillary reaction, etc.). Nurse document subjective and objective information that supports the focus.

Action reflects planning and implementation and includes immediate and future nursing actions. It describes interventions performed (e.g. administration of medication).

Response reflects the evaluation phase of nursing process and describes clients response to any nursing and/or medical care. The focus charting system provides a holistic perspective of client and client needs by using following format.

Date	Hour	Focus	Progress notes
18-04-2007	09.00	Pain	D: Guarding abdominal incision, facial grimacing, severe pain A: Administered Pethidine Hgl
	09.30	Pain	R: Client states pain reduced

Charting by Exception

Charting by exception (CBE) is a documentation in which only abnormal or significant finding or exceptions to norms are recorded. CBE uses preprinted flowsheets to document most aspects of care. Normal responses for various assessment are defined on the form. It is system of documentation using standardized protocols stating what the expected course of the illness is and only significant findings (exceptions) are documented in a narrative form. It assumes that client care needs are routine and predictable and that client responses and outcomes are also routine and predictable.

The advantages of CBE system is elimination of lengthy, repetitive notes and it makes client changes in condition more obvious, which means that it reduces the time required to chart, reduces repetitive charting of routine care, provides a record that is easily read and understood and clearly highlights any variations from the expected plan of care. Usually CBE records at the bedside, facilitate to promote timely documentation.

Computerized Documentation

Computerized clinical record system are being developed as a way to manage the huge volume of information required an health care delivery. Health care facilities have been using computers for many years to order diagnostic tests and medications and to receive results of diagnostic tests. Total computerization system were adopting slowly in health care delivery system.

Nurses use computers to stone the client data base, add progress. Nursing information system are various software program. That allow nursing documentation in an electronic record. These system generally follow the components of the nursing process.

Computers make care planning and documentation relatively easy. To record nursing actions and client responses, the nurse either chooses from standardized lists of terms or types narrative information into the computer. Automated speech recognition technology now allows nurses to enter data by voice for conversion to written documentation. Multiple flowsheets are not needed in computerized record system, because information can be easily retrieved in a variety of formats.

The selected pros and cons of computer documentation are given below:

Pros

- Computer records can facilitate a focus on clients outcomes.
- Bedside terminals can synthesize information from monitoring equipment.
- Allows nurses to use their time more efficiently.
- The system links various sources of client information.
- Client information, requests, and results are sent and receive quickly.
- Links to monitors improve accuracy of documentation.
- Bedside terminals eliminate need to take notes on worksheets before recording.
- Information is legible.
- The system incorporates and reinforces standards of care.
- Standard terminology improves communication.

Cons

- Clients privacy may be infringed on if security measures are not used.
- Break downs make information temporarily unavailable.
- System is expensive.
- Extended training periods may be required when a now or updated system installed.

Confidentiality of Computer Records

Since there is an increased use of computerised client records, health care agencies have developed policies to ensure the privacy and confidentiality of client information stores in computers. The following are some suggestions for ensuring the confidentiality of computerised records.

- A personal password is needed to enter and sign off computer files.
- Do not share this password with anyone, including other health team members.
- After logging on, never leave a computer terminal unattended.
- Don not leave client information displayed on the monitor where others may see it.
- Stored all unneeded computer-generated worksheets.
- Know the facility's policy and procedures for correcting any entry error.
- Follow agency procedures for documenting sensitive material, such as diagnosis of HIV/AIDS.

In computerised documentation decision-support system are available to alert nurses and other health team member of client drug incompatibility, appropriate antibiotics based on culture and antibiotic susceptibility results, and adverse drug reactions. Another decision-support system uses assessment data to suggest possible nursing diagnosis, goals and outcomes criterion and interventions from which the nurse selects those appropriate for a specific client. Bedside computer terminals allow the nurse to immediately documents client assessments, medication given, and interventions performed; the nurse can also check care plans and revise if necessary, check test results, and many other functions. Timeliness, completeness, and the quality of nursing documentation are improved. In addition computerised charting increases legibility; stores and retrieves information quickly and easily; helps link diverse sources of client information and uses standardised terminology, which helps improve communication and departments.

Forms of Documentation

KARDEXES

The kardex is a concise method of organising and recording data about a client, making information quickly accessible to all health profession. It is a brief worksheet with basic client care information that traditionally is not part of the medical record. This system consists of a series of cards kept in a portable index file or on computer generated forms. The kardex is used as a reference throughout the shift and during change-of-shift reports. The kardex usually contain the following information:

- Client information – Name, age, religion, marital status, admission date, time, ward number, family contacts with phone number, physician name, diagnosis.
- List of medical diagnosis on priority.
- List of nursing diagnosis on priority.
- List of medications with date of order, and times of administration.
- List of intravenous fluids with dates of infusions and dosage.
- List of daily treatments, procedures and measurement of vital signs.
- List of diagnostic procedure order, such as X-ray and lab tests.
- Allergies.
- Activities permitted: functional limitations, assistance needed in ADL, and safety precautions, diet.
- Special instruction if any.

FLOW SHEETS

Flow sheets, with vertical or horizontal columns for recording date, time and assessment data and intervention information make it easy to track the client changes in condition. The flow sheets enables nurses to record nursing data quickly and concisely and provides an easy-to-read record of clients condition overtime. Flow sheets includes the following:

- Graphic records: Temperature, pulse, respiration, blood pressure, etc.
- Fluid balance record: Intake and output charts.
- Medication administration record.
- Wound assessment record, etc.

Flow sheets are used as supplement in many documentation system. Nurses still must document observations, client responses and teaching, details, interventions, and other significant data in the progress notes.

PROGRESS NOTES

Progress notes made by nurses provide information about the progress a client is making toward achieving desired outcome. Nurses progress notes are used to document the client condition, problems, and complaints, interventions, the client response to achievement of outcomes, standardised flow sheets can be used in the progress notes.

DISCHARGE SUMMARY

A discharge summary or referral summary are completed when the client is being discharged and referred to another institution or to a home. A narrative discharge summary in the progress notes includes:
- Client status on admission and discharge or referral
- A brief summary of the clients care
- Intervention and education outcome
- Resolved problems and continuing care needs unsolved problems including referrals
- Client instructions about medication, diet, food-drug interactions, activity, treatments, follow-ups and other special needs.

Do's and Dont's of Documentation

Do's
- Chart a change in a clients condition and show that follow-up action were taken.
- Read the nurses notes prior to care to determine if there has been a change in the client condition.
- Be timely state entry is better than no entry, however, the longer the period of time between actual care and charting, the greater the suspicion.
- Use objective, specific and factual description.
- Correct charting errors.
- Chart all teaching.
- Record the clients actual words by putting quotes around the words.
- Chart the clients response to interventions.
- Review your notes – are they clear and do they reflect what you want to say.

Dont's
- Leave blank space for a colleague to chart later.
- Chart in advance of the event (e.g. procedure, medication).
- Use vague terms (e.g. appears to be comfortable, had a good night).
- Chart for someone else.
- Use patient or client as it is in the chart.
- After a record even if requested by a superior or a physician.
- Record assumption or word reflecting bias (e.g. complainer, disagreeable).

REPORTING

A record is a written or computer based. The process of making an entry on a client record is called recording, charting or documenting. A clinical record is a formal, legal document that provides evidence of a client care.

A report is oral, written or computer-based communication intended to convey information to others. The purpose of reporting is to communicate specific information to a person or group of people. A report, whether oral or written, should be concise, including pertinent information but no extraneous detail.

Reporting summarizes the current critical information pertinent to clinical decision making and continuity of care. Reporting, like recording, is based on the nursing process, standard of care, and legal and ethical principles. To verbally report in a well-organised efficient manner the nurse should consider questions like – what to say, what to say not and how to say it.

Critical element in reporting is listening. Reports require everyone to participate when receiving a report, enhance listening skill by eliminating distractions, putting thoughts and concerns aside, concentrating on those things being said, and not anticipating the presenters next statements. Reporting process is an integral part to promoting continents of client care. Types of report include summary reports, walking rounds, or nursing round, telephone reports and orders, incidents reports, care plan conference reports.

Reporting summarizes the current critical information pertinent to clinical decision making and continuity of care. Reporting, like recording, is based on the nursing process, standards of care, and legal and ethical principles. To verbally report in a well-organized efficient manner the nurse should consider the following questions:

- What to say
- Why to say it
- How to say it

Another critical element of reporting is listening. Reports require everyone present to participate. When receiving a report, enhance listening skills by eliminating distractions, putting thoughts and concerns aside, concentrating on those things being said, and not anticipating the presenter's next statements. The reporting process is integral to promoting continuity of client care. Some facilities tape record the end-of-shift report. Summary reports, walking rounds, telephone reports and orders, and incident reports are all types of reporting.

Information for Shift Report

- Client name, room and bed, age, and gender
- Physician, admission date and diagnosis, and any surgery
- Diagnostic tests or treatments performed in the past 24 hours; results, if available
- General status, any significant change in condition
- New or changed physician's orders
- Nursing diagnoses and suggested nursing orders
- Evaluation of nursing interventions
- Intravenous fluid amounts, last PRN medication
- Concerns about the client.

Summary Reports

Information pertinent to the client's needs and identified by the nursing process is outlined in summary reports. Summary reports commonly occur either at the change of shift when new caregivers arrive or when the client is transferred to another area. A summary report should include the following information in the order indicated:

- Background data obtained from client interactions and assessment of the client's functional health patterns
- Prioritized medical and nursing diagnoses
- Identified client risks
- Recent changes in condition or in treatments (e.g. new medications, elevated temperature)
- Effective interventions or treatments of priority problems, inclusive of laboratory and diagnostic results (e.g. client's response to pain medication)
- Progress toward expected outcomes
- Adjustments in the plan of care
- Client or family complaints.

This logical and time-sequenced format follows the nursing process and thus provides structure and organization to the data. In order to provide continuity of care, the new caregiver must receive an accurate, concise report about those things that happened during the previous shift. Because client and family complaints usually generate questions and discussion, they should be addressed last.

Walking Rounds

Walking rounds can take the form of nursing rounds, instructor-student rounds, physician-nurse rounds, or multidisciplinary rounds. Walking rounds is when the members of the care team walk to each client's room and discuss progress and care with each other and with the client.

Nursing rounds are used most frequently by charge nurses as their method of report. The oncoming nurse is introduced to the client and the offgoing nurse discusses with the client and the oncoming nurse any changes in the plan of care. This is more time-consuming than a summary report, but gives the nurses and the client time to evaluate the effectiveness of care together.

Nursing rounds are also used for teaching when the instructor introduces the client to the student and they discuss the client's care together. The student's observation, communication, and decision-making skills can also be assessed by the instructor.

Nurse-physician rounds involve the physician and either staff nurse or the charge nurse. These rounds usually occur daily and allow the nurse, the physician, and the client to evaluate the effectiveness of care.

Multidisciplinary rounds involving all disciplines occur less frequently than other types of rounds, primarily because it is difficult to schedule everyone. Multidisciplinary rounds are done most commonly to discuss discharge planning or to supplement case conferences.

Telephone Reports and Orders

Nurses are expected to exhibit courtesy and professionalism when using the telephone.

When initiating a phone call, the nurse should organize the information to be reported or received. For example, the nurse should:

- Ensure that all lab results are back: if they are not, identify those that are missing and telephone the lab or check the computer to ascertain whether the results are available. Spell the client's name and provide the client's medical record number when calling the lab to minimize the chances of receiving results for the wrong client. Write down the tests and the results.
- Have the client's assessment data available, especially any significant data related to abnormal results.
- Minimize the chance of being interrupted during the call by informing the charge nurse or someone else at the nurses' station of the call.

State the reason for the call, for example. "I am calling Dr Dhanyakumar regarding the blood culture results for Mrs Basanth." Be brief, listen carefully, and repeat the test results and any orders received from the physician.

The date and time the phone call was placed, the client data reported by the nurse, the name of the person with whom the nurse spoke, and whether an order was obtained should be recorded accurately in the client's record. Telephone orders should be charted and the nurse's progress notes updated immediately after the call to prevent another caregiver from writing an entry before the telephone orders have been written.

Physician's Order Sheet

DATE	HOUR	ORDERS
07-07-07	12.00	Give pethidine/2 ml TO Dr Dhanyakumar, Lalitha RN

Above table shows how to write a telephone order on the physician's order sheet: the entry is dated and timed; the order as given by the physician is recorded; the order is signed beginning with TO (telephone order); the physician's name is written; and the nurse's name is signed. If another nurse witnesses the phone order, that nurse's signature should follow the first nurse's signature.

The physician must countersign the order within a time frame specified by the facility's policy. The use of fax machines has decreased the need for lengthy or complicated telephone orders, saving time and minimizing errors. The physician should be phoned to confirm the physician's identity as the initiator of the fax orders. The physician must countersign the fax orders according to agency policy.

Incident Reports

Incident reports, also called occurrence reports or variance reports, document any unusual occurrence or accident in the facility. Incident reports are not a means of punishment, but ethical practice requires that an incident report be filed to protect the individual involved.

Incident reports are not only an internal device for the facility; they are required by federal, national, and state accrediting agencies. For legal reasons, nurses are often advised not to document the filing of an incident report in the nurse's notes.

An incident report serves two functions:

- It informs the facility's administration of the incident and allows risk management personnel to consider ways to prevent similar occurrences in the future.
- It alerts the facility's insurance company to a potential claim and the possible need for investigation.

Incident report forms vary from one facility to another, but the following information must be recorded on the report:

- The date, exact time, and place the nurse discovered the occurrence.
- The person(s) involved in the occurrence, including witnesses.
- The exact occurrences witnessed by the nurse (e.g. "Found the client sitting on the floor, client stated that. . . ," rather than "Client fell.").
- The exact details and time sequence of what happened and the consequences for the persons involved.
- The nurse's actions to provide care and the results of the nurse's assessment for injuries and client complaints.
- The supervisor on duty who was notified and the time and name of the physician notified; if telephone orders were received from the physician, these should be documented as previously discussed and the orders implemented.
- Never record personal opinions, assumptions, judgments, or conclusions about what happened; point blame; or suggest ways to prevent similar occurrences. Forward the incident report to the designated person defined in the facility's policy.

It has been suggested writing a brief, accurate description of the incident and keeping it at home. The description should include details of the incident and the names of the people who were involved. Because lawsuits may take several years until the case goes to court, personal notes will help accurate recall of the incident. The notes may be read by the plaintiff's attorney and should reflect the same elements as the incident report.

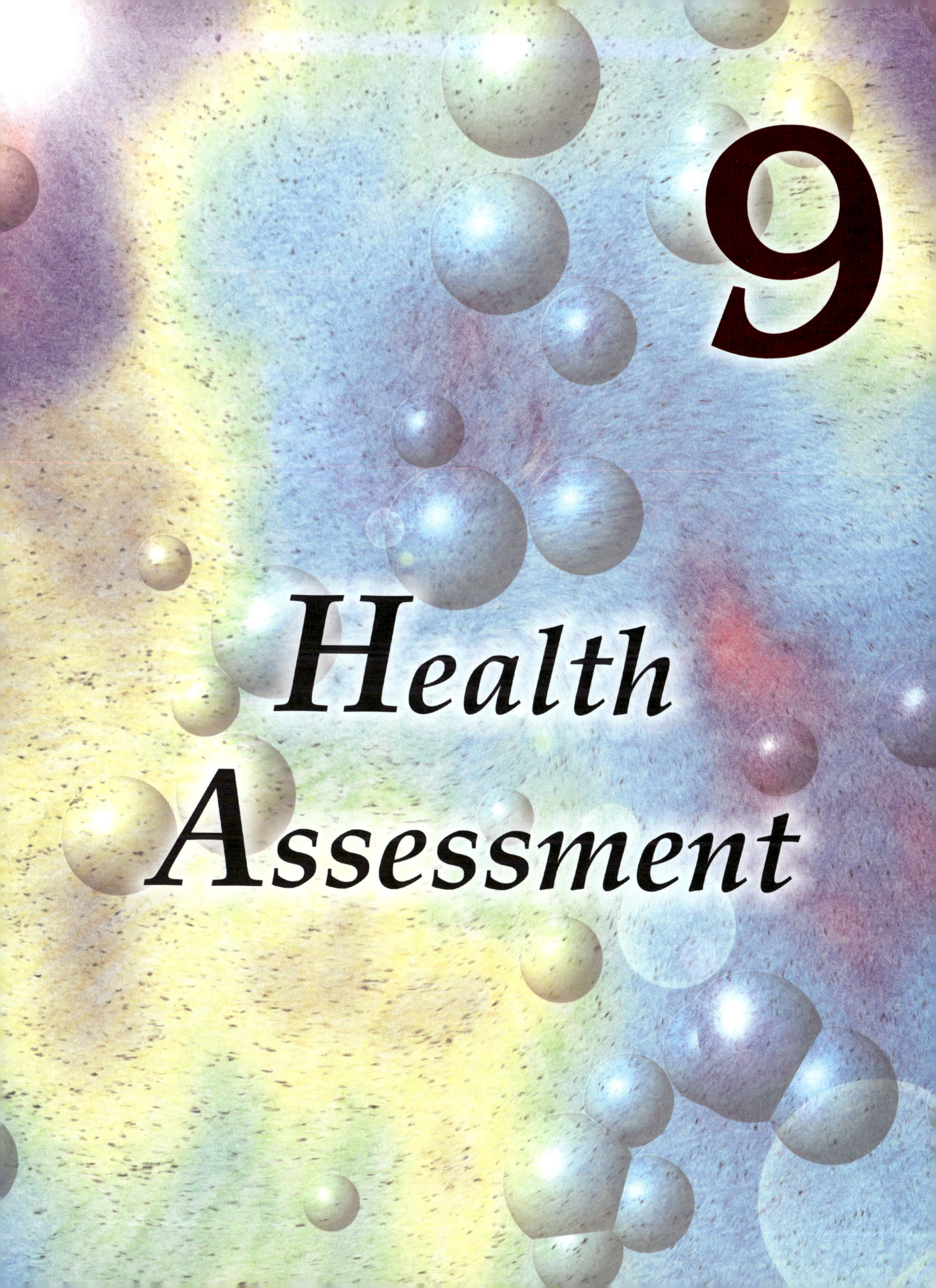

9
Health
Assessment

Introduction

Health assessment is a process where, the nurse, can obtain data that describe a persons responses to actual or potential health problems and then analyze that data to form pertinent diagnoses. Health assessment also enables nurses to determine a persons strengths that promote health behaviors and wellness.

The two phases of health assessment are the *measurement phase,* when nurses obtain data about a person, and the *judgment phase,* when nurses evaluate the data. A number of methods are used to obtain health assessment data, including interviewing, observing, listening, physical examination, reviewing records, and reviewing results of diagnostic tests. During the judgment phase, nurses cognitive abilities are involved in formulating diagnostic statements about the person whose health that are evaluating.

Evolution of Health Assessment in Nursing

Florence Nightingale considered health assessment an essential nursing function, and referred to this process as "observation of the sick" (Seymer, 1954). Nightingale believed nurses needed to develop health assessment skills, including technical skills such as measuring and recording vital signs and observing vital functions. Nightingale also emphasized the importance of interviewing patients to obtain pertinent information about health and illness states. Moreover, she believed that assessing the environment and living conditions of the patient should be a component of health assessment. Nightingale stressed that effective assessment required judgment rather than mere data accumulation.

Nursing historians state that Florence Nightingale was well ahead of her time, for although her nursing peers had begun to discuss the importance of nurses observational skills, patient assessment and related judgments were considered more within the domain of medicine than nursing.

Expanded Nursing Roles: Nursing roles continued to expand in the later part of last century as more hospitals were built in response to urban and industrial growth. As the need for nurses in hospitals increased, so did the number of nurse training programs. Public health nursing, which developed in the early 1900s and focused on health assessment and preventive health care, also provided new opportunities for nurses. Public health nurses practiced in homes and in the community, especially in rural areas, to promote health and identify problems requiring intervention. Consequently, they needed additional skills to screen people for health problems. As public health nursing expanded in scope, postgraduate courses were developed to teach nurses additional skills, including health assessment of environments, families, groups, and individuals.

During the 20th century roles continued to develop. Some nurses began to specialize in primary care, acute care, long-term care and intensive care, each requiring greater health assessment skills. In the 1970s the development of nurse-staffed intensive care units expanded nursing roles to include surveillance of patients with acute pathological conditions. Nurses were expected to make on-the-spot diagnostic judgments about patient status, often without physician consultation until the physician could be notified by telephone or in person.

The nurse practitioner role emerged during the same period, as a result of two programs: a nurse-run ambulatory clinic program at the University of Kansas Medical Center and the first pediatric nurse practitioner program, established at the University of Colorado. The nurse practitioners responsibilities evolved to include providing primary health care to certain underserved groups, especially children and women, rural communities, and the elderly. In providing primary health care, nurse practitioners, began performing health assessment to identify problems traditionally addressed by nurses, as well as physical diagnosis, a service that traditionally had been considered a medical function. Increasingly, nurses used physical examination skills to obtain data pertinent to patient care.

Whether nurses should use physical examination skills and whether such skills contributed to nursing goals were debated during this time by both nurses and physicians. Many nurses believed they should use physical examination skills while maintaining a nursing focus.

In response to expanding nursing roles, health assessment competencies, including the ability to conduct physical examinations, were incorporated into undergraduate nursing education programs in the 1970s. Influenced by nurse practitioner programs, most undergraduate nursing programs used a medical model to teach health assessment. This model included a specific interview format (chief complaint, history of the present illness, general health history, family health history, review of systems) and physical examinations according to body systems. Although a medical model of assessment enabled nurses to formulate diagnoses relevant to medicine, it did not provide a means of systematically assessing client's conditions to formulate nursing diagnoses. Nevertheless, the medical assessment model dominated nursing education literature during the 1970s and into the present.

The Nursing Process: Lydia Hall first conceptualized nursing as a process in the 1950s. Thereafter, many nurse scholars began to describe nursing activities in the context of a nursing process. Yura and Walsh defined the nursing process in phase: assessing, planning, implementing and evaluating. Since then, each nursing process component has been extensively discussed and developed, and assessment has been divided into assessment and diagnosis. During a 1967 conferences on the nursing process, tow scholars presented papers dealing extensively with assessment. It has been stated that a nursing assessment was focused on assessing "patient needs". Nursing needed grater guidance, however, if such assessments were to be useful and accurate. Merely saying that patients had physical, psychological, social, and spiritual needs….. fails to point to particulars that are specific enough to guide us in a detailed assessment of needs. Instead, Black advocated referring to Maslow's hierarchy of needs (1968) as a framework for nursing assessment, and specified assessment parameters for each of Maslow's example, the nurse should collect data about food and fluid intake, oxygenation, rest, physical activity, waste elimination, and sexual satisfaction. (Details of Nursing Process, see Chapter 10).

At the same conference, Harpine (1967) emphasized that nursing assessment should actively involve the client whenever possible. Only after making observations about the client, and then exploring those observations with the client as a means of validating the nurse's perceptions, should the nurse enter the judgment phase of assessment. Consequently, certain aspects of nursing assessment have been established:

- Nursing assessment is crucial if the nurse initiates the nursing process.
- Nursing assessment is a systematic, deliberate, and interactive process.
- Nursing assessment focuses on specific client characteristics, especially functional abilities and the ability to perform activities of daily living.
- Data are collected from several sources by various methods
- Nursing assessment includes data collection, validation of perceptions, and diagnostic judgment.

Nursing diagnosis is a more recent addition to the nursing process. Before the early 1970s, when nurses began to classify nursing diagnoses, diagnosis was implicitly understood to be part of assessment. The judgment phase of assessment does imply diagnosis, in that data analysis enables the nurse to identify a problem. During assessment, however, the nature of the problem is not precisely described. Nursing diagnosis specifically refers to a definitive problem statement expressed in standard terminology. Nursing diagnosis labels, each representing a health problem, provide the current impetus for the evolution of health assessment in nursing. As nurses analyze be natural to ask what facts or client characteristics must be detected and analyzed to cause the nurse to select a particular nursing diagnosis. The skills required for physical diagnosis of pathological problems probably will not be sufficient for nursing diagnosis.

Nursing Process Models: A model of the nursing process illustrates the assessment phase (Fig. 9.1). It presents the measurement and judgment components of health assessment and emphasizes additional assessment aspects. And views assessment as a circular and continuous process, the nature of which is especially evident as the nurse evaluates the client's response to nursing intervention. Moreover, the initial assessment has a broad scope: the nurse must detect and label states amenable to nursing therapy as well as states that require collaborative intervention from multiple care providers or primary intervention from others. In this capacity, the nurse must rely on traditional assessment methods such as the medically oriented interview and especially physical examination. Finally, so that nurses may better identify those states amenable to nursing therapy. Further it proposes a conceptual framework to guide the manner in which nurse's think about nursing and the nursing client.

It has been argued that conceptual nursing models may be too abstract to guide the structural areas of nursing assessment or to identify what information should be obtained to generate a clinical database. Regardless of nursing models, every nursing client should be assessed for health behaviors, level of wellness, and actual or potential health problems. After establishing a clinical database, the nurse may further interpret the client's status by applying a conceptual model of framework (Gorden, 1987).

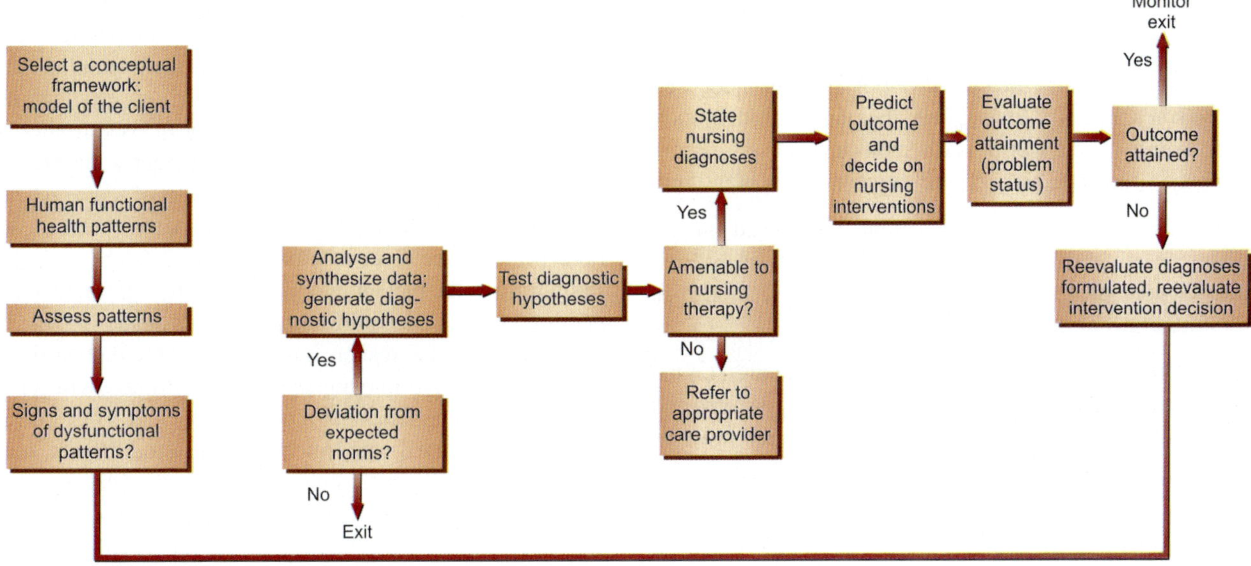

Figure 9.1: Nursing process model advocating the use of a nursing conceptual framework and functional health patterns, and diagnostic reasoning

Functional Health Patterns

Gordon proposed the typology of human functional health patterns as a guide establishing a comprehensive nursing data base. Theses 11 categories make possible a systematic and standardized approach to health assessment data collection, and enable the nurse to determine the following aspects of health and human function:

Health-Perception-Health-Management Pattern: Assessment is focused on the persons perceived level of health and well being, and on practices for maintaining health. Actual or potential related to safety an health management advice may be identified.

Nutritional-Metabolic Pattern: Assessment is focused on the pattern of food and fluid consumption relative to metabolic need. The adequacy of local nutrient supplies is evaluated. Actual or potential problems related to fluid balance, tissue integrity, and host defenses may be identified.

Elimination Pattern: Assessment is focused on excretory patterns (bowel, bladder, skin). Excretory problems such as incontinence, constipation, diarrhea, and urinary retention may be identified.

Activity-Exercise Pattern: Assessment is focused on the activities of daily living requiring energy expenditure, including self-care activities, exercise, and leisure activities. The status of major body systems involved with activity and exercise is evaluated, including the respiratory, cardiovascular, and musculoskeletal systems.

Cognitive-Perceptual Pattern: Assessment is focused on the ability to comprehend and use information and on the sensory functions. Sensory experiences such as pain and altered sensory input may be identified and further evaluated.

Sleep-rest Pattern: Assessment is focused on the persons sleep, rest, and relaxation practices. Dysfunctional sleep patterns, fatigue, and responses to sleep deprivation may be identified.

Self-perception and Self-concept Pattern: Assessment if focused on the person's attitudes toward self, including identity, body image and sense of self-worth. The persons level of self-esteem and response to threats to his or her self-concept may be identified.

Role-Relationship Pattern: Assessment is focused on the persons roles in the world and relationships with others. Satisfaction with roles, role strain, or dysfunctional relationships may be further evaluated.

Sexuality-Reproductive Pattern: Assessment is focused on the persons satisfaction or dissatisfaction with sexuality patterns and reproductive functions. Concerns with sexuality may be identified.

Coping-Stress Tolerance Pattern: Assessment is focused on the persons perception of stress and on his or her coping strategies. The effectiveness of a persons coping strategies in terms of stress tolerance may be further evaluated.

Value-Belief Pattern: Assessment is focused on the persons values and beliefs (including spiritual beliefs), or on the goals that guide his or her choices or decisions.

The Outcomes of the Health Assessment Process: Analyzing health assessment data leads to one or more of the following conclusions:

- The persons state of wellness is affirmed
- No problem exists
- The persons strengths are identified
- Nursing diagnoses are formulated
- Problems that can be treated collaboratively by the nurse and other health professionals are identified.

Types of Nursing Health Assessment

The nurse must obtain pertinent information about all parameters specified by a particular standardized assessment tool or structures. A comprehensive database using the functional health pattern typology, for example, requires the nurse systematically to collect data on all 11 health patterns. Realistically, we cannot always generate a comprehensive nursing data base that identifies all human responses to all health problems. Nurse may not have time for such comprehensive assessment or may need to focus attention on the clients most threatening problem. The scope of health assessment, including the frequency of reassessment, is influenced by our goals and by the clients state. Assessment may be comprehensive, screening, or focused.

(i) Comprehensive Health Assessment: When initiating a comprehensive health assessment, our goal should be to collect data that will verify wellness and strengths and suggest nursing diagnoses or collaborative clinical problems. Often, this type of assessment is a prerequisite to establishing a nursing care plan.

Nurse should consider the clients condition before initiating a comprehensive assessment. If he or she is in pain, in need of sleep or rest, or physiologically or psychologically threatened, postpone the comprehensive assessment or use an alternative approach. For example, for a patient recently admitted to a coronary care unit with the medical diagnosis of acute myocardial infraction, pain relief and other illness management measures take precedence over comprehensive health assessment. Furthermore, the patient may find a lengthy interview intrusive and irrelevant in such a life-threatening context.

Nurses have the responsibility for, and the patient the right to, comprehensive nursing assessment. Rather than omit the comprehensive assessment, modify the format. For example, if uses a standardized assessment form to establish the nursing data base, may fill in selected parts of the form with data collected during ongoing nurse-client interaction. Nurse may collect data while providing care. While giving the patient a dinner tray, for example, she may ask several questions about usual diet or special problems with eating or digestion. While assisting the patient with a bedpan or commode, she may ask questions about usual patterns of bowel or bladder elimination. Considerable skill is data to collect when standardized questionnaires and forms, which might be intrusive during routine nursing care, are not at hand, and remember the information in order to record it on the data base later.

(ii) Screening health assessment: Screening health assessments have several purposes:

- Primary prevention (wellness promotion)
- Case finding for secondary prevention
- Ongoing surveillance.

The scope of a screening is limited. Usually data collection is specific and brief. A lengthier screening might be aimed at detecting a number of potential problems. (Such a screening might take place during a routine annual physical examination). Screening assessments are typically conducted to detect hypertension, various forms of cancer, and sensory deficits. Screening for the purpose of primary prevention is often client-initiated, and the client usually perceives the process as relevant and essential.

Screening assessments may also be appropriate for ill or injured persons. For example, an emergency room nurse assessing the condition of a trauma victim may conduct a screening assessment to determine the status of vital functions, such as circulation and oxygenation, and the extent of injury. A nurse caring for a patient who has undergone coronary artery bypass surgery routinely screens for significant alterations in hemodynamic status and other physical functions.

Several data collection tools have been developed to facilitate monitoring the condition of ill or injured persons. Generally, nurses use a head-to-toe or body systems approach to data collection. These are convenient, time-saving approaches to data collection. You should become skilled at rapid screening, talking 5 minutes or less, for cases where detecting life-threatening problems is a priority. A more detailed assessment may be performed later.

Focused Nursing Assessment

A focused nursing assessment involves collecting data relevant to a particular health problem. The amount and type of information elicited form the client will be limited. If the clients problem appears to be activity intolerance, for example, you should focus on the signs and symptoms he or she exhibits in response to activity. A focused nursing assessment may be informal and may be initiated as you perform other aspects of care. it may involve eliciting the clients verbal or nonverbal response to questions about his or her condition, or evaluating the effect of a nursing intervention. When administering pain relief medications, for example, you may initiate a focused assessment to evaluate the clients response.

Sources to obtain data: The client should be considered the primary data source, and other sources, such as family members,

medical records, and other health care professionals, should be considered secondary sources. Nurses should attempt to elicit data from the client and then validate information as needed through secondary sources.

Data is usually classified as subjective or objective.

Subjective data represents the clients perspective and is communicated to the nurse by the client. You cannot measure or directly observe subjective aspects of the clients condition, however, based on his or her statements. Examples of subjective data include the client's descriptions of pain, nausea, dizziness, and fear.

Objective data is information obtained by observation, measurement, or physical examination. Such data can be verified by another observer. The nurse can collect objective data by observing, listening, feeling, smelling, or measuring. Examples of objective data include a grimace during a dressing change, a potassium level measurement of 4 mEq, crackles heard during lung auscultation, and a decubitus ulcer measuring 4 cm in diameter.

The Physical Examination/Assessment

The physical examination is performed to gather objective information and also as a screening device. Four common methods used during the physical examination are inspection, palpation, percussion, and auscultation. These techniques incorporate the senses of sight, hearing, touch and smell. For the data collected during the physical examination to be meaningful, it is vital to know the normal physical and emotional characteristics of human beings sufficiently well enough to be able to recognize deviations. To gain as much information as possible from the assessment procedure, the same format should be used each time a physical examination is performed to lessen the possibility of omissions.

Physical assessments are necessary to obtain the objective data needed to complete the assessment phase of the nursing process. A complete database of both subjective and objective data allows the goals and intervene to promote health and prevent disease.

The physical assessment is carried out systematically. It may be organized according to the examiners preference, in a heal-to-toe approach or as a body systems approach. During the physical assessment, the nurse assesses all body parts and determines anthropometrics measurements. Instead of giving a complete examination, the nurse may focus on a specific problem area noted from the nursing assessment, such as the inability to urinate. On occasion, the nurse may find it necessary to resolve a client complaint or problem prior to completing the examination, e.g. if the client appears short of breath. Alternatively, the nurse may perform a screening examination, a brief review of essential functioning of various body parts or systems. Data obtained from this examination are measured against norms or standards, such as ideal height and weight standards or norms for body temperature or blood pressure levels.

To obtain data systematically the nurse needs to use an organized assessment framework or structure. This systematic method of collecting desired data about the client is referred to as a nursing health history or, more recently, a nursing assessment. The purpose of the nursing assessment is to gather as much information as possible about the client in order to identify problems for nursing interventions. The data collected during the nursing health history between the nurse and client largely constitute a *subjective assessment*. The nurses obtains information about the client, nurses perceptions, it clears the way for new ideas, and it helps the client to note progress and forward direction. Sometimes clients may spontaneously offer a summary; at other times the nurse must initiate it or ask the client to do so. Summaries are particularly helpful for clients who are anxious or who have difficulty staying with the topic, the clients health, response to illness, sociocultural factors, health beliefs and practices, coping patterns, and day to day activities.

There are many nursing models and frameworks that guide data collection through structured assessment tools. An example is Newman's tools, an assessment/intervention tool that has been seven categories; intake summary, stressors as perceived by the client, stressors as perceived by the caregiver, intrapersonal factors, interpersonal factors, extrapersonal and formulation of the problem.

Abdellah (1961) and Henderson (1966) developed earlier frameworks used or adapted in many settings. More recently, Gordon (1857) established a framework of 11 functional health patterns. Gordon used the word pattern to signify a sequence of behavior. The nurse collects data about dysfunctional as well as functional behavior. Thus, using Gordon's framework to analyze data, nurse are able to discern emerging patterns.

Roy (1984) outlines the data to be collected according to the Roy Adaption model and classifies observable behavior into four categories physiologic, self-concept, role function and interdependence. Orem (1985) delineates eight universal self-care requisites of humans (Table 9.1).

Other framework and models from other disciplines are also helpful for data collection, including Maslow's hierarchy of needs, Piaget's assessment of cognitive development, and Sely's stress theory. These framework are narrower than the model required in nursing, the nurse usually needs to combine these with other approaches to obtain a complete history.

The physical examination is usually conducted in a head toe-to-toe sequence, but can be adapted to meet the need of the

Table 9.1: Areas of Data Collection According to Theories of Orem and Roy

Orem (1985)	*Roy (1984)*
Universal self-care requisites	*Adaptive modes*

1. The maintenance of a sufficient intake of air	1. Physiologic needs
	   a. Exercise and rest
	   b. Nutrition
	   c. Elimination
	   d. Fluid and electrolytes
	   e. Oxygen and circulation
	   f. Regulation: temperature
	   g. Regulation: the senses
	   h. Regulation: endocrine

2. The maintenance of a sufficient intake of water	2. Self-concept
	   a. Physical self
	   b. Moral-ethical self
	   c. Self consistency
	   d. Self ideal and expectancy
	   e. Self-esteem

3. The maintenance of a sufficient intake of food	3. Role function
4. The provision of care associated with elimination processes and excrements	4. Interdependence
5. The maintenance of a balance between activity and rest	
6. The maintenance of a balance between solitude and social interaction	
7. The prevention of hazards to human life, human functioning and human well being	
8. The promotion of human functioning and development within social groups in accord with human potential known human limitations and human desire to be normal. (Normalcy is used in the sense of that which is essentially human and that which is in accord with the genetic and constitutional characteristics and the talents of individuals).	

client being examined. It offers objective information about the client. The nurse uses the skills of physical assessment to make clinical judgment. The clients condition and response affects the extent of the examination. The accuracy of physical assessment influences the choices of therapies a client receives and the determination of the response to those therapies. Continuity in health care improves when the nurse makes ongoing, objective and comprehensive assessment. An examination should be designed for the clients needs. If a client is acutely ill, the nurse may assess only the involved body system. A more comprehensive examination conducted when the client feels more at ease and the nurse learns about the clients health status.

Preparation for Physical Assessment

It is very important that some preparation needed for client while conducting physical assessment in the physical environment. Physical examination requires privacy. An examination room should be well-equipped for all necessary procedures. Adequate lighting is needed for proper illuminations of body parts. The room should be sound proof, well-ventilated and should be warm enough to maintain clients comfort. There should be proper examination table or bed with pad or mattress with necessary articles and linen including small pillow and others.

Client or Patient

Preparation of the client, both psychologically and physiologically also is very important. By which nurse explains to client that body structures will be examined, and asks the client to use toilet to void. For employing the bladder and bowel, if needed, instruct to collect the specimen required. Physical preparation involves being sure that client is dressed and draped properly.

Equipment

The equipment or instrument needed for examination should be readily available and arranged in order for easy use (Figs 9.2A and B).

Instruments	Equipment and supplies
• Blood pressure apparatus or sphygmomanometer • Stethoscope • Ophthalmoscope • Snellen's chart • Otoscope • Nasal speculum • Scale with height measurement • Vaginal speculum • Tuning fork • Percussion hammer • Thermometer • Tongue or depressor	• Alcohol swabs • Cotton applicators • Disposable pad • Drape or sheet • Gauze dressing (4 and 4) • Gloves (sterile or non-sterile) • Lubricants • Penlight • Flash light and spot light • Safety pin • Substance for testing smell • Tap measure • Wrist watch with second hand • Paper towels • Swabs and sponge forceps • Specimen container

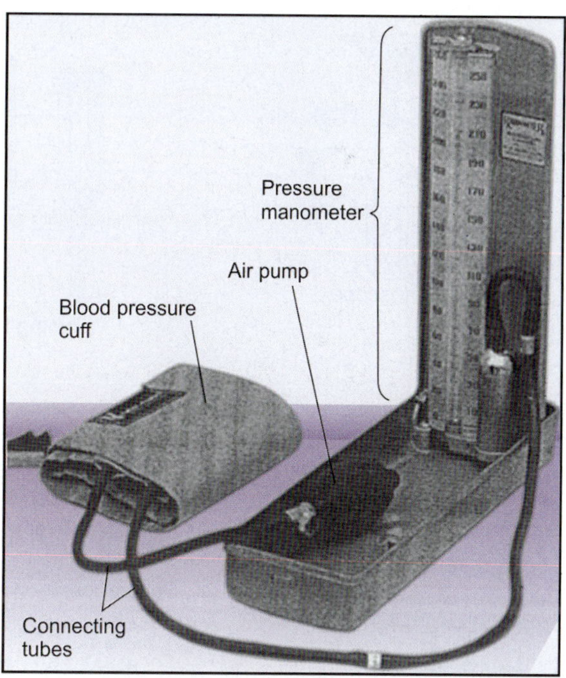

Figure 9.2A: Sphygmomanometer

Positions for Physical Examination

A number of positions are used during physical assessment, because during examination, the nurse asks client to assume proper positions so that the body parts are accessible and clients stay comfortable. The positions and their uses during physical assessment are as follows.

Sitting Positions (Fig 9.3A)

The client may sit upright in a chair or on the side of the examining table or bed. Sitting upright provides full expansion of lungs and provides better visualization of symmetry of upper body parts and facilitates full-lung expansion. It is used to assesses the head and neck, posterior and anterior thorax, and lungs, breasts, axillae, heart and upper extremities, and also to take visual signs. If physically weakened, client may be unable to maintain an upright position, may be supine in the bed with the head elevated.

Supine Position (Fig 9.3B)

In supine position, the client lies flat on the back with legs together but extended and slightly bent at the knees. The head may be supported with a small pillow. This is most normally relaxed position. It prevents contracture of abdominal muscles and provides easy access to pulse sites. This position can be used to assesses the head and neck, anterior thorax and lungs, breasts, heart, abdomen extremities and peripheral pulses. In this position client becomes short of breath easily, examiner may need to raise the head of the bed.

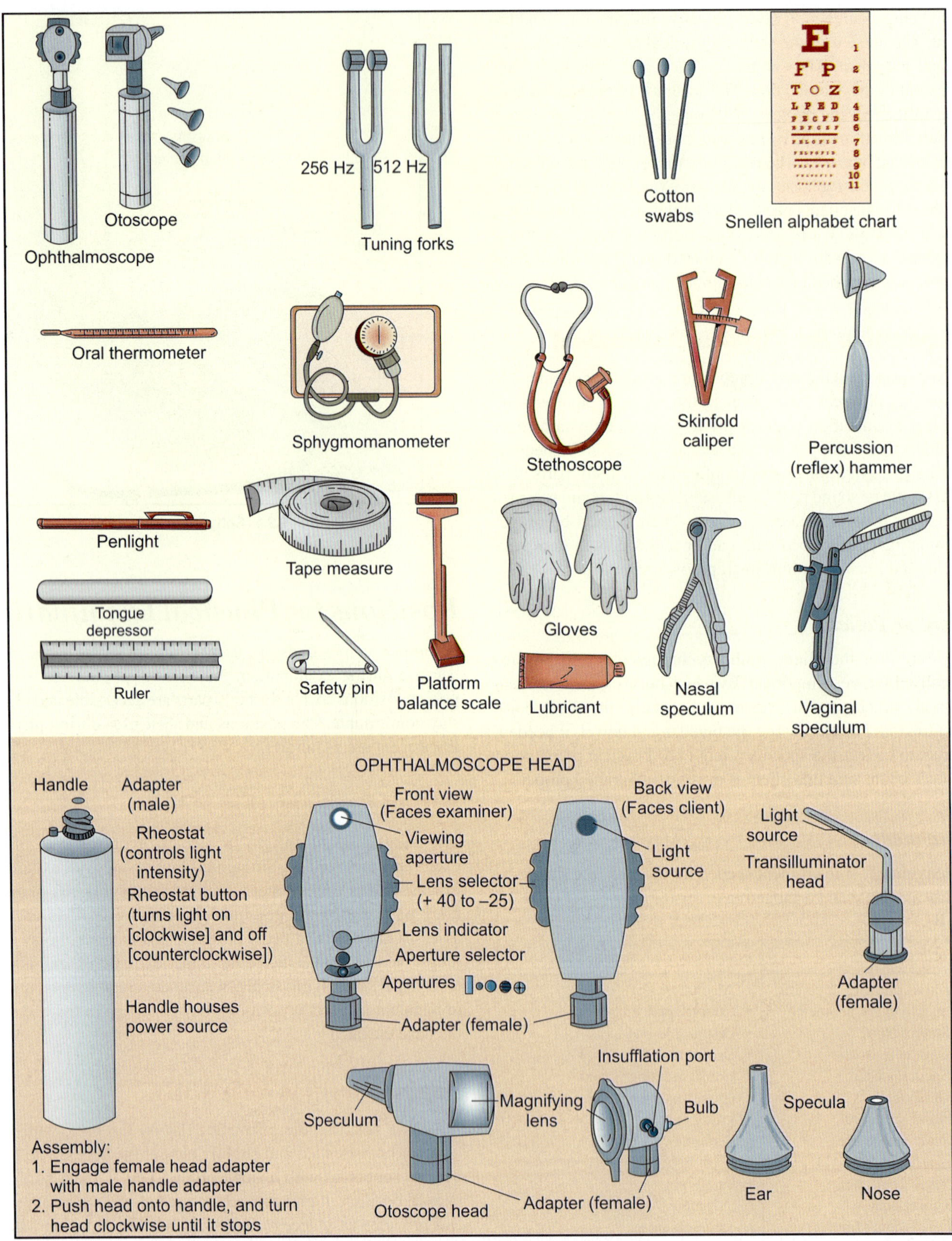

Figure 9.2B: Equipments used for physical examination

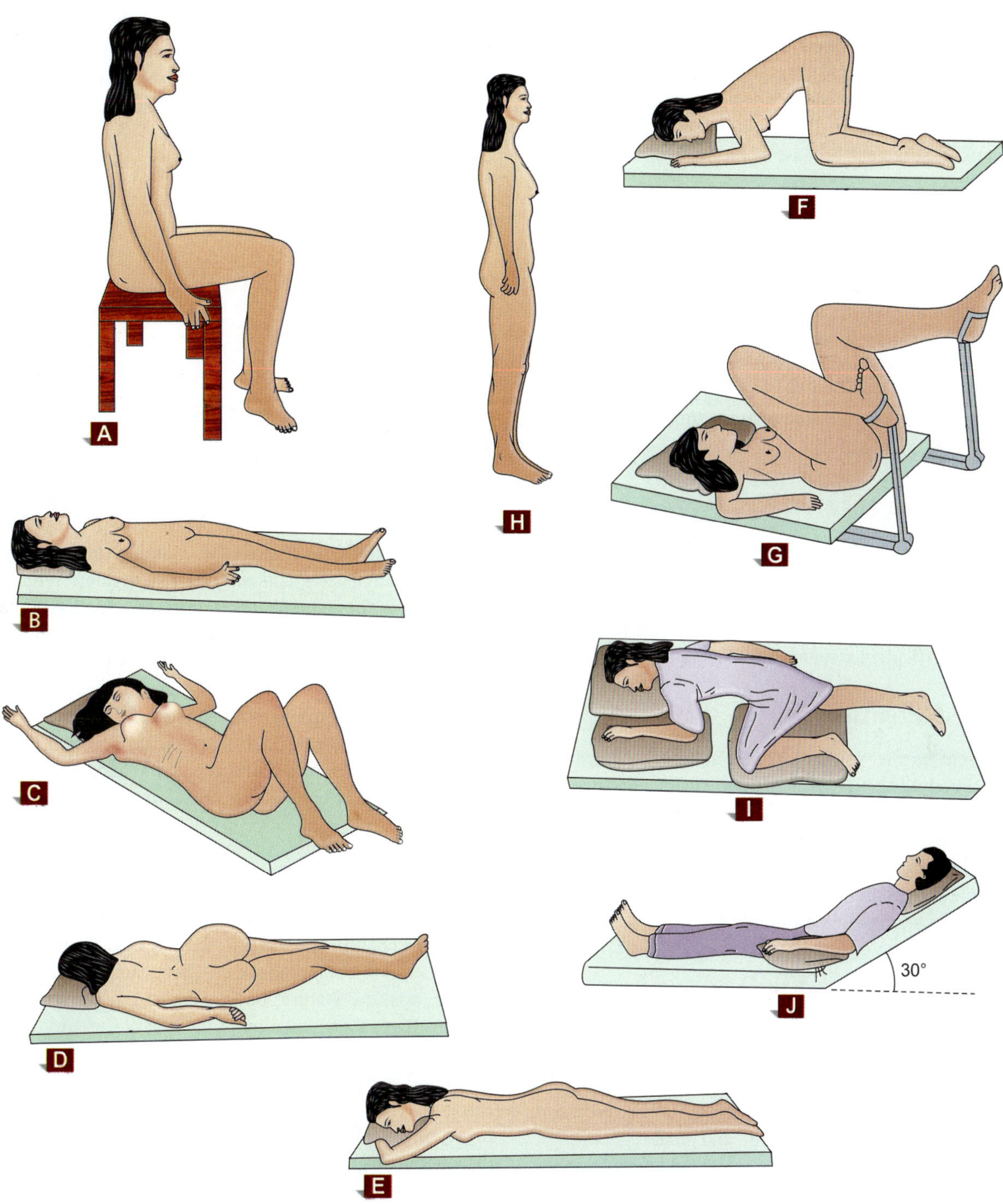

Figures 9.3A to J: Various client positions used during the nursing examination: (A) Sitting position, (B) Supine position, (C) Dorsal recumbent position, (D) Sims' position, (E) Prone position, (F) Knee-chest position, (G) Lithotomy position, (H) Erect or standing position, (I) Lateral side lying position (J) Semi Fowler's position

Dorsal Recumbent Position (Fig 9.3C)

In the dorsal recumbent position, the client lies on the back with legs separated, knee bent, and soles of the feet flat on the bed. In this position clients with painful disorders are more comfortable with knees flexed. This position also is used to assess the head and neck, anterior thorax, and lungs, breasts, heart, extremities and peripheral pulse. It is used for client who have difficulty in maintaining supine position. This position should not be used for abdominal assessment because it promotes contraction of abdominal muscle.

Sims Position (Fig 9.3D)

In this, the client lies on either the right and left side. The lower arm behind the body and upper arm is bent at the shoulder and elbow. The knees are both bent, with the uppermost leg more acutely bent. Here the flexion of hip and knee improves exposure of rectal area. This position is used to assess the rectum and vagina. It should not be used for person with joint deformities which may hinder clients ability to bend hip and knee.

Prone Position (Fig 9.3E)

In this, the client lies on the abdomen, flat on the bed, with the head turned, to one side. This position is used only to assess extension of hip joint; and can be used to assess the posterior thorax. This position is intolerable for client with respiratory difficulties and difficult in assuming this position for older adults.

Knee-chest Position (Fig 9.3F)

Here, the client kneels, using the knees and chest to bear the weight of the body. The body is at 90° angle to the hips, with the back straight, the arm above the head, and the head turned to one side. This position provides maximal exposure to rectal area, used to assess rectal area. This position is embarrassing and uncomfortable. Clients with arthritis or other joint deformities may be unable to assume this position.

Lithotomy Position (Fig 9.3G)

In this position, the client is in the dorsal recumbent position with the buttocks at the edge of examining table and the feet supported in stirrup. This position provides maximum exposure of genitalia and facilitates insertion of vaginal speculum, so used to assess rectum and the area of female genitalia and genital tract.

Lithotomy position is also embarrassing and uncomfortable, so examiner minimizes time that the client spends in it. Client is kept well draped. It is uncomfortable for older persons and difficult for clients with severe arthritis or other deformities.

Standing Position (Fig 9.3H)

The standing or erect position may be used to assess posture, gait and balance. Clients abilities to assume positions will depend on their physical strength and degree of wellness. As stated earlier, some positions may be embarrassing and uncomfortable. Therefore, clients should be kept in these positions and assist clients necessary. The examiners explain the positions and assist clients in attaining them. The drapes are adjusted to be sure that the area to be examined is accessible and that no body part is unnecessarily exposed. The nurse chooses the position according to part of body of the client examined on priority wise.

Lateral Side Lying Position

See Figure 9.3I.

Semi Fowler's Position

See Figure 9.3J.

Techniques of Physical Examinations

Observation

The basic techniques of physical examination are inspection, palpation, percussion, and auscultation, together referred to as *Observation*. These skills enable you to collect data systematically using the senses of sight, touch, hearing and smell. Physical appearance, behavior, communication patterns and activity abilities can all be observed, as can a persons environment and events that effect him or her. Observing facial expression for signs of discomfort, detecting odors that indicate infection, listening to chest sounds to determine airway patency, and touching the skin to determine body temperature are all examples of observation.

Inspection

Inspection is systematic and deliberate visual observation determine health status. Begin the physical examination with general survey or inspection of the client, including an assessment of age, posture, stature, body weight, grooming at mobility patterns. Next carry out a more thought observation a head-to-toe fashion. Note the shape and size of the head, its distribution, general skin condition and facial expression. Inspect the face for symmetry of eyes and balance of face expression. While inspecting the neck note visible pulsation bulges or venous distension. Inspect the chest and abdomen noting symmetry, masses, pulsations, skin condition and visible signs of discomfort, such as holding the abdomen. Inspect the lower extremities, noting especially ankle swelling and its integrity.

Following the general survey, more detailed observation are made as the physical examination progresses to specific body parts or systems. Inspection always precedes palpate percussion, or auscultation of a particular area. More specific guidelines on examination skills are provided in subsequent chapters.

Effective inspection is facilitated by good lighting and exposure. Occasionally, instruments such as the ophthalmoscope and the otoscope may be used as well.

Palpation

With palpation you rely on the sense of touch to make judgments about (1) the size, shape, texture and mobility of structure and masses (2) the quality of pulses (3) the condition of bone and joints (4) the extent of tenderness in injured areas or structures (5) skin temperature and moisture (6) fluid accumulation and edema and (7) chest wall vibrations.

Different parts of the hand are used to palpate different type of structures. Breasts, lymph nodes and pulses should be palpated with the fingertips, where nerve endings are most concentrated. The thumb and index fingertips are used to evaluate tissue firmness. Temperature can be quickly assessed with the back of the hand, where temperature sensory nerves are more concentrated and the skin is thin. Vibrations can be felt more strongly with the palm of the hand especially along the met carpal joints.

Palpation should be carried out in such a way as to avoid discomfort. Your hands should be warm and the client relaxed to avoid muscle tensing. Palpate painful areas last. The amount of pressure you apply is governed by the type of structure you are examining and the degree to which palpation may cause discomfort. Any expression of distress or pain should prompt you to palpate lightly.

Palpation may be light, deep or bimanual. *Light palpation* the safest and least uncomfortable involves exerting gentle pressure with the fingertips of your dominant hand, moving them in a circular motion. Place your hand parallel to the part of the body surface you are examining and extend your fingers to depress the skin surface approximately 0.5 to 0.75 inches (1 to 2 cm). Exert and release fingertip pressure several times over an area. Exerting continuous pressure would tend to dull the tactile discrimination senses (Figs 9.4 and 9.6).

Deep Palpation, which is done after light palpation, is used to detect abdominal masses. The technique is similar to light palpation except that the fingers are held at a greater angle to the body surface and the skin is depressed about 1.5 to 2 inches (4 to 5 cm). A variation of this technique involves placing the fingertips of one hand over the fingertips of the palpating hand. The top hand should press and guide the bottom hand to detect underlying masses (Figs 9.5 and 9.7).

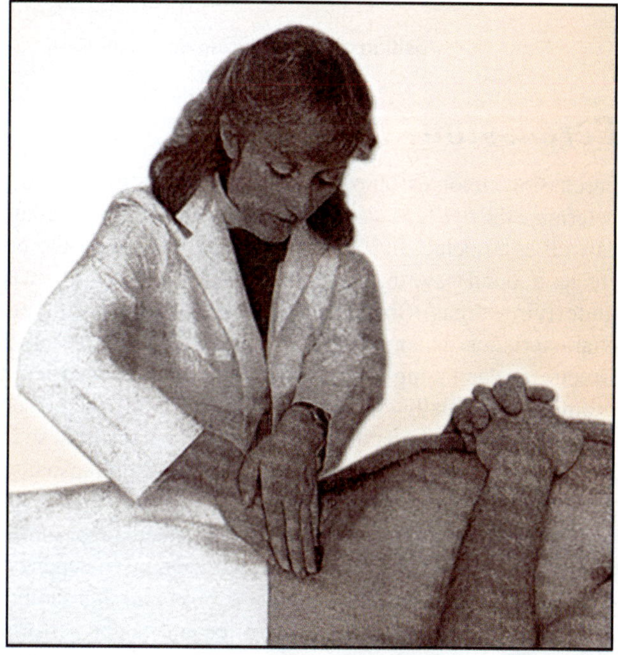

Figure 9.5: Deep palpation

Bimanual Palpation, involves using both hands to trap a structure between them. This technique can be used to evaluate the spleen, kidneys, breasts, uterus and ovaries.

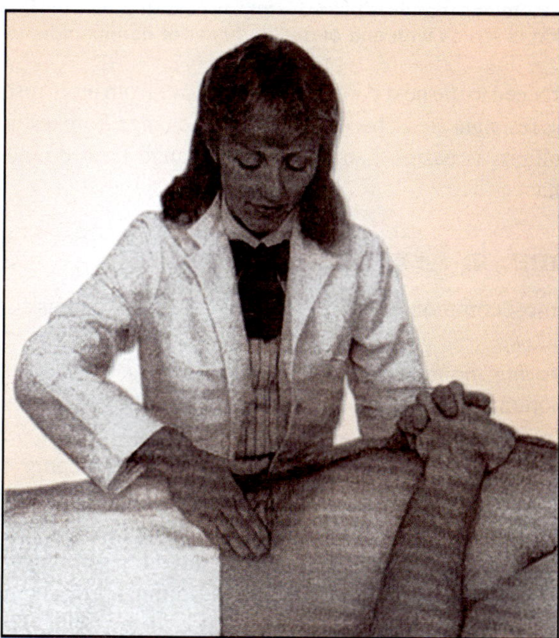

Figure 9.4: Light palpation

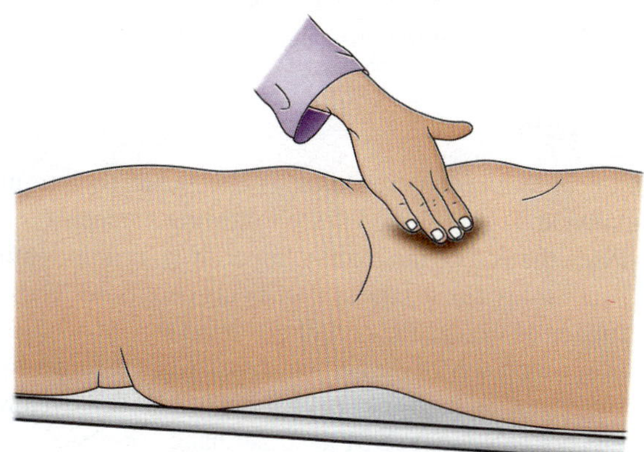

Figure 9.6: Position of the hand during light palpation

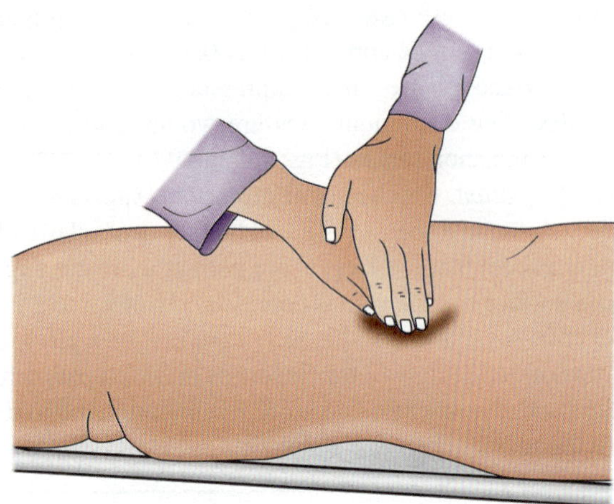

Figure 9.7: Position of hands during deep palpation

Percussion

Percussion involves tapping the body lightly but sharply to determine the position, size and density of underlying structures, as well as to detect fluid or air in a cavity. Tapping the body creates a sound wave that travels 2 to 3 inches (5 to 7 cm) towards underlying areas. Sound reverberations assume different characteristics depending on the features of the underlying structures. Percussing the right upper abdominal quadrant, for example will usually elicit dull sounds, including the presence of the liver, tapping over the lungs should reveal resonant sounds associated with air filled spaces. Percussion should usually be performed after an area has been palpated.

Three percussion methods can be used: mediate or indirect, immediate and fist percussion. The method chosen depends on the area to be perused. *Mediate or indicate percussion* should be used to percuss the abdomen and thorax, and can be performed by using the finger of one hand as a plexor (striking finger) and the middle finger of the other hand as a pleximeter (the finger being struck). *Immediate percussion,* used mainly to evaluate the sinuses or an infant's thorax, involves striking the surface directly with the fingers of the hand only. *Fist percussion* is used to evaluate the back and kidneys for tenderness, involves placing one hand flat against the body surface and striking the back of the hand with a clenched fist of the other hand (Figs 9.8A and B).

Procedure

Mediate or indirect percussion is the basic technique of percussion and is performed in the following manner.

1. Place the pad of the middle finger of your non-dominant hand firmly against the surface being percussed. The other fingers as well as the heel of this hand should be raised to avoid contact with the body surface. Hold the finger firmly against the body surface throughout percussion, even when it is not begin tapped by the other hand.
2. Use the meddle finger of your dominant hand as the plexor. Hold the forearm horizontal to the surface being percussed.

Keep the forearm stationary and use wrist motion to make striking movements.

3. Quickly strike the distal phalanx of the finger that is positioned on the body surface with the tips of the finger of the other hand. Use only the wrist to generate motion, and quickly remove the striking hand after percussing to avoid muffling the percussion sound. You may percuss a single area two or three times before moving to the next area. Light tapping is more effective than heavy tapping.
4. Identify the percussion sound. Skillful percussion reveals one of the five percussion sounds, flatness, depending on the density of underlying structures, flatness, dullness, resonance, hyperresonance, and tympany, (Table 9.2). A *Flat sound* is elicited by percussing over solid masses such as bone or muscle. *A Dull sound* which has a lower pitch than a flat sound, is elicited when high density structure, such as the liver, are percussed. *Resonance* is a hollow sound heard for example, by percussing the lung. *Hyperresonance* is an abnormal sound with a pitch between resonance and tympany and may indicate an emphysematous lung or pneumothrorax. *Tympany* is a drum-like sound heard over air filled body parts such as the bowel or stomach.

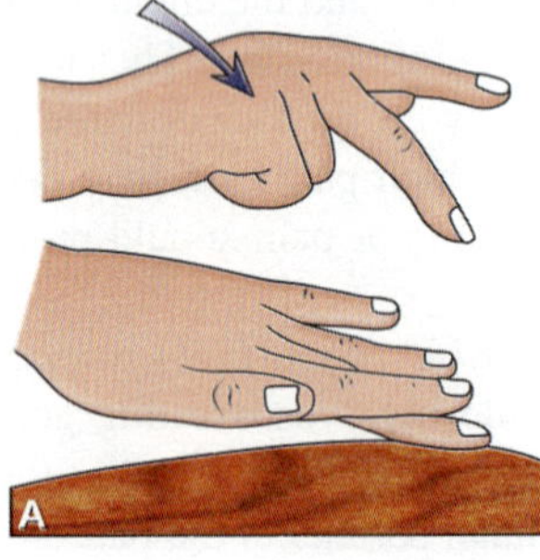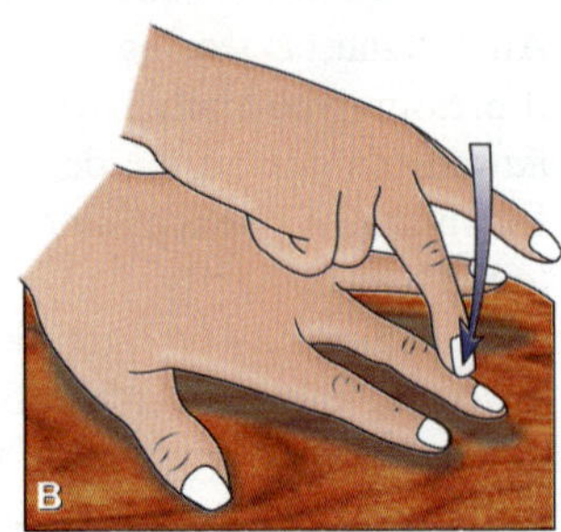

Figures 9.8A and B: Percussion. (A) First phalanx of middle finger of nondominant hands is placed firmly on person's skin. (B) Phalanx on skin is struck with end of middle finger of dominant hand

Proceed to the next percussion area. Move from more resonant to less resonant areas, because detecting a change from resonance to dullness is easier than detecting a change from dullness to resonance.

Common Errors in Percussion

The most common errors in performing mediate percussion are as follows:

- *Moving the forearm of the dominant hand:* Remember, all motion should be generated from the wrist.
- *Pressing the striking finger into the positioned finger:* Remove the striking finger immediately after tapping
- *Causing injury to oneself or the client:* By inadvertently striking the client or your own hand with a long fingernail. The fingernail of the plexor finger should be kept short.
- *Falling to hear the percussion note:* Eliminate environmental noise including noise caused by bracelets or loose fitting watches. If the note is still difficult to hear, check your technique.

Table 9.2: Percussion Sounds

Sound	Pitch	Intensity	Quality	Location
Flatness	High	Soft	Extreme dullness	Normal: Sternum, thigh Abnormal: Atelectatic lung
Dullness	Medium	Medium	Thud like	Normal: Liver, diaphragm Abnormal: Pleural effusion
Resonance	Low	Loud	Hollow	Normal: Lung Abnormal: Emphysematous lung
Hyper-resonance	Lower than reso-nance	Very loud	Booming	Normal: Gastric air bubble, puffed out check Abnormal: Air-distended abdomen
Tympany	High	Loud	Musical, drum-like	

Auscultation

Auscultation is the skill of listening to body sounds created in the lungs, heart, blood vessels, and abdominal viscera. Auscultation is usually the last technique used during the examination. The sequence usually progresses from inspection to palpation, percussion, and auscultation, except during the abdominal examination, when auscultation is the second step (following inspection).

Immediate auscultation involves placing ones ear directly on the skin, such as over the lung. This method is rarely used because environmental noise frequently interferes with hearing. The usual method is *Mediate auscultation*, for using a stethoscope to detect sounds. The best results are gained using a good quality stethoscope. You should eliminate extraneous poise such as televisions, voices and equipment sounds before performing auscultation. Do not create noise by moving the stethoscope over the body hair or clothing or by touching the stethoscope tubing.

Auscultated sounds are described in terms of pitch, intensity, duration and quality. *Pitch* is determined by the frequency of sound vibrations and should be classified as high or low. *Intensity* refers to the loudness of the sound. *Duration* refers to how long the sound lasts or how long it takes to occur in relation to a physiological event such as systole. Quality of sound must be desorbed using subjective terms such as tinkling, harsh or blowing. Specific ausultatory guidelines are discussed throughout the test.

Symptoms Analysis

Symptom are detected during the physical examination or identified during the interview. Symptom that indicate a possible change in physical status include pain, nausea, dizziness, dysphagia, and dyspnea. Such symptoms are systematically evaluated to aid in diagnosing physiological alterations. Evaluate each reported physical symptom according to the following criteria (elicited by questioning the client).

- *Onset:* When you first notice the symptom (time and date)was the onset sudden or gradual? Has this symptoms occurred at other times in the past? What circumstances precipitated the symptom?
- *Location (may be relevant only when the symptom is pain):* Where did the pain occur? (ask the client to point to exact location). Does the pain radiate?
- *Quality:* How did you feel when it occurred? How would you describe it?
- *Quantity:* How intense was the symptom (mild or sever or rated on a scale of 1 to 10)? Did the symptom interfere with your usual activities, such as: walking, sleeping or talking?
- *Frequency and duration:* How frequently did the symptom occur and how long did it last?
- *Aggravating or alleviating factors:* What makes the symptom worse or better?
- *Associated factors:* Did you notice any other changes when you noticed this symptom? (ask about factors normally associated with the symptom, such as nausea with chest pain)
- *Course:* How the symptom changed or progressed over time?

Physical Examination Instruments

The physical examination is conducted with the aid of several instruments. Some are simple, such as safety pins and cotton wisps used to evaluate sensory function. Others are complex such as stethoscopes, which are used to evaluate heart tones. Some of the more complex, commonly used physical examination instruments are discussed in this chapter as well as in other chapters. During a complete physical examination, the instruments and equipment listed in display may be used.

Stethoscope

A stethoscope is used to evaluate sounds that are difficult to hear with the human ear, such as: heart, bowel, vascular and lung sounds. The stethoscope transmits sound to the ears while blocking out environmental noise (Fig. 9.9).

The chest piece of the stethoscope is designed to detect high or low-frequency sounds and consists of two main part the diaphragm and the bell. The flat, closed diaphragm filters out low-pitched sounds and is used to detect high-pitched sounds such as lung sounds. Best results are obtained by placing the diaphragm evenly and firmly over the persons exposed skin. Because the diaphragm has a relatively large surface, it transmits acute sounds over a wide area. The diaphragm should be at least 1.5 inches in diameter. Smaller diaphragm pieces are available for examining children.

The open bell portion of the chest piece is used to detect low-frequency sounds such as diastolic heart murmurs. The bell should be at least 1 inch in diameter. The bell is placed gently on the persons skin. If too much pressure is applied, the bell will function as a diaphragm. Pain sounds may be difficult to detect with the bell because of its relatively small size.

The stethoscope tuning is made of flexible rubber or plastic that is thick enough to block environmental sounds. Double tubes that are less than 12 inches long further enhance sound transmission.

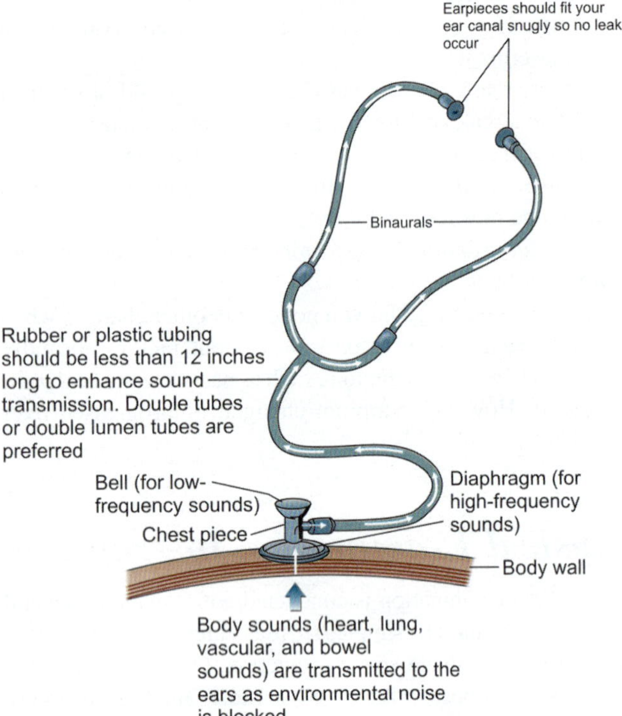

Figure 9.9: The stethoscope

The binaural are placed in the ears and are positioned to project sound towards the tympanic membrane. The tips of the earpieces approximate the angle of the ear canal and should fit snugly and comfortably. Manufacturers usually supply several earpieces so that a comfortable pair can be selected.

Doppler Probe

The Doppler probe is used to evaluate blood flow, especially when traditional methods such as pulse palpation or auscultation are inappropriate or ineffective. Common clinical applications include evaluating fetal heart sounds and peripheral pulses such as brachial, radial, femoral, peripheral, dorsalis pedis and posterior tibial pulses. The Doppler probe or transducer is placed on the skin in order to send a low-energy, high-energy sound beam (ultrasound beam) towards underlying red blood else. Ultrasound waves are reflected off moving objects, in this case, the red blood cells and return to the Doppler transducer, which

also functions as a receiver. The Doppler probe detects the change in sound frequency as found is returned and converts the sound into an audible signal. When blood is flowing through the vessel that is being evaluated, a pulsatile sound can be heard.

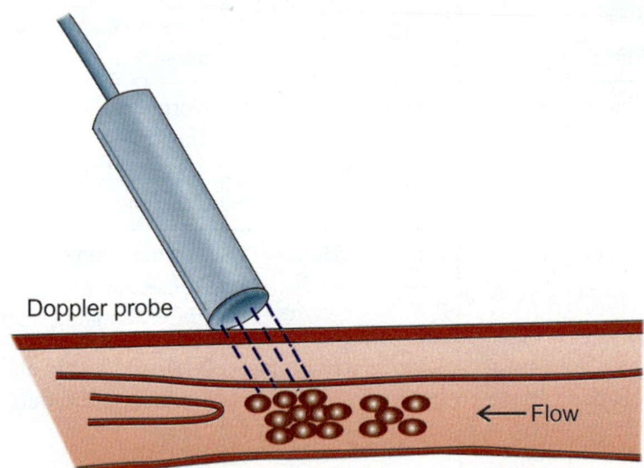

Figure 9.10: Doppler sound generation. The transmitting crystal emits an ultrasound beam through the skin to a vessel and moving red blood cells. The red cells reflect the ultrasound beam to the receiving crystal

Doppler probes (Fig. 9.10) are available as pencil-shaped probes, flat disks or stethoscope-like units. Each device usually has an on/off switch and a volume control dial. A small amount of gel can be applied between the end of the Doppler transducer and the clients skin to eliminate air interference. The probe is then placed gently on the skin over the vessel at approximately a 60° angle to the flow within the vessel. Excessive pressure applied to the skin may occlude the vessel.

Ophthalmoscope

An ophthalmoscope is used inspect internal eye structures. The had of the ophthalmoscope is placed on a battery base, and may be exchanged for an otoscope head. To understand the effective use of this instrument, it is important to become familiar with the structures of the ophthalmoscope head (Figs 9.11A and B).

Internal eye structures can be viewed by directing a light source toward the persons pupil and looking through the viewing aperture. Light is directed away from the headpiece by a front mirror window. The viewing aperture may be adjusted by turning the aperture selection dial. To see the different apertures available on the ophthalmoscope model, shine the light towards a piece of paper and adjust the aperture selection dial. Usually, the large aperture is selected if pupils are dilated and the small aperture chosen if pupils are constricted. The slit aperture may be used to examine the anterior portion of the eye and evaluate fundal lesion levels. The grid aperture may be used to characterize, locate and measure fundal lesions. The red-free filter or green beam may be used to evaluate the retina and disc, especially for any hemorrhaging, which appears black with this filter, while melanin pigments usually appear gray.

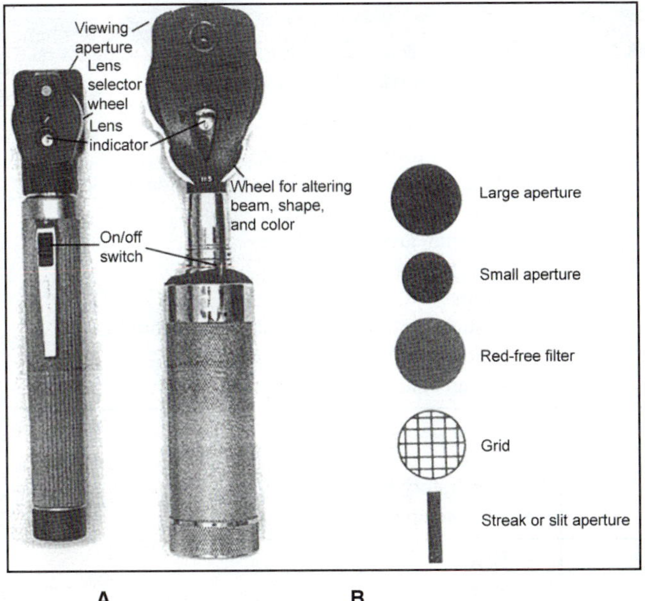

Figures 9.11A and B: (A) Front views of two different ophthalmo-scopes (B) Five apertures contained within the viewing aperture

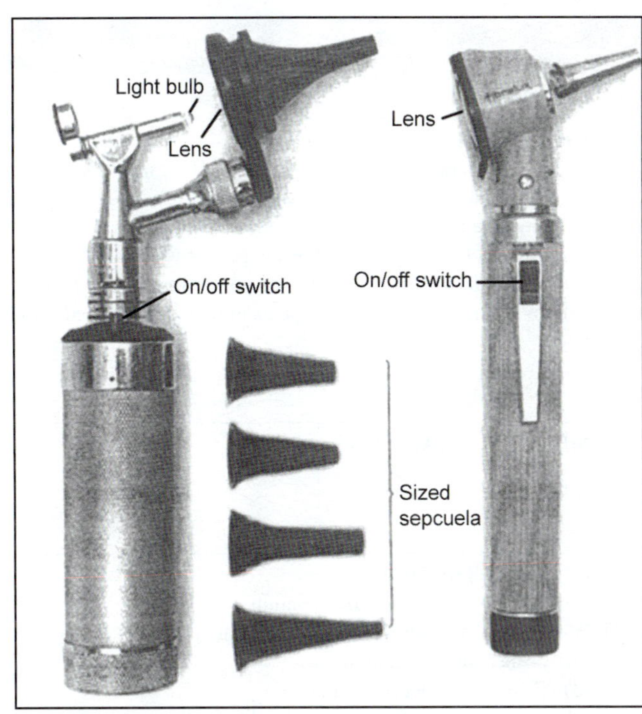

Figure 9.12: The otoscope

The ophthalmoscope lens can be adjusted to bring the internal eye structures into sharp focus, compensating for near sightedness or farsightedness of the client or examiner. If necessary, you may wear contact lenses or glasses during the examination if the lens adjustment does not provide sufficient compensation. The lens can be adjusted by rotating the lens selection dial with the index finger while looking through the viewing aperture. At the zero diopter setting on the lens indicator, the lens neither converges or diverges light. The black numbers, obtained by moving the lens selection dial clockwise, have positive values (+1 to +40) and improve visualization if the client is farsighted. The red numbers obtained by counter-clockwise rotation, have negative values (1 to 20) and improve visualization if the client is nearsighted.

Otoscope

An otoscope is used to inspect the structures of the internal ear. The head of the otoscope should be placed on a battery base and may be exchanged for an ophthalmoscope head (Fig. 9.12).

Internal ear structures should be viewed by looking through the illuminated magnifying lens and speculum. The lens may be displaced to the side so that instruments can be inserted or foreign bodies removed. The size of the speculum should allow maximal visualization with minimal discomfort to the client.

Some otoscopes are equipped with pneumonic devices to introduce a small amount of air against the tympanic membrane, and may be used to evaluate the flexibility of the tympanic membrane.

Guidelines for Head-to-Toe Approach to Physical Examination

General Approach

The physical examination is performed in a systematic manner, such as in a head-to-toe fashion. The guidelines presented here (Table 9.3) apply to the comprehensive examination of an ambulatory adult. The examination sequence may be modified depending on your preference and the clients condition. Variations are usually recommended when examining persons who are seriously ill or injured, or when examining infants, children and frail elderly patients. The different examination positions used in physical examination shown in Figures 9.3A and 9.13.

Preliminary Evaluation

At the beginning of the examination, while the person is ambulatory and before he or she changes into an examining gown, you may evaluate the following:

- Height and weight
- Posture and gait
- Sneellen visual acuity
- Cerebellar function

Sensory Testing

Sensory testing may be performed throughout the examination.

Table 9.3: Examination Guidelines Head-to-Toe Examination

	Procedures	What to observe and record
1.	**INITIATE THE GENERAL SURVEY** (a) The general survey begins when you first meet the client, in the waiting room or examination room, or while delivering bedside care (b) Survey mobility and gait as the person walks into the room (c) Continue the general survey as you examine each body region (d) With the client seated on the examination table, bed, or chair	• General state of health • Signs of distress such as breathing difficulty, pain • Awareness, behavior, facial expression, mood • Height, weight, nutritional status • Hygiene, grooming, clothes • Skin condition • Odors • Postures, motor activity, physical deformities • Speech pattern • Apparent age vs. actual age.
2.	**MEASURE VITAL SIGNS**	• Blood pressure • Pulse • Respiratory rate • Body temperature
3.	**EXAMINE THE HEAD** (a) Inspect and palpate the cranium (b) Palpate and auscultate the temporal arteries (c) Inspect and palpate the face (d) Test cranial nerves V and VII (e) Inspect the nose and test cranial nerve I	• Hair • Size, shape and symmetry • Tenderness • Scalp smoothness • Thickening • Tenderness • Bruits • Symmetry • Movements • Tenderness • Nodules • Sinus tenderness • Motor and sensory response • Patency • Septum • Mucosa • Sense of smell
4.	**EXAMINE THE EYES AND TEST VISION** (a) Inspect and palpate to evaluate external eye structures. (b) Evaluate visual acuity. Perform near vision new or snellerjacger chart testing of far vision at the beginning of the examination. (c) Test extraocular muscle function (cranial nerves III, IV and VI). (d) Test papillary reflexes. (e) Inspect internal eye structure with the ophthalmoscope; darken the room if possible.	• Shape and symmetry • Eyelids and eyelashes • Lacrimal glands, puncta, and lacrimal functions. • Upper and lower conjunctiva • Eye chart readings. • Peripheral vision. • Extraocular eye movement • Eye movements during cover uncover test. • Eye alignment and symmetry. • Reaction to light • Accommodation • Retina • Optic disc • Mascula
5.	**EXAMINE THE EARS AND TEST HEARING.** (a) Inspect and palpate the external ear (b) Evaluate hearing (c) Inspect the ear canal and tympani membrane with the otoscope	• Skin integrity • Structure, alignment and symmetry • Tenderness • Ability to distinguish sound varying in pitch and intent • Sound lateralization • Perception of air conduct of sound vs. bone conduction. • Skin integrity.

Contd...

Table 9.3: *Contd...*	
Procedures	*What to observe and record*
	• Obstructions, foreign body • Color, light reflection. Landmark, and configure of the tympanic member

6. EXAMINE THE ORAL CAVITY
  (a) Inspect and palpate the outer structures of the oral cavity.
  (b) Inspect and palpate the inner structures of the oral cavity.
  (c) Test cranial nerves V, IX and XII.
	• Lips
	• Jaw
	• Temporomandibular joint
	• Parotid glands
	• Oral mucosa
	• Tongue
	• Inner check
	• Hard and soft palates
	• Oropharynx
	• Uvula
	• Motor responses

7. EXAMINE THE NECK
  (a) Inspect musculoskeletal structures
  (b) Palpate the lymph nodes
  (c) Inspect and palpate the thyroid gland
  (d) Test neck musculoskeletal function and cranial nerve XI.
  (e) Palpate and auscultate the carotid arteries
  (f) Test neck musculoskeletal function and cranial nerve XI.
  (g) Palpate and auscultate the carotid arteries
	• Alignment
	• Symmetry
	• Consistency
	• Enlargement
	• Nodules
	• Tenderness
	• Consistency
	• Enlargement
	• Nodules
	• Tenderness
	• Muscle strength and tone
	• Range of motion
	• Pulsation
	• Vascular sounds

8. EXAMINE THE UPPER EXTREMITIES
  (a) Inspect the musculoskeletal structure skin and nails
  (b) Test musculoskeletal function
  (c) Palpate branchial and radial arteries
  (d) Test deep tendon reflexes
	• Skin integrity
	• Muscle mass
	• Alignment and symmetry
	• Muscle strength and tone
	• Range of motion
	• Pulsations
	• Motor response

9. EXAMINE THE ANTERIOR CHEST
  (a) Inspect the palpate the breasts and axillae
  (b) Inspect, palpate, percuss, and auscultate the thorax
  (c) Inspect, palpate and auscultate the precordium
	• Skin integrity
	• Size, shape and symmetry
	• Consistency
	• Skin integrity
	• Ventilatory pattern
	• Shape and symmetry
	• Chest excursion
	• Vibrations
	• Percussion tones
	• Breath sounds
	• Pulsations
	• Vibrations
	• Heart sounds

10 EXAMINE THE BACK
  (a) Inspect and test musculoskeletal structures
  (b) Perform fist percussion over the spine and kidneys
  (c) Inspect, palpate, percuss and auscultate the posterior thorax
	• Spinal alignment
	• Muscle tone
	• Range of motion
	• Tenderness
	• Same as anterior thorax

Position client supine of the examining table or bed. Elevate the head 30 degrees to inspect the neck veins

Contd...

<table>
<tr><td colspan="3" align="center">Table 9.3: Contd...</td></tr>
<tr><td colspan="2">Procedures</td><td>What to observe and record</td></tr>
<tr><td>11.</td><td>INSPECT THE NECK VEINS</td><td>• Jugular venous pulsations
• Central venous pressure</td></tr>
<tr><td>12.</td><td>EXAMINE THE ANTERIOR CHEST
(as above, adding palpation of glandular breast tissue and precordial auscultation in the left lateral position)</td><td></td></tr>
<tr><td>13.</td><td>EXAMINE THE ABDOMEN
(a) Inspect, auscultate, palpate and percuss the four abdominal quadrants
(b) Palpate and percuss specific organs (liver, spleen, kidneys)</td><td>• Contour and symmetry
• Skin integrity
• Bulges
• Bowel sounds
• Vascular stands
• Muscle tone
• Masses
• Organ characteristics
• Percussion tones
• Tenderness
• Size
• Consistency
• Tenderness</td></tr>
<tr><td>14.</td><td>EXAMINE THE LOWER EXTREMITIES
(a) Inspect musculoskeletal structures, skin and toenails
(b) Test musculoskeletal function
(c) Palpate political, posterior, tibial and pedal arteries
(d) Test deep tendon reflexes and plantar reflex</td><td>• Skin integrity
• Muscle mass
• Alignment and symmetry
• Muscle strength and tone
• Range of motion
• Pulsations
• Motor response</td></tr>
<tr><td colspan="2">Position the female client in the lithotomy position with stirrups.</td><td></td></tr>
<tr><td>15.</td><td>EXAMINE THE GENITALS AND PELVIS
(a) Inspect the external genitals
(b) Inspect the vagina and cervix
(c) Palpate the vagina, uterus, and cervix</td><td>• Skin integrity
• Contour and symmetry
• Discharge
• Skin integrity
• Masses
• Discharge
• Muscle tone
• Position
• Size
• Consistency and masses</td></tr>
<tr><td>16.</td><td>EXAMINE THE RECTUM</td><td>• Muscle tone
• Stool
• Tenderness
• Masses
• Bleeding, discharge</td></tr>
<tr><td colspan="2">Assist the male client to a standing position</td><td></td></tr>
<tr><td>17.</td><td>EXAMINE THE EXTERNAL GENITALS
(a) Inspect and palpate the penis
(b) Inspect and palpate the scrotum
(c) Inspect and palpate for hernias</td><td>• Skin integrity
• Masses
• Discharge
• Skin integrity
• Size and shape
• Testicular descent and mobility
• Mosses
• Tenderness
• Bulges</td></tr>
<tr><td>18.</td><td>EXAMINE THE RECTUM (for male patients, different positions may be used and special attention is given to prostate palpation)</td><td></td></tr>
</table>

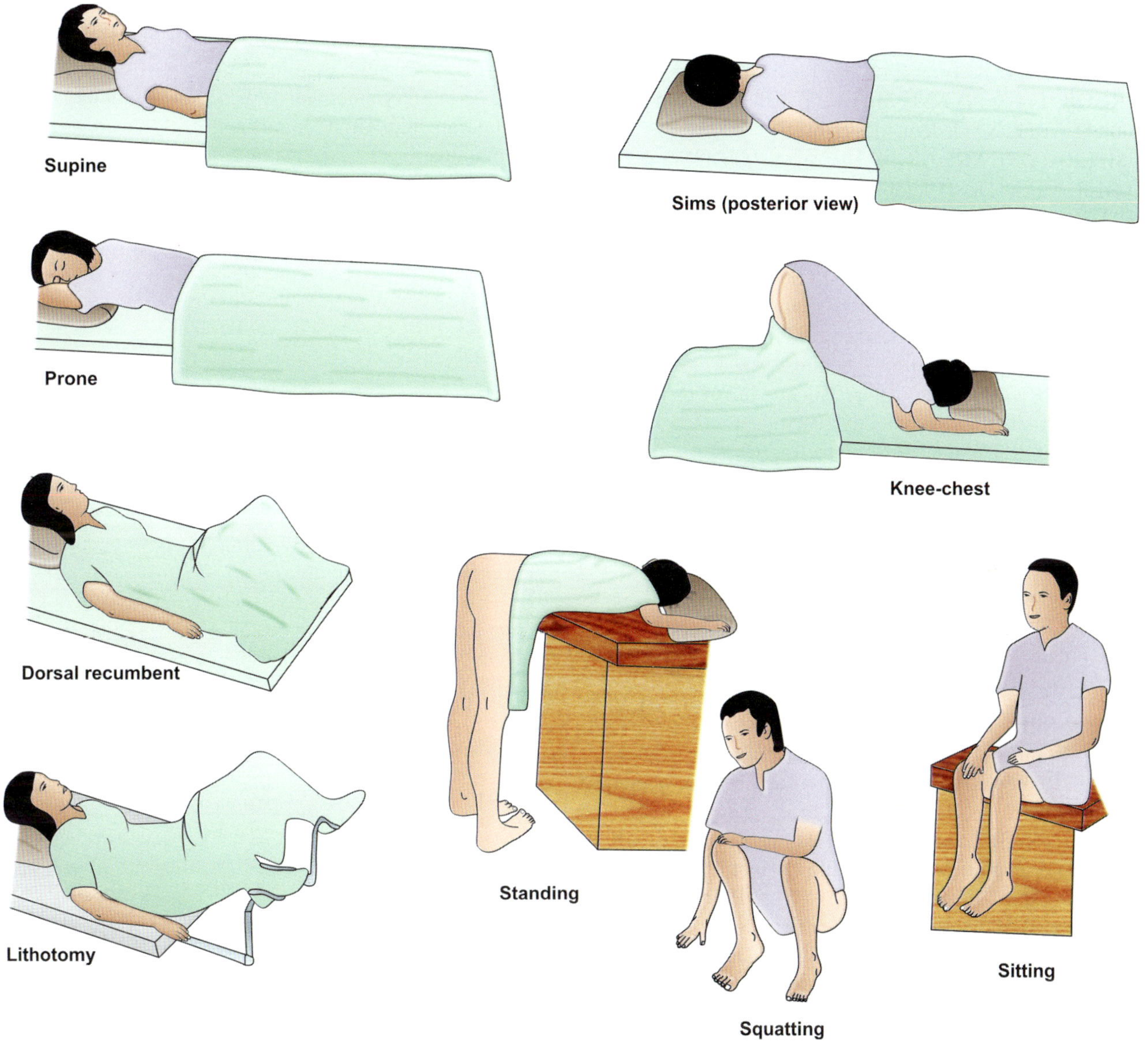

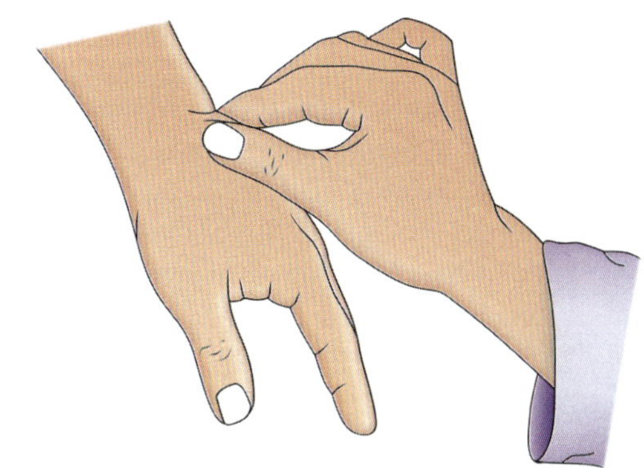

Figure 9.13: Different examination positions

Descriptive Terminology for Documentation

After examination, documentation is necessary; this should be specific, descriptive and objective. The following descriptive terminology suggested for documentation.

OVERALL APPEARANCE INSPECTION

SEX: male/female

GENERAL GROOMING: Clean? Hair combed? Make-up?

POSITION/POSTURING: Supine? Prone? Rigid? Opisthotonos? Erect? Slumped?

BODY SIZE: Thin? Fat? Obese? Emasciated? Flabby? Weight proportionate to height? Mesomorph? Endomorph? Ectomorph?

FACIAL EXPRESSIONS: Eye contact? No eye contact? Arms folded over chest?

OTHER OBSERVATIONS: Restless? Fidgeting? Lying quietly? Listless? Trembling? Tense?

Figure 9.14: Assessing skin turgor

SKIN INSPECTION AND PALPATION

COLOR AND VASCULARITY: Pink? Tan? Brown? Dark brown? Grayish? Pasty? Yellowish? Flushed? Jaundiced?

TURGOR (Fig. 9.14) AND MOBILITY: Elastic? Non-elastic? Tenting? Wrinkles? Oedematous tight?

TEMPERATURE AND MOISTURE: Cold? Cool? Warm? Hot? Feverish? Moist? Dry? Clammy? Oily? Sweating? Diaphoresis?

TEXTURE: Smooth? Rough? Fine? Thick? Coarse? Scaly? Pully?

NAILS: Clean, manicured? Smooth? Rough? Dry? Hard? Brittle? Splitting? Cracking? Angle of nail bed? Clubbing? Curved? Flat? Thick? Yellowing? Paronychia?

NAIL BEDS AND LUNULE: Pale? Pink? Cyanotic? Red? Shape of lumule? Blanching? Spooning?

BODY HAIR GROWTH: Color? Thick? Thin? Coarse? Fine? Location and distribution on body? Hirsutism?

SKIN INTEGRITY: Intact? Not intact?

LESIONS, BIRTH MARKS, MOLES, SCARS AND RASHES: (describe shape, size and location) Nevi? Fissures? Maculas? Papules? Pustules? Nodules? Vullae? Eysts? Carbuncle? Wheals? Crythema? Excoriation? Desquamotion? Abrations? Cherry angiomas? Senile lentigines? Senile purpura? Senile keratoses? Seborrheic keratoses? Bruises? Inset bites? Crusts? Warts? Pimples? Blackheads? Bleeding? Drainage? Lacerations? Scaly? Lichenificaiton?

HEAD INSPECTION AND PALPATION

SHAPE: Round? Oval? Square? Pointed? Normocephalic?

FACE: (TRGEMINAL CN V): Sensation on three branches? Clenched teeth?

FACIAL CN VII: Facial expressions, smiles?

HAIR: Color and growth coarse? Fine? Thick? Thin? Sparse? Alopecia? Long? Short? Curly? Straight? Premed? Glossy? Shiny? Greasy? Dry? Brittle? Stringy? Frizzy?

CONDITIONS OF SCALP: Clean? Scaly? Dandruff? Rashes? Sores? Drainage?

MASSES AND LUMPS: (describe location and shape, measure size).

EYES INSPECTION AND PALPATION

EYE DROPS: Color and shape: alignment? Straight? Curved thick? Thin, sparse? Plucked? Scaly?

EYE LASHES: Long? Short? Curved? None? Artificial?

EYE LIDS: Dark? Swollen? Inflamed? Red? Style? Infected? Open and close simultaneously? Ptosis? Entropion? Extropion? Itlag? Xanthomas?

SHAPE AND APPEARANCE OF EYES: Almond? Rounded squinty? Prominent? Exophthalmia? Sunken? Symmetrical bright? Clear? Dull? Tearing? Discharge (serous) purulent? Exotropia? Esotropia? Nystigmus? Strabismus?

SCLERA: White? Cream? Yellowish? Jaundiced? Injected? Pterygium?

CONJUNCTIVA: Pale pink? Pink? Red? Inflamed? Nodules? Swelling?

IRIS: Color and shape: Round? Not round? Colobona? Areasenilis?

CORNEA: Clear? Milky? Opaque? Cloudy?

PUPILS (OCULOMOTOR-CN III) (PERRLA): SIZE AND SHAPE: (measure in mm) Round? Notround? (describe EQUALITY: Symmetrical? Anisocoria? Right larger than left? Left large than right?convergence? Reaction to light and accomondation? Consensual reaction?

EXTRAOCULAR MOVEMENT (OCULOMOTOR), TROCHLEAR, ABDUCENS, CN III, IV, VI: Intact?

LACRIMAL GLANDS: Tender? Non tender? Inflamed? Swollen tearing?

AIDS: Glasses? Contact lenses? Prosthesis?

VISUAL FIELDS (OPTIC-CNII): Intact?

VISION (OPTIC-CNII): reads newsprint? Reports objects across room?

EARS INSPECTION AND PALPATION

PINNAE: Size and shape: Large? Small? In proportion to fact protruding oval? Large lobes? Small lobes? Symmetrical? Right larger than left? Left larger than right? Pinnae irregular? Color skin intact? Redness? Swelling? Tophi? Cauliflower ear? Furuncle darwin's tuburcle?

LEVEL IN RELATION TO EYES: Top of pinnae level with outer canthus of eyes? Top of pinnae lower than outer canthus of eyes? Top of pinnae higher than outer canthus of eyes?

CANAL: Clean? Discharge? (serous? Bloody? Purulent?) nodules? Inflammation? Redness? Foreign object?

CILIA: Present? Absent?

CERUMEN: Present/absent? Color? Consistency?

TYMPANIC MEMBRANE: Color? Pearly white? Injected? Red inflamed? Discharge? Cone of light? Landmarks? Scarring bubbles? Fluid level?

HEARING (AUDITORYT-CN VII): Right-present/absent? Left present/absent? Hears watch tick? Hears whisper? Respond readily when spoken to?

WEBER (Fig. 9.15): Laterlizes equally? To left right side?

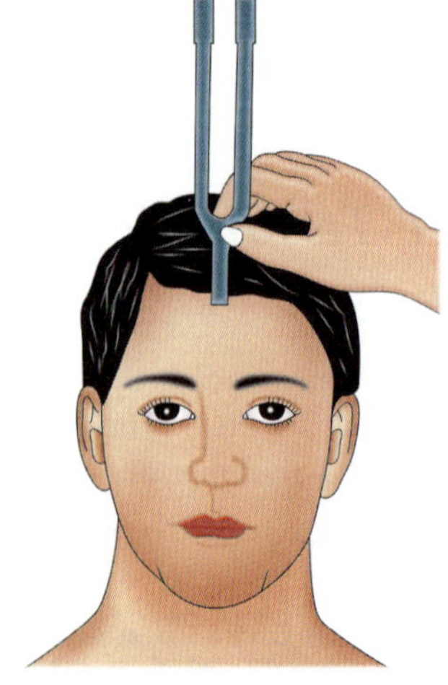

Figure 9.15: Weber lateralization test

RINNE (Fig. 9.16): Air condition: Bone conduction 2:1? Hearing aid: right/left?

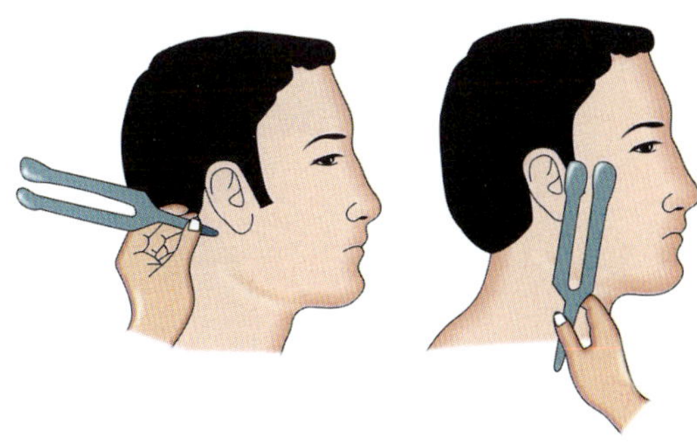

Figure 9.16: Rinne air and bone conduction test

NOSE AND SINUSES INSPECTION AND PALPATION

SIZE AND SHAPE: Long? Short? Large? Small? In proportion to face? Flat? Broad? Based? Thick? Thin? Enlarged? Nares symmetrical/asymmetrical? Pointed? Swollen? Bulbous? Flaring of nostrils?

SEPTUM: Midline? Deviated right? Left? Perforated?

NASAL MUCOSA AND TURBINATES: Pink? Pale? Bluish? Red? Dry? Moist? Discharge? (purulent? Clear? Watery? Mucus?) cilia present/absent? Rhinitis? Epistaxis? Polyps?

POTENCY OF NARES: (close each side and ask client to breathe) right-patient/partial obstruction/obstructed? Left? Patent/partial obstruction and obstructed?

OLFACTORY (CN I): Correctly identifies odors?

SINUSES: Tender? Non-tender? Transillumination?

MOUTH AND PHARYNX INSPECTION

LIPS: COLOR: Pink? Red? Tam? Pale? Cyanotic?

SHAPE: Thin? Thick? Enlarged? Swollen? Symmetrical? Asymmetrical? Drooping left side? Drooping right side?

CONDITION: Soft? Smooth? Dry? Crackled? Fissured? Blisters? Lesions? (describe)

TEETH: Color and condition: white? Yellow? Grayish? Spotted? Stained? Darkened? Pitting? Notched? Straight? Protruding? Separated? Crowded? Irregular? Broken? Notching? Peglike? Loose? Dull? Bright? Dentulous? Malocclusion?

CARRIES AND FILLINGS: Number and location? DENTAL HYGIENE: Clean ? Not clean? Breath odor: sweet? Odorless? Haliltosis? Musty? Acetone? Foul? Fetid? Odor of drugs or food? Hot? Sour? Alcohol?

GUMS: Pink? Firm? Swollen? Bleeding? Sensitive? Gingivitis? Hypertrophy nodules? Irritated? Receding? Moist? Ulcerated? Dry? Shrunken? Blistered? Spongy?

FACIAL AND GLOSSOPHARYNGEAL (CN VII and IX): Identifies taste? Or note?

TONGUE: Macroglossia? Microglossia? Glossitis? Geographic? Red? Pink? Bluish? Brownish? Swollen? Clean? Thin? Thick? Fissured? Raw? Coated? Moist? Dry? Cracked? Glistening? Papillae?

HYPOGLOSSAL (CN XII) TONGUE MOVEMENT: Symmetry? Lateral? Fasciculation?

MUCOSA: Color? Leukoplakia? Dry? Moist? Intact? Not intact? Masses? (describe size, shape and location) Chancre?

PALATE: Moist? Dry? Color? Intact? Not intact?

UVULA: Color? Midline? Remains at midline when saying "ah"? Gag reflex present?

PHARYNX: Color? Petechia? Injected? Beefy? Dysphagia?

TONSILS: Present/absent? Cryptic? Beefy? Size 1+ to 4+?

TEMPOROMANDIBULAR JOINT: Fully mobile symmetrical? Tenderness? Crepitus?

NECK INSPECTION AND PALPATION

APPEARANCE: Long? Short? Thick? Thin? Masses? (describe size and shape) symmetrical? Not symmetrical?

THYROID: Palpate? Nodules? Tender?

TRACHEA: Midline? Deviated to right/Left?

LYMPH NODES: (Occipital-preauricular, postauricular, submental, sub-maxillary, tonsilar, anterior cervical, posterion cervical, superficial cervical, deep cervical, supraclavicular) non-palpable? Tender? Lymphadenopathy? Shotty? Hard? Firm?

THORAX AND LUNGS INSPECTION, PALPATIONS, PERCUSSION AND AUSCULTATION

RESPIRATIONS: Rate? Tachypnea, eupnea, bradypnea? Apnea? Orthopnea? Laboured? Stertorous?

RHYTHM: Regular/irregular? Inspiration time greater than expiration time? Expiration time greater than inspiration time? Spasmodic? Gasping? Orthopnic? Gasping? Deep? Eupnic? Shallow? Flaring of nostrils with respirations? Symmetrical asymmetrical? Right thorax greater than left? Left thorax greater than right? Ratio of diameter to lateral diameter between 1:2 and 5:7? Ribs sloped downward at 45° diameter angle? Well? Defined costal space? Accessory muscles used? Pigeon chest? Funnel chest? Barrel chest? Abdominal or chest breather? Skin intact? Lesions? Color? Thin? Muscular? Flabby?

POSTERIOR THORAX: Tenderness? Masses?

RESPIRATORY EXCURSION: Symmetrical? Asymmetrical? No respiratory movements on right/left? Subcutaneous emphysema? Crepitus? Fremitus? Estimation of level of diaphragm? Spine alignment? Tenderness? Cavy tenderness? Resonance? Dull? Hyperresonance? Diaphragmatic excursion 3-5 cm? Comparison of one side to the other? Suprasternal north located? Costochondral junctions tender? Chest wall stable? Vocal fremitus?

LUNG AUSCULTATION: Vesicular? Bronchovesicular? Bronchial? Whispered pectoriloquy? Adventitious sounds? Rales? Thonchi? Wheezes? Crackles? Rub? Bronchophony? Egophony?

BREASTS AND AXILLAE INSPECTION (Figs 9.17 to 9.19)

BREASTS: Male? Female? Present/absent? Color? Large? Small? Well developed? Firm? Pendulous? Flat? Flabby? Symmetrical? Asymmetrical? Dimpling? Thickening? Smooth? Retraction? Peau'd orange? Venous pattern? Tenderness? Masses? (describe gynecomastia)

NIPPLES: Present? Absent? Circular? Symmetrical? Asymmetrical? Inverted? Everted? Pale? Brown? Rose? Extranipples? Discharge? Deviation? Supernumerary?

AXILLA: Shaved/unshaved/odor? Masses or lumps? (describe size and shape)

LYMPH NODES (Fig. 9.20): (Lateral, central, subscapular, pectoral, epitrochlear) Palpable? Tender? Snotty?

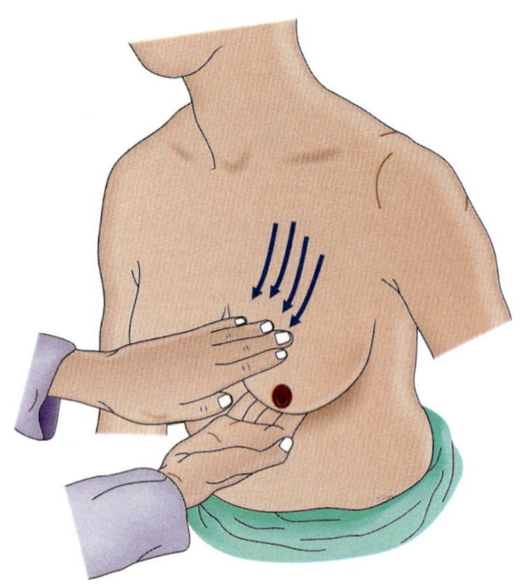

Figure 9.17: Bimanual breast palpation

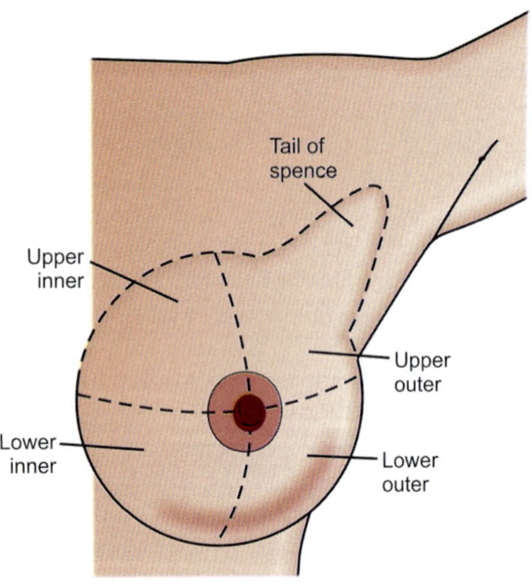

Figure 9.18: Breast quadrants used for assessment

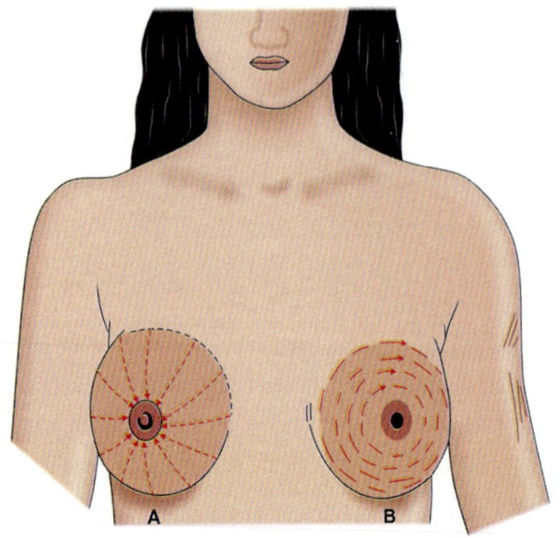

Figure 9.19: Patterns for breast palpation

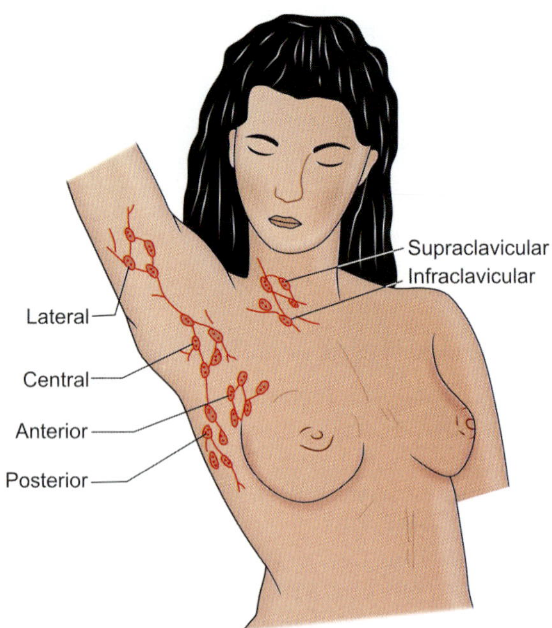

Figure 9.20: Lymph nodes the breast and axillary area

Breast Self-Examination (Figs 9.21A to G)

Procedure

1. Examine the breasts in the tub or shower when skin is wet and hands move easily over breast tissue (Figs 9.21A and B). Use the right hand to examine the left breast as you raise the left arm over the head to expose more breast tissue.

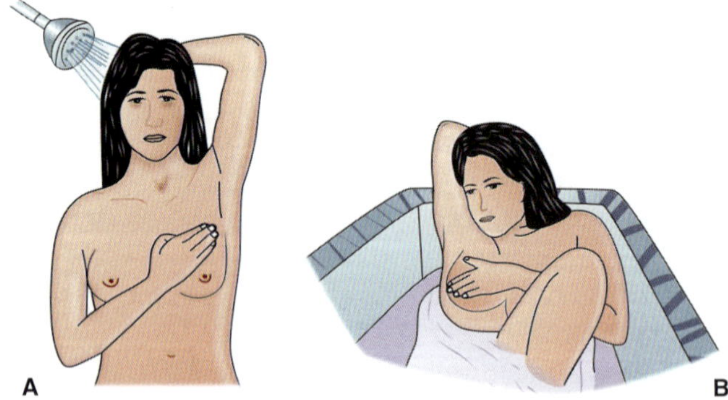

Figures 9.21A and B

2. Examine the breast in front of a mirror to detect unusual contours or changes in the skin appearance, such as puckering, dimpling, or retraction of the nipple. Note the appearance of the breasts in three different positions: Arms at the sides (Fig. 9.21C), arms over the head (Fig. 9.21D), and hands on the hips while flexing the chest muscle (Fig. 9.21E).

3. Examine the breasts lying down. Place a small pillow or blanket under your shoulder on the side being examined, to expose more breast tissue (Fig. 9.21F). Use the right hand to examine the left breast. Be thorough, proceeding in a circular

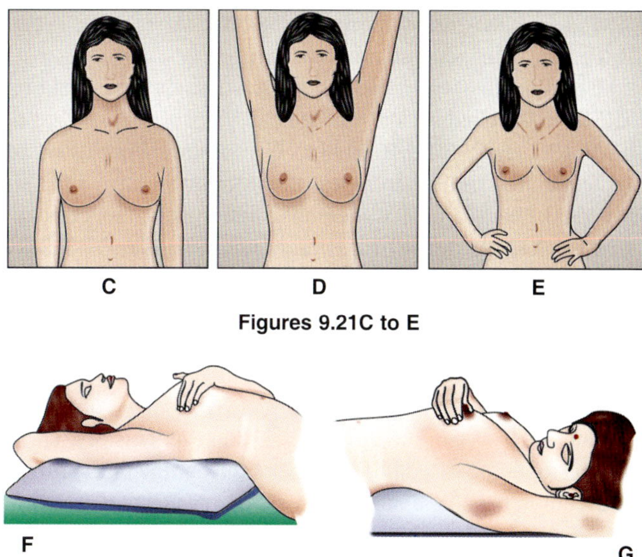

Figures 9.21C to E

Figures 9.21F and G

Figures 9.21A to G: Breast self-examination

pattern from the center of the breast outward, feel the breast tissues that extend to the armpit. Squeeze the nipple to detect any discharge (Fig. 9.21G). Any hard lumps, clear or bloody nipple discharge, or skin changes should be reported to a health professional.

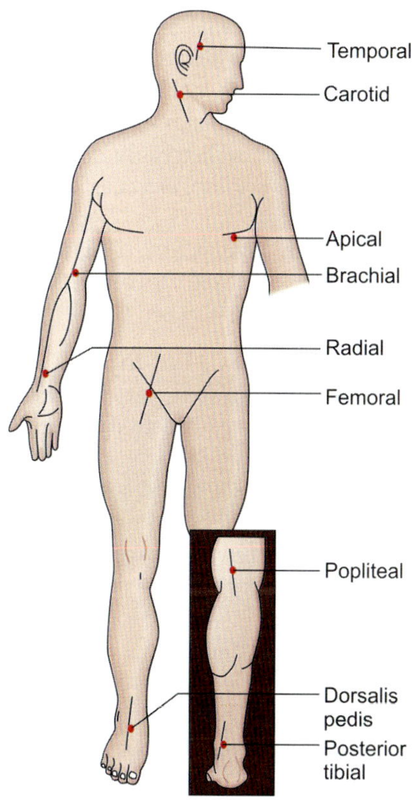

Figure 9.22: Pulse sites

Heart and Peripheral Vascular Inspection, Percussion, Auscultations and Palpation

HEART: Precordial bulge? Abnormal palpations? PMI? Thrills? Heave or lift with pulsation? S_1 loudest at apex? S_2 loudest at base? S_3? S_4? Splits? Clicks? Snap? Rub? Gallop?

MURMURS: Systolic? Diastolic? Holosystolic? Harsh? Soft? Blowing? Rumbling? Grading 1 through 6? High pitch? Medium pitch? Low pitch? Radiating?

CAROTID PULSE: Note: Do not check both right and left carotid pulses simultaneously.

VOLUME: Bounding? Forceful? Strong? Full? Weak? Feeble? Thready? Symmetrical? Right less than left? Left less than right? Rhythm: regular? Irregular? Symmetrical? Asymmetrical? Bruits present? Absent?

APICAL PULSE: Record rate; tachycardia? Bradycarda? Pounding? Forceful, weak? Moderate? Regular? Irregular?

PERIPHERAL PULSES (Fig. 9.22): (Do not count rate of these pulses except radial) record character, volume, rhythm and symmetry of brachial, radial femoral, popliteal, dorsalis pedis, and posterior tibial pulses. volume: full? Strong? Forceful? Bounding? Perceptible? Imperceptible? Weak? Thready? Symmetrical? Asymmetrical? Right greater than left? Left greater than right?

RHYTHM: Regular? Irregular? Symmetrical? Asymmetrical?

SYMMETRY: Record as symmetrical? Right greater than left or left greater than right? Pulse deficit, pulse pressure, BP in both arms, BP lying, sitting and standing if applicable. jugular venous distention? (record cm above level of sternal angle).

ABDOMEN INSPECTION, AUSCULTATION, PERCUSSION, PALPATION

CONTOUR: Irregular? Protruding? Enlarged? Distended? Scaphoid? Concave? Sunken? Flabby? Firm? Flat? Flaccid?

SKIN: Color; intact? Not intact? Shiny? Smooth? Scars? Lesions? (describe size, shape and type of lesion) striate? Umbilicus?

BOWEL SOUNDS: Present? Absent? Hyperactive? High-pitched tickling? Gurgles? Borborygmus?

PERCUSSION: Tympanic? Dull? Flat? (describe where) liver size 6-12 cm? Splendid dullness (6-10th rib? Ascites?

PALPATION: Splenomegaly? Hepatomegaly? Organomegaly? Masses? Aortic pulse? Diastasis recto? Tenderness? Bulges? Lower pole of kidneys palpable? Inguinal or femoral hernia? Inguinal nodes? (describe).

MUSCULOSKELETAL INSPECTION AND PALPATION

BACK: Shoulders level? Right shoulder higher than left? Left shoulder higher than right? Alignment? Lordosis? Seoliosis? Hypnosis? Ankylosis?

VERTEBRAL COLUMN ALIGNMENT: Straight? Lordosis? Scoliosis? Kyphosis?

JOINTS: Redness? Swelling? Deformity? (describe) crepitation? Size? Symmetry? Subluxation? Separation? Bogginess? Tenderness? Pain? Thickening? Nodules? Fluid? Bulging?

RANGE OF MOTION: Describe as full, limited or fixed, estimate degree of limitation, assess range of motion of neck, should elbows wrists, fingers, back, hips, knees, ankles, toes.

EXTREMITIES: Compare extremities with each other; describe color and symmetry, temperature; hot, warm, cool, cold, clammy, dry; muscle tone descriptors are firm, muscular, flaccid, atrophy? Fasciculation? Tremor?

LOWER EXTREMITIES: Symmetry? (describe any variety from normal abrasions? Bruises? Swollen? Edema? Rash lesions? (describe) prosthesis? Varicose veins?

GENITOURINARY AND RECTUM INSPECTION

RECTUM: Haemorrhoids? Inflammation? Lesions? Skin fissures? Excoriation? Swelling? Mucosal bulging? Retraced fissures?

FEMALE GENITALIA: Public hair distribution and color? Pediculosis? Lesions? Nodules? Inflammation? Swelling pigmentation? Dry? Moist? Shriveled, atrophy or full discharge? (describe) odor? Asymmetry? Varicosities? Utoprolapse? Smegma? Rash?

MALE GENITALIA (Fig. 9.23): Public hair distribution and color? Pediculosis? Circumcised? Uncircumcised? Phimosis? Epedius? Hypospadius? Smegma? Priapism? Varicocele? Crypchism? Hydrocele? Swelling? Redness? Chancre? Crusing? Discharge? (describe) edema? Scrotal sack rugated? Atrophy?

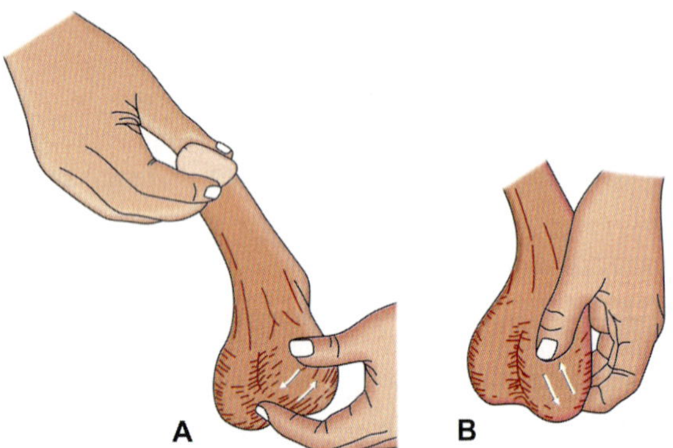

Figures 9.23: Male genitalia. (A) Along horizontal plane
(B) Along vertical plane

NEUROLOGIC

Describe ties, twitches paresthesia, paralysis, co-ordination.

GAIT: Balanced? Shuffling? Unsteady? Ataxic? Parkinson swaying? Scissor? Spastic? Wadding? Staggering? Falter swaying? Slow? Difficult? Tottering? Propulsive?

ACCESSORY-CN XI: Shrugs shoulder? Symmetry?

REFLEXES: Report as present or absent

CO-ORDINATION: Report as to test done

CRANIAL NERVES: May be reported here.

MENTAL STATUS

LEVEL OF ALERTNESS: Alert? Stuporous? Semicomatose comatose?

ORIENTATION: Oriented to time, place, and person? Confuse disoriented?

If confused, check orientation as follows:
TIME: Ask client year, month, day, date.
PLACE: Ask clients residence address, where she/he is residing
PERSON: Ask clients name, birthday.
MEMORY: RECENT MEMORY: Give client short series of numbers and ask client to repeat those numbers later. LONG-TIME: Ask client to recall some event, that happened several ago.
LANGUAGE AND SPEECH: Language spoken? SPELL: Slurred? Slow? Rapid? Difficulty forming words? Aphasis?
RESPONSIVENESS: Responds appropriately to verbal sting responds readily? Slow to respond?

It is probable that all of the questions in each system will be included every time you take a history. Nevertheless, questions regarding each system should be included in every history. These essential races are listed in bold type in the outline that follows. More comprehensive and detailed areas for questions relating to each systems are listed afterward and should be included whenever the patient gives positive responses to the first group of questions for that system. Keep in mind that these list of not represent an exhaustive enumeration of questions that might be appropriate within an organ system. Even more detailed questions may be required, depending on the patients problems.

General Constitutional Symptoms

Fever, chills, malaise, fatigability, night sweats; weight (average, preferred, present, change, appetite).

Skin

Rash or eruption, pruritus, pigmentation or texture change; excessive sweating, abnormal nail or hair growth.

Skeletal

Joint stiffness, pain, restriction of motion, edema erythema, heat, bony deformity.

Head

1. General: Frequent or unusual headaches, dizziness, syncope, sever injuries
2. Eyes: Visual acuity, blurring, diplopia (double vision), photophobia (abnormal sensitivity to light), pain, recent change in appearance or vision, glaucoma, use of eyedrops or other eye mediations, history of trauma or familial eye disease
3. Ears: Heating loss, pain, discharge, tinnitus, vertigo
4. Nose: Sense of smell, frequency of colds, obstructions, epistaxis, postnasal discharge, sinus pain
5. Throat and mouth: Hoarseness or change in voice; frequent sore throats, bleeding or edema of guma; recent tooth abscesses or extractions; soreness of tongue or buccal mucosa ulcers, disturbance of taste.

Endocrine

Thyroid enlargement or tenderness, heat or cold intolerance, unexplained weight change, diabetes, polydipsia (excessive thirst), polyuria, changes in facial or body hari, increased fat and glove size, skin striac.

Respiratory
Pain relating to respiration, dyspnea, cyanosis, wheezing, cough, sputum (character and quantity), hemoptysis (expectorating blood from respiratory tract, night sweats, exposure to TB, date and result of last chest X-ray examination.

Cardiac
Chest pain or distress, recipitating causes, timing and duration, relieving factors, palpations, dyspnea, orthopnea (number of pillows needed), edema, claudication (weakness of legs accompanied by cramp-like pain), hypertension, previous myocardial infarction, estimate of exercise tolerance, past ECG or other cardiac tests.

Hematological
Anemia, tendency to bruise or bleed easily, thromboses, thrombophlebitis, any known abnormality of blood cells, transfusions.

Lymph Nodes
Enlargement, tenderness, suppuration to produce purulent(pus) material.

Gastrointestinal
Appetite, digestion, intolerance for any class of foods, dysphasia, heartburn, nausea, vomiting, hematemises, regularity of bowels, constipation, diarrhea, change in stool color or contents (clay-colored, tarry, fresh blood, mucus, undigested food), flatulence, hemorrhoids, hepatitis, jaundice, dark urine, history of ulcer, gallstones, polyps, tumor; previous X-ray examinations (where, when, findings).

Genitourinary
Dysuria, flank or suprapubic pain, urgency, frequency, nocturia, hematuria, polyuria, hesitancy, dribbling, loss in force of stream, passage of stone, edema of face, stress incontinence, hernias, sexually transmitted disease inquire what kind and symptoms, and list results of serological test for syphilis (STS), if known.

Neurological
Syncope (brief lapse in consciousness caused by transient cerebral hypnosis), weakness or paralysis, abnormalities of sensation or co-ordination, tremors, loss of memory unusual frequency, distribution, or severity of headaches, serious head injury in past.

Psychiatric
Depression, mood changes, difficulty concentrating, nervousness, tension, suicidal thoughts, irritability, sleep disturbances.

Advice to purlic: An advice to public by nurses after assessment of client will include the following:

Taking charge of your own health care, deciding when to see a doctor, when an alternative practitioner might be more appropriate, and what you can handle yourself, is an intelligent, perhaps even necessary approach these days. Unfortunately, there are no easy guidelines – many physicians with years of training and experience often find such decisions difficult. Still the more you know about how diseases can be treated, the more likely you are to make appropriate choices in managing your own and your family's medical care.

When to Call Doctor?
Thousands of people will die needlessly each year because of denial and delay. Among them are heart attack victims who wait an average of six hours to call a doctor, and other people who ignore for months the common warning signs of a major disease such as cancer.

By contract, those who run to a medical specialist for every ache, pain, and sniffed not only drive up medical costs, but also increase their risk of adverse reactions from over treatment. The ideal is to find a middle ground based on common sense and knowledge.

Whom to See?
Everyone should have a primary-care physician to oversee and co-ordinate medical care. This might be a family practitioner, an internist, and osteopath, a pediatrician (for children), or a gynecologist (for women). The doctor may have his or her own practice or be part of a group practice or a client. The important thing is that your practitioners know your medical history and have a stake in maintaining your health.

When you are injured or acute illness strikes, always turn first to a conventionally trained medical doctor. These practitioners are the best qualified to treat trauma and other emergencies, infections, diabetes, heart disease, cancer, and other serious illnesses.

If you suffer from a chronic pain syndrome or some other conditions for which conventional medicine can do little, you might be better off seeing an alternative practitioner. And in many cases, you may be the best person to manage your illness, often under the guidance of a medical professional.

In the box to the right and on the next two pages is a listing of medical signs and symptoms and their possible causes.

Conditions that Demand Prompt Medical Attention

Call your local emergency service or get to the nearest emergency room if any of the following develop;

Possible Heart Attack

- Severe pain, light-headedness, fainting, sweating, nausea or shortness of breath
- Feeling of pain, pressure, fullness, or squeezing in the center chest that lasts more than two minutes
- Pain spreading from the center chest to the shoulders, neck, or arms.

Possible Stroke or Mini-stroke

- Sudden weakness or numbness on one side of the body usually affecting the face, an arm or leg
- Sudden loss of speech or difficulty speaking or understanding speech

- Loss of vision or dimness, usually in one eye or half of both eyes
- Unexplained dizziness, unsteady gait, lack of co-ordination or falling
- Sudden severe headache unlike any experienced in the pain
- Abrupt loss of memory or altered mental abilities.

Possible Shock

- Cold, clammy and pale skin
- Weakness and light headacheness
- Rapid, weak pulse
- Rapid, shallow and irregular breathing
- Agitation and feeling of apprehension.

Possible Anaphylactic Reaction

- Severe swelling, especially around the eyes, mouth, and face
- Weak, rapid pulse
- Difficulty breathing
- Possible nausea, vomiting, and abdominal cramps
- Bluish tinge to skin and nails
- Confusion, dizziness, possible loss of consciousness.

Possible Internal Bleeding

- Coughing or vomiting up blood, which may look like coffee grounds
- Blood in the stool or urine
- Bleeding from a body opening, such as the ears, nose and mouth
- Abdominal swelling and tenderness
- Excessive thirst.

Fever

See a doctor as soon as possible if:
- Body temperature rises to 100.5° F (38°C) in a baby younger than 3 months
- Body temperature rises to 103°F (39.4°C) in a child or adult of any age
- Body temperature rises to 101°F (38.3°C) and stays there for three days
- Low-grade fever recurs or persists for two or more weeks
- Fever of any degree is accompanied by severe headache stiff neck, swelling of the throat, or mental confusion.

Table 9.4: Common Signs or Symptoms and Possible Causes	
Signs or symptoms	*Possible causes*
Anxiety	Alcoholism, panic attack, premenstrual syndrome, stress, a thyroid disorder
Belching	Gallbladder disease, indigestion, a malabsorption syndrome
Bleeding and bruises Gums	Periodontal disease, leukemia, vitamin deficiency
Eye	Diabetes, high blood pressure
Nose	A clotting disorder, high blood pressure, injury, nasal polyps or tumors
Rectal	Anal fissure, colon cancer or polyps, diverticulitis or other intestinal disorder, hemorrhoids, ulcers
Skin	Allergic reaction, anemia, a blood or clotting disorder, Cushing's syndrome, drug reaction, hemophilia, injury, leukemia
Sputum	Bronchitis, lung cancer, pneumonia, pulmonary embolism, throat infection, tubeculosis
Urine	Bladder infection, urinary tract cancer, kidney stone, prostate disorder
Vagina	Abortion or miscarriage, cancer, a hormonal disorder, infection, menstrual abnormalities, injury, polyps
Vomit	Cirrhosis of the liver, esophageal tear, ulcers
Breathlessness	Anemia, anxiety, asthma, heart disease, hyperventilation, a lung disorder
Confusion	Addiction, alcoholism, Alzheimer's disease or other dementia, drug reaction, head injury, stroke
Constipation	Appendicitis, colon cancer or other bowel disorder, diabetes, diet, drug side effects, inactivity, pregnancy, a thyroid disorder
Coughing	Asthma, bronchitis, common cold, croup, cystic fibrosis, flu, pneumonia
Cyanosis (bluish skin)	A circulatory disorder, congenital heart defect, cystic fibrosis, heart failure, respiratory failure, Raynaud's disease
Delirium	Alcohol or drug abuse, brain tumor or abscess, encephalitis, head injury, heat stroke, meningitis, mountain sickness, poisoning, psychosis, Reye's syndrome

Contd...

Table 9.4: *Contd...*

Signs or symptoms	Possible causes
Diarrhea	AIDS, allergies, celiac disease, food poisoning, inflammatory bowel disease, irritable bowel syndrome or other colon disorder, infection, a malabsorption syndrome, traveler's diarrhea
Dizziness	Alcohol or drug, abuse, anemia, a brain disorder, cardiae arrhythmia, drug reaction, ear infection, Meniere's disease, stroke or mini-stroke, tumor
Fatigue	Anemia, cancer, chronic fatigue syndrome, depression, flu or other infectious disorders, heart disease, hepatitis, mononucleosis, premenstrual syndrome, respiratory disorders
Fever	Abscess, AIDS, appendicitis, cancer, infection (bacterial or viral), medication side effects, rheumatoid arthritis or other autoimmune diseases
Fainting	Anxiety, blood loss, cardiac arrhythmias, heart attack or other heart condition, hyperventilation, hypoglycemia, stroke
Gait changes	Arthritis, a back disorder, multiple sclerosis or other neuromuscular disorder, Parkinson's disease, stroke
Hallucinations	Alcoholism, drug reaction, fever, schizophrenia or other psychotic disorder
Hirsutism	Cancer, Cushing's syndrome, drug side effects, hormonal imbalances, polycystic ovaries or other ovarian disorder
Hoarseness	Anxiety, asthma, bronchitis, cancer, common cold, croup, polyps, smoking, thyroid deficiency
Impotence	Alcoholism, depression, diabetes, drug reaction, multiple sclerosis, hormonal abnormalities, a nerve disorder, surgery for prostate tumors or disease, a thyroid disorder
Insomnia	Alcohol and caffeine use, anxiety or depression, drug side effects, a thyroid disorder
Intestinal gas	Colic, colon cancer or other bowel disorder, diet, indigestion, a malabsorption syndrome
Itching	Allergies, chickenpox or other rash, dry skin, eczema, fungal or other infection, liver disease, stress, vaginitis
Jaundice	Anemia, blocked bile duct, cirrhosis, hepatitis or other liver disorder, gallbladder disease, a pancreatic disorder, infant prematurity
Loss of appetite	AIDS, anemia, cancer, depression, a digestive disorder, drug reaction, an eating disorder, infection, loss of taste
Mood changes	Alcohol or drug abuse, depression or other psychological disorder, drug reaction, a hormonal disorder, menopause, premenstrual syndrome, psychological stress
Nausea and vomiting	Alcohol abuse, appendicitis, brain injury, drug reaction, ear infection, gallbladder disease, food poisoning, gastritis, glaucoma, heart attack, hepatitis, indigestion, infection, intestinal obstruction Meniere's disease, morning sickness, motion sickness, ulcers, vertigo
Nightmares	Alcohol or drug abuse, anxiety, depression fever, posttraumatic stress syndrome
Numbness or tingling	Bell's palsy, carpal tunnel syndrome, a circulatory disorder, neuropathy, Raynaud's disease, shingles
Pain abdomen	Appendicitis, a digestive disorder, gallstones, hepatitis, intestinal disorders menstrual cramps, pelvic inflammatory disease, tubal pregnancy
Back	Arthritis, muscle spasms or strain, osteoporosis, ruptured disk
Chest	Angina, an esophageal disorder, heart attack, heartburn, pleurisy, peneumonia, pneumothorax
Ear	Infection, foreign body
Eye	Conjunctivitis, glaucoma, foreign body, iritis, sinus infection, injury, sty, tumors
Face	Bell's palsy, dental disease, headache, shingles, sinus infection, temporomandibular joint disorder
Foot	Arthritis, bunions, corns or calluses, gout, neuromas, warts
Generalized aches	Flu, lupus, mononucleosis, rheumatoid arthritis, shingles
Head	Brain tumor, migraine or other type of headache, muscle tension, sinusitis, stroke
Knee	Arthritis, chondromalacia patella, infection, Lyme disease, strain or

Contd...

Table 9.4: *Contd...*	
Signs or symptoms	*Possible causes*
Leg	A circulatory disorder, fracture, muscle injury, phlebitis, shin splints
Mouth	Canker sores, cold sores, dental cavities, gum disease, infection
Neck	Arthritis, meningitis, muscle injury slipped disk, stress
Joint/muscle throat	Arthritis, lupus, strain or sprain, tendonitis cold, flu, laryngitis, strep infection, tonsillitis, quinsy
Painful intercourse: **In males** **In females**	Penile warts, prostatic or urethral infection Menopausal dryness, vaginitis, premenstrual syndrome
Papitations	Anemia, anxiety, caffeine, heart disease, hypoglycemia, menopause, medications, premenstrual syndrome, a thyroid disorder
Rashes	Allergies, drug reactions, eczema, an infectious disease, lupus, rosacea, toxic shock syndrome
Runny nose seizures	Allergies, common cold, sinus infection Brain tumor, drug side effect, cerebral palsy, epilepsy, fever, head injury, hypoglycemia, toxemia of pregnancy, meningitis, poisoning
Speech problems	Alcohol abuse, Alzheimer's disease, Bell's palsy, multiple sclerosis, stroke, Parkinson's disease
Swallowing problems	Anxiety, diphtheria, an esophageal disorder, pharyngitis, strep throat, throat cancer, tonsillitis, quinsy
Sweating	Anxiety, drug reaction, fever, heart attack, infection, menopause, stress, a thyroid disorder
Swelling and lumps : **Abdominal**	Cancer, heart failure, hernias, internal bleeding, intestinal gas, kidney failure liver disease, pregnancy, uterine tumor
Breast generalized	Cancer, fibrocystic condition, mastitis Anaphylactic reaction, drug reaction, heart failure, kidney disease, phlebitis, a liver disorder, thyroid disease
Joints **Skin or body surface**	Arthritis, sprains Abscess, cysts or other benign growths cancer, edema, enlarged or obstructed lymph glands, ganglion, hives, infection moles, warts
Taste changes	Bell's palsy, cancer, drug reaction gum or dental disease, liver disease, loss of smell pregnancy, a salivary disorder
Thirst **Tinnitus** **(ringing in the ears)**	Diabetes, fever, heat exhaustion Brain injury or tumor, cold or flu, drug side effects, ear infection, exposure to loud noise, Meniere's disease, earwax build-up otosclerosis, vertigo
Tremor	Alcoholism, anxiety, Parkinson's disease, a thyroid disorder
Urinary problems **Discoloured urine**	Bladder or kidney infection, kidney stone, liver or gallbladder disease, urinary tract cancer
Incontinence	Aging, Alzheimer's disease, a bladder disorder, nerve deterioration, spinal injury, stoke
Urgency	Bladder infection, bladder tumor, diabetes, interstitial cystitis, drug reaction, pregnancy
Painful urination	Bladder infection, gonorrhea or other sexually transmitted disease, kidney infection, kidney or bladder stones, prostatitis, urethritis, vaginitis
Vaginal discharge	Cancer, cervicitis, gonorrhea, vaginitis pregnancy, premenstrual syndrome
Vision problems	Cataracts, detached retina, glaucoma, iritis, macular degeneration, mini-stroke, retinopathy
Weakness	Anemia, cancer, Guillain-Barre syndrome, heart disease, infection, liver disease, multiple sclerosis, muscular dystrophy, myasthenia gravis, rheumatoid arthritis
Weight changes: **Unexplained gain**	Heart failure, kidney disease, liver disease, medications, toxemia of pregnancy, underactive thyroid
Unexplained loss	AIDS, anemia, cancer, diabetes, an eating disorder, infection, an intestinal disorder, malabsorption syndrome, ulcers
Wheezing	Allergies, asthma, bronchitis, emphysema, heart failure, lung disorders

Common Signs and Symptoms

In medical terms, a sign is any visible indication of disease bleeding, a rash, or swelling, for example. A symptom is some thing you can feel, such as pain, fever or nausea, and it may not be accompanied by a physical change. Below are common signs and symptoms and their possible causes (Table 9.4).

Laboratory and other diagnostic studies are (See Chapter 23) a part of the information-gathering stage providing supportive evidence. These studies aid in the management, maintenance, and restoration of health. In reviewing and interpreting laboratory tests, it is important to remember that the origin of the test material does not always correlate to an organ or body system (e.g. a urine test to detect the presence of bilirubin and urobilinogen could indicate liver disease, biliary obstruction, or hemolytic disease). In some cases the results of a test are *nonspecific* because they only indicate a disorder or abnormality and do not indicate the location of the cause of the problem (e.g. an elevated erythrocyte sedimentation rate suggests the presence but not the location of an inflammatory process).

In evaluating laboratory tests, it is advisable to consider which medications (e.g. heparin, promethazine) are being administered to the client, including over-the-counter and herbal supplements (e.g. vitamin E), because these have the potential to alter, blur, or falsify results, creating a misleading diagnostic picture.

Documenting and Clustering the Data

Data gathered during the interview, the physical examination, and from other records/sources are organized and recorded in a concise systematic way and clustered into similar categories. Various formats have been used to accomplish this, including a review of body systems. This approach has been used by both medicine and nursing for many years, but was initially developed to aid the physician in making medical diagnoses. Currently nursing is developing and fine-tuning its own tools for recording and clustering data. Several nursing models available to guide data collection include Doenges and Moorhouse Diagnostic Divisions Gordon's Functional Health Patterns, and Guzzetta's Clinical Assessment Tool.

The use of a nursing model as a framework for data collection (rather than a body systems approach [assessing the heart, moving on to the lungs] or the commonly known head-to-toe approach) has the advantage of focusing data collection on the nurse's phenomena of concern – the human responses to health and illness. This facilitates the identification and validation of *nursing* diagnosis labels to describe the data accurately.

Assessment Tool for Adults

General Information

Name: ____

Age : _________________________________ DOB: ___________________ Gender: ___________________________

Race: _______________________________________ Admission date: _______________________________

Time: _______________________________________ From: ____

Source of information: ___________________________ Reliability (1-4 with 4 being very reliable: _______________

Activity/Rest
Subjective (Reports)

Occupation: ___________________________________ Usual activities: _______________________________

Leisure time activities/hobbies: ____

Limitations imposed by condition: ____

Sleep: Hours: _________________________ Naps: _________________________ Aids: ________________ Insomnia:

Related to: _________________________ Rested on awakening: ____________ Excessive grogginess: _____________

Feelings of boredom/dissatisfaction: ____

Circulation
Subjective (Reports)

History of: Hypertension: _________________ Heart trouble: _________________ Rheumatic fever: _____ Ankle/leg edema:

Phlebitis: _________________________ Slow healing: ____Claudication: ___Dysreflexia: _______________

Bleeding tendencies/episodes: ____

Palpitations: _________________________ Syncope: ____

Extremities: Numbness: _________________ Tingling: ____

Cough/hemoptysis: _________________ Change in frequency/amount of urine: _______________________

Objective (Exhibits)

Observed response to activity:

Cardiovascular: _________________________ Respiratory: _______________________________________

Mental status (e.g. withdrawn/lethargic): ____

Neuromuscular Assessment:

    Muscle mass/tone: _________________ Posture: _________________ ROM: _________________

    Strength: _________________ Tremors: _________________ Deformity: _________________

BP: R and L: Lying/sit/stand: _________________ Pulse pressure: _________________

Auscultatory gap: _________________

Pulses (palpation): _________________ Carotid: _________________ Temporal: _________________

Jugular: _________________ Femoral: _________________ Popliteal: _________________

Radial: _________________ Positibial: _________________ Dorsalis pedis: _________________

Heart sounds: _________________ Rate: _________________ Rhythm: _________________ Quality: _________________

Murmur: _________________ Vascular bit: _________________

Jugular vein distention (JVD): _________________

Breathe sounds: _________________

Extremities: Temperature: _________________ Color: _________________

Capillary refill: _________________ Homans' sign: _________________

Varicosities: _________________ Nail abnormalities: _________________

Edema: _________________

Distribution/quality of hair: _________________

Tropic skin changes: _________________

Color: General: _________________

    Mucous membranes: _________________ Lips: _________________

    Nail beds: _________________ Conjunctiva: _________________

    Sclera: _________________

Diaphoresis: _________________

Ego Integrity
Subjective (Reports)

Stress factors: _________________

Ways of handling stress: _________________

Financial concerns: _________________

Relationship status: _________________

Cultural factors/ethnic ties: _________________

Religion: _________________ Practicing: _________________

Lifestyle: _________________ Recent changes: _________________

Sense of connectedness/harmony with self: _________________

Feeling of: Helplessness: _________________

Hopelessness: _________________ Powerlessness: _________________

Elimination
Subjective (Reports)

Usual bowel pattern: _________________

Laxative use: _________________

Character of stool: _________________ Lat BM: _________________

Constipation: _________________ Diarrhea: _________________

History of bleeding: _________________ Hemorrhoids: _________________

Usual voiding pattern: _________________

Incontinent/when: _________________ Urgency: _________________

Frequency: _________________ Retention: _________________

Character of urine: _________________

Pain/burning/difficulty voiding: _________________

History of kidney/bladder disease: _________________

Diuretic use: _________________

Food/Fluid
Subjective (Reports)

Usual diet (type): _________________ Last meal/intake: _________________

Cultural/religious restrictions: _________________

Dietary pattern/content: B: _________________ L: _____________________ D: _____________________

Carbohydrate/protein/fat intake: g/d ____

Number of meals daily: ____

Vitamin/food supplement use: ____

Last meal/intake: ____

Loss of appetite: _______________________ Nausea/vomiting: ___________________________

Heartburn/indigestion: __________________ Related to: _______________________________

____ Relieved by: ______________________________

Food preferences: _______________________ Food prohibitions: _________________________

Allergy/food intolerance: ____

Objective (Exhibits)
Emotional status (check those that apply):

Clam: _____________________________ Anxious: _____________________ Angry: _____________________

   Withdrawn/Fearful: _________________ Irritable: ______________________________

   Restive: _________________________ Euphoric: _____________________________

Observed physiological response(s): ____

Changes in energy field: ____

   Temperature: ____________________ Color: ______________________________

   Distribution: ____________________ Movement: ___________________________

   Sounds: ____

Objective (Exhibits)

Abdomen: Tender: __________________ Soft/firm: ________________________________

   Palpable mass: __________________ Size/girth: ______________________________

   Bowel sounds: Local/type: ____

Hemorrhoids: _____________________ Stool guaiac: _____________________________

Bladder palpable: ____

Overflow voiding: ____

CVA tenderness: ____

Objective (Exhibits)

Current weight: __________________ Height: __________________________________

Body build: _____________________ Skin turgor: ______________________________

Mucous membranes: Moist/dry: ____

Breath sounds: Crackles: ____

Wheezes: ____

Edema: General: _______________ Dependent: ___________ Periorbital: _________ Ascites: _________________

Jugular vein distention (JVD): ____

Thyroid enlarged: ____

Condition of teeth/gums: ____

   Appearance of tongue: ____

   Mucous membranes: _______________ Halitosis: ___________________________

Mastication/swallowing problems: ____

   Dentures: ____

Usual weight: __________________ Changes in weight: _________________________

Diuretic use: ____

Hygiene
Subjective (Reports)

Activities of daily living: Independent/ dependent (level):

   Mobility: ________________ Feeding: __________________ Hygiene: _______________

   Dressing/grooming: ______________________ Toileting: _______________

Preferred time of personal care/bath: ____

Equipment/prosthetic devices required: ____

Assistance provided by: ____

Neurosensory
Subjective (Reports)
Fainting spells/dizziness: ____
Headaches: Location: _______________________________________ Frequency: _________________
Tingling/numbness/weakness (location): ____
Stroke/brain injury (residual effects): ____
Seizures: ___________________________________ Type: ________________ Aura: ______________
Frequency: _________________ Postictal state: ____
How controlled: ____
Eyes: Vision loss: ________________________________ Last exam: _________________________
    Glaucoma: ___________________________________ Cataract: _________________________
Ears: Hearing loss: _______________________________ Last exam: _________________________
Sense of smell: __________________________________ Epistaxis: __________________________

Pain/Discomfort
Subjective (Reports)
Primary focus: ____________________________ Location: _______________________________
Intensity (0-10 with 10 being most severe): ____
Frequency: ____________________________ Quality: __________________________________
Duration: ______________________________ Radiation: _______________________________
Precipitating/aggravating factors: ____
How relieved ____
Associated symptoms: ____
Effect on activities: ______________________________ Relationships: ______________________
Additional focus: ____
Bowel sounds: ____
Hernia/masses: __________________________________ Urine S/A or Chemstix: ______________
Serum glucose (Glucometer): ____

Objective (Exhibits)
General appearance: ____
Manner of dress: ____
Personal habits: ____
    Body odor: _____________________________________ Condition of scalp: _______________
    Condition of scalp: ______________________________ Presence of vermin: ______________

Objective (Exhibits)
Mental status (Note duration of change): ____
    Oriented/disoriented: Person: _
    Place: _________________________________ Time: ___________________ Situation: _________
Check all that apply:
    Alert: ___________________________________ Drowsy: ________________ Lethargic: _________
    Stuporous: _______________________________ Comatose: ______________________________
    Cooperative: _____________________________ Combative: _____________________________
    Delusions: _______________________________ Hallucinations: _________________________
    Affect (describe): ____
    Memory: Recent: __________________________ Remote: _______________________________
Glasses: ___________________________________ Contacts: _________________ Hearing aids: __________
Pupil: Shape: ______________________________ Size/reaction: R/L: _______________________
Facial droop: ______________________________ Swallowing: _____________________________

Hand grasp/release, R/L:
Deep tendon reflexes: ____
Posturing: _________________________________ Paralysis: ______________________________

Objective (Exhibits)

Facial grimacing: ____

Guarding affected area: ____

Emotional response: ____

Narrowed focus: ____

Change in blood pressure: ____ Pulse: ______________

Subjective (Reports)

Dyspnea/related to: ____

Cough/sputum: ____

History of bronchitis: ________________________________ Asthma: ______________________

    Emphysema: ______________ Tuberculosis: ______________________________________

    Recurrent pneumonia: ____

    Exposure to noxious fumes: ____

Smoker:____ Pack/day: ______________________

No, of pack years: ____

Use of respiratory aids: ___________________________ Oxygen: _________________________

Safety
Subjective (Reports)

Allergies/sensitivity: __________________________ Reaction: __________________________

Exposure to infectious diseases:____

Previous alteration of immune system: ____

  Cause: ____

History of sexually transmitted disease:

    Date/type: __________________________________ Testing: _______________________

    High-risk behaviors: ____

Blood transfusion/number: ________________________ When: _________________________

    Reaction: ___________________________________ Describe: _____________________

Geographic areas lived in/visited: ____

Seat belt/helmet use: ____

Workplace safety/health issues: ____

History of accidental injuries: ____

    Fractures/dislocations: ____

Arthritis/unstable joints: ____

Back problems: ____

Changes in moles:____________________________ Enlarged nodes: _____________________

Delayed healing: _____________________________ Cognitive limitations: __________________

Impaired vision/hearing:____

Prosthesis:________________________________ Ambulatory devices: ___________________

Objective (Exhibits)

Respiratory: ___________________________ Rate: _______________ Depth: ______________

Symmetry:____

Use of accessory must by: ____

Nasal flaring: ____

Fremitus: ____

Breath sounds: _________________________________ Egophony: _____________________

Cyanosis: ____

Clubbing of fingers: ____

Sputum characteristics:____

Mentation/restlessness: ____

Temperature:_____________________________ Diaphoresis: _________________________

Skin integrity: Scars: _______________________ Rashes: ____________________________

    Lacerations: ___________________________ Ulcerations: _________________________

Ecchymosis: _______________________   Blisters: _________________________________
Burns:(degree/percent): _______________   Drainage: ________________________________
Mark location of the above on diagram:
General strength: ____
  Muscle tone: ____
  Gait: _________________________________   ROM: _______________________________
  Paresthesia/paralysis: ____
Result of cultures: ____
  Immune system testing: ____
  Tuberculosis teaching: ____

Sexuality

Component of Ego Integrity and Social Interaction

Subjective (Reports)
Sexually active: ___________________________   Use of condoms: _____________________
Birth, control method: ____
Sexual concerns / difficulties: ____
Recent change in frequency / interest: ____

(i) Female
Subjective (Reports)
Age at menarche: __________________________   Length of cycle: _____________________
  Duration: _____________________________   Number of pads used/d: ________________
  Last menstrual period: ___________________   Pregnancy now: _____________________
Bleeding between periods: ____
Menopause: ______________________________   Vaginal lubrication: ________________
Vaginal discharge: ____
Surgeries: ____
Hormonal therapy/calcium use: ____
Practices breast self-exam: ____
  Last mammogram: _______________________   PAP smear: _________________________

(ii) Male
Subjective (Reports)
  Penile discharge:________________________   Prostrate disorder: __________________
  Circumcised: ______________ Vasectomy: _________   Practice self-exam: Breast: ___ Testicles: ___________
  Last proctoscopic/prostate exam: ____

SOCIAL INTERACTIONS
Subjective (Reports)
Marital status: ____________________________   Years in relationship: ______________
Living with: ______________________________   Concerns/stresses: _________________
Extended family: ____
Other support person(s):____
Role within family structure: ____
Perception of relationships with family members:_______________________________________
Ethnic affiliation: ____
Strength of ethnic identity: ____
Length in ethnic community (y/n):
Feelings of: Mistrust: _____________________   Rejection: _________________________
  Unhappiness: ____________________________   Loneliness/isolation: ________________
Problems related to illness/condition: ____
Problems with communication: ____

Objective (Exhibits)
Comfort level with subject matter: ____

Speech: Clear: ___________________________________ Slurred: _______________________________________
Unintelligible: _______________________________________ Aphasic: _______________________________________
Usual speech pattern/impairment: ____
Use of speech/communication aids: ____
Laryngectomy present: ____
Verbal/nonverbal communication with family / SOs: ____
Family interaction (behavioral) pattern: ____

Teaching / Learning

Objective (Exhibits)
Dominant language (specify): ____
  Second language: ____
  Literate: ___________________ Education level _______________________________________
  Learning disabilities: (specify): ____
  Cognitive limitations: ____
Where born: _______________________________ If immigrant how long in this country: _______________
Health and illness beliefs/practices (e.g. complementary therapies/customs): _______________________
Which family member makes health care decisions/is spokesperson: _________________________________
Presence of Advance Directives/Durable Medical Power of Attorney: _________________________________
Special health care concerns (e.g. impact of religious/cultural practice): ___________________________
Health goals: ____
Familial risk factors (indicate relationship):
  Diabetes: ___________________________ Thyroid (specify): _______________________________
  Tuberculosis: _________________________ Heart disease: _______________________________
  Strokes: _____________________________ High BP: _______________ Epilepsy: _______________
  Kidney disease: _______________________ Cancer: _______________________________
  Mental disease: _______________________ Other: _______________________________
Prescribed medications:
  Drug: _______________________________ Dose: _______________________________
  Times (circle last dose): ____
  Take regularly: _______________________ Purpose: _______________________________
  Side effect/problems: ____
Nonprescription drugs: OTC drugs:
  Herbal supplements (specify): ____
  Street drugs: _________________________ Tobacco: _______________________________
  Smokeless tobacco: ____
Alcohol (amount/frequency): ____
Admitting diagnosis per provider: ____
Reason for admission per client: ____
History of current complaint: ____
Client expectations of care: ____
Previous of failure to improve: ____
Surgeries: ____
Evidence of failure to improve: ____
Last complete physical exam: ____

Discharge Plan Considerations
DRG projected mean length of stay: ____
Date information obtained: ____
Anticipated date of discharge: ____
Resources available: Persons: ____
Financial: ___________________________ Community: _______________ Support groups: _______________
Socialization: ____
Areas that may require alteration/assistance: ____
Food preparation: _______________________________ Shopping: _______________________________

Transportation: ________________________________ Ambulation: ________________________________
Medication/IV therapy: ____
Treatments: ________________________________ Wound care: ________________________________
Supplies: ________________________________ Self-care (specify): ________________________________
Homemaker/maintenance (specify): ____
Physical layout of home (specify): ____
Anticipated changes in living situation after discharge: ________________________________
Living facility other than home (specify): ____
Referrals (date, source, services): ____
Social services: ____
Rehabilitation services: ____
Dietary: ________________________________ Home care: ________________________________
Resp/O_2: ________________________________ Equipment: ________________________________
Supplies: ________________________________ Other: ________________________________

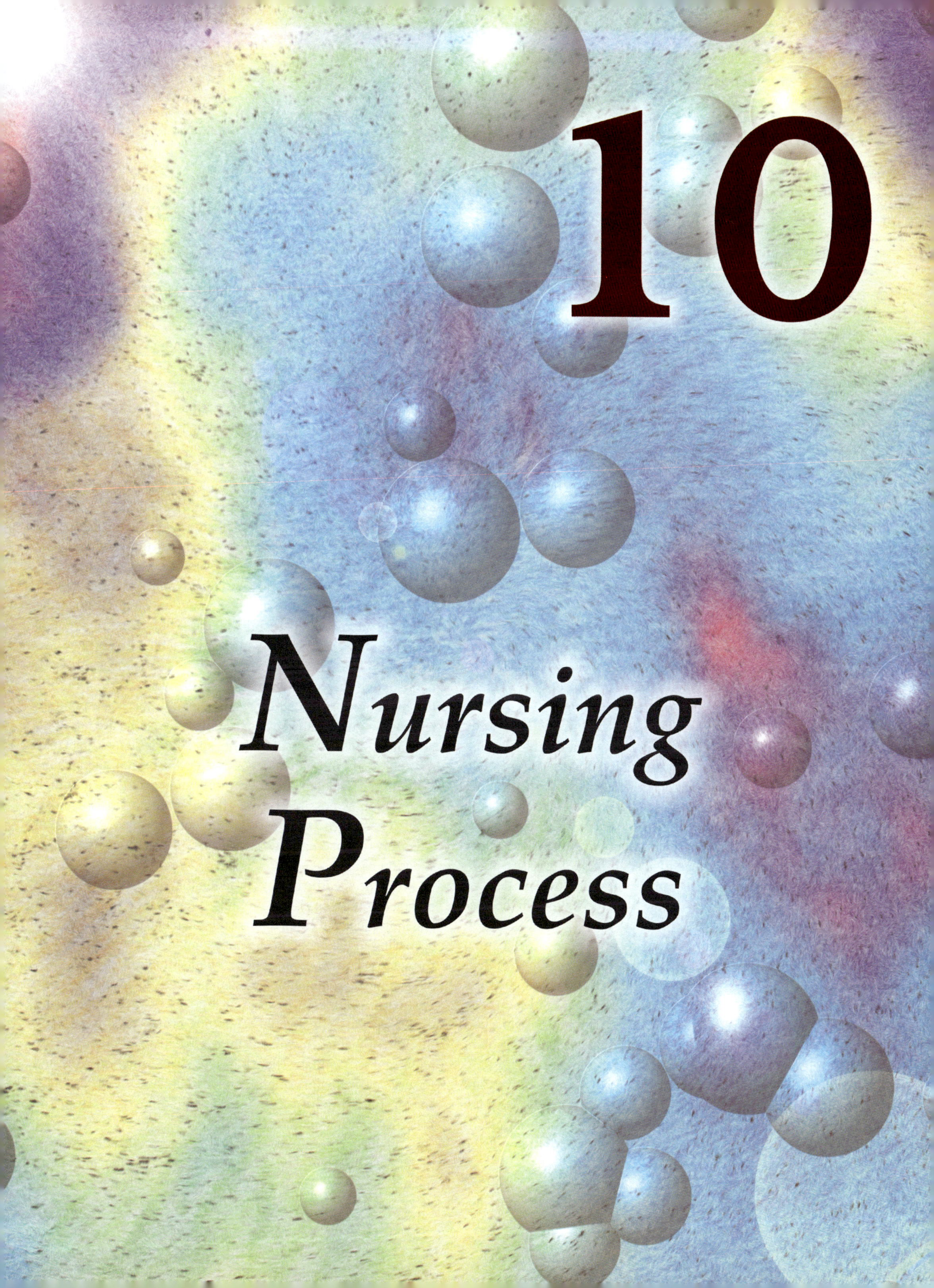
10
Nursing Process

Introduction

Nurses and health care consumers agree that nursing care is a key factor in achieving positive outcomes and enhancing client satisfaction. Nursing care is instrumental in all phases of acute care as well as in the maintenance of general well being (i.e. prevention of illness, rehabilitation and maximization of health), or where a return to health to health is not possible, the relief of pain and discomfort and a peaceful death. To this end, the nursing profession has identified a problem-solving process that "combines the most desirable elements of the art of nursing with the most relevant elements of systems theory, using the scientific method."

The original concept of assessment, planning, and evaluation based on the scientific method observing, measuring, gathering data and analyzing the findings. Over time, this process became part of the conceptual framework of all nursing curricula and is included in the legal definition of nursing in the nurse practice acts of most states. After years of study, use, and refinement, the three-step process was expanded. The five-steps are as follows:

1. Assessment (systematic collection of data relating to client and their problems/needs),
2. Problem identification (analysis and interpretation of data)
3. Planning (prioritizing needs, identifying goals and choosing solutions)
4. Implementation (putting the plan into action) and
5. Evaluation (assessing the effectiveness of the plan and changing the plan as indicated by current needs).

These are central to nursing actions and the delivery of high-quality, individualized client care in any setting.

When a client enters the health care system, the nurse uses the steps of the nursing process to work toward achieving the desired outcomes and goals identified for the client. The effectiveness of the plan of care is evaluated by ascertaining whether or not the desired outcomes and goals have been attained (clients problems/needs have been resolved) or whether problems remain at the tune if discharge. If problems are unresolved, plans need ot be made for further follow-up including assessment, additional problem/need identification, alteration of desired outcomes and goals, and/or changes of interventions in the next care settings.

Although some nurses view the nursing process as separate, progressive steps, in reality, the elements are interrelated. Together they form a continuous circle of thought and action throughout the clients contact with the health care system. The process combines all the skills of critical thinking and good nursing care because it created a method of active problem solving that is dynamic and cyclic. As we learn more abut diagnostic reasoning and critical thinking, some scholars are proposing a new model of describing what nurses do. With the emphasis on outcomes and new research into the nature of thinking and reasoning, the nursing process continues to be redefined.

Critical thinking is defined as the "intellectually disciplined process of activity and skillfully conceptualizing, applying, analyzing, synthesizing and evaluating information gathered from or generated by observations, experience, reflection, reasoning or communication, as a guide to belief and action". Critical thinking requires cognitive, psychomotor and affective skills to use the tools of a comprehensive knowledge base, the nursing process and established standards of care, as well as nursing research to analyze data and plan a course of action based on new insights and conclusions nursing practice, they are most evident when assessment data are analyzed to identify relevant information, make decisions about client needs and develop and individualized plan of fare. Therefore, client assessment is the foundation on which identification of individual needs, responses and problems is based. Nurses of the future will need to manage and interpret data and evaluate nursing activities and interventions. They will also need competencies in case and financial management, health are policy and economics, legislative outcomes and research methods. Additionally, they will need skills of delegation and the ability to think and reason across a diversity of settings in which they will practice.

To facilitate the steps of assessing and diagnosing in the nursing process and to aid in the critical thinking process, assessment database have been developed that use a nursing focus instead of the traditional medical approach of review of systems. To achieve this nursing focus, we have grouped the NANDA International nursing diagnoses into related categories titled Diagnostic Divisions which reflect a blending of theories, primarily Maslow's Hierarchy of Needs and a self-care philosophy. These divisions serve as the framework or outline for collection of data ad direct the nurse to the corresponding nursing diagnosis labels. Because these divisions are based on human responses/needs and are not specific "systems", data may be recorded in more than one area. For this reason, the nurse is encouraged to keep an open mind and to collect as much information as possible before choosing the nursing diagnosis label. The results (synthesis) of the collected data are written concisely (client diagnostic statements) to best reflect the clients situation.

From the specific data recorded in that database, the related/risk factors (etiology) and signs and symptoms can be identified, and individualized client diagnostic statement and be formulated according to the problem, etiology, and signs/symptoms (PES) format to accurately represent the clients situation. For example, the diagnostic statement may read: ineffective peripheral Tissue Perfusion related to decreased arterial flow, evidenced by decreased pulses, pale/cool feet, thick brittle nails, numbness/tingling of feet when walks ¼ mile. Objectives or outcomes are identified to facilitate choosing appropriate interventions and to serve as evaluators of both nursing care and client response. In addition to being measurable, outcomes also from the framework for documentation.

Nursing Interventions are designed to specify the action of the nurse, the client, and/or significant other(s).they are not all inclusive because such basic nursing actions as "bathe the client" or "notify the physician of change" have been omitted. It is expected that these actions are included in routine client care. Sometimes controversial issues or treatments are presented for the sake of information and/or because different therapies may be used in different care settings or geographic locations. Interventions need to promote the clients movement toward health and independence. This requires involvement of the client in his or her own care, including participation in decisions about the care activities and projected outcomes. This promotes client responsibility, negating the idea that health care providers control client's lives.

Critical Thinking

Nursing is an applied science and activity oriented. In which major part of nursing is about doing and relied emphasis on thinking. So nursing involves both thinking and doing. The scientific bases for providing health care changes daily. According to changes nurses have update their knowledge by adopting lifelong learning. It needs to develop critical thinking skills.

Critical thinking as the term is generally used, roughly means reasonable and effective thinking focused on deciding what to believe or do. Critical thinking is the disciplined, intellectual process of applying skillful reason as a guide to belief or actions; Critical thinking is careful and deliberate determination of whether to accept, reject or suspend judgment. Critical thinking is dynamic purposeful, analytical process that results in reasoned decisions and judgment; It is disciplined, self-directed, rational thinking than supports what we know and makes clear we do not know. So critical thinking is combination of reasoned thinking openness to alternative, ability to reflects, and desire to seek truth.

In nursing, critical thinking for clinical decision-making in the ability to think in a systematic and logical manner with openness to question and reflect on the reasoning process used to ensure safe nursing practice and quality of care. Critical thinking skills refer to the cognitive (intellectual) activities and processes used in complex thinking process such as problem solving and decision-making clinical reasoning.

- *Problem-solving:* Identifying a problem and finding reasonable solutions to it. Requires critical thinking skills such as organizing data, identifying relevant data and important data, making inferences, making decisions, projecting consequences of actions, and applying theoretical knowledge to a specific patient complex. The nursing process is a problem-solving process.
- *Decision-making:* Choosing the best action to take. In nursing this is usually the action likely to produce the desired patient outcomes. Requires thinking skills such as making judgment (e.g. about what is important) and making choices. Important in problem-solving; however, many decisions are made than are not related to problem-solving.
- *Clinical reasoning:* Reflective, concurrent, creative thinking about patients and patient care. Clinical reasoning is used in nursing process. Reasoning is logical thinking than links thoughts together to create meaning.

Nurses use complex critical-thinking process stated above to sum up the following are the few examples of critical thinking skills:

- Objectively gathering information on a problem or issue
- Recognizing the need of more information
- Recognizing gaps in ones own knowledge
- Listening carefully, reading thoughtfully
- Separating relevant from irrelevant data, important from unimportant data
- Organizing or grouping information in meaningful ways
- Making inferences (tentative conclusions) about the meaning of the information
- Integrating new information with prior knowledge
- Visualizing potential solutions to a problem
- Objectivity evaluating the likelihood that each potential solution will work
- Exploring the advantages, disadvantages and consequences of each potential action
- Evaluating the credibility and usefulness of sources of information.

Critical thinking needs to have something to think about and with one's knowledge base. Nurses use various kinds of knowledge as given below:

- **Theoretical knowledge:** Consists of information, facts, principles, and theories in nursing and related discipline (e.g. anatomy and Psychology). This kind of knowledge consists of research finding and rationally constructed explanation of the phenomena.
- **Practical knowledge:** Knowing what to do and how to do it consists of processes (e.g. decision-making process and nursing process) and procedures (e.g. how to give an injection or oxygen).
- **Personal knowledge:** That is self-understanding. To think critically the persons must be aware of their beliefs, values, cultural and religious biases, and so on. This helps to find errors in thinking and enable to tune into clients.
- **Ethical knowledge:** That is knowledge of obligation or right and wrong. Ethical knowledge consists of information about moral principles and processes for making moral decisions.

Evolution of the Nursing Process

In earlier days before the *nursing process* was developed, nurses tended to provide care that was based on medical orders written by physicians and focused on specific disease conditions rather than on the person being cared for. Nursing practice that was provided independently of the physician was often guided by intuition and experience rather than it scientific method.

In 1955, Lydia Hall originated the term *nursing process.* Since then, various nurses have described the process of nursing in different ways. Wiedenbach (1963) described three steps in nursing: Observation, ministration of help and validation. Later, Knowles (1967) suggested "five Ds" necessary for the practice of nursing: discover, delve, decide, do and discriminate. During the first two stages, the nurse collects data about the client. During the third stage, (decide), the nurse determines a plan of action; and during the fourth stage (do), the nurse implement the plan. In the fifth stage, (discriminate), the nurse assesses the clients reaction to the nursing actions.

In 1967, the Western Interstate Commission on Higher Education (WICHE) identified a nursing process with five steps; perception, communication, interpretation, intervention and evaluation. WICHE defined the nursing process as "the interrelationship between a patient and a nurse in a given setting; it incorporates the behaviors of patient and nurse and the resulting interaction". Also in same year, the nursing faculty of the catholic University of America proposed four components of the nursing process: assessment, planning, intervention and evaluation.

In 1973, the use of the nursing process in clinical practice gained additional legitimacy when the American Nurses Association (ANA) published *Standards of Nursing Practice,* which describes the five steps of the nursing process, assessing, diagnosing, planning, intervention and evaluation. Subsequently, a number of states revised their nurse practice acts to reflect these aspects of nursing.

As the nursing process developed both theoretically and clinically, the term *nursing diagnosis* gained considerable recognition in the nursing literature. The concept of a nursing diagnosis, as it evolved in the 1950s and 1960s, applied to the identification of client problems or needs. The term was not easily accepted, although many nursing authors regarded the nursing diagnosis as basic to professional nursing. Nearly a decade later, Bloch (1974) defined the terms that were crucial in nursing, an found that the term diagnosis – in relation to nursing practice – was still quite controversial.

In 1973, St. Louis University School of Nursing helped to form the first national conference on the classification of nursing diagnoses. The participants at this conference defined the nursing diagnosis as the "conclusion or judgment which occurs as a result of nursing assessment" (Gebbie and Lavin 1975). Subsequently, conferences have been held every two years and have gained support and interest. In 1982, the conference group accepted the name North American Nursing Diagnosis Association (NANDA), thus reorganizing the participation and contributions of Canadian nurses. This group has currently established and accepted about 100 diagnostic categories (NANDA 1990).

In 1980, ANA declared that "Nursing is the diagnosis and treatment of human responses to actual or potential health problems". Clearly, the ANA saw diagnosis as a nursing function even though it was not unusual of some people to believe diagnosis was the unusual for some people to believe diagnosis was the prerogative of the physician. In 1982, the National Council of State Boards of Nursing defined and described the five-step nursing process in terms of nursing behaviors: assessing, analyzing, planning, implementing and evaluating (National Council of State Boards of Nursing 1982). Table 10.1 lists some of the nurses and groups who contributed to the development of the nursing process and nursing diagnosis movements.

The "what" and "how" of the work of nursing have been explained in part in a number of existing publications that help operationalize the work of nursing. The ANA Social Policy Statement (1980) defined nursing as the "diagnosis and treatment of human responses to actual and potential health problems". It represents a framework for understanding nursing relationship with society and nursing obligations to those who receive nursing care. In 1991, the ANA *Standards of Clinical Nursing Practice* described the client care process and standards for professional performance, providing impetus and support for the use of nursing diagnosis in the practice setting. The work of NANDA International (formerly North American Nursing Diagnosis Association) has been ongoing for more than 25 years, beginning with efforts to identify client problems/needs for which nurses are accountable. NANDA continues to develop nursing diagnostic labels, which are now being complemented by the Lowa Intervention Project: Nursing Interventions Classification (NIC) and the Lowa Outcomes Project: Nursing Outcomes Classification (NOC). NIC directs our focus to the content and process of nursing care by identifying and standardizing the care activities nurses perform while NIC describes client outcomes that are responsive to nursing intervention and developing corresponding measurement scales.

Concepts of Nursing Process

The nursing process is a method used by nurses in solving patient problems in professional practice. It is an outgrown of scientific method and can be used as a framework for approaching almost any problem. Yura and Walsh (1983) defined nursing process as "a designated series of action intended to fulfill the purposes of nursing – to maintain the patients wellness and if this states changes, to provide the amount of quality of nursing care the situation demands to direct the patient back to wellness. They went on "if wellness cannot be achieved the purpose of the nursing process is to contribute to the patient quality of life, maximizing his source as long as life is a reality". Nursing is continuing to evolve into a well defined profession with a more clearly delineated definition and phenomena of concern. Fundamental philosophical beliefs and qualities have been identified that are important for the nurse to possess to provide quality care.

The nursing profession has developed a body of knowledge that contributes to the growth and well being of the individual and the community, the prevention of illness and the maintenance and/or restoration of health (or relief of pain/discomfort and provision of support when a return to health is not possible). The nursing process is the basis of all nursing actions and is the essence of nursing providing a flexible, orderly, logical problem-solving approach for administering nursing care so that client (whether individual, community, or population) needs for such care are met comprehensively and effectively. It can be applied in any health care or educational setting in any theoretical or conceptual framework, and within the context of any nursing philosophy. Each step of the nursing process builds on and interacts with the other steps, ensuring an effective practice model. Inclusion of the standards of clinical nursing practice

Nurse expert/Institutions	Contributions to nursing process
	Table 10.1: Evolution of the Nursing Process
Nurse expert/Institutions	*Contributions to nursing process*
Peplau H, 1952	Identified four phases in an interpersonal relationship orientation, identification, exploitation and resolution. The phases are sequential and focus on interpersonal therapeutic interaction
Hall L, 1955	Originated the term nursing process
Kreuter FR, 1957	Described steps in a nursing process as coordinating, planning, and evaluating nursing care and directing the family and the nursing auxiliary as they give nursing care. Theses were considered to promote the quality of professional practice
Johnson DE, 1959	Saw the nursing process as assessing situations, arriving at decisions, implementing a course of action designed to resolve nursing problems, and evaluating
Orlando IJ, 1961	Saw the nursing process as interactive stated that the process included three phases, clients behavior, reaction of the nurse, and nursing actions
Henderson V, 1965	Stated that the nursing process was the same as the steps of the scientific method
Wiedenbacch E, 1963, 1970	Introduced a three-step nursing process model: identify help needed, minister help, validate that help was given
Heidgerken L, 1965	Described steps of professional nursing care as evaluating behavior and situations recognizing physical symptoms; diagnosing, planning and meeting nursing needs, and coordinating the clients regimen through all stages of care
McCain RA, 1965	Was the first to use the term assessment in an article published and used the functional abilities of the client as the framework for assessment. Collected and recorded objective and subjective data in assessment
Knowles L, 1967	Introduced a process model called the "five Ds" discover, delve, decide, do and discriminate
WICHE, 1967	Listed the steps of the nursing process as perception and communication; interpretation; intervention and discrimination
Catholic University of America, 1967	Proposed four components of the nursing process; assessment, planning, intervention and evaluation (Yura and Walsh 1988,)
Orem C, 1971	Stated that there were three steps in nursing care: (a) initial and continuing determination of need for nursing care: (b) designing nursing actions for the client that will contribute to the clients achievement of health goals; and (c) the initiating conducting, and control of assisting actions
ANA Standards of Nursing Practice, 1973	Referred to a five-step process, assessing, diagnosing, planning, evaluation and intervention.
Bloch D, 1974	Suggested a five-step nursing process that similar to the four-step model: collection of data, definition of problem, planning of intervention, implementation of the intervention, and evaluating of the intervention
Gebbie K and Lavin MA, 1975	Initiated first national conference on the classification of nursing diagnosis in 1973, which led to the use of a five-step nursing process model; assessment, nursing diagnosis, planning, intervention a devaluation
Roy Sr. C, 1976	Used six-step nursing process: assessment of client behaviors, assessment of influencing factors problem identification, goal setting, intervention, and selection of approaches a devaluating. Advocated the use of the term nursing diagnosis

provides additional information to reinforce understanding and opportunities to apply knowledge.

The term 'client' is used in this title rather than patient to reflect the philosophy that the individuals or groups you work with are legitimate members of the decision-making process with some degree of control over the planned regimen and as able, active participants in the planning and implementation of their care.

Nursing is both a science and art concerned with the physical, psychological, sociological, cultural and spiritual concerns of the individual. The science of nursing is based on a broad theoretical framework; its art depends on the caring skills and abilities of individual nurse. The importance of the nurse within the health care system is being recognized in many positive ways, and the profession of nursing is itself acknowledging the needs for its practitioners to be professional and accountable.

Nursing leaders have identified a process than combines the most desirable elements of the art of nursing with the most relevant elements of systems theory, using the scientific method.

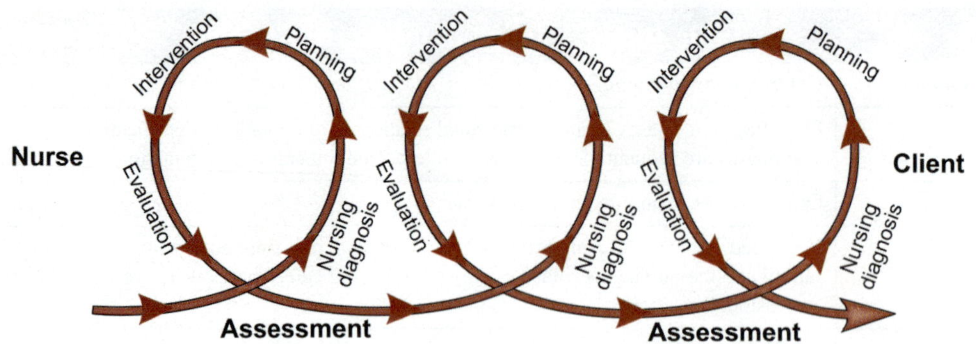

Figure 10.1: The nursing process

This process incorporates an interactive interpersonal approach with a problem solving and decision-making process.

The process is a series of steps or acts that lead to accomplishing some goal or purpose. According to Bevis "Processes have three characteristics:"

- Inherent purposes
- Internal organizations
- Infinite creativity

These characteristics have found in the nursing process. The nursing process is a systematic method of providing care to clients. The purpose is to provide individualized, holistic, effective client care efficiently. Although the steps of the nursing process build on each other, they are not linear. Each step overlaps (Fig. 10.1) with the previous or subsequent steps. The nursing process is dynamic and requires creativity in its application. The steps of the same for each client situation, but the correlation and results will be different. The nursing process can be used with clients of all ages and in any care setting.

"Nursing process is an orderly, systematic manner of determining the patients, problems, making plan to solve them, initiating the plan or assigning others to implement it, and evaluating the extent to which the plan was effective in resolving the problems identified" (Yura and Walsh 1978).

"The nursing process is a method of organizing and delivering nursing care to understand its functions, components and interactions, the nurse should have a working knowledge of the nature of the process. A process is series of steps or components leasing to achievement of a goal. The three characteristics of a process or purpose, organization and creativity" (Bevis 1978). Purpose is the goal or specific aim of the process. Organization is the series of steps or components needed to achieve the goal. Creativity is the process in a continuous progression from one point to another to achieve a specific goal.

In every discipline the process is used to their professional practice differently using various names. Nurses currently call this process the nursing process. Physicians call it patient evaluation and management, health planners all it health planning, researchers all it the research method and other disciplines call it problem-solving.

The science of nursing is based on a broad theoretical framework. The nursing process is the method by which this framework is applied to practice nursing. It is a deliberative problem-solving approach that requires cognitive, technical and interpersonal skills and is directed to meeting the needs of the patient.

The nursing process is one of the scientific methods used by the nursing personnel of modern era. It is a deliberate intellectual activity whereby the practice of nursing is approached in an orderly, systematic manner to patient care in a dynamic, continuous method to assist the patient to achieve and maintain health. It is basically a problem solving approach to nursing that involves interaction with the patient, making decisions, and carrying out nursing actions based on an assessment of an individual followed by an evaluation of the effectiveness of action. Therefore, nursing process can be applicable to any setting or system with any patient regardless of his/her place on the health illness continuum.

Health care workers use the process to focus on the individuals, others it to focus on family or a community.

Nature of Nursing Process

In the past, nurses prided themselves on comforting those, who are ill and on executing with precision such tasks as dressing wounds administering medications and bathing, feeding and ambulating client. Many of these tasks were ordered by doctors and few nurses would have characterized their 'job' on being independent, scientifically based or creative. Now health care delivery system has changed, and nursing has changed with it. Nurses now work with well and ill clients in all settings. In addition to their role as caregiver, nurses fill specialized roles as care managers – co-coordinators, teachers, counselors, advocates, nursing administrators, nurse-educators and nurse researchers. Nurses are responsible of a unique dimension of health care "the diagnosis and treatment of human responses to actual or potential health problems" and as such are knowledgeable, competent and independent professionals who work collaboratively with other health care professionals to design and deliver holistic care.

As the practice of nursing became more complex, nurses began to study the process of nursing to both understand and improve the means nurses used to accomplish their aims. It has been assumed that professional nursing practice is interpersonal in nature. Recognizing the importance and effect of the nurses relationships with the client/patient professional nurses use this knowledge throughout the nursing process. It is also assumed that professional nurses view human being as holistic, thereby acknowledging that mind and body are not separate but function as a whole. People respond as unique whole beings. What happens is one part of mind or body affects the person as a whole. These assumptions give clue that nursing is interpersonal in nature and the professional nurses view human beings as holistic, give guidance and directions to the use of the nursing process.

As stated earlier, "nursing is the diagnosis and treatment of human responses to actual or potential problems". The fundamental basis of nursing practice "Process". Every aspect of practice is affected by a understanding and utilization of nursing practice.

Nursing process is an organized approach to problem-solving and decision making that describes the intellectual activity of the nurse. It is the accepted methodology for nursing practice. The nursing process is the underlying scheme that provides order and direction of nursing care. It is the essence of profession – Nursing practice. It is the 'tool' and methodology of the nursing profession and as such it helps nurses in arriving at decisions and in predicting and evaluating consequences.

The nursing process is a "*deliberate, intellectual* activity by which the practice of nursing is approached in an orderly *systematic* manner. Each of these terms for defining the process can be further delineated as follows:

- 'Deliberate' refers to careful, thoughtful and intentional process
- 'Intellectual' refers to the process has rational, knowledgeable, reasonable and conceptional
- 'Activity' refers to state or condition of functioning, initiating, changing and behaving
- 'Orderly' refers to that it is methodological, efficient, and has logical arrangement
- 'Systematic' means to purposeful and pertaining to classification.

The nursing process is a method of making clinical decisions. It is a way of thinking and acting in relation to the clinical phenomena of concern to nurses. Classifically the nursing process comprises of five phases or dimensions: assessment, nursing diagnosis, planning, implementation and evaluation. The nursing process is a systematic decision-making model that is cyclic not lineal (Fig 10.1). By virtue of evaluational phase, the nursing process incorporates a feedback loop that maintains quality control of its decision-making outputs.

The nursing process is indeed a method of solving clinical problems but it is not merely a problem-solving method. Similar to a problem-solving method, the nursing process offers an organized, systematic, approach to clinical problems. Unlike a problem solving method, the nursing process is continuous, not episodic. The five phases constitute a continuous cycle throughout the nurse's moment-to-moment data interpretation and management of patient care. The phases of nursing process

being not only continuous, but "interactive" in other words, all phases of the nursing process operate and influence each other and the patient simultaneously. This illustrates interactive nature of the nursing process, wherein each phase represented by a line that intersects with others and converges at point in time to which the nurse attends.

The nursing process was developed as a specific method for applying a scientific approach or a problem-solving approach to nursing practice. Problem-solving approaches are not unique to nursing. For example, health planners have long used a health planning process that is a problem-solving approach aimed at planned social change. Physicians use a specific process for gathering assessment data to make a medical diagnosis. The nursing process deals with problem specific to nurses and their clients/patients. In nursing client/patient may be an individual, family or community and the nursing process has been adapted for use with each type of client/patient. Students of nursing using the nursing process are learning to behave as professional nurses in practice behave. Since the nursing process is the essence and tool (methodology) of professional nursing practice, student must become familiar with and adopt at using it as their basis of practice. The nursing process also provides, a means for evaluating the quality of nursing care given by nurses and assures their accountability and responsibility to the client/patient.

To use the nursing process effectively, nurses need to understand and apply appropriate concepts and theories from nursing, the theological, physical and behavioral sciences and the humanities. These concepts and theories provide a rationale for decision making, judgments, interpersonal relationships and actions. These concepts provide the framework for nursing care.

Definition of Nursing Process

The nursing process is often defined as the application of critical thinking to client-care activities. In addition, because nursing is a human-caring discipline, other styles of thinking influence nursing decision. Four ways of thinking which include ritual, random, appreciative, and critical thinking. Ritual thinking underlies the development of habits-actions we perform so often or regularly, that we do them automatically, without conscious decisions. Random thinking is the free association of ideas at the unconscious level that can lead to impulsive implementation of the first problem solving solution that comes in mind it comes to mind it can also be creating source of new problem solving ideas and approaches. Appreciative thinking reflects awareness of human values and respect for clients individual needs. Critical thinking is based on the scientific method, i.e. the deliberative and systematic use of rational informed thought processes in problem finding and problem solving. It is the key stone of sensible decision-making using the nursing process and it yields predictable, repeatable results.

The nursing process can be defined in terms of three major dimensions which include purpose, organization and properties.

Purpose

The primary purpose of the nursing process is to help manage each client care scientifically, holistically and creatively. To do this successfully the nurse needs many intellectual, technical and interpersonal and ethical/legal competencies as well as the willingness to use them creatively when working with the clients to promote wellness, to prevent disease, or illness, to restore health and to facilitate coping with altered functioning.

Organization

The nursing process has traditionally defined as a systematic method for assessing health status, diagnosing health care needs, formulating a plan of care, initiating and implementing plan and evaluating the effectiveness of plan of care. The nursing process consists of five sequential steps or inter-related phases, i.e. assessment, nursing diagnosis, planning, implementation and evaluation. These are considered as organized steps or components or nursing process.

Properties

The nursing process has seven properties, that is, systematic dynamic, interpersonal, flexible, theoretically-based, goal-oriented and universally applicable. Here the various words and phrases have been used to describe the nursing process.

1. *Systematic:* The nursing process is a systematic method that directs the nurse and client as together determine the need for nursing care, plan and implement the care and evaluate the results. The steps in this client-centred, goal-oriented process are interrelated each of the five steps preceding it. The process provides a framework that enables the nurse and client to do the following:
- Collect systematically clients data (assessing)
- Clearly identify client strengths and problem (diagnosis)
- Develop holistic plan of individualized care that specified the desired client goals and related outcomes and the nursing interventions most likely to assist the client to meet those expected outcomes (planning)
- Execute the plan of care (implementing)
- Evaluate the effectiveness of the plan of care in terms of the client goal and achievement (evaluation).
  The nursing process directs each step of nursing car in a sequential order/manner. So it is systematic.

2. *Dynamic:* The nursing process is dynamic, because it involves continuous change. It is an ongoing process focused on the changing responses of the client that are identified throughout the nurse-client relationship.

3. *Interpersonal:* The nursing process is interpersonal. Always at the heart of nursing is the human being. It is interactive because the interactive nature is based on the reciprocal relationship that occurs between the nurse and the client, family and other health professionals.

4. *Flexible:* The nursing process is flexible, because the flexibility of the process may be demonstrated in two contexts.
- It can be adapted to nursing practice and any setting or area of specialization dealing with individuals, groups or communities.
- Its phrases may be used sequentially and concurrently, i.e. the nursing process is most frequently used in sequence, however, the nurse may use more than one step at a time.

5. *Theoretically based:* The nursing process is theoretically based because the process is devised from a broad-based knowledge including the sciences and humanities and can be applied to any other theoretical models of nursing.

6. *Goal-oriented:* The nursing process is goal oriented because it offers a means for nurses and clients to work together to identify specific goal related to wellness promotion, disease and illness prevention, health restoration and coping with altered functioning, which are most important to client and to match them with appropriate nursing actions. Once these are recorded in the plan of care, each nurse can quickly determine the client's priorities and begins nursing with a clear sense of how to proceed. The client benefits from continuity of care and each nurse can move the client close to good achievement.

7. *Universally applicable:* The nursing process is universally applicable the one constant in health care is changed. Once nurses have a working knowledge of the nursing process, they find that they can practice nursing with well or ill persons, young or old, in any type of practice setting. Efforts made by the nurses to master nursing process will result in their possession of a valuable tool that can be used with ease in any nursing situation.

Advantages of the Nursing Process

The use of the nursing process has many advantages:
- The nursing process provide a framework for meeting the individual needs of the client, the clients family/significant other(s), and the community.
- The steps of the nursing process focus the nurses attention on the individual human responses of a client/group to a given health situation, resulting in a holistic plan of care addressing their specific needs.
- The nursing process provides an organized, systematic method of problem solving, which may minimize dangerous errors or omissions in care giving and avoid time-consuming repetition in care and documentation.
- The use of nursing process promotes the active involvement of the client in his or her own health care, enhancing consumer satisfaction. Such participation increases the clients sense of control over what is happening to him or her, stimulates problem-solving and promotes personal responsibility all of which strengthen the clients commitment to achieving identified goals.
- The use of the nursing process enables nurses to have more control over their own practice. This enhances the opportunity

for nurses to use their knowledge, expertise and intuition constructively and dynamically to increase the likelihood of a successful client outcome. This inturn promotes greater job satisfaction and professional growth.

- The use of the nursing process provides a common language for practice, unifying the nursing profession. Using a system that clearly communicates than plan of care to coworkers and clients enhances continuity of care, promotes achievement of client goals, provides a vehicle for evaluation and aids in the development of nursing standards. In addition, the structure of the process provides a format for documenting the clients response to all aspects of the planned care.
- The use of the nursing provides a means of assessing nursing economic contribution to client care. The nursing process supplies a vehicle for the quantitative and qualitative measurements of nursing care than meets the goal of cost effectiveness and still promotes holistic care.

Nursing Process and Philosophy of Nursing

Beliefs about nursing shape the way nurses practice. Consider the nature of nursing when it is based on a model of dependence on medical practice. Much of nursing as taught and practiced, is standardized according to medical diagnoses and supports medical intervention. The physician does the assessment needed for the medical diagnosis, and the planning is the basis for the medical orders. The focus of nursing is on supporting the medical regimen to cure the client's disease. In this model, the so called nursing knowledge is actually borrowed from medicine and includes detailed knowledge of pathopysiology, symptoms of disease, and standard medical interventions, as well as single "best" way to perform treatments and procedures.

In contrast, consider the nature of nursing when it is based on a model of autonomous professional practice. In an autonomous nursing model, the focus is on supporting the client to improve well being status and potential. *Nursing knowledge* includes detailed understanding of:

- The client as a whole person
- Health and the factors that promote health
- The environment and the mutual and ongoing interaction between environment and humans
- The purpose and functions of nursing.

The nurse does her own assessment of the client, gathering information about the clients well being status, including the:

1. Individual strengths as well as his weaknesses
2. Individual whole response to his health concerns
3. Individual analysis of the circumstances associated with his well being status
4. Individual knowledge related to health and well being
5. Individual beliefs and values about health
6. Individual life style
7. Individual health related goals
8. Individual support systems.

Because the nurses views the client as a whole person and views nursing and professional nurses as collaborative with other health care professions and providers, the nurse will also gather information about the regimens of the other providers, such as physicians, pharmacists, physical therapists and others. Understanding other regimens helps the nurse more fully appreciate the whole client, who is continually interacting with the whole environment. Understanding the impact of nursing, medical and other regimens on her client helps the nurse to assume mutual and equal responsibility for the health teams effectiveness in assisting the client to achieve his health goals. If a nurse practices from a belief in an autonomous model for nursing, she uses nursing knowledge in applying the nursing process and perceives herself to be both an independent and interdependent health care provider.

The model of nursing accepted by the practitioner can have a major impact on the knowledge needed and the nature of practice. Acceptance of the professional model mandates the acceptance of responsibility for nursing knowledge based on a rationale for practice. The nursing process provides a systematic approach to nursing practice. The logical elements of the process remain the same regardless of which framework or model is used to integrate theoretical formulations.

The nursing process has been defined as "a set of actions leading to a particular goal". All parts of the process are interrelated and influence the whole. The parts or phases of the nursing process occur sequentially, but they are not linear. Planning may lead to intervention, or evaluation during planning may result in more assessment. The nursing process viewed from an interactional perspective.

Nursing Paradigms and the Nursing Process

The central concepts of the discipline of nursing, regardless of the paradigm, or model that is used, are person, environment, health and nursing, the nursing process provides a logical way for the nurse to participate with the client in a purposeful way that reflects her analysis of the interrelationship among the concepts. These four concepts constitute the domain of nursing. The conceptual models present diverse views of the meaning and interrelationships of the four concepts of the discipline of nursing. It has been agreed that there is a more global perspective of a discipline within which conceptual structures develop. This more global perspective is referred to as the "paradigm for the discipline". The *paradigm* presents the major proposition on which the nursing model is founded. That proposition declares how the nurse will view man and health. The paradigm structure of nursing has been presented in at least three ways: Parses totality and simultaneously paradigms, Fawcett's growth and stability of change paradigms, and Newman, Sime and Corcoran-Perry particulate deterministic, interactive-integrative, and urinary transformative paradigms.

Parse (1987) asserted that the discipline of nursing now has two major paradigms from which conceptual models have emerged: totality and simultaneity. The totality paradigms major proposition is that "man, as a total summative organism whose nature is a combination of bio-psycholosocial spiritual features…..interacts with the environment to maintain balance and achieve goals". In this paradigm, nursing focuses on the wholeness of human beings and recognizes the continuous interaction of human with their environment; however, the analyses that take place regarding the human are organized around interrelated parts of the whole. The simultaneously paradigm major proposition is that "man is a unitary being in continuous mutual interrelationship with the environment and whose health is a negentropic unfolding" negentropic unfolding refers to constant exchanges of the energy that generate the ongoing life process. Within the simultaneity paradigm, "the goals of nursing…focus on quality of life from the person's perspective". Analyses are grounded in the human environment mutuality and in the equal responsibility of the nurse and client in the relationship. According to Parse the totality paradigm differs from the simultaneity paradigm in two ways that affect the nursing process (among other differences): its goals for nursing and its implications for practice, she states that the goals "focus on health promotion, care and cure of the sick and prevention of illness", and that the "prime decision maker…. is the nurse". The view of the client is focused on the interacting parts of the whole person. The major implication for practice in the totality model is that the nurse client relationship is primarily a problem solving one.

Newman, Sime and Corcoran-Perry (1991) propose three paradigms: the particulate-deterministic, the interactive-integrative, and the unitary-transformative. Believing that caring, health and health experience are concepts central to the discipline of nursing, they submit that "nursing is the study of caring in the human health experience". In the *particulate deterministic* view, human beings are viewed as isolatable, reducible entities with definite properties that can be measured. Change is the consequences of antecedent conditions, however, there can be control and prediction of the antecedent conditions in the change. Relationships are linear and casual. Caring is shown in the therapeutic interventions affecting a client's health, and the clients responds to these interventions in measurable responses. In the interactive-integrative view, human beings are perceived as multiple interrelated parts in relation to a specific context. Change is a function of multiple antecedent factors and probabilistic relationships. Relationships may be reciprocal. Caring is shown through the nurses interactive–integrative functions within a special relational context. In the unitary-transformative view, human beings are seen as unitary self-organizing fields embedded in larger self-organizing fields. Change is unidirectional and unpredictable as systems move through stages of organization and disorganization to more complex organizations. Relationships ad knowledge are personal, and patterns can be recognized in both. Caring is a unitary-transformative process of mutuality and creative unfolding.

Fawcett (1989) described how change and persistence can reflect different world views for nursing. It is the nature of the person- environment relationships that differentiates these two views. In the change view, the metaphor for the person-environment process in life is growth. Change is believed to be natural, inherent in living, and continuous. In the persistence view, the metaphor is stability. Stability, not change, is natural and normal; change occurs only for survival purposes. In the change view, progress and realization of potential are valued. In the persistence view, conservation is emphasized and solidarity is valued.

The way the nurse views the client, the client's environment, health and the purpose of nursing directs how she will implement the nursing process. Assessment, goals, and planned interventions are guided by the nurses understanding of both the cognitive and interpersonal aspects of the nursing process. This understanding is developed by integrating knowledge inherent in the conceptual model(s) in which the nurse has been educated.

Models derived from the change paradigm (the growth model of change) do not emphasize illness as the most significant factor with which the nurse is concerned. The direction of the nursing process is determined by the clients and the nurses view of the health situation and their belief in change. The nurse-client relationship focuses on the potential for growth. We believe that this paradigm guides the nurse to view the client predicament through the clients perceptions, and that change toward higher levels of wellness are achieved best by the nurse and the client mutually sharing the responsibility of the nursing process. Change is facilitated by the nurse focusing the client on his strengths. The plans for nursing care emerge from identifying strengths (abilities) rather than from identifying problems alone (the usual direction of the persistence paradigm). Nurses serve as facilitators of change.

Components of the Nursing Process

A process is a series of planned actions or operations directed toward a particular result. The nursing process is a systematic, rational method of planning and providing nursing care. Its goal is to identify a client health status, actual or potential health care problems to establish plans to meet the identified needs and to deliver specific nursing interventions to meet those needs. The nursing process is cyclical; that t is the components of the using process follow a logical sequence, but more than one component may be involved ay any on time (Fig. 10.2).

To carry out the nursing process most effectively and individualize approaches to each person's particular needs, the nurse must collaborate with the client. An individual, a family or a community may be considered a client. If the client is unable to take part in the planning and decision making process, a family member may be asked to participate on the clients behalf. Application of the nursing process requires that the nurse have a variety of skills, including interpersonal, technical and intellectual. Interpersonal skills include communicating, listening, conveying interest, compassion, knowledge and information, developing trust and obtaining data in a manner that enhance the individually of the client promotes the integrity of the family and contributes to the viability of the community.

Technical skills are manifested in the use of equipment and the performance of procedures. Intellectual skills required by a nurse include problem solving. Decision making is involved in every component of the nursing process.

The nursing process consists of a series of four or five components or steps. The four step process is assessing, planning, implementing and evaluating. In this system, diagnosing is included in the assessing phase. The five step nursing process is assessing, diagnosing, planning, implementing and evaluating. Some authorities believe the five step nursing process gives greater prominence to diagnosing than the four step process.

Both the four and five-step nursing process provide an organizational structure for achieving the goals of the process. In both nursing process, interaction between the client and the nurse is essential, as illustrated in Figure 10.2.

Nursing theorists may use different terms to describe these steps. In spite of these differences, the activities of the nurse using the process are similar. To avoid misunderstanding, nurses should be familiar with alternate terms that describe steps in process. For example, *nursing diagnosis* may be called analysis,

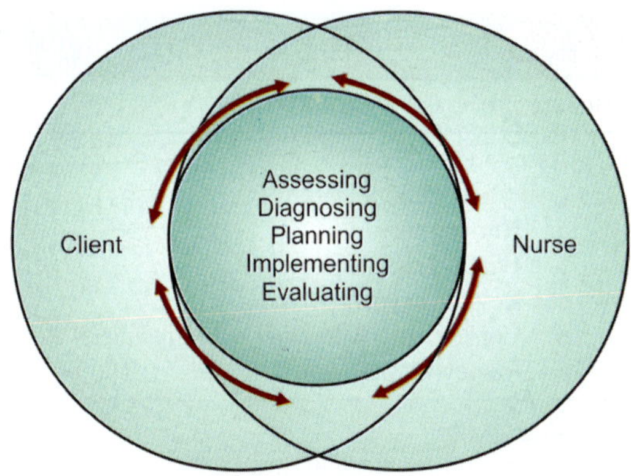

Figure 10.2: The interrelationship of the client, the nurse, and the nursing process

and *implementation (implementing)* may be called intervention or intervening.

An overview of the five-step nursing process may be found in Table 10.2. Each of the five components of the nursing process is discussed in depth in subsequent chapters of this unit.

Table 10.2: Purposes and Activities of the Nursing Process According to Components	
Component and purpose(s)	*Activities*
Assessing: To establish a database	Obtain health history Perform physical assessment Review records, i.e. laboratory records, other health care records Interview support persons Review literature Validate assessment data
Diagnosing: To identify the clients health care needs and to prepare diagnostic statements	Organize data Compare data against standards Cluster or group data (generate tentative hypotheses) Identify gaps and inconsistencies Determine the clients health problems, risks, and strengths Formulate nursing diagnosis statements
Planning: To identify the clients goals and appropriate nursing interventions	Set priorities in collaboration with client Write evaluation goals and outcome criteria in collaboration with client Select nursing strategies Consult other health personnel Write nursing orders Write nursing care plan
Implementing To carry out planned nursing interventions to help the client attain goals	Reassess client Update database Review and revise care plan Perform or delegate planned nursing interventions
Evaluating To determine the extent to which goals of nursing care have been achieved	Collect data about the clients response Compare the clients response to evaluation (outcome) criteria Analyze the reasons for the outcomes Modify the care plan

Table 10.3: Comparison of the Nursing Process and the Medical Process

Nursing process	Medical process

1. Assessing
Collection of data from:
  a. Nursing history
  b. Health examination
  c. Review of records
  d. Consultation with other team members
  e. Review of literature
	1. Assessing
	Collection of data from:
	  a. Medial history
	  b. Physical examination
	  c. Diagnostic tests
	  d. Review of literature

2. Diagnosing
  a. Analysis and synthesis of data
  b. Identification of the health problems
  c. Formulation of nursing diagnosis
	2. Medial diagnosis
	  a. Organization of data
	  b. Analysis and interpretation of the data
	  c. Formulation of a diagnosis

3. Planning
  a. Establishment of priorities
  b. Establishment of goals
  c. Development of objectives
  d. Written nursing care plan
  e. Delegation of nursing activities
	3. Medical planning
	  a. Establishment of priorities
	  b. Establishment of goals for therapy
	  c. Written plan of therapy

4. Implementing
  a. Preimplementation interventions
  b. Implementation
  c. Postimplementation strategies: update database, review, and revise care plan
	4. Therapy
	  a. Physician's orders
	  b. Medical therapy
	  c. Referrals

5. Evaluating
  a. Collection of data about the clients response
  b. Comparison of the data to the established objectives and goals
  c. Determination of the effectiveness of the nursing plan
  d. Analysis of variables affecting the outcomes
  e. Modification of the care plan
	5. Evaluating
	  a. Establishment of the effectiveness of the medical therapy in terms of the goals
	  b. Analysis of variables
	  c. Revision of the plan of therapy as necessary

The nursing process is an adaptation of problem-solving techniques and systems theory. It can be viewed as parallel to but separate form the medical process. Table 10.3 lists the two processes for comparison. The focus of the medical process examining, diagnosing, planning treating or curing disease processes, and evaluating the effectiveness of the treatment. The focus of the nursing process is gathering data, diagnosing (analyzing), planning, implementing, and evaluating the degree to which the client's goals have been met.

Generally medical diagnosis has four or five phases:

1. Suspected diagnosis following the patients initial complaint
2. Tentative diagnosis following the medical history
3. Provisional diagnosis following the physical examination
4. Definitive diagnosis following diagnostic tests
5. Anatomic diagnosis following a postmortem.

Both processes begin with data gathering and analysis and base action (interventions or treatment) on a problem statement (nursing diagnosis or medical diagnosis). Both processes include an evaluative component. Where the focus of the medical process is on the disease process, however, the nursing process is directed towards a client's response to illness.

The nurse can be highly creative when using nursing process. Nurse are not bound by standard response but may apply problem-solving skills, creativity, critical thinking, and their own knowledge and skills to assist clients. The nursing process is universally. It can be used with individuals of all ages, groups, and communities.

The five steps of nursing process are not discrete entities but overlapping, continuing subprocesses for example, assessing, the first step of the nursing process, may also be carried out during implementing and evaluating. Each step must be continually updated as the situation changes. Just as client's health, is never static but constantly changing. Nursing process, because it is responsive to the client's health, is also dynamic.

Each step or phase of the nursing process affects the others; they are closely interrelated. For example, if an inadequate database is used during assessment, the nursing diagnoses will be incomplete or incorrect; this will be reflected in the planning, implementing, and evaluating phases. Incomplete or incorrect assessment necessarily means equivocal evaluation because the nurse will have incomplete or incorrect criteria against which to evaluate changes in the effectiveness of intervention.

The nursing process individualized the approach to each client. In the assessment phase, data are collected to determine the habits, routines, and needs of the client. These data about normal health patterns of the client allow the nurse to write a care plan that incorporates these prior routines whenever possible. The nursing process is also interpersonal. To assure the delivery of quality nursing care, the nurse and client must share concerns and problems and participate in continuous evaluations of the plan. The success of the nursing process depends on open and meaningful communication and the development of rapport between the client and the characteristics of the nursing process.

Characteristics of the Nursing Process

- The system is open, flexible, and dynamic.
- It individualized the approach to each client's particular needs.
- It is planned.
- It is goal directed.
- It is flexible to meet the unique needs of client, family or community.
- It permits creativity for the nurse and client in devising ways to solve the stated health problem.
- It is interpersonal. It requires the nurse to communicate directly and consistently with clients to meet their needs.
- It is cyclical. Since all steps interrelated, there is no absolute beginning or end.
- It emphasizes feedback, which leads either to reassessment of the problem or to revision of the care plan.
- It is universally applicable. The nursing process is used as a framework for nursing are in all types of health care settings, with clients of all age groups.

Accountability and Nursing Process

Accountability: It is the condition of being answerable and responsible to someone for specific behaviors that are part of the nurse professional role. The nursing process provides a framework for accountability and responsibility in nursing and maximizes accountability and responsibility for standards of care. Nurses are accountable to the client (public), to their professional statutory nursing body, to colleagues, to the employing agency and to themselves. The nursing process provides a framework for accountability in all areas. The professional nurse is accountable for activities in all five phases of the nursing process.

Assessing: The nurse is accountable for collecting information, encouraging client participation and for judging the validity of the collected data. When assessing, the nurse is accountable for gaps in data or conflicting data, inaccurate data and biased data.

Diagnosing: During the second phase, nurse are accountable for the judgments made abut the client's health problems, i.e. the diagnostic statements. Is the health problem recognized by the client or only by the nurse? Did the nurse consider the clients values, beliefs and cultural practices when determining the health problems? When making judgments, nurses are accountable for considering a broad spectrum of client sociocultual backgrounds.

Planning: Accountability at the planning stage involves determining priorities, establishing client goals and objectives, predicting outcomes and planning nursing activities. Theses are all incorporated into a written nursing care plan available to all involved nurses. In this phase, nurses are also accountable for ensuring that the clients priorities are considered as well as the nurses.

Implementing: Nurses are accountable for all their actions in delivering nursing care. These actions may be performed directly or in collaboration with others, or they may be delegate to another. Even though a nurse delegates an activity to another person, the nurse is still accountable for the delegated action as well as for the act of delegating. The nurse should be able to give reasoned answers as to why the activity was delegated, why the person was chosen to perform the activity, and how the delegated action was arrived out. Nursing actions must be charged after being carried out, thereby providing a written record.

Evaluating: By establishing the degree to which the goals have been attained, the nurse is accountable of the success or failure of the nursing actions. The nurse must be able to explain why a client goal was not met and what phase or phase of the nursing process requires changing and why.

The nursing process provides the framework for nurses to help clients with their health needs and to produce a record of the actions and their effectiveness. The nursing process makes nurses responsible primarily to the client. An implicit part of applying the nursing process is having the knowledge and skills to make the required decision to implement the required nursing actions. Therefore, nurses are also accountable to themselves for heaving the knowledge and skills to use the nursing process in a specific situation.

The integrated use of cognitive, interpersonal and psychomotor skills in client care is basic to the practice of professional nursing. The nursing process provides a logical and rational way for the nurse to organize information so that the care given is appropriate and effective. Although the process is a scientific one, it is conducted by human beings who can carry it out in a sensitive and caring manner. Thus, the nursing process is both scientific and humane, just as nursing is perceived as both a science and an art. Torres (1986) states that "it is impossible to provide nursing care without processing knowledge in some way". Noting that theory is the knowledge or content for nursing practice, Torres also says that "process is the way of using that content".

Nursing process is defined as the method or operational procedure that the nurse uses to accomplish the specific result of maximal client well being. Nursing process is not the focus of nursing; it is simply a logical and dynamic method for practice.

Operationally, nursing process is the systematic:

1. Assessment of the clients health status
2. Specification of the clients strengths and problems
3. Determination of the nursing diagnosis
4. Development of a plan to maximize the clients strengths and resolve the problems ro reduce the concerns associated with the problems
5. Utilization of the nurse client relationship characterized by empathy, genuineness and respect to implement the plan
6. Engagement in an ongoing evaluation process to measure the effectiveness of the process.

It is a logical method in which the nurse sensitively and systematically approaches practice to achieve mutually determined health goals with the client.

Nursing Care and Nursing Process

Nursing leaders have identified a process that "combines the most desirable elements of the art of nursing with the most relevant elements of systems theory, using the scientific method". This nursing process incorporates an interactive/interpersonal approach with a problem-solving and decision-making process which serves as a framework for the delivery of nursing care.

As stated above, the concepts of nursing process was first introduced in the 1950s as a three-step process of assessment, planning and evaluation based on the scientific method of observing, measuring, gathering data and analyzing the findings. Years of study, use, and refinement have led nurses to expand the nursing process to five distinct steps that provide an efficient method of organizing thought processes for clinical decisions-making, problem-solving and delivery of higher quality, individualized client care. The nursing process now consists of:

- Assessment or the systematic collection of data relating to clients
- Diagnosis/need identification involving the analysis of collected data to identify the clients needs or problems
- Planning, which is a two part process of identifying goals and the clients desired outcomes to address the assessed health and wellness needs along with the selection of appropriate nursing interventions to assist the client in attaining the outcomes
- Implementation or putting the plan of care into action and
- Evaluation by determining the clients progress toward attaining the identified outcomes, and the clients response to and effectiveness of the selected nursing interventions for the purpose of altering the plan as indicated.

Because these five steps are central to nursing actions in any setting the nursing process is now included in the conceptual framework of nursing curricula and is accepted as part of the legal definition of nursing in the Nurse Practice Acts of most states.

When a client enters the health care system, whether as an inpatient, client outpatient or a home care client, the steps of the nursing process are set into motion. The nurse collets data, identifies client needs (nursing diagnoses), establishes goals, creates measurable outcomes and selects nursing interventions to assist the client in achieving theses outcomes and goals. Finally, after the interventions have been implemented the nurse evaluated the clients responses and the effectiveness of the plan of care in reaching the desired outcomes and goals to determine whether or not the needs or problem have been resolved and the client is ready to be discharged from the care setting. If the identified needs or problems remain unresolved, further assessment, additional nursing diagnoses, alteration of outcomes and goals, and/or changes of interventions are required.

Although nurses use the terms assessment, diagnosis/need identification, planning, implementation and evaluation as separate, progressive steps, in reality they are interrelated. Together these steps form a continuous circle of thought and action, which recycles throughout the client's contact with the health, care system and the nursing process used and the nursing diagnosis (the clinical judgment product of critical thinking). Based on this judgment, nursing interventions are selected and implemented. Now we will discuss the details of steps of Nursing Process.

Assessment

Assessment is the systematic gathering of information related to the physical, mental, spiritual, socio-economic and cultural states of an individual group or community although various definition exists, all definitions of assessment include from the following features:

- Collecting data—data collection form a variety of sources
- Using a systematic and ongoing process—data collection, verification, validation
- Categorizing the data—data organization and interpretation
- Recording data—documentation.

Hence assessment is the first in the nursing process, includes systematic collection, verification, organization and documentation of data. The completeness and correctness of this data relate directly to the accuracy of the steps than follow. Assessment steps involves – data collection, data validation, data organization, data interpretation and data documentation.

The purpose of assessment is to organize a data base regarding a client physical, psychosocial and emotional health so than health-promoting behavior and actual and/or potential health problems can be identified. The nurse ascertains the client, functional abilities, the absence or presence of dysfunction, normal activities of daily living and lifestyle patterns through assessment.

Assessment is the first phase of the nursing process. Data must be accurate and complete, because the remainder of the nursing process rests on this foundation of data. Assessment is related to other nursing process, steps are shown in Figure 10.1.

Identifying the clients strengths give the nurse information bout the abilities, behaviors ad skills the client can be during th treatment and recovery process. Assessment also provides an opportunity to form a therapeutic interpersonal relationship with the client. During assessment, the clients can discuss health concerns and goals with the nurse.

Types of Assessment

The information needed for assessment is usually determined by the health and setting and needs of the client. Three types of assessment are comprehensive, focused, and ongoing. A comprehensive assessment is must desirable when first determining a clients need for nursing care. Time limits or special circumstances may require an abbreviated data collection, as shown in a focused assessment. The assessment data base can then be broadened through ongoing assessment.

1. *Comprehensive assessment:* It provides baseline client data including a complete health history and current needs assessment. It is usually completed upon admission to a health care agency. Changes in the client's health status can be measured against this database. It should include assessment of the client's physical and psychological health. Perception of health, presence of health risk factors, and coping patterns.
2. *Focused assessment*: It is limited to potential health are risks, a particular need, or health care concern. They are not as detailed as comprehensive assessment and are often used when short stays are anticipated (e.g. outpatient surgery centers and emergency departments). In specialty areas such as mental health settings, labor and delivery or for screening for specific problems or risk factors (e.g. well-child clinics).
3. *Ongoing assessment*: When problems are identified during a comprehensive or focused assessment, follow-up is required. An **ongoing assessment** includes systematic monitoring of specific problems. This type of assessment broadens the database and allows the nurse to confirm the validity of data obtained during the initial assessment. Systematic monitoring allows the nurse to determine the client's response to nursing interventions and to identify any other problems.

Sources of Data Collection

Although data are collected from a variety of sources, the client is considered the **primary source** of data (the major provider of information about a client). As much information as possible should be gathered from the client, using both interview techniques and physical examination skills. Sources of data other than the client are considered **secondary sources** and include family member, other health care providers, and medical records.

Types of Data

Two types of information are collected through assessment; subjective and objective.

- **Subjective data** are data from the clients (sometimes family's) point of view and include perceptions, feelings and concerns. The primary method of collecting subjective data (also called symptoms) is the interview. The **health history,** a review of the clients functional health patterns prior to the current contact with the health care agency, provides much of the subjective data.
- **Objective data** (also called signs) are observable and measurable data that are obtained through both standard assessment techniques performed during the physical examination and the results of laboratory and diagnostic testing.

Validating the Data

Objective data may add to or validate subjective data. Validation is a critical step that prevents misunderstandings, omissions and incorrect inferences and conclusions. This process is particularly important if data sources are considered unreliable, such as when a client is confused or unable to communicate. If two sources provide conflicting data, further information or clarification must be sought. Findings should also be compared with norms, and grossly abnormal findings should be rechecked and confirmed.

Organizing the Data

Collected data must be organized so as to be useful to the health care professional collecting the data and to others involved in the clients care. After being organized into categories, the data are clustered into groups of related pieces. **Data clustering** is the process of putting data together in order to identify areas of the client's problems and strengths. Many health care agencies use an admission assessment format, which assists the nurse in collecting and organizing data.

An **assessment model** is a framework providing a systematic way to organize data. A few of the many assessment models available to nurses are described following:

1. **Hierarchy of needs:** Maslow's hierarchy of needs proposed that an individual basic needs (physiological) must be met before higher-level can be met. An initial assessment of all physiological needs followed by assessment of the higher-level is necessary when using this model.
2. **Body systems model:** The body systems model organizes data collection according to tissue and organ function in the various body systems (e.g. respiratory, cardiovascular, gastrointestinal). Physicians frequently use this model, so it is sometimes called the "medical model".
3. **Functional health patterns:** Gordon's Functional Health Patterns (Gordon 1998) provides a framework for data collection focusing on 11 functional health patterns. These functional health pattern areas cluster information about a clients habitual patterns and any recent changes to determine if the client's current response is functional or dysfunctional. For example, the elimination pattern is assessed for a client who now has diarrhea several times a week. Data collection would be focused on elimination habits, diet and fluid intake before the diarrhea began, and the effect of any changes on the client's functional ability and lifestyle.

The 11 patterns are:

- Health perception /health management pattern
- Nutritional/metabolic pattern
- Elimination pattern
- Activity/exercise pattern
- Cognitive/perceptual pattern
- Sleep/rest pattern
- Self-perception/self-concept pattern
- Role/relationship pattern
- Sexuality/reproductive pattern
- Coping/street-tolerance pattern
- Value/belief pattern (Gordon, 1998).

4. **Theory of self-care:** Orem (2001) developed the theory of self-care based on a client's ability to perform self-care activities. Self-care, learned behavior with deliberate actions responding to need, includes activities an individual performs to maintain health. This theory focuses on the assessment of the client's ability to meet self-care needs and identifying existing self-care deficits. The theory is primarily concerned with illness states.

The self-care essentials are:

- Maintenance of a sufficient intake of air
- Maintenance of a sufficient intake of water
- Maintenance of a sufficient intake of food
- Provision of care associated with elimination processes and excrements
- Maintenance of a balance between activity and rest
- Maintenance of a balance between solitude and social interaction
- Prevention of hazards to human life, human functioning, and human well-being
- Promotion of human functioning and development within social groups in accord with human potential, known human limitations, and the human desire to be normal (Orem 2001).

Interpreting the Data

After data have been collected, the nurse can begin developing impressions or inferences about the meaning of the data. Organizing data in clusters helps the nurse recognize patterns of response or behavior. When data are placed in clusters, the nurse can:

- Distinguish between relevant and irrelevant data
- Determine whether and where there are gaps in the data
- Identify patterns of cause and effect.

Documenting the Data

Assessment data must be recorded and some reported. The nurse must decide which data should be immediately reported to the head nurse and/or physician and which data can just be recorded. Data reflecting a significant change form the normal (e.g. BP 180/100, severe difficulty in breathing, or a high level of anxiety) would need to be reported as well as recorded. Data that need only be recorded include the fact that prescribed medication relieved a headache and that an abdominal dressing is dry and intact.

It is essential for accurate and complete recording of assessment data to communicate information to other health care team members. The basis of determining quality of care is documentation, which includes data to support identified problems.

As stated earlier is the first phase of the nursing process. It involves data collection and validation and is necessary before a nursing diagnosis can be made. "Assessment is part of each activity the nurse does for and with the patient". In effect, assessing, is a continuous process carried out during all phases of the nursing process. It may be used during the diagnosis phase to validate diagnoses. During the planning and implementing stages, data collection may be used before writing a nursing intervention or in obtaining information about a client's response to the nursing strategies. In the evaluation phase, assessment is done to determine the outcomes of the nursing strategies and to evaluate goal achievement. All phases of the nursing process depend on the accurate and completer collection of data (information).

The American Nurses Association states that nursing is "the diagnosis and treatment of human responses to actual or potential health problems". Thus the focus of assessment is to establish a database about client's response to health concerns or illness in order to determine the clients the nursing care needs. Client's responses include areas of daily living, health, and biophysical, emotional, socioeconomic, cultural and religious concerns. In contrast to other health professionals, the nurse is concerned with human needs that affect the total person rather than one problem or segment of need fulfillment.

A database (baseline data) is all the information about a client; it includes the nursing health history and physical assessment, results of laboratory and diagnostic tests, and material contributed by other health personnel. Data collection is the process of gathering information about a clients health status. It must be both systematic and continuous. Systematic collection can largely prevent the omission of significant data, and continuous data collection maintains the currency of the data, reflecting a clients changing health.

Assessing involves participation by both the client and the nurse. The nurse may be one or more individuals, a family, or even a community. Both the nurse and the client enter the relationship with specific knowledge and previous experiences that influence their perceptions and interpretations. It is important for nurses to be aware that their interpretations or assumptions may not be fact. For example, a nurse seeing a man holding his arm to his chest might assume that he is experiencing chest pain when in fact he has a painful hand. Another example of mistaking interpretation for fact is assuming that a client who states that her husband died three weeks ago feels sadness when in fact the death was a great relief.

This acceptance of assumptions as fact is called *premature closure*. To build an accurate database and avoid premature closure, nurses must validate assumptions regarding the clients physical or emotional behavior. In the first of the previous two examples, the nurse should question the client as to why he is holding his arm to his chest. The response of the client may validate the assumptions of the nurse or lead to further questioning. In the second example, the nurse should ask the client how she feels about her husbands death. Failure to validate or verify leads to the acceptance of assumptions as fact, and an inaccurate or incomplete nursing assessment, if the nursing process is to be a successful framework for nursing care, the information gathered during the assessment phase must be complete, factual, and accurate. To collect data accurately, nurses need to be aware of their own biases, values, and beliefs and separate fact from inference.

Assessment is the first phase in the nursing process and has two sub phases which include data collection and data analysis or synthesis. Assessment consists of the systematic and orderly collections and analysis of data about the health status of the client/patient for the purpose of making the nursing diagnosis. If incorrect or insufficient assessment leads to incorrect nursing diagnosis which could mean inappropriate planning, implementation, and evaluations. Therefore, the importance of accurate assessment cannot be over emphasized. It is vital to the process and is the basis for all other phases. Although assessment is the first phase, it may also occur as reassessment during any other phase of the process when new data are obtained.

The systematic and orderly collection of data is essential for the nurse to know if sufficient data have been collected. It also provides a method of quick retrieval of information about the client/patient for auditing professional practice and for doing research. In addition, it serves as a means of communicating information to their health care providers, assessing involves a thorough, ongoing, comprehensive collection, of subjective and objective data of the patient-family-environment, interactions. Such data are obtained via history-taking, observation, physical examination, laboratory data, X-rays, and other diagnostic studies. Use of *functional health* pattern assists in eliciting information concern in nursing. A holistic view during assessment phase ensures that the biological, psychological, social, cultural and spiritual spheres of the client are considered. Any assessment guidelines include the following:
* Biographical data
* A health history including family members
* Subjective data and objective data about current health status including physical examination and reason for contact with health care professional, medical diagnosis, if the client/patient has a medical problem, and results of diagnostic studies.
* Social, cultural, and environmental data
* Behaviors that may place a person at risk for potential disease/problems

By using these guidelines, the data collected are classified into discrete areas that can be compared, contrasted for relationships and clustered during the analysis of data. The current health status of the client is also ascertained through interviewing the client or the person responsible for the client (subjective data) and thorough examination and observation of the client to obtain that can be seen or measured objectively (objective data). For example, client's description of pain is considered subjective data, whereas vital signs are an example of objective measurement.

The standard of clinical nursing practice addresses the assessment process. The standard stipulates the data collection process is systematic and ongoing. The nurse collects client health data from the client, significant others, and health care providers when appropriate. The priority of the data collection activities is determined by the clients immediate condition or needs. Pertinent data are collected using appropriate assessment techniques and instruments. Relevant data are documented in a retrievable form.

The assessment step of the nursing process is focused on eliciting a profile of the client that allows the nurse to identify client problems or needs and corresponding nursing diagnoses, plan care, implement interventions, and evaluate outcomes. This profile, or *client database,* supplies a sense of the clients overall health status, providing a picture of the clients physical, psychological, sociocultural, spiritual, cognitive, and developmental levels; economic status, functioning abilities, and lifestyle. It is a combination of data gathered from the history-taking interview (a method of obtaining SUBJECTIVE information by talking with the client and/or significant other(s) and listening to their responses), the physical examination (a "hands-on" means of obtaining OBJECTIVE information), and data gathered from the results of laboratory/diagnostic studies. To be more specific, subjective data are what the client/significant others perceive and report, and objective data are what the nurse observes and gathers from other sources.

Assessment involves three basic activities:
* Systematically gathering data
* Organizing or clustering the data collected
* Documenting the data in a retrievable format.

By virtue of nursing unique orientation and commitment to holism, nurses collect an enormous amount of data about a patient's biopsychosocial health status. And by virtue of an array of techno-physiologic monitoring devices, nurses process and additional layer of data in the form of physiologic parameter measurements. Consequently, assembling this database, nurses need some place to file the information as it is collected. Ideally, this storage would contain compartments, whish could keep the data separated and organized. Such system is called as *assessment or organizational framework.*

Organizational framework can also serve as guides for assessment and their compartments consists of headings corresponding to the attributes the nurse accepts as constituting the nature of human health illness and nursing. In this way, framework helps guide the identification of diagnosis that are within the domain of nursing.

Assessment framework are neither new nor unique to nursing. Traditionally nursing used medical assessment framework for the collection and organization of data, but a nursing knowledge base and conceptual orientations become increasingly differentiated and complex, the biologic mechanistic scheme of medicine was found to be insufficiently comprehensive for its use by nurses as a tool for holistic assessment.

- The assessment framework for the generalist medical practice include body systems like cardiovascular, respiratory, neurologic, endocrine metabolic, hematopoietic, integumentory, gastrointestinal, genitourinary, reproductive and psychiatric.
- The functional health pattern typology developed by *Majority Gordon* are categories of human biologic, psychologic, developmental, cultural, social and spiritual assessment has gained wide acceptance in nursing service and education systems as assessing framework which includes:

1. Health perception – health management
2. Nutritional – metabolic
3. Eliminations.

And nine human responses revised by NANDA (1986) named NANDA (North America Nursing Diagnostic Association).

Taxonomy I (system of classification that organizes known phenomena into a hierarchic structure and helps direct the discovery of new phenomena). The specifications of a nomenclature and its successor, a taxonomy, is an important preliminary step in building nursing theory and science. The Nine human responses patterns of taxonomy I revised are as follows:

1. Exchanging: A human response pattern involving mutual giving and receiving.
2. Communicating: A human response pattern involving sending messages.
3. Relating: A human response pattern involving establishing bonds.
4. Valuing: A human response pattern involving the assigning of relative worth.
5. Choosing: A human response pattern involving selection of alternatives.
6. Moving: A human response pattern involving activities.
7. Perceiving: A human response pattern involving reception of information.
8. Knowing: A human response pattern involving the meaning associated with information.
9. Feeling: A human response pattern involving the subjective awareness of information.

The selection of any one framework over another, as long as it is designed to organize nursing data is an individual choice.

Methods of Data Collection

The major methods of collecting data are observing, interviewing, and examining. Although these nursing activities are often carried out during the implementing and evaluating phases of the nursing process, they are the main nursing activities during the assessing phase. During assessment, observation occurs whenever the nurse is in contact with the client or support persons. The primary interviewing process during the assessment phase is the nursing health history. Examining during the assessment phase is the major method used in the physical health assessment. Consulting, another nursing activity.

Observing

To *observe* is to gather data by using the five senses. Although nurses observe mainly through sight, all of the senses are engaged during careful observations. Observation has two aspects: (a) noticing the stimuli and (b) selecting, organizing, and interpreting the data, i.e. perceiving them. A nurse who observes that a client's face is flushed must relate that observation to, for example, body temperature, activity, environmental temperature, and blood pressure. Because observation involves selecting, organizing, and interpreting data, there is a possibility of error. For example, a nurse might not notice certain signs simply because they are unexpected in a certain client or situation or because they do not conform to preconceptions about a client's illness. Another source of error is faulty organization and misinterpretation of data. A nurse may interpret a clients wish not to talk as depression when in fact the clients is very tired.

Observation is a conscious, deliberate skill that is developed only through effort and with an organized approach. Nurses often need to focus in specific stimuli in a clinical situation; otherwise they are overwhelmed by a multitude of stimuli. Observing, therefore involves discriminating among stimuli, that is separating stimuli in a meaningful manner. Nursing observations must also be organized so that nothing significant is missed.

Health assessment is an integral part of holistic nursing. It provides the basis for nursing process. The nurse works in a variety of settings, seeking information about clients health status. The purposes of the health assessment are to:

- Establish a nurse-client relationship
- Gather data about the clients general health status, integrating physiologic, psychologic, cognitive, socio-cultural, developmental and spiritual dimensions
- Identify clients strengths
- Identify actual and potential health problems
- Establish a base for the nursing process.

There are two components of health assessment which includes health history and physical assessment.

Health History

Health history is a collection of subjective and objective data that provides a detailed profile of the client's health status. The subjective data are the symptoms which are indication of illness that are perceived by the patient or client for example (pain nausea feeling nervous, etc.) the objective data are ate signs of illness as perceived by ate examiner, i.e. doctor or nurse for example, rashes altered vital drainage. etc.

The nurse collects information thought interview with the client. An interview is planned communication. During the assessment, the nurse conducts the interview in a relaxed unhurried manner in a quiet private well lighted settings. To conduct an effective and informative interview the nurse must develop interviewing skills, gain the patients trust, and convey feelings of compassion whole remaining objective. The patient must feel the information being given is important to the nurse, the nurse must demonstrate and interest in the patients state of wellness. The nurse initially establishes trust by introducing himself or herself and asking what name the patient wishes to be called by and then using the name during the interview. An accepting posture in which the nurse is sitting in a relaxed manner at eye level with the patient, will foster trust. A pleasant facial expression will help and eye contacts make the patient feel he has the nurse's full attention. The nurse can enhance communication by using non-judgmental language. The tips of maintaining effective communication are as follows:

1. Promoting Effective Communication

Maintaining silence: Silence can help the nurse and patient to organize their thoughts. It also enables the nurse to observe the patient more closely.

Listening attentively: Attentive listening allows one to understand an entire message conveyed, verbally and non-verbally. It also facilitates trust.

Conveying acceptance: Acceptance means that one is non-judgmental. Acceptance is not synonymous with agreement; rather, it is a willingness to hear the persons message. One conveys acceptance through positive feedback and making sure verbal and non-verbal cues match.

Asking related questions: Questioning is a direct method of communicating. Asking related questions allows the patient to give information logically. Open-ended questions are useful for eliciting more information from the patient about a subject.

Paraphrasing: Paraphrasing sends feedback to tie patient that information has been accurately received.

Clarifying: Clarifying helps retain important information. Using examples can clarify abstract ideas. All clarification should be specific.

Focusing: When a discussion becomes vague or ill-defined, focusing directs conversation to a specific topic or issue. It limits the area of discussion to which the patient an respond. The nurse seeks meaning in the patients message.

Stating observation: Describing a patients observed behavior can provide feedback as to whether an intended message was received. It can clarify conflicts between verbal and non-verbal cues.

Offering information: Offering information provides a patient with relevant data and prevents one-sided conversations. It is useful for health teaching and helps in decision making.

Summarizing: Summarizing is a concise review of main ideas from a discussion. It sets the tone for interactions. By reviewing a conversation the participants can focus on key issues and any relevant information previously deleted.

2. Inhibiting Effective Communication

Giving an opinion: Giving an opinion takes decision making away from the patient. It inhibits spontaneity, stall problem solving and creates doubt. If offering suggestions, the nurse should stress that they are only options.

Offering false reassurance: Offering false reassurance can do more harm than good. False reassurance may allow the nurse to promise something that will not occur or is unrealistic.

Being defensive: Defensiveness in the face of criticism implies that the patient has no right to an opinion. The patients concerns often becomes ignored. Attentive listening helps the patient open up but does not imply agreement.

Showing approval or disapproval: Showing approval or disapproval is judgmental and may halt a conversation. It inhibits the patient's ability to share ideas and make decisions independently. Disapproval can indicate rejection.

Asking why: Asking why may imply an accusation. It can cause resentment, insecurity and mistrust. If additional information is needed, the nurse can phrase a question to avoid use of "why".

Changing the subject inappropriately: Changing the subject inappropriately is rude and shows a lack of empathy. It stalls communication. The patient may then give incomplete or inadequate information.

Forming communication barriers: Forming communication barriers by saying something inadvertently that blocks a patients communication can break down communication. By acknowledging the mistake, the nurse can start the communication process anew.

The health assessment interview also provides information about how the client perceives his or her health status or problems. Although you may not agree with the clients perceptions, it is important to understand these perceptions when planning nursing care.

Any uncertainty about the client's perceptions should be clarified during the interview. Communication techniques such as: direct questioning or reflecting, or restating the clients comments, may enhance understanding. For example, you can say, I am not understand. Did you mean…?

Interviewing

An interview is a planned communication or a conversation with a purpose. Some possible purposes are to gather data, to give information to identify problems of mutual concern, to evaluate change, to teach, to provide support and to provide counseling or therapy. Interviewing can be viewed as a process that is applied in most phases of the nursing process. One example of the interview is the nursing health history, which is the primary tool for data collection during the assessment phase of the nursing process.

There are two approaches to interviewing directive and nondirective. The direct interview is highly structured and elicits specific information. The nurse establishes the purposes of the interview and controls the interview, at least at the outset, by asking closed questions (see the next section) that call for a specific amount of data. The client responds to questions but may not heave an opportunity to ask questions or discuss concerns. Directive interview are frequently used to gather and to give information in a limited amount of time. During a nondirective or rapport building interview, the nurse allows the client to control the purpose, subject matter and pacing. Rapport is an understanding between two or more people. The nurse encourages communication by using open-ended questions and empathetic responses. Nondirective interviewing is used for problem solving counseling and performance appraisal.

A combination of directive and nondirective approaches is usually appropriate during the information gathering interview. The goals of the information gathering interview are to collect data and to begin to establish rapport. The nurse begins by using open ended questions to determine areas of concern for the client. As the interview evolves, the nurse may use closed questions to obtain needed data and to complete the nursing to obtain needed data and to complete the nursing health history. It has been suggest using as little authority or structure as possible to obtain the data within the allotted time frame.

When interviewing a client nurse has to ask many questions

Although there are many ways to categorize questions, in this usually they are classified as open-ended or closed, and neutral or leading. The type a nurse chooses depends on the needs of the client at the time. For example, the nurse asks closed questions in an emergency or other acute situation when information must be obtained quickly. Closed questions used in the directive interviewers, are restrictive and generally require only short answers giving specific information. Thus the amount of information gained is generally limited. Closed questions often begin with "when", "where", "who", "what", "do (did, does)", "is (are, was)", and sometimes "how". Examples of closed questions are: "What medication did you take?" "Are you having you pain now? Show me where it is". The highly stressed person and the person who has difficulty communicating will find closed questions easier to answer than open questions (Table 10.4).

Open-ended questions, associated with the non-directive interview, are ones that leas or invite clients to explore (elaborate, clarify, or illustrate) their thoughts or feelings. They allow clients the freedom to talk about what they wish. They also place responsibility on clients to explore and to understand themselves, in contrast to receiving advice frrom another. An open-ended question is broad, specifies only the topic to be discussed, and invites answers longer than one or two words. Such questions give the client the freedom to divulge only information he or she is ready to disclose. The response may also convey attitudes and beliefs the client holds. The chief disadvantage of the open-ended question is that the client may spend time conveying irrelevant information. However the open-ended question is useful at the beginning of an interview or to change topics.

Examples of open-ended questions are: "How have you been feeling lately?" "What brought you to the hospital?" How do you feel about coming to the hospital?" These questions or statements require more than a "yes" or "no" or other short, response, such as "yesterday" or "I don't know". They encourage clients to discover what their thoughts and feelings truly are. Such questions usually begin with "what" or "how".

The nurse often finds it necessary to use a combination of directive and indirective techniques throughout an interview to accomplish the goals of the interview and obtain needed information.

A client can answer a neutral question without direction or pressure from the nurse. Examples are: "How do you feel about that?" "Why do you think you had the operation?" A leading question directs the clients answer. Examples are: "You're stressed about surgery tomorrow aren't you?" "You don't think this illness is fair?" "You will take your medicine, won't you?" The leading question does not give the client an opportunity to decide if the answer is true or not. The interviewer suggests the expected answer by the way the question is asked. Leading questions create problems if the client, in an effort to please the nurse, gives inaccurate responses.

Information in the client database is obtained primarily from the client (who is the most important source) and than form family members/significant others (secondary sources), as appropriate, through conversation and by observation during a structured interview. Clearly the interview involves more than simply exchanging and processing data. Nonverbal communication is as important as the client's choice of words in providing the data. The ability to collect data that are meaningful to the client's health concerns depends heavily on the nurses knowledge base; the choice and sequence of questions; and the ability to give meaning to the clients responses, integrate the data gathered, and priorities the resulting information. Insight into the nature and behavior of the client is essential as well.

The nurse's initial responsibility is to observe, and record data without drawing conclusions or making judgment/assumptions. Personal self-awareness is a crucial factor in the interaction, because perceptions, judgments and assumptions can easily color the assessment findings unless they are recognized.

The quality of a history improves with experience with the interviewing process. Tips for obtaining a meaningful history include:

- Be a good listener
- Listen carefully and attentively for whole thoughts and ideas, not merely isolated facts
- Use skills of active listening, silence and acceptance to provide ample time for the person to respond. Be as objective as possible
- Identify only the clients and/or significant others contribution to the history.

Table 10.4: Selected Advantages and Disadvantages of Open and Closed Questions	
Advantages	*Disadvantages*
Open Questions	
1. They let the interviewee do the talking 2. The interviewer is able to listen and observe 3. They are easy to answer and non threatening 4. They reveal what the interviewee thinks is important 5. They may reveal the interviewees lack of information, misunderstanding of words, frame of reference, prejudice or stereotypes 6. They can provide information the interviewer may not ask for 7. They can reveal the interviewees degree of feeling about an issue 8. They can convey interest and trust because of the	1. They take more time 2. Only brief answers may be given 3. Valuable information may be withheld 4. They often elicit more information than necessary 5. Responses are difficult to document and require skill in recording 6. The interviewer requires skill in controlling an open-ended interview 7. Responses require psychologic insight and sensitivity from the interviewer
Closed Questions	
1. Questions and answers can be controlled more effectively 2. They require less effort from the interviewee 3. They may be less threatening, since they do not require explanation or justifications 4. They take less time 5. Information can be asked for before the information is volunteered 6. Responses are easily documented 7. They are easy to use and can be handled by unskilled interviewers	1. They may provide too little information and require follow-up questions 2. They may not reveal how the interviewee feels 3. They do not allow the interviewee to volunteer possibly valuable information 4. They may inhibit communication and convey lack of interest by the interviewee 5. The interviewer may dominate the interview with questions

The interview question is the major tool used to obtain information. How the question is phrased is a skill that is important in obtaining the desired results and getting the information necessary to make accurate nursing diagnoses. Note: Some questioning strategies to be avoided include closed-ended and leading questions, probing and agreeing or disagreeing that implies the client is "right" or "wrong". It is important to remember, too, that the client has the right to refuse to answer any question at all, no matter how reasonably phrased.

Nine effective data collection questioning techniques include:

- Open-ended questions allow the client maximum freedom to respond in his or her own way, impose no limitations on how the question may be answered, and can produce considerable information
- Hypothetical questions pose a situation and ask the client how it might be handled
- Reflecting or "mirroring responses" are useful techniques in getting at underlying meanings that might not be verbalized clearly
- Focusing consists of eye contact (within cultural limits) body posture, and verbal responses
- Giving broad openings encourages the client to take the initiative in what is to be discussed
- Offering general leads encourages the client to continue
- Exploring pursues a topic in more depth
- Verbalizing the implied give voice to what has been suggested
- Encouraging evaluation helps the client to consider the quality of his or her own experiences.

The client's medial diagnosis can provide a starting point for gathering data. Knowledge of the anatomy and physiology of the specific disease process/severity of condition also helps in choosing and prioritizing specific portions of the assessment. For example, when examining a client with severe chest pain, it may be wise to evaluate the pain and the cardiovascular system in a focused assessment before addressing other areas, possibly at a late time. Likewise, the duration and length of any assessment depend on circumstances such as the condition of the client and the urgency of the situation.

The data collected about the client and/or significant others contain a vast amount of information, some of which may be repetitious. However, some of it will be valuable for eliciting information that was not recalled or volunteered previously. Enough material needs to be noted in the history so that a complete picture is presented, and yet not so much that the information will not be read or used.

Planning the Interview and Setting

It is important to plan an interview beginning it. The nurse reviews what information is already available such as a postoperative record, information about the current illness, or literature about the client's health problem. The nurse also reviews the data collection form to make sure that the data to be collected are really needed and will serve some purpose related to the clients care. If a form is not available, most nurses prepare an interview guide to remember areas of information and determine what questions to ask. The guide includes a list of topics and subtopic rather than a series of questions.

Each interview and its setting is influenced by time, place and seating arrangement. In all instances, the clients should be made to feel comfortable and unhurried. Interviews with clients need to be scheduled for a time when the client is physically comfortable and free of pain and when interruptions by friends, family and other health professional are absent and minimal. The place of the interview must have adequate privacy to promote communication. A room that is relatively free of noise, movements, and interruptions encourages communication. A seating arrangement in which the parties sit on two chairs placed at right angles to a desk or table or a few feet apart with no table between creates a less formal atmosphere and the nurse and client tend to feel on equal terms. Avoid a superior or head-of-the-table position.

Most people feel uncomfortable when talking to someone who is too close or too far away. Generally, people feel comfortable 3 to 4 ft apart during an interview. A distance of 5 to 6 ft encourages a client to talk longer. Height also affects communication. By standing and looking down at a client, the nurse may intimidate the client. The client may perceive the nurse who stands during an interview as having greater status.

Stages of an interview: An interview has three major stages; the opening or introduction, body or development, and the closing.

The opening: The opening can be the most important part of the interview since what is said and done at that time sets the tone for the remainder of the interview. An inadequate opening can be misleading and create problems during and following the interviews. The opening is two-process: establishing rapport and orienting the interviewee. Either step can come first depending on the situation, the relationship between the two parties, or the interviewer's choice. The rapport and orientation stages may occur at the same time as they are often indistinguishable.

Establishing rapports is process of creating good will and trust. It can begin with a greeting or self-introduction accompanied by non-verbal gestures such as a smile, a handshake, and a friendly manner. Next the rapport stage is developed by asking questions about the person and proceeding with some small talk about the weather, sports, families, and the like. The nurse must be careful nit to overdo this stage since too much superficial talk can arouse anxiety about what is to follow and may appear insincere.

The orientation steps consist of explaining the purpose and nature of the interview, e.g. what information is needed, how long it will take, and what it expected of the client. For instant, the nurse might state that the client has the right not to provide data or might tell the client how the information will be used.

The body: In the body of the interview, the client communicates what he or she thinks, feels, knows and perceives in response to questions from the nurse. Transition from the opening stage to this stage can often be facilitated by the use of an open-ended question that is related to the stated purpose, is easy to answer, and does not embarrass or place stress on the person. For example, "what brought you to the hospital today?"

Effective development of the interview demands that the nurse use communication techniques that make both parties feel comfortable and serve the purpose of the interview.

The closing: The interview is usually terminated by the nurse, although in some cases the client terminates it. Nurses normally terminate interviews when they have obtained the information they need. Clients terminate interviews when they decide not to give any more information or are unable to offer more information for some other reason – fatigue, for example, the closing is important in maintaining the rapport and trust established during the interview and in facilitating future interactions. The following ways are commonly used to close and an interview.

1. Signal that the interview is coming to an end by offering to answer questions. Be sure to allow time for the person to answer, or the offer will be regarded as insincere.
2. Declare completion of the purpose or task by saying, "Well, that's about all I need to know for now" or "Well, those are all the questions I have for now". Preceding a remark with the word well generally signals that the end of the interaction is near.
3. State appreciation or satisfaction about what was accomplished: "Well – those are all the questions I have. I really enjoyed meeting you and I think we accomplished a great deal".
4. Express concern for the person's welfare and future: "I hope all goes well for you. If you run into additional problems, be sure to get in touch with me".
5. Plan for the next meeting, if there is to be one. Include the day, time, place, topic and purpose.
6. Reveal what will happen next. For example: "I will be responsible for giving you care each Monday, Tuesday and Wednesday between eight 0' clock and noon while you are here. At those times, we can adjust you if we need to".
7. Signal that the time is up if a time limit was agreed upon or explain why the interview must close at that time: "Well, I see our time is up; I'm sorry, but we're going to have to end our discussion.
8. Provide a summary to verify accuracy and agreement. Summarizing serves several purposes: it helps to terminate the interview, it reassures the client that the nurse has listened, it checks the accuracy of the schedule.

The Interview Proceses

The health assessment interview may be formal and structured to collect a wide range of information or informal and focused on a specific area of concern. In a formal interview, your primary concern is to establish a comprehensive data base. In an informal interview, you may discuss specific questions with the client while giving nursing care. Assessment through interviewing and questioning should be continuous, ongoing process lasting as long as you and the client interact.

The health care setting may influence the choice of interview topics. In well-child clinics, for example, the interview usually focuses on routine health practices, nutrition and normal growth and development, whereas in the intensive care unit, data collection focuses on physiological or psychological stability and on maintaining vital functions.

Three interrelated phases constitute an effective interview; the introductory phase, working phase and the termination phase.

A. *The Introductory Phase*

The introductory phase sets the tone and direction of the interview and establishes a mutual understanding of the purpose of the exchange. The purpose of the introductory phase are as follows:

(i) *Establishing rapport:* Establishing rapport begins with demonstrating respect for the client as a person with problems, rather than regarding the person as a problem to be solved.

You should demonstrate respect at the beginning of the interview by extending a cardial greeting, addressing the client by name and then introducing yourself by name. You should not address an adult client with his or her first name unless invited. Offering to shake hands is one way of demonstrating warmth and acceptance.

Non-verbal behaviors, especially on your part, may also help build rapport. Mutual respect best can be express when you and the client face each other and maintain eye contact. If possible you should avoid standing over the person, because this may be intimidating. Of course, such a position may be appropriate if your are informally interviewing the person while providing care. If the interview is conducted at the bedside, you should sit beside the bed with the siderail down, leaning slightly toward the person. Non-verbal behaviors such as expressions of disgust, boredom, or impatience may interfere with establishing rapport or may imply lack of interest.

Beginning the interview with a brief, casual conversation that focuses on the client may help dispel tension or awkwardness. If your comments are predominantly self-center, the person may feel neglected or unimportant.

(ii) *Ensuring Comfort:* If possible, you should conduct the interview in a private setting, free from interruptions. When privacy is difficult to maintain, such as in acute care settings, you can at least close the door or wait until other people have left the room before initiating the interview. Pulling the curtains or moving to the corner of the room also helps to promote a sense of privacy, even though these gestures may not necessarily prevent others from hearing what is said.

It is also helpful to demonstrate concern about physical comfort by asking how the clients is feeling, whether he or she is comfortable or needs to use the bathroom before proceeding. If the client is in pain or is fatigued, consider postponing the interview.

Clinical guidelines for communicating during an interview are:
- Listen attentively, using all your sense, and speak slowly and clearly
- Use language the client understands and clarify points that are no understood, for instance, by asking the person to describe what a word means to him or her
- Plan questions to follow a logical sequence
- Ask only one question at a time. Double questions limit the client to one choice and may confuse both the nurse and the client
- Allow the client the opportunity to look at things the way they appear to him or her not the way they appear to the nurse or someone else
- Do not impose your values on the client
- Avoid using personal examples, such as saying, "If I were you....."
- Nonverbally convey respect, concern, interest and acceptance
- Use and accept silence to help the client search for more thoughts or to organize them
- Use eye contact and be calm unhurried and sympathetic

(iii) *Defining expectations:* It is important to clarify what both you and the client expect from the interview and to establish an agreement about the rules and norms of the interview. This process is known as *CONTRACTING.* You should explain how discussing the person's health concerns will help in planning nursing care and encourage the person to participate in the interview. The client who answers questions, responds honestly, and shares relevant personal information is most likely to benefit from the health assessment interview.

In addition, you should inform the client about other professionals who will see the written account of the interview and the way in which the information will be used. To ensure confidentiality, you should ask if the client does not want certain information recorded.

You may also discuss the length of time the interview will run and the possibility that future sessions may be needed. Finally, you and the client should discuss decision-making. For example, if you intend to make some decisions for the client, the client should be so informed. If you intend to encourage the client to make his or her own decisions, the client should be made aware of the expectation.

B. *The Working Phase*

During the working phase of the interview, which is the most time-consuming phase, you should collect data that are pertinent to the clients overall health status. Such information will be invaluable in forming an appropriate care plan. Both verbal responses and non-verbal behavior should be recorded. The purposes of the working phase are:
- To collect the biographic data
- To collect data pertinent to the clients health status
- To identify and respond to the clients needs.

The structured interview: A structured interview may be used to facilitate data collection during the working phase. Familiarity with the forms before the interview will enable you to concentrate on the clients responses. Formats for structured interviews vary. Traditionally, nurses have followed a medical model in conducting health assessment interviews. However, nursing models are not being used in many settings. The structured interview usually begins with biographic information including name, age and birth date, sex, address, birth place, marital status, and occupation. Although asking about previously recorded biographic information is unnecessary, you should always review such data, because it is relevant to the persons social identify and self concept.

The next portion of the structured interview concentrates on determining the persons functional status, (subsequent chapters discuss specific interview guidelines for each functional area). You can proceed smoothly from on topic to the next by using transitional phrases such as "Now I'd like to discuss how you feel about your sleep habits", or "Now I'd like to ask some questions about your bowel and bladder functions".

The structural interview should proceed from general to specific. Gather general biographic information and data pertaining to health perceptions before discussing sexuality, personal values and relationships. You must establish trust and rapport before discussing intimate topics.

If the client is reluctant to discuss specific topics, you should provide an opportunity to talk about what he or she feels most important. Use broad opening statements, such as, "Why don't you begin by telling me what brings you here", or "What troubling you today?" Once the client has expressed immediate concerns, he or she is more like lot discuss other subjects.

You should view the structured interview as a guide rather than a rigid series of questions that must be asked in a set orders. Excessive questioning may undermine rapport, inhibit responses, and encourage the client to assume a passive role, merely answering questions. Applying principles of therapeutic communication rather than direct questioning may results a more productive interview, as is discussed in more detail the next section. Such techniques encourage free expression about the topics raised.

Communication is also enhanced when both you and the client speak the same 'language'. The terminology you use should be simple and appropriate and not based on medical jargon. When necessary, definite terms and structure questions to allow time for the client to respond thoughtfully and meaningfully.

C. *The Termination Phase*

The termination phase serves to end the interview. Saying how long interview will last at the beginning will prevent the client experiencing a sense of premature closure at the end of the interview.

Presummary, summary and follow-up techniques may help incorporated into the termination phase. Presummary involved providing cues to indicate that the interview is coming to an end. For example, you could say, "I see that we only have minutes left. Is there anything else you would like to discuss before our time is up?" or "There are three more questions I like to as". Planning additional interview sessions may be necessary if all topics have not been adequately discussed.

Next, a brief summary of the points covered will allow both you and the client a chance to validate perceptions. Specify plans for follow-up or additional interviewing are discussed at this time.

Diagnosis

Diagnosis is the second steps of the nursing process. It is the phase in which nurses determine the meaning of assessment data. Second step in the nursing process involves further analysis (breaking down the whole into parts that can be examined) and synthesis (putting data together in a new way) of the collected data (list of nursing process).

Nursing process is a clinical judgment about individual, family or community responses to activate or potential health problems/life process. A nursing diagnosis provides the basis for selection of nursing interventions to achieve outcome for which the nurse is accountable (NANDA 2003).

- A health problem is any condition than requires intervention to promote wellness or to prevent or resolve disease or illness. When once identified by a health problem, then it should be decided how to treat it, independently or in collaboration with other health professionals. The health problems may be nursing diagnosis, or medical diagnosis or a collaboration problems.

- A nursing diagnosis is a statement of client health status than nurses can identify, prevent or treat independently. It is stated in terms of human responses (reactions) to disease, injury or other stressors, and it can be either a problems or a strength. Human responses can be biological, emotional, interpersonal, social or spiritual.

- A medical diagnosis describes a disease, illness or injury. The purpose of a medical diagnosis is to identify a disease process or pathology so that appropriate treatment can be given. It is more narrowly focused than a nursing diagnosis.

- Collaborative problems are certain physiologic complications (of diseases, medical treatment, or diagnostic studies) than nurses monitor to detect onset or changes in status. Collaborative problems can be found in certain disease or treatment are at risk for developing the same complication and may be a potential problems to become actual problems.

- To diagnose is to identify the type and cause of a health conditions. Diagnosis is a clinical judgment about the client's response to actual or potential health conditions or problems or needs. The diagnosis provides the basis for determination of a plan of care to achieve expected outcomes.

A problem is any health care condition that requires diagnostic, therapeutic or educational action. When the patient has a problem or a potential problem, cues are usually present will that that will help the nurse identify the area of concern. Several guidelines help the nurse identify the cues that have significance for nursing care. The nurse considers any of the following to be important.

- A deviation from population norms. Example TPR & BP
- Changes in usual health patterns that are not explained by developmental or situational changes example, any change in the patient's usual health status.
- Indirections of delayed growth and development. Example milestones of child
- Changes in usual behaviors in roles and relationships
- Non-productive or dysfunctional behavior.

The second step in the nursing process involves further **analysis** (breaking down the whole into parts that can be examined) and **synthesis (**putting data together in a new way) of the collected data. A list of nursing diagnoses is the result of this process. According to NANDA, a **nursing diagnosis** is a clinical judgment about individual, family or community responses to actual or potential health problems/life processes. A nursing diagnosis provides the basis for selection of nursing intervention to achieve outcomes for which the nurse is accountable. The nursing diagnoses provide the basis for client care through the remaining steps.

Clients have both medical and nursing diagnoses; Table 10.5 compares the two categories of diagnoses. It is important to have a clear understanding of the nurse of a nursing diagnosis as compared to a **medical diagnosis** (clinical judgment by the physician that identifies or determines a specific disease, condition, or pathological state) (Table 10.6).

Table 10.6: Comparison of Select Nursing and Medical Diagnoses

Nursing diagnosis	Medical diagnosis
Decreased **C**ardiac Output	Congestive heart failure
Ineffective **B**reathing	
Risk for Imbalanced **F**luid Volume	
Impaired Physical **M**obility	Meniere's disease
Death Anxiety	Lung cancer
Ineffective **A**irway Clearance	Chronic obstructive pulmonary disease
Ineffective **B**reathing Pattern Anxiety	

and anticipate treating, is rapidly evolving in clinical and educational settings. Critical attention is being focused on aspects of nursing practice and education that either foster or inhibit the establishment of the discipline nursing as a profession. A traditional reliance on the language and therapeutics of other sciences is inhibiting the establishment of nursing as a free-standing profession. Effort to identify and name the conditions that nurses study and treat, on the other hand, foster nursing professional identity by clarifying its distinct services to society and providing a vehicle for the building of its science.

Nursing diagnosis has provided the profession with an appropriate focus on the content and the diagnostic categories that were in the domain of nursing. The term *diagnosis,* according to the dictionary, is derived from the greek word *diagignoskein,* which means "to distinguish." Definitions include (a) the art of identifying a disease from its signs and symptoms, (b) a statement or conclusion concerning the nature of some phenomenon, and (c) analysis of the course or nature of a condition, situation, or problem. Although the first definition pertains to physicians, diagnosis is not restricted to one particular profession and must be qualified by a professional designation. In fact, anyone who makes a statement or conclusion about the nature of a condition or problem is diagnosing.

The term *nursing diagnosis* refers to both the process of making a diagnosis and to the clinical judgment reached and expressed in a category name or label. Several definitions of nursing diagnosis have been stated since the early 1950s. Each has a different emphasis, but all have many similarities. The earliest definition of nursing diagnosis was formulated by Abdellah (1957) who stated that it was the "determination of the nature and extend of nursing problems presented by the individual patients or families receiving nursing care."

In 1973, the First National Conference on the Classification of Nursing Diagnosis accepted this definition: A *nursing diagnosis* "is the judgment or conclusion [that] occurs as a result of nursing assessment". To Gordon (1976), *nursing diagnoses,* or clinical diagnoses made by professional nurses, describe a combination of signs and symptoms that indicate actual or

Table 10.5: Comparison of Nursing and Medical Diagnosis

Nursing diagnosis	Medical diagnosis
Recognizes situations that the nurse is licensed and qualified to treat	Recognizes conditions the physician is licensed and qualified to treat
Concentrates on the clients responses to health problems or life processes	Concentrates on injury, illness or disease processes
Varies as the clients responses and/or health problems change	Stays the same until a cure is realized or client dies
Example:	**Example:**
Nausea	Cholelithiasis
Acute **P**ain	Surgery
Acute **P**ain	Cholocystectomy
Impaired Physical **M**obility	

The nurse uses critical thinking and decision-making skills in developing nursing diagnoses. Nursing diagnosis, the second phase of the nursing process is recognized in ANA definition of nursing as the diagnosis and treatment of human responses to actual or potential health problems. The concept of nursing diagnosis, a process whereby nurses interpret assessment data and apply standardized labels to health problems they identify potential health problems that nurses by virtue of their education and experience are able, licensed, and accountable to treat. To Edel (1982), a *nursing diagnosis* is the statement of a potential or actual altered health status of a client, which is derived from nursing assessment and which requires intervention from the domain of nursing. Edel's definition emphasizes that the entity to be diagnosed is *health status,* which avoids the negative connotation of problem and allows for positive diagnoses of clients (Health status is the health of a person at a given time). The strengths and the problems of the person are considered. To Shoemaker (1984), a *nursing diagnosis* is a clinical judgment about an individual family or community that is derived through a deliberate, systematic process of data collection and analysis. The diagnosis is the basis for prescriptions of definitive therapy for which the nurse is accountable. It is expressed concisely and includes the etiology (when known) of the condition.

In March 1990, the Ninth Conference on the Classification of Nursing Diagnoses in Orlando, Florida accepted the working definition of nursing diagnosis. "Nursing diagnosis is a clinical judgment about individual, family, or community responses to actual and potential health problems/life processes. Nursing diagnoses provide the basis for selection of nursing interventions to achieve outcomes for which the nurse is accountable."

Characteristics of Nursing Diagnosis

Implied in these definitions are the following characteristics:

- Professional nurses (registered nurses) are the persons responsible for making nursing diagnoses. Even though other nursing personnel may contribute data to the process of diagnosing and may implement specified nursing care, the formulation of a diagnostic statement lies within the realm of the professional nurse.
- A health problem is any condition or situation in which a client requires help to promote, maintain, or regain a state of health or to achieve a peaceful death. It does not always refer to an undesirable state but does refer to a situation for which the client needs nursing assistance.
- Nursing diagnoses describe (a) actual health problems (deviations from health), (b) potential health problems (risk factors that predispose persons and families to health problems), and (c) areas of enriched personal growth. Examples of actual health problems are *Ineffective airway clearance, Fluid volume deficit, and knowledge deficit.* Examples of potential health problems are *High risk for infection and High risk for injury.* Examples of areas of enriched personal growth are self-development, health maintenance management, and parenting.
- The domain of nursing diagnosis includes only those health states that nurses are able and licensed to treat. For example, nurses are not educated to diagnose or treat diseases such as diabetes mellitus; this task is defined legally as within the practice of medicine. Yet they can diagnose a *Knowledge deficit, Ineffective individual coping, Altered nutrition,* and *High risk for injury*, all of which may accompany diabetes mellitus. These problems are within the nurse's capabilities and the scope of the nurse's licensing laws; thus, the nurse is responsible and accountable for the treatment provided for these nursing diagnoses.
- A nursing diagnosis is a judgment made only after a thorough, systematic process of data collection.

A nursing diagnosis is a statement of a nursing judgment, and refers to a condition that nurses are licensed to treat. In contrast, a medical diagnosis is made and treated by a physician. Nursing diagnosis is made and treated by a physician. Nursing diagnoses refer to physical, sociocultural, psychologic, and spiritual conditions, whereas medical diagnoses refer to disease.

Nursing diagnoses relate to the nurse's independent functions, i.e. the areas of health care that are unique to nursing and are separate and distinct from the care included in medical management. Even though the nurse is obligated to carry out medical orders, i.e. dependent functions, the nurse is also obligated to diagnose and prescribe within the limits of nurse practice acts.

Advantages of Using Nursing Diagnoses

Some of the advantages of using nursing diagnoses are outlined as given below:

- Nursing diagnoses facilitate communication among nurses and with other health team members. A diagnosis identifies a client's health status, strengths, and health problems.
- They strengthen the nursing process and provide direction for planning independent nursing interventions.
- They help the nurse focus on independent nursing actions.
- They help identify the focus of a nursing activity and thus facilitate peer review and quality assurance programs. Peer review is the appraisal of a nurse's practice, education, or research by coworkers of equal status. Quality assurance is the evaluation of nursing services provided and the results achieved against an established standard.
- They facilitate nursing intervention when a client moves from one hospital unit to another or from hospital to home. The nursing diagnoses guide the planning of the nursing interventions that the client requires after discharge.
- They facilitate comprehensive health care by identifying, validating, and responding to specific health problems.

The Diagnostic Process

Diagnosis is a process of analysis and synthesis. Analysis is the separation into components, i.e. breaking down the whole into its parts. Synthesis is the opposite, i.e. putting together the parts into the whole.

The cognitive skills required for analysis and synthesis are objectivity, critical thinking, decision making, and inductive and deductive reasoning. To be objective is to be without bias; i.e. the values and beliefs of the nurse do not affect how data are viewed and analyzed. To be objective, nurses must be aware of their own values and beliefs. *Critical thinking* is a cognitive process during which data are reviewed and explanations considered before an opinion is formed. In this process, nurses use all the subjective and objective data acquired and validated during the assessment phase as well as their knowledge to develop a nursing diagnostic statement.

The diagnostic process is used continuously by most nurses working in hospitals, ambulatory care settings, clients' homes, and long-term care facilities. An experienced nurse may enter a client's room and immediately observe significant data about the client. The nurse is able to do this because of knowledge, skill, and expertise in the practice setting. The outcome of the diagnostic process, the statement of the nursing diagnosis, is recorded in the care plan. This conclusion or statement provides nurse colleagues with a common language and direction for individualized interventions.

Although experienced practitioners are able to perform these mental processes automatically, the novice needs guidelines to understand and formulate diagnoses. The diagnostic process has the following steps:

1. Data processing – interpreting collected data
2. Determining the client's health problems, health risks, and strengths
3. Formulating nursing diagnoses.

Data Processing

Data processing, the first aspect of analyzing, is the act of interpreting collected data. It involves the following steps:

1. Organize data
2. Compare data against standards (identify significant cues)
3. Cluster data (generate tentative hypotheses)
4. Identify gaps and inconsistencies.

These activities occur continuously rather than sequentially.

Organizing the Data: Once the data are collected, they need to be organized into a usable framework for the nurse and others who may need access to them. Theoretical frameworks and conceptual models often guide the format of the assessment tool, thus facilitating the organization of data. The nurse may choose one or more nursing models and develop skill by using them consistently.

To illustrate data organization, a summary of the nursing assessment data using a functional health pattern assessment format is shown in the Table 10.7.

Comparing Data Against Standards: The nurse compares the client's data to a wide range of standards, such as normal health patterns, normal vital signs, laboratory values, basic food groups, growth, and development. The nurse also uses personal knowledge, e.g. physiology, psychology, and sociology – as well as past experience when comparing the data. A *standard* or *norm* is a generally accepted rule, model, pattern, or measure. To be used in comparing, however, a standard must be both relevant and reliable. To be relevant, it must be of the same class as the data to which it is compared. The nurse compares the client data

against standards and norms in order to identify significant and relevant cues. A *cue* is a piece of information or data that influences decisions. Cues are acquired through the use of the five senses (taste, touch, smell, hearing, and sight). Gordon (1987) suggests the following guidelines to assist in determining significant cues.

1. *Cues that point to change in a client's health status or pattern:* These may be positive or negative. For example, the client states: "I have recently experienced shortness of breath while climbing stairs" or "I have not smoked for three months."
2. *Cues that vary from norms of the client population:* The client's pattern may fit within cultural norms but vary from norms of the general society. The client may consider a pattern – for example, eating very small meals and having a poor appetite – to be normal. This pattern, however, may not be productive and may require further exploration.
3. *Cues that indicate a development delay:* Changes in health patterns occur as the person grows and develops. By age 9 months, the infant is usually able to sit alone without support, stand while holding on, and turn the wrists to examine objects. The infant who has not accomplished these tasks needs further assessment for possible developmental delays. To identify significant cues, the nurse must be aware of normal patterns and changes.

The nurse must always consider the client's interpretation of the situation. Making diagnostic decisions without eliciting the perceptions of the client or family may lead to missed diagnoses or misdiagnoses. The client's perceptions are an important aspect of the decision-making process.

Clustering Data: Clustering or grouping data is a process of determining the relatedness of facts and finding patterns in the facts. This is the beginning of synthesis. Data are examined to determine whether any patterns are present, whether the data represent isolated incidents, and whether the data are significant. The process of data clustering is influenced by the nurse's background of scientific knowledge, past nursing experiences, and concept of nursing.

Together, these factors are a mental reference file of facts and principles the nurse uses to verify the significance of the data. The nurse may cluster data inductively by combining data from different assessment areas to form a pattern, or the nurse may begin with a framework, such as Gordon's functional health patterns, and cluster the subjective and objective data into the appropriate categories. The latter is a deductive approach to data clustering, or pattern formation.

To relate and group data, the nurse must consider nursing diagnostic categories or areas of nursing responsibility. Gordon (1987) states that clustering information involves a search in the nurse's memory stores for previously learned meaningful groups of clinical cues that are associated with a diagnostic category. Gordon believes that clustering occurs in conjunction with data collection and interpretation, as evidenced in remarks or thoughts such as, "I'm getting a picture of" or "This cue doesn't fit the

Table 10.7: Organization of Data for Mr Venkatesh

Health Perception/Health Management	*Value/Belief*
• No energy	• Religion/spirituality is important to him
• Shortness of breath	• Wants to see hospital chaplain
• Had left hip replacement 2 years ago	*Medication/History*
• Eats a good diet	• Tolazamide (Tolinase) 250 mg daily
• Does not smoke	• Furosemide (Lasix) 20 mg daily
• Does not drink	• Slow K 20 mEq daily
Nutritional/Metabolic	• Nitroglycerin 1/150 gr prn for angina
• Has diabetes	*Nursing Physical Assessment*
• Does not eat sugar	• 81 years old
• Lost 5 pounds over past year	• Height 95.3 kg
Elimination	• TPR 36.5, 80, 16
• Urinates frequently	• Blood pressure 124/80 mm Hg
Activity/Exercise	• Large, slightly obese
• Lacks energy to do daily ranch chores	• Joint stiffness
• Moves more slowly since hip surgery	• Slight limp
Cognitive/Perceptual	• No pedal edema
• Slightly hard of hearing	• Femoral pulses very strong (R) and bounding (L)
• Wears glasses	• Popliteal, dorsalis pedis, posterior tibial pulses absent in left leg
• Doesn't read much, prefers to be told how to do things	• Left leg cooler than right leg
Roles/Relationship	• Heart rhythm is regular
• Lives with wife and 6 of 13 children	• Loud heart murmur in aortic area
• Family "scared" about his illness	• History of angina (6 months)
• Cattle rancher and farmer	• Rales in bases of both lungs cleared by coughing
Self-perception/Self-concept	• Urinary frequency because of Lasix
• Too weak to do day work on the farm	• No allergies
Coping/Stress	
• Usually too busy to worry about things	
• Perceives his son Tom as helpful in talking things over	
• Wants family to visit	

picture." The novice nurse does not have the knowledge base or the clinical experience that facilitates the recognition of cues related to diagnostic categories. Thus, the novice must take careful assessment notes, search data for abnormal cues, and use textbook resources for comparing the client's cues with the defining characteristics and etiologic factors of the accepted nursing diagnoses. After comparing the client cues against available resources, the nurse can group data into clusters.

Data clustering involves making inferences. An *inference* is the nurse's judgment or interpretation of cues. Inferences are made throughout the diagnostic process. During data clustering, the nurse interprets the possible meaning of the cues and labels the cue clusters with tentative diagnostic hypotheses. Data clustering or grouping for Mr Venkatesh is illustrated in Table 10.8. The data are clustered according to nursing diagnostic categories.

Identifying Gaps and Inconsistencies in Data Gaps: These are missing information needed to determine a data pattern. For example, during the assessment phase, the nurse needs data about a client's definition of health to interpret his statement "I am sick all the time." Data may be completely missing or incomplete. For example, information about a 15 months old childs mobility

may not specify whether the child crawls or walks. This information is essential for establishing the child's developmental stage.

Inconsistencies are conflicting data. Possible sources of conflicting data include: measurement error, expectations, and conflicting or unreliable reports. For example, if the client reports a history of high blood pressure but the nurse obtains a low reading, the nurse should check the equipment and procedure for possible error. All inconsistencies must be clarified before a valid pattern can be established.

Nursing diagnostic statements are derived from the nurse's *inferences* which are based on the assessed and validated data coupled with nursing, scientific and humanistic concepts and theories. The term 'inference' is very useful in defining nursing diagnosis, because it emphasizes the tentative and assumptive nature of diagnoses. *Inference* refers to the process of arriving at a conclusion by reasoning from evidence" and warns that "if the evidence is slight the term comes close to surmise". In recognizing that *element* of both judgement and inference are part of nursing diagnosis, one can appreciate the need to limit or control the influence of bias on the part of the nurses and in the act of diagnosing so that the diagnostic conclusion reached is as logical and factually based as possible.

Table 10.8: Formulating Nursing Diagnoses for Mr Venkatesh

Diagnostic category	Data clustering / Grouping data	Determining strengths and health problems	Formulating nursing diagnostic statements
Activity intolerance	Shortness of breath Lacks energy to do daily chores Does not smoke	Does not smoke (strength) Activity intolerance (problem)	**Activity intolerance** related to shortness of breath and lack of energy secondary to decreased strength of cardiac contraction
Ineffective airway clearance	Rales in bases of both lungs relieved by coughing	Able to expel secretions by coughing (strength) Secretions in lung bases (problem)	**Potential ineffective airway clearance** postoperatively related to chest incision
High risk for injury	Left hip replacement Movement slightly limited Joint stiffness Slight limp	Carries out daily activities independently (strength) Movement slightly limited (problem)	**High risk for injury (trauma)** related to joint stiffness and limp from hip replacement surgery
Altered nutrition	Is diabetic Takes tolazamide (Tolinase) daily "No sugar" in diet "Eats a good diet" Overweight for height Weight loss of 5 pounds in past year	Controls diabetes with Tolinase and "no sugar" (strength) Weight loss of 5 pounds in past year (strength) Overweight (problem)	**Altered nutrition: More than body requirements** related to imbalance of intake versus activity expenditure
Knowledge deficit	Takes furosemide (Lasix) daily Takes slow K daily Urinates frequently	Complies with medical regime (strength) Does not relate urinary frequency to diuretic (problem)	**Knowledge deficit:** Side effects of diuretic therapy
Altered peripheral tissue perfusion	Vital signs normal Heart rhythm regular Loud heart murmur (aortic area) Femoral pulses stronger than normal Absent pulses (popliteal, dorsalis pedis, posterior tibial) in left leg Left leg cooler than right leg Integument pink and intact	Vital signs within normal range (strength) Skin intact and of good color (strength) Impaired circulation in left leg (problem)	**Altered peripheral tissue perfusion** (left leg) related to impaired arterial circulation
Fear	Hospitalized for cardiac catheterization and possible aortic valve replacement States family "scared" about illness Wants to see chaplain Wants family to visit Perceives son Tom as helpful Says is usually too busy to worry about things	Perceives family as supportive (strength) Says family anxious about illness. Did not indicate own feelings (problem)	**Fear** related to cardiac catheterization, possible surgery, and its outcome
Pain	History of angina (6 months) Takes nitroglycerin for angina	Has not needed nitroglycerin for 2 months (strength)	**Potential pain (angina)** related to excessive activity or stress

The human response to health and illness situation constitutes the focus of phenomenon, of concern to nurses, and it is the object of nurse's diagnostic activities. As one proceeds through the analysis of data, certain patterns develop and the use of relevant concepts and theories become appropriate. Nursing diagnosis can be considered a client-related behavioral statement that identifies the area for focus of nursing action. A diagnosis may deal with an actual (present-oriented) or a potential (future-oriented) health problem. It is based on conclusions reached in the assessment phase.

Formulating Nursing Diagnosis Statements

Guidelines for use of the taxonomy of approved nursing diagnosis: It is important to recognize that classification of the phenomena to which a profession addresses itself is a sizable and ongoing task. The development and refinement of nursing's nomenclature of health status are in their earliest stages and subject to much revision based on the reserved and clinical reports presented and reviewed at each of NANDA's conferences and by the Diagnosis Review Committee. Work on existing diagnoses also is incomplete. Several have etiologies and defining characteristics yet to be developed, making clinical use difficult and frustrating. Other diagnosis may be deleted from the approved list from conference to conference. Such changes are both necessary and usual in the process of taxonomy development. One has only to look at the system of names describing health problems treated by physicians not many years ago (for example, chilblain's consumption, dropsy) to appreciate nursing's progress to date.

Guidelines for Diagnostic Labels

Definitions of health problems: Nearly all approved diagnoses have accompanying definitions to better explain the health state they represent. These definitions are important for the student of nursing diagnosis to consider, because they clarify more about the health state than is apparent from the label alone. For example, the definition accompanying the diagnoses fear and anxiety draw a particularly useful distinction between the two problems. Fear is an emotion that has an identifiable source or object that the patient validates, whereas anxiety is an emotion whose source is non-specific or unknown to the patient. Other good examples of such definitions accompany the diagnoses social isolation, powerlessness, altered parenting, and caregiver role strain.

Until definitions accompany all approved diagnoses, it is important for nurses collaborating in care to establish consensus about the meaning and scope of the health problems stated.

Making diagnostic labels specific: Some nursing diagnoses need accompanying qualifiers or specifies based on the characteristics of the health problem as it manifests itself in a particular patient. For example, the diagnosis fear needs specification as to the object of the patient's particular fear, such as death, pain, disfigurement, or malignancy. Similarly, the diagnosis knowledge deficit needs specification about the content of the deficit, such as use of incentive spirometer, counting the pulse rate or respiratory muscle strengthening exercise. Following is a list of nursing diagnoses needing specification, each with an example of a particular patient circumstance so specified:

Fear: Postoperative pain.
Knowledge deficit: Self-monitoring of oral anticoagulation therapy.
Altered peripheral: Tissue perfusion.
Altered nutrition: Less than body potassium requirements.
Altered nutrition: More than body *kilocalorie* requirements.
Self-care deficit: Bathing and feeding.
Non-compliance: Prescribed activity restrictions.

Guidelines for Etiologic/Related Factors

Making etiologies specific: In many instances, NANDA's etiologies are broad categories or examples needing to be made specific based on characteristics of the health state and the patient being treated. For example, one of several possible etiologies for the diagnosis fluid volume excess is **Compromised Regulatory Mechanism**. Considering this, the cause of the fluid excess in a particular patient, the nurse needs to specify which regulatory mechanism and in what way compromised (for example, inappropriate ADH secretion by the neurohypophysis) before the diagnosis can be formally stated (disregarding the question of whether the problem is treatable by nurses or needs referoal).

Several etiologies needing to be made specific follow-up along with examples of such specification in parenthesis;

- Situational crisis (recent diagnosis of terminal illness).
- Psychologic injuring agent (hurtful relationship, verbal abuse).
- Development factors (developmental arrest, extremes of age).

Nursing diagnoses as etiologies: Nursing diagnostic labels may rightfully serve as etiologies for other diagnoses. Examples are anxiety R/T knowledge deficit and activity intolerance R/T decreased cardiac output.

Etiologies as the focus of treatment: The treatment plan formulated for a given diagnosis must include interventions aimed at resolution or management of the etiologic factors, as well as the health state. In fact, in some instances nursing treatment is directed exclusively at the etiology of a diagnosis, with the logical expectation that, if the causative factors are reduced in influence, the problem should begin to resolve. This is true especially in instances where a nursing diagnosis has as its etiology another nursing diagnosis, consider treatment approaches to the diagnosis. In effective breathing pattern R/T there is high abdominal incision pain. Predictably, little effectiveness is shown if the interventions are focused solely on reviewing the rationale for slow, deep symmetrical, breathing; demonstrating the technique; and encouraging the patient in its performance without some plan for manipulation of the pain variable.

Medical diagnoses as etiologies: Because, as mentioned, the etiology of a nursing diagnosis becomes a focus of intervention in the management of the overall health state, citing a medical condition or diagnosis as the etiology is conceptually inadvisable if the diagnosis statement is to retain its identity as a health problem primarily resolved by nursing therapies. And yet, many health states of concern to critical care nurse and amenable to their treatment are consequent to medical conditions. Examples are the ineffective airway clearance that results from chronic obstructive pulmonary disease (COPD), and sensory-perceptual alterations that result from coronary artery bypass grant surgery. In these instances the nurse should isolate those aspects of the contributing pathologic state that are modifiable by nursing intervention and cite these factors as etiologic, for instance, ineffective airway clearance R/T thick tracheobronchial secretions, respiratory muscle weakness, and knowledge deficit; effective cough and hydration techniques, and sensory-perceptual alterations R/T sensory overload, sensory depression, and sleep pattern disturbance. These diagnostic statements are more clearly worded and provide a much sharper focus for nursing intervention.

Guidelines for Defining Characteristics

Making defining characteristics specific: As with diagnostic labels and statements of etiology, defining characteristics cited for diagnoses are in non-specific form and often need to be modified to reflect the particular situation presented by the patient being diagnosed. For example, the diagnosis impaired gas exchange has as one of the possible defining characteristics ***abnormal blood gases***. In the nurses' formulation of this diagnostic statement for clinical use, the specific blood gas value used to diagnose the problem should be cited in the statement (e.g. PO_2: 54 mm Hg and/or PCO_2: 50 mm Hg) versus the non-specific sign category, abnormal blood gases.

Several defining characteristics are cited as following non-specific form with accompanying examples of proper specification:

- Respiratory depth changes (hypoventilation)
- Blood pressure changes (hypotension)
- Autonomic responses (dilated pupils, tachycardia)
- Altered electrolytes (hypokalemia)
- Change in mental state (confusion, obtundation, apprehension).

Major or critical defining characteristics: Major or critical defining characteristics are designated signs and/or symptoms that must be present for the health problem to be considered present. Major defining characteristics, when applicable, must be present in the nurse's assessment profile to diagnose the corresponding health state with any degree of certainty. For example, the diagnosis unilateral neglect has as its major defining characteristic *Consistent in attention to stimuli* on *affected side*. It is essential, the, that the characteristic be present in the patient's situation (in addition, perhaps, to several other non-critical signs)

for the diagnosis of the problem. The assignment of major or critical status to a defining characteristic is based on research or extensive clinical experience in which the signs and symptoms of a health problem are tested for their ability to meet reliably predict the presence of the diagnosis and can therefore be used with confidence by the nurse diagnostician.

Guidelines for Diagnosing High-Risk States

Determining a risk state for diagnosis: Predicating a potential health problem in a given patient involves an estimation of probability. The potential for an event, or pattern of response, to occur can truly be said to exist in almost any situation. Consider the high-risk health problems facing the postoperative patient. This risk state includes high-risk for non-compliance with the rehabilitative regimen, high-risk for body image disturbance, high-risk for sleep pattern, disturbance, high-risk for ineffective airway clearance, high-risk for constipation and high-risk for aspiration, to name only a few. To state each of these diagnoses on a treatment plan without regard for probabilities and develop desired patient outcomes and interventions for each is pointless.

What should occur is an appraisal of the patient's health status and the identification of risk factors that place him or her at higher risk for the health problem than the general population. For example, all persons recovering from abdominal surgery have high-risk for constipation because of the effects of general anesthesia and narcotic analgesics, manipulation of abdominal viscera, and postoperative immobility. All nurses have a tacit understanding of this risk, and monitoring and Intervention are carried out as part of routine nursing care to avert the problem. Hence there is no need to state the problem.

Identifying the Client's Health Problems, Health Risks, and Strengths

After data are processed, the nurse and the client can together identify strengths and problems. This is primarily a decision-making process.

Health Problems and Risks: During data processing, the nurse groups data according to categories and labels the clusters with tentative diagnoses. However, for health problems (existing or potential) to have a successful outcome, the client must accept the existence of the problem. The nurse, by contrast, determines whether the client needs help dealing with the problem. The nurse and the client can then make any of the following judgments:

1. No problem exists, and the client's health status is confirmed.
2. No problem exists, but there is a potential problem.
3. A problem exists, but the client is coping effectively.
4. A problem exists, and the client needs help in handling it.
5. A problem exists, but the client cannot deal with it at this time.

6. A problem requires further study and diagnosis.
7. A problem is not presently incapacitating but will be at a later date.
8. A problem places heavy demands on the client's ability to cope.
9. A problem is critical to the client.
10. The problem is long-term and permanent.

See Table 10.8 for examples of Mr Venkatesh is problems.

Strengths: At this stage, the nurse and client also establish the client's strengths, resources, and abilities to cope. Generally, people have a clearer perception of their problems or weaknesses than of their strengths and assets, which are often taken for granted. By taking an inventory of strengths, the client can develop a more well-rounded self-concept and self-image. Strengths can be an aid to mobilizing health and regenerative processes.

A client's strengths might be that his weight is within the normal range for his age and height, thus enabling him to cope better with surgery. In another instance, a client's strengths might be that she is allergy-free and a non-smoker. The same client's resources could be a supportive family and an ability to cope. Coping is a learned pattern or response that helps an individual deal with crises and stressful events. Nurses must remember, however, that because of the magnitude of an event, the number of stressful events occurring at one time, or the unfamiliarity of the situation, a client may be unable to cope and require assistance of the nurse.

A client's strengths can be found in the nursing assessment record (health, home life, education, recreation, exercise, work, family and friends, religious beliefs, and sense of humor, for example), the health examination, and the client's records. See Table 10.8 for examples of Mr. Venkatesh, strengths.

At this final stage, the nurse formulates causal relationships between the health problems and the factors related to them. These factors may be, for example, environmental, sociologic, psychologic, physiologic, or spiritual. More than one factor may be related to one health problem. It is also important to determine at this time that the problem can be resolved by independent nursing interventions. If it cannot, the nurse should refer the client to the appropriate health team member. By including the causal factors in diagnostic statements, the nurse can tailor a plan of care for the client. For example, the diagnosis ***Impaired physical mobility*** tells the nurse the problem but does not suggest the direction the nursing intervention should take, whereas ***Impaired physical mobility related to neuromuscular impairment*** suggests a direction for plans and interventions to deal with the problem. Obviously, the causative factor *neuromuscular impairment* suggests a different direction than the factor *fear of falling* would.

Nurses can refer to a list of accepted nursing diagnoses to select a diagnostic category. The causal factors are obtained form the data. If no causal factor appears in the data, the nurse may wish to make a tentative diagnosis based on scientific nursing knowledge and experience. The nurse should then review the database for inconsistencies and gaps and the analysis/synthesis for error. Once the causal relationships have been established, the nurse is ready to write the diagnostic statements.

Prior to writing the diagnostic statement in the care plan, the diagnostician reviews the following checkpoints:

1. Do I understand client data, and have I verified any questionable data? Have I been careful and objective regarding my observations?
2. Have I recognized diagnostic cues accurately?
3. Have I processed data and reports accurately? Did I test data with standards and compare data from different sources to ensure accuracy?
4. Have I considered several tentative diagnoses to explain the cues, and ruled out incorrect ones?
5. Have I reviewed all the *major* and *minor* defining characteristics for the tentative diagnostic statements? See *Nursing Diagnosis Format* below. Have I accurately assessed the client for these signs and symptoms?
6. Do I have adequate cues to support the formulation of the nursing diagnoses?

See Table 10.8 for Mr Venkatesh nursing diagnostic statements.

Nursing Diagnosis Format

There are three essential components of nursing diagnostic statements; they are referred to as the **PES format**. Nurses need to consider these components when developing new diagnostic categories and writing diagnoses for specific clients. The components are:

1. *The terms describing the problem (P):* This component, referred to as the *diagnostic category label* or *title,* is a description of the client's (individual, family, community) health problem (actual or potential) for which nursing therapy is given. The state of the client is described clearly and concisely in a few words. To be clinically useful, category labels need to be specific. When the word *specify* follows a category label in the list on the inside backcover, the nurse states the area in which the problem occurs. For example, a knowledge deficit may be in the area of medication prescription, dietary adjustments, or disease process and therapy.
2. *The etiology of the problems (E)* or contributing factors. This component identifies one or more probable causes of the health problem and gives direction to the required nursing therapy. Etiology may include behaviors of the client, environmental factors, or interactions of the two. For example, the probable causes of alteration in health maintenance include perceptual or cognitive impairment, lack of gross or fine motor skills, lack of material resources, and ineffective individual coping. Several authors have identified etiologies for many diagnoses. Differentiating among possible causes in the nursing diagnosis is essential because each may require different nursing therapies.

3. *The defining characteristics or cluster of signs and symptoms (S):* The defining characteristics provide information necessary to arrive at the diagnostic category label (component 1). Each nursing diagnostic category is associated with signs and symptoms that occur as a clinical entity. *Major* signs and symptoms are those that must be present to make a valid diagnosis. *Minor* characteristics may or may not be present. Nursing diagnostic categories are similar to medical diagnostic categories. For example, the medical diagnostic category myocardial infarction (heart attack) is associated with a standard set of signs and symptoms that are universally understood and accepted. Likewise, the nursing diagnostic category **Activity intolerance** is associated with a standard cluster of signs and symptoms. For most nursing diagnoses the list of defining characteristics is still being developed and refined. Partial listings have been published to assist nurses in developing and validating nursing diagnoses (Table 10.9).

Writing a Diagnostic Statement

A nursing diagnostic statement (nursing diagnosis) is a clear statement about a client's actual or potential health problem that is within the scope of independent nursing intervention. It is the outcome of the diagnostic process: the second phase in the nursing process.

Nurses may write diagnoses as either two-part or three-part statements. The two-part nursing diagnostic statement includes

1. Problem (P) – Statement of the client's response
2. Etiology (E) – Factors contributing to or probable causes of the responses.

The two parts are joined by the words *related to or associated with* rather than *due to*. The phrase *due to* implies a cause-and-effect relationship; one clause causes or is responsible for the other clause. By contrast, the phrases *related to* and *associated with* merely imply a relationship. The phrase *related to* is most commonly used. If one part of the diagnostic statement changes, the other part may change as well. Legal hazards are thus avoided. Here are some examples of nursing diagnoses containing two parts:

* **Ineffective breathing pattern** (problem) related to *pain* (etiology)
* **Self-esteem disturbance** (problem) related to *altered body image (loss of arm)* (etiology)
* **Anticipatory grieving** (problem) related to *anticipated loss* (etiology) secondary to *husband's illness* (etiology).

A three-part nursing diagnosis statement includes:

1. Problem (P) – Statement of the client's response
2. Etiology (E) – Factors contributing to or probable causes of the response
3. Signs and symptoms (S) – Defining characteristics manifested by the client

The three-part diagnostic statement includes the problem, the etiology, and the observed signs and symptoms (PES). Actual nursing diagnoses can be documented by using the three-part statement (using *related to* and *manifested by*), since the signs and symptoms have been identified. Several alternatives for writing the PES format have been suggested.

1. Nurses learning to write diagnoses may find it helpful to list the signs and symptoms before (even though the S is last) or after the two-part diagnostic statement in a care plan format. The defining characteristics may include both objective and subjective data.

	Table 10.9: Components of a Nursing Diagnostic Category		
Diagnosis	*Definition*	*Etiology*	*Defining characteristics*
Activity intolerance	A state in which an individual has insufficient physiologic or psychologic energy to endure or complete required or desired daily activities	Sedentary life-style Generalized weakness Prolonged bedrest or immobility Sensory deficits Impaired motor function Fatique Alterations in oxygen transport system Lack of motivation Obesity Acute or chronic pain	*Major* (must be present) Altered response to activity, For example, Dyspnea, shortness of breath, tachypnea, rapid shallow respirations Weak, thready pulse, tachycardia, irregular pulse, failure to return to resting after 3 minutes, EKG changes during activity Failure of blood pressure to increase with activity, hypotension, increased dialtolic pressure of 15 mm Hg Weakness and fatique *Minor* (may be present) Pallor, cyanosis, vertigo, diaphoresis, confusion

2. Signs and symptoms may be written after the diagnostic statement joined by the words *manifested by* or *evidenced by*.

Here are some examples of three-part statements:

- **Self-esteem disturbance** (problem) related to *altered body image* (*loss of arm*) (etiology) manifested by *crying and hostility* (signs and symptoms)
- **Anticipatory grieving** (problem) related to *husband's terminal illness* (etiology) manifested by *anorexia and withdrawn behavior* (signs and symptoms)
- **Altered family processes** (problem) related to *mother's hospitalization* (etiology) manifested by son's *unmet physical and emotional needs* (signs and symptoms).

Characteristics of a Diagnostic Statement

- A diagnostic statement is clear and concise.
- It is specific and client centered.
- It relates to one client problem.
- It is accurate.
- It is based on reliable and relevant assessment data.

A patient is at higher risk than the general population of postoperative patient if there is, for example, a history of dependence on laxatives, fluid volume deficit, prolonged immobility, or non-compliance with nursing prescriptions for ambulation. The diagnosis indicating this potential and its risk factors could be stated so that additional and/or more intensified interventions, over those that are routine, can be planned.

Stating high-risk diagnosis: Several of the approved diagnoses address potential dysfunctional status and cite risk factors. Examples of such diagnoses are the following.

Altered Nutrition

High-risk for more than body requirements
High-risk for aspiration
High-risk for disuse syndrome
High-risk for impaired skin integrity
High-risk for infection
High-risk for injury
High-risk for poisoning
High-risk for suffocation
High-risk for trauma
High-risk for violence.

In addition to those diagnoses formally listed as high-risks, any diagnosis from the approved list can be stated as an at risk problem by simply adding the modifier high-risk to the label. For example, self-esteem disturbance can be written high-risk for self-esteem disturbance by virtue of the presence of factors but not yet the actual health problem.

High-risk nursing diagnoses have only two parts to the statement: the *HEALTH PROBLEM AT RISK* and the *RISK FACTORS* (e.g. High-risk for ineffective individual coping, risk factors, malignant biopsy results, absence of inter personal support system, and history of alcohol abuse).

Guidelines for Stating Wellness Diagnoses

Wellness nursing diagnoses represent clinical judgements regarding an individual, family, or community in transition from a specific level of wellness and functioning to a higher level of wellness and functioning. The terms potential for enhanced (specify) is the designated diagnostic label. Wellness diagnoses are one-part statements, for example, potential for enhanced parenting, potential for enhanced coping.

Diagnostic reasoning: Diagnostic reasoning is the critical thinking process through which the nurse moves to arrive at a nursing diagnosis. Like any process, it is often orderly and systematic, However, unlike a process, not all of its factors and operations exist in one's conscious awareness. The challenge of refining one's diagnostic reasoning is to bring into awareness the factors and operations that influence the process and are necessary in arriving at an accurate "answer" or diagnosis. Four key components of diagnostic reasonings are collecting and organizing the data base, identifying cues, making inferences, and validating inferences.

Collecting and organizing the data-base: Collecting and organizing a data-base was discussed earlier.

Identifying cues: A cue is a piece of information, a raw fact. Nurses notice and seek cues regarding patients' health status and functioning. Sweaty palms, restlessness, and a heart rate of 102 beats/min are cues. In the process of diagnostic reasoning, cues are the units of information that are collected and recorded for later analysis.

Making inferences: An inference is the assignment of meaning to cues. A nursing diagnosis is an example of an inference. When individual cues are clustered and interpreted collectively, they begin to assume an identity different from what each represents individually. Sweaty palms, restlessness, and a heart rate of 102 beats/min when interpreted as a cluster could now represent anxiety, shock, fear or pain.

Inferences are created, whereas cues exist. The process of creating inferences from cues, therefore, carries with it the risk of error in logic. If the cues sweaty palms, restlessness, and a heart rate of 102 beats/min were grouped and interpreted in a patient, who also manifested gargling respiratory sounds and a rapid shallow breath in pattern and these additional cues were overlooked or ignored by the person assigning meaning to the cluster – the inference might be erroneous, the more probable inference now might be erroneous the more probable inference now being ineffective airway clearance. Nursing diagnoses are inferences, and defining characteristics and risk factors are the cues that lead to these inferences.

Validating inferences: Once a diagnostic inference is formulated, the nurse will develop and implement a treatment plan designed to resolve or reduce the problem represented by that inference. Erroneous inferences carry, an obvious implication in terms of potential patient harm resulting from treatment of a non-existent health problem or from treatment withheld for a missed diagnostic nursing malpractice. Consequently, it is essential to seek validation of diagnostic interferences before implementing treatments.

Four approaches to the validation of interferences are recommended. First, consult with an authoritative source. This may be a clinical nurse specialist, nurse educator, textbook or published research, for example, Seek confirmation of the logical and scientific integrity of your diagnostic statement. Second, re-exam the cues; could the ones in the diagnostic statement support and other diagnosis or only the one chosen? Could the cues from the data-base believe not to be a part of the cluster supporting this diagnosis belong to some other cluster, or could several of them, together different diagnosis? Third, validate inferences with the patient. Nurses may share with the patient the cluster of cues identified and what is represented.

Patients often have remarkable insight into what underlies their pattern of response and can be a great resource in validating the nurse's conclusions. Additionally, people benefit significantly from having their situations reflected back to them. Indeed, collaborating with the patient in this way may be all the interversion that is necessary. Fourth seek evidence of the reliability of the diagnostic inference from within the appropriate reference group. Do most professional peers conclude the same explanation for the available cues?

These approaches are workable strategies for seeking validation of diagnostic references before the institution of treatment, however the only way to achieve or confirm validation of a diagnosis is to treat the problem and evaluate the outcome. If favourable and predicted outcomes result, strong evidence exists that the problem and its etiology or risk factors and defining characteristics were accurately inferred.

Source of diagnostic error: Much scientific curiosity exists within the nursing profession regarding the diagnostic reasoning process, strategies employed by experts and those used by notices. The following discussion focuses only on the most common type of diagnostic error. ***The Inferential Leap***, and several of the sources. For more in-depth examinations of the skills of clinical problem solving and decision-making.

Inferential leap: As the term implies, the inferential leap involves a jump to a conclusion based on premature termination of the data gathering/data analysis phase of the nursing process. Numerous studies show that this jump to an erroneous conclusion is most frequently made because not all of the variables are known or examined at the time the inference is formulated. Of interest, the novice often closes the *SEARCH* for cues prematurely, whereas the expert will more often prematurely terminate the *ANALYSIS* of cues.

The novice may close the search for cues prematurely because of a lack of understanding of the scope of the problem to be diagnosed. Diagnose such as disturbance in self-concept and infective individual coping are reported to be at the highest level

of abstraction among nursing diagnoses and are, therefore, more difficult to fully grasp, let along discriminate from other diagnostic possibilities. The expert has an advantage in this regard by virtue of a greater breadth of experience, both with the label and the clinical presentation of patients demonstrating the diagnosis.

Professional advantages of nursing diagnosis: Baer assembled from the literature the following statements in advocacy of nursing diagnosis. They are presented here to highlight the advantages nursing diagnosis brings to the profession. Nursing diagnosis does the following:

- Assists in organizing, defining and developing nursing knowledge or scope.
- Aids in identifying and describing the domain and scope of nursing practice.
- Focus as nursing care on the patient's response to problems.
- Prescribes diagnosis-specific nursing interventions that should increase the effectiveness of nursing care.
- Facilitates the evaluation of nursing practice.
- Provides a framework for testing the validity of nursing interventions.
- Provides a standardized vocabulary to enhance intraprofessional and interprofessional communication.
- Prescribes the content of nursing curricula.
- Provides a framework for developing a system to direct third party reimbursements for nursing services.
- Indicates specific rationales for patient care based on nursing assessment.
- Leads to more comprehensive and individualized patient care.

Nursing diagnoses are standardized labels that represent clinical judgements made by professional nurses and describe health states resolved primarily by nursing therapies. Nursing diagnosis focuses on nursing assessment and intervention on the human response to altered health states thus constituting a unique, distinct, and imperative component to critical health care. Diagnosing involves the identification of the patients' actual or potential problem, and the artiology or cause of the problem that nurses can independently treat. The most essential and distinguishing feature of any nursing diagnosis is to describe a health condition primarily resolved by nursing intervention or therapies. Nursing diagnosis is a pivotal component of nursing process. On the one hand it is the judgement, conclusion or decision determined by the nurses as a result of the assessing and problem-solving process. It reflects the process involved in gathering analyzing and interpreting the assessment data. On the other hand, nursing diagnosis provides the basis from which patient outcomes are derived and a plan of appropriate nursing interventions is developed and implemented. Put another way, nursing diagnosis emerges from the collection, analysis and interpretation of assessment data, and provides the framework from which the patient's plan of nursing care involves.

Nursing, as a diagnosis-based practice, demands the nurses become expert at assessing patient's needs and problems formulating nursing diagnosis based on that assessment, evolving and implementing, a plan of care and documenting this nursing care process in a manner reflective of the professional, skilled nursing care rendered. It is the only documenting nursing activities that professional practice can be validated and financially rewarded. Nursing diagnosis reflects a patient's problems or unhealthful response and the problem or etiology that nurses can treat independently. It is a definitive statement of an actual or potential problem, alteration or deficit in the life process (i.e. physiologic, psychologic, sociologic, and spiritualism) of an individual. After the nursing diagnosis are identified, they should be ranked in order of priority. This ranking should both the clients' and the nurses' opinion. Those areas that have the greatest impact on the client, the family or both should receive particular attention. The nurse should also determine priorities based on past nursing experience and on scientific knowledge of the needs and functions of human beings. Therefore, a continuum of priorities of nursing diagnosis is developed that is based on the degree of threat to the level of wellness of the client.

The nursing diagnosis can be considered a decisive statement concerning the client's nursing needs. It is important to remember that diagnoses are based on the client's concerns as well as an actual or potential problems that may be symptoms of physiological disorder or of behavioral psychosocial or spiritual problem.

Nurses are encouraged to use the nursing diagnostic categories (as listed) in their daily practice when formulating nursing diagnosis. But it should be remembered and noted that nurses need not feel restricted to the use of NANDA's list but rather should be motivated to develop in practice. Other nursing diagnosis which may be submitted included in NANDA's list or to make separate better list of nursing diagnosis. In this way, nurses are able to share their ideas, experiences, logic and creativity. The procreation of nursing language, along with an ever-increasing awareness of the intellectual activity involved in its process and implementation is every nurse's professional responsibility.

Common Diagnostic Errors

Clear, concise, client-centered nursing diagnoses can be written by following the guidelines presented in Table 10.10. Some common errors in writing diagnostic statements are:

1. Writing the client's response as a need instead of a problem
2. Using judgmental statements
3. Placing the etiology before the client's response
4. Using statements that provide no specific direction for planning independent nursing interventions
5. Using medical rather than nursing terminology
6. Starting the diagnosis with a nursing intervention
7. Using a single symptom as the client's response.

The accuracy of nursing diagnostic statements also depends on a complete database and appropriate data processing. If data are omitted, a diagnosis can be missed. If data are not processed properly, e.g. are not clustered appropriately, a diagnosis can be made prematurely or incorrectly, or be missed. Gordon (1987), categorizes diagnostic errors as (a) errors of omission, i.e. failure to diagnose a problem and (b) errors of commission, i.e. diagnosing a problem when no problem exists. Both errors can occur during data collection, data interpretation, and data clustering.

To avoid such errors during assessment, the nurse needs to ensure that relevant data are not missed and that large quantities of irrelevant data are not obtained. The nurse can prevent data omissions by using an organized assessment plan, striving for accuracy, and drawing on personal knowledge. Collecting irrelevant data can be avoided if the nurse asks appropriate questions. An overload of irrelevant data hinders the nurse's capacity to process information.

Data interpretation errors occur when the meaning of cues is misinterpreted. The nurse can avoid inaccurate interpretation of cues by determining how the client perceives the health problem, its probable cause, and actions taken to remedy it. For example, the nurse observes that a client repeatedly gets out of bed after the physician has ordered complete bed rest. The nurse may interpret this behavior as noncompliance. However, the client may be experiencing diarrhea and may be embarrassed to use the bedpan or may be refusing to accept a dependent sick role. Obviously, inaccurate interpretation of cues leads to diagnostic errors. Another source of diagnostic errors in data interpretation is overgeneralization from one isolated observation of client behavior. For example, one episode of angry behavior does not mean that the client is hostile.

A diagnosis may be made prematurely, before all relevant data have been considered or collected. For example, a nurse, learning of a client's history of angina and his prescription for nitroglycerin, may write this diagnostic statement: **Pain (anginal).** Additional data, however, reveal that angina has not been a problem since the client had cardiac bypass surgery as year ago and that pain is therefore not a current problem.

Incorrect clustering of data also leads to diagnostic errors. For examples, by clustering "urinary frequency" and "has diabetes," the nurse could erroneously begin a diagnostic statement for Mr. Frederick Smith with **Altered urinary elimination pattern.** However, clustering other data such as "takes furosemide (Lasix, a diuretic) daily," "shortness of breath," "no energy," and "aortic valve insufficiency," changes the diagnostic focus from a urinary problem to **Activity intolerance** or **decreased cardiac output.**

Taxonomy of Nursing Diagnoses

A **taxonomy** is a classification system of groups, classes, or sets. The first taxonomy of nursing diagnoses was done in 1973, at the First National Conference on the Classification of Nursing Diagnoses. Following the approval of the 31 diagnostic categories, the diagnoses were then grouped alphabetically. The nonhierarchic alphabetically ordering was considered unscientific by some, and a hierarchic structure was sought.

Table 10.10: Common Errors in writing Nursing Diagnosis

	Guideline	*Correct statement*	*Incorrect and/or ambiguous statement*
1.	State in terms of a problem. Not a need	**Fluid volume deficit** (problem) related to fever	**Fluid replacement** (need) related to fever
2.	State so that it is legally advisable	**Impaired skin integrity** related to immobility (legally acceptable)	**Impaired skin integrity** related to improper positioning (implies legal liability)
3.	Use nonjudgmental statements	**Spiritual distress** related to inability to attend church service secondary to immobility (nonjudgmental)	**Spiritual distress** related to strict rules necessitating church attendance (judgmental)
4.	Make sure that both elements of the statement do *not* say the same thing	**High risk for impaired skin integrity** related to immobility	**High risk for impaired skin integrity** related to ulceration of sacral area (response and probable cause are the same)
5.	Make sure that the client's response precedes the contributing or causal factor	**Noncompliance with diet** (response) related to lack of knowledge (contributing factor)	**Knowledge deficit** (contributing factor) related to noncompliance with diet (response)
6.	Use statements that provide guidance for planning independent nursing interventions	**Social isolation** related to loss of speech (loss of speech provides direction for planning alternative communication methods)	**Social isolation** related to laryngectomy (the nurse can do nothing about the laryngectomy)
7.	Word diagnosis specifically and precisely to provide direction for planning nursing intervention	**Impaired tissue integrity (oral mucous membrane)** related to decreased salivation secondary to radiation of neck (specific)	**Impaired tissue integrity (oral mucous membrane)** related to noxious agent (vague)
8.	Use nursing terminology rather than medical terminology to describe the client's response	**Potential ineffective airway clearance** (nursing terminology)	**Potential pneumonia** (medical terminology)
9.	Use nursing terminology rather than medical terminology to describe the probable cause of the client's response	**Potential ineffective airway clearance** related to accumulation of secretions in lungs (nursing terminology)	**Potential ineffective airway clearance** related to emphysema (medical terminology)
10.	Do not start the nursing diagnosis with a nursing intervention	**Altered nutrition: less than body requirements** related to inadequate intake of protein (directs but does not state nursing intervention)	Provide high protein diet because of **potential altered nutrition** (stars with nursing intervention)
11	Avoid using a symptom such as nausea as the client's response. A symptom does not reflect a pattern and requires additional data collection	Insufficient data for a diagnosis	**Nausea** related to medication

NANDA's Taxonomy I, Revised In 1978, the Nurse Theorist Group of NANDA proposed the utilization of the "nine patterns of unitary man" as an organizing principle. This proposal was accepted by NANDA in 1982. An initial taxonomic tree was generated. One of the major reasons for classifying and coding nursing diagnosis is to facilitate computer storage and access of information.

In 1984 NANDA renamed the "patterns of unitary man" as "human response patterns." In 1986, NANDA accepted the system as *Taxonomy I* (McLane, 1987). In 1988, some refinements and revisions were made after the acceptance of new diagnoses, and the new taxonomy was called *Taxonomy I, Revised*. All nursing diagnoses, once accepted, now become subcategories of these nine human response patterns. For example, the human response patterns *Feeling* includes:

* Anxiety
* Pain or chronic pain
* Grieving (anticipatory, dysfunctional)
* Fear
* High risk for violence (self-directed or directed at others)
* Post-trauma response
* Rape-trauma syndrome (compound reaction, silent reaction).

Human Response Patterns

1. Exchanging: mutual giving and receiving
2. Communicating: sending messages
3. Relating: establishing bonds
4. Valuing: assigning relative worth
5. Choosing: selection of alternatives
6. Moving: activity
7. Perceiving: reception of information
8. Knowing: meaning associated with information
9. Feeling: subjective awareness of information.

The taxonomy is numerically coded and organized from the most abstract (Level I) to the most concrete (Level IV or V). Each of the nine human response patterns constitute Level I concepts, which are the most abstract. Level II concepts refer to alterations in the human response patterns, and subsequent levels refer to more specific responses.

Translating Taxonomy I Revised into ICD Code: To prepare the taxonomy for possible inclusion into the World Health Organization's 10th revision of the *International Classification of Diseases* (ICD 10), the NANDA Taxonomy Committee, in liaison with the American Nurses' Association, made further revisions to conform to the ICD framework (Fitzpatrick et al. 1989).

These revisions approved by the NANDA board include:

1. Arranging the nine human response patterns in alphabetical order: choosing, communicating, exchanging, feeling, knowing, moving, perceiving, relating, and valuing.
2. Decreasing the levels of abstraction from four, five, or six levels to only two levels.
3. Modifying the diagnostic coding to meet ICD criteria. A four character code is used: an alphabetical character (Y) is placed first, followed by three numerical characters. For example Y27.1 is the code for **Skin integrity, impaired.**

Advantages of Nursing Diagnosis Taxonomy

- *Nursing diagnosis promotes professional accountability and autonomy by defining and describing the independent area of nursing practice:* It provides a standardized terminology for categorizing clusters of signs and symptoms for specific conditions. These category names, such as **Knowledge deficit** or **self-care deficit** focus the nursing interventions needed to achieve the desired outcomes.
- *Nursing diagnoses provide an effective vehicle for communication among nurses and other health care professionals:* Because a nursing diagnosis consolidates a great deal of information into concise statements and includes assessment parameters, it provides a shorthand method of communication. A nurse who knows that a client has a certain nursing diagnosis known about that client's problem, the causal or contributing factors, and the necessary nursing actions.
- *Nursing diagnoses provide an organizing principle for the building of meaningful research:* A valid nursing diagnosis taxonomy would more clearly define the scope of nursing practice. This ability to access such client data in relation to their nursing diagnoses would provide a framework for testing the validity of nursing interventions and also provide feedback for further development of nursing's unique body of knowledge. In addition, the organization of data in this manner would facilitate retrieval and analysis by computer-based information systems.

The evolution of nursing diagnostic categories is in its early developmental stages, and the list of diagnoses is not to be considered a comprehensive guide for nursing practice. Although some nurses feel constrained and frustrated with the existing list of diagnoses, it is well to remember that disciplines with well-established taxonomies, such as medicine, have taken many decades to develop. Each NANDA publication emphasizes that the existing list is not at all definitive. McLane (1987) states that this taxonomy "is an investment by NANDA which can be tested, refined, revised and expanded. A major task of all nurses is to locate diagnoses that are neglected, to test and develop them, and to present them for inclusion in future listings." A relationship between the nursing diagnosis taxonomy and theoretical frameworks for nursing is yet to be demonstrated. The diagnostic focus of proposed conceptual frameworks for nursing depends on the concepts outlined in the nursing theory. For this reason, such frameworks do not necessarily fit the taxonomy of nursing diagnoses. Dialogue between nursing practitioners and theorists is essential for continued development in this area.

The taxonomy needs to be tested for reliability and validity. Although it has been approved and accepted by participants at the national NANDA conferences, the usefulness of each diagnostic category must still be validated by appropriate research. *Validation* is the determination that the diagnosis accurately reflects the problem of the client, that the methods used for data gathering were valid, and that the conclusion or diagnosis is justified by the data. There is some concern that the use of nursing diagnoses may lead to stereotyping by the nurse and lessen the client's role in the decision-making process. Nurses must ensure that the client's perception of the problem is the focus of care. They need to be aware of the problems involved in professional labeling and make every effort to provide individualized client care. Henderson (1987) suggests the use of client questionnaires to maintain a consistent approach.

A weakness of the present nursing diagnoses taxonomy is the lack of focus on health promotion and health education. Nationally and internationally there is now an emphasis on consumer education and activities to promote a healthy life-style. However, the present taxonomy of nursing diagnoses is mainly focused on client problems. Assessing the strengths of the client and promoting wellness activities are also important nursing functions and should be more visible in the nursing diagnoses taxonomy.

The development of *Taxonomy I, Revised* based on the nine human response patterns is receiving some criticism. Porter (1986), points out that the human response patterns provide a theoretical or conceptual framework for the diagnostic categories rather than a true taxonomic structure that is based on principles of classification. Modifications therefore may need to be made to *Taxonomy I, Revised,* or an alternative taxonomy may have to be developed.

One of the major purposes of nursing diagnoses is to establish a method of validating independent nursing functions that would define nursing's unique role. A major task that is yet to be considered is the development of nursing interventions specific to each nursing diagnosis. Nurses will be accountable for these prescribed interventions. To date, a taxonomy of accepted clinical nursing interventions does not exist. However, lists of independent nursing functions are being developed. The nursing diagnoses accepted for use and research through 2006 are given below:

Nursing Diagnoses Accepted for Use and Research Through 2006

Activity intolerance (specify level)
Activity intolerance, risk for
Adjustment, impaired
Airway clearance, ineffective
Allergy response, latex
Allergy response, risk for latex
Anxiety (specify level)
Anxiety, death
Aspiration, risk for
Attachment, risk for impaired parent/infant/child
Autonomic Dysreflexia
Autonomic Dysreflexia, risk for

Body image, disturbed
Body temperature, risk for imbalanced
Bowel incontinence
Breastfeeding, effective
Breastfeeding, ineffective
Breastfeeding, interrupted
Breathing pattern, ineffective

Cardiac output, decreased
Caregiver role strain
Caregiver role strain, risk for
Communication, impaired verbal
Communication, readiness for enhanced
Conflict, decisional (specify)
Conflict, parental role
Confusion, acute
Confusion, chronic
Constipation
Constipation, perceived

Constipation, risk for
Coping, compromised family
Coping, defensive
Coping, disabled family
Coping, ineffective
Coping, readiness for enhanced
Coping, ineffective community
Coping, readiness for enhanced community
Coping, readiness for enhanced family

Death syndrome, risk for sudden infant
Denial, ineffective
Dentition, impaired
Development, risk for delayed
Diarrhea
Disuse syndrome, risk for
Diversional activity, deficient

Energy field, disturbed
Environmental interpretation syndrome, impaired

Failure to thrive, adult
Falls, risk for
Family Processes: alcoholism, dysfunctional
Family Processes, interrupted
Family Processes, readiness for enhanced
Fatigue
Fear (specify focus)
Fluid Balance, readiness for enhanced
(Fluid Volume, deficient hyper/hypotonic)
Fluid Volume, deficient (isotonic)
Fluid Volume, excess
Fluid Volume, risk for deficient
Fluid Volume, risk for imbalanced

Gas Exchange, impaired
Grieving, anticipatory
Grieving, dysfunctional
Grieving, risk for dysfunctional
Growth, risk for disproportionate
Growth and Development, delayed

Health Maintenance, ineffective
Health-Seeking Behaviors (specify)
Home Maintenance, impaired
Hopelessness
Hyperthermia
Hypothermia

Identity, disturbed personal
Infant Behavior, disorganized
Protection, ineffective

Rape-Trauma Syndrome
Rape-Trauma Syndrome: compound reaction
Rape-Trauma Syndrome: silent reaction

Religiosity, impaired
Religiosity, risk for impaired
Religiosity, readiness for enhanced
Relocation Stress Syndrome
Relocation Stress Syndrome, risk for
Role Performance, ineffective

Self-Care Deficit, bathing/hygiene
Self-Care Deficit, dressing/grooming
Self-Care Deficit, feeding
Self-Care Deficit, toileting
Self-Concept, readiness for enhanced
Self-Esteem, chronic low
Self- Esteem, situational low
Self- Esteem, risk for situational low
Self- Mutilation
Self-Mutilation, risk for
Sensory Perception, disturbed (specify: visual, auditory, kinesthetic, gustatory, tactile, olfactory)
Sexual Dysfunction
Sexuality Pattern, ineffective
Skin Integrity, impaired
Skin Integrity, risk for impaired
Sleep, readiness for enhanced
Sleep Deprivation
Sleep Pattern, disturbed
Social Interaction, impaired
Social Isolation
Sorrow, chronic
Spiritual Distress
Spiritual Distress, risk for
Spiritual Well-Being, readiness for enhanced
Suffocation, risk for
Suicide, risk for
Surgical Recovery, delayed
Swallowing, impaired

Therapeutic Regimen Management, effective
Therapeutic Regimen Management, ineffective
Therapeutic Regimen Management, ineffective community
Therapeutic, Regimen Management, ineffective family
Therapeutic Regimen Management, readiness for enhanced
Thermoregulation, ineffective
Though Processes, disturbed
Tissue Integrity, impaired
Tissue Perfusion, ineffective (specify type: cerebral, cardiopulmonary, renal, gastrointestinal, peripheral)
Transfer Ability, impaired
Trauma, risk for

Urinary Elimination, impaired
Urinary Elimination, readiness for enhanced
Urinary Incontinence, functional
Urinary Incontinence, reflex
Urinary Incontinence, risk for urge

Urinary Incontinence, stress
Urinary Incontinence, total
Urinary Incontinence, urge
Urinary Retention (acute/chronic)

Ventilation, impaired spontaneous
Ventilatory Weaning Response, dysfunctional
Violence, (actual/) risk for other-directed
Violence, (actual/) risk for self-directed

Walking, impaired
Wandering (specify sporadic or continual)

After data are collected and areas of concern/need identified, the nurse is directed to the Diagnostic Divisions to review the list of nursing diagnoses that fall within the individual categories. This will assist the nurse in choosing the specific diagnostic label to accurately describe the data. Then, with the addition of etiology or related/risk factors (when known) and signs and symptoms, or cues (defining characteristics), the client diagnostic statement emerges.

Activity/Rest – Ability to engage in necessary/desired activities of life (work and leisure) and to obtain adequate sleep/rest
- Activity Intolerance
- Activity Intolerance, risk for
- Disuse Syndrome, risk for
- Diversional Activity, deficient
- Fatigue
- Lifestyle, sedentary
- Mobility, impaired bed
- Mobility, impaired physical
- Mobility, impaired wheelchair
- Sleep Deprivation
- Sleep Pattern, disturbed
- Sleep, readiness for enhanced
- Transfer Ability, impaired
- Walking, impaired

Circulation – Ability to transport oxygen and nutrients necessary to meet cellular needs
- Autonomic Dysreflexia
- Autonomic Dysreflexia, risk for
- Cardiac Output, decreased
- Intracranial Adaptive Capacity, decreased
- Tissue Perfusion, ineffective (specify type: renal, cerebral, cardiopulmonary, gastrointestinal, peripheral)

Ego Integrity – Ability to develop and use skills and behaviors to integrate and manage life experiences
- Adjustment, impaired
- Anxiety (specify level)
- Anxiety, death
- Body Image, disturbed

- Conflict, decisional (specify)
- Coping, defensive
- Coping, ineffective
- Coping, readiness for enhanced
- Denial, ineffective
- Energy Field, disturbed
- Fear
- Grieving, anticipatory
- Grieving, dysfunctional
- Grieving, risk for dysfunctional
- Hopelessness
- Personal Identity, disturbed
- Post-Trauma Syndrome
- Post-Trauma Syndrome, risk for
- Powerlessness
- Powerlessness, risk for
- Rape-Trauma Syndrome
- Rape-Trauma Syndrome: compound reaction
- Rape-Trauma Syndrome: silent reaction
- Religiosity, readiness for enhanced
- Religiosity, impaired
- Religiosity, risk for impaired
- Relocation Stress Syndrome
- Relocation Stress Syndrome, risk for
- Self-Concept, readiness for enhanced
- Self-Esteem, chronic low
- Self-Esteem, situational low
- Self-Esteem, risk for situational low
- Sorrow, chronic
- Spiritual Distress
- Spiritual Distress, risk for
- Spiritual Well-Being, readiness for enhanced

Elimination – Ability to excrete waste products
- Bowel Incontinence
- Constipation
- Constipation, perceived
- Constipation, risk for
- Diarrhea
- Urinary Elimination, impaired
- Urinary Elimination, readiness for enhanced
- Urinary Incontinence, functional
- Urinary Incontinence, reflex
- Urinary Incontinence, stress
- Urinary Incontinence, total
- Urinary Incontinence, urge
- Urinary Incontinence, risk for urge
- Urinary Retention (acute/chronic)

Food/Fluid – Ability to maintain intake of and utilize nutrients and liquids to meet physiological needs
- Breastfeeding, effective
- Breastfeeding, ineffective
- Breastfeeding, interrupted
- Dentition, impaired

- Failure to Thrive, adult (Fluid Volume, deficient hyper/hypotonic)
- Fluid Volume, deficient (isotonic)
- Fluid Volume excess
- Fluid Volume, risk for deficient
- Fluid Volume, risk for imbalanced
- Infant Feeding Pattern, ineffective
- Nausea
- Nutrition, less than body requirements, imbalanced
- Nutrition, more than body requirements, imbalanced
- Nutrition, risk for more than body requirements, imbalanced
- Nutrition, readiness for enhanced
- Oral mucous Membrane, impaired
- Swallowing impaired

Hygiene – Ability to perform activities of daily living
- Self-Care Deficit: bathing/hygiene, dressing/grooming, feeding, toileting

Neurosensory – Ability to perceive, integrate, and respond to internal and external cues
- Confusion, acute
- Confusion, chronic
- Infant Behavior, disorganized
- Infant Behavior, risk for disorganized
- Infant Behavior, readiness for enhanced organized
- Memory, impaired
- Peripheral Neurovascular Dysfunction, risk for
- Sensory Perception, disturbed (specify: visual, auditory, kinesthetic, gustatory, tactile, olfactory)
- Thought Processes, disturbed
- Unilateral Neglect

Pain/Discomfort – Ability to control internal/external environment to maintain comfort
- Pain, acute
- Pain, chronic

Respiration – Ability to provide and use oxygen to meet physiological needs
- Airway Clearance, ineffective
- Aspiration, risk for
- Breathing Pattern, ineffective
- Gas Exchange, impaired
- Ventilation, impaired spontaneous
- Ventilatory Weaning Response, dysfunctional

Safety – Ability to provide safe, growth-promoting environment
- Allergy Response, latex
- Allergy Response, risk for latex
- Body Temperature, risk for imbalanced
- Environmental Interpretation Syndrome, impaired
- Falls, risk for
- Health Maintenance, ineffective
- Home Maintenance, impaired

- Hyperthermia
- Hypothermia
- Infection, risk for
- Injury, risk for
- Injury, risk for perioperative positioning
- Mobility, impaired physical
- Poisoning, risk for
- Protection, ineffective
- Self-Mutilation
- Self-Mutilation, risk for
- Skin Integrity, impaired
- Skin Integrity, risk for impaired
- Suffocation, risk for
- Suicide, risk for
- Surgical Recovery, delayed
- Thermoregulation, ineffective
- Tissue Integrity, impaired
- Trauma, risk for
- Violence, (actual/) risk for other-directed
- Violence, (actual/) risk for self-directed
- Wandering (specify sporadic or continual)

Sexuality (Component of Ego Integrity and Social Interaction)—Ability to meet requirements/characteristics of male/female role
- Sexual Dysfunction
- Sexuality Pattern, ineffective

Social Interaction – Ability to establish and maintain relationships
- Attachment, risk for impaired parent/infant/child
- Caregiver Role Strain
- Communication, impaired verbal
- Communication, readiness for enhanced
- Coping, ineffective community
- Coping, readiness for enhanced community
- Coping, compromised family
- Coping, disabled family
- Coping, readiness for enhanced family
- Family Processes, interrupted
- Family Processes, alcoholism, dysfunctional
- Loneliness, risk for
- Parental Role Conflict
- Parenting, impaired
- Parenting, risk for impaired
- Parenting, readiness for enhanced
- Role Performance, ineffective
- Social Interaction, impaired
- Social Isolation

Teaching/Learning – Ability to incorporate and use information to achieve healthy lifestyle/optimal wellness
- Development, risk for delayed
- Growth and Development, delayed
- Growth, risk for disproportionate

- Health-Seeking Behaviors (specify)
- Knowledge, deficient (specify)
- Knowledge (specify), readiness for enhanced
- Noncompliance [Adherence, ineffective] [specify]
- Therapeutic Regimen Management, effective
- Therapeutic Regimen Management, ineffective community
- Therapeutic Regimen Management, ineffective family
- Therapeutic Regimen Management, ineffective

Grouping on NANDA Nursing Diagnoses Grouped by Gordon's Functional Health Patterns

Health-perception-health

Management pattern
- Health-Seeking Behaviors (Specify)
- Altered Health Maintenance (Specify)
- Ineffective Management of Therapeutic Regimen (Specify Area)
- Risk for Ineffective Management of Therapeutic Regimen (Specify Area)
- Effective Management of Therapeutic Regimen
- Ineffective Family Management of Therapeutic Regimen
- Ineffective Community Management of Therapeutic Regimen
- Health-Management Deficit (Specify Area)
- Risk for Health-Management Deficit (Specify Area)
- Non-compliance (Specify Area)
- Risk for Non-compliance (Specify Area)
- Risk for Infection (Specify Area/Type)
- Risk for Injury (Trauma)
- Risk for Perioperative Positioning Injury
- Risk for Poisoning
- Risk for Suffocation
- Altered Protection (Specify)
- Energy Field Disturbance

Nutritional – Metabolic Pattern
- Altered Nutrition: More than Body Requirements or Exogenous Obesity
- Altered Nutrition: Risk for More than Body
- Requirements or Risk for Obesity
- Altered Nutrition: Less than Body Requirements or Nutritional Deficit (Specify Type)
- Adult Failure to Thrive
- Ineffective Breastfeeding
- Interrupted Breastfeeding
- Effective Breastfeeding
- Ineffective Infant Feeding Pattern
- Impaired Swallowing (Uncompensated)
- Nausea
- Risk for Aspiration
- Altered Oral Mucous Membrane (Specify Alteration)
- Altered Dentition
- Fluid Volume Deficit

- Risk for Fluid Volume Deficit
- Fluid Volume Excess
- Risk for Fluid Volume Imbalance
- Impaired Skin Integrity
- Risk for Impaired Skin Integrity or Risk for Skin Breakdown
- Pressure Ulcer (Specify Stages)
- Impaired Tissue Integrity (Specify Type)
- Latex Allergy Responses
- Risk for Latex Allergy Responses
- Ineffective Thermoregulation
- Hyperthermia
- Hypothermia
- Risk for Altered Body Temperature

Elimination Pattern
- Constipation
- Perceived Constipation
- Intermittent Constipation Pattern
- Risk for Constipation
- Diarrhea
- Bowel Incontinence
- Altered Urinary Elimination Pattern
- Functional Urinary Incontinence
- Reflex Urinary Incontinence
- Stress Incontinence
- Urge Incontinence
- Risk for Urinary Urge Incontinence
- Total Incontinence
- Urinary Retention

Activity-Exercise Pattern
- Activity Intolerance (Specify level)
- Risk for Activity Intolerance
- Fatigue
- Impaired Physical Mobility (Specify level)
- Impaired Bed Mobility (Specify level)
- Impaired Transfer Ability (Specify level)
- Impaired Wheelchair Mobility
- Impaired Walking (Specify level)
- Risk for Disuse Syndrome
- Risk for Joint Contractions
- Total Self-Care Deficit (Specify level)
- Self-Bathing-Hygiene Deficit (Specify level)
- Self-Dressing-Grooming Deficit (Specify level)
- Self-Feeding Deficit (Specify level)
- Self-Toileting Deficit (Specify level)
- Developmental Delay: Self-Care Skills (Specify level)
- Delayed Surgical Recovery
- Altered Growth and Development
- Risk for Altered Growth
- Risk for Altered Development
- Diversional Activity Deficit
- Impaired Home Maintenance Management (Mild, Moderate, Severe, Potential, Chronic)
- Dysfunctional Ventilatory Weaning Response
- Inability to Sustain Spontaneous Ventilation

- Ineffective Airway Clearance
- Ineffective Breathing Pattern
- Impaired Gas Exchange
- Decreased Cardiac Output
- Altered Tissue Perfusion (Specify)
- Dysreflexia
- Risk for Autonomic Dysreflexia
- Disorganized Infant Behavior
- Risk for Disorganized Infant Behavior
- Potential for Enhanced Organized Infant Behavior
- Risk for Peripheral Neurovascular Dysfunction
- Decreased Intracranial Adaptive Capacity

Sleep-Rest Pattern
- Sleep-Pattern Disturbance (Specify Type)
- Sleep Deprivation
- Delayed Sleep Onset
- Sleep Pattern Reversal

Cognitive-Perceptual Pattern
- Pain (Specify Location)
- Chronic Pain (Specify Location)
- Pain Self-Management Deficit (Acute, Chronic)
- Uncompensated Sensory Loss (Specify Type/Degree)
- Sensory Overload (Sensory-Perceptual Alteration)
- Sensory Deprivation (Sensory-Perceptual Alteration)
- Unilateral Neglect
- Knowledge Deficit (Specify Area)
- Altered Thought Processes

Attention-Concentration Deficit
- Acute Confusion
- Chronic Confusion
- Impaired Environmental Interpretation Syndrome
- Uncompensated Memory Loss
- Impaired Memory
- Risk for Cognitive Impairment
- Decisional Conflict (Specify)

Self-Perception-Self-Concept Pattern
- Fear (Specify Focus)
- Anxiety
- Mild Anxiety
- Moderate Anxiety
- Severe Anxiety (Panic)
- Anticipatory Anxiety (Mild, Moderate, Severe)
- Death Anxiety
- Reactive Depression (Specify Situation)
- Risk for Loneliness
- Hopelessness
- Powerlessness (Severe, Moderate, Low)
- Low Self-Esteem
- Chronic Low Self-Esteem
- Situational Low Self-Esteem
- Body Image Disturbance
- Risk for Self-Mutilation
- Personal Identify Disturbance

Role-Relationship Pattern

- Anticipatory Grieving
- Dysfunctional Grieving
- Chronic Sorrow
- Altered Role Performance (Specify)
- Unresolved Independence-Dependence Conflict
- Social Isolation or Social Rejection
- Social Isolation
- Impaired Social Interaction
- Developmental Delay: Social Skills (Specify)
- Risk for Self-Directed Violence
- Risk for Other -Directed Violence
- Relocation Stress Syndrome
- Altered Family Processes (Specify Process)
- Altered Family Processes: Alcoholism
- Altered Parenting (Specify Alteration)
- Risk for Altered Parenting (Specify Alteration)
- Parental Role Conflict
- Weak Parent-Infant Attachment
- Risk for Altered Parent-Infant/Child Attachment
- Parent-Infant Separation
- Caregiver Role Strain
- Risk for Caregiver Role Strain
- Impaired Verbal Communication Skills (Specify Type)
- Risk for Violence

Sexuality-Reproductive Pattern

- Ineffective Coping (Individual)
- Avoidance Coping
- Defensive Coping
- Ineffective Denial or Denial
- Compromised Family Coping
- Disabling Family Coping
- Ineffective Community Coping
- Family Coping: Potential for Growth
- Potential for Enhanced Community Coping
- Impaired Adjustment
- Post-trauma Syndrome
- Risk for Post-trauma Syndrome
- Support System Deficit

Value-Belief Pattern

- Spiritual Distress (Distress of Human Spirit)
- Potential for Enhanced Spiritual Well-being
- Risk for Spiritual Distress

Guidelines for Good Diagnosis Statements

- When choosing a label (NANDA) do not rely on the label definition alone. Always compare patient data to the defining characteristics of the label do well as to the definition.
- Include both problem and etiology, with cause and effect stated correctly, e.g. Ineffective Breast feeding r/t deficient knowledge (specify)
- Be sure that the etiology does not merely restate the problem,e.g. impaired physical mobility, inability to walk r/t weakness and pain in legs

- Avoid using medical diagnosis and treatments as etiological factor risk for impaired skin integrity (ulcers, infection) r/t lack of knowledge of self-care measures for trimming nails and inspecting fact
- Risk for impaired or skin integrity (pressure ulcers) r/t improved physical mobility (total) secondary to high spinal injury
- Write the statement clearly: avoid abbreviations and jargons as much as possible, e.g. Impaired physical mobility (inability to get out of bed without assistance) r/t muscle weakness and pain in left leg
- Write the statement concisely use complex etiology instead of listing numerous etiological factors or describe the signs and symptoms in the nurses notes, e.g. constipation r/t complex factors (see nurses notes)
- Be sure the statements is descriptive and specific
  - Being sure to include all appropriate etiological factors
  - Reviewing the label definition
  - Using PES format to add the patients signs and symptoms
  - Adding qualifying wards (e.g. mill, severe, occasional, or constant) to the label, e.g. severe abdominal pain r/t peptic ulcer
  - Adding secondary to the etiology
  - Adding a colon and descriptors to the label, e.g. impaired mobility: inability to walk r/t pain in legs
- State the problem as a potential response, e.g. deficient fluid volume r/t………
- Use non-judgmental language, e.g. risk for infection r/t lack of information about sanitation and hand washing
- Avoid legally questionable language

Planning

In general, planning is designing or arranging the parts of something to achieve an end or goal. In nursing, planning is the third step of the nursing process. In this context, **Planning** is the process of designing the nursing strategies or interventions required to prevent, reduce, or eliminate those client health problems identified and validated during the diagnostic phase. The following people can be involved in planning nursing strategies, one or more nurses, the client, family members, support persons, and/or caregivers, and sometimes members of other health professions. Although the planning process is basically the responsibility of the nurse, input from the client and support persons is essential if a plan is to be effective. It is no longer sufficient that nurses plan for the client, whenever possible, the client must participate actively.

Medicine and nursing as well as other health care disciplines are interrelated, and therefore the actions for each discipline have implications for the others. This interrelationship allows for exchange of information and ideas and for development of plans of care that include all data pertinent to the individual client and/or family. In this book, the plan of care contains not only the actions initiated by medical an nursing orders, but also the coordination of care provided by all related health care disciplines. The nurse is often the person responsible for coordinating theses various activities into a comprehensive functional plan, essential in providing holistic care for the client. Although independent nursing actions are an integral part of this process, collaborative actions are usually present based on the medical regimen or orders from other disciplines participating in the care of the client. We believe that nursing is an essential part of collaborative practice, and, as such, nursing has a responsibility and accountability in every collaborative problem in which the nurse interacts with the client. The educational background and expertise of the nurse, standing protocols, delegation of tasks, the use of care partners and the area of practice (rural or urban, acute care or community care settings) influence whether and intervention is actually an independent nursing function or requires collaboration.

The well-written plan of care communicates the clients past and present health status and current needs to all members of the health care team involved in providing care. It identifies problems solved and those yet to be solved, can inform of approaches that have been successful, and notes patterns of client responses to interventions. In legal terms, the plan of care documents client in areas of liability, accountability, and quality improvement. It also provides a mechanism to help ensure continuity of care when the client leaves a care setting while still needing services.

For a client in a home setting, the home health care nurse needs to involve the client, if the clients health permits, as well as the clients support person and/or the caregiver. With the nurse guidance, these people can implement the plan of care, thus, its effectiveness depends largely on them. They can also provide information about problems previously unknown to the nurse.

When a client is admitted to the hospital or long-term care setting, it is important for the nurse to know if the person required care at home prior to admission. If care was necessary, input from the family and other caregivers assists the nursing staff in continuing to implement appropriate interventions and thus provide the client optimum continuity of care.

Planning is a deliberative, systematic process that is critical to the attainment of quality nursing care. It is a process in which decision making and problem solving are carried out. The planning process uses (1) data obtained during assessing (2) the diagnostic statements that present the clients health problems (potential and actual). Accurate nursing diagnoses provide direction for determining client goals and developing a plan of care.

The critical element for providing effective planned nursing care is its relevance a identified in client assessments. Client assessment is required in the following areas; physical, psychologic, sociocultural, spiritual, cognitive, functional abilities, developmental, economic and lifestyle. These assessments, combined with the results of medical findings and diagnostic studies, are documented in the client database and form the foundation for development of the clients plan of care. For each plan of care presented in this book, a client assessment database is created from information that would likely be

obtained from the history, physical examination, and related diagnosis studies. Nursing priorities are then determined and ranked. Priorities are simply stated and represent a general ranking system for the nursing diagnoses in the plan of care. They can be rewarded and/or reorganized along with their timelines to create short- and long-term goals. Next, the nursing diagnosis statements, which include possible related factors (etiology) and corresponding signs and symptoms (cues) when appropriate are presented. Desired client outcomes are then identified and followed by appropriate independent and collaborative interventions with accompanying rationales. Each selected medical condition has an accompanying client database that includes subjective ("may report") and objective ("may exhibit") data that would likely be collected through the history-taking interview, physical assessment, diagnostic studies, and review of prior records.

Interviewing the client and/or significant other(s) provides data that the nurse obtains through conversation and observation. This information includes the individual's perceptions, that is, what the client perceives to be a problem and typically what he or she wants to share. Data may be collected during one or more contact periods and should include all relevant information. All participants in the interview process need to know that collected data are used in planning the client's care. Organizing and updating the data assists in the ongoing identification of client care needs and nursing diagnoses. During information gathering, the nurse exercises perceptual and observational skills, assessing the client through the senses of sight, hearing, touch and smell. The duration and depth of any physical assessment depend on the current condition of the client and the urgency of the situation, but it usually includes inspection, palpation, percussion and auscultation. In this book, the physical assessment data are presented within the client database as objective data. Interpretation of diagnostic test results is integrated with the history and physical findings as part of objective findings. Some tests are used to diagnose disease, whereas others are useful in following the course of a disease or in adjusting therapies. The nurse needs to be aware of significant test results.

Nursing diagnoses are a uniform way of identifying, focusing on, and dealing with specific client needs and responses to actual and high-risk problems. Nursing diagnosis labels provide a format for expressing the problem identification portion of the nursing process. The definition of nursing diagnosis developed by NANDA is "Nursing diagnosis is a clinical judgment about individual, family or community responses to actual and potential health problems/life processes. Nursing diagnoses provide the basis for selection of nursing interventions to achieve outcomes for which the nurse is accountable".

There are several steps involved in the process of problem/need identification. Integrating these steps provides a systematic approach to accurately identifying nursing diagnoses using the process of critical thinking.

1. Collecting a client database (nursing interview, physical assessment, and diagnostic studies) combined with information collected by other health care providers.

2. Reviewing and analyzing the client data.

3. Synthesizing the gathered client data as a whole and then labeling your clinical or high-risk problems/life processes.

4. Comparing and contrasting the relationships of your clinical judgments against related factors and defining characteristics for the selected nursing diagnosis. This step is crucial to choosing and validating the appropriate nursing diagnosis label that will be used to create a specific client diagnostic statement.

5. Combining the nursing diagnosis with the related factors and defining characteristics to create the client diagnostic statement. For example, the diagnostic statement for a paraplegic client with a decubitus ulcer could read: impaired skin integrity related to pressure, circulatory impairment, and decreased sensation evidenced by draining wound, sacral area.

The nursing diagnosis is as correct as the present information allows because it is supported by the immediate data collected. It documents the client's situation at the present time and should reflect changes as they occur in the client's condition. Accurate need identification and diagnostic labeling provide the basis for selecting nursing interventions.

The nursing diagnosis may be a physical or a psychosocial response. Physical nursing diagnoses include those that pertain to physical processes, such as circulation (ineffective renal Tissue Perfusion), ventilation (impaired Gas Exchange) and elimination (Constipation). Psychosocial nursing diagnoses include those that pertain to the mind (acute Confusion), emotions (Fear), or lifestyle/relationships (ineffective Role Performance). Unlike medical diagnoses nursing diagnoses change as the client progresses through various stages of illness/maladaption to resolution of the problem or to the conclusion of the condition. Each decision the nurse makes is time dependent, and, with additional information gathered at a later point in time, decisions may change. For example, the initial problems/needs for a client undergoing cardiac surgery may be acute pain, decreased Cardiac Output, ineffective Airway Clearance, and Risk for Infection. As the client progresses, problems/needs are likely to shift to Activity Intolerance, deficient Knowledge, and Ineffective Role of Performance.

Diagnostic reasoning is used to ensure the accuracy of the client diagnostic statement. The defining characteristics and related factors associated with the chosen nursing diagnosis are reviewed and compared with the client data. If the diagnosis is not consistent with a majority of the cues or is not supported by relevant cues, additional data may be required or another nursing diagnosis needs to be considered.

A desired client outcome is defined as the result of achievable nursing interventions and client responses that is desired by the client and/or caregiver and attainable within a defined time period, given the present situation and resources. These desired outcomes are the measurable steps toward achieving the previously established discharge goals and are used to evaluate the client's response to nursing interventions. Useful desired client outcomes must:

- Be specific
- Be realistic
- Be measurable
- Indicate a definite time frame for achievement
- Consider clients desires and resources.

Desired client outcomes are created by listing items and/or behaviors that can be observed or heard. They are monitored to determine whether an acceptable outcome has been achieved within a specified time frame. Action verbs and time frames are used, for example, "client will ambulate, using cane, within 48 hours of surgery". The action verbs describe the client's behavior to be evaluated. Time frames are dependent on the clients projected or anticipated length of stay, often determined by diagnosis-related group (DRG) classification and considering the presence of complication or extenuating circumstances (e.g. age, debilitating disease process). The ongoing work of NOC in identifying 330 outcomes now also addresses client groups or aggregates. Although the NOC outcomes are listed in general terms such as Ambulation: Walking, 12 indicators are included for this outcome that can be measured by a five point Likert-type scale ranging from "dependent, does not participate" to "completely independent". This facilitates tracking clients across care settings and can demonstrate client progress even when outcomes are not met.

When outcomes are properly written, they provide direction for planning and validating the selected nursing interventions. Consider the two following client outcomes: "Client will identify individual nutritional needs within 36 hours" and " …..formulate a dietary plan based on identified nutritional needs within 72 hours". Based on the clarity of these outcomes, the nurse can select nursing interventions to ensure that the clients dietary knowledge is assessed, individual needs identified, and nutritional education presented. Often, the client outcomes identified are not unique to nursing because we provide care in a team approach with other disciplines. However, the NOC indicators for outcomes are more sensitive to interventions. Other team members can use the majority of NOC labels and identify different indicators relative to their speciality focus to demonstrate their contribution to client improvement or to track deterioration (See Appendix ——for NIC & NOC).

Nursing in interventions are prescriptions for specific behaviors expected from the client and actions to be carried out/facilitated by nurses. These actions/interventions are selected to assist the client in achieving the stated desired client outcomes and discharge goals. The expectation is that the prescribed behavior will benefit the client/family in a predictable way related to the identified problem/need and chosen outcomes. These interventions have the intent of individualizing care by meeting a specific client need an should incorporate identified client strengths when possible.

Nursing interventions should be specific and clearly stated, beginning with an action verb. Qualifiers of how, when, where, time/frequency and amount provide the content of the planned activity, for example, "Assist as needed with self-care activities each morning". "Record respiratory and pulse rates before, during and after activity", and "Instruct family in postdischarge care".

The NIC project has identified 514 interventions (Both direct and indirect) that are stated in general terms, such as Respiratory Monitoring. Each label has a varied number of activities that may be chosen to accomplish the intervention. The interventions encompass a broad range of nursing practice, with some requiring specialized training/advanced certification. Others may be appropriate for delegation to other care providers, (e.g. licensed practical nurses [LPNs], nursing assistants, unlicensed personnel) but still require planning and evaluation by registered nurses. In this next, these NIC labels are boxed to help the user begin to identify how they can be used.

This divides the nursing interventions/actions into independent (nurse initiated) and collaborative (initiated by/ performed in conjunction with other care providers) under the appropriate NIC labels. Examples of these two different professionally initiated actions are:

- Independent: Provide calm, restful surroundings, minimize environmental activity/noise, and limit numbers of visitors and length of stay.
- Collaborative: Administer antianxiety medication as indicated

Although rationales do not appear on regular plans of care, they are included in this book to assist the student and practicing nurse in associating the pathophysiologic and/or psychologic principles with the selected nursing intervention. This will help the nurse determine whether an intervention is appropriate for a specific client.

Phases of Planning

Planning may be formal or informal; Formal planning is a conscious, deliberate activity involving decision-making, critical thinking and creativity, while performing other nursing process steps we will include something in the plan called informal planning. Planning phase of the nursing process the nurse establishes priorities of care, selects and converts nursing interventions into nursing orders, and communicates the plan of care using standardized language or recognized terminology to document the plan. After the nursing diagnosis and the clients strength have been identified, planning begins the nurse must decide what can be done to lessen or solve an actual problem or prevent a risk problem from becoming actual problem. The decision about what interventions will likely be effective is made during the planning phase.

The planning occurs in three phases: initial, ongoing and discharge.

- *Initial planning:* Involves development of a preliminary plan of care by the nurse who performs the admission assessment and gathers the comprehensive admission assessment data. Progressively shorter stays in the hospital make initial planning very important to ensure resolution of the problems
- *Ongoing planning:* Updates the client's plan of care. New information about the client is collected and evaluated and revisions made to the plan of care

- *Discharge planning:* Involves anticipation and planning for the clients needs after discharge.

The planning phase involves several tasks, which includes:
- Prioritizing the nursing diagnosis
- Identifying and writing client centered long and short-term goals, objectives/outcomes
- Identifying specific nursing interventions
- Recording the entire nursing care plan in the clients record

1. *Prioritizing the Nursing Diagnosis***:** Once a list of nursing diagnosis has been developed, the problems can be ranked in order to importance for the patient's life and health. A useful framework to guide the prioritization is Maslow's hierarchy of Needs. The structure is based on the principle that lower-level needs must be met before higher-level needs can be satisfied. The physiological needs are more vital than the safety and security needs and the safety and security needs are more critical than the love and belonging needs. Life threatening and health-threatening problems are ranked before other types of problems.

2. *Identifying and Writing Goals and Objectives:* A goal is an aim, intent or end. Goals are broad statements than describe the desired or intended change in the client's conditions or behavior. Goals are important for planning, implementation and evaluation. A goal statement is a statement about the purpose to which effort is directed. The nurse would then carry out activities to accomplish the goals. Here goals may be long-term goals or short-term goal. Long-term goals are changes in health status than nurse with to achieve over a long period – a week, a month, or more. They describe the optimum level of functioning than nurse expect the patient to achieve, given health status and available resources. A long-term goal is a statement than profiles the desired resolution of the nursing diagnosis over a longer period of time, usually weeks or months.

Short-term goals are those that nurse expect the patient to achieve within few hours or days. A short-term goal is a statement that profits the desired resolution of the nursing diagnosis over a short period of time, usually a few hours or days (less than a week). After the goals have been established, the objectives can be identified based on the goals. Objectives are the short statements of precise, descriptive, clearly stated goals or expected outcomes, which will form the criteria for evaluation; provide a guide for selection of nursing intervention and motivate the client and nurse by providing a sense of achievement when the goals are met.

A well-written objective does the following:
- Uses the word patient or a part of the patient as subject of the statement
- Uses a measurable verb
- Is specific for the patient and the patient problem
- Is realistic for the patient and the patient problem
- Includes a time frame for patient reevaluation.

The statement of the objectives should have subject, action verbs, performance criteria, target time and special conditions:
- The subject is undertake to be the client/patient, but it can also be a function or part of the client. The statements should begin with the words, "the client will............".

- Use an action verb to indicate the action than client will perform: which the client will learn, do or say. Use concrete or measurable verbs than describe actions and indicates the precise behavior than the nurse anticipates, seeing, hearing, smelling, and feeling. Following are the examples of action verbs".

Apply	Explain	Select
Choose	Eat	Transfer
Define	List	Turn
Demonstrate	Measure	Verbalize
Drink	Prepare	
	Report	

- There are some standards of evaluating the client performance, which describes the extent to which nurse expect to see the action or behavior. So write them in concrete, observable terms, performance criteria specify: How, what, when and where something to be done. And also amount, quality, accuracy, speed, distance and so far.
- The target time is the 'When' part of the performance criteria. The realistic data or time by which performance/behavior should be achieved. Time frame helps to provide a disorders for evaluation of the patient progress.
- Include special conditions which it important for other nurses to know then that is describe the amount of assistance of resources needed or the experiences/treatment the client should have to perform the behavior.

3. *Identifying the Specific Nursing Intervention:* Nursing intervention are actions based on clinical judgment and nursing knowledge than nurses perform to achieve client outcomes. Interventions are also referred to as nursing actions, measures, strategies, and activities. Nursing interventions include a broad range of activities as given below:

- A direct care intervention is one performed through the interactions with the client(s). Direct care activities include physical care, emotional support and patient teaching.
- An indirect care, an intervention is an activity performed away from the client but on behalf of a client or group of clients. Indirect care activities include advocacy, managing the environment, consulting with other members of the health care team, and making referred.

Nursing interventions include independent, dependent and collaborations actions.

- *Independent:* Nursing interventions (Nurse prescribed intervention) is one than nurses are authorized to prescribe perform or delegate based on their knowledge and skill. These are initiated by the nurse and do not require directions or an order from another health care professional. For example, elevating the clients edematan extremity, knowing how, when and why to the perform an activity makes action independent. For example, providing a back massage, changing positions, monitoring complication.
- *Dependent:* Nursing intervention (physical prescribed intervention) are one that is prescribed by the physicians or another health care profession. Dependent nursing interventions are usually orders for diagnostic tests, medications, treatments, intravenous therapy, diet and activities. Dependent interventions must be governed by appropriate knowledge and judgment by the nurse.
- *Inter-dependent or collaborative intervention:* It is carried out collaboration with other health care team members, since nurses care for the whole person, their responsibilities often overlap with other team members. Ex, assist the client to perform exercises taught by physiotherapist.

4. *Recording the Nursing Care Plan:* The nursing care plan is a written guide of strategies implements to help the client achieve optimal health. Nursing care plans usually include components such as assessment, nursing diagnosis, objectives and nursing interventions. The nursing care plan is begin on the day admission and is continually updated until discharge.

After completing the initial assessment, analyzing the data, writing the nursing diagnosis and selecting appropriate nursing interventions, than are then made more specific by nursing orders, the nurse must communicate the detailed plan of care for the patient. The written nursing care plan is the product of the nursing process.

Format for the written nursing care plan vary from institution to institution.

Nursing care plan may be prepared for each patient, be standardized for a group of patients with common illness or be computerized. Individually prepared care plans are the most time consuming but after provide the most individualized care. Some comprehensive system print and updated nursing care plan for each shift.

Components of Planning

The six components of planning are:
1. Setting priorities
2. Establishing client goals and outcomes criteria or objectives
3. Planning nursing strategies
4. Writing nursing orders
5. Writing the nursing care plan
6. Consulting

Setting Priorities

Priority setting is the process of establishing a preferential order for nursing strategies. To set priorities, the nurse and the client first order the nursing diagnosis preferentially, i.e. they decide which deserves attention first, which second, and so on. Diagnoses can be grouped as having high, medium, or low priority. This priority setting, however, does not mean that all the high-priority diagnoses must be resolved before any others are considered. A high-priority diagnoses may be dealt with. In addition, the nurse may address more than one diagnosis at a time. Because client problems are usually multiple, this is often the case. (See Table 10.11 for the assignment of priorities to the diagnostic statements for Mr Venkatesh.)

Setting priorities is made easier by using a framework such as nursing model or theory. One frequently used framework is Maslow's hierarchy of needs. Maslow's physiologic needs, such as air, food and water, are basic to life and receive higher priority than the need for security or activity.

Life threatening problems, such as loss of respiratory or cardiac functioning, have the highest priority. Health threatening problems, either actual or potential, such as acute illness and decreased coping ability, may result in delayed development or impaired functioning. Health threatening problems usually have medium priority. Growth needs, such as self-esteem are not necessary for sustaining life. Thus, when the nurse plans care for a client with unmet physiologic needs and unmet growth needs, the basic or physiologic needs are the first priority.

The importance of the clients involvement in setting priorities cannot be overemphasized. Although a nurse may believe she or he knows a client, the clients values may be different than the nurse supposes, one nursing diagnosis may relate to smoking and another to nutrition. The nurse may give the smoking problem a higher priority than the problem of obesity, but the client may see the problem of obesity as more important. When there is such a difference of opinion, the client and nurse should discuss it openly or resolve the conflict. However, in a life-threatening situation, the nurse needs to take the initiative.

The priorities assigned to problems should not remain fixed. Nursing priorities must change as a client's health problems and therapy change.

Nursing priorities are listed in a certain order to facilitate the linking/ranking of selected associated nursing diagnoses that appear in the plan of care guidelines. In many given client situation, nursing priorities are based on the clients specific needs and can vary from minute to minute. A nursing diagnosis that is a priority today may be less a priority tomorrow, depending on the fluctuating physical and psychosocial condition of the client or the clients changing responses to the existing conditions.

An example of nursing priorities for a client diagnosed with severe hypertension would include (Table 10.11).

1. Maintain/enhance cardiovascular functioning
2. Prevent complications
3. Provide information about disease process, prognosis, and treatment regimen
4. Support active control or management of condition.

Once the nursing priorities are determined, the next step is to establish goals of treatment. In this book, each medical condition has established discharge goals, which are broadly stated and reflect the desired general status of the client on discharge or transfer to another care setting.

Discharge goals for a client with severe hypertension would include:

1. Blood pressure within acceptable limits for individual
2. Cardiovascular and systemic complications prevented/minimized
3. Disease process/prognosis and therapeutic regimen understood
4. Necessary lifestyle/behavioral changes initiated.

Values concerning health may be very important to the nurse but not to the client. For example, a client may see attendance at school or being home for the children as more urgent than a health problem. Offering the client the opportunity to set priorities allows client participation in care planning and enhances cooperation between the nurse and client. Sometimes, however, the clients perception of what is important conflicts with the nurses knowledge of potential future problems or complications. For example, an elderly female may not regard ambulation or turning and repositioning every 2 hours as important, preferring to be undisturbed. The nurse, however, aware of the potential complications of prolonged bed rest (e.g. muscle weakness and decubitus ulcers), needs to inform the client and implement necessary interventions to prevent such debilitating effects. If money, equipment or personnel are scarce, then a health problem may be given a lower priority than usual. Nurses in a home setting, for example, do not have the resources of a hospital, therefore, if the resources needed for specific nursing strategies are not available, the solution of that problem might need to be postponed, or the client may need referral.

Client resources, such as finances or coping abilities, may also influences the setting of priorities. For example, a client who is unemployed may defer dental treatment; a client whose husband is terminally ill and dependent on her may consider nutritional guidance directed toward weight loss as too much to handle. Each client feels comfortable with a certain pace of action. Some clients may want to discuss the problem with family members or think about it overnight. Others may want "to get on with it". The nurse must allow adequate time for the necessary strategies resulting from the nursing diagnosis.

Life-threatening situations require that the nurse establish priorities quickly. This also applies to situations that affect the integrity of the client, i.e. that could have a negative or destructive effect on the client. Such health problems as drug abuse and radical alteration of self-concept due to amputation can be destructive not only to the individual but also to the family. These health problems should receive high priority. The priorities for treating health problems must be congruent with treatment by other health professionals. For example, a high priority for the client might be to become ambulatory; however, if the physician's therapeutic regimen calls for extended bed rest, then ambulation must assume a lower priority in the nursing strategy plan. In such a case, however, the nurse can provide strategy plan. In such a case, however, the nurse can provide or teach exercises to facilitate ambulation later, provided the clients health permits. The diagnostic statement related to ambulation is not ignored; it is merely deferred.

Establishing Client Goals and Outcome Criteria (Objectives) Planning is the third phase of the nursing process. The plan for providing nursing care plan can be described as the determination of what can be done to assist the client. Planning involves the mutual setting of goals and objectives judging priorities an designing methods to resolve actual or potential problems. Two things are accomplished in the planning phase of nursing process, which includes:

Table 10.11: Assigning Priorities to Diagnostic Statements for Mr. Venkatesh (Before Cardiac Catheterization)

Diagnostic statement list	Priority rating	Rationale
Activity intolerance Related to shortness of breath and lack of energy secondary to decreased strength of cardiac contractions	Medium priority	Lack of energy is the clients stated major concern. Too much activity can create excessive cardiac demands, resulting in further decreased cardiac output with lowered blood pressure and inadequate circulation. However, because Mr. Venkatesh is able to handle basic activities of daily living, strategies to deal with this diagnostic statement can be deferred until after cardiac catheterization and/or cardiac surgery
Potential ineffective airway clearance Postoperatively related to chest incision	Low priority	Until surgery is performed, ineffective airway clearance is not likely since he is currently able to clear his airways by coughing
High risk for injury (trauma) related to joint stiffness and limp from hip replacement surgery	High priority	The client is independent and moves slowly to accommodate his limitations. However, new surroundings and a sedative given before cardiac catheterization increase his risk of injury
Knowledge deficit Side effects of diuretic therapy	Medium priority	Although the client complies with his medical regime, he does not seem to understand the side-effects of the prescribed diuretic, e.g. as relation to increased urination
Altered peripheral tissue perfusion (left leg) related to impaired arterial circulation	High priority	Decreased circulation and tissue perfusion to the clients left leg can result in damage to the tissues of the limb
Fear related to cardiac catheterization, possible heart surgery, and its outcomes	High priority	Extreme fear could impair his coping capacity
Potential pain (angina) related to excessive activity or stress	Medium priority	Angina has not been a problem for 2 months, but it could recur with the stress of hospitalization and planned treatments

- Establishing goals and objectives
- Selection of nursing intervention.

Goals: A client goal is desired outcome or change in client behavior in the direction of health. Goal attainment reflects the resolution of the client concern or health problem that is specified in the nursing diagnosis. The nursing diagnosis guides the type of goal statements: goals may reflect health restoration, health maintenance or health promotion. In the past, nursing goals were often written to direct care. For example, a nursing goal might have been stated as follows: "Increase the clients exercise", or "Teach client about diabetic diet". From theses nursing goals, specific nursing activities were derived, such as ambulating the client at specified intervals, offering instruction about needed dietary adjustments, and ensuring that the correct diet was provided. Recently, however, nurses have begun to state goals in terms of desired client behavior, not in terms of nursing activities. The term outcome means the result of an activity rather than the activity itself.

The concept of goals varies in nursing literature. In nursing education, goals are often referred to as objectives. In nursing process literature, some nurses separate goals from objectives; others use the terms synonymously. Still others use the term outcomes or outcome criteria synonymously with objectives. In this book, the terms goal and outcome criteria are differentiated, whereas outcome criteria and behavioral objectives are used synonymously. Goals are broadly stated and require further specification. Outcome criteria are specific and measurable.

A client goal, then, is a broad statement about the expected or desired change in the status of the client after he or she receives nursing interventions. Since goals are broad indicators of performance, the use of such verbs as increase, decrease, improve, develop and restore is appropriate. See examples of client goals in the accompanying.

Examples of Client Goals are as given below:

The client/clients will:

- Increase activity tolerance
- Maintain urinary elimination pattern
- Restore fluid volume
- Decrease potential for injury
- Develop coping abilities
- Improve nutritional pattern
- Increase parenting knowledge
- Establish change in family roles.

The purpose of client goals is to:

1. Provide direction for planning nursing interventions that will achieve the anticipated changes in the client.
2. Provide direction for establishing evaluation criteria to measure the effectiveness of the interventions

Client goals are derived from the first clause of the nursing diagnosis, i.e. from the identified client response. For example, if the first clause of the nursing diagnosis or problem (P) is **Feeding self-care deficit,** the goal might be stated as follows: "Client will demonstrate increased ability to feed self". More specific client outcomes (criteria) are then set form this goal; these criteria form the basis of evaluation. For example, if the goal is "The client will demonstrate increased ability to feed self", tow criteria might be, "Will drink from a glass through a straw" and "Will feed self using utensils with sponge-wrapped handles".

Long-term and short-term goals: Goals may be short-term or long-term. A short-term goal might be, "Client will raise right arm to shoulder height by Friday. "In the same context, a long-term goal might be, "Client will regain full use of right arm in 6 weeks. "Because a great deal of the nurses time is focused on the immediate needs of the client, most goals are short-term. In addition, the nurse is better able to evaluate the clients progress or lack of it with short-term goals.

Long-term goals are often used for clients living at home and having chronic health problems or clients in nursing homes, extended care facilities, and rehabilitation centers. Short-term are useful (a) for clients who require health care for only a short time and (b) for persons who are frustrated by long-term goals that seem difficult to attain and who need the satisfaction of achieving short-term goal.

Goals and objectives which are derived from the nursing diagnoses evolve from and predicated by the portion of the nursing diagnoses, and are established for each nursing diagnosis listed. Goals are stated in broad terms to identify effective criteria for evaluating nursing action. These goals pertain to rehabilitation, prevention of complication associated with stressors, the ability of the client to adapt to these stressors, or all three goals may deal with the achievement of the highest health potential for a client. For example, client will have and adequate understanding of basic food groups and their relationship to RDA (Recommended Daily Allowance) requirements within one month.

Objectives are the short statement of desired or expected outcomes of the client/patient. Objectives are determined from the goals and need to be stated in terms of observable behavior. Objectives should define the conditions under which the expected or desired end behaviors are to occur and should specify the performance level and specific behaviors that will be accepted as evidence that desired outcomes have been met. The behavior in question refers to psychological, physiological, social, cultural and intellectual activities and other observable response. The desired behavioral outcomes (objectives) should be stated in a manner that everyone can understand without having to seek clarification. The criteria for stating objectives include the following:

- Be written as the patient behaviors or goals. Patient's outcomes reflect those human responses (physiologic, psychologic, emotional) that must occur if the patient problems is to be resolved. Patient outcomes do not reflect goals that the nurse will achieve. The nurse's role is to support and assist the patient to identify and use his/her capabilities and coping mechanisms more effectively in dealing with the problem.
- Be written in precise and concise terms using action verbs
- Provide directions for care
- Specify appropriate time frame within which the patient is reassessed and the care plan is revaluated. This serves to determine the effectiveness of the nursing intervention in assisting the patient to achieve the desired outcomes (s).
- Be realistic
- Be measurable. It is crucial that patient outcomes be stated in measurable terms so that nurses caring for the patient can use the same criteria to evaluate the patient's response to therapy.

Establishing Goals from Nursing Diagnosis

Client goals are derived from the first clause of the nursing diagnosis, which is the client problems (P) as examples shown below:

(1) Nursing diagnosis	**Impaired physical mobility** related to pain
Client response or problem	Impaired physical mobility
Client goal	Client will demonstrate increase in physical mobility
(2) Nursing diagnosis	**Self-care deficit: Inability to feed self** related to depression
Client response or problem	Self-care deficit: inability to feed self
Client goal	Client will perform self-feeding

Outcome Criteria: Outcome criteria or objectives are needed to add specificity to the broad goal statements. A criterion is a standard or model that can be used in judging. Outcome criteria are statements that describe specific, observable and measurable responses of the client. They determine whether the stated goals have been achieved and are therefore essential to the evaluation phase of the nursing process.

Outcome criteria serve four purposes:

- They provide direction for nursing interventions
- They provide a time span for planned activities
- They serve as criteria for evaluation of progress toward goal achievement
- They enable the client and nurse to determine when the problem has been resolved.

Outcome criteria are derived form and relate to the client goals. Client goals, as described previously, are derived from the first clause of the nursing diagnosis. For example, if the nursing diagnosis is **High Risk for impaired skin integrity** related to imposed bed rest, and the client goal is "Maintain intact skin, particularly over bony prominences", the outcome criteria might be as follows. The client:

- Demonstrates correct technique for positioning and turning and the use of pillows to prevent pressure, within two days
- Discusses two methods for reducing pressure over bony prominences, within two days
- Has an absence of redness or irritation to skin when discharged from the hospital.

Generally, three to six outcome criteria are needed for each goal. Some nurses consider outcome criteria to be part of goals and add criteria directly to the goal statement, as follows: "Clients hydration status will be maintained (goal) as evidenced by (outcome criteria): (a) fluid intake of at least 2500 ml daily, (b) urinary output in balance with fluid intake, (c) normal skin turgor, (d) moist mucous membranes". Other nurses find this method cumbersome and separate the goal statement from the criteria statements.

Whichever method is used, the process of developing outcome criteria is the same. The nurse needs to ask two questions:

- How will the client look or behave if the desired goal is achieved?
- What must the client do and how well must the client do it before the goal is attained?

Characteristics of well-stated outcome criteria are shown here as follows:

- Each outcome criterion related to the established goal.
- The outcome stated in the criterion is possible to achieve
- Each criterion is a statement of one specific outcome
- Each criterion is as specific and concrete as possible, to facilitate measurement
- Each criterion is appraisable or measurable, i.e. the outcome can be seen, heard, felt or measured by another person.

Components of outcome criteria: Outcome criteria generally have all or some of the following four components:

- *Subject:* The subject, a noun is the client any part of the client, or some attribute of the client, such as the clients pulse or urinary output. Often, the subject is omitted in nursing care plan goals; it is assumed that the subject is the client unless indicated otherwise.
- *Verb:* The verb denotes an action the client is to perform, e.g. what the client is to do, learn, or experience. Verbs that denote directly observable behaviors, such as *administer, demonstrate, show, walk, drink, tell, list, state, etc. are used.*
- *Conditions or modifiers:* Conditions or modifiers may be added to the verb to explain the circumstances under which the behavior is to be performed. They explain what, where, when, or how.

For example: *walks with the help of a walker* (how),

After attending two group diabetes classes, lists signs and symptoms of diabetes (when),

When at home, maintains weight at existing level (where),

Discusses *four food groups and recommended daily servings* (what).

Conditions need not be included if the standard of performance clearly indicates what is expected.

- *Criterion of desired performance:* The criterion indicates the standard by which a performance is evaluated or the level at which the client will perform the specified behavior. These criteria may specify time or speed, accuracy, distance and quality. To establish a time achievement criterion, the nurse needs to ask "how long?" To establish an accuracy criterion. The nurse asks, "how far?" and "what is the expected standard?" to establish distance and quality criteria, respectively. Examples are:

Weighs 75 kg by *April* (time)

Lists *five out of six* signs of diabetes (accuracy)

Walks *one block per day* (time and distance)

Administers insulin *using aseptic technique* (quality)

See Table 10.12 for other examples of outcome criteria.

Table 10.12: Components of Outcome Criteria			
Subject	*Verb*	*Conditions/Modifiers*	*Desired performance standard*
Client	Drinks	2500 ml of fluid	Daily (time)
Client	Administers	Correct insulin dose	Using aseptic technique (quality standard)
Client	Lists	Three hazards of smoking (after reading literature)	(accuracy indicated by number of hazards)
Client	Recalls	Five symptoms of diabetes before discharge	(accuracy indicated by number of symptoms)
Client	Walks	The length of the hall without a walker	By date of discharge (time)
Client ankle	Measures	Less than 10 inches in circumference	In 48 hours (time)
Client	Carries out	Leg ROM exercises as taught	Every 8 hours (time)
Client	Identifies	Foods high in salt from a prepared list	Before discharge (time)
Client	States	The purposes of his medications	Before discharge (time)

Guidelines for Writing Goals and Outcome Criteria

The following guidelines can help nurses write goals and outcome criteria:

1. Write goals and outcomes criteria in terms of client behavior. Begin each goal and outcome criteria with "the client". This helps to focus on what the client will be able to do when the outcome criteria are achieved. Outcome criteria should focus on what the client will accomplish, *not what the nurse will do.* For example, a postoperative client may have the following goal (and outcome criteria): The client will maintain clear, open airways (goal) and manifest normal breath sounds (e.g. no wheezing or rales), normal rate of respirations, and absence of dyspnea and cyanosis (outcome criteria) allow, let, permit or similar verbs followed by the word client. These verbs indicate what the nurse hopes to accomplish, not what the client will do. For example, the statement "assist the client to deep breathe and cough every two hours" is a nursing action, not an observable behavior.

2. Make sure the goal statement is appropriate for the nursing diagnoses and that the outcome criteria are appropriate for the goal. Validate the outcomes. If the outcomes are accomplished, will the goal be achieved? Validate the goal statement. If the goal is accomplished, will the clients nursing diagnosis be resolved?

3. Make sure that the outcome criteria are realistic for the clients capabilities, internal and external limitations and designated time span, if it is indicated. *Internal limitations* refer to the person's physical and mental health status and coping mechanisms. *External limitations* refer to finances, equipment, family support, social services, and time. For example, the goal" The client will walk with crutches on level surfaces and on stairs" may be unrealistic for an elderly woman with a heavy leg cast. "The client will walk with crutches from bed to bathroom with assistance" may be more realistic. The goal "Measures insulin accurately" may be unrealistic for a client who has poor vision due to cataracts.

4. Make sure the client considers the goals important and values them. Outcomes are value decisions. Some outcomes, such as those for problems related to self-esteem, parenting, and communication, involve choices that are best made by the client or in collaboration with the client. Whenever possible, clients should be given information that will allow them to make informed choices with regard to goals. Some clients may know what they wish to accomplish with regard to their health problem. For instance, the client's goal may be "relief of pain". Other clients may not know all the outcome possibilities for their specific problem. The nurse must actively listen to the client to determine personal values, goals, and desired outcomes in relation to current health concerns. Then, discuss the nursing diagnosis and goals to determine if the client agrees with the stated problem and goals. Clients are usually motivated and expend the necessary energy to reach a goal if they consider it important.

5. Ensure that the goals and outcome criteria are compatible with the work and therapies of other professionals. The goal "Increase the clients activity tolerance" and the attending criterion "Will increase the time spent out of bed by 15 minutes each day" are not compatible with a physicians prescribed therapy of bed rest for 3 days.

6. Make sure that each *goal* is derived from only one nursing diagnosis. For example, the goal "The client will increase the amount of nutrients ingested and show progress in the ability to feed self" is derived from two nursing diagnoses. **Feeding self-care deficit** related to neuromuscular impairment and **Altered nutrition less than body requirement** related to anorexia. Keeping the goal statement related to only one diagnosis ensures that outcomes criteria and planned nursing interventions are clearly related to the diagnosis.

7. When writing *outcome criteria*, use observable, measurable terms; avoid words that are vague and require interpretation or judgment by the observer. For example, such phrase as "increase daily exercise", "increase participation in social activities", and "improve knowledge of nutrition" can mean different things to different people. If used in criteria, theses phrases can lead to disagreements about whether the criterion was met. These phrases may be suitable for a broad client goal but are not sufficiently clear and specific for use in outcome criteria used to evaluate the client's response. Examples of client goals and outcome criteria associated with the diagnostic statements for Mr. Venkatesh are shown in Table 10.13. Note that the diagnostic statements have been reordered according to established priorities.

Planning Nursing Interventions

Nursing interventions, are nursing actions chosen to treat a specific nursing diagnosis in order to achieve client goals. The specific strategies chosen for actual nursing diagnoses should focus on eliminating or reducing the cause of the nursing diagnosis, which is the second clause of the diagnostic statement. When nurses determine strategies for potential nursing diagnosis, the interventions should focus on measures to reduce the clients contributing factors, i.e. signs and symptoms.

The correct identification of the etiology during the nursing assessment provides the framework for choosing successful nursing interventions. For example, **Activity intolerance** may have several etiologies – pain, weakness, sedentary life-style, anxiety or cardiac arrhythmias. The interventions will vary depending on the cause of the problem.

Selecting nursing strategies is a decision-making process. Planning nursing strategies involves generating a number of alternative nursing actions likely to solve the clients problem,

Table 10.13: Goals and Outcomes Criteria for Mr Venkatesh
(Before Cardiac Catheterization)

	Diagnostic statement	*Client goals*	*Outcome criteria*
1.	**Fear** related to cardiac catheterization, possible heart surgery and its outcome	Experience increased emotional comfort and feelings of control	Verbalizes specific concerns Communicates thoughts clearly and logically Facial expressions, voice tone, and body posture correspond to verbal expressions of increased emotional comfort or feelings of control
2.	**Altered peripheral tissue perfusion (left leg)** related to impaired arterial circulation	Improve circulation to left leg and foot	Skin intact, pink, and moist Skin temperature warm (as other foot) Left dorsalis pedis, posterior tibial, an popliteal pulses palpable and of same strength as corresponding right pulses Verbalizes factors that improve and inhibit peripheral circulation Capillary refill of left toe nails within 1 to 3 seconds
3.	**High risk for injury (trauma)** related to joint stiffness and limp from hip replacement surgery	Prevent injury	Moves in and out of bed and ambulates without falling or injuring self
4.	**Activity intolerance** related to shortness of breath and lack of energy secondary to decreased strength of cardiac contraction	Avoid performance of activities causing shortness of breath and excessive cardiac workload	Rests after meals No shortness of breath during activities Pulse and blood pressure remain stable at 80 beats per minute and 124/80 mm Hg

considering the consequences of each alternative action, and choosing one or more nursing strategies.

Alternative Nursing Interventions

The client and nurse can use several methods of generating alternative nursing strategies at this stage; brainstorming, hypothesizing, and extrapolating.

Brainstorming is a technique used by more than one person, usually a group of people. In this process, one persons idea elicits an idea form another, and so forth. The ideas should not be evaluated while they are being generated. An idea is expressed, developed by another, modified by another, and so on, until a solution acceptable to all is established. The results of this process are often creative solutions.

Hypothesizing is a technique of predicting which actions will solve a problem or meet a goal. Hypothesized alternatives are the result of knowledge and experience, and each of the proposed alternatives is likely to be effective. Hypothesizing is not guessing because the alternatives have been tried successfully in the past.

Extrapolating is inferring facts or data from known facts or data. In this technique, the individual suggests an action because everything that is known about the problem suggests the action will be effective.

Often, the nurse and the client can establish a number of nursing strategies for each problem statement. Too many alternatives can be confusing. Usually three to five alternative nursing strategies for each health problem are satisfactory (Table 10.14).

And the nurse has to consider the consequences of each action, including the risks. Often, each action will have more than one consequence. For example, the strategy "Provide" accurate information" could result in the following client behaviors:

1. Increased anxiety
2. Decreased anxiety
3. Wish to talk with the physician
4. Desire to leave hospital
5. Relaxation.

Establishing the consequences of each strategy requires nursing knowledge and experience. The nurses experience may suggest that providing information before the clients bedtime may increase the clients worry and tension and that maintaining the usual rituals before sleep is more effective. Perhaps some alternative nursing actions should be implemented during the day to facilitate sleep at night, e.g. providing accurate information during the day and increasing daytime activity.

Selecting Nursing Interventions

After considering the consequences of the alternative nursing strategies or interventions the nurse selects one or more that are likely to be most effective. Although the nurse bases this decision on knowledge and experience, the clients input is very important. For example, a client may say: "I always have a sandwich and glass of milk before going to bed when I am home. I know I'll sleep if I can have that, "Maintaining the clients routine may indeed help the client sleep, and this action might be the first choice as a nursing strategy.

Table 10.14: Developing Alternative Nursing Strategies		
Diagnostic statement	*Client goal*	*Alternative nursing strategies*
Sleep pattern disturbance related to anxiety	Obtain 6 to 9 hours of sleep	Provide warm milk and a snack in the evening. Provide more activity during daytime Encourage client to decrease activity 2 hours before bedtime Assess diet for stimulants, i.e. caffeine Provide soft music Encourage verbalization of worries

The following criteria can help the nurse choose the best nursing strategy. The planned action must be:

1. Safe and appropriate for the individuals age, health, and so on.
2. Achievable with the resources available (e.g. in the previous example, sandwiches and milk must be available)
3. Congruent with the clients values and beliefs
4. Congruent with other therapies (e.g. if the client is not permitted food, the strategy of an evening snack must be deferred until health permits)
5. Based on nursing knowledge and experiences or knowledge from relevant sciences, Example: *Clients Diagnosis.* **High risk for impaired skin integrity** related to immobility. *Nursing Strategies:* Assess skin integrity over bony prominences q2h. Turn and change position q30 minutes. Pad pressure points. Use egg crate mattress on bed. *Rationale:* Continuous pressure on a body area compresses tissue, obstructs blood flow to and from an area, and can result in damaged tissue.
6. Within established standards of care as determined by state laws, professional association (Trained Nurses Associations, Government Nurses Associations), and the policies of the institution.

Each state has nurse practice acts that govern the scope of nursing practice. What nurses can do varies somewhat from state to state. Nurses should know the laws of the state where they practice and remain aware of current changes.

The second subphase in nursing care planning is the identification of nursing actions. For each nursing diagnosis, i.e. nursing interventions, nursing interventions evolve from the etiology position of the nursing diagnosis. For learning experiences (learning by doing) each nursing action is based on carefully thought out scientific rationale and specifies what kind of nursing care is to be done to meet the clients problems effectively. Nursing action should be spelled out precisely. These actions are part of the scheme for providing good nursing care. The characteristics of nursing interventions will include the following.

- Determining the nursing intervention requires that the nurses have a strong theoretical and experiential knowledge base. The nurse must be able to establish appropriate rationale for each nursing intervention implemented.
- Nursing interventions need to be specific. Their implementation is directed towards treating the cause and resolving the patients problems.
- Nursing interventions prescribe nursing treatments, that is, what it is, the nurse must do to treat the etiology (cause) of the patients problem. Behaviors described by nursing interventions reflect those of the nurse and not necessarily those of the patient.
- Clear and concise documentation of nursing interventions on the patient care plan is essential to communicate the activities and behaviors of the nurses to colleagues and other healthy care providers.
- In writing the nursing interventions, the care plan needs to be revised systematically in terms of patient's responses and outcomes. Decisions can then be made as to when specific interventions should be revised, updated, renewed or discontinued. Specific dates and time frames should be documented accordingly (Please note that specific dates and times are not included in the nursing care plan presented in this text because they need to be individualized for the specific patient).
- Each documented nursing intervention should be dated and signed by the nurse. The nurse's signature is particularly important in terms of accountability and in the sharing of information (feedback), including clarification of goals and rationales underlying care.

Interventions are the power of nursing and a distinct strength, also known as nursing orders or nursing prescriptions which constitute the treatment approach to an identified health alterations. Interventions are selected to satisfy the outcome criteria and prevent or resolve the nursing diagnosis or problem. Planned interventions should provide clarity, specificity, and direction to the spectrum of nurses implementing care of the patients, e.g. "Check vital signs", "measure intake and output", "Monitor heart state", etc.

Nursing interventions are said to be hypotheses established for testing if they contribute to the solution of the problem. It is upto the nurse with the client, the family or both to select appropriate action to produce desired results. In selecting nursing action, it is important to analyze the available options and to determine the probability of success in reaching the objective. Sometimes compromises must be made to provide the best care for the clients, and the nurse needs to be aware of this when specifying nursing actions.

The nursing care plan deals with actual or potential problems. Nursing interventions are based on scientific principles and theories of nursing and they need to be specific. The plan serves as a means of resolving the problems and for meeting established goals in an orderly fashion. Also it provides a means for organization, giving direction and meaning to the nursing action used in helping the client, the family or both to resolve the health problem. A plan of action is necessary, because it aids in the efficient use of time. It saves both time and energy by providing essential data for those individuals who are responsible for giving care. Since the clients condition is continuously changing, the written nursing care plan needs to reflect these change. Therefore, planning becomes a continuous process based on evaluation and reassessment. The written plan is the most efficient way of keeping all individuals involved in the clients care informed of modification in the plan of nursing care.

Documentation of the patients nursing care plan reflects the culmination of the problem-solving/decisions-making activities of the professional nurse. Such documentation demonstrates the ability of the nurse to apply nursing knowledge to clinical situations and to integrate this knowledge in the implementation of the nursing process.

Nursing Care Plan

The nursing care plan (NCP) format is used throughout this text to afford the reader the opportunity to examine the interrelatedness of the components of the process which includes problem, reason, objectives, nursing intervention (with rationale) and evaluation.

Problem refers actual or potential problems, stated in the form of nursing diagnosis, which is the product of assessment.

Reason refers to an inference in the diagnostic reasoning. Diagnostic reasoning is the critical thinking process through which the nurse moves to arrive at a nursing diagnosis, which includes the key point of subjective data (client complaints) and objective data.

Objectives refer to short statement of desired or expected outcomes of the patient, in the subpahse of planning component of nursing process.

Nursing Intervention refers to planned interventions which will provide clarity, specificity and direction to the spectrum of nurses implementing care for a patient. Implementation of nursing intervention is the action component of the planning. It is the phase of the nursing process in which the nursing treatment plan is carried out.

Evaluation of the attainment of the expected patient outcomes occurs formally at intervals designated in the outcome criteria. Please note that evaluation column is not included in the nursing care plans presented in this text, because they need to be individualized for each patient.

Please see nursing care plan based on 'PRONE' format (Table 10.15).

Author used the following 'PRONE' format for nursing care plans when 'P' stands for **problem**, 'R' stands for **reason** and 'O' stands for **objectives.** This is where and 'N' stands for nursing

intervention and 'E' stands for evaluation. The sample of nursing care plan with 'PRONE' format are in the end of this chapter.

Table 10.15: Nursing Care Based on PRONE Format

Problem	Reason	Objective	Nursing intervention	Evaluation

Many agencies have policies to guide nursing activities and the activities of other health professionals. Policies are usually intended to safeguard clients, ex., rules for visiting hours, procedures to follow when a client has cardiac arrest, and so on. If a policy does not benefit clients, nurses have a responsibility to bring this to the attention of the appropriate people.

Writing Nursing Orders (Table 10.16)

Carnevali (1983) says the term nursing order is preferable to the terms approaches, activities, actions and interventions because order connotes a sense of accountability for the nurse who gives the order and for the nurse who carries it out.

The degree of detail included in the nursing orders depends to some degree on the health personnel who will carry out the order. It is advisable, however, to be exact in writing orders.
- Date when they are written
- Precise action verb to start the order [e.g. *Explain* (to the client) the action of insulin]. Two examples of imprecise verbs are shown in the box below.
- Content area, or the *where* and *what* at the order (e.g. Apply *spiral bandage* to the *left lower leg).*
- Time element (e.g. Assist client to change position every 2 hrs *between* 0700 and 2100 hrs).
- Signature of the nurse prescribing the order.

Order for *nursing therapy* include those activities that maintain or restore the clients usual patterns, alleviate symptoms, and prevent additional problems. These make-up the majority of orders.

The *collection of additional data* is often necessary to define a nursing diagnosis better or to learn how to manage a problem. For example, if the nurse notices that a client appears withdrawn, worried and tense, the nurse needs additional data from the client to clarify the contributing causes of this behavior. The nurse may write a tentative nursing diagnosis of **Anxiety** and then write nursing orders that guide interventions toward confirming the cause. For example, a nursing order may state, "Talk with client to determine cause of anxiety".

Examples of Imprecise Action Verbs

Imprecise Verbs	Suggested Alternatives
Have the client	Ask the client if he will _________
	Request the client to ___________
	Remind the client to ___________
Reassure the client	Inform the client of ____________
	Listen to the client _____________
	Stay with the client ____________

Table 10.16: Nursing Orders for Mr Venkatesh

	Diagnostic statement	*Goals*	*Nursing orders*	*Outcome criteria*
1.	**Fear** related to cardiac cauterization, possible heart surgery, and its outcome	Experience increased emotional comfort and feelings of control	Establish a trusting or relationship with the client and family Encourage client and family to express feelings and concerns Discuss the cardiac catheterization procedure and what is expected of him before and after the procedure Encourage conversation with another client who has recuperated from similar surgery	Verbalize specific concerns Communicates thought clearly and logically Facial expressions, voice tone and body posture correspond to verbal expressions of increased emotional comfort or feelings of control After instruction, describes the cardiac catheterization procedure and what is expected of him before and after the procedure.
2.	**Altered peripheral tissue perfusion (left leg)** related to impaired arterial circulation	Improve circulation to left leg and foot	Consult with physician about exercise program, such as walking and range-of-motion exercises to hip, knee and ankle Keep the extremity in a *dependent* position (i.e. lower than the heart) Use Doppler ultrasound stethoscope (DUS) to assess blood flow in left dorsal pedis, posterior tibial and popliteal arteries q2h Instruct client to keep his leg warm, e.g. wear warm socks but discourage use of external heat sources	Skin intact, pink, and moist Skin temperature warm (as other foot) Left dorsalis, posterior tibial, and popliteal pulses palpable and of same strength as corresponding right pulses Capillary refill of left toenail within 1 to 3 seconds
3.	**High risk for injury (trauma)** related to joint stiffness and limp from hip replacement surgery	Prevent injury	Closely assess ambulation and transfers during first few days Keep bed at lowest level Encourage to request assistance to ambulate during the night Closely attend or put side rails up when client is sedated	Moves in and out of bed and ambulates without falling or injuring self
4.	**Activity intolerance** related to shortness of breathe and lack of energy secondary to decreased strength of cardiac contraction	Avoid performance of activities causing shortness of breath and excessive cardiac workload	Organize client care and provide undisturbed rest periods Discuss energy conservation methods such as taking periodic test periods Tell the client to reduce the intensity duration and frequency of activity if he experiences chest pain, shortness of breath, dizziness or abnormal pulse and blood pressure after activity Monitor vital signs q2h and report decreasing blood pressure, increasing heart rate or increasing respiratory rate	Rests after meals No shortness of breath during activities Pulse and blood pressure remain stable at 80 beats per minute and 124/80 mm Hg

If the nurse needs information about how to manage a problem, data may be collected from many sources. One example is the order "Nurse to consult physician about method of cleaning ulcer". The nurse may consult with a pharmacist about the side-effects of a medication, a dietician about the foods allowed on a certain diet, a physical therapist about appropriate exercise, and so on.

Nursing orders may specify the need to distribute information about continuing management of a problem to the clients support persons or other health team members. For example, a family member may need to learn how to help the client manage a long-term illness, or a visiting a nurse association may need information about follow-up nursing care requirements for a client who is being discharged.

Writing the Nursing Care Plan

The nursing care plan organizes information about a clients health into a meaningful whole; it focuses on the actions nurses must take to address the clients identified nursing diagnoses and meet the stated goals. It is also referred to as the *client care plan,* since its focus is the client.

The purposes of a written care plan are:
* To provide direction for *individualized care* of the client. The plan is organized according to each clients unique nursing care needs.
* To provide for *continuity of care.* The written plan is a means of communicating and organizing the actions of a constantly changing nursing staff.
* To provide *direction about what needs to be documented* on the clients progress notes.
* To serve as a *guide for assigning staff* to care for the client. Certain aspects of the client care may need to be delegated to someone who can make necessary judgments about the clients responses
* To serve as a *guide for reimbursement* from medical insurance companies (third-party reimbursement). The medical record is used by the insurance companies to determine what they will pay in relation to the hospital care received by the client. If nursing care has not been documented precisely in the care plan, the nurse has no way to prove that it was done, and the insurers will not pay for care that is not documented.

Format: Although formats differ form agency to agency, the plan is generally organized into four columns or categories: (a) nursing diagnosis or problem list, (b) goals, (c) nursing strategies/interventions/nursing orders, and (d) outcome or evaluation criteria. Some agencies have a five-column plan that includes a column for assessment data before the nursing diagnoses column. Others use a three-column plan that subsumes the evaluation (outcome criteria) column under the goal column. Author designed and used 'PRONE' format of his own on the basis of his experience (Tables 10.15 and 10.17).

Nursing students are required to write care plans to demonstrate their ability to apply their knowledge to client situations. For this reason, educators often modify the standard care plan by adding a column headed "Rationale" after the nursing intervention column. A rationale is the scientific reason for selecting a specific nursing action. Students may also be required to cite supporting literature for this stated rationale. These care plans are called instructional care plans and differ in purpose from the care plans developed by practicing nurses.

Many agencies use a nursing Kardex or Rand system for organizing and storing nursing care plans. Some agencies have adopted 8½-by-11-inch nursing care plan records that correspond to the standard chart size and require that the plan be written in ink so that it can be retained as part of the clients permanent legal record. In other agencies, problem-oriented medical records (POMR) are used; in this situation, the nursing care plan is documented in a SOAP format. In still other agencies, medical orders are not included on the nursing care plan.

Guidelines for Writing Nursing Care Plans

In addition to following the earlier suggestions for writing nursing orders, the nurse can use the following guidelines when writing nursing care plans.
* Date and sign the plan. The date the plan is written is essential for evaluation, review, and future planning
* Indicate that goals are met or revised by a signature or some other method specified by the agency
* List the nursing orders for each goal in order of priority
* Use standardized medical or English symbols and key words rather than complete sentences to communicate your ideas
* Refer to procedure books or other sources of information rather than including all the steps on a written plan. For example, write: "See unit procedure book for tracheotomy care", or attach a standard nursing plan about such procedures as radiation-implanation care and preoperative care
* Tailor the plan to the unique characteristics of the client by ensuring that the clients choices, such as preferences about the times of care and the methods used, are included. This reinforces the clients individually and sense of control
* Ensure that the nursing plan incorporates preventive and health maintenance aspects as well as restorative aspects
* Include collaborative and coordination activities in the plan
* Include plans for the clients discharge and home care needs. It is often necessary to consult and make arrangements with the community health nurse, social worker, and specific agencies that supply client information needed equipment.

Consulting Process in Nursing

Consulting is deliberating two people. Nurses consult a variety of personnel, including other nurses, throughout the nursing process. Consulting implies that the nurse involved in the care seeks advice of clarification regarding client goals. Also, the nurse may serve as a resource to provide assistance in health or client-related issues. Increasingly nurses consult with other nurses within the agency about a variety of specialized nursing practice areas. Nurses may also consult with other health care personnel including physicians, nutritionists, and physical therapist and social workers. Some agencies have a protocol to be followed by those consulting a health professional not presently involved in the clients care. For example, if a nurse wants to discuss a client's depression with an agency psychiatrist, the nurse may need to send a form to the psychiatrist requesting a consultation. However, many consultations are done on an informal basis. For example, the nurse may discuss a clients skin problem with the physician during the physician's rounds.

Nurses generally consult to verify findings, implement change, and obtain additional knowledge. Nurses frequently ask other nurses to verify assessment data, such as extremely low blood pressure or exceptionally fast pulse, when their findings are unexpected or they are uncertain about them. Sometimes nurses discuss a clients care plan with another nurse, often to make sure the best possible plan has been arranged, or to implement change in the plan. A second persons ideas can often generate new approaches to the clients care. Consultation to obtain knowledge is desirable. No nurse can know everything about nursing, and another nurse may have knowledge and experience about a particular problem.

The consulting process has seven steps:
1. Identify the problem
2. Collect pertinent data about the client
3. Select the consultant
4. Communicate the problem and pertinent information
5. Discuss the recommendations with the consultant
6. Include the recommendations in the clients nursing care plan.

Identify the Problem: Before consulting another person, the nurse must have the problem clearly in mind, including circumstances surrounding the problem. For example, a nursing student is unsure how to place the dressings on a draining wound to catch all the drainage because the student did not see the previous dressing before the physician removed it. The problem is clearly described, i.e. how to place the dressing, and the circumstances include the site of the source of the drainage, the amount of drainage, and the present absence of a correct dressing.

Collect Pertinent Data about the Client: When planning to consult a health professional who is unfamiliar with the client, collect all the data relevant to the problem.

Select the Consultant: The nurse who has identified a problem regarding nursing care should consult a recognized health professional who has the skills or knowledge required – a nurse with special knowledge and skills.

Communicate the Problem and Pertinent Information: This information often varies with each client and each problem. However, it is important to convey information about the client's strengths and problems. Convey the information clearly and objectively so that the consultant does not become biased yet obtains a clear picture of the situation. Make sure the data provided are factual and not interpretive.

Discuss the Recommendation with the Consultant: The consultant may provide recommendations at the time nurse describes the problem, or a later meeting may be necessary.

Include the Recommendations in the Clients Nursing Care Plan: Once recorded, the recommendation become part of the clients record and are available to all health professionals involved in the clients care. After implementing the recommendations, the nurse needs to evaluate their effectiveness and to record these. If they are not effective, it may be necessary to see the consultant again and make further adjustments in the clients nursing plan

Implementation

Implementing, also called intervening, is putting the nursing strategies listed in the nursing care plan into action; it is the nursing action taken to attain the desired outcome of the clients goals. Implementing involves carrying out nursing orders. Within the context of the nursing process, nursing intervention (implementation as "an autonomous action based on scientific rationale that is executed to benefit the client in a predicted way related to the nursing diagnosis and stated goals." By this definition, nursing interventions do not include those strategies resulting from a physicians order.

The client is always the primary participant in implementing the nursing care plan, although the nurse may act on the clients behalf, e.g. referring the client to a community health nurse for home care. The client degree of participation often depends on the clients health status. For example, because an unconscious man is unable to participate in his care, he needs to have care given to him. By contrast, an ambulatory client may require very little care from the nurse and carry out health care activities independently. The nurse or nurses, other health professionals, support persons, and/or caregivers can all be involved in implementing nursing.

Implementation is the action phase of the nursing process which involves both thinking and doing, but the emphasis doing. Nursing process are independent. Each affects and is affected by others. Without the assessment, diagnosis and planning steps, implementation would reflects only dependent functions, such as carrying out policies, protocols and medical orders. The autonomous nursing activities performed during implementation are built on the nurses reasoning in the previous three steps. Implementation overlaps in something with every other phases of the nursing process.

Implementation phase includes ongoing activities of data collection, prioritization, performance of nursing interventions and documentation. It also involves the delegation of some nursing intervention to staff members or assigning specific task to assertive personnel capable of competently performing specific task. The nurse is accountable for appropriate delegation and supervisions of care provided by the assertive personnel.

Implementation involves many skills including assessing the client condition before, during and after each nursing

Table 10.17: Nursing Care Plan (PRONE Format)

Name: Revanna Age: 50 Years Medical Diagnosis: Benign prostate hypertrophy

	Problems	Reason	Objectives	Nursing interventions	Evaluation

1	Anxiety related to unfamiliar disease condition	Patient expresses fear about hospital for surgery. On behavior:
		• Patient looks worried
		• Restlessness
		• Elevated BP
		• Looks pallor
		• Tachycardia
			Relieve anxiety	• Assess the patient for signs and symptoms of fear and anxiety like change in facial expressions, elevated BP, tachycardia, etc.
				• Place the patient in a comfortable bed
				• Implement measures to reduce anxiety
				• Encourage verbalization of fear and provide feedback
				• Establish good rapport with the patient
				• Orient to hospital environment, equipment and routine
				• Be a good listener and adviser
				• Explain about the diagnostic tests to gain cooperation
				  - Explain the need for surgery
				  - Possible results of surgery
				• Reassure the patient
				• Encourage the pertinent participating indiverse activities
					Anxiety is relieved

2	Urinary retention related to obstruction of urethra due to prostrate enlargement	Patient complains of difficulty of maturation, pain on abdomen. On observation: • There is retention of urine • Distended bladder • Tenderness of abdomen	Overcome retention of urine	• Gather baseline data regarding patients usual urinary elimination pattern. • Provide comfortable bed • Assess for signs and symptoms of urinary retention, i.e. frequent voiding of small amount of urine • Implement measures of treat urinary retention • After catheterization, gradually decompress the bladder • Keep the drainage tube free of kinks • Allow patient to assume normal position while voiding. If measures fail, then catheterization is done. • Give plenty of oral fluids • Monitor vital signs • Monitor intake and output chart	The patient will experience resolution of urinary retention

3	Knowledge deficit regarding hospital, routine, associated to preparation	Patient asks number of questions regarding hospital physical preparations On observation:
		• Patient looks dull, fearful
			Impart knowledge regarding physical preparation of postoperative exercises	• Provide information about usual preoperative routines
				• Explain the need for surgery
				• Take consent from patient or relatives
				• Provide psychological support
				• Explain about physical preparation like skin preparation, giving bath, preparation of bowel
				• Teach postoperative exercises like:
				  – Deep breathing exercises
				  – Perineal exercises
				  – Urethral exercises
					Patient has understood the purpose of preparation

Contd...

	Problems	Reason	Objectives	Nursing interventions	Evaluation
				Table 10.17: *Contd...*	
Postoperative nursing care plan					
4	Alteration in fluid and electrolyte balance related to nil to orally	Patient is operated and kept nil by mouth, On observation: • Dry lips and tongue	To maintain fluid and electrolyte balance	• Place the patient in a comfortable bed • Start IV fluids as per instructions • While administering IV fluids. Check for IV infiltration rate and flow • Maintain fluid intake of 3000 to 4000 mL/day • Record vital signs • Maintain intake and output charts	Maintained fluid and electrolyte balance

5	Altered comfort related to postoperative pain	Patient complains of pain on the site of surgery, On observation: • Patient is restless • Change in facial expressions, etc.	To reduce pain	• Place the patient in a comfortable position.
				• Implement measures to reduce pain
				  - Assess the nature and duration of pain
				  - Instruct the patient to avoid straining to save bowel movements
				  - Observe the operated site for any oozing and tightness of the dressing
				  - Observe urine for change of color
				  - Give plenty of oral fluids
				  - Administer analgesics as per dose order
					Pain is reduced

6	Alteration in nutritional status due to less intake due to surgery	Patient was kept not orally for two days. Patient complains of fatigue, loss of appetite, On observation: • Patient looks weak, easily tired	Maintain normal nutritional status	• Assess the patient for signs and symptoms of malnutrition
				  – Weight, abnormal, BUN, weakness and fatigue
				• Implement measures to maintain adequate nutritional status
				  – Provide oral care before feeds
				  – Instruct patient to ingest food an fluids slowly
				  – Instruct to avoid spicy foods
				  – Encourage early ambulation
				  – Provide clean environment
					Maintained adequate nutritional status

7	Anxiety related to sexual dysfunction due to surgery	Patient asks number of questions regarding sexual life	To relive anxiety	• Determine the patients and knowledge and concerns about the prostatectomy and relation to sexual dysfunction • Provide accurate information about effects of prostatectomy • Encourage questions and clarify misconceptions • Provide information as necessary • Assure the patient that these 'do not' reduce the level of sexual performance of satisfaction	Anxiety is relieved
8	Potential for • Wound infection • UTI	There is presence of surgical wound and presence of indwelling catheter. So patient is liable for infection	Prevent wound infection and UTI	• Assess for and report signs and symptoms of infection like chills, fever, redness swelling of wound area, etc. • Obtain culture of wound drainage • Implement measure to prevent wound infection • Use good handwashing technique • Instruct patient not to touch the wound • Maintain aseptic technique before any procedure • Teach the importance of personal hygiene • Encourage to take adequate fluid about 2500 mL/day • Encourage deep breathing exercises • Monitor vital signs	No sign of infection

Contd...

Table 10.17: *Contd...*

	Problems	Reason	Objectives	Nursing interventions	Evaluation
9	Knowledge deficit related to follow-up care	Patient asks many questions regarding follow-up care	To impart knowledge regarding follow-up care	• Impart knowledge regarding personal hygiene • Instruct the client to prevent pressure on surgical area • Avoid prolonged sitting and standing • Avoid long walking, long automobile trips • Avoid heavy lifting • Avoid consumption of alcohol and smoking • Avoid straining at defecation • Fluid maintenance of at least 2500 mL/day • Take nutritious diet • Instruct to do exercises	

interventions. Positive responses add information to the database to use where evaluating the interventions. Negative responses must be dealt with immediately.

Psycholomotor, interpersonal and cognitive skills are also needed to perform the planned nursing interventions.

- Psychomotor skills are used when handling medical equipment and performing skills such as changing dressings, giving infections, and helping client to perform range-of-motion (ROM) exercises
- Interpersonal skills are used when collecting data, providing information in teaching sessions, and offering support in times of grief
- Cognitive skills enable the nurse to make appropriate observations, understand the rationale for the activities performed, ask appropriates questions and make decisions about those things than need to be done. Critical thinking is an important element within the cognitive domain. It helps nurse to analyze data, organize observations, and apply prior knowledge and experience to current client situation.

Nursing interventions are written as orders in the care plan and may be initiated by nurses, doctors or from collaboration with other health care professionals. Interventions can be implemented on the basis of specific orders, standing orders or protocols.

- **Specific orders** is an order written in a clients medical record by physician or nursing care plan by the nurse especially for that individual client it is not used by any other client.
- **Standing order** is a standardized intervention written, approved and signed by a physician that is kept on file within the health care agencies to be used in predictable situations or in circumstances requiring immediate attentions. Nurses implement standing order after assessing the client and identifying problems. A physicians initiates standing order on an inpatient unit might be specific medication.
- **Protocol** is a series of standing orders or procedures that should be followed under certain specific conditions. It defines interventions that are permitted and circumstances under which the nurse can implement the measures. Health

care agencies or individual physician often use standing orders or protocol for preparing client for diagnostic tests or for immediate interventions in life-threatening circumstances. Protocols prevent needlessness writing the same orders for different clients, saving valuable time.

In emergency situations, the nurse proceeds directly from assessment of the problem to intervention. For example the nurse initiates CPR for a patient whose respiratory or cardiac function, has failed.

Daily contact with the patient and patient's family provides opportunities for additional data collection. Increasing pain, fatigue or changes from the patient's initial health status may be noted. As a result of this ongoing assessment, priorities of care may need to be altered. Activities may need to be delayed or canceled as the patient condition warrants.

Nursing intervention include both independent and dependent activities. Interventions that the nurse may perform includes the following:

- Performing an activity for a patient
- Assisting the patient to perform an activity
- Teaching the patient or family about health maintenances
- Counseling the patient and family
- Monitoring for problems or complication
- Administering medications and monitoring for therapeutic and non-therapeutic effects
- Referring the patient for care and following activities.

Documentation is vital components of the implementation phase. The written documentation of the nursing process is a legal record of what has transpired while the patient was in the health care facility. The implementation step involves documentation and reporting. Data to the recorded include the client's condition before the interventions, the specific intervention and client outcomes.

Documentation provides valuable communication among health care team members to ensure continuity of care and evaluate toward expected outcomes. Written documentation also provides data necessary for reimbursement.

Verbal communication between nurses generally occurs in the change of shift, when care responsibility changes. Nursing students also must report relevant information to the nurse responsible for their clients when they leave the unit. Information than should be shared in the verbal report includes:

- Completes activities and those not completed
- Statues of current relevant problems
- Assessment changes and abnormalities
- Results of treatments
- Diagnostic tests scheduled or completed (and results).

Communication must be objective, descriptive and completes. Communication of implementation activities is basic to client care and evaluation of progress toward goals.

Types of Nursing Actions Interventions

The terms *independent, dependent, and collaborative* (interdependent) are often used to describe nursing actions. An action, in this context, is an activity strategy. An independent nursing action is an activity that the nurse initiates as a result of the nurses own knowledge and skills. It is better to prefers the term *autonomous nursing practice to independent nursing practice.* She states "Knowing why, when and how to position clients and doing it skillfully makes the function an autonomous therapy". In this instance, the nurse determines that the client requires certain nursing interventions, either carries that these out or delegates them to other nursing personnel, and is accountable for the decision and the actions. To be accountable is to be answerable. Independent nursing actions are receiving increasing attention from nurses today.

Experts have identified a taxonomy of independent nursing interventions. A *taxonomy* is a set of classification that are ordered and arranged on the basis of a single principle or consistent set of principles. See Table 10.18 for a beginning taxonomy of nursing interventions. Dependent nursing interventions are those activities carried out on the order of the physician, under the physicians supervision, or according to specified routines. The dependent activity in nursing practice is usually directly related to the clients disease, and its importance should not be minimized. In addition to the task of carrying out the physicians order, the nurse who performs a dependent nursing action also conducts the appropriate nursing activities associated with the order, e.g. monitoring the client for signs of improvement.

Collaborative nursing interventions are those activities performed either jointly with another member of the health care term or as a result of a joint decision by the ensure and another health care team member. Collaborative nursing activities sometimes illustrate the overlapping responsibilities of health personnel and reflect the collegial relationship between health professionals. For example, a nurse and a respiratory therapist together may decide on a schedule of bathing exercises for a woman. The therapist may initially teach the exercises to the clients and the nurse reinforces the learned behavior and assists the clients in the therapists absence. Collaboration refers to "true partnership in which the power on both sides is valued by both, with recognition an acceptance of separate and combined spheres of activity and responsibility, mutual safeguarding of legitimate interests of each party and a commonality of goals that is recognized by both parties". To achieve effective collaborative nursing practice, nurse must heave clinical competence, feel confident of their knowledge and skills, and assume responsibility for their own actions.

The amount of time that the nurse spends in an independent versus a collaborative or dependent role will vary according to the clinical area. It has been estimated that the critical care nurse spends only about 10% of the day functioning in the independent nursing role. In other settings, e.g. home health care, nurses may find that they function independently 50% of the time. Clinical nurse specialists may work independently 100% of the time. Often, so many activities are integrated into a clinical day that it is difficult for many nurses to assess how much of their time is spent in an independent practice role.

After planning, implementation is the next, or fourth phase of the nursing process. Implementation refers to the actions initiated to accomplish the defined goals and objectives. Implementation is often considered as the actual giving of nursing care. It is putting the plan into action. Other terms used to describe this part of the process are action or intervention. The words implementation and intervention are not synonymous. Implementation refers to putting a plan into action; intervention speaks to involvement in the affairs of another, a coming between the other and a problematic situation. Therefore, the term implementation seems more appropriate to describe this phase of the process if nursing actions directed towards resolving the problem and meeting the health care needs of the client. It is an ongoing process through which the nurse is reassessing reviewing and modifying the plan of care, and if necessary, a seeking assistance in meeting the client's health care needs.

Since the nursing process is interpersonal in nature, it must take place between the nurse and the client. The client may be a person, a group, a family or even a community. The beliefs that the nurse and the client have about human beings, nurses and clients and about interactions between nurses and clients will affect the types of actions that both consider appropriate. If human beings are considered unique, then nursing actions that he or she uses in meeting the needs of clients. It has been indicated that the implementation phase of the nursing process draws heavily on the intellectual, interpersonal, and technical skills of the nurse. Experts support the importance of critical thinking throughout the nursing process. Although the focus is on action, the action is intellectual, interpersonal, and technical in nature.

The implementation phase begins when the nurse considers various alternative actions and selects those most suitable to achieve the planned goals and objectives. Just as goals and objectives have priorities. Nursing actions may he carried out by the nurse who developed the nursing care plan or by other nurses or nursing assistants. Nursing actions may also be carried out by the client or family. To carry out a nursing action, the nurse refers to the written plan for specific information. Many

Table 10.18: Taxonomy of Nursing Interventions

Most abstract *Level 1*	*Level 2*	*Level 3*	*Most concrete* *Level Nth*
Stress management	Relaxation training Cognitive reappraisal Music therapy		
Life-style alteration	Self-modification Patient contracting Counseling Nutritional counseling Sexual counseling Reminiscence therapy Role supplementation Patient teaching Values clarification Support groups Exercise programs Group psychotherapy Assertiveness training		
Acute care management	Preparatory sensory information Crisis intervention Preoperative teaching Surveillance Presence		
Self-care assistance	Ambulation Bathing Bladder training Bowel training Feeding Oral hygiene Positioning Skin care		
Communication	Active listening Advocacy Cultural brokerage Truth telling Discharge planning		

nursing actions fall into the broad categories of counseling, teaching, providing physical care, carrying out delegated medical therapy, coordination of resources, referral to other sources of help, and therapeutic communication (verbal and non-verbal). According to the goals and objectives for client, as discussed earlier, several nursing actions could be implemented. For example, under objective 1 (identify the basic food groups from a chart), the following actions could be considered.

1. Establish and agreed upon time when client and her family could meet with the nurse in their home during the next week.
2. Establish a baseline knowledge about the client and the family members understanding of basic food groups
3. Take chart and booklets containing information about the basic food groups to client home
4. Teach family about using the basic good groups for good nutrition (base teaching on information gained from baseline knowledge)
5. Focus on the value of the food groups for each family member based on age, height, weight and activity
6. Request a return demonstration in which client and other family members will identify foods by planning the food in a food group and will state why each food group is important.

A study of nursing diagnoses and nursing actions, seven categories of nursing actions were developed. These are assertive, hygienic, rehabilitative, supporting, preventive, observational and educative. In Campbell's (1980), Wilkinson (1992) speaks to doing, delegating and recording. Both point out that almost all nursing actions are initiated by nurses without medical direction. Nurses initiate and carry out all activities that fall within the nursing domain. In the hospital setting, nurses are also asked to assist physicians in carrying out medical prescriptions and to follow institutional policies. Therefore, nurses need to be clear about their dependent and independent functions.

For every nursing action, the client responds as a total person, that is, as a whole, the concept of HOLISM, which states that a person is more than the sum of that persons parts, means that the nurse may be treating a persons leg but the person will respond as a whole person. The concept is used in thinking about the consequences of any nursing actions. For example, the simple action of turning the patient every two hours will have a variety of consequences. Some of these consequences could or should be (1) increased circulation, (2) improved muscle tone, (3) improved breathing, (4) less flatus (gas) in the intestinal track, (5) prevention of pressure sores, (6) increased or decreased pain (7) opportunity for communication with caregiver, (8) increased ability to socialize with patient in next bed, and (9) increased or decreased ability to reach articles at bedside. There may be other consequences that could not have been predicted, such as an opportunity to express values or beliefs. Therefore, in planning nursing actions, it is important to consider the cluster of consequences of both positive and negative value that can be expected to occur with and following each action. Using this knowledge will help the nurse select the most appropriate actions. Although not all consequences are predictable for a specific client, it is possible to develop a general knowledge of expected consequences. Knowledge of consequences is an important aspect of the implementation phase of the nursing process. The implementation phase is completed when the nursing actions are finished and the results are recorded against each diagnosis.

Process of Implementing

The process of implementing normally includes reassessing the client, validating the nursing care plan, determining the need for nursing assistance, implementing the nursing strategies and communicating the nursing actions. Reassessing the client and validating the nursing care plan are subprocesses that operate continuously throughout the implementing phase.

- **Reassessing the Client:** As was mentioned earlier, assessing or reassessing is carried out throughout the nursing process, i.e. during assessing, implementing, and evaluating – in fact, whenever the nurse has contact with the client. While providing care, nurses must continue to collect data about changes (subtle or acute) in the clients level of wellness, i.e. health problems as well as reactions, feelings and strengths.

Following an extensive assessment during the first phase of the nursing process, reassessing in later phases usually focuses on more specific needs or responses of the client, i.e. fluid intake, pain, pulse rate, an during output. Through this mechanism, nurses are able to determine whether planned nursing strategies are currently appropriate for the clients.

It should never be assumed that once nursing strategies are established or ordered they must be implemented without assessing the client first. New data may, in the nurse judgment, indicate a need to change the priorities of care or the nursing strategies. For example, a nurse begins to teach a client, Miss Anitha who has diabetes, how to give herself insulin injections. Shortly after beginning the teaching, the nurse realizes that Miss. Anitha is not concentrating on the lesson. Subsequently discussion reveals that she is worried about her eyesight and fears she is going blind. The nurse ends the lesson because the client's level of stress is interfering with her learning and makes arrangement for a physician to examine the client's eyes. The nurse also provides supportive communication to alleviate the clients stress and revises the nursing care plan appropriately.

Validating the Nursing Care Plan

A nursing care plan cannot be fixed; it must be a flexible tool. When new data are collected, they should be compared with the database. Sometimes, the new data are incongruent with baseline data. The nurse must judge the value of the new data and determine whether the nursing plan is still valid. When a clients health status changes, i.e. when physical or psychosocial responses change, the nursing care plan needs to be adjusted. If the client regarding the clients health status are unchanged, the nurse proceeds with the implementing process. For information on modifying or changing the nursing care plan.

- **Determining the Need for Assistance:** When implementing some nursing strategies, the nurse may require assistance for one of the following reasons: The nurse is unable to implement the nursing strategies safely alone (e.g. turning an obese client in bed) and to reduce stress upon a client (e.g. turning a person who has acute pain when moved). In addition, nurses should obtain assistance if they lack the knowledge or skills to implement a particular nursing activity. For example, a nurse who is not familiar with a particular model of oxygen mask needs assistance the first time it is applied.

- **Implementing Nursing Strategies:** Nursing strategies are implement to help the client meet his or her health goals.

There are four primary areas of nursing practice: health promotion, health maintenance, health restoration and care of the dying. Nursing actions in each of these areas can be independent, dependent or collaborative.

Six important considerations for implementing nursing strategies are:

1. *The clients individually:* Individualized actions are needed, while care is taken not to violate the scientific basis of the activity. For example, a client may prefer to have an oral medication after meals rather than before. However, this might not be justified if the medication will not act in the stomach in the presence of food.

2. *The clients need for involvement:* Some clients want to be totally involved in their care, while others prefer little involvement. The amount of desired involvement is often

related to the client's energy, severity of illness, number of stressors, fear, understanding of the illness, and understanding of the intervention.

3. *Prevention of complication:* When changing a sterile dressing, for example, the nurse must observe sterile technique to prevent the complication of infection.

4. *Preservation of the body defenses*: For example, when turning a client, the nurse protects the clients skin from abrasions, which could permit microorganisms to enter the body and establish an infection.

5. Provision of comfort and support to the client.

6. Accurate and careful implementation of all nursing activities. The nurse takes care to administer the correct dosage of a medication by the ordered route, for example:

- ***Communicating Nursing Actions:*** Nursing actions are often communicated verbally as well as in writing. When a clients health is changing rapidly, the charge nurse and/or the physician may want to be kept up to date with verbal reports. Verbal reports are given to another nurse or other health professionals. Nurses often give verbal reports regarding clients at a change of shift and upon a clients discharge to another unit or health agency.

Evaluation

To evaluate is to judge or to appraise. In the context of the nursing process, evaluation is the fifth and last phase. Here to evaluate means to identify whether or to what degree the clients goals have been met. Evaluation is an exceedingly important aspect of the nursing process because conclusions drawn form the evaluation determine whether the nursing interventions can be terminated or must be reviewed or changed.

Evaluating is a concurrent and a terminal process. It is concurrent in that the nurse normally evaluates during the implementing phase of the process. How is the client reacting to this nursing action? Is the reaction expected or unexpected? At this stage, the nurse may change a nursing action to help the client meet the planned goals. It is a terminal process because after completing the nursing activity, the nurse evaluates whether the clients goals have been met. Often the time (if stated) in the outcome criteria is used.

Evaluating is a purposeful and organized activity. Through evaluating, nurses accept responsibility for their actions, indicate interest in the results of the nursing actions, and demonstrate a desire not to perpetuate ineffective actions but to adopt more effective ones.

Evaluation is a determination made about the extent to which the established outcomes have been achieved. Evaluation, is the final step of the nursing process, is a planned. Ongoing, systematic activity in which nurse will make judgment about:

- The elements progress toward desired outcomes
- The effectiveness of the nursing care plan
- The quality of nursing care in the health care setting.

The nurse takes several steps to complete the evaluating phase as follows:

- The nurses reviews the patient centered objectives that were established earlier. These outcomes statement present standards and criteria than are observable and measurable

- The nurse reassess the patient to gather data indicating the patient actual response to the nursing interventions

- The nurse compares the actual outcomes with the desired outcomes and makes critical judgment about the patient centered objectives were achieved

- Here nurse determine, whether client objectives have been met, partially met or not met or achieved. When an objective is achieved, the nurse decides whether nursing interventions should stop or continue for the status to be maintained. When an objective is partially achieved or not achieved, the nurse reassesses the situation and find out the reason for not area modify the nursing care plan by collecting some more data. The possible reason for not meeting or partially meeting objective includes:
  - Initial assessment data were incomplete
  - Goals and objectives were unrealistic
  - Time frame was not adequate
  - Nursing interventions were not appropriate for the client or situation.

Evaluation is a fluid process than depends on all the other components of the nursing process.

Types of Evaluation

Evaluation is classified according to criteria and frequency and time

- Structure, Process, and Outcomes (criteria)
- Ongoing, Intermittent and Terminal (frequency and time).

1. Evaluation according to criteria

Structure, process and outcomes all work together affect care. However each requires different criteria and methods of evaluation.

- **Structure evaluation:** Focuses on the setting in which care is provided. It explores the effect of organizational characteristics an the quality of care. It requires data about policies, procedures, fiscal resources, physical facilities and equipment, and number and qualification of personnel.

- **Process evaluation:** Focuses on the manner in which care is given – the activities performed by nurses and other personnel. It explore whether the care was relevant to the patient needs, appropriate, complete and timely.

- **Outcome evaluation:** Focuses on demonstrable or measurable changes in the patient health status than result from the care given.

2. Evaluation according to frequency and time

- **Ongoing evaluation:** It will be performed while implementing, immediately after an evaluation or at each patients contact.

- **Intermittent evaluation:** It is performed at specific times, which enables nurse to judge the progress toward goal achievement and to modify the care plan as needed.

- **Terminal evaluation:** It describes the clients health status and progress toward goals at the time of discharge…Most hospitals have special discharge forms for terminal evaluate which includes instructions about medications, treatment and follow-up care.

Evaluation is the fifth and final phase of the nursing process. It may be defined as the appraisal of the clients behavioral changes that are a result of the action of the nurse. Although evaluation is considered to be the final phase, it frequently does not end the process. As mentioned earlier in this chapter, evaluation may lead to reassessment, which in turn may result in the nursing process beginning all over again. The main question to ask in evaluation are: Were the goals and objectives met? Were there identifiable changes in the clients behavior? If so, why? If not, why not? Where the consequences of nursing actions predict. These questions help the nurse to determine which problems need to be reassessed and replanned. Unsolved problems cannot be assumed to reflect faulty or inadequate data collection: rather, each part of the nursing process may need to be evaluated to determine the cause ineffective actions.

The key to appropriate evaluation of nurse-client actions lies in the planning phase of the nursing process. When objectives are described in behavioral terms with clearly stated expected outcomes, it is easy to determine whether or not the nurse-client actions were successful. These objectives become the criteria for evaluating nurse client actions. Just as goals should be mutually set with a client whenever possible, it is also important for the nurses and client to mutually establish the objectives (criteria for evaluation).

Evaluation consists of the following five steps:
- Review the goals or predicted outcomes
- Collect data about the clients responses to nursing action
- Compare actual outcomes to predicated outcomes and decide if goals have been met
- Record the conclusion
- Relate nursing plans to client outcomes.

The first three steps are specific to client outcomes. Step 1 has been briefly discussed relation to the planning phase of the process. In addition to stating the desired behaviors change. It is also important for the nurse to decide how the change will be measured (predicted outcome) and when it will be measured.

Step 2 involves the collection of evidence (data). Although data are collected in both assessment and evaluation, the data collected during evaluation are used differently from data collected during assessment. In assessment, data are collected for the purpose of making a nursing diagnosis. In evaluation, data are collected as evidence to determine whether the goals and objectives were met. This is an important difference to note in using the nursing process.

Step 3 in evaluation is the one that is often the most difficult because it is easy to use different measurements in making judgments. For example, if an nurse observed that a client "ate well", would this mean the same thing the client or to another nurse? "Ate well" could be interpreted to mean that the client was able to chew, swallow, and digest the food consumed.

Therefore, in evaluation, it is not only important to determine the criteria (objectives) and be specific in predicting outcomes, it is also important to determine the exact ways, in which evidence is gathered and interpreted to ascertain whether the criteria were met.

When predicted outcomes are not reached, reassessment should occur, and the process begins again. If the evaluation shows that the nurse-client objectives have been met, the nursing process is complete.

Evaluating Process

The evaluation process has six components:
1. Identifying the outcome criteria (standards for measuring success) that will be used to measure achievement of the goals
2. Collecting data related to the identified criteria
3. Comparing the data collected with the identified criteria and judging whether the goals have been attained
4. Relating nursing actions to client outcomes
5. Reexamining the clients care plan
6. Modifying the care plan.

Identifying Outcome Criteria

The identification of outcome criteria used to evaluate the clients response to nursing care is already discusses. This criteria serve two purposes: They establish the kind of evaluative data that need to be collected, and they provide a standard against which the data are judged. Criteria that are clearly stated, precise, and measurable guide the next step of the evaluation process: data collection.

Collecting Data

Data are collected so that conclusions can be drawn about whether goals have been reached. The nurse collects data in relation to the specified criteria, either by observation, direct communication, and purposeful listening or from reports of other health professionals.

Collection of both objective and subjective data may be necessary. Objective, measurable data are preferred for evaluation purposes; for example, "Respirations increased from 12 to 16 breaths per minute, and pulse rate increased from 70 to 90 beats per minute after client walked around the corridor". However, the nurse often needs to collects subjective data and some objective data that require interpretation. Examples of objective data requiring interpretation are the degree of tissue turgor of a dehydrated client or the degree of restlessness of a client with pain. Examples of subjective data include complaints of nausea or pain by the client.

When objective data require interpretation, the nurse may obtain the views of one or more other nurses to substantiate changes. When subjective data are required, the nurse must rely upon either (a) the clients statements (e.g. "My pain is worse now than it was after breakfast") or (b) objective indicators of the subjective data, even though these indicators may require interpretation (e.g. decreased restlessness, decreased pulse and respiratory rates, and relaxed facial muscles as indicators of pain relief). Data collected must be recorded concisely and accurately to facilitate the third part of the evaluating process. Flowsheets and problem oriented medical records in the SOAP format are recoding aids.

Judging Goal Achievement

If the first two parts of the evaluation process have been carried out effectively, determining whether a goal has achieved is relatively simple. Both the nurse and the client play active roles in this. The data collected are compared with established criteria. There are three possible outcomes of evaluation:

1. The goal was met: i.e. the client responded as expected
2. The goal was partially met: i.e. a short-term goal was achieved, but the long-term goal was not: or, some, but not all, of the outcome criteria were attained
3. The goal was not met.

See Table 10.12 on page 288 for evaluation examples of Mr Venkatesh outcome criteria.

Relating Nursing Actions to Client Outcomes

The fourth aspect of the evaluation process is determining whether the nursing actions had any relation to the outcomes. It should never be assumed that a nursing action was the cause of or the factor in meeting, partially meeting or not meeting a goal. For example, Mrs. Bharathi, Bharathi was obesed and needed to lose 14 kg (30 lb). When the nurse and client drew up a care plan, one outcome criterion was "Lose 14 kg (3 lb) by 07/07/07". A nursing strategy in the care plan was "Explain how to plan and prepare a 900-calorie diet". On 07/07/07, the client weighed herself and had lost 1.8 kg (4 lb). The goal had been met, in fact, exceeded. It is easy to assume that the nursing strategy was highly effective. However, it is important to collect more data before drawing that conclusion. Upon questioning the client the nurse could find any of the following: (a) the client planned a 900 calorie diet and prepared and ate the food; (b) the client planned a 900-calorie diet but did not prepare the correct food; (c) the client did not understand how to plan a 900-caloried diet so she did not bother with it. If the first possibility is found to be true, the nurse can safely judge that the nursing strategy "Explain how to plan and prepare a 900-calorie diet" was effective in helping the client lose weight. However, if the nurse learns that either the second or third possibility actually happened, then it must be assumed that the nursing strategy did not affect not outcome. The next step for the nurse is to collect data about what the client actually did to lose weight. It is important to establish the relationship (or lack thereof) of the nursing actions to the outcomes.

Reexamining the Clients Care Plan

Evaluating goal achievement provides the feedback necessary to determine if the care plan was effective in resolving, reducing or preventing the clients problems. It is then necessary for the nurse to reexamine all aspects of the care plan, whether or not the goals have been met. Reexamining is a process of reasoning and replanning. (See Table 10.19, for an example of evaluating goal achievement for Mr Venkatesh.)

When Goals are Met: If a goal have been met, one of the following decisions may be made:

- The nurse may decide that the problem stated in the diagnosis no longer exists. In this instance, the nurse must document that the goal was met and that the care planned to meet this goal is discontinued.
- The nurse may decide that the problem still exists even though the goal was met. For example, if the criterion is: Client will ingest 3000 ml of fluid daily", and the goal is "Client state of hydration will be maintained", nursing interventions need to continue even though the goal and criterion have been met.

When Goals are not Met: When goals are not met or only partially met, the nurse needs to reexamine the clients database, nursing diagnoses statements, goal statements and nursing strategies.

Database: An incomplete or incorrect database influences all subsequent steps of the nursing process and care plan. In some instances, new data may invalidate the database, necessitating new nursing diagnoses, new goals, and new nursing actions.

Diagnostic statements: If the database is incomplete, new diagnostic statements are required. If the database is complete, the nurse's needs to analyze whether the problem was identified correctly and whether the nursing diagnoses are relevant to that database.

Goal statements: If the nursing diagnostic statement is inaccurate and requires correcting, it is obvious that the goal statement needs revision. If the nursing diagnostic statement is appropriate, the nurse then checks that the goal statement are realistic an attainable. Unrealistic, unattainable goals require correction. The nurse should also determine whether priorities have changed and whether the client and nurse still agree on the priorities. For example, a priority for the nurse may be to increase the clients fluid intake but a priority for the client may be to decrease intake because of nausea.

Nursing strategies: Last, the nurse investigates whether the nursing strategies are related to the goals and whether the best nursing strategies were selected. Even when the diagnoses and goals are appropriate, the nursing strategies selected may not have been the best ones to achieve the goal. Before selecting new strategies, the nurse should check whether the ordered nursing actions have been carried out. Other personnel may not have carried them out, either because the orders were unclear or because the orders were unreasonable in terms of such external constraints such as money, staff and equipment.

Table 10.19: Evaluating Goal Achievement for Mr Venkatesh

Assessment data	*Diagnostic statement*	*Goal*
Hospitalized for cardiac catheterization and possible aortic valve replacement States family scared about illness Wants to see chaplain Wants family to visit Perceives son Tom as helpful Says is usually too busy to worry about things	**Fear** related to cardiac catheterization possible heart surgery, and its outcome	Experience increased emotional comfort and feelings of control
Vital signs normal Heart rhythm regular Loud heart murmur (aortic area) Femoral pulses stronger than normal Absent pulses (popliteal, dorsalis, pedis, posterior tibial) in left leg Left leg cooler than right leg Integument pink and intact	**Altered peripheral tissue perfusion (left leg)** related to impaired arterial circulation	Improve circulation to left leg and foot
Left hip replacement Movement slightly limited Joint stiffness Slight limp	**High risk for injury (trauma)** related to joint stiffness and limp form hip replacement surgery	Prevent injury
Shortness of breath Lacks energy to do daily chores Does not smoke	**Activity intolerance** related to shortness of breath and lack of energy secondary to decreased strength of cardiac contraction	Avoid performance of activities causing shortness of breath and excessive cardiac workload
Nursing orders	*Outcome criteria*	*Evaluation*
Establish a trusting relationship with the client and family Encourage client and family to express feelings and concerns Discuss what the cardiac catheterization procedure entails and what is expected of him before and after the procedure Encourage conversation with another client who has recuperated from similar surgery	Verbalizes specific concerns Communicates thoughts clearly and logically Facial expressions, voice tone and body posture correspond to verbal expressions of increased emotional comfort or feelings of control After instruction, describes the cardiac catheterization procedure and what is expected of him before and after the procedure	*Goal met* Verbalized concerns: "I'm worried about how my wife support the family especially if anything bad happens during surgery? Asked questions about cardiac catheterization and surgery Nonverbal and verbal communication are congruent Described what to expect and what is expected of him before and after the cardiac catheterization procedure, e.g. "I know I will be taking a pill to help me relax before the procedure".
Consult with physician about exercise program, such as walking and range-of-motion exercises to hip, knee, and ankle Keep the extremity in a dependent position (i.e. lower than the heart) Use Doppler ultrasound stethoscope (DUS) to assess blood flow in left dorsalis pedis, posterior tibial, and popliteal arteries q2h. Instruct client to keep his legs warm, e.g. by wearing socks, but discourage use of external heat	Demonstrates intact, pink, and moist skin Exhibits warm skin temperature (as other foot) Demonstrates palpable left dorsalis pedis, posterior tibial, and popliteal pulses of same strength as corresponding right pulses Verbalizes factors that improve and inhibit peripheral circulation Demonstrates capillary refill of left toenails within 1 to 3 seconds	*Goal partially met:* Skin of left foot and ankle intact but pale Skin temperature still cooler in left than right foot Left popliteal pulse palpable but weak Left dorsalis pedis and posterior tibial pulses not palpable Blood flow evident only by DUS Capillary refill in left toenails within 7 seconds

Contd...

Table 10.19: *Contd...*

Assessment data	Diagnostic statement	Goal
Closely assess ambulation and transfers during first few days Keep bed at lowest level Encourage client to request assistance to ambulate during the night Closely attend client or put side rails up when client is sedated	Moves in and out of bed and ambulates without falling or injuring self	*Goal met:* Ambulated and moved in and out of bed safely
Organize client care and provide undisturbed rest periods Discuss energy conservation methods, such as taking periodic rests Tell the client to reduce the intensity, duration and frequency of activity if he experiences chest pain, shortness of breath, dizziness or abnormal pulse and blood pressure after activity Monitor vital signs q2h and report decreasing blood pressure, increasing heart rate, or increasing respiratory rate	Rests after meals No shortness of breath during activities Shows stable pulse rate and blood pressure at 80 bpm and 124/80 mm Hg	*Goal met:* Rested after meals and activities Experiences no shortness of breath while performing ADLs Pulse rate and blood pressure remained stable at 80 bpm and 124/80 mm Hg

Table 10.20: Modified Care Plan for Mr Venkatesh after Cardiac Surgery (Selected Examples Only)

Assessment data	Diagnostic statement	Goal
Rales in bases of both lungs relieved by coughing before surgery Painful chest incision	**Potential ineffective airway clearance** related to chest incision	Maintain a clear airway
Aortic valve replacement (7/15) Heart rhythm regular at rest Pulse: 80 beats per minute (bpm) BP: 110/80 mm Hg	**Potential decreased cardiac output** related to physical exertion and/or shock	Maintain cardiac output and blood volume
Left dorsalis pedis pulse and posterior tibial artery not palpable Skin of left extremity cool and pale	**Altered tissue perfusion** related to impaired arterial circulation	Improve arterial circulation
Aortic valve replacement	**High risk for activity intolerance** related to reduced strength of cardiac contraction	Increase activity tolerance

Modifying the Care Plan

When it is determined that the care plan needs revising, the nurse follows five steps:

1. Change the data in the assessment column to reflect the more recent findings. The new data should be dated and flagged in some way to indicate they are new. Follow agency practice: Some nurse's use ink of a different color; others put a colored tab at the edge of the paper.
2. Revise the nursing diagnoses to reflect the new data. The new nursing are also dated.
3. Revise the client's priorities, goals, and outcome criteria to reflect the new nursing diagnoses. These are also dated.
4. Establish new nursing strategies to correspond to the new nursing diagnoses. New nursing strategies may reflect increased or decreased of the client for nursing care, scheduling changes, and rearrangement of nursing activities to group similar activities or to permit longer rest or activity periods for the client.
5. Change the outcome criteria to reflect the other changes in the plan. These changes should project the desired level of wellness indicated by the client. Criteria that apply to outdated nursing diagnoses should be deleted (Table 10.20).

Table 10.21: Nursing Orders and Outcome criteria

Nursing orders	Rationale	Outcome criteria
Administer analgesics during first 48 hours Splint incision with pillows or hands during coughing Turn q2h during first 48 hours Assist with deep breathing and coughing (DB & C) exercises q2h	Pain relief makes coughing on comfortable and more effective Splinting minimizes pain Turning prevents the accumulation of secretions in one lung area DB & C exercises help to move and expel assertions	Normal breath sounds auscultated in all areas of both lungs
Assess vital signs 11h for first 24 hours, q2h if stable for next 48 hours, and q4h thereafter if stable Asses apical pulse and heart rhythm, not radial pulse Report an increase in resting pulse rate above 110 bpm and below 100 mm Hg.	A lowered blood pressure and rapid pulse indicate lowered blood volume or inadequate cardiac output	Stable vital signs Pulse: 80-100 bpm Respirations not more than 15 balance per minute
Keep clients legs warm (especially left leg) with blankets or socks Assess blood flow in left dorsalis, pedis artery and posterior tibial artery q2h using DUS Keep left leg in dependent position	Warmth increases circulation The DUS detects and indicates movement of blood through the arteries A dependent position facilities arterial blood flow by gravity	Left posterior tibial and dorsalis pedis pulses palpable and of same strength as corresponding right pulses Skin warm, intact, pink Capillary refill of left toenails within 1 to 3 seconds
Consult physician about a schedule for increasing activity Monitor and later show the client how to monitor his response to increased activity by: 1. Taking a resting pulse before activity 2. Taking pulse immediately after activity 3. Taking pulse 3 minutes after activity 4. Nothing rate decreases, rates about 110, rates not within 6 bpm of resting pulse after 3 minutes. Monitor blood pressure after activity Starting on 7/19, discuss factors contributing to increased cardiac workload, such as stress, excessive weight, blood pressure, large minutes.	A gradual increase in activity helps the heart muscle and new valve accommodate increased demands Pulse rate monitoring provides awareness of activities that do not overly exert the heart A drop is blood pressure indicates a reduction in cardiac output Knowledge of factors contributing to increased cardiac workload may facilitate such as eating smaller meals, losing weight, and altering activity patterns Knowledge of the effects of reduced cardiac output may motivate him to avoid excessive activity	After activity, heart rate remains below 110 bpm and within 6 bpm of resting pulse after 3 minutes

Evaluation based on behavioral changes is outcome evaluation. There are two other types of evaluation, both of which are reflected in evaluation steps. *Structure evaluation* relates to such things as appropriate equipment to assess the client or to carry out the plan and to record evaluation conclusions (Step 4). For example, if the scales were inaccurate, then correct data could not be obtained. Structure evaluation may also relate to the organization within which the nurse works. Then nurse may be unable to carry out the nursing process appropriately because of agency limitations on time: this must be considered a part of the evaluation. *Process evaluation* which focuses on the activities of the nurse, can be done during each phase of the nursing process, or it may be carried out at the end of the process (Step 5). The following are examples of process evaluation questions that can be used in evaluating each phase of the process.

Assessment
1. Were historical data that might be related to health problems collected?
2. Was a physical examination carried out and the problems corded?
3. Was the analysis logical? Did it make use of the collected data? Were significant findings mentioned in the analysis?

Diagnosis
1. Was the diagnosis based on the analysis?
2. Is the diagnosis a logical conclusion from the data collected?

Planning
1. Are goals and objectives stated?
2. Does the plan rationally follow from the diagnosis?

3. Were goals and objectives mutually established with the client?

Implementation

1. What activities did the nurse carry out?
2. What activities did the client carry out?
3. Were the activities consistent with the objectives?

Evaluation

1. Were the predicted outcomes achieved?
2. What evaluation methods were used?
3. Were the conclusions recorded?

The nurse and the client are responsible for carrying out outcome evaluation. Structure and process evaluations are typically carried out by the nurse, others in nursing administration, or both within and agency.

Evaluating the Quality of Nursing Care

There has been considerable work on the evaluation of the quality of nursing care to determine what good care is, whether the care nurses give is appropriate and effective, and whether the quality of care provided is good. Evaluating the quality of nursing car is an essential part of professional accountability. Other terms used for this measurement are quality assessment and quality assurance. Quality assessment is an examination of services only; quality assurance implies that efforts are made to evaluate and ensure quality health care.

Evaluation of the quality of care is not a new concept. Florence Nightingale's Note on Hospitals, published in 1859, included an evaluation of medical and nursing care. Since that time, evaluation has progressed through a number of stages. Initially, it focused on the environment, e.g. whether equipment was available at the time it was developed. Later, organizational standards in agencies were developed. For example, the ratio of nurses to clients was studied and evaluated in terms of clients needs. Since 1952, Accreditation of organization, has surveyed hospitals. Objective criteria were applied to evaluate a clients record after discharge from the hospital. This was called a retrospective audit. A nursing audit is a review of client's charts to evaluate nursing competence or performance. And revised its standards to include the requirement that hospitals be subjected to medical and nursing audits before receiving accreditation. The maximum length of accreditation is three years, with reports submitted periodically to determine the institutions progress toward the recommendations submitted by the surveyors at the last visit.

Since that time a national and state wide system of professional review organizations (PROs) has been developed. The purposes of the PROs include developing standards and monitoring the quality of, cost of, and access to care. Hospitals are required to contract with a PRO for utilization review. The objective of these procedures is to ensure that the care given under federal programs was necessary, and that the appropriate facilities were chosen to provide the care. Once problems are identified, an education process may be suggested to facilitate the correction of unacceptable staff practices, or penalties may be imposed on noncompliant care providers.

The PROs are based on the concept of peer review, an encounter between two persons equal in education, abilities and qualifications, during which one person critically reviews the practices that the other has documented in a clients record. These evaluative processes may be concurrent audits, that is reviews of present practices.

Approaches to Quality Evaluation

Three aspects of care – structure, process and outcome – can be evaluated. Standards of care for each type of evaluation have been developed based on nursing and health-related research and expert opinion.

- ***The Structure in Which Client Care Takes Place:*** Structure evaluation focuses on the organizations of the client care system, for instance, administrative and financial procedures that direct the provision of care, staffing patterns, management styles, availability of equipment, and physical facilities. Information about these support structures can be obtained easily. All of these factors indirectly influence care. For example, the hospital administration determines the number of nursing positions that the hospital can afford. Quality care cannot be delivered without adequate staff and resources. However, adequate staffing patterns and adequate facilities do not ensure quality care.

- ***The Process of Care:*** The focus of process evaluation is the activities of the nurse, i.e. the performance of the caregiver in relation to the clients needs. This approach may be the most effective in determining the quality of care provided. The care given by the nurse is evaluated by talking with the client, auditing the clients record, and observing the nursing activities. Evaluators may seek answers to questions such as these: Are medications recorded properly? Was client teaching documented? Is the care plan complete? This type of evaluation is time consuming and requires the judgment of expert practitioners. *Standards of Practice* are process standards the provide the nursing profession with a framework for the delivery and evaluation of care.

- ***Outcomes of the Care:*** The focus of outcome evaluation is the client's health status, welfare, and satisfaction, or the results of care in terms of changes in the client. Its advantages is that outcomes may be easily observed, especially in relation to medical care, which focuses on disease entitles. In nursing, however, outcomes are more difficult to determine, since nursing takes a holistic view of the client. Defining emotional, social, and behavioral outcomes is more complex than defining medical outcomes. In addition, client outcomes cannot be wholly attributed to nursing care. the clients own physical and psychologic mechanisms and contributions by family and other health professionals collectively produce outcomes. Outcome evaluation can focus on the clients change in behavior toward goal achievement prior to discharge (concurrent audit), or the clients record may be reviewed after discharge for evidence of goal attainment (retrospective audit).

Tools and Methods for Measuring Quality Care

Measuring the quality of care is a complex task. Development of tools involves four steps:

1. Defining and clarifying the nature of nursing
2. Deciding what approach to take (structure, process, outcome)
3. Developing standards and criteria. Standards are optimum levels of care against which actual performance is compared. Criteria are predetermined indicators of measures of health care, the presence, absence, and completeness of which indicate the quality of services. Here is an example of a standard and its criteria:

Standard IV: Each client has a written nursing care plan
Criteria: The nursing care plan is initiated within 8 hours of admission. It is based on information from the nursing health history and physical assessment. Goals are mutually set with the client and family, and the nursing care plan is evaluated and modified according to the clients needs.

4. Testing the criteria. Criteria must be valid and reliable. A valid criterion measures what it is intended to. A reliable criterion produces consistent results when used by the same person over time or by a different person.

Several established tools are available for measuring the quality of care. Some are process tools, some are outcome tools, and others are process-outcome tools. Each tool consists of standards and criteria. Developing effective quality care evaluation tools is a challenge for the nursing profession. Much work is continuing even on established tools.

Methods of using these tools also vary. Some evaluate by retrospective audits of nursing records using nursing audit committees. Others evaluate using a concurrent audit of process, i.e. direct observation of the nurse or nurses providing the nursing care by educated observers or by peers. Data may also be obtained by questioning and observing clients, questioning the family, and observing the client's environment and the general environment. The time period for measurement also varies. Some tools are designed for use over a 2-hour period, some are designed to evaluate the whole process of care given to the client from admission to discharge.

Scoring system differ among tools. Levels of care may be rated as *excellent, good, incomplete, poor, and unsafe*. Some tools require only simple person responses. Nurse's performance may be rated on a scale of 5 (best nurse) to 1 (worst nurse).

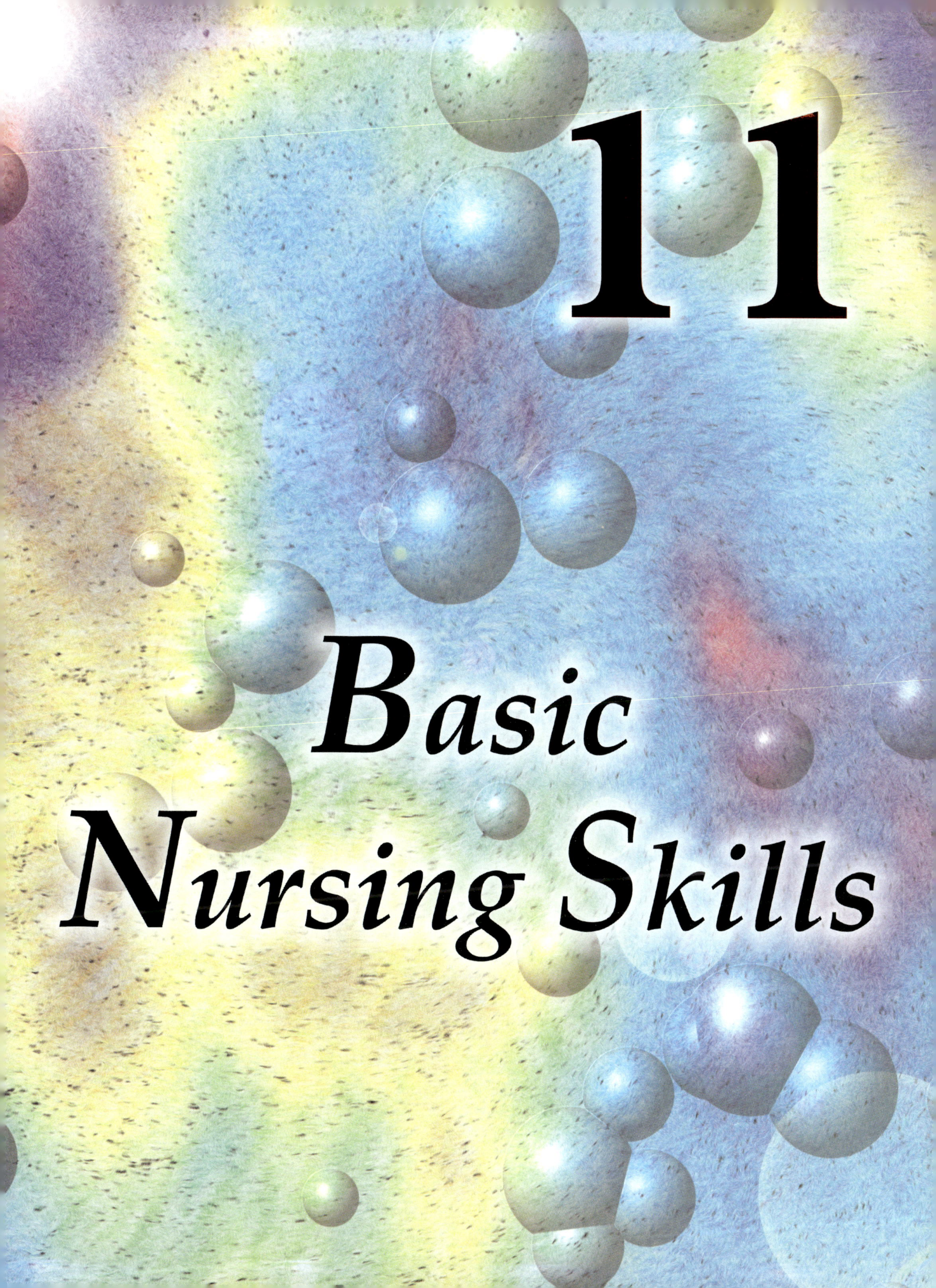
11
Basic
Nursing Skills

Helping Relationship Skill (Nurse-Patient Relationship)

Introduction

A helping relationship exits among people who provide and receive assistance in meeting human needs. A helping relationship sets the climate for the participants to move toward common goal, which arises from human needs. Therefore need gratification occur as the result of successful helping relationship.

The helping relationship between the nurse and client is sometimes called "nurse-client relationship". The nurse-client relationship is more than a mutual partnership. It is a process in which the helper asked to intervene in the life of the client to help the client engage in more effective behavior. **The nurse-client relationship is a dynamic process involving collaborative effort of nurse and client to resolve a problem and to promote the clients health and adaption abilities.** When a nurse and client are involved in helping relationship, the nurse assists the client to achieve goals that allow the client human needs to be satisfied. The nurse is the helper and the client is the person being helped.

The nurse uses skills of interpersonal communication to develop a relationship with clients that allows understanding of them as total persons. This helping relationship is therapeutic, promoting psychological climate that brings positive client change and growth. This relationship also focuses on meeting client needs.

A helping relationship between the nurse and client does not just happen. It is built with care as the nurse uses therapeutic techniques. The essential feature of helping relationships, the nurse has to develop to build, are trust, empathy, sympathy, caring autonomy and mutuality.

Phases of Helping Relationships

The helping relationships is established and maintained by a professional nurse and consists of the preinteraction orientation, working and terminal phases.

Preinteraction Phase: In the preinteraction phase, before a first meeting with a client, the nurse ideally reviews information pertaining to the client by going through the records such as medical and nursing history, an entry in the nurse's notes or discussion with another nurse who is providing care for the client. In this phase, nurse plans approach to meet the client for the first time.

Orientation Phase: Orientation phase begins when the nurse and the client first meet. It sets the tone for the rest of the nurse-client relationship. The orientation phase is superficial and is often marked by uncertainty and exploration. In this phase, nurse and client meet and identify each other by name. The client will accurately describe the role of the participant in the relationship. The client often test, the nurse by posing many questions, acknowledging need for help. The nurse who is aware of the client's concern attempts to display confidence and competence. She/he develops trusting relationships by confidence, dependability, confidentiality and credibility, by genuine caring. Here the client and nurse will establish an agreement about goal of the relationship; location, frequency, and length of contact; and duration of the relationships. During this initial encounter nurse begins to identify the problem and goals, clarifying the framing contact with the client.

Working Phase: Working phase is usually longest phase of helping relationships. In the phase nurse strives to meet goals set during orientation phase. The nurse and the client work together to meet the client's needs. The nurse-client interactions occur in this stage are purposeful in that they have been designed to ensure achievement of mutually agreed upon health goals and objectives. The nurse encourages the client open expression of feelings. This may be best achieved by listening. In the phase the nurse provides whatever assistance may be needed to achieve each goal. The nurse demonstrates conformation, i.e. the nurse makes clients aware of inconsistencies and behavior oar thought that interfere with self-understanding. This technique helps client recognize growth or deal with important issues. The nurse make self disclosure, i.e. she/he reveals personal experiences, thoughts, ideas, values or feelings and context of relationship. It shows clients that their experience can be understood.

In this phase, nurse integrating communication with nursing action. The nursing action can generally be divided into four groups, i.e. physiological, psychological, spiritual, and socio-economic. Physiological action includes nutrition, elimination and comfort; psychological action serve emotional needs; socioeconomic action includes referral agencies and assisting client to adapting invent; and spiritual action help client gain support for their belief system. In this phase client will actively participate in the relationship and co-operate in activities that work toward achieving mutually accepted goals. The client also will express feelings and concerns to the nurse.

Termination Phase: Termination phase occurs when the conclusion of the initial agreement acknowledges. This may happen at change-of-shift time, when the client discharged or when a nurse leaves on vocation or for transfer. The client will participate in identifying the goals accomplished or the progress made toward goals. The client will verbalize feelings about the termination of the relationships.

Role of Communication in Helping Relationship

Communication is the transmission and receiving information, feelings and or attitudes with the overall purpose of having understood producing a response. In short it is the process of passing messages, ideas, facts, opinions, attitudes, information and understanding from one person to another. Communication is an enabling process that allows information to be transferred and ideas to be translated into action. Communication is the exchange of meaning between and among individuals through a shared system of symbols that have the some meaning for both the sender and receiver of the message. The symbols include both verbal and non-verbal. In highly complex society and profession, and in an ever increasing environment of technological expansion, the need for more effective communication is clear. Nurses in particular must develop effective writing, speaking and listening skills to perform their job effectively in the large, complex organization in which they work. As professionals, most of the professional time (95%) of nurses is spent in dealing with human beings whether that is with a patient, patient's relatives, colleagues, seniors, subordinates or somebody visiting hospital or in the community setting. So nurses are constantly communicating with their environment. Effective communication can improve the working relationship, which will lead to higher job satisfaction. The importance of building relationships is one of the most important communication activities that nurse face and becoming more important with the growth trend of providing quality patient care. And also communication is very essential for administration and management of aim-related aspects. Our success in any field will largely depend on our ability to communicate effectively.

Advantages of Communication

Communication is the basic element of human interaction that allows people to establish, maintain and improve contacts with others. It constitutes the foundation of interaction among human beings. Nursing is a communicative intervention and the foundation of nursing lies in the "Communicative attitude". This attitude is manifested in striving for mutual understanding, co-ordination, and co-action. Instead of striving for control over clients by manipulating, them to behave in specific ways or by defining success as setting and meeting predetermined, definite goals, communicative interaction emphasizes clients as co-subjects, and is oriented at reaching a shared understanding.

A critical component of nursing practice is the ability to communicate effectively. Communication skills help the nurse in many ways.

- Communication skills help to generate trust between the nurse and clients
- Communication skills provide the nurse with professional satisfaction, i.e. it provides job satisfaction
- Communication is also a means for bringing about change, i.e. nurse listens, speaks and acts to negotiate change that promotes client's well being
- Communication is the foundation of all relationship between the nurse and other members of the health team. It induces human beings to put forth greater efforts in their worm performance
- Communication serve as a lubricant fostering the smooth operation of the management process, i.e. it helps promotion of managerial efficiency
- Communication provides basis for leadership action
- It provides means of co-ordination.

The nurse manager/supervisor can achieve work goals only by working through others. Therefore, she or he must be able to communicate ideas, opinions, requests, and directions effectively with coworkers. Effective communication consists of transmitting and accurate message to the proper recipient at the appropriate time in a manner that conserves the senders and receivers energy, followed by checking to ensure that intended message was received.

Elements of Communication

Studies supports the crucial contribution positively, perceived communication makes to both nurses' morals and their productivity. Communication theories contain communication elements as follows (Fig. 11.1).

1. Sender – refers to a person who initiates and transmits message. The sender is also called the encoder
2. Message – refers to information, opinion, effect that are directed to target, i.e. the information that is sent or expressed by the sender
3. Signal – refers to sign that symbolizes message contents
4. Channel – refers to route through which a message is transmitted; channels are means of conveying messages, such as through, visual, auditory, and tactile senses
5. Receiver – refers to an intended perceiver, interpreter of message. The receiver also is called the decoder
6. Noise – refers to a stimulus that blocks signal transmission
7. Feedback – refers to an information relayed from later to earlier stage. Feedback helps to reveal whether the meaning of the messages received.

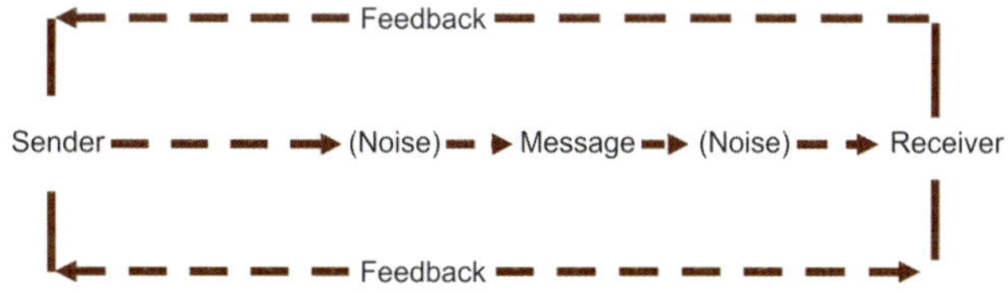

Figure 11.1: Effective communication

Level of Communication

Communication occurs at the intrapersonal, interpersonal, and public levels.

Intrapersonal Communication

Intrapersonal communication occurs within the individual. It is a self-talk or an internal dialogue that occurs constantly and consciously. The senders' motivation is transmitting a message and the receivers' mind-set in interpreting the message are conditions by a continuous stream of 'self-talk', a process through which the persons trust in the other's intentions, her/his feeling of being valued, and fixed views in target subjects acquired from precious experience are taken into account. For example, nurse supervisor can detect intrapersonal messages that insulate a worker from supervisor-initiated messages by asking workers opinion about controversial work issues.

Interpersonal Communications

Interpersonal communications is the interaction occurs between two people or in small group. Healthy interpersonal communications allows problem solving, sharing of ideas, decision-making and personal growth. In administration challenges the nurse's ability to express ideas clearly and decisively. Interpersonal communication is the heart of nursing practice.

Public Communication

Public communication is the interaction with large groups of people, e.g. giving lecture to students and speaking to a consumer group on health education.

Modes of Communication

Messages are communicated in number of ways, i.e. verbal, nonverbal.

(i) Verbal Communication

Verbal communication is an exchange of information's using words and includes both the spoken and the written word. Words are signs or symbols used to express ideas or feelings, arouse emotional responses, or describe objects, observations, memories and influences. Words may also be used to convey hidden meanings, test the others interest or degree of concern, or express hostility of fear.

Verbal communication depends on language. Language is prescribed way of using words so that people can share information effectively. Language is a code that conveys meaning. A single word can change a phrase or sentence. Language includes a common definition of words as well as method of arranging the words in certain order. Languages is effective only when each person communicating, understanding the message clearly.

Verbal communication is used tentatively by nurses when speaking with clients, giving oral reports to others, writing care plans and recording nursing progress notes. To make a message clear, the nurse uses effective verbal communication techniques; clear and concise phasing of words, a proper pacing of statements, and understandable vocabulary.

Clarity and brevity: Clarity can be achieved by speaking slowly and enunciating clearly. Using examples can make an explanation easier to understand. Brevity in best achieved by using words that express an idea simply, i.e. "tell me what is your problem."

Vocabulary: Instead of using purely technical words, use local words, synonyms to technical words for better understanding.

Denotative and connotative meaning: A denotative meaning is one shared by individuals who use a common language that is used to define a word so that it means the same to everyone. The connotative meaning of a word is the thoughts, feelings of ideals that people have about to word.

Pacing: Verbal communication is successful when expressed at an appropriate speed or pace.

Timing and relevance: Timing is critical to reception. For example if the supervisor/manager is in bad mood, the time is wrong to ask for a raise. And relevance is also important, i.e. that communication is most likely; to have an impact when messages pertain to an individual interest and needs.

Humor: It can be a powerful tool in promoting all aspects in management, and also for well being. Laughter is the best medicine. When it is used in good sense according to circumstances and events.

The written communication must be based on four essential 'C's, i.e. clear, correct, complete and concise. It should be written in such a language as it becomes easily intelligible to those fore show benefit the writing is made. It must be known words and familiar phrase and avoid official jargons or ambiguous terms.

(ii) Nonverbal Communication

Nonverbal communication is the exchange of information without the use of words; it is what is not said, i.e. action. Actions often speak louder than words.

So nonverbal communication is transmission of messages without the use of words. It is one of the most powerful ways people convey messages to others, i.e. nonverbal language delivers powerful messages. It is usually motivated by subconscious feelings and is therefore a more reliable indication of true feelings than the spoken word. Observation of nonverbal clue is an important skill. Nonverbal cues add meaning to the verbal message.

The nurse needs to be alert to nonverbal messages accompanying verbal message sent to clients. Meta communication is a message within a message that conveys a senders attitudes toward the self and the message and the attitudes, feelings and intentional toward the listener. It can explicit (verbal) statement or an implicit (nonverbal) demonstration of feelings. For example, when a nurse initially greets a client, maintaining eye contact and speaking in a calm voice can relay a sense of security to the client.

There are various forms of nonverbal communication are as follows:

Personal appearance: It is one of the first things noticed during an interpersonal encounter. This time general impression formed of another person influences the response to that person. People form an impression about another person within 20 seconds to 4 minutes.

The impression is based mostly on appearance, physical characteristics, dress, grooming and the presence of jewellery and adornment provide clues to the persons physical well being, personality, social status, occupation, religion, culture and self-concept. Paying attention to one's appearance can contributes to positive self-image and professional image.

A person's clothing and grooming (make up, combing hair) practices easy significant nonverbal messages. Personal clothes and grooming give sense of physical recovery and mental alertness. Healthy people with good self-esteem tend to pay attention to details of dress and grooming whereas those with low esteem show much less interest in personal appearance and it is often a sign of returning health when interest in mode of dress and appearance resumes.

Most illness cause atleast some alterations in general physical appearance. Observing for changes in appearance is an important nursing responsibility in detecting a particular illness or in evaluating such as the condition of hair, color of skin, weight, energy level and the presence of physical deformity, also communicate information about level of health.

The nurse's physical appearance influences the clients perception of care received. Each client has preconceived image of a nurse. The traditional white uniform can be a symbol of cleanliness and competence.

Intonation: The tone of a speakers voice can have a significant effect on a message's meaning. Depending on intonation, a message can express enthusiasm, concern, hostility or indifference. The intonation of the message is affected by the personal emotions. It is important for nurses to be aware of how they are sending a message. Voice tone can be a cue to a client's emotional state and energy level. Crying, moaning, gasping and sighing are oral but nonverbal forms of communication. Such sounds can be interpreted in numerous ways. For example, cry indicates joy and sadness; gasping indicates fear, pain or surprise. A sigh may be a sign of reluctant agreement to do something or of relief.

Periods of silence during communication often carry important nonverbal messages. The silence between two people may indicate complete understanding of each other, or it may mean they are angry with each other.

Facial expression: The face is the most expressive part of the body and it has rich communication potential. Communication often begins with eye contact. Eyes are windows to personal soul. A glance, e.g. is often and attention getting method to open conversation. Eye contact also suggests respect and willingness to listen and to keep communication open. Absence of eye contact means many things. Eye contact is an important facial expression. Wide eyes are associated with frankness, terror and naiveté; downward glances reflect modesty or shyness. Raised upper eyelids reveal displeasure and a stare is often associated with anger and coldness. Facial expressions convey various messages such as anger, joy, suspicion, sadness, fear and contempt. Nurses need to learn some control or looking away may indicate embarrassment dislike, withdrawal or possibly an attempt to remember of process what is being said.

Posture and gait: Body movement or motion may add significant meaning to a verbal statement or total communication. Total body movement or posture may indicate strong emotions.

The way that people holds the body carries nonverbal message and the person's stand on move is visible form of self-expression. Posture and gait reflect attitudes, emotions, self concept and physical wellness. Learning forward or toward a person conveys attention to that person leaning backward in a more relaxed manner shows less interest and caution. As erect posture and a quick purposeful gait communicate a sense of well-being and assuredness. A bouncy, purposeful walk usually carries a message of well-being. A less purposeful, shuffling gait often means the person is sad or discouraged. Certain gaits associated with illness are as follows:

Squirming, rocking back and forth, or extreme rigidity may indicate worry, tension, or anxiety. Slouching or sitting at an angle may show unwillingness to interact. As stated earlier facing the other person directly and learning forward in a relaxed manner usually indicate openness. Nurses can receive useful information by observing clients posture and gait. Specific illness can cause identifiable gait, e.g. neuromuscular disorder. Gait may be altered by many physical factors such as pain, drugs or fractures.

Gestures: These are used to illustrate an idea that is difficult or inconvenient to describe in words. Gestures using various parts of the body are capable of carrying numerous messages. For example, thumbs up means victory whereas thumbs down carries negative connotation; a wave of a hand, a salute and shifting of feet are gestures. They are visual enhancers that emphasize, punctuate, and clarify the spoken word. Pointing to an area of pain may be more accurate than describing the pains location. Gestures may reveal specific meanings or with other communication cues, they may send messages, e.g. kicking in object often express anger; wringing hands or tapping foot usually indicates anxiety or anger; a waving hand serves to back on someone to come, or if waved in another way signified that someone should leave. The arms and hands may indicate a persons emotional state. Relaxed hands and arms indicate openness. Arms that are rigid with hands clenched indicate anger, tension to explosiveness.

Touch: It is a powerful expression of communication. It is a meaningful personal mode of communication and it's meaning is different to different people. Touch can convey warmth and interest. Touch expresses personal behavior, various messages, such as affection, emotional support, encouragement, tenderness, security and personal attention, are conveyed through touch. Touch is an important part of nurse-client relationship but it must be used with discrimination because strong social norms govern its use. Who, when, why and where people touch are determined by unwritten sociocultural guidelines. The nurses must always be aware of the appropriate use of touch in varied situations and settings. Nurses rely on touch when carrying out interventions.

Factors Influencing Communication (Fig. 11.2)

Development: The rate of speech and language development varies and is directly related to neurological and intellectual

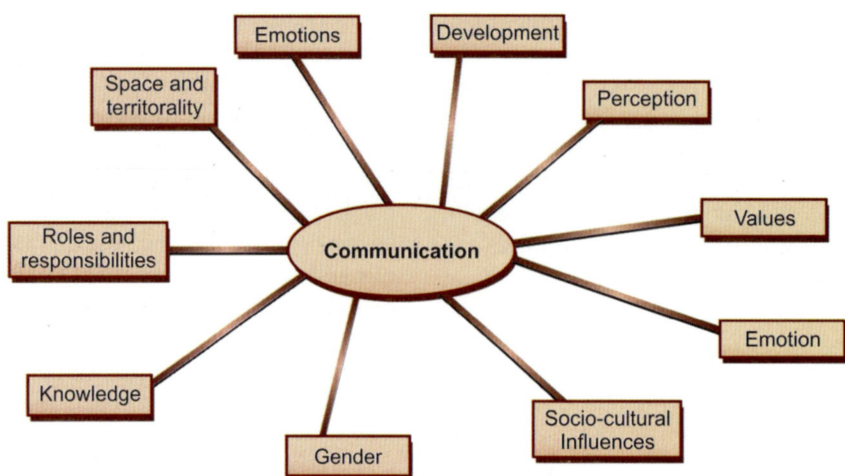

Figure 11.2: Factors influencing communication

development. Most children are born with the physical mechanism and capacity to develop speech and languages skills. It is helpful for nurses to understand the process of language development as well as the stages of intellectual and psychosocial development, so they can communicate appropriately with clients of all ages. To communicate effectively with children, the nurse must understand the influence of development of languages and thought process. Both affect the way children communicate and the manner in which the nurse can successfully interact with them.

Perception: Each person senses, interprets and understands events differently. Perception is the personal view of events. Perceptions are formed by expectations and experiences. Difference in perceptions between people who are interacting, can be a barrier of communication.

Values: Communication is influenced by the way people value themselves one another, and the purpose of any human interaction. Values are standards that influence behavior. They are what a person considers important in life and thus influences expression of thoughts and ideas. Values also affect interpretation of messages. Because values are a general guide to behavior, it is important for a nurse to develop awareness in them. Knowing and clarifying values are important to clinical decision-making and interaction. A nurse does not allow personal values to interfere with professional relationship.

Emotions: The degree to which people are physically comfortable and mentally and emotionally free to engage in interaction will also influence communications. Emotions are person's subjective feelings about events. Emotions influence the ability to receive a message successfully. They can also cause misinterpretation or not to hear message. Nurses can assess clients emotions by observing their interaction with family, physicians or other nurses. When nurses care for clients they must be aware of their own emotions. It is helpful for nurses to develop sensitivity to the physical, mental, and emotional barriers to effective communication.

Socio-cultural influences: Culture is the sum total of learned ways of doing, feeling and thinking. It is a form of conditioning that shows itself thought behavior. Language, gestures, values, and attitudes reflects cultural origin. Nurses need to develop skills in recognizing ways in which culture, economic condition, and overall lifestyle influence a clients preferred mode of communicating.

Gender: Men and women demonstrate different communication styles and each influences the communication process, or may give different interpretations to the same conversation. Since these sex differences affect the communication process, the nurses need to be aware of these differences when working with clients and other health team members of the opposite sex. Active listening and seeking clarification will help prevent misperception and misunderstandings.

Knowledge: It is difficult to communicate when the person communicating have different levels of knowledge. A message will not clear if the words or phrases are not part of the listener's vocabulary. Nurses communicate with clients and professional, who have different levels of knowledge. A common language is essential when communicating across different levels. Nurses assess client's knowledge, by noting their responses to questions, abilities to discuss health problems and questions that they ask. After that, nurses use terms and phrases that client understand to promote attention and interest.

Roles and responsibilities: A person's occupation may give the nurse a general idea of his or her abilities, talents, interests, and economic status. People communicate in a style appropriate to their roles, relationship and responsibilities. Nurses may feel comfortable communicating with colleagues, but when communication with clients who is entering clinic or hospital for the first time requires a different role. People feel more comfortable when expressing ideas to individuals with whom they have developed positive, satisfying relationships. As a nurse-client relationships develops and client gains confidence in relating ideas and feelings communication is more effective when the participants remain aware of that roles in a relationship and the challenge for the nurse caregiver is to respect the roles and responsibilities of clients, especially in their influence, their preferred manner of communicating without denying the client needed care.

Space and Territoriality: Territoriality defines the meaning of person's right to an area and surroundings. People are generally most comfortable in areas they claim as their own. Territory is important because it provides people with a sense of identify, security and control. In other words, individuals feels threatened when others invade their territory because it disrupts psychological homeostasis, creates anxiety, and produce feelings of loss of comfort. Most people comfortable talk at distance of 3 to 5 feet. Nursing procedures often require less distance; nurses must realize this invading the client's personal space and might make them uncomfortable. During social interaction, people consciously maintain a distance between themselves.

Environment: Communication happens best when the environment facilitates an easy exchange of needed information. People tend to communicate better in a comfortable environment. A warm room, free of noise and distractions is best. Noise and lack of privacy or space may create confusion, tension or discomfort.

Principles of Communication

The principles of communication which are helpful and useful for communication are as follows:
- Systematic analysis of the message, i.e. the idea, should be so communicated, that one is clear about it
- Selection and determination of appropriate languages and medium of communication in accordance with the purpose of communication
- Timing, physical setting and the organizational climate for communication need to be appropriated to convey the desired meaning of the communication conveyed by words
- Consultation with others for planning of communication
- The basic content and overtones of messages as well as the receptiveness to the viewpoint of the receiver influences effectiveness of communication
- The messages should convey something of value to the receiver in the light of his needs and interests, whenever possible
- Feedback from receivers, follow-up of communication through expression of the receivers, reactions and their performance review help in effective communication
- Communication while meeting the needs of immediate situations should be consistent with long-term goals and interest of the organization

- The communicators action following a communication is important in effective communication as this speaks more than his words
- The sender has to understand the receiver's attitude and reaction by careful, alert and proper listening to ensure that the desired meaning of the message has been comprehended by the receiver.

Barriers of Effective Communication

Blocks are verbal techniques and attitudes that jeopardize communication. The following are the block of communication.

Asking why: When people disagree with or fail to understand others, they are tempted to ask why the others believe or have acted in such a way. Clients frequently interpret 'why' question as accusations. They may also think that the nurse knows the reasons and simply testing them. Regardless of clients perceptions of the nurses motivation 'why' questions can cause resentment, insecurity and mistrust.

Changing the subject inappropriate: It might be harmful. A nurse might inadvertently stop client from discussing a subject of importance by changing the subject. Abruptly interpreting conversation is rude and shows a lack of empathy. It is important to avoid changing the subject during assessment.

Excessive questioning: It place too much pressure on the client and is upsetting particularly when more than one question is asked at a time. It becomes an interrogation rather than an interaction.

Giving opinion: It takes decision-making away from the client. It inhibits spontaneity stalls problem solving and creates doubt. Often client simply needs an opportunity to express feelings. Giving opinion the client from developing solutions to problem. At times client may require suggestion.

Offering false assurance: It is nonfactual information that makes the nurse feel good but may harm the client. It is patronizing and actually devalues client's feelings. Genuine and truthful reassurance is important and helps validate a client self worth and sense of hope.

Being defensive: Defensiveness, is response to criticism, suggests that the client has no right to an opinion. When a nurse becomes defensive the clients concerns are often ignored.

Stereotyping: Everyone is unique, stereotyped responses inhibit uniqueness and oversimplify the situation. Stereotyped and generalized beliefs held about people. The use of stereotypes inhibits communication and can threaten nurse-client relationship.

Using highly emotional words (angry, crazy, hostile and guilty: These should be avoided because many clients will not admit to having these strong feelings.

Showing approval or disapproval: Expressing excessive approval can be harmful to a nurse-client relationship, as stating disapproval. Offering excessive praise implies that the behavior being praised is the only acceptable one. Often the client shares a decision with the nurse, not in an effort to seek approval but to provide a means to discuss feelings.

Focusing on self: It is one way; some nurses maintain distance from client.

In addition the language differences, deafness, suffering, and blindness, are the physical barriers to communication.

Therapeutic Communication in Nursing

Therapeutic communication is the process in which the nurse, utilizing a planned approach, learns about the client. This process focuses on the client but is planned and directed by the professional. Therapeutic communication develops an interpersonal relationship between the client and nurse. This process involves significant skills, since the nurse must pay attention to multiple interacting and nonverbal behaviors. It conveys confidentiality. Since the client knows all information shared with the nurse remains part of the medical record and is not shared as gossip, the client feels comfortable disclosing pertinent health information, concerns, fears and family issues. In ideal situations the nurse is alert to the need to share information to the benefit of the client and maximize the plan of care. Only members of the health team directly involved with the clients plan of care are privileged to the information. Therapeutic communication ultimately enables the nurse to establish a working relationship with client and family.

Therapeutic communication is goal directed, client centered, time limited, structured, content specific (to patient need) and deliberative, planned and purposeful; whereas non- therapeutic communication has no set goals, task limited, superficial and has no structures, casual, intuitive, unplanned and superficial contact.

The following techniques assist the nurse to develop therapeutic communication.

Social interaction: It is first attempt at communicating with a client. A nurse often uses superficial social interaction at the beginning conversation with a client to lay a foundation for a closer relationship. The skillful nurse does not allow social interaction to dominate a conversation but does maintain a congenial and warm style to build the clients trust. The goal is to help the client to feel comfortable in sharing attitudes and feelings.

Active listening: Listening is one of the most effective technique of therapeutic communication. It is a listening with all senses and requires energy and concentration. It is a nonverbal method to convey interest in the clients needs, concerns and problems. It is trying to understand the complete message. As an attentive and active listener, the nurse can convey in attitude of active listening by the following:
- Face client while they speak
- Maintaining good eye contact without staring

- Leaning forward, showing interest, maintaining non defensive posture
- Avoid destructing body movement such as writing hands, tapping feet, and such others
- Nod in acknowledgement when clients talk about important points or look for feedback
- Lean toward speakers to communicate involvement.

The nurse listening skillfully during a nursing procedure is beneficial and efficient use of time.

Acceptance and understanding: These are often conveyed through active listening. Showing acceptance means not judging another person and demonstrates the interviewers willingness to listen to the client's beliefs, values and practices. Acceptance is a willingness to hear the person without conveying doubt or disagreement. To show acceptance the nurse remains aware of personal nonverbal expressions. The nurse avoids facial expressions and gestures that suggest disapproval, such as frowning, rolling and eyes upward or shaking the head in disbelief. The following show that the nurse accepts what a client has to say:
- Listening without interrupting
- Providing verbal feedback that demonstrates understanding
- Being sure that nonverbal cues match verbal communication
- Avoiding arguing, expressing doubts, or attempting to change the clients mind.

Questioning: It is an acceptable direct method of obtaining information. Questions used during a conversation set the tone of the verbal interaction and control its direction. Questions are most effective when they relate to the topic or subject being discussed and use words and work patterns in the clients, normal sociocultural context. During assessment of the client's health status, questions follow a logical sequence.

There are several types of questions being used to obtain client information. The open ended question requests information but does not specify the exact consent. It requires an explanation and is not easily answered with a one word or 'yes' or 'no' answer. The closed question asks for specific information and can be answered with a one word or 'yes' or 'no' answer. This type of questions is included in most hospital health history forms. The nurse wants the client to elaborate, open ended questions are more effective. They give a client to talk more completely about problems or concerns. Open-ended questions are most helpful for the nurse obtaining depth of information about the health status of the client.

Paraphrasing and reflection: Reflection is demonstrated when the nurse restates the connective part of the messages, the effective part of the message or both. Reflection is used to indicate the nurse hears what is being said and encourages the client to continue. Paraphrasing is similar to reflection except the clients message is rephrased in the nurse own words. Usually a paraphrased statement uses fewer words than the original statement. Through paraphrasing the nurse send feedback that lets client know whether their messages were understood and prompts further communication. More practice is required to paraphrase accurately, otherwise leads to ineffective communication.

Clarification: It is the act of restating what has been stated or sent to the receiver of the message. Without clarification, valuable information can be lost. Despite efforts are paraphrasing, the nurse; may not understand the clients message, clarification is asking the client to rephrase or add to message to correct a misunderstanding. When the nurse is unclear about the message, a client is conveying, it is appropriate to ask clarification, usually clarification is requested in the form of a question.

Focusing: It may be defined as centering information on the key elements or concept of the message that has been sent. Focusing is used to keep the communication specific and concrete. Some clients have difficulty in staying with the subject matter. Focusing is used to keep the clients responses relevant to the issue. Focusing eliminates vagueness in communication by limiting the area of discussion. As clients discuss topics related to health, their messages often become vague. To focus the discussion, the nurse might respond to client saying, relevant words.

Stating observation: It often leads to the client to communicate more clearly without the need for extensive questioning, focusing of clarification. When communicated, people are often unaware of the way that their messages are received. Feedback from others tells them whether they communicated the intended message, one way the nurse can provide feedback is by sharing with client observation of their behavior during communication. The nurse describes the impressions created by nonverbal cues; the nurse does not state observation that might embarrass or anger the client.

Offering information: It is a method of supplying the client with information, often used in conjunction with the other techniques for health teaching. When two people communicate the process is rarely one sided. In an interaction with a client, the nurse frequently offers information that gives the client additional data or insight. Providing the client with additional information encourages further response. Offering information on an ongoing, timely basis not only facilitates communication but also promotes health teaching.

Maintaining silence: There are several ways to use silence. Silence allows the nurse and client to organize their thoughts or gain control of their emotions. Silence may be combined with touch to show concern or support. It may be used to place some of the responsibility of the interaction on the client. The use of the silence requires skill and timing. Silence allows the client an opportunity to communicate interpersonally, organize thoughts and process of information. It gives clients time to search for words of feelings. Silence is particularly useful when clients are confronted with difficult decisions that they are not sure how to share with the nurse. For example, silence may help clients gain confidence needed to share the decision to refuse medical treatment.

The use of silence can be effective but is difficult because pauses in conversation that last several seconds or minutes can cause unease. In the beginning, nurses may need to practice this technique before feeling comfortable. When silence used for reflection or reminiscence, caution must be used so that the client can keep thoughts in perspective. Silence allows the nurse to observe clients. The nurse pays particular attention to nonverbal messages, such as worried expressions, or loss of eye contact. Remaining silence demonstrates the nurses willingness to wait for a response. When clients become emotionally upset, then helps them gather thoughts. A quiet period may diffuse an emotionally tense situation. A nurse silence acknowledges client's are ready to talk again, they will more likely to express feelings clearly.

It is standing up for one's rights without violating those of others. Through assertiveness people express feelings and emotions confidently, spontaneously and honestly. Assertive persons make choices are decisions and are able to control their lives more effectively than nonassertive individuals. Nurses can teach client assertiveness skills and how to use them to promote their own health. Assertiveness skills include speaking clearly, dealing with manipulation and protecting against criticism. Constructive criticism can promote growth, but manipulative criticism makes people vulnerable. A clear message is complete and specific and includes all information that client needs to understand. The nurse should have been more specific when transmitting the message and should have given the client more information. To avoid being manipulated, nurse acquires skills to protect themselves from others who consciously or unconsciously use them.

Summarization: It is a concise statement reviewing the content of the interview or series of interviews. It sets the tone for further interactions between the nurse and client. Summary can be used to identity key issues to be discussed during next interview, or it can be used to progress toward a goal.

Therapeutic Communication during Interview

During the interview, nurse should attempt to elicit as much relevant information as possible within a limited time frame. Therapeutic communication techniques, nonverbal as well as verbal, will promote a free flow of information. The effectiveness of the techniques used will vary from person to person and will depend on nurse skill as an interviewer. Overuse or forced use may actually stifle communication. Practice is the key to using therapeutic communication effectively.

Verbal therapeutic communication techniques are most effective, is the questions asked are open-ended rather than closed-ended. A closed ended question elicits a one-word answer, such as "yes", "no", or "okay". For example,

Nurse: How are you today?
Client: Fine.
Nurse: That's good. Do you need anything?
Client: No.

Obviously, closed-ended questions limit interaction. In certain instances, however, such questions may be appropriate. Questions aimed at eliciting biographic information such as name, occupation, address and marital status, for example, are closed-ended. This type of questioning is also appropriate in an emergency situation. For example, if a person arrives in the emergency room wheezing and out of breath, you would ask, "Do you have asthma? Are you allergic to anything?" rather than say, "Tell me about your shortness of breath".

Open-ended questions usually prompt full answers and provide more information. For example,

"Tell me about your family"

"What are some of your concerns about caring for your new baby?"

"What do you go to stay healthy?"

Open-ended questions that ask "why" – should be avoided because such questions may be threatening and could elicit a defensive response. For example, questions such as, "why did you stop taking your medication?" may convey judgment or criticism, which inhibit constructive communication.

Therapeutic Communication Techniques

Make broad opening statements: These statements may be especially helpful in the earliest stages of the interview, but may be used at any time. This technique allows the client to play an active role in the interview and to establish the priorities for discussion. Examples of this kind of statement are as follows:

"Tell me about your accident".

"What brings you to the clinic today?"

"What would you like to discuss today?"

Use reflection: Reflection is the technique of repeating or paraphrasing a person's words of questions in order promotes further explanation and discussion. For example,

Client: My skin is driving me crazy.

Nurse: Driving you crazy?

Client: Yes. For the last week it's been itching and burning.

Nurse: Well not constantly. And it seems to itch more than burn. I think it burns only after I've been scratching it.

Verbalize implied ideas: This technique involves restating what the client has said, and adding some interpretation. As with reflection, the purpose is to encourage further discussion in order to amplify the problem being explored. This technique also gives the client an opportunity to verify the meaning of what he or she has said.

For example,

Client: I don't know what's wrong with me. I used to sleep 6 to 7 hours a night without awakening.

Nurse: You're concerned because you've notice a change in your sleeping habits?

Client: Yes, I've always been a good sleeper. Now I'm up and down all nights.

Nurse: This seems unusual to you.

Client: Yes, even though I don't feel tired or take naps during the day.

Nurse: You're getting enough sleep but you are still bothered by night time awakenings?

Client: Yes. The nights are so long – just lying there, awake in bed, when I should be sleeping.

Provide general leads: Another method for keeping the conversation going in a specific direction is to inject certain leading phrases or responses, such as, "Go on", "Um – hmm" "oh?". "And then what happened" or "How did you feel about that?"

Seek clarification: Occasionally, the person being interviewed will make a vague or confusing statement. In such instances, it is important to clarify what has been said before continuing with the interview. A suitable response might be, "I'm not sure I understand what you're trying to say", or "what do you mean by unbearable?"

Use silence: At times during the interview the most appropriate response is silence. Silence allows you a moment to organize your thoughts and also indicates that talking is not necessarily a criterion of nurse-client interaction. Some interviewers however feel uncomfortable when nothing is being said. Self-confidence is needed to use this technique effectively. Periods of silence offer an opportunity to observe nonverbal cues such as posture, facial expressions, and body movements.

Use open body language: Nurse should also use nonverbal cues as a method of communication. Maintaining eye contact or sitting in a relaxed, no threatening posture conveys a sense of interest in what the client is saying. Sit with your arms unfolded and your body slightly relaxed, and lean toward the client. Keep your facial expression interested but neutral, avoiding expressions of disgust, anger or boredom.

Listen actively: Listening is a communication skill that enhances assessment because it concentrates attention on what the client is saying and enables you to consider subtle messages that the client may be conveying. Effective listening involves blocking out environmental distractions as well as your own prejudices. Attentive behavior and occasional verbal responses assure the client that you are listening.

Share perceptions: It often helps to share your observation with the client in order to prompt further discussion. Statements such as "You appear to have some physical discomfort today" or "I notice that you bring you your boyfriend frequently or It seem to me that you…" may open the conversation to a greater expression of feelings.

Confront contradiction: When inconsistencies arise between the client's statements and behavior, you should explore the contradiction directly, as, for example, in the following statements: "You tell me that you are not upset about it, but you look like you're about to cry" or "You tell me that you are not tired but it looks like it's becoming more of an effort to keep talking".

Review the discussion: Therapeutic interactions, especially health assessment interviews, should always close with some type of summary. The main points should be discussed and reviewed in relation to the goals of the interview. For example, you could briefly review the person's health strengths, perceptions, and any identified health problems.

Barriers to Therapeutic Communication

Offering advice: Giving the client advice or voicing opinions is generally not helpful and may discourage decision-making. Often when the client asks, "What would you do?", he or she is seeking assurance that you would do the same thing in the same situation. If your advice differs from what the client wants to hear, it may stir feelings of ambivalence. A request for advice can be turned into a therapeutic exchange, with a response such as, "What would you like to do?" or "It sounds like you need more information to make this decision. Let's talk about it some more".

Abruptly changing subjects: It is generally not a good idea to change subjects too quickly. Doing so can be disconcerting and can disrupt rapport. Pausing frequently during the interview and using transitional phrases when moving from one subject to another provide opportunities to think through responses and reactions.

Acting defensively: If the person being interviewed lashes out at other members or friends, it is better not to defend the people being criticized. To do so would imply judgment and inhibit further expression of feelings.

Minimizing feelings: Disagreeing with a person's feelings about a situation succeeds only in denying the person the right to his or her feelings. It is equally nonproductive to insist that there is nothing to worry about when, in fact, the person in expressing concern. Such a response demonstrates a lack of understanding or empathy.

Offering false assurance: Offering false hope or promising a quick solution to complicated problems is unfair and unrealistic. Saying, "Everything will be okay", denies the reality of the situation and frequently forces the person to hide fear and anxiety, which are human responses that require nursing intervention.

Jumping to conclusions: Nurse should never make an assumption and act on that assumption without first checking out the facts. For example, you should not assume that a person who is over-weight wants to lose weight. Neither is it wise to assume that a person who has breast cancer will automatically agree to the traditional treatment. Such conclusions represent your personal values and judgments, and may serve to antagonize the client.

Cultural Considerations

Culture has a profound effect on the way people communicate. Therefore, sensitivity to culture should influence how an interview is conducted. Cultural differences that have the greatest impact on communication are language, verbal communication patterns, and nonverbal communication that exists in that culture. People from two different cultures, however, may have different "rules" for interaction, and therefore may misunderstand each other.

Nurse should keep in mind that cultural differences may influence how verbal and nonverbal messages are interpreted. For example, Indian woman may avoid eye contact when talking to a man. An American women, on the other hand, may have no such compulsion and may look directly at anyone with whom she is talking.

Culture also influences health beliefs and behaviors. Members of some cultures believe that disease can be cured by magic or rituals or by eating certain foods. Therefore, it is important to determine the person's ethnic or cultural orientation and to ask about health beliefs.

Languages and meaning: Language barriers will obviously affect the length of the interview and may necessitate the presence of a translator. Allowing enough time for the interview, arranging for a translator and maintaining a relaxed and unhurried attitude will facilitate communication. Family or friends may serve as ready translators but may not always be objective in what they communicate. Furthermore, when family is involved, confidentiality may be a problem.

Even when there is no language barrier, misunderstandings may arise, depending on how certain words are interpreted. For example, for today's teenagers, the word "Bad" often means something that is respected or valued.

One way to determine if concepts or words must be clarified during the interview is to watch for nonverbal and verbal cues, such as a frown or a blank stare, which indicate misunderstanding in such a case, you may say, "I'm not sure you understand what I mean when I ask if you have been dieting. Let me explain". To prevent misunderstanding, avoid slang expressions, especially when cultural differences exist.

Verbal communication patterns: Cultural traditions and norms also influence verbal communication patterns. Some cultures consider direct questioning to be the best way to gain information, while others view direct questioning as intrusive, rude, or embarrassing. Some cultural groups will respond to interview questions in a vague manner to avoid embarrassment and confrontation.

Verbal response to pain also varies among cultures. For example, many Anglo-Americans and native-Americans are taught not to cry in the face of pain because crying is considered to be childish or self-indulgent. On the other hand, Latin-Americans are permitted by their culture to respond to pain in a physical and vocal manner.

Nurse may have to adapt the interview style to account for such cultural variations. At the same time, you should make a special effort to maintain a nonjudgmental attitude toward different communication styles.

Nonverbal communication patterns: Gestures, body movements, and personal space area all influenced by culture and personal space are all influenced by culture and upbringing. In many Western cultures, direct eye contact may indicate interest and attention. In other cultures, eye contact may be viewed as an intrusion. Touching may be an accepted part of everyday interactions in some cultures; others consider touching among casual acquaintances to have a sexual connotation. Similarly, how close people stand or sit to one another is determined by the way their culture defines personal space. In many Middle Eastern cultures, people stand close when talking to one another, whereas Anglo-Americans prefer to maintain a greater distance when engaged in conversation.

Developmental Considerations

The age of the person being interviewed can affect the way you should conduct the interview, especially if the person is very young or very old. For a child under 6, it is usually necessary to interview a parent or guardian, although the child's behavior should be observed for relevant verbal and nonverbal cues. Interviewing apparent or guardian similar to those used when interviewing any adult. The feelings and concerns of the parents must be taken into consideration. Parents frequently feel guilty if their child becomes sick or injured, and may actually blame themselves for the child's illness. In such instances, you should use nonjudgmental questions to elicit pertinent data. Questions such as, "When did you first notice signs of fever?" is much more appropriate then asking, "Why didn't you bring him to the clinic sooner?" Providing support and reassurance by empathizing with the parent's concern (You seem very worried) may encourage a more open response and result in additional information.

A child over 6 years old can be interviewed directly. Play and picture-drawings are alternative means to elicit data. Asking the child to draw a picture illustrating his or her experience in the hospital, a picture of a family member or a self portrait can serve as a basis for discussion. Children over 6 years should not be "talked down to" or treated as if they were babies. As when interviewing adults, you should maintain eye contact and assume a position that does not intimidate the child.

Parents may or may not be present, when you interview a child. If a parent is present, you are afforded an opportunity to observe family interaction. If the parent is dominating the conversation, or coaching or coercing the child to make certain responses, you should address the child directly with comments such as, "Now I'd like to hear how your feel about the situation".

Similar considerations are necessary when interviewing an elderly person. Sensory problems need to be recognized. However, avoid raising your voice even if the person has a hearing problem. Loud voices can be distressing and even offensive. In the elderly person with a hearing loss, it is usually the high-pitched sounds that are not perceived, and raising our voice usually raises the pitch. Instead, to minimize sensory problems, make sure before the interview begins that the person is wearing his or her eyeglass or hearing aid. Facing the person and speaking slowly and clearly can help improve communi-

cation by making it easier for the hard-of-hearing person to lip-read. Making sure the area is well lit so that the speaker's face can be seen, and eliminating extraneous sounds such as from televisions and radios will facilitate better interactions.

Allow more time when interviewing an older person; more than interview session may be necessary to collect all the appropriate data.

An elderly person usually has more information to share than a younger person. On the other hand, older people tend to underreport or refrain from revealing pertinent symptoms, because they may consider the symptoms to be part of aging and therefore unimportant. Older people may also hesitate to share information if they consider you to be too young or the information to be too personal. Establishing rapport and credibility is one way to overcome this reluctance. One effective way to establish rapport is to encourage older clients to reminisce and to take pride in their past accomplishments.

Teaching and Learning Skill

Introduction

Teaching is an interaction process between a teacher and one or more learners (Redman 1988). It consists of a deliberate set of actions that help individuals gain knowledge or perform new skills. A teacher provides information that prompts that learners to participate in or initiate activities that lead to desired cognitive or behavioral change. Teaching is a planned method or series of methods used for someone to learn.

Learning is a dynamic and fluid and is a shared, lifelong, even (Redman et al 1986). To learn is to acquire knowledge or skills through reinforced practice and experience. Learning is the process by which a person acquires or increases knowledge or changes behavior in a measurable way as a result of an experience.

Generally, teaching and learning begin when a person identifies a need for knowing or acquiring an ability to do something. According to Knowles (1970), adults can learn; learning is an internal process, and there are superior conditions of learning and principles of teaching. Teaching is most effective when it responds to a learner's needs. The teacher identifies these needs by asking questions and determining the learner's interests. Teaching relies on principles of interpersonal communication. On other words, teacher must send messages of significance to the learner and receive the learner's feedback.

Many of the developmental concerns related to teaching and learning are exacerbated by age. As people age, their personalities as well as their learning abilities a change. Most psychologists who have studied the teaching-learning process have based their work on children and adolescents, because a large amount of learning occurs in early life.

The science of teaching-pedagogy-generally refers to the teaching of children and adolescents. Androgogy refers to the teaching of adults, which emphasizes that adults need to be taught differently.

Knowles (1984) lists the following four assumptions concerning to adult learners:

- As a person matures, his or her self-concept is likely to move from dependence to independence
- The previous experience of the adult is a rich resource for learning
- The readiness to learn an adult often related to a developmental task or a social role
- The adults orientation to learning is that material should be useful immediately, rather that at sometime in the future.

Teaching-Learning and the Nursing Process

Teaching involves a behavioral method for facilitating another person's learning. Learning is an internal experience for the receiver. It denotes an integration of thoughts, ideas, theory, and experience (past and present).

Keeping the focus of teaching and learning in mind while using the nursing process and interacting with a client and the client's system, two functions are involved. First, the nurse assesses the learning needs of the client; these become the teaching responsibilities of the nurse. Second, to carry out teaching responsibilities, the nurse must assess learning needs of self relative to teaching the client – does the nurse have the background to know what should be taught and the best method for doing so? The teaching-learning process can therefore to conceptualized as a two-way interaction between learner and teacher, each dimension being dependent on the other with both parties learning.

It follows that nurse becomes involved in two diagnostic steps.

1. Assessing the learning needs of the client-nursing diagnosis, and
2. Assessing the nurse's own learning needs to carry out teaching responsibilities–self-diagnosis.

It is deemed essential that the professional nurses consider both steps to provide comprehensive nursing care. The experience of the author has found that learning needs infinitely exist. This open-end must be clothed with the variables of priority, time and space, reflective of a given purpose. Further, the author admonishes continual consideration of these steps so as not to close doors before realizing what is being shut out. With this rhetoric, learning needs should be considered in light of past and present educational theory.

Theory of Learning

Conley (1973) explicates eight generalizations from the literature on learning theories. She has synthesized a wealth of theory and research. Each principles is discussed separately and applied into the framework of the chapter.

Learning requires perceiving: Many years ago Dewey (1938, 1961) interpreted learning as a sociologic phenomenon between an organism and the organism's environment. It is important that learners perceive a situation or subject manner as something that is important for themselves and is relevant and/or needed. Bruner (1977) calls this learning as readiness.

Unique characteristics of the learner govern the extent of what is integrated: Differences between learners have been noted by many theorists in education. Pagiet understood intellectual variations based on the developmental maturation of a human being (Ginsburg and Opper, 1969, Wadsworth, 1971). Thorndike noted individual differences while developing "connection" as a theory (Hilgard, 1956) and Wertheimer (1945), Gestalt a psychologist, earmarked the importance of phase experience in learning. Research has consistently proved that learning differences exist between individuals and the disparity can be attributed to a variety of factors.

The degree of learning is influenced by one's environment: Again coming from a sociological framework, behaviorists such a Watson (1916, 1928), Dewey, (Hilgard, 1956) in his functionalist perspective, and von Bertalanffy (1968) in systems theory have shown that the environment is an important learning variable.

Learning is dependent upon the activity of the learner: This principle involves problem solving and behavior toward goal accomplishment by the learner. Hull (1942) discussed this in terms of his drive reduction theory. When one has a need or drive to learn, problem solve or accomplish, one is so motivated to satisfy this need.

Motivation of the learner influences what is learned: Internal motives such as achievement, esteem, and self-actualization (Maslow, 1954) as well as external drives an incentives must be considered. Both play a key role in determining that one learns.

Reinforcement of desired behavior increases the probability that the behavior will reoccur in another situations: Behaviorist theories have long documented this principle; positive reinforcements of those behaviors that one desires is effective.

Transfer of learning occurs when similar conditions are present in old and new situations: Thorndike (Hilgard, 1956) was very early in documenting this principle. Guthrie (1952) later reaffirmed that stimulus pattern that produces a certain response will tend to replicate the response if after a similar pattern is repeated. Bruner (1977) underscored the importance of transfer in learning through the principle.

Practice determines the effectiveness and efficiency in learning: Repetition is of primary importance in learning but the learner must possess knowledge of practice at each point. Thorndike (Hilgard, 1956) was early in noting this effect. Research has found that time between practice periods and evaluation between intervals facilitates learning.

Understanding and use of general principles developed by learning theorists must ground a nurse's teaching processes. Within this frame-work, there are a variety of instructional modes and media that the nurse can employ to meet the learning needs of client and self.

Principles of Teaching and Learning

- The teaching-learning process is facilitated by the existence of a helping relationship
- Teacher needs to be able to communicate effectively with individuals small groups and in some instances, large groups
- Knowledge of the communication process is necessary for the assessment of verbal and nonverbal feedback
- A thorough assessment of students/clients and the factors that affect learning helps to diagnose their learning needs accurately
- The teaching-learning process is more effective when the student/client is included in the planning or the learner's objectives
- Unless the client/student values these objectives, little learning is likely to occur
- The implementation of teaching plan should include various strategies for sensory stimulation, which apparently promote learning
- Relating new learning material to students/clients past life experiences is effective in helping to assimilate new knowledge
- Proposed behavioral changes must always be realistic and explored in the context of the clients/students resources and every day lifestyle
- Careful attention should be paid to time constraints, scheduling, and physical environment
- Learners objectives provide the basis for evaluating whether learning has occurred
- When learning objectives have not been met. Careful reassessment provides ideas for changing the teaching plan for subsequent implementation.

Teaching Strategies

The use of teaching strategies must based on principles of learning, as well as dimensions of the learner and the teacher. The term strategy implies a means or method for achievement of a goal. It is not the aim of teaching but rather the vehicle through which teaching occurs. This vehicle should reflect the best way to accomplish teaching objective synchronized with the perceived best means by which the learner will integrate new knowledge and the experience and ability of the teacher in using the strategy.

There are no absolutes in choosing a teaching strategy and the instructor is limited only by personal ingenuity and creativity in composing a variety of modes and media around teaching objectives and what is known about the client and self. If is with this background that this portion of the chapter broadly discusses teaching strategies – modes and media – as they apply in nursing practice. They can be considered as a resource pool from which a nurse can draw but not be limited.

Conley (1973) distinguishes modes from media by designating modes as types of conversations between teacher and learner; media are devices or props used in instruction to extend what is discussed. Conley provides the types of modes and media; the author amplifies each in nursing practice, when appropriate and when nurse acting as a teacher and patient considered as learner or student.

Teaching Modes

Lecture: This is the most widely used mode in education systems and consists mainly of one-way communication – teacher to learner. In one to one teaching situation, this framework has little application. It is useful, however in reaching large groups of clients who share a particular learning need and remains best when followed by group discussion, thus reinforcing the intended learning.

Group discussion: This is a group-learning format that facilitates integration of new material by enabling two-way conversation between teacher-learners and learner-learners. It is one of the best means for development and discussion of ideas, feelings, beliefs, and experiences around a particular content area. In this mode, the teacher is often seen as a facilitator or learning with expertise in the topic. This has been found as most beneficial when learners shared a particular problem or disability and support can be given and shared. It tends to destroy the myth of being alone and can build bonds of assistants between clients, staff and colleagues.

Panel discussion: Again, this is a more formal method and can be used in teaching client groups as can the lecture. An interplay or mini-group discussion can occur between panel members on a topic with the audience being listeners and occasionally raisers of questions addressed to members of the presenting panel.

Seminar: Respecting nursing practice, the seminar is most useful for self-learning situations in groups of pears. The typical format involves one or two members presenting an idea, problem, or two members presenting an idea, problem, or issue, with everyone then discussing it. The team conference as discussed can be equated this mode.

Demonstration: The demonstration involves use of media by the teacher to personify what is intended for learning by the audience. This can occur with any number of participants from large groups. An example is a nurse demonstrating the act of giving insulin, using the necessary equipment, plus an arrange, doll, or self. Steps and procedures of the task are the foci and learners may then be given the opportunity to practice also. This latter aspect is reflective of the next mode.

Laboratory instruction: Instruction in a laboratory is usually used in formal student learning where self-discovery is the primary basis for learning. Simulations may be involved and didactic presentation may precede or follow the event. In nursing practice, laboratory instruction may follow teacher demonstration, thereby providing the opportunity for "trying on" the new behaviors in a safe environment with assistance if this is required.

Team teaching: Team teaching occurs when two or more professionals carry the responsibility for fulfilling specific teaching objectives with a client or group. In reality, this is most often the case in nursing practice situations, especially with a team of nursing model of delivery. Communication between teachers on the team is under scored as essential and the learner has the opportunity to experience several perspectives in a given area. Learning can be enhanced if the team concept is put into operation but two separate people doing the same thing can be oppressive; team teaching mandates coordination and integration of all efforts.

Teaching Media

Media are devices chosen and used to amplify the aforementioned modes of teaching.

Programmed instruction and computer-assisted instruction: Both media comprise teaching machines or books that carry a learner step by step through content. They offer immediate feedback to the learner in terms of correct responses to questions that usually follow theory. Tow-way communication indirectly occurs between the author of the material on the learner. This method has benefit as an augmenter of learning in nursing practice environments. It is best when preceded and followed by group discussion or one to one talks with the teacher.

Television: Closed circuit and public television is becoming increasing popular in education. Closed-circuit television can employ videotapes prepared by teachers on a given content area for teaching a specified audience. It is commonly found in medical and dental offices for use by clients in a learning. Public television involves many areas, some are specific in content and others provide vicarious experience of direct health education. Hospital situation dramas are prime example of the latter; television specials addressing such topics as life after death or rape, for instance, are examples of the former.

Motion pictures: These can be useful in learning when they are specific to the content requiring teaching. Conley (1973) describes motion pictures as similar to demonstration when the films amplify content.

Simulations: This is primarily involved with laboratory learning and demonstration. Everything that must be achieved is presented in a hypothetical situation. With low-risk and a safe environment provided by the teacher, cognitive, affective, and psychomotor aspects of learning are all amplified and group of one-to-one discussion usually precedes and follows the simulation. Further, these simulations can be videotaped and used as media in future endeavors. The humanistic exercises in this book are examples of simulations.

Pictorial presentations and printed language: These forms of media are most often employed by nurses. Pictures and figures with adjacent explanations are helpful in reinforcing learning that has occurred via a specific mode. They should be used to augment learning. Filmstrip and slides are other examples of this teaching mode.

Tape and disc recording: These can be helpful in self-learning, group discussions, and seminars when what is recorded focuses on a situation or presentation that talks to the topic in focus, often, tape or disc recordings provide narration or an explanation of slides.

Models: These are usually representations of objects needed in demonstration. A model may be a female pelvis that can be taken apart in order to portray childbirth. Again, as with other media, models illustrate what one wishes to teach.

It should be recognized that whatever mode or method is chosen for teaching objectives, personality aspects of both the learner and teacher should be considered. If the client is observed as shy and uncomfortable with groups, that mode is contraindicated. Moreover, if the nurse is inexperienced or nervous demonstrating with groups, another mode is indicated. The decision of using modes and media must portray the best possible learning environmental for all the interacters in the situation.

Role of the Nurse in Teaching and Learning

The basic purpose of teaching is to help clients and families develop the self-care abilities, i.e. knowledge, attitudes and skills that enable them to maximize their functioning and quality of life (or dignified death). When skillfully used by nurses, teaching is a powerful tool for nursing goals or nursing, which includes promoting wellness, preventing illness restoration of health and facilitating coping.

Nurses assume the role of teacher when clients have identifiable learning needs. The teacher-learner relationship is enhanced by the continuance of the helping relationship, in which mutual respect and trust have been established. This nurse build on this trust by sharing information the nurse and client have mutually identified as impertinent. The client may ask for the information or the nurse may initiate teaching as the result of assessment and diagnostic factors. Clients often ask nurse for information about their health. A client may request information about what will happen during an X-ray procedure. Family members may question the reason for their client's pain. A school may ask for information about childhood immunization. Identification of the need for teaching is easy when clients request information.

The nurse is frequently able to anticipate clients needs for information. Clients physical conditions or treatment plans established by the physicians often require that clients acquire new knowledge or skills. It is the responsibility to teach information that clients and their families need. Although the physician is ultimately responsible for providing information about diagnosis, treatment and prognosis, the nurse must help clients understand their responses to illness. A nurse clarifies information provided by physicians and becomes the primary source of information that assists clients adjustments to their health problems.

To be an effective teacher, nurse must do more than just pass on facts, the nurse must engage the client in learning. Nurses have numerous opportunities to pass on facts and nurses must carefully determine what clients need to know and find time when they are ready learn. The goal of client education is to change client behavior and to maintain or improve the clients health.

The techniques used by a teacher to promote learning are teaching strategies. Teaching strategies are planned before the actual teaching sessions so that every content area can be matched with an effective teaching technique. The strategies chosen depend upon the teacher familiarity and teaching aids such as audiovisual and printed materials, the facilities using audiovisual (AV) materials and factors in the client learning such as educational level and cultural background and also age-appropriate methods. The commonly used teaching strategies by the nurses will include the following:
- Role modelling
- Lecture
- Discussion
- Panel discussion
- Demonstration
- Discovery
- Role playing
- AV material
- Printed material
- Programmed instruction
- Computer–assisted instruction.

Skills of Monitoring Vital Signs

Introduction

Vital signs are a person's temperature, pulse, respiration and blood pressure (TPR and BP). Monitoring vital signs is a basic nursing function in assessing the health status of an individual. It is necessary for the nurse to be able to obtain accurate measurement of vital signs are an indication of basic body functioning. It is appropriate to begin the physical assessment by obtaining this information. This physiologic status of the body reflected by these indicators of body functions, which are normally regulated by body through homeostatic mechanism and fall within normal ranges. A change from a person's normal pattern is considered indication of a change in health. Measurement of vital signs provides data that can be used to determine a clients usual state of health as well as the response to physical and psychological stress and medical and nursing therapy. An alteration from normal may signal the need for medical and nursing intervention.

Vital signs are taken and compared with accepted normal values and to the clients usual pattern in wide variety of instances as given below:

- In the patients admission to a health care facility
- In a hospital on a routine schedule according to a physician's order or hospital policy
- Before and after an invasive diagnostic procedure
- Before and after the administration of certain medications that affect cardiovascular, respiratory and temperature control functions
- When the patients general physical condition changes (as with loss of consciousness or increased intensity of pain)
- Before and after nursing interventions influencing visual signs/ vital signs
- When the patient reports nonspecific symptoms of physical distress
- In an emergency situation.

It is an independent nursing action to take and record visual signs as often as possible, the condition of a client requires such intervention.

Temperature Monitoring

Introduction

Temperature is hotness or coldness of a substance. Body temperature is the heat of the body, measured in degrees. The degree of body temperature reflects the difference between health production an heat loss. The core body temperature of a healthy person is maintained within a fairly constant range by the thermoregulatory center in the hypothalamus. This center receives messages from thermal receptors located throughout the body either to produce or conserve body heat or increase heat loss. Temperature regulatory mechanisms keep the body's core temperature (temperature of deep tissues) in a relatively constant range, 37°C (98.6°F).

Core body temperature reflect the temperature of viscera and the muscles, which are insulated by the adipose tissue and skin to prevent heat loss. Heat is lost when heat from the body increase is transferred to the skin surface by circulating blood. The normal body temperature according to sites are as follows:

1. Oral 98.6°F or 37.0 °C
2. Rectal 99.5°F or 37.5°C
3. Axillary 97.6° F or 36.4°C
4. Tympanic 98.6° F or 37.0° C
5. Forehead 94.0° F or 34.4°C

Body temperature is regulated by the hypothalamus, which is located in brain, forming the floor and part of the lateral wall of third ventricle. The hypothalamus helps maintain a balance between heat produced by the body. The primary source of heat in the human body is metabolism, with heat produced as a by-product of metabolic activities that general energy for cellular functions various mechanisms increase body metabolism including hormone (e.g. thyroid), muscle movements (activity) and exercises and sympathetic stimulation (epinephrine and nor-epinephrine). The skin is the primary source of heat loss. The circulating blood brings heat to the skin surface, where small connections between the arterioles to the venules lie directly below the surface. These connections, called artereovenous stunts, may remain open to allow heat to dissipate to the skin and thus to the external environment or they may close and retain heat in the body, construction of peripheral vessels helps conserve heat by preventing heat lost and heat produced through the skin surface.

Factors Affecting Body Temperature

To assess temperature variations and evaluate the significance of changes from normal, the nurse must be aware of several factors the affect body temperature are given below.

Circadian rhythm: Body temperature normally change 0.5° to 10°C (0.9° to 1.8° F) during 24-hour period due to many environmental and physiological processes. Some events in human appear to recur at 24-hour intervals. This cycling pattern is referred to as 'circadian rhythm'. During the day body temperature steadily rises until 6 pm and then declines to early morning level. This is also called diurnal variations.

Age: Both the very young and the very old are more sensitive to changes in the environmental temperature. The neonate's temperature normally ranges from 35.5°to 37.5°C (96° to 99.5°F).

Temperature regulation is liable during infancy because of physiological mechanism. This can continue until puberty. The normal temperature range gradually drops as individual approach older adulthood, with aging sensitivity to temperature extremes develops because of deteriorating control mechanisms.

Exercise: Any form of exercise can increase the body temperature, prolonged strenuous exercises can increase temperature to as high as 41° C (105° F).

Sex: Women tend to have more fluctuations in body temperature than to men. This is most probably the results of changes in the hormones, the increase in progesterone secretion at ovulation increases body temperature as much as 0.5° to 1°F. Hormonal changes during ovulation and menstruation cause body temperature fluctuation.

Stress: Physical and/or emotional stress, such as anxiety may raise body temperature.

Smoking: Smoking cigarettes or cigars may alter body temperature measurement.

Ingestion of hot/cold liquids: Drinking hot and cold liquid can cause slight variations in actual oral temperature reading, e.g. coffee, tea, cool drinks, etc.

Environment: Environment temperature extremes can raise or lower the body temperature. The changes depend on the extent of exposure, air humidity and the presence of convection currents.

Hypothermia: When the person exposed to cold without adequate protective clothing, heat loss may be increased to the point of hypothermia. Similarly, if exposed to extreme of heat for long periods of time in a point of hypothermia, a cause, effects and treatment of hypothermia and hypothermia are as follows:

Temperature less than 35° C leads to hypothermia—the causes and effects or hypothermia–the causes and effects or hypothermia are given in Table 11.1:

Table 11.1: Causes and Effects of Hypothermia	
Causes	*Effects*

• Exposure to prolonged cold
• Older age
• Contributing factors
  - Acute alcoholism
  - Cardiovascular disease
  - Cerebrovascular disease
  - Malnutrition
  - Homelessness
  - Hypothyroidism
	• Intense shivering
	• Increased heartbeat
	• Deep breathing
	• Rigid muscles
	• Decreasing blood pressure
	• Poor cardionation
	• Slurred speech
	• Skin blue, puffy
	• Dilated pupils
	• Weak, irregular pulse
	• Loss of consciousness
	• Death

Treatment of hypothermia includes following:
- Realming – Depends on degree, and may involve applying blankets, giving warm fluids, immersing in warm water, applying heat pads or hot water bottles, instilling warmed fluids, supplying warmed oxygen, using extra corporeal blood warming
- Supporting vital function
- Preventing and treating complications.

Hyperthermia: More than normal body temperature considered according to various conditions of hypothermia. The cause, effects and treatment of hyperthermia and as follows (Table 11.2).

Table 11.2: Causes and Effects of Hyperthermia	
Causes	*Effects*
• Exposure to prolonged heat • Prolonged muscular exertion • Older age • Cardiovascular disease • Drugs that increase muscle tone or reduce heat loss • Leaving children in closed ear in hot weather • Damage to spinal cord or brain	• Heat cramps in heavily used following vigorous activity • Heat syncope – sudden onset of unconsciousness with a fall in BP and cold dump skin • Health exhaustion – thirst, fatigue, nausea, delirium, moist skin, rapid pulse, core temperature more than 37. 8°C (100°F) • Heat stroke – core temperature greater that 40°C (104°F), absence of sweating, nausea, dizziness, blurred vision, convulsion, coma, death

Treatment of hypothermia includes:
- Heat cramps – drink fluids containing salt and rest in cool place

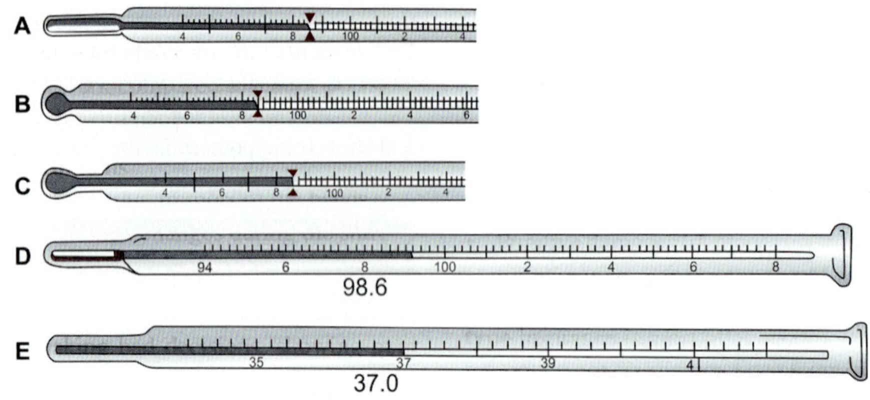

Figures 11.3A to E: Types of glass thermometers: (A) Long or slender tip. (B) Stubby tip (the rectal thermometer). (C) Pear-shaped tip. (D) Slender tip – Fahrenheit: the mercury level is at 99.2°F, (E) Slender tip – centigrade: the mercury level is at 37°C.

- Heat syncope – replace fluids (oral or IV) and rest in cool place
- Heat exhaustion – replace fluids and salt, rest in cool place
- Heat stroke – rapidly cool core temperature by submersing in cold water or applying ice packs.

Temperature elevation may be the first sign of illness. When body temperature is also above normal, the patient is said to be pyrexia, febrile or hypothermia. Pyrexia is an increase in body temperature above normal. The lay term is 'fever'. Fever is actually a body defense. Elevated temperature will destroy invading bacteria. Unfortunately, if temperature exceeds 105°F, normal body cells will be damaged. A person with an increased body temperature is said to be febrils, normal body temperature is said to be febrils, normal body temperature referred to a febrile. Hyperpyrexia is a high fever usually above 41°C (105.8°C). The common courses of pyrexia are as follows:

1. Intermittent fever refers to the body temperature alternates between a period of fever and a period of normal or subnormal temperature.
2. Remittent fever refers to the body temperature fluctuates several degrees, more than 2°C (3.6°F) above normal but does not reach normal between fluctuations.
3. Constant fever refers to the body temperature remains consistency elevated and fluctuates little, less than 2°C.
4. Relapsing fever refers to the body temperature returns to normal at least a day, but then fever recurs.
5. Resolution of pyrexia by crisis is elevated by temperature returns to normal suddenly.
6. Resolution of pyrexia by lyses is an elevated body temperature returns to normal gradually.

Assessment of Body Temperature

The common sites for measuring body temperature are mouth, rectum axilla. Body temperature may be assessed by using a variety of devices. These are glass thermometers (Fig. 11.3), electronic thermometer, tympanic membrane thermometer, disposable thermometer, temperature sensitive patches or tapes and automated monitoring devices.

The advantages and disadvantages and common site of measuring temperature are as follows (Fig. 11.4):

Mouth: It is the most accessible site and more comfortable for clients. Mouth should not be used for clients who could be injured by thermometer, who are unable to hold thermometer properly

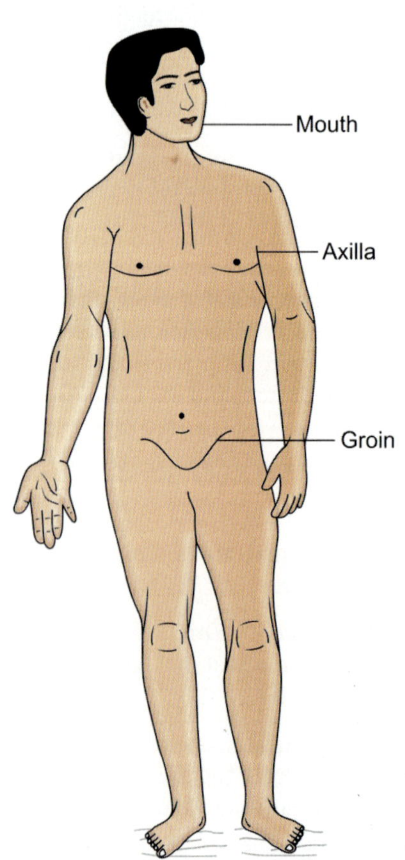

Figure 11.4: Sites for taking temperature

or who might bite thermometer, including infants or small children; conscious or unconscious patients; patients who has oral surgery, trauma to face for mouths, oral pains, who breath only with mouth open; clients with history of convulsions, who experiencing chills.

Rectum: It is thought to provide most reliable measurement. Rectum should not be used for clients who has rectal surgery, who have a rectal disorder (tumor, piles) who cannot be positioned for proper thermometer placement (who had traction), newborn, cardiac patients, who have diarrhea.

Axilla: It is the safe because of noninvasiveness. It requires nurse to hold thermometer in position in less accurate.

Tympanic membrane: It is easy to access to vascular tympanic membrane which reflects care temperature. It is costly device and less accessible.

Preparation for Taking a Temperature

The nurses should determine the need for temperature data based on a physician's guideline or nursing judgment. Patient data indicating feelings of being chilled or hot, confusion, sweating, shivering, cold extremities or a flushed face may indicate an altered thermal state and the need for assessment. Check the patients last recorded temperature for unusually elevated or low readings. These patients should be assessed every 1 to 2 hours for temperature readings until they are consistently within the normal range and determine the best route for taking a particular patient's temperature, as stated earlier.

Measuring body temperature by oral methods with glass thermometer: Equipments needed and steps for oral method of taking temperature with glass thermometer are as follows (Table 11.3).
- Oral thermometer
- Soft tissues
- Pencil or pen
- Paper or flowsheet
- Disposable gloves (optional).

Measuring body temperature by oral method with electronic thermometer: Equipments needed and steps for oral method of taking temperature with electronic thermometer are as follows (Table 11.3).
- Thermometer with probe
- Disposal probe cover
- Soft tissues
- Pencil or pens
- Paper or flow sheet.

Electronic thermometer measure body temperature in 25 to 50 seconds. Most have unbreakable temperature probes, one for oral and one for rectal. They are equipped with disposable covers, a feature that minimizes changes for cross infection and decreases clearing chores. This helps the nurse avoid washing time (Figs 11.5A to F).

Measuring body temperature by rectal method with glass thermometer: Equipments needed and steps for oral method of taking temperature with glass thermometer are as follows (Table 11.3).
- Rectal thermometer
- Soft tissues
- Pencil or pen
- Paper or flow sheet
- Storage container
- Lubricant
- Disposable gloves.

Measuring body temperature by tympanic membrane thermometer: Tympanic membrane thermometer used in traced sensors to detect heat given off by the tympanic membrane. The probe of the thermometer is covered with a probe cover, and the probe is inserted into the ear canal tightly enough to seal the opening. The reading is obtained in less than 2 seconds.

The procedures for assessing a temperature using a tympanic membrane thermometer are as follows:
- Wash hands and attach tympanic probe cover to thermometer
- Insert probe into ear canal with gentle but firm pressure
- Remove thermometer after reading I s displayed on digital unit
- Remove probe cover and dispose in proper container
- Return thermometer to storage area
- Wash hands and document temperature by tympanic membrane.

Measuring body temperature by axillary method with glass thermometer: Equipment needed and steps for oral method of taking temperature with glass thermometer are as follows (Table 11.3).
- Thermometer
- Soft tissues
- Pencil or pen
- Paper or flow sheet

Taking a Temperature

Monitoring body temperature is basic skill necessary in nursing and medical decision-making. When heat production exceeds heat loss, and body temperature rises above the normal range, pyrexia (fever) occurs. Pyrexia can accompany any inflammatory response, loss of body fluid, or prolonged exposure to high temperatures. When the body is exposed to temperatures lower than normal for a prolonged length of time, hypothermia occurs. Hospitalized clients are at particular risk for infection and accompanying fever. Clients are stressed by their presenting conditions and their bodies are further stressed by the hospital environment; thus they are more susceptible to the infectious agents found there. Hypothermia generally occurs in response to prolonged exposure to cold weather or as a result of being immersed in cold water. Accurate monitoring and recording of a client's temperature is essential for diagnosis, treatment, and monitoring of the client.

Prior to taking temperature nurse should:

- Assess body temperature for changes when exposed to pyrogens (endogenous or exogenous substances that cause fever) or to extreme hot or cold external environments because such environments may indicate the cause of an infection.
- Assess the client for the most appropriate site to check temperature to obtain an accurate reading.
- Confirm that the client has not consumed hot or cold food or beverage nor smoked for 15 to 30 minute before the measurement because these activities may alter the oral reading.
- Assess for month breathing and tachypnea because both can cause an inaccurate oral reading
- Assess for oral lesion, especially herpetic lesions, because herpes viruses are extremely contagious and require implementation of Standard Precautions of the Centres for Disease Control and Prevention. Clients with herpetic lesions should have their own glass thermometer or disposable thermometer to prevent transmission to others.

Equipment Needed

- Thermometer (one of the following)
  - Electronic thermometer with disposable protective sheath
  - Tympanic membrane thermometer with probe cover
  - Disposable, single-use chemical strip thermometer
  - Glass (mercury free): oral or rectal at clients bed side, usually color coded to avoid cross use
- Lubricant for rectal and glass thermometer
- Two pairs of non sterile gloves
- Tissues

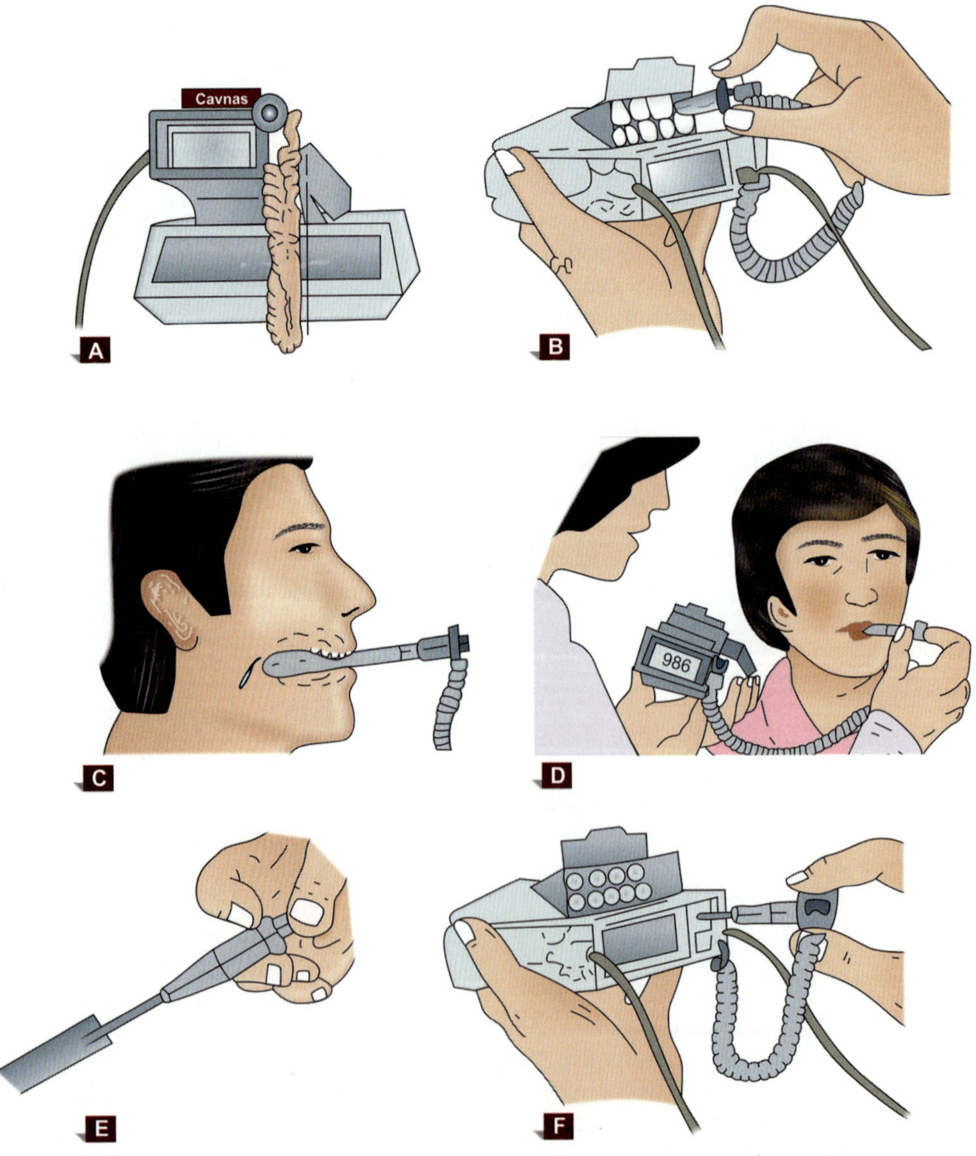

Figures 11.5 A to F: Procedures for using and electronic thermometer

Table 11.3: Taking Temperature

	Nursing actions		*Rationales*
	Check clients identification band Explain procedure before beginning		To identity right patient To reduce anniets and reassure patient
1.	Review medical record for baseline data and factors that influence vital signs.	1.	Establishes parameters for clients normal measurements, provides direction in device selection and helps determine site to use for measurement. Vital signs are measured in the order of temperature, pulse, and respiration (TPR) and blood pressure (BP), usually without interruptions, to provide the nurse with an objective clinical database to direct decision-making.
2.	Explain to the client that vital signs will be assessed. Encourage the client to remain still and refrain from drinking, eating and smoking, and to avoid mouth breathing, if possible.	2.	Encourages participation, allays anxiety, and ensures accurate measurements. Cold or hot liquids and smoking alter circulation and body temperature. Mouth breathing can alter temperature.
3.	Assess clients toileting needs and proceed as appropriate.	3.	Prevents interruptions during measurements, communicates caring and promotes client comfort.
4.	Gather equipment.	4.	Facilitates organization.
5.	Provide for privacy.	5.	Decreases embarrassment
6.	Cleanse hands and apply gloves when appropriate.	6.	Hands are cleansed before and after every contact with a client to reduce the transmission of microorganisms. Gloves are worn to avoid contact with bodily secretions and to reduce transmission of microorganisms.

Oral temperature – electronic thermometer

7.	Repeat Actions 1 to 6	7.	See Rationales 1 to 6
8.	Place disposable protective sheath over probe	8.	Reduces transmission of microorganisms
9.	Grasp top of the probe's stem. Avoid placing pressure on the ejection button.	9.	Pressure on the ejection button releases the sheath from the probe
10.	Place tip of thermometer under the client's tongue and along the gum line to the posterior sublingual pocket lateral to center of lower jaw (Fig. 11.5)	10.	Sublingual pocket contains superficial blood vessels.
11.	Instruct client to keep mouth closed around thermometer	11.	Maintains thermometer in proper place and decreases amount of time required for an accurate reading
12.	Thermometer will signal (beep) when a constant temperature registers (Fig. 11.5)	12.	Signal indicates final temperature reading
13.	Read measurement on digital display of electronic thermometer. Push ejection button to discard disposable sheath into receptacle and return probe to storage well	13.	Reduces transmission of microorganisms. Ensure that the electronic system is ready for next use
14.	Inform client of temperature reading	14.	Promotes clients participation in care
15.	Remove gloves and cleanse hands	15.	Reduces transmission of microorganisms
16.	Record reading according to institution policies	16.	Accurate documentation by site allows for comparison of data
17.	Return electronic thermometer unit to charging base, checking that it is plugged in	17.	Ensures charging base is plugged into electrical outlet and thermometer is ready for next use
18.	Cleanse hands	18.	Reduces transmission of microorganisms

Contd...

<table>
<tr><th colspan="2" align="center">**Table 11.3:** *Contd....*</th></tr>
<tr><td align="center">*Nursing actions*</td><td align="center">*Rationales*</td></tr>
</table>

Tympanic Temperature: Infrared Thermometer

	Nursing actions		Rationales
19.	Repeat Actions 1 to 6	19.	See Rationales 1 to 6
20.	Position client in Sims' or sitting position	20.	Promotes access to ear.
21.	Remove probe from container and attach probe cover to tympanic thermometer unit (Fig. 11.5)	21.	Prevents contamination.
22.	Turn clients head to one side. For an adult, pull pinna upward and back; for a child, pull down and back. Gently insert probe with firm pressure into ear canal (Fig. 11.5)	22.	Provides access to ear canal. Gentle insertion prevents trauma to external canal. Firm pressure is needed to ensure probe will record an accurate temperature.
23.	Remove probe after the reading is displayed on digital storage unit (usually 2 seconds)	23.	Reading is displayed within seconds.
24.	Discard probe cover into receptacle and replace probe in storage container	24.	Reduces transmission of microorganisms. Protects reusable probe from damage.
25.	Return tympanic thermometer to storage unit.	25.	Recharges batteries of unit for future use.
26.	Record reading according to institution policy.	26.	Promotes accurate documentation for data comparison.
27.	Cleanse hands.	27.	Reduces transmission of microorganisms

Using a "Tempa-Dot"

	Nursing actions		Rationales
28.	Repeat Actions 1 to 6	28.	See Rationales 1 to 6
29.	Position the client to a sitting or lying position	29.	Promotes clients comfort, and promotes site access for all measurement.
30.	Prepare Tempa-Dot according to directions (Fig. 11.6). • Oral measurement: Place Tempa-Dot under tongue as far back as possible. Have client press tongue down on thermometer and keep mouth closed for 60 seconds. Remove thermometer, read the last blue dot: Ignore any skipped dot. • Axillary's measurement: Place thermometer high in the armpit, vertical to the body, with dots against the torso. Lower clients arm to hold thermometer in place. Remove thermometer after 3 minutes.	30.	Promotes accurate measurement and client safety.
31.	Record temperature. Indicate the method, and discard the thermometer.	31.	Nursing documentation, practice clean technique.
32.	Cleanse hands.	32.	Reduces transmission of microorganisms.

Contd...

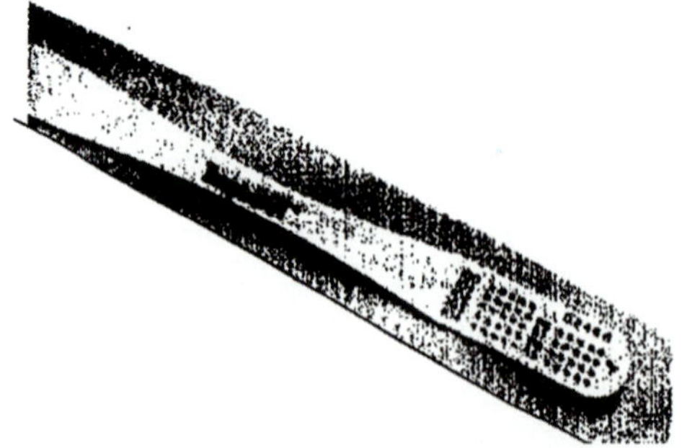

Figure 11.6: 'Tempa-dot' single-use disposable thermometer

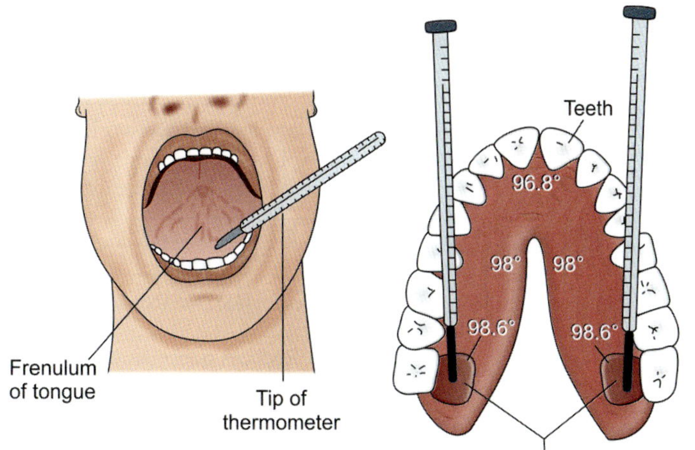

Figure 11.7: Thermometer placement in the mouth

	Table 11.3: *Contd....*		
	Nursing actions		*Rationales*
Oral Temperature: Glass Thermometer			
33.	Repeat Actions 1 to 6	33.	See Rationales 1 to 6.
34.	Select correct color tip of thermometer from clients bedside container (Fig. 11.3)	34.	Identifies correct device: a blue tip usually denotes an oral thermometer.
35.	Remove thermometer from storage container, hold at end away from bulb and cleanse under cool water.	35.	Cleansing removes disinfectant, which can irritate oral mucosa. Cool water prevents expansion of the colored solution/ mercury. Touching the bulb will heat the solution and cause an inaccurate reading.
36.	Use a tissue to dry thermometer from bulb's end toward fingertips.	36.	Wipe from area of least contamination to most contaminated area.
37.	Read thermometer by locating colored solution or mercury level. It should read 35.5°C (96°F)	37.	Thermometer must be below normal body temperature to ensure an accurate reading.
38.	If thermometer in not below normal body temperature reading, gasp thermometer with thumb and forefinger and shake vigorously by snapping the wrist in a downward motion to move mercury to a level below normal.	38.	Shaking briskly lowers level of mercury in column. Because glass thermometer break easily, make sure that nothing in the environment comes in contact with the thermometer when shaking it.
39.	Place thermometer in clients mouth under the tongue and along the gum line to the posterior sublingual pocket. Instruct client to hold lips closed (Fig. 11.7)	39.	Ensures contact with large blood vessels under the tongue. Prevents environmental air from coming in contact with the bulb.
40.	Leave in place as specified by institution policy, usually 3 to 5 minutes	40.	Thermometer must stay in place long enough to ensure an accurate reading.
41.	Remove thermometer and wipe with a tissue away from fingers toward the bulbs end (Fig. 11.7)	41.	Mucus on thermometer may interfere with the effectiveness of the disinfectant solution. Wisps from area of least contamination to most contaminated area.
42.	Read at eye level and rotate slowly until mercury level is visualized.	42.	Ensures an accurate reading

Contd...

Table 11.3: *Contd....*

	Nursing actions		Rationales
43.	Shake thermometer down, cleanse glass thermometer with soapy water, rinse under cold water, and return to storage container.	43.	Mechanical cleansing removes secretions that promote growth of microorganisms. Hot water may cause coagulation of secretions and cause expansion of mercury in the thermometer.
44.	Remove and dispose of gloves in receptacle. Cleanse hands.	44.	Reduces transmission of microorganisms
45.	Record reading according to institution policy.	45.	Accurate documentation by site allows for comparison of data.
46.	Cleanse hands.	46.	Reduces transmission of microorganisms
Rectal Temperature (Fig. 11.8 and Table 11.4A)			
47.	Repeat Actions 1 to 6	47.	See Rationales 1 to 6.
48.	Place client in the shims position with upper knee flexed. Adjust sheet to expose only anal area.	48.	Proper positioning ensures visualization of anus.
49.	Place tissues in easy reach. Apply gloves.	49.	Tissue is needed to wipe anus after device is removed.
50.	Prepare the thermometer	50.	Ensures a smooth procedure an accurate reading.
51.	Lubricate tip of rectal thermometer or probe (a rectal thermometer usually has a red tip or cap).	51.	Promotes ease of insertion of thermometer or probe.
52.	With dominant hand, grasp thermometer. With other hand, separate buttocks to expose anus (Fig. 11.8)	52.	Aids in visualization of anus.
53.	Instruct the client to take a deep breath. Insert the thermometer or probe gently into anus: infant, 1.2 cm (0.5 inches); adult, 3.5 cm (1.5 inches). If resistance is felt, do not force insertion.	53.	Relaxes anal sphincter. Gentle insertion decreases discomfort to client and prevents trauma to mucous membranes.
54.	Hold in place for 2 minutes.	54.	Prevents trauma to mucosa and breakage of glass thermometer
55.	Wipe off secretions on the glass thermometer with a tissue. Dispose of tissue in a receptacle.	55.	Removes and fecal material for visualization of mercury level. Prevents transmission of microorganisms.
56.	Read measurement and inform the client of the temperature reading	56.	Promotes clients participation in care.
57.	While holding glass thermometer in one hand, use other hand to wipe anal area with tissue to remove lubricant or feces. Dispose of soiled tissue. Cover client.	57.	Prevents contamination of clean objects with soiled thermometer, decreases skin irritation, and promotes client comfort. Prevents embarrassment.
58.	Cleanse thermometer.	58.	Reduces transmission of microorganisms.
59.	Remove and dispose of gloves in receptacle. Cleanse hands.	59.	Reduces transmission of microorganisms
60.	Record reading according to institution policy.	60.	Accurate documentation by site allows for comparison of data.
Axillary Temperature (Figs 11.9A and B and Table 11.4B))			
61.	Repeat Actions 1 to 6	61.	See Rationales 1 to 6
62.	Remove clients arm and shoulder from one sleeve of gown. Avoid exposing chest.	62.	Exposes axillary area
63.	Make sure ancillary skin is dry: if necessary, pat dry.	63.	Removes moisture and prevents a false low reading.
64.	Prepare thermometer.	64.	Ensures accurate use of thermometer.

Contd...

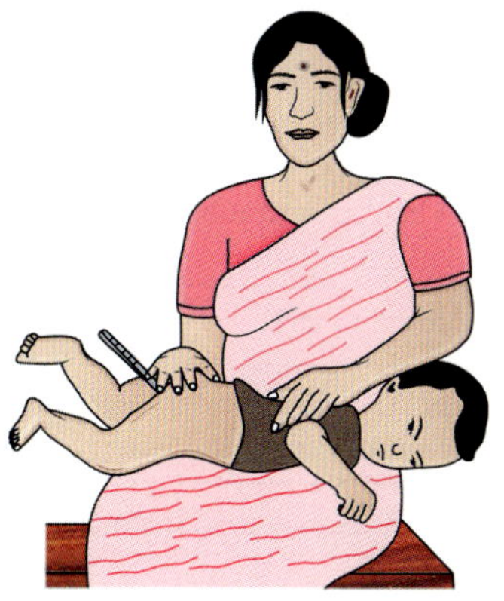

Figure 11.8: Taking rectal temperature in child

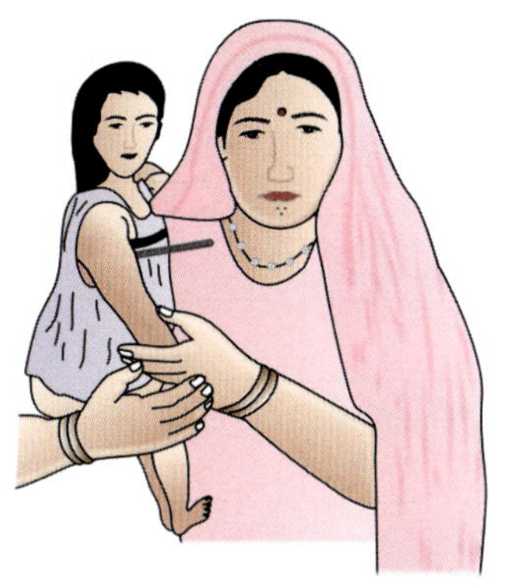

Figure 11.9A: Taking axillary temperature in child

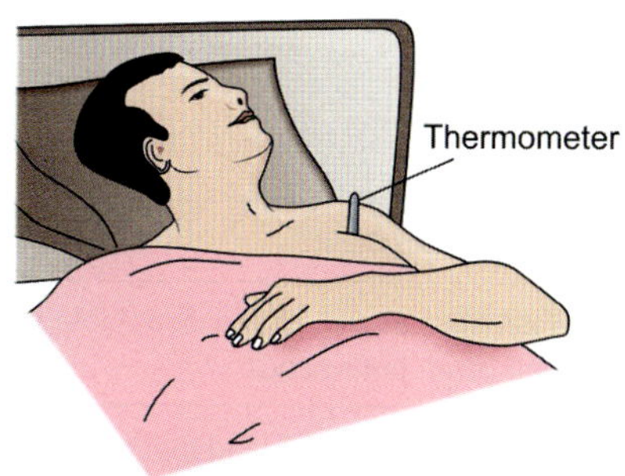

Figure 11.9B: Taking axillary temperature in adult

Table 11.3: *Contd....*

	Nursing actions		Rationales
65.	Place thermometer or probe into center of axilla. Fold the client's upper arm straight down, and place arm across the client's chest.	65.	Puts device in contact with axillary blood supply. Maintains the device in proper position.
66.	Leave glass thermometer in place as specified by institution policy (usually 6 to 8 minutes). Leave an electronic thermometer in place until signal is heard.	66.	Device must stay in place long enough to ensure an accurate reading. Signal indicates final temperature reading.
67.	Remove and read thermometer.	67.	Allows accurate reading of temperature
68.	Inform client of temperature reading.	68.	Promotes clients participation in care.
69.	Shake down thermometer, cleanse glass thermometer with soapy water, rinse under cold water, and return to storage container.	69.	Prevents breakage of glass thermometer and transmission of microorganisms.
70.	Assist the client with replacing the gown.	70.	Promotes comfort.
71.	Record reading according to institution policy.	71.	Promotes accurate documentation for data comparison.
72.	Cleanse hands.	72.	Reduces transmission of microorganisms
Disposable (Chemical strip) Thermometer			
73.	Repeat Actions 1 to 6	73.	See Rationales 1 to 6.
74.	Apply tape to appropriate skin area, usually forehead.	74.	Tape must be in direct contact with the clients skin.
75.	Observe tape for color changes.	75.	Color indicates temperature reading (refer to the manufacturer's instructions).
76.	Record reading and indicate method.	76.	Promotes accurate documentation for data comparison.
77.	Cleanse hands.	77.	Reduces transmission of microorganisms

Table 11.4A: Steps for Rectal Method of Taking Temperature with Glass Thermometer

	Nursing actions		*Rationales*
1.	Explain the procedure to patient.	1.	An explanation encourage client cooperation and reduces client his apprehension.
2.	Gather equipment.	2.	It provide for organized approach to task.
3.	Wash your hands. Don a disposable glove on your dominant hand or on both hands.	3.	Hand wash deters the spread of the organism disposable glove, protected the nurse from microorganism in the faces.
4.	Wipe and shake and read the rectal thermometer (RT).	4.	RT requires the same preparation as in oral thermometer.
5.	Lubricate the mercury bulb and an area approximately 2.5 cm (1 inch) above the bulb.	5.	Lubrication reduces friction and thereby facilitates insertion, minimizing irritation or injury to the mucus membrane of anal canal.
6.	Provide for privacy, with the client on his or her side, fold back the bed linen and separate the buckles so that and sphincter is seen clearly.	6.	It not placed directly through the anal opening, the bulb of the thermometer may injure the adjacent tissue or cause discomfort for the client.
7.	Insert the thermometer for approximately 3.8 cm (1.5 inch) in an adult, 2.5 cm (1 inch) in a child, and 1.25 cms (0.05 inch) in an infant (Fig. 11.8).	7.	Insertion length must be adjusted according to the anatomical size of the clients return.
8.	Permit the clients buttocks to fail, in place while holding the thermometer in place for 2 to 3 minutes.	8.	The thermometer may become displaced internally or externally if it is not held in place.
9.	Remove thermometer and wipe it once with soft tissue from the fingers to the mercury bulb, using a firm, twisting motion.	9.	Cleaning from an area where there are few organisms to an area where there are numerous organisms minimizes the spread of organism Friction, helps to loosen the lubricant and fecal matter from the surface.
10	Wipe any residue of lubricant or stool remaining about the anus.	10.	Removing lubricant and stool promotes the cleanliness and comfort to the client.
11.	Read the thermometer and dispose of the tissue in a rectable used for contaminated items.	11.	Items containing organisms should be placed in containers for disposal to avoid transmitting them to other people.
12.	Wash thermometer in lukewarm water. Rinse in cold water. Dry and replace the thermometer on container marked (Rectal thermometer) at the bedside. Remove disposable gloves from the inside out and discard the glove.	12.	Mechanical action of washing aids in removal of organic material and organisms.
13.	Wash your hands.	13.	Hand washings deters the spread of microorganisms.
14.	Record temperature on flow sheet or paper. Indicate that rectal route was used. Report any abnormal finding to the appropriate person.	14.	Recording the temperature provides accurate documentation.

The skill of temperature measurement is often delegated to ancillary personnel: however the nurse retains responsibility for knowledge of the clients temperature and appropriate actions. The expectation is that ancillary personnel will have documented instruction and competency validation of their ability to:
- Select the correct route for measurement of the temperature
- Correctly position the client for measurement.
- Correctly perform the measurement according to established guidelines and record on the appropriate flow sheet (clinical record).
- Recognize and report abnormal findings to the nurse.

Taking Pulse/Monitoring Pulse

Pulse

The pulse is the palpable bounding of blood flow noted at various points on the body. It is perceptible sensation as a wave of blood is pumped into the arteries by the contraction of the left ventricle. It is a rhythmic beating or vibrating movement. It is the regular recurrent expansion and contraction of an artery produced by waves of pressure caused by the ejection of blood from the left ventricle of the heart as it contracts. It corresponds to each beat

Table 11.4B: Steps for Axillary Method of Taking Temperature with Glass Thermometer			
	Nursing actions		*Rationales*
1.	Explain the procedure to patient.	1.	It encourages client cooperation and reduces anxiety, apprehension.
2.	Gather equipment.	2.	It provide for organized approach to task.
3.	Wash your hands.	3.	Hand washing deters the spread microorganism.
4.	Provide for privacy and move down to expose axilla.	4.	Moving down to expose axilla ensures accurate placement of the thermometer.
5.	Wipe the thermometer with a clean tissue if it has been stored in a chemical solution. Use a firm, twisting motion to remove the moisture.	5.	Chemical solution may irritate the skin. The presence of solution may after skin temperature. Soft tissue and friction help remove the solution.
6.	Shake and read the thermometer.	6.	The mercury must be below the calibrations of the previous recording to assess the current temperature accurately.
7.	Place the bulb of the thermometer into the center of the axilla.	7.	The deepest area of the axilla provides the most accurate temperature measurement.
8.	Bring the clients arm down close to his or her body, and place the clients forearm over his or her chest.	8.	Surrounding the bulb with the skin surfaces of the axilla reduces the amount of surrounding air and ensures reliable measurement.
9.	Remain with the client and leave the thermometer in place for 3 to 5 minutes.	9.	Additional time is required because the thermometer has not been placed in a body cavity and it takes longer for the mercury to risk to the maximum level of clients temperature.
10	Remove and read the thermometer. Clean the thermometer and replace it in its location for reuse.	10.	A thermometer that has been used for an axillary temperature should be cleaned before using it for another route and vice versa..
11.	Wash your hands.	11.	Hand washing deters the spread microorganism.
12.	Record temperature on flow sheet or paper. Indicate axillary route, report any abnormal findings to the appropriate person.	12.	Recording the temperature provides accurate documentation.

of the heart. It is an indicator of circulatory state. Circulation is the means by which cells receives nutrients and remove waste products of metabolism.

The heart is a pulsatile pump, ejecting blood intermittently into the arterial system. Each time the left ventricle of the heart contacts to eject blood into an already full aorta, the arterial walls in the blood system expands to compensate of the aorta sends a wave through walls of the arterial system that, on palpation can be felt as a light tap. The pulse is regulated by the autonomic nervous system through the sino-artial node. Parasympathetic stimulations decreases the heart rate and sympathetic decreases the heart rate and sympathetic stimulation increases the heart rate. The quantity of blood forced out of the left ventricle with each contraction is called 'stroke volume'. The average amount of blood per contraction is 70 mL for an adult. The cardiac output is the amount of blood pumped per minute. The volume is determined by using the following formula. Cardiac output + Stroke volume x pulse rate. Thus the cardiac output of an adult with a stroke volume 70 mL. Many factors can affect both the heart rate and the volume are exercise, fever, acute pain, anxiety, drugs, hemorrhage, postural drainage.

Character of the Pulse

Plus rate: The pulse rate is the number of palpation felt over a peripheral artery of heart over the apex of the heart in one minute. The normal pulse rate per minute varies according to age as given in Table 11.5.

Pulse rate varies, depending on age, level of activity and a variety of other factors. The factors that influence pulse rate are as follows:

1. *Exercise:* Short-term exercise increases pulse rate. Long-term exercises strengthen heart muscles, resulting in a lower than normal rate at rest and a quicker return to the resting rate after exercise.

Table 11.5: Normal Pulse Rate According to Age

Age	Range	Average
Newborn	120-160	140
1 to 12 months	80-140	120
1 to 2 years	80-130	110
2 to 6 years	76-120	100
6 to 12 years	76-110	96
Adolescent to adult	60-100	80

2. *Fever and heart:* These both increase the pulse rate because of increased metabolic rate.
3. *Acute pain and anxiety:* These increase the pulse rate because of sympathetic stimulation.
4. *Unrelieved severe and chronic pains:* These are decreases the pulse rate because of parasympathetic stimulation.
5. *Medications:* Some medications alter pulse rate. For example, digitals and beta blockers decrease pulse rate, where as atrophic increases the pulse rate.
6. *Age:* Pulse rate decreases on the aging process progresses from infancy, through puberty, to adulthood.
7. *Metabolism:* Certain diseases such a hyperthyroidism or cardiomyopathy can cause a chronic elevated pulse rate; hypothyroidism can cause a slowing of the pulse.
8. *Hemorrhage:* Loss of blood increases the pulse rate because sympathetic stimulation.
9. *Postural changes:* Lying down decreases the pulse rate; standing or sitting increases it, e.g. bed rest.

If the pulse is faster than 100 beats per minute, the patient has Tachycardia, if it is slower than 60 beats per minute the patient has bradycardia. Tachycardia can result from shock, hemorrhage, strong emotions, exercise, fever, pain, prolonged application of heat, decreased blood pressure and some medication, i.e. adrenaline. Bradycardia can result from unreleased severe pain, drugs such as digitalis, resting in a supine position, and heart block.

Pulse rhythm: It is the pattern of pulsation and the pauses between them. This rhythm is normally regular that is the beat and the pauses occur similarly throughout the time of pulse being obtained. An irregular pattern of heartbeats is called dysarrythmia.

Pulse amplitude: It describes the quality of pulse in terms of its fullness and reflects the strength of the left ventricular contraction. It is assessed by the feel of the blood flow through the vessel. The variation of pulse volume/amplitude are termed as following:

1. *Absent pulse:* No pulsation is felt despite extreme pressure
2. *Thready pulse:* Pulsation is not easily felt and slight pressure caused, it to disappear.
3. *Weak pulse:* Stronger than a thready pulse; light pressure causes it to disappear.
4. *Normal pulse:* Pulsation is easily felt, takes moderate pressure to cause it to disappear, i.e. but not palpable when moderate pressure applied.
5. *Bounding pulse:* Pulsation is strong and does not disappear with moderate pressure. It feels full and spring like even under moderate pressure.
6. *Normal pulse:* Pulsation is easily felt, takes moderate pressure to cause it to disappear, i.e. but not palpable when moderate pressure applied.
7. *Bounding pulse:* Pulsation is strong and does not disappear with moderate pressure. It feel full and spring like even under moderate pressure.

Assessment of Pulse

There are two ways of measuring pulse rate. One is by using a stethoscope and listening over the apex of the heart. This is called as 'apical pulse'. The other way of taking a pulse involves palpation of an artery between your (nurses) fingers and a bony surface within the patient. By trapping the pulsing artery between your fingers and a hard surface, the heart rate can be determined in a peripheral site. The pulse that is palpated at any number of sites on the body is caused by the contraction of the left ventricle which forces bolus of blood into the aorta. The aorta distends to accommodate the surge of blood an then recoils as the ventricles relax and the blood moves on down the artery. The surge of blood action the elastic arteries to cause a wave like distention and recoil all the way down the artery. This is what is palpated as the pulse. The pulse is normally easily palpated and feels strong and regular.

The radial and apical pulses are most common sites for assessment of vital signs. The local assessment criteria for pulse sites are as give below (Fig 11.10.).

Temporal: Located over temporal bone of the head, above and lateral to the eye, it is easily accessible sites used to assess pulse in children.

Carotid: Located along medical edge of sternocledomastoid muscle in the neck, it is also easily accessible site used to assess character of pulse peripherally and is used during shock and cardiac arrest when other sites are not palpable.

Apical: Location is fourth to fifth intercostals space at midclavicular line. This site is used for auscultation of heart sounds.

Brachial: Location is groove between biceps and triceps muscle at anticubital fossa. This site is used to assess status of circulation to lower arm and auscultate blood pressure.

Radial or thumb side of forearm at wrist: It is a common site used to assess character of pulse peripherally and status of circulation to hand.

Ulnar: Ulnar side of forearm at wrist is used to assess status of circulation to ulnar side of hand and assess Allerns test.

Femoral: Location is below inguinal ligament, midway between symphysis pubis and antero-superior iliac spine. The site is used to assess character of pulse during physiologic shock or cardiac arrest when other pulses are not palpable and to assess status of circulation to leg.

Popliteal: Location is behind knee in propliteal fossa. This site is used to assess status of circulation to lower leg.

Posterior tibial: It is the inner side of each ankle below medial malleolus. This site is used to assess status of circulation to foot.

Dorsalis pedis: It is along top of foot between extension tendency of great and first toe. This site is used to assess status of circulation of foot.

Preparation for Obtaining a Pulse

The nurse has to determine need for measuring a patients pulse may be an independent nursing bases on the patients condition, or it may be ordered by the physician or another nurse on a set schedule, such as every four hours whenever there is any change in the patient condition based on objective or subjective data, taking blood pressure, respiration, and temperature since many changes will be reflected these measurements. Remember that an order for vital signs on a set schedule is not based on the patient current condition but on a previous evaluation. It is the responsibility of the nurse caring for the patient at the bed time to decide if more frequent measurement of pulse and other vital signs are needed. And determine which method is appropriate for taking a patient pulse according to the condition of the patient. After taking pulse, the words can be used to describe a pulse are as follows.

- *Regular interval*: The interval between the beat is equal.
- *Irregular interval*: The interval between each beat is uneven.
- *Tachycardia*: Pulse rate is above normal range for patients stage of growth and development (as explained earlier) rapid heart rate.
- *Bradycardia*: Pulse rate is below normal range for stage of growth and development (slow heart rate).
- *Weak, feeble, thready*: All indicate a reduced force or volume in peripheral pulse; difficult to obliterate by pressure.
- *Bigeminal pulse*: Pulse has occasional premature beats, resulting in a shorter interval between beats followed by longer interval. Beats in group of two with pause before next beat.
- *Paradoxiacal pulse:* The force or volume of the peripheral pulse is reduced when the patient inhales (if pronounced, may indicate coritical situation called cardiac temponade where blood fills the sac around the heart, the pericardial sac and interferes with the pumping action of the heart).
- *Chrotic pulse*: The pulse is completely irregular with no pattern to the irregularity.
- *Sinus arrhythmia:* Pulse speeds up at peak of inspiration and slows down as the person exhales, common in children, disappears if pulse takes while child holds breath.
- *Intermittent pulse*: A pulse with normal rhythm intermixed with periods of irregular rhythm.
- *Pulse deficit:* The difference in number of beats each minute between the apical and radial pulse (or peripheral) when measured simultaneously; apical rate is always higher if there is a pulse deficit.
- *Pical radial pulse:* One nurse takes the radial pulse, while another nurse simultaneously takes apical pulse; taken whenever pulse rates are known or suspended or being different. Record pulse deficit in chart.

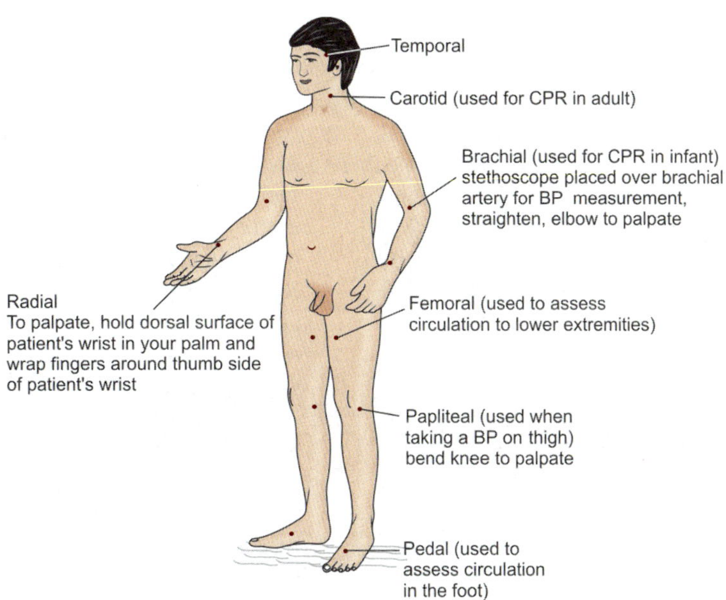

Figure 11.10: Common peripheral sites for measuring pulse

Obtaining a radial pulse rate: Equipments needed and procedures for obtaining a radial pulse rate are as given in Table 11.7.
- Watch with second hand or digital readout
- Pencil or pen
- Paper or flow sheet.

Obtaining the apical pulse rate: Equipments needed and procedures for obtaining the apical pulse rate are as given in Table 11.7.
- Watch the second hand or digital read out
- Stethoscope
- Pencil or pen
- Paper or flow sheet
- Alcohol swab

Pulse assess is the measurement of a pressure pulsation created when the heart contracts and ejects blood into the aorta. The amplitude of the pulse reflects the stroke volume with each ejection. Assessment of pulse characteristics provides clinical data regarding the hearts pumping action and the adequacy of peripheral artery blood flow. The radial pulse is most often used for basic assessment; however, other site areas are used in total assessment and when specific areas of circulation are to be determined.

Pulse-Monitoring Techniques

Palpation

Palpation of a pulse involves the index and middle fingers of one hand. Start with gentle pressure to locate the strongest pulsation and then use firmer palpation for the counting. When counting, also assess the rhythm and quality of the pulse. Measure the pulse for 30 and 60 seconds, and then multiply the counts if need be to obtain the one-minute reading.

Auscultation

Auscultation is usually used to assess the apical pulse. The apical pulse is the most accurate pulse, especially when the peripheral pulse is difficult to locate. Auscultation requires the stethoscope. The stethoscope should be equipped with a bell and a diaphragm. The diaphragm side is normally used for low-pitch sound, such as normal heart sound, bowel sound or breath sound; the bell side is used for high-pitch sound, such as murmur and abnormal heart sound.

Doppler

- An ultrasonic Doppler device is usually used when the pulse cannot be detected by palpation (Fig. 11.11). The Doppler can detect the peripheral pulses in situations such as cardiopulmonary collapse in obese clients, infants with small arms, or clients with edema in which palpation of the pulse is difficult.

- A vendor-recommended conductive gel should be applied to the skin as a coupling medium for ultrasound transmission. The transmitting device (probe) is then placed over the artery to be assessed. The Doppler usually is equipped with both high and low frequency probes. A high frequency (8 to 10 Hz) probe is usually used on the surface vessel sites. A low frequency (2 to 3 Hz) probe of ten is used for deeper sites, such obstetric assessment.

- The sounds can be amplified and heard through an earpiece or speaker attached to the device, assessing with low volume initially. Tilt the back of the probe toward the hand at an angle of about 45 degrees. Search the area of the assessed artery and tilt the probe for best Doppler sounds. Adjust the sound volume control to a comfort level for counting.

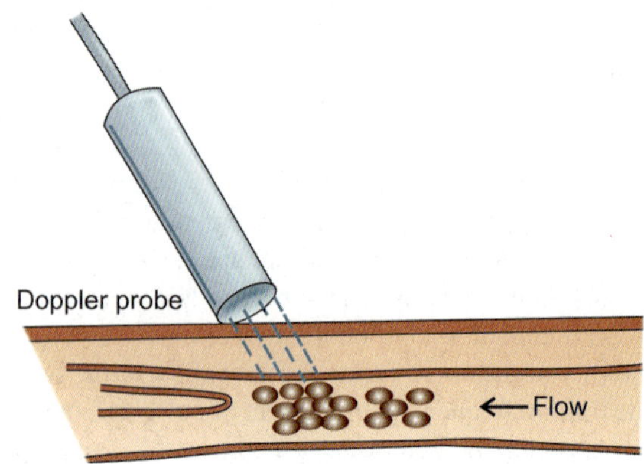

Figure 11.11: Doppler sound generation

Before taking pulse nurse should:
- Assess client for need to monitor pulse because certain diseases or conditions, such as history of heart disease or cardiac dysrhythmias, chest pain, invasive cardiovascular diagnostic tests, infusion of large volume of IV fluids or hemorrhage, can cause an increased risk for alterations in pulse.
- Assess the pulse for rate, amplitude contour and regularity.
- Assess for signs and symptoms of cardiovascular alterations, such as dyspnea, chest pain, orthopnea, syncope, palpations, edema of extremities, cyanosis, or fatigue, because these signs may indicate deficient cardiac or vascular function.
- Assess client for factors that may affect the character of the pulse, such as age, medications, exercise, change in position or fever. This enables the nurse to accurately assess for the significance of an alteration in pulse.
- Assess for the appropriate site for measuring pulse so the pulse will be accurate.
- Assess the baseline heart rate and rhythm in the clients chart to compare it with the current measurement.
- Assess circulatory status by using appropriate site (Table 11.6) because pulses may be affected by surgery, medical condition, arterial blood draws, or poor circulation.

Table 11.6: Pulse Point Assessment (Please see Figure 11.10)

Sl. No.	Pulse Point	Location	Assessment Criteria
1.	Temporal	Over the temporal bone, lateral to the eye, upper to the ear	Accessible, used routinely for infants and when radial is inaccessible
2.	Carotid	Bilateral, under the lower jaw, beneath the sternomastoid muscles. Carotid pulse best presents the aortic pulse for its close location to the central circulation. Palpation of the artery on the neck may cause stimulation of the carotid sinus and result in decrease of the pulse rate.	Accessible, used routinely for infants and during shock or cardiac arrest when other peripheral pulses are too weak to palpate; also used to assess cranial circulation. Take a carotid pulse on only one side of the apical-radial deficit.
3.	Apical	Left ventricle, fourth to fifth intercostal space, on the midclavicular line	Used to auscultate heart sounds and assess apical-radial deficit
4.	Brachial	Inner side between the groove of bicep and tricep muscles at the antecubital fossa	Used in cardiac arrest for infants, to assess lower arm circulation, and to auscultate blood pressure
5.	Radial	On the thumb side, outer aspect of the wrist	Accessible; used routinely in adults to assess character of peripheral pulse
6.	Ulnar	On the little finger side, outer aspect of the wrist	Used to assess circulation to ulnar side of hand and to perform the Allen test
7.	Femoral	Below the inguinal ligament, in the anterior medial aspect of the thigh, midway to the anterior-superior iliac spine and symphysis pubis	Used to assess circulation to legs and during cardiac arrest
8.	Popliteal	Behind the knee, Medical or lateral to the popliteal fossa	Used to assess circulation to legs and to auscultate leg blood pressure
9.	Posterior Tibial	Inner side of the ankle, between the Achilles tendon and tibia	Used to assess circulation to feet
10.	Pedal/Dorsal Pedal	Lateral to the extension tendon, from the great toe toward the ankle	Used to assess circulation to feet

Equipment Needed

- Watch with a second hand
- Stethoscope
- Alcohol swab
- Gloves.

The radial pulse assessment is often delegated to trained ancillary personnel; however, the nurse is responsible for knowing the results. Assessment of the apical pulse may be delegated to specially prepared staff. The assessment of peripheral circulation is delegated after proper training in the monitoring of peripheral sites for the presence of abnormal color, motion, or sensation in the extremity. The absence of pulses must be immediately reported for further assessment by the nurse, and the nurse is responsible for reviewing the data collected in a timely manner and revalidating the results, if indicated. The institutions policy should clearly indicate the training and validation requirements before the nurse delegates the monitoring of apical pulses and peripheral vascular assessments on stable clients. These tasks should not be delegated if the client is unstable.

After procedure nurse should:
- Compare client's pulse with baseline rate, amplitude and rhythm to detect any changes.
- If pulse is irregular or abnormal, ask another nurse to check the pulse and then report to health care provider.
- Evaluate pulse site as required by client's condition and compare bilateral pulses. Example: For clients with poor peripheral circulation in the lower extremities, compare both pedal/dorsal or both posterior tibial pulses.

Nurses Notes on Flow Sheet
- Pulse rate
- Observations regarding regularity, volume, or rate
- New irregularities in pulse reported to the clients health care provider.

Respiration Monitoring

Human survival depends on the ability of oxygen to reach and of carbon dioxide to remove out from the body cells. Respiration involves several physiologic events which includes the following:

Table 11.7: Taking Pulse/Pulse Monitoring

	Nursing Action		Rationale
	Check clients identification band Explain procedure before beginning		To Identity right Patient To reduce anniets and reassure patient
Taking Radial (Wrist) Pulse			
1.	Cleanse hands	1.	Reduces transmission of microorganisms
2.	Inform client of the site(s) at which you will measure pulse	2.	Encourages participation and always anxiety
3.	Flex clients elbow and place lower of arm across chest.	3.	Maintains wrist in full extension and exposes artery for palpation. Placing clients hand over chest will facilitate later respiratory assessment without undue attention to your action. (It is difficult for any person to maintain a normal breathing pattern when someone is observing and measuring).
4.	Support clients wrist by grasping outer aspect with thumb	4.	Stabilizes wrist and allows for pressure to be exerted.
5.	Place your index and middle fingers on inner aspect of clients wrist over the radial artery and apply light but firm pressure until pulse is palpated 0	5.	Fingertips are sensitive, facilitating palpation of pulsating pulse. The nurse may feel his or her own pulse if palpating with thumb. Applying light pressure prevents occlusion of blood flow and pulsation.
6.	Identify pulse rhythm	6.	Palpate pulse until is determined. Describe as regular or irregular.
7.	Determine pulse volume	7.	Quality of pulse strength is an indication of stroke volume. Describe as normal, weak, strong or bounding.
8.	Count pulse rate by using second on watch. For a regular rhythm, count number beats for 30 seconds and multiply by 2. For an irregular, count number of beats for a full minute, nothing number of irregular beats.	8.	An irregular rhythm requires a full minute of assessment to identify the number of inefficient cardiac contractions that fail to transmit a pulsation, referred to as a "skipped" or irregular beat.
Taking an Apical Pulse			
9.	Cleanse hands	9.	Reduces transmission of microorganisms
10.	Raise clients gown to expose sternum and left side of chest	10.	Allows access to clients chest for proper placement of stethoscope
11.	Cleanse earpiece and diaphragm of stethoscope with an alcohol swab	11.	Decreases transmission of microorganisms from one health care practitioner to another (earpiece) and from one client to another (diaphragm)
12.	Put stethoscope around your neck	12.	Ensures stethoscope is nearby for frequent use.
13.	Locate apex of heart: • With client lying on left side, locate suprasternal notch • Palpate second intercostal space to left of sternum • Place index finger in intercostal space, counting downward until fifth intercostal space is located • Move index finger along fourth intercostals space left of the sternal border and to the fifth intercostal space left of the midclavicular line to palpate the point of maximal impulse (PMI). • Keep index finger of non-dominant hand on the PMI.	13.	Identification of landmarks facilitates correct placement of the stethoscope at the fifth intercostal space in order to hear point of maximal impulse. • Ensures correct placement of stethoscope
14.	Inform client that you are going to listen to his or her heart. Instruct client to remain silent.	14.	Elicits client support, stethoscope amplifies noise
15.	With dominant hand, put earpiece of the stethoscope in your ears and grasp diaphragm of the stethoscope in palm of your hand for 5 to 10 seconds.	15.	Dominant hand facilitates psychomotor dexterity for placement of earpiece with one hand. Heat warms metal or plastic diaphragm and prevents starting client.

Contd...

	Table 11.7: *Contd...*		
	Nursing Action		*Rationale*
16.	Place diaphragm of stethoscope over the PMI and auscultate for sounds S_1, and S_2 to hear lub-dub sound	16.	Movement of blood through the heart valves creates S_1, and S_2 sounds. Listen for a regular rhythm (heartbeats are evenly spaced) before counting.
17.	Note regularity of rhythm	17.	Establishment of a rhythmic pattern determines length of time to count the heartbeats to ensure accurate measurement.
18.	Start to count while looking at second hand of watch, count lub-dub sound as one beat • For a regular rhythm, count rate for 30 seconds and multiply by 2. • For an irregular rhythm, count rate for a full minute, nothing number of irregular beats.	18.	Ensures sufficient time to count irregular beats
19.	Share your findings with client.	19.	Promotes client participation in care
20.	Record by site the rate, rhythm, and if applicable, number of irregular beats	20.	Record rate and characteristics at bedside to ensure accurate documentation
21.	Cleanse hands	21.	Reduces transmission of microorganisms

- *Pulmonary ventilation or breathing:* Movement of air in and out of the lungs; inspiration or inhalation is the act of breathings in and expiration or exhalation is the act of breathing out.
- *External respiration:* The exchange of oxygen and carbon dioxide between the alveoli of the lungs and the circulating blood.
- *Internal respiration:* The exchange of oxygen and carbon dioxide between the circulation blood and tissue cells.

Breathing is generally a passive process. The respiratory center of a person is in the brainstem that regulates the voluntary control of respiration. During inspiration the respiratory center, sends impulses along the phrenic nerve, causing the diaphragm, a thin dome shaped muscle connected to the lower ribs, to contract. As diaphragm contract the abdominal organs move downward, and forward, increasing the length of the chest cavity. At the same time, the ribs lift upward, and outward causing transverse expansion of the lungs. During expiration, the diaphragm relaxes in the elevated position, and abdominal organs returns to their original positions. The elastic lungs and chest will also returned to a relaxed state. Inspiration is more active than expiration. Expiration becomes active only during exercises.

The nurses assess the respiration by observing for normal thoracic and abdominal movements and symmetry in chest wall movement. Under normal conditions, healthy adults breath about 16 to 20 times each minute, the normal respiratory rates by age are as follows (Table 11.8).

Assessment of Respirations

The respiratory rate is the number of ventilation occurring each minute. One inspiration plus one expiration equals one respiration, more accurately called a ventilation. Respiration rate

Table 11.8: Normal Respiration According to Age	
• Newborn – 35/min	• 8 years – 20/min
• 1-11 months – 30/min	• 12 years – 18/min
• 2 years – 26/m	• 14 years – 18/min
• 4 years – 24/min	• 16 years – 16-18/min
• 6 years – 22/min	• Adult – 16-20/min

may be over 100 breaths each minute or as slow as 12 breath or less each minute, depending on the age and health status of the patient. Respiration can be assessed by visual inspection, watch the chest rise an fall. The respiratory rate can also be obtained by auscultation of air movement in the lungs while listening with stethoscope. Respiration can be counted by palpation if the movement. Mostly, respiratory rate is assessed by visual inspection because this method makes the patient least consciousness of what nurse is doing. When people know some one is counting their respiration, they find difficult to breath normally and will often alter the rate an depth of their breathing efforts.

For this reason nurses tries to assess respirations without making the patient aware of the observation, of rate, depth, pattern or character and rhythm. The rate is the number of breath in one minute. The dept of respirations refers to the volume of air being exchanged with each breath, compared to the normal volume of 500 cc per breath, at rest. Depth is usually described as normal, shallow, or deep. The rhythm of respiration refers to the time interval between each breath. When respiration is regular, the time interval is similar between each breath. When respiration is irregular, the time interval varies. The character or pattern of the respiration refers to an observable repetitive pattern of respirations.

These patterns are described at the end of nursing skill and are used in documenting respiratory character. The following terms are commonly used to describe respirations:

- *Eupnoea* – normal respirations; normal rate; depth and rhythm for age.
- *Dyspnea* – difficult or labored breathing; may be accompanied by other signs of labored breathing, such as nasal flaring, retraction of skill around the ribs and above and below the sternum; noisy breathing and increased rate of breathing.
- *Tachypnea* – increased rate of breathing about normal for age group.
- *Bradypnea* – decreased rate of breathing below normal for age group.
- *Appea* – absence of breathing; may he periodic, so respirations occur with periods of apnea lasting 10 seconds or more.
- *Hyperventilation* – increases in rate and depth of respirations.
- *Hypoventilation* – decrease in rate and depth of respiration.
- *Hyperpnoea* – increased depth of breathing with normal rate.
- *Cheyne stokes breathing* – a cycle of ventilation with increasing rate and depth to a point, than decreasing rate and depth, followed by period of apnea (20 seconds or more). The breathing cycle lasts approximately 30 to 4o seconds before each apnea episode; related to increased intracranial pressure, congestive heart failure, renal disease, meningitis and drug overdose.
- *Kussmaul's breathing* – increased rate and depth; appears labored and similar to panting; related to renal failure and metabolic acidosis.
- *Biots breathing* – similar to Cheyne-strokes breathing because of intermittent period of apnea; breathing episodes are the same depth; related to central nervous system problems.
- *Orthopnea* – discomfort in breathing in any but exact sitting or standing position.
  The factors which affect/influence are as follows:
- *Exercise* – increases rate and depth to meet the body's greater oxygen needs.
- *Acute pain* – increases rate and depth as a result of sympathetic stimulation.
- *Anxiety and stress* – increases rate and depth as a result of sympathetic stimulation. An anxious or fearful patient is likely to have increased the rate and depth of respiration and as a result hypoventilation occurs.
- *Age* – with growth from infancy to adulthood, the lungs capacity increases and respiratory rate gradually declines, with old age lungs elasticity and depth of respiration decrease, and respiratory rate increases.
- *Sex* – men have a greater lungs capacity than women.
- *Body positions* – straight, erect postures promote full chest expansion. Slumped or stopped position impairs ventilatory movements.
- *Medications* – narcotic, analgesics and selectives depress rate and depth. Amphetamines and cocaine may increase rate and depth.
- *Brainstem injury* – impairs the respiratory center and inhibits respiratory rate and rhythm.

When assessing respirations, the nurse counts the respiratory rate and listens to breath sounds. Breath sounds are heard by listening various locations over the chest with a stethoscope. The terms used to describe the nature of breath sounds are as follows:

- *Stertorous breathing* – is a general term used to refer to noisy respirations.
- *Stridor* – is harsh, high-pitched sound heard on inspiration when there is a narrowing of the upper airway, such as larynx or trachea. Infant or young children with croup often manifests stridor.
- *Wheeze* – is a continuous, high pitched squeak or musical sound made as air moves through a narrow or partially obstructed airway.
- *Crackles (Rales)* – are fine crackling sounds made as air moves through wet secretions; they are most often heart on inspiration.
- *Gurgles (Rhonchi)* – are coarse wheezing or whistling sounds as air moves through thick mucous or narrowed airways, they are best heads on expiration.

Preparation for Obtaining Respiratory Rate

While obtaining respiratory rate, nurse has to determine the need for measuring respiratory rate based on the patient condition or symptoms, a physicians' guideline or the recommendations of more experienced nurse. Generally whenever pulse is measures, the respirations are checked; since oxygen-need satisfaction is dependent on the both the respiratory and cardiovascular system. Patients in unstable condition, febrile, strongly medicated or recovering from anesthesia require frequent monitoring of their respiratory status for signs of hypoventilation.

To make sure that patient is resting and has not just been involved in muscular activity that would increase the pulse rate and respiratory rate: Wash your (nurse) hands and explain the procedure as necessary to patient. Provide privacy if needed. Start obtaining respiratory rate as follows in Tables 11.9 and 11.10.

Equipments

1. Watch with a second hand or digital read-out
2. Pencil or pen
3. Paper or flow sheet.

Document and report data on temperature pulse and respiration as requested by institution, report any unusual data to responsible nurse and nursing instructor or nursing superintendent and recheck any unusual finding related to TPR. It helps communication among members of the health team; legal responsibility and verifies competent nursing care.

Counting of Respiration

Respiratory assessment is the measurement of the breathing pattern. Assessment of respirations provides clinical data regarding the pH of arterial blood. Normal breathing is slightly observable, effortless, quiet, automatic, and regular. It can be assessed by observing chest wall expansion and bilateral symmetric movement of the thorax or by placing the back of the hand next to the clients nose and mouth to feel the expired air. When assessing respiration, ascertain the rate, depth and rhythm of ventilatory movement. Assess the rate by counting the number of breaths taken per minute. Note the depth and rhythm of ventilatory movements by observing for the normal thoracic and abdominal movements and symmetry in chest wall movement. Normal respirations are characterized by a rate ranging from 12 to 20 breaths per minute.

One inspiration and expiration cycle is counted as one breath. The nurse can observe the rise and fall of the chest wall and count the rate by placing the hand lightly on the chest to feel it rise and fall. Count the number of respirations for a 30 second interval and multiply by 2 if respirations are regular and even. If the client is experiencing any respiratory difficulty, count the rate for a full minute. Also observe alterations in the movement of the chest wall: Costal (thoracic) breathing occurs when the external intercostal muscles and the other accessory muscles are used to move the chest upward and outward; diaphragmatic (abdominal) breathing occurs when the diaphragm contracts and relaxes as observed by movement of the abdomen. Dyspnea refers to difficulty in breathing as observed by labored or forced respirations through the use of accessory muscles in the chest and next to breathe. Dyspnea clients are acutely aware of their respirations and complain of shortness of breath.

Respiratory alterations may cause changes in skin color as observed by a bluish appearance of the nail beds, lips and skin. The bluish color (cyanosis) results from reduced oxygen level in the arterial blood. Changes in the level of consciousness (restlessness, anxiety, and dyspnea) may also occur with decreased oxygen level. Clients assume a forward-leaning position or may have to stand to increase the expansion capacity of the lungs. Metabolic alterations such as diabetic ketoacidosis can cause Kussmaul's respirations, which are abnormally deep but regular.

Apnea is the cessation of breathing for several seconds. Persistent apnea is called respiratory arrest. Irregular rhythm with alternating periods of apnea and hyperventilation is called Cheyne-stokes respirations. The cycle begin with slow, shallow breaths that gradually increase to abnormally deep and rapid respirations, which then gradually slow and return to shallow breathing following by apnea. This is common in clients who are dying.

Before counting respiration nurse should:

1. Assess the movement of clients chest wall to see if it is equal bilaterally, if the movement is labored, or if the client is using accessory muscles to breathe.
2. Assess the rate of respirations to identify slow, rapid, or irregular respirations or even periods of apnea.
3. Assess the depth of the clients breaths to monitor shallow, deep or uneven respirations. Think if there might be something influencing the clients respirations. Is the client in pain, frightened, talking or smoking?
4. Assess for risk factors such as fever, pain, anxiety diseases, or trauma to the chest wall that may alter the respirations because certain conditions may cause increased risk of alterations in respirations.
5. Assess for factors that normally influence respirations such as age, exercise, anxiety, pain, smoking, medications or postural changes so that an accurate assessment can be made.

Equipment Needed

- Watch with a second hand
- Stethoscope if needed.

The skill of respiratory rate measurement is often delegated to properly trained ancillary personnel: the nurse is responsible for this information and appropriate action. Respiration counts over 30 (adult) or 60 (child should be immediately reported to the nurse for further assessment.

After procedure nurse has to evaluate clients respirations as a baseline value and compare respirations with baseline to detect any alterations.

Recording the Respiratory rate vital signs flow sheet.

Note the following:
- Depth, rhythm and character of respirations
- Respiratory rate outside the normal age range, an irregular rhythm, inadequate depth, or any abnormal characteristics such as dyspnea.

Blood Pressure Monitoring

Blood pressure is the force exerted by the blood against a vessel wall. In other words, it is the pressure exerted by the circulating volume of blood on the arterial walls, veins and chambers of the heart. The standard unit of measuring blood pressure is millimetre of mercury (mm Hg). The measurement indicates the height to which the blood pressure can raise a column of mercury in the sphygmomanometer (BP apparatus). A blood pressure consists of two measurements, i.e. a systolic pressure and a diastolic pressure.

The systolic pressure is the maximum pressure to which the arteries are subjected during left ventricular contraction of the heart (systole). The diastolic pressure is the remaining pressure within I = the arterial system when the ventricles are relaxed and filling with blood (diastole). A pulse pressure is the numerical difference between the systolic and diastolic pressure measurement. Normally the systolic, diastolic and pulse pressure are in the ratio of 3:2:1 for example, in a blood pressure of 120/80, the ratio is 120/80/40 or 3:2:1. The pulse pressure is an indicator of adequate cardiac stoke volume.

Blood pressure reflects the balance between various factors including cardiac output, blood volume and peripheral resistance (resistance with the blood vessels in the periphery of the body) and blood viscosity (thickness). Each factor can affect another, e.g. an increase in blood volume increases cardiac output. Blood

Table 11.9: Counting Respiration/Monitoring Respiration

	Nursing Action		*Rationale*
	Check clients identification band Explain procedure before beginning		To Identity right Patient To reduce anniets and reassure patient
1.	Cleanse hands.	1.	Reduces transmission of microorganisms
2.	Be sure chest movement is visible. Client may need to remove heavy clothing	2.	Facilitates observation of chest wall and abdominal movements
3.	Observe one complete respiratory cycle. If it is easier, place the clients hand across the abdomen and your hand over the clients wrist.	3.	Helps determine what constitutes a breath. Helps to determine what to count. Hand rises and falls with inspiration and expiration.
4.	Start counting with first inspiration while looking at the second hand of a watch • Infants and children: Count a full minute. • Adults: Count for 30 seconds and multiply by 2. if an irregular rate or rhythm is present, count for one full minute.	4.	Respiratory rate is one complete cycle (inspiration and expiration). • Infants and children: have usually have an irregular rate.
5.	Observe character of respirations: • Depth of respirations by degree of chest wall movement. (shallow, normal or deep) • Rhythm of cycle (regular or interrupted)	5.	Reveals volume of air movement into and out of the lungs
6.	Observe skin color and level of consciousness	6.	Reveals reduced oxygen level in arterial blood.
7.	Replace clients gown if needed	7.	Prevents embarrassment and chilling
8.	Record rate and character of respirations	8.	Record rate and characteristics at bedside to ensure accurate documentation
9.	Cleanse hands	9.	Reduces transmission of microorganisms

Table 11.10: Simple Procedures to Obtain a Respiratory Rate

	Nursing actions		*Rationales*
1.	While your finger tips are still in place after counting the pulse rate, observe the clients respirations.	1.	Counting respiration while presumably still counting the pulse helps to keep the client from becoming conscious of own breathing and possibly altering usual rate.
2.	Note the rise and fall of the clients chest with each inspiration and expiration.	2.	A complete cycle of inspiration and expiration constitute one act of respiration.
3.	Using a watch with a second hand, count the number of respiration for a 30 seconds. Multiply this number by two to obtain clients respiratory rate per minute.	3.	Sufficient time is necessary to observe rate, depth and other characteristics.
4.	If respirations are abnormal in any way, count the respiration rate for a full minute. Repeat if necessary to determine rate and characteristics of breathing.	4.	Full minute counting allow the detection of unequal timing between intervals
5.	Record respiratory rate on flow sheet or paper. Report any abnormal finding to the appropriate persons.	5.	Recording the respiratory rate provides accurate documentation.
6.	Wash your hands.	6.	Hand washing deters the spread microorganism.

pressure does not stay constant. Many factors influence throughout the day. An understanding of theses factors ensures a more accurate interpretation of blood pressure reading.

Factors Influencing Blood Pressure

Age: A persons age influences the blood pressure, with reading being lowest at birth, peaking at adolescence and then slightly decreasing with aging. However, the older adult has decreased elasticity of the arteries, which increases peripheral resistance and therefore, increases blood pressure. An average blood pressure and hypertensive blood pressure according to age are give in Table 11.11.

Table 11.11: Average BP and Hypertensive BP According to Age		
Age	*Average Bp*	*Hypertensive BP*
Newborn	40 mm Hg systolic	Undetermined
1 month	85/54 mm Hg	Undetermined
1 year	95/65 mm Hg	= 110/75 mm Hg
6 years	105/65 mm Hg	= 120/80 mm Hg
10-13 years	110/65 mm HG	= 125/85 mm Hg
14-17 years	120/80 mm Hg	= 135/90 mm Hg
18 + years	120/80 mm Hg	= 140/90 mm Hg

Sex: Women usually have a lower BP than men of the same age before menopause.

Diurnal: Normal fluctuations occur during the day. The usually lowest in the morning. The blood pressure has been noted to rise as much as 5 to 10 mm Hg by late afternoon and it gradually fails again during sleep/night.

Hormones: Variations in blood pressure may be manifested as persons ages because of hormonal alterations. Pregnancy may cause mild to severe elevations in blood pressure.

Food: Blood pressure increases after eating food; obesity tends to increase blood pressure.

Anxiety, fear, pain, and emotional stress: These factors may increase blood pressure because of increased heart rate and increased peripheral resistance.

Medications: These also may increase or decrease blood pressure depending on their pharmacological action.

Position: A persons blood pressure tends to be lower when in a prone or supine position than sitting or standing.

The conditions which causing alteration in blood pressure are hemorrhage, increased inrtracranial pressure, acute pain chronic, renal failure, essential hypertension and general anesthesia. The patient with a blood pressure below normal is hypotensive. It is considered healthy to have a low blood pressure provided there is no ill effects such as vertigo or syncope.

Orthostatic hypo tension occurs when a person rises too quickly from a supine position.

Assessment of Blood Pressure

Blood pressure readings are taken with a sphygmomanometer an stethoscope. A sphygmomanometer consists of an inflatable cuff and a gauge. The cuff is inflated around the patients arm to compress the artery which will occlude blood flow, then it is slowly deflated, which were allow blood flow to resume. While performing this, the stethoscope and hears pulsating sounds. These are called Korotkoff's sounds. When the first sound is heard nurse makes a mental note of that point on the sphygmomanometer gauge and again note when the sound is disappears. The point when first sound heard is the systolic pressure, the point at when last sound is heard is diastolic pressure.

Blood pressure may be measure by palpatory method. The nurse applies BP cuff as in the angulatory method. The radial pulse is then palpated on that arm. The radial pulse is then palpated on that arm. The cuff is inflated until pulse is obliterated. As the cuff is slowly deflated the nurse notes the point at which the pulse is again felt, than corresponds to systolic pressure.

Preparation for Taking Blood Pressure

Determining the need to take a blood pressure reading is guided by the patients current conditions, the physician's guidelines and advice from the experienced nursing personnel. Generally, a patient's blood pressure is taken at least once or twice a day, but is the patient is unstable, it may be taken every few minutes. One blood pressure reading in isolation is not as helpful in assessing the patient condition as a series of readings. The patients normal blood pressure, usually considered to be an admission BP unless the patient was unstable when admitted, provides a baseline value for comparison of current and future readings.

Obtaining blood pressure: Equipments needed and procedures for obtaining BP are as follows (Table 11.12)

Equipments

- Stethoscope
- Sphygmomanometer/BP apparatus
- Blood pressure cuff of appropriate size
- Pencil or pen.

Taking Blood Pressure

Blood pressure measurement is performed during a physical examination, at initial assessment and as pat of routine vital signs assessment. Depending on the clients condition, the blood pressure is measured by either a direct or indirect technique.

The indirect method requires use of the sphygmomanometer and stethoscope of auscultation and palpation as needed. The most common site for indirect blood pressure measurement is the clients arm over the brachial artery. When the client's

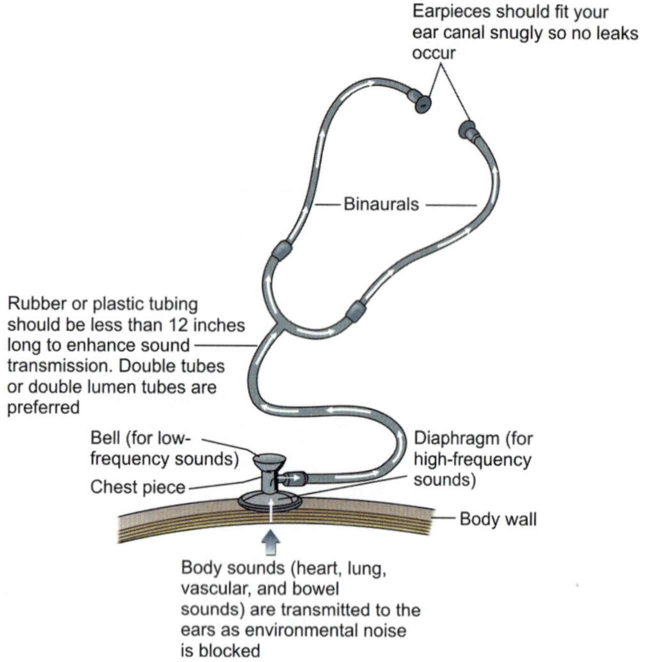

Figure 11.12: The stethoscope

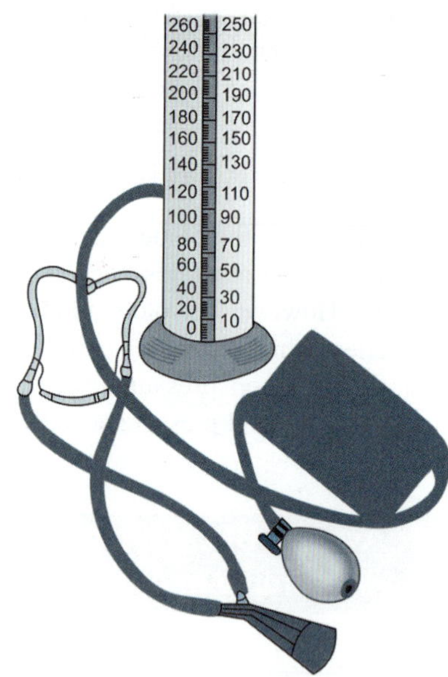

Fig 11.13: Blood pressure equipment: Equipment needed to measure a person's blood pressure includes a stethoscope, a blood pressure cuff of the correct size, and a manometer (Mercury manometer as pictured) or aneroid manometer. Digital display models are also available

conditions prevents auscultation of the brachial artery, assess the blood pressure in the forearm or leg sites. When pressure measurements in the upper extremities are not accessible, the popliteal artery, located behind the knee, is the site of choice. Blood pressure can also be assessed in other sites, such as radial artery in the forearm and the posterior tibial or dorsalis pedis artery in the lower leg. Because it is difficult to auscultate sounds such as the radial artery in the forearm and the posterior tibial or dorsalis sites are usually palpated to obtain a systolic reading.

Before taking Blood Pressure nurse should:
- Assess the condition of the potential blood pressure (BP) site so that a site with an injury or surgery proximal to the site can be avoided.
- Assess the artery for any compromise to it so that compressing the artery briefly will not cause decrease in circulation.
- Assess the distal pulse to check if it is intact and palpate.

- Assess the circumference of the extremity for the right size cuff to be used so an accurate reading can be obtained.
- Assess for factors that affect blood pressure, such as age, anxiety, fear, medications, smoking, eating or exercising within 30 minutes before BP assessment, and postural changes so an accurate reading can be obtained.
- Determine client's baseline blood pressure by reading the medical record so a comparison can be made with each BP reading.

Equipment Needed

- Stethoscope (Fig. 11.12)
- Sphygmomanometer/bladder with mercury column or aneroid dial (Fig. 11.13)
- Gloves, if required
- Alcohol swabs.

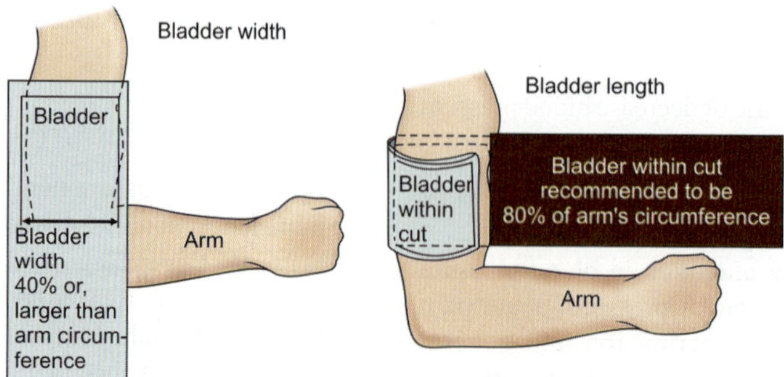

Fig 11.14: The blood pressure cuff is measured to match the size of the patients arm for maximum accuracy in blood pressure assessment

Table 11.12: Taking Blood Pressure

Check clients identification band	To Identity right Patient
Explain procedure before beginning	To reduce anniets and reassure patient

	Nursing action		*Rationale*
1.	Cleanse hands.	1.	Reduces transmission of microorganisms.
2.	Determine which extremity is most appropriate for reading. Do not take a pressure reading on an injured or painful extremity or one in which an intravenous line is running.	2.	Cuff inflation can temporarily interrupt blood flow and compromise circulation in an extremity already impaired or a vein intravenous fluid.
3.	Select a cuff size appropriate for the client. Estimate by inspection or measure with a tape, the circumference of the bare upper arm at the midpoint between the shoulder (acromion) and the elbow (olecranon process) (Fig. 11.14).	3.	The bladder inside the cuff should encircle 80% of the arm in adults and 100% of the arm of children less than 13 years old. If in doubt, use a larger cuff to ensure equalization of pressure on the artery and accurate measurement.
4.	Have the clients bared arm resting on a support so the midpoint of the upper arm is at the level of the heart. Extend the elbow with palm turned upward.	4.	Blood pressure increases when the arm is below the level of the heart and decreases when the arm is above the level of the heart.
5.	Make sure the bladder cuff is fully deflated and the pump valve moves freely. Place the manometer so the center of the merc	5.	Equipment must be visible and function properly to obtain an accurate reading.
6.	Palpate the brachial artery. In the antecubital space, and place the cuff so that the midline of the bladder is over the arterial pulsation. Next, wrap and secure the cuff snugly around the client's bare upper arm. The lower edge of the cuff should be 1 inch (2 cm) above the antecubital fossa (bend of the elbow), where the head of the stethoscope is to be placed.	6.	Ensures even pressure distribution over the brachial artery. Rolling up the sleeve may form a tourniquet around the upper arm. Always use a bare arm.
7.	Inflate the cuff rapidly to 70 mm Hg and increase by 10 mm increments while palpating the radial pulse. Note the level of pressure at which the pulse disappears and subsequently reappears during deflation.	7.	The palpatory method provides the necessary preliminary approximation of systolic blood pressure to ensure an accurate reading. When frequent measurements are required, such as every 15 minutes, the palpatory method is generally not incorporated with each pressure check.
8.	Insert the earpieces of the stethoscope into the ear canals with a forward tilt to fit snugly.	8.	The bell, the low-frequency position of the stethoscope, enhances sound transmission from chest piece to ears.
9.	Relocate the brachial artery with your nondominant hand, and place the bell of the stethoscope over the brachial artery pulsation. The bell should be held firmly in place, ensuring that the head is in direct contact with the skin and not touching the cuff.	9.	Sound is heard best directly over the artery. Wedging the head of the stethoscope under the edge of the cuff results in considerable extraneous noise and may cause an inaccurate reading.
10.	With the dominant hand, turn the valve clockwise to close. Compress the pump to inflate the cuff rapidly and steadily until the manometer registers 20 to 30 mm Hg above the level previously determined by the palpation.	10.	Prevents air leaks during inflation. Ensures the cuff is inflated to a pressure greater than the clients systolic pressure.
11.	Partially unscrew (open) the valve counterclockwise to deflate the bladder at 2 mm/sec while listening for the appearance of the of the five phases of the Korotkoff sounds. Note the manometer reading for these sounds. • A faint, clear tapping sound that increases in intensity • Swishing sound • Intense sound • Abrupt, distinctive muffled sound • No sound	11.	Maintains constant release of pressure to ensure hearing first systolic sound. Identify manometer readings for each of the five phases. • Identify two consecutive tapping sounds to confirm systolic reading • The American Heart Association (2002) recommends using Phase IV as the diastolic level in children less than 13 years old. Even though 5 phases of Korotkoff sounds have been identified, most clients have only 2 clearly distinct sounds (phase I and IV), identified as the systolic and diastolic sounds.

Contd...

Table 11.12: Contd...

	Nursing Action		*Rationale*
12.	After the last Korotkoff sound is heard, deflate the cuff slowly for at least another 10 mm Hg to ensure that no other sounds are audible: then, deflate rapidly and completely.	12.	Prevents arterial occlusion and client discomfort from numbness or tingling.
13.	Allow the client to rest for at least 30 seconds and remove cuff. (A measurement should be repeated after 30 seconds and the two readings averaged. It may be done in the same or opposite arm).	13.	Releases trapped blood in the vessels. Ensures accurate measurement.
14.	Inform the client of the reading.	14.	Promotes clients participation in health care.
15.	The systolic (Phase I) and diastolic (Phase V) pressure should be immediately recorded, rounded off (upward) to the nearest 2 mm Hg. (In children and when sounds are heard nearly to the level of 0 mm Hg, the Phase IV pressure should also be recorded).	15.	Ensures accuracy.
16.	If appropriate, lower bed, raise side rails and place call light in easy reach.	16.	Promotes clients safety.
17.	Put all equipment in proper place.	17.	Fosters maintenance of equipment.
18.	Cleanse hands.	18.	Reduces transmission of microorganisms.

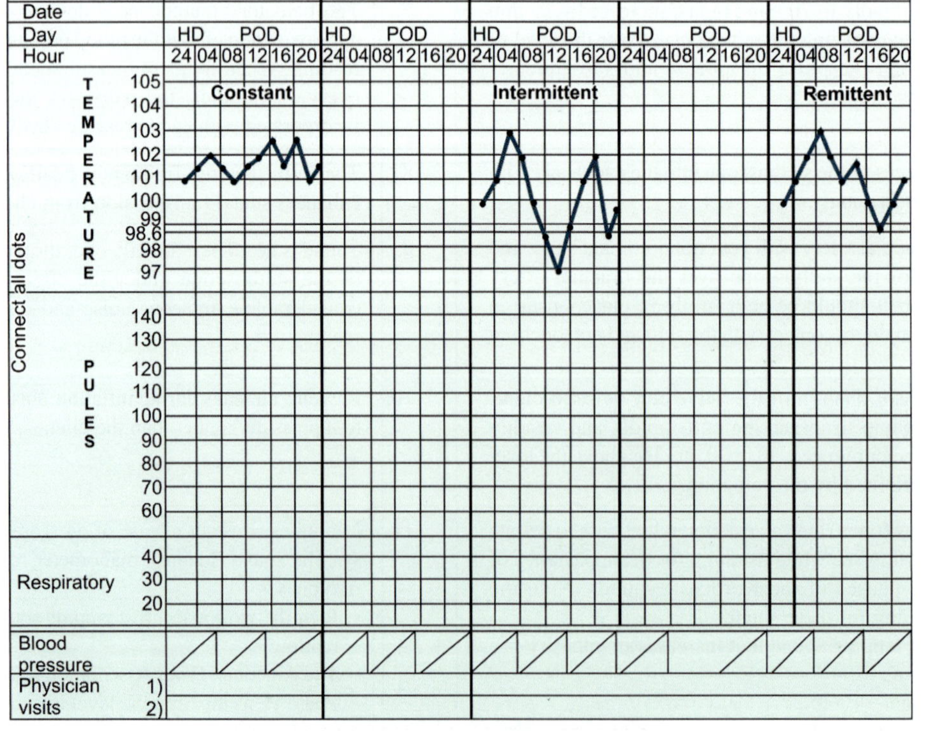

Figure 11.15: Graphic record of vital signs
Note: Temperature graphic showing types of fevers

Table 11.13: Weighing the Client

Check clients identification band
Explain procedure before beginning

To Identity right Patient
To reduce anniets and reassure patient

	Nursing actions		*Rationales*
1.	Cleanse hands.	1.	Reduces transmission of microorganisms.
2.	Place the scale near the client.	2.	Reduces risk of fall or injury.
3.	Turn on the scale and calibrate it to zero.	3.	Ensures accurate reading.
4.	Ask client to remove shoes, step up on the scale and stand still *Electronic scale*: Slide the larger weight into the notch most closely approximating the clients weight. Slide the smaller weight into the notch so the balance rests in the middle. Add the two numbers for the clients weight.	4.	Obtains weight. Reading is not accurate when the numbers are still fluctuating. Weights on scale must be balanced to obtain accurate reading.
5.	Ask the client to step down. Assist the client back to the bed or chair, if necessary.	5.	Reduces risk of injury if client needs assistance.
6.	Wipe the scale with appropriate disinfectant.	6.	Reduces risk of spread of infection.
7.	Cleanse hands.	7.	Reduces transmission of microorganisms.

Sling Scale

8.	Cleanse hands and put on gloves if needed.	8.	Reduces risk of nosocomial infection.
9.	Place plastic covering on sling if available (can usually be ordered in bulk from the manufacturer).	9.	Reduces risk of spreading infection between clients.
10.	Remove pillows. Turn the client to one side and place half of sling on bed next to the client, with remaining half rolled up against the clients back.	10.	Most accurate weight will be obtained by leaving no other bedding between the client and sing.
11.	Turn the client to the other side, and unroll the rest of the sling so it lays flat beneath the client.	11.	Turning in this manner maximize client comfort.
12.	Roll the scale over the bed such that the legs of the scale are underneath the bed. Open and lock the legs of the scale.	12.	Ensures equipment is being used safely to reduce risk of injury.
13.	Turn on scale and calibrate to zero.	13.	Ensures accurate reading.
14.	Lower arms of the scale and slip hooks through holes in sling.	14.	Reading is not accurate when the numbers are still fluctuating.
15.	Pump scale until sling rests completely off the bed.	15.	Prepares for removal of sling.
16.	Remind the client to remain still. Read weight after digital numbers have stopped fluctuating.	16.	Reading is not accurate when numbers are still fluctuating.
17.	Lower the client back to bed and remove arms of the scale from sling.	17.	Prepares for removal of sling.
18.	Unlock scale legs, return to their original position, and remove scale from bed.	18.	Allows for removal of equipment that obstructs proximately to the client, thereby facilitating removal of the sling.
19.	Turn the client on his or her side, roll up sling, turn client to the other side.	19.	Facilitates removal of the sling.
20.	Realign the client with pillows and covers.	20.	Ensures comfort and privacy.
21.	Remove gloves and cleanse hands.	21.	Reduces risk of spread of infection and nosocomial infection.
22.	Remove gloves and cleanse hands.	22.	Reduces transmission of microorganisms.

After procedure nurse should:
- Evaluate the blood pressure reading for accuracy by comparing with the medical record.
- Evaluate the clients blood pressure for being within the normal range.
- Identify variations in the clients blood pressure of more than 5 to 10 mm Hg from one arm to the other.
- Evaluate if the clients blood pressure changes significantly when he or she stands up.
- Report abnormal measurements to charge nurse or health care provider.

Recording Vital Signs Flow Sheet
- Blood pressure measurement
- Site where recording was done
- Method of obtaining the pressure – auscultation or palpation.

Weighing a Client, Mobile and Immobile (Table 10.13)

A clients weight is an essential piece of data used in monitoring his or her response to a variety of therapies. Changes in a clients weight could necessitate an alteration in the assessment and intervention plans. An accurate weight is important.

Prior to weighing a client, mobile or immobile, nurse should:
1. Assess the child's ability to stand independently and safely on a scale. Consider factors requiring the use of a sling scale. The client is somnolent or comatose: paralyzed: too weak to stand: or unsteady when standing.
2. Determine if clothing is similar to that worn during previous weight measurement to help determine accuracy of the new weight.

Equipment Needed

- Scale; standing electronic or balance scale or sling scale
- Recommended disinfectant
- 1 to 3 other staff members to assist when using sling scale
- Plastic cover for sling scale
- Gloves (when applicable).

The skill of weighing the mobile and immobile client is routinely delegated to trained personnel.

The personnel should be instructed to do the following:
- Select the correct scale for measurement
- Property and safely position the client for measurement
- Correctly and safely perform the measurement according to established guidelines and record on the appropriate flow sheet (clinical record)
- Recognize and report abnormal findings promptly to the nurse.

After Procedure Nurse should:
- Compare weight obtained to previously recorded weight. Repeat weight if large discrepancy is noted.
- If large discrepancy still remains, notify appropriate health care team members.

Recording Vital Signs Flow Sheet

- Date, time of day and the weight of the client on the appropriate flow sheet. Graphical record of temperature showing different types of fever is shown in Fig. 11.15.

12

Safety, Comfort and Body Mechanics

A fundamental concern of nurses, which extends from the bedside to the home to the community, is prevention of accidents and injury, as well as assisting the injured. Motor vehicle accidents, falls, drowning, fire and burns, poisoning, inhalation and ingestion of foreign objects, and firearm use are major causes of accidental injury and death.

Nurse need to be aware of what constitutes a safe environment for a particular person or for a group of people in home and community settings. Accidents are often caused by human conduct and can be prevented.

Factors Affecting Safety

The ability of people to themselves from injury is affected by such factors as age and development, lifestyle, mobility and health status, sensory-perceptual alterations, cognitive awareness, psychological state, ability to communicate, safety awareness, and environmental factors. Nurses need to assess each of these factors when they plan care or teach clients to protect themselves.

Age and development through knowledge and accurate assessment of the environment, people learn to protect themselves from many injuries. Children walking to school learn to stop before crossing the street and wait for oncoming traffic. They also learn not to touch a hot stove. For the very young, learning about the environment is essential. Only through knowledge and experience do children learn what is potentially harmful.

Elders can have difficulty with movement and diminished sensory acuity that contributes to the likelihood of injury. Specific age related potential hazards and preventive measures are discussed later in this chapter.

- *Developing fetus:* Exposure to material smoking, alcohol consumption, addictive drugs, X-rays (first trimester) certain pesticides.
- *Newborns and infants:* Falling, suffocation in crib, choking from aspirated milk or ingested objects, burns from hot water or other spilled hot liquids, automobile accidents, crib or playpen injuries, electric shock, poisoning.
- *Toddlers:* Physical trauma from falling, banging into objects, or getting cut by sharp objects; automobile accidents; burns; poisoning; drowning and electric shock.
- *Preschoolers:* Injury from traffic, playground equipment, and other objects; choking, suffocation and obstruction of airway or ear canal by foreign objects; poisoning; drowning; fire and burns; harm from other people or animals
- *Adolescents:* Vehicular (automobile, bicycle) accidents, recreational accidents, firearms, substance abuse.

Lifestyle: Lifestyle factors that place people at risk include unsafe work environments; residence in neighborhood with high crime rates; access to guns and ammunition; insufficient income to buy safety equipment or make necessary repairs, and access to illicit drugs, which may also be contaminated by harmful additives. Risk-taking behavior is a factor in some accidents.

Mobility and Health Status: People who have impaired mobility due to paralysis, muscle weakness, and poor balance or coordination are obviously prone to injury. Clients with spinal cord injury and paralysis of both legs may be unable to move even when they perceive discomfort. Hemiplegics clients or clients with leg casts often have poor balance and fall easily. Clients weakened by illness or surgery are not always fully aware of their condition.

Sensory–Perceptual Alterations: Accurate sensory perception of environmental stimuli is vital to safety. People with impaired touch perception, hearing, taste, smell, and vision are highly susceptible to injury. A person who does not see well may trip over a toy or not see an electric cord. Deaf people do not hear a siren in traffic and people with impaired olfactory sense may not smell burning food or the sulfar aroma of escaping gas.

Cognitive Awareness: Awareness is the ability to perceive environmental stimuli and body reactions and to respond appropriately through thought and action. Clients with impaired awareness include people lacking sleep; unconscious or semiconscious persons; disoriented people (i.e., those who may not understand where they are or what to do to help themselves); people who perceive stimuli that do not exist; and people whose judgment is altered by disease or medications, such as narcotics, tranquilizers, hypnotics, and sedatives. Mildly confused clients may momentarily forget where they are, wander from their rooms, misplace personal belongings, and so forth.

Emotional State: Extreme emotional states can alter the ability to perceive environmental hazards. Stressful situations can reduce a persons level of concentration, cause errors of judgment, and decrease awareness of external stimuli. People with depression may think and react to environmental stimuli more slowly than usual.

Ability to Communicate: Individuals with diminished ability to receive and convey information are also at risk for injury. Aphasic clients, people with language barriers, and those unable to read are among them. For example, the person unable to interpret the sign "No smoking–oxygen in use" could cause a fire.

Safety Awareness: Information is crucial to safety. Clients in unfamiliar environments frequently need specific safety information. Lack of knowledge about unfamiliar equipment, such as oxygen tanks, intravenous tubing, and hot pack is a potential hazard. Healthy clients need knowledge about water safety, car safety, fire prevention, ways to prevent the ingestion of harmful substances, and many preventive measures related to specific age-related hazards.

Environmental Factors: A safe home requires well-maintained flooring and carpets, a nonskid bathtub or shower surface, functioning smoke alarms that are strategically placed, and knowledge of fire escape routes. Outdoor areas, such as swimming pools, need to be safely secured and maintained. Adequate lighting, both inside and out, will minimize the potential for accidents.

In the workplace, machinery, industrial belts and pulleys, and chemicals may create danger. Worker fatigue, noise and air pollution, or working at great heights or in subterranean areas may also create occupational hazards. The work environment of the nurse may also be unsafe. The health care worker needs to maintain an awareness of potential risk.

Adequate street lighting, safe water and sewage treatment, and regulation of sanitation in food buying and handling all contribute to a healthy, hazard-free community. A safe and secure community strives to be free of excess noise, crime, traffic congestion, dilapidated housing, or unprotected creeks and landfills.

Safety Measures during the Life Span

Following safety measures can be followed during their stages of life as given below:

Newborns and Infants

- Use a federally approved car seat at all times (including coming home from hospital). It should be in the back seat, facing backward.
- Never leave the infant unattended on a raised surface.
- Check the temperature of the infants bath water and formula prior to using.
- Hold the infant upright during feeding. Do not prop the bottle. Cut food in small pieces, and do not feed the infant peanuts or popcorn.
- Investigate the infants crib for compliance with federal safety regulations; slats no more than $2^3/_8$ inches apart, lead-free paint, height, of crib sides, tight fit of mattress of crib.
- Use a playpen with sides made of small-size netting. Never leave playpen sides down.
- Provide large soft toys with no small detachable or sharp-edged parts.
- Use guard gats on stairs and screens on windows. Supervise the infant in swings and highchairs.
- Cover electric outlets. Coil cords out of reach.
- Place plants, household cleaners and wastebaskets out of reach. Lock away potential poisons, such as medicines, paint, and gasoline.

Toddlers

- Continue to use federally approved car seats at all times. Place children in back seat when travelling in a car.
- Teach children not to put objects in the mouth, including pills (unless given by parent).
- Keep objects with sharp edges (such as furniture and knives) out of children's reach.
- Place hot pots on back burners with handles turned inward.
- Keep cleaning solutions, insecticides and medicines in locked cupboards.
- Keep windows and balconies screened.
- Supervise toddlers in the tub.
- Fence in pools, and supervise toddlers, at all times when in or near pools. Do not overfill bathtub. Do not overfill bathtub. Do not let toddlers play near ditches or wells.

- Teach children not to run ride a tricycle into the street.
- Obtain a low when the child begins to climb.
- Cover outlets with safety covers or plugs.

Preschoolers

- Do not allow children to run with candy or other objects in the mouth.
- Teach children not to put small objects in the mouth, nose, and ears.
- Remove doors from unused equipment such as refrigerators.
- Always supervise preschoolers crossing streets and begin safety teaching about obeying traffic signals and looking both ways.
- Check Halloween treats before allowing children to eat them. Discard loose or open candy.
- Teach children to play in "safe" areas, not on streets and railroad tracks.
- Teach preschoolers the dangers of playing with matches and playing near charcoal, fire and heating appliances.
- Teach children to avoid strangers and keep parents informed of their whereabouts.
- Teach preschoolers not to walk in front of swings and not to push others off playground equipment.

School-age Children

- Teach children safety rules for recreational and sports activities; never swim alone, always wear a life jacket when in a boat, and wear a protective helmet and knee and elbow pads when needed.
- Supervise contact sports and activities in which children aim at a target.
- Teach children to obey all traffic and safety rules for bicycling, skateboarding and roller skating.
- Teach children safe ways to use the stove, garden tools, and other equipment.
- Supervise children when they use saws, electric appliances tools, and other potentially dangerous equipment.
- Teach children not to play with fireworks, gunpowder, or firearms. Keep firearms unloaded, locked up, and out of reach.
- Teach children to avoid excavations, quarries, vacant buildings, and playing around heavy machinery.
- Teach children the health hazards of smoking. If you smoke, stop.
- Teach children the effects of drugs and alcohol on judgment and coordination.

Adolescents

- Have adolescents complete a drivers education course, and take practice drives with them in various kinds of weather.
- Set firm limits on automobile use, namely, never to drive after drinking or using drugs, and never to ride with a driver who has some so. Encourage adolescents to call home for a ride if they have been drinking, assuring them they can do so without a reprimand.

- Restrict number of passengers in car during the first year of driving.
- Teach adolescents to wear a safety helmet when riding motorcycles, scooters and other sports vehicles. Teach safety rules for water sports.
- Teach adolescents to wear a safety helmet when riding motorcycles, scooters, and other sports vehicles. Teach safety rules for water sports.
- Encourage adolescents to use proper equipment when participating in sports. Schedule a physical examination before participation, and be certain there is medical supervision for all athletic activities.
- Encourage adolescents to swim, jog and go boating in groups so they can obtain help in case of an accident.
- Teach safety measures for use of powder tools.
- Teach rules for hunting and the proper care and use of firearms.
- Inform the adolescent of the dangers of drugs, alcohol, an unprotected sex. Include teaching about date rape prevention and defense.
- Teach dangers of sunbathing and tanning beds, as well as use of sun block and protective clothing when doing outdoor activities.
- Be alert to changes in the adolescents mood and behavior. Listen to and maintain open communication is a powerful preventive measure.
- Set a good example of behavior that the adolescent can follow.

Young Adults

- Reinforce motor vehicle safety: Drive defensively, use "designated drivers" if alcohol is consumed, routinely check brakes and tires, and use seat and shoulder belts or car seats for all passengers.
- Remind the young adult to repair potential fire hazards, such as electric wiring.
- Reinforce water safety: Know the depth of a pool or lake before diving; supervise backyard pools and other water activities.
- Discuss evaluating the potential for work phase injuries or death when making decisions about a career or occupation.
- Encourage the young adult to participate actively in programs that reduce occupational hazards.
- Discuss avoiding excessive sun radiation by limiting exposure, using sun-blocking agents, and wearing protective clothing. Explain the skin changes that may indicate a cancerous condition.
- Encourage young adults who are unable to cope with the pressure, responsibilities, and expectations of adulthood to seek counselling.

Middle-aged Adults

- Reinforce motor vehicle safety: Use seat belts and drive within the speed limit, especially at night. These visual acuity periodically.

- Make certain stairways are well lighted and uncluttered.
- Equip bathrooms with hand grasps and nonskid bath mats.
- Test smoke detectors and fire alarms regularly.
- Keep all machines and tools in good working condition at work and at home. Follow safety precautions when using machinery.
- Reinforce safety measures taught earlier in life, such as the hazards of excessive sun exposure.

Elders

- Encourage the client to have regular vision and hearing tests.
- Assist the client to have a home hazard appraisal.
- Encourage the client to keep as active as possible.

Preventive Measures: To Enhance Safety in Hospitals

- Ensure eyeglasses are functional.
- Ensure appropriate lighting.
- Mark doorways and edges of steps as needed.
- Keep environment tidy and uncluttered.
- Set safe limits of activities.
- Remove unsafe objects.
- Wear shoes or well-fitted slippers with nonskid soles.
- Use ambulatory devices as necessary (cane, crutches, walker, braces, wheelchair).
- Provide assistance with ambulation as needed.
- Monitor gait and balance.
- Adapt living arrangements to one floor if necessary.
- Encourage exercise and activity as tolerated to maintain muscle strength, joint flexibility and balance.
- Ensure uncluttered environment with securely fastened rugs.
- Encourage client to request assistance.
- Keep bed in the low position.
- Install grab bars in bathroom.
- Provide raised toilet seat.
- Instruct client to rise slowly from a lying to sitting to standing position, and to stand in place for several second before walking.
- Provide a bedside commode as needed.
- Assist with voiding on a frequent and scheduled basis.
- Encourage client to summon help.
- Monitor activity tolerance.
- Attach side rails to the bed.
- Keep rails in place when the bed is in the lowest position.
- Monitor orientation and alertness status.
- Encourage annual or more frequent review of all medications prescribed.

Comfort

Every nursing procedure is aimed for the comfort of the patient. It should give the satisfaction to the patient, relatives and the nurse on completion of the work. Here we are starting with bed that is making a bed provides comfort.

Bedmaking

The process of bedmaking includes to provide comfort; to maintain clean environment to reduce transmission of microorganisms; to stimulate and refresh; to observe and prevent complications; to save time, effort and materials; to provide good neat appearance to ward; to adopt according to comfort needs of patient and to create an effective nurse-patient relationship.

Bed making is a responsibility of the nurse. Making bed that is suitable and comfortable and appropriate for hospitalized patient. Bed making is an expected part of the care of the hospitalized patient. The nurse needs to know specific concepts, principles and activities associated with bedmaking. The patients bed is usually made in the morning. The nurse keeps the bed clean and comfortable. It is usual procedure to change bed linens after the bath but some hospitals change linens only when soiled. It is the responsibility of nurses to keep bed as clean and comfortable as possible. This may require frequent inspection to be sure that linen is clean, dry and wrinkle free. The nurse will check the linens for food particles after meals, and for urine incontinence or involuntary stool. If linens are soiled with urine, feces, blood or emesis, they should be changed.

A bed is an article or furniture to take rest or sleep, which helps to keep a patient for providing comfort, performing physical examination and procedure for treatment as nursing care.

The common bed positions used by nurses are as follows:

1. *Fowler's position* In this position the bed is raised to angle of 45° or more; semisitting position. It is used during nasotrachial suctioning. It helps promotion of lung expansion. It is preferred while client sits.
2. *Semi-Fowler's position* Head of the bed is raised approximately 30°, inclination less than Fowler's position. It also promotes lungs expansion helps breathing.
3. *Trendelenburg position* Entire bedframe tilted with head of the bed down. It is used for postural drainage. This position also facilitates venous return in clients with poor peripheral perfusion.
4. *Reverse Trendelenburg position* Entire bedframe tilted with foot and bed down, it is used infrequently helps to promote gastric emptying and prevents esophageal reflux.
5. *Flat position* In this position entire bedframe tilted horizontally parallel with floor. It is used for clients with vertebral injuries and in cervical traction and also used for clients who are hypotensive. It is generally preferred by clients for sleeping.

While making all bedmaking procedures, the nurse will follow certain principles to maintain asepsis:

- Hold clean and soiled linen away from uniform
- Place soiled linen in special bags before discarding it in hamper or plastic bag
- Never fan linen in air, to avoid air currents can spread microorganism
- Dirty linen should never be placed on the follow to prevent transmitting microorganism
- Wash your hands before you begin bedmaking
- Handle linen carefully, avoid shaking it, tossing it into the laundry hamper or throwing on the floor

A clean, fresh, comfortable bed is very important for people who have to spend time in bed. A comfortable bed uplifts one mentally, is physically relaxing, and may prevent serious complications.

Without proper attention to the bed and bed linens, the following problems can occur:

- Skin irritation form laundry dyes and bleaches
- Abraded skin on heels form rubbing on linen, especially on seams
- Pressure sores form lying on wrinkles sheets
- Skin irritation and discomfort from wet linen.

Bed Linens

Need for linen change: Change linen according to client need. Linen may be changed with morning hygiene care and at other times as it becomes soiled, damp or excessively wrinkled. In addition to changing, linen often requires tightening to keep it wrinkle-free. For a restless person, linen may need tightening several times a day. Straightening linen at bedtime is one means of promoting a comfortable night sleep.

Types of Bed Linens and their Uses

Full sheets: Regular full-length sheets or contour sheets can be used.

Draw sheets: A draw sheet is about half the size of a regular sheet and is placed across the middle section of the bed. Draw sheets may be rubber, plastic or linen. Plastic or rubber draw sheets protect the mattress or the bottom sheet from becoming wet. Always cover plastic or rubber with a linen draw sheet to protect the persons skin and absorb moisture.

Linen draw sheets should not be relied upon for lifting (pull sheets).

Mattress pads: Mattress pads are usually made of thick, soft cotton and have bound edges. When used, the pad, with or without contour corners, is placed lengthwise on the bed between the mattress and sheet. The mattress pad decreases movement of the sheet, reduces heat generated between a plastic mattress and the persons body, and absorbs moisture. All of these enhance comfort. (A bath blanket can be used in place of a mattress pad) Change mattress pads only when excessively wrinkled, damp or soiled.

Blankets: A bed blanket of wool, cotton, or synthetic material may be used for warmth. Thermal bed blankets are used in many facilities. These are made of a porous, synthetic material and have the advantage of being relatively lightweight yet warm. The bed blanket is usually not changed unless it becomes soiled or wet.

Bedspreads: Bedspreads are usually light weighted cotton or synthetic material. They are changed only when soiled, wet or excessively wrinkled.

Pillow cases: A standard pillow case is one of the most frequently changed bed linens. To reduce the need for a clean pillow case, turn the pillow with a tuck. A clean, smooth pillow case can be very refreshing.

The nurse must use proper body mechanics during bed making. Nurses can apply following principles of body mechanics to all bed making procedures:

- Raising the bed to a working level to avoid bending down or stretching over the mattress
- When you (nurse) bend, bend your knees, not your back
- Point your toes and face in the direction that you are moving, avoid twisting
- Conserve steps by making as few trips around the bed as possible.

When making an occupied bed, the nurse should also use principles of body mechanics while turning and repositioning the patient. And when making a bed, the nurse also keep in mind that providing privacy, comfort, and safety for the clients. Using side rails, keeping call lights.

Bedmaking: Unoccupied Bed

After the client takes a bath, clean linens are placed on the bed to promote comfort and decrease transmission of micro-organisms. If the client is able to get out of bed, assist the client to a chair and proceed with making the bed. After surgery, the client should be returned to a clean bed with linens folded to the foot of the bed to promote easy client transfer.

Before making an unoccupied bed the nurse should:

1. Assess your equipment. Check for all linens necessary to change the bed. Check for a dirty linen hamper which helps to facilitates a smooth procedure.
2. Assess whether the bed needs cleaning before placing clean sheets on it which helps to reduce the transmission of microorganisms.
3. Assess the client's needs in the bed. Check for profuse drainage, incontinence, or special needs for comfort or skin integrity and determines how the procedure will be performed.
4. Take care the client's ability to be out of the bed in a safe place while changing linens.

Equipment Needed

- Bottom sheet (fitted, if available)
- Top sheet
- Draw sheet (regular top sheet may be used)
- Pillowcase (each pillow on the bed)
- Mattress pad
- Antiseptic solution, washcloth, and towel
- Linen bag hamper outside the room
- Nonsterile gloves.

Proper safety precautions for nursing personal themselves and the client and understanding the appropriate use of Standard Precautions would be followed while making bed.

For performing any procedure including bedmaking nurses and ancillary personnel (if needed), prior to procedure follow standing instruction like:

- Cleanse hands – to reduce spreading of microorganisms
- Check clients identification band – proper identity of patient
- Explain procedure before beginning – promote cooperation.

After unoccupied bed making nurse should: Confirm that fresh linens were placed on the bed in a manner appropriate to the client's needs.

And document in the Nurses Notes as follow: Client's tolerance to being out of bed. (Linen changes are not generally documented.)

Procedures for unoccupied bed making please refer Table 12.1.

Bedmaking: Occupied Bed

After the client takes a bath, clean linens are placed on the bed to promote comfort and decrease the transmission of microorganism. If the client is unable to get out of bed, change the linens around the client. Assistance will be needed if the client is in traction or cannot be turned. Care must be taken to avoid disturbing the traction weights. If the client cannot be turned change the linens from head to toe. Place a waterproof draw sheet on the beds of clients who are incontinent or have profuse drainage. The type and amount of linens placed on the bed will vary based on the type of bed the client is using. Air beds and Clinitron beds, for example, use only minimal linens under the client. Procedures for making an occupied bed please refer Table 12.2.

Before making an occupied bed nurse should:

1. Assess your equipment. Check for all the linens necessary to change the bed. Check for a dirty linen hamper. Facilitates a smooth procedure.
2. Assess whether the bed needs cleaning before placing clean sheets on it. Reduces the transmission of microorganisms.
3. Assess the client's needs in the bed. Check for profuse drainage, incontinence, or special needs for comfort or skin integrity. Determines how the procedure will be performed.
4. Assess the client's ability to assist with the procedure including mobility, mental status, and muscle strength. Determines whether assistance will be needed to change the client's linens.
5. Assess for the presence of dressings, IV lines, tubes, or any equipment that may be attached to the client.

Equipment Needed

- Linen hamper
- Top sheet, draw sheet, bottom sheet
- Pillowcase
- Blanket
- Bath blanket
- Gloves (if needed).

Table 12.1: Making an Unoccupied Bed

	Nursing action		Rationale
1.	Place hamper by client's door if linen bags are not available. Assess condition of blanket and/or bedspread.	1.	Provides for proper disposal of soiled linens. Allows for organization of supplies.
2.	Gather linens and gloves. Place linens on a clean, dry surface in reverse order of usage at the client's bedside (pillowcases, top sheet, draw sheet, bottom sheet).	2.	Provides easy access to items.
3.	Inquire about the client's toileting needs and attend as necessary.	3.	Provides for client comfort and prevents interruptions during bed making.
4.	Assist client to a safe, comfortable chair.	4.	Increases client's comfort and decreases risk of falls.
5.	Apply gloves.	5.	Reduces risk of infection from soiled, contaminated linens.
6.	Position bed: flat, side rails down, adjust height to waist level.	6.	Promotes good body mechanics and decreases back strain.
7.	Remove and fold blanket and/or bedspread. If clean and reusable, place on clean work area.	7.	Keeps reusable bed linens clean.
8.	Remove soiled pillowcases by grasping the closed end with one hand and slipping the pillow out with the other. Place the soiled cases on top of the soiled sheet, and place the pillows on clean work area.	8.	Allows easy removal of the pillowcases without contamination of uniform by soiled linens and keeps pillows clean.
9.	Remove soiled linens: start on the side of the bed closest to you; free the bottom sheet and mattress pad (if used) by lifting the mattress and rolling soiled linens to the middle of the bed. Go to the other side of the bed, repeat action.	9.	Prevents tearing and fanning of linens. Linens are folded from cleanest area to most soiled to prevent contamination.
10.	Fold (do not fan or flap) soiled linens: head of bed to middle, foot of bed to middle. Place in linen bag or hamper, keeping soiled linens away from uniform.	10.	Fanning or flapping linens increases the number of microorganisms in the air. Folding linens reduces the risk of transmission of infection to others.
11.	Check mattress. If the mattress is soiled, clean it with an antiseptic solution and dry it thoroughly.	11.	Reduces the transmission of microorganisms.
12.	Remove gloves, cleanse hands, and apply a second pair of clean gloves (when appropriate).	12.	Reduces the transmission of microorganisms to clean linens.
13.	Open the clean mattress pad lengthwise onto the bed. Unfold half the pad's width to the center crease and smooth the pad flat. If there are elastic bands to hold the pad in place, slide them under the corners of the mattress.	13.	Facilitates making bed in an organized, time-saving manner by not having to go from one side of the bed to the other.
14.	Proceed with placing the bottom sheet onto the mattress. Linens differ from facility to facility. Bottom sheets may be fitted or they may be flat. Proceed to the appropriate action for the linen available.	14.	Use linen available at the facility.
Fitted Bottom Sheet			
15.	Position yourself diagonally toward the head of the bed.	15.	Ensures good body mechanics and efficient procedure.
16.	Start at the head with seamed side of the fitted sheet toward the mattress.	16.	Placement of seamed side toward mattress prevents irritation to the client's skin.
17.	Lift the mattress corner with your hand closest to the bed; with your other hand, pull and tuck the fitted sheet over the mattress corner; secure at the head of the bed.	17.	Prevents straining of back muscles; decreases the chance that the sheet will pull from under the mattress.

Contd...

Table 12.1: *Contd...*

	Nursing action		Rationale
18.	Pull and tuck the fitted sheet over the mattress corners at the foot of the bed.	18.	Prevents straining of back muscles; decreases the chance that the sheet will pull out from under the mattress.
Flat Regular Sheet			
19.	Unfold the bottom sheet with the seamed side toward the mattress. Align the bottom edge of the sheet with the edge of the mattress at the foot of the bed.	19.	Placement of the seamed side toward the mattress prevents irritation to the client's skin. Ensure proper placement of the sheet so that it can be tightly secured at the top and on both sides of the bed.
20.	Allow the sheet to hang 10 inches (25 cm) over the mattress on the side and at the top of the bed.	20.	Proper placement of linens ensures adequate sheeting for all sides of the bed.
21.	Position yourself diagonally toward the head of the bed. Lift the top of the mattress corner with the hand closest to the bed and smoothly tuck the sheet under the mattress.	21.	Prevents straining of back muscles; decreases the chance that the sheet will pull out from under the mattress.
22.	Miter the corner at the head of the bed using the following technique (Fig. 12.4).	22.	Secures sheet tightly to the mattress, with the triangular fold providing a smooth tuck to keep the linen in place.
23.	Face the side of bed and lift and lay the edge of the sheet onto the bed to form a triangular fold.	23.	Forms the base for the tuck.
24.	With your palms down, tuck the lower edge of sheet (hanging free at the side of the mattress) under the mattress.	24.	Forms the first half of the tuck.
25.	Grasp the triangular fold, bring it down over the side of the mattress. Allow the sheet to hang free at the side of the mattress.	25.	Will form the final portion of the mitered corner when tucked in.
26.	Place the draw sheet on the bottom sheet and unfold it to the middle crease.	26.	Provides a sheet to lift and move the client in bed without having to use the bottom sheet and remake the bed. Helps to keep the bottom sheet clean.
27.	Face the side of the bed, palms of hands down. Tuck both the bottom and draw sheets under the mattress. Ensure that the bottom sheet is tucked smoothly under the mattress all the way to the foot of the bed.	27.	Keeps sheet taut, in place, and wrinkle-free, thereby decreasing the risk of skin irritation.
28.	Go to the other side of the bed, unfold the bottom sheet, and repeat the actions used to apply the mattress pad and bottom sheet.	28.	Unfolding decreases air current; air currents can spread microorganisms.
29.	Unfold the draw sheet, if used, and grasp the free-hanging sides of both the bottom and draw sheets. Pull toward you, keeping your back straight, and with a firm grasp (sheets taut) tuck both sheets under the mattress. Use your arms and open palms to extend the linen under the mattress. Place the protective pad on the bottom sheet.	29.	Uses your body's weight in pulling the sheet taut and prevents strain on your back muscles.
30.	Place the top sheet on the bed and unfold lengthwise, placing the center crease (width) of the sheet in the middle of the bed. Place the top edge of the sheet (seam up) even with the top of the mattress at the head of the bed then pull	30.	Saves time and movement, making one side of the bed at a time. Seam will be folded down to prevent contact with the client's skin, which can result in irritation.
31.	Unfold and apply the blanket or spread. Follow the same technique as used in applying the top sheet.	31.	Provides warmth.

Contd...

Table 12.1: Contd...

	Nursing action		Rationale
32.	Miter the bottom corners. With your palms down, tuck the lower edge of the sheet under the mattress. Grasp the triangular fold and bring it down over the side of the mattress. Allow the sheet to hang free at the side of the mattress.	32.	Secures linen at the foot of the bed.
33.	Face the head of the bed and fold the top sheet and blanket over 6 inches (15 cm). Fanfold the sheet and blanket (from the foot to the middle of the bed).	33.	Allows the client easy access to the bed.
34.	Apply a clean pillowcase on each pillow. With one hand, grasp the closed end of the pillowcase. Gather the pillowcase and turn it inside out over hand. With same hand, grasp the middle of one end of the pillow. With other hand, pull the case over the length of the pillow. The corners of the pillow should fit snugly into the corners of the case. *Change pillow case* • Remove soiled pillow case and place in laundry bag. • Grasp closed end of clean pillow case at center with one hand (Fig. 12.1A). Next, maintaining grasp, use other hand to grasp open end of case (Fig. 12.1B). invert case over hand and forearm (at closed end) by pulling open end of case back over hand at close end. Maintain grasp at closed end. • Grasp pillow end with hand holding case (Fig. 12.1C). Maintaining grasp, use other hand to pull case down over pillow (Fig. 12.1D).	34.	Keeps clean pillowcase away from your uniform.
35.	Return the bed to the lowest position and elevate the head of the bed 30 to 45 degrees. Put side rails up on side, farthest from client.	35.	Provides for client safety.
36.	Inquire about toileting needs of the client; assist as necessary.	36.	Saves client energy and provides time to care for the client's needs.
37.	Assist the client back into the bed and pull up the side rails; place call light in reach; take vital signs.	37.	Promotes client safety and a means to call for assistance. Sitting up in a chair and movement may cause changes in the client's vital signs.
38.	Remove gloves and cleanse hands.	38.	Reduces the transmission of microorganisms.
39	Adjust bed as necessary (Fig 12.2).	39.	Promoter comfort and safety.

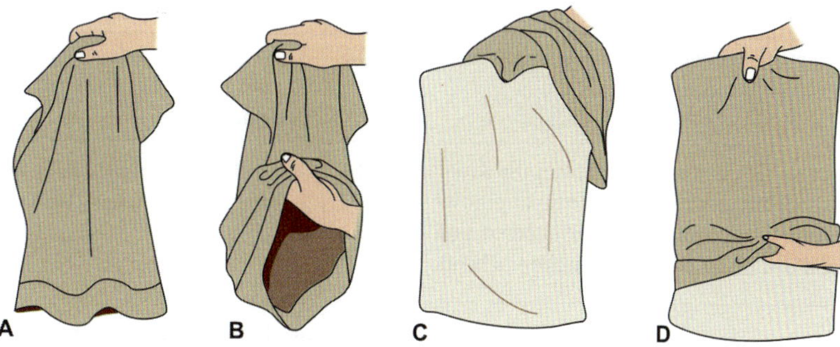

Figures 12.1A to D: Change pillow case

Table 12.2: Making an Occupied Bed

	Nursing action		*Rationale*
1.	Explain procedure to client.	1.	Promotes client cooperation.
2.	Bring equipment to the bedside.	2.	Facilitates procedure organization.
3.	Cover client with a bath blanket. Remove top sheet and blanket. Loosen bottom sheet at foot and sides of bed. Lower side rail nearest the nurse, if necessary for access.	3.	Bath blanket prevents exposure and chills. Facilitates easy removal of linens. Lowering only side rail close to nurse reduces client's risk of falls.
4.	Position client on side, facing away from you. Reposition pillow under head.	4.	Provides space to place clean linens.
5.	Fanfold or roll bottom linens close to client toward the center of the bed.	5.	Keeps soiled linen together. Promotes comfort when client later rolls to other side.
6.	Place clean bottom linens with the center fold nearest the client. Fanfold or roll clean bottom of mattress (Fig 12.3).	6.	Provides for maximum fit of sheets and decreases chance of wrinkles.
7.	Miter bottom sheet at head of bed. To miter, lift the mattress and tuck the sheet over the edge of the mattress, lift edge of sheet that is hanging to form a triangle, and lay upper part of sheet back onto bed; tuck the lower hanging section under the mattress. Repeat for each corner. Tuck the sides of the sheet under the mattress (Fig 12.4).	7.	Holds linens firmly in place.
8.	Fold the draw sheet in half. Identify the center of the draw sheet and place it close to the client. Fanfold or roll draw sheet closest to client and tuck under soiled linen, smoothen the linen. Add protective padding if needed. Tuck draw sheet under mattress, working from the center to the edges. Draw sheet should be positioned under the lower back and buttocks.	8.	Draw sheet facilitates moving and lifting clients while in bed.
9.	Move to other side of bed. Remove soiled linens by rolling into as bundle and place in linen hamper without touching uniform.	9.	Positions client off soiled linen. Protects client from falling.
10.	Move to other side of bed. Remove soiled linens by rolling into a bundle and place in linen hamper without touching uniform.	10.	Prevents cross-contamination.
11.	Unfold/unroll bottom sheet, then draw sheet. Look for objects left in the bed. Grasp each sheet and pull tightly while leaning back with your body weight. Client may be positioned supine.	11.	Tight sheets keep linens wrinkle-free and decrease the risk of skin irritation. Leaning back uses body weight for good body mechanics.
12.	Place top sheet over client with center of sheet in middle of bed. Unfold top of sheet over client. Remove bath blankets left on client. Place top blanket over client, same as the top sheet.	12.	Provides client with top sheet and blanket to prevent chilling.
13.	Raise foot of mattress and tuck the corner of the top sheet and blanket under. Miter the corner. Repeat with other side of mattress. Bend knees and not the back for proper mechanics.	13.	Secures top sheet and blanket in place.
14.	Grasp top sheet and blanket over client's tows and pull upward, then make a small fanfold in the sheet.	14.	Provides room under the tight top sheet and blanket for client to move feet. Prevents toe decubitus and sheet burns from pressure.
15.	Remove soiled pillowcase. Grasp center of clean pillowcase and invert pillowcase over hand/arm. Maintain grasp of pillowcase while grasping center of pillow. Use other hand to pull pillowcase down over pillow. Place pillow under client's head.	15.	Provides clean pillowcase without shaking pillow or pillowcase. Promotes comfort.
16.	Cleanse hands.	16.	Reduces the transmission of microorganisms.

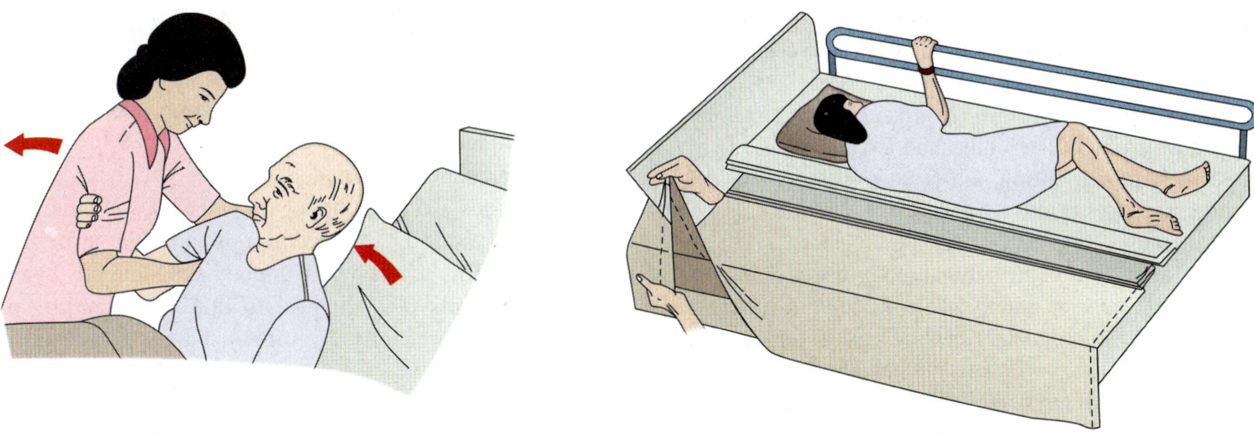

Figure 12.2: Adjust the bed as necessary

Figure 12.3: Placing the clean bottom linens with the center fold nearest the client

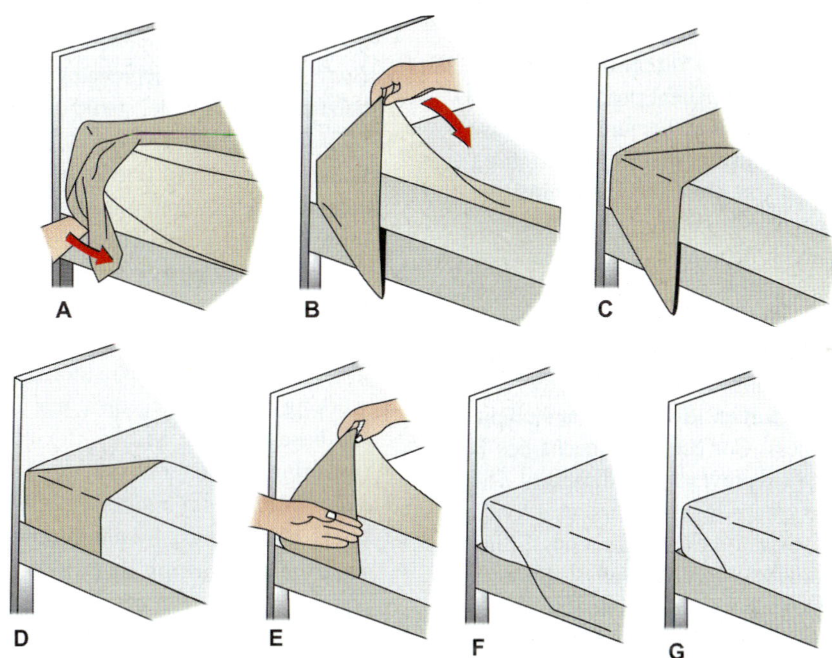

Figure 12.4: Miter bottom sheet at head of bed

While Bed making proper instruction should include the appropriate use of Standard Precaution and safety precautions for themselves and the client, such as the proper movement of the client in bed, how to manage drains and dressings, and the use of proper body mechanics. In certain situations where the client is in critical condition and multiple tubes, especially chest tubes, are present, the nurse should assist and use clean hands, and check the identity of patient before starting procedure.

After bed making nurse should see that the client has clean, unwrinkled linen, the linen placed on the bed is suitable for the client's special needs and the linen was changed with a minimum of path and trauma to the client.

And document on Nurses' Notes that how the client tolerated the bed change, and any unusual findings. (Bed change is not generally documented.)

Body Mechanics

Body mechanics are the coordinated effort of the musculoskeletal and nervous systems to maintain balance, posture and body alignment during lifting bending, moving and performing activities of daily living. Use of proper body mechanics reduce risk of injury to the musculoskeletal system. Proper body mechanics also facilitates body movement allowing physical mobility without muscle strain and excessive use of muscle energy.

Body alignment and postures are analogous terms and refer to the positioning of the joints, tendors, ligaments and muscles while in standing, sitting and lying positions. Correct body alignment reduces strain on musculoskeletal structures, maintain adequate muscle tone and contributes balance.

Body alignment contributes to body balance. Without this balance the center of gravity is displaced which increases the force of gravity, consequently creating a risk of falling and getting injury. Body balance is achieved when a wide base of support exists, the center of gravity falls within the base of support. Body balance is also enhanced by posture and lowering the center of gravity which can be achieved by a squatting position. The more aligned the posture the greater the body balance. Body balance is required for maintaining a position, remaining stable while moving one position to another, performing acts of daily living and moving freely in the community.

Friction is a force that occurs in a direction to oppose movement. A passive or immobilized patient produces greater friction to movement. Whenever possible the nurse should use some of the clients strength and mobility when lifting, transferring or moving the client. This can be done by explaining the procedure and telling the client when to move so that the client can then participate and friction is decreased. Friction can also be reduced by lifting rather than pushing a client. Lifting has an upward component and decreases the pressure between the client and the bed or chair. Pulling along with a sheet reduces friction because the client is more easily moved along the surface.

Proper body mechanics is important to the nurse and client. It affects their levels of wellness. Correct body mechanics is necessary for health promotion and prevention of disability. The nurse uses a variety of muscle groups for each nursing activity, such as walking during rounds, administering medications, lifting and transferring clients, and moving objects. The physical forces of weight and friction can influence body movement. If correctly used, these forces increases the nurses efficiency. Incorrect use can impair the ability of the nurse to lift, transfer and position clients. The nurse also incorporates knowledge of physiological and pathological influences on mobility and body alignment.

Nursing requires the nurse to incorporate knowledge and skills into practice. One component of knowledge and skill is 'body mechanics'. Body mechanics is the coordinated effort of the musculoskeletal and nervous system to maintain balance, posture and body alignment during lifting, bending, moving and performing activities of daily living. Using appropriate body mechanics or movement protects the nurses large muscle groups from injury and provides safety for the patient when ambulating. Proper mechanics also facilitated body movement, which allows physical mobility, without muscle strain and excessive use of muscular energy.

The nurse uses body mechanics daily in making beds, assisting the patient to walk, carrying supplies and equipment, lifting, providing patient care and carrying out other procedures.

Concepts of Body Mechanics

Body mechanics is the efficient use of the body as a machine and as a means of locomotion. Body mechanics is directly related to the effective functioning of the body. The correct use of body mechanics should be evident of every activity and even during rest periods. Because correct use of the body is another phase of illness prevention and health promotion; the nurse has major responsibility to teach both directly and indirectly by example. The concepts most helpful to the understanding of body mechanics are body alignment, balance and coordinated movement.

1. *Body alignment:* It refers to the positioning of the joints; tendons, ligaments and muscles while in standing, sitting and lying positions. Correct body alignment reduces strain on musculoskeletal structures maintains adequate muscle care and contributes to balance. A person in correct alignment is experiencing no undue strain on the joints, muscles, tendon or ligaments while balance maintained.

2. *Body balance:* It is achieved when the center of gravity is balanced over a wide, stable of supports and vertical line falls from the center of gravity and base of support. In human the center of gravity when standing located in the center of pelvis admit midway between the umbilicus and the symphysis pubis. The line of gravity is a vertical line that passes through the center of gravity. The base of support is the foundation that provides for an object's stability. The wider the base of support and the lander the center of gravity. The nurses can increase body balance when working by spreading their feet further apart (breathing the base support) and by flexing their hips and knees (lowering the center or gravity).

3. *Coordinated body movement:* While giving care to the client nurses must frequently use the body to assist in positioning, turning and lifting body of clients and equipment, it is important to do this knowledgeably to avoid musculoskeletal strain and injury.

Principles of Body Mechanics

- The wider the base of supports, the greater the stability of the nurse
- The lower the center of gravity, the greater the stability of the nurse
- The equilibrium of an object is maintained as long as the line of gravity passes through its base of support
- The stronger the muscle group, the greater amount of work can be safely done by it
- Facing the direction of movement prevents abnormal twisting of the spine
- Dividing balanced activity between arms and legs reduces the risk of back injury
- Leverage, rolling, turning or pivoting requires less work than lifting

- When friction is reduced between the object to be moved and the surface on which it is move, less force is required to move it
- Reducing the force to work reduced the risk of injury
- Maintaining good body mechanics, reduces fatigue of the muscle groups
- Alternating periods of rest and activity help reduce fatigue.

Using Proper Body Mechanics (Table 12.3)

Skills needed to care for clients often require physical strength to provide individuals with assistance required to remain mobile. Nurses/caregivers may need to carry, pull, push, or lift clients and/or equipment to accomplish daily care. It is imperative to know and use proper lifting techniques and seek assistance as needed to avoid injury to self and clients. Body mechanics is the term used when referring to lifting techniques. Correct body mechanics are essential to avoid work-related musculoskeletal injuries, diminish excessive strain and fatigue, and minimize the potential for injury.

Body mechanics involve pushing, pulling, stooping, carrying, and lifting correctly. Knowledge of various client transfer techniques, the use of a team as needed, and the use of proper supportive equipment are included in this skill. Proper techniques of body mechanics, specialized lifting skills of transfer from bed to stretcher and from bed to chair or wheelchair, and the use of the bed transfer board and a hydraulic lift are reviewed. Specific tips for client and staff safety are highlighted. Promotion of client independence and self-help behavior as an intervention to reduce the risk of client and nurse injury is discussed.

While using proper body mechanics, nurses should:

1. Assess the need and degree to which the client requires assistance to achieve physical movement. Identifies client's ability to attain maximum level of self-help before initiating intervention.
2. Identify the type of physical movement required to ensure the use of proper body mechanics such as pushing, pulling, or lifting.
3. Identify the potential need for assistive equipment to accomplish the goal of safe lifting to minimize the risk of client/nurse injury.
4. Identify any unusual risks to safe lifting, such as an extra-heavy client or a home care setting. Allows nurse to plan modifications to ensure good body mechanics and reduce the risk of injury.
5. Assess the client's vital signs, pain status, and need for pain medications before ambulating. Assess incisional areas and/or areas of injury.
6. Check equipment to ensure that it is in working order to facilitate a safe and uninterrupted transfer. Especially check locks on wheelchair.
7. Identify all equipment and tubes connected to the client and take appropriate preventive measures.

Equipment Needed

- Transfer or gait belts
- Wheelchair equipped with working locks
- Transfer board
- Draw or lift sheet
- Nonslip shoes or slippers
- Safety or gait belt
- Stretcher equipped with working locks
- Hydraulic lift.

After procedure nurse should see than:

- The client or object is lifted and/or moved without sustaining injury or damage.
- The nurse who is lifting and moving clients or objects is not injured.

And document in the Nurses' Notes

- Type of lift or transfer in the progress notes
- Client's tolerance of the lift or move.

Using Appropriate Body Mechanics (Table 12.4)

The nurse uses appropriate body mechanics for the following purposes:

- To prevent strain and injury to the patient
- To prevent strain and injury to the nurse
- To use appropriate technique when moving the patient
- To provide safety for the patient.

The equipment needed is chair. Procedures are given in Table 12.4.

Positioning the Patient on Bed

Positioning patients on bed performed daily by the nurse. There are many positions a nurse must learn to prevent the patient from developing complications. Different types of nursing positions are shown in Figure 12.7 (A to J). Permanent disability can occur from unappropriate positions certain nursing actions with rationale are given in Table 12.5.

Equipment and Supplies are as Follows

- Pillows
- Hand roles
- Foot board
- Restraints
- Trachanter rolls
- Siderails
- Sandbags.

Moving and Lifting Patient

Nurses often provide care for immobilized patients whose position must be changed, who must be moved in the bed (Fig. 12.8), or who must be transferred from a bed to chair or bed to a stretcher. Moving includes lifting the patient up in the bed, turning, dangling and assisting the patient in and out of bed

Table 12.3: Using Proper Body Mechanics

	Nursing Action		*Rationale*
	Check clients identification band Explain procedure before beginning		To identify right patient To get cooperation and reduce anxiety
1.	Cleanse hands.	1.	Reduces the transmission of microorganisms.
2.	Assess the situation for obstacles, heavy clients, poor handholds, or equipment or objects in the way. Reduce or remove safety hazards prior to lifting the client or object. Assess for any tubing or equipment connected to the client.	2.	Good planning helps prevent accidental injury.
3.	Assess the situation for slippery surfaces, including wet floors; slippery shoes on client, helper, or nurse; and towels, linen, or paper on the floor. Resolve the slippery surface before lifting the client or object.	3.	Removes the cause of many falls and slips.
4.	Assess the situation for hidden risks, including client confusion, combativeness, orthostatic hypotension, drug effects, pain, or fear.	4.	Allows the nurse to anticipate and plan for unexpected events.
5.	Maintain low center of gravity by bending at the hips and knees, not the waist. Squat down rather than bend over to lift and lower.	5.	Provides for the equal distribution of body weight and assists in maintaining safe balance.
6.	Establish a wide support base with feet spread apart.	6.	Provides stability and lowers the center of gravity.
7.	Use feet to move, not a twisting or bending motion from the waist.	7.	Assists in maintaining correct body alignment, which increases strength to lift, push, pull, and carry.
8.	When pushing or pulling, stand near the object and stagger one foot partially ahead of the other.	8.	Provides a safety net for avoiding potential back injuries.
9.	When pushing a client or an object, lean into the client or object and apply continuous light pressure. When pulling a client or an object, lean way and grasp with light pressure. Never jerk or twist your body to force a weight to move.	9.	Firm pressure will provide continuous movement of the object and will avoid abrupt movements that require the expenditure of increased energy.
10.	When stooping to move an object, maintain a wide base of support with feet, fleck knees to lower body, and maintain straight upper body.	10.	Provides the appropriate mechanics for the strength and endurance to achieve the task and to stand up straight upon completion.
11.	When lifting or carrying an object, squat in front of the object, take a firm hold, and assume a standing position by using the leg muscles and keeping the back straight.	11.	This stance will avoid the use of the back, diminish the potential for spinal twisting, and provide the lifter with a firm center of gravity and strength to lift the required weight.
12.	When rising up from a squatting position, arch your back slightly. Keep the buttocks and abdomen tucked in and rise up with your head first.	12.	Keeps the back from bowing and increasing the strain on the back muscles.
13.	When lifting or carrying heavy objects, keep the weight as close to your center of gravity as possible.	13.	Reduces the strain on arm, leg, and back muscles.
14.	When reaching for a client or an object, keep the back straight. If the client or object is heavy, do not try to lift the client or object without repositioning yourself closer to the weight.	14.	Avoids straining the back and arm muscles.
15.	Use safety aids and equipment. Use gait belts, lifts, drawsheets, and other transfer assistance devices. Encourage clients to use handrails and grab bars. Wheelchair, cart, and stretcher wheels should be locked when they are not actually being moved.	15.	Reduces the strain on the nurse and improves the safety for the client.

Table 12.4: Procedures for Using Appropriate Body Mechanics

	Nursing actions		*Rationales*
1.	Position feet 6 to 8 inches apart.	1.	Provides adequate base support.
2.	Align and balance weight on both feet.	2.	Distribute weight evenly.
3.	Flex knees slightly.	3.	Prevents hyperextension.
4.	Tilt pelvis forward by pulling buttocks inward.	4.	Helps straighten curve of spine.
5.	Hold abdomen in and up.	5.	Provides support and reduces muscle strain.
6.	Hold chest up.	6.	Allows better lung expansion.
7.	Keep head erect.	7.	Helps maintain appropriate alignment of spine.
8.	Use appropriate body mechanics in all activities: (a) Standing (b) Sitting (c) Bending (d) lifting	8.	- - - (a) Demonstrate appropriate body movement (b) – do – (c) – do – (d) – do -

Table 12.5: Procedures for Positioning the Patient on Bed

	Nursing actions		*Rationales*
1.	Assess the need for positioning patient.	1.	Determines patient need for movement.
2.	Choose appropriate position.	2.	Rotating position prevents pressure areas.
3.	Gather equipment.	3.	It provide organization approach to task.
4.	Explain the procedure.	4.	Seeks cooperation and decreases anxiety.
5.	Wash hands.	5.	Hand washing deters spreading microorganism.
6.	Provide for client privacy.	6.	Ensuring clients mental comfort.
7.	Put bed in flat position and move client to head of bed, slide patient and matters to head of bed and remove pillow. (Fig. 12.5)	7.	Provides easy access to client and allows nursing personnel to reposition client without working against gravity. Allows room for proper positioning. Helps mechanics proper body alignment.

Contd...

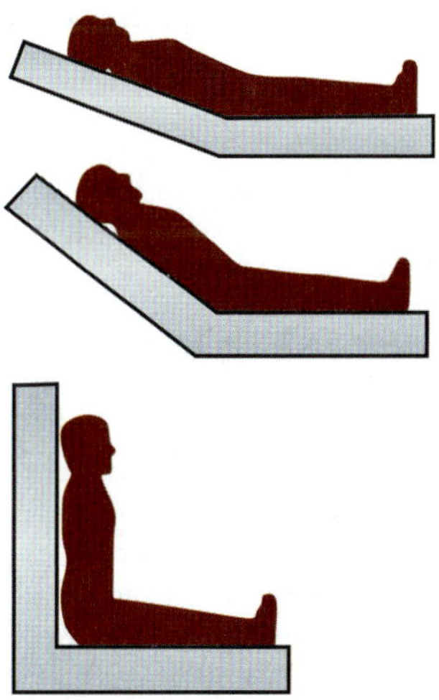

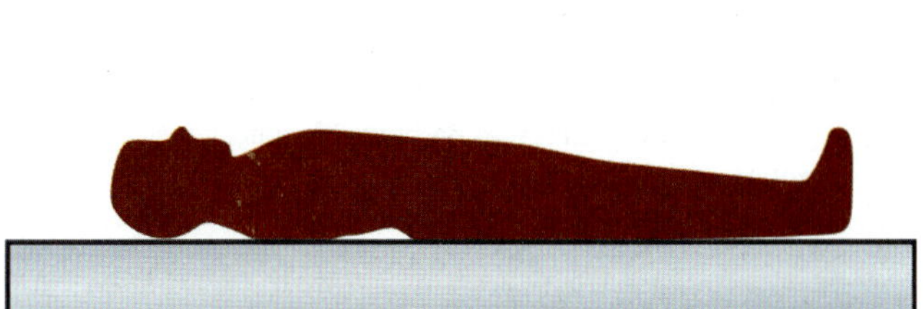

Figure 12.5: Flat position

Figure 12.6: Flat position

Table 12.5: *Contd...*	
Nursing actions	*Rationales*
8. Positioning patient is supported by Fowler's position (Fig. 12.6) (a) Elevate head of bed 45-60° opportunity to increases. (b) Rest head against mattress or on small pillow. (c) Use pillows to support arms and hand if client does not have voluntary control or use of hands and arms. (d) Position pillow at lower back. (e) Place small pillow or roll under thigh. (f) Place small pillow or roll under ankles. (g) Place foot board at bottom of clients feet.	8. - - - (a) Increases comfort, improves ventilation, and socialize or relax. (b) Prevents cervical flexion contractures. (c) Prevents shoulder dislocation from effect of downward gravitation pull of unsupported arms, promotes circulation by preventing venous polling, and prevents flexion contracture of arms and wrists. (d) Supports lumber vertebral and decrease flexion of vertebral. (e) Prevents hyperextension of knee and occlusion of artery political from pressure from body weight. (f) Prevents prolonged pressure on heals from mattress (g) Maintain dorsal reflexion and prevents foot drop.
9. Positioning patient in supine position [Fig. 12.7(B)] (a) Place patient on back with head of bedflat. (b) Place small rolled towel under lumbar area back. (c) Place pillow under upper shoulders, neck and head contractures of cervical vertebral. (d) Place trochanter roll or sandbags parallel to lateral surface of tights. (e) Place small pillow or roll under ankle to elevate heals. (f) Place footboards or soft pillows against bottom of feet. (g) Place the pillow under pronated forearms, maintaining upper arms parallel to clients body [Fig. 12.7(B)] (h) Place hand rolls in hand.	9. - - - (a) Necessary for positioning in supine position. (b) Provides support for lumberspine. (c) Maintain correct alignment and prevents flexion, (d) Reduces extended rotation of hip. (e) Reduces pressure on heals, helping prevents pressure ulcers. (f) Maintain feet in dorsiflexion prevents foot drop. (g) Reduces internal rotation of should and prevents extension of elbows. Maintain correct body alignment. (h) Reduces extension of fingers and abduction of thumb. Maintain thumb slightly abducted and in opposition.
10. Positioning patient in prone position [Fig. 12.7(E)]: (a) Roll patient over arm positioned closed to body with elbow straight and hand under hip. Position on abdomen in center of bed with bedflat. (b) Turn patient's head to one side and support with small pillow. (c) Place small pillow under the abdomen below level of diaphragm. (d) Support arms in flexed position level at shoulder. (e) Support lower legs with pillow to elevate toes.	10. - - - (a) Position patient so that alignment can be maintained. (b) Reduces flexion of hyperextension of cervical vertebral. (c) Reduces pressure on breasts of some women. Decreases hyperextension of lumber vertebrae and stain on lower back. Improves breathing by reducing mattress pressure on diaphragm. (d) Maintain proper body alignment. Support reduces risk of joint dislocations. (e) Prevents foot drop. Reduces external rotation of legs. Reduces mattress pressure on toes.
11. Positioning patient in lateral (side-lying) position [Fig. 12.7(I)]: (a) Lower the head of the bed completely or as low as patient can tolerate. (b) Position client to side of bed. (c) Turn patient onto side. (d) To turn helpless patient onto side, flex patients knees that will not be next to mattress. Place one hand on patients hip and one hand on shoulder. (e) To roll patient onto side. (f) Place pillow under patients head and neck (g) Bring shoulder blade forward. (h) Position both arms in slightly flexed position. Uppermost arm is supported by pillow level with shoulder. (i) Place tuck-back pillow behind patient back. (j) Place pillow under semiflexed upper leg level at hip to foot. (k) Place sand bag parallel to plantar surface of dependent foot.	11. - - - (a) Provides position of comfort for patient and removes pressure from bones prominences on back. (b) Provides room for patient to turn to side. (c) Prevents injury to joints as patient is rolled to side. Leverage on hip makes turning easy. (d) Maintains alignment. Reduces later neck flexion. (e) Prevents weight from resting directly on shoulder joint. (f) Decreased internal rotation and adduction of shoulder. Protects joint. Ventilation is improved because chest can expand more easily. (g) Provides support maintain patient on side. (h) Prevents hyperextension of leg. Maintains leg in proper alignment. Prevent pressure on bony prominence. (i) Maintains dorsiflexion of the foot. Prevent foot drop.

Contd...

Table 12.5: Contd...

Nursing actions	Rationales
12. Positioning patient in Sims (semiprone) position [Fig. 12.7(D)]: (a) Place head of bed flat. (b) Place patient in supine position. (c) Position patient in lateral position lying partially on abdomen. (d) Place small pillow under head. (e) Place pillow under flexed upper arm, supporting other arm on mattress. (f) Place pillow under flexed upper legs, supporting by level with hip. (g) Place sandbags parallel to plantar surface of foot.	12. - - - (a) Provides for proper body alignment while patient is lying. (b) Prepares patient for Sims position. (c) Patient is rolled only partially on abdomen. (d) Maintains proper alignment and prevents lateral neck flexion. (e) Prevents internal rotation of shoulder. Maintain proper alignment. (f) Prevents internal rotation of hip and abduction of leg, prevents hyperextension of leg. Reduces mattress pressure on knees and ankles. (g) Maintain foot is dorsiflexion. Prevent foot drop.
13. Positioning patient in knee-chest position [Fig. 12.7(F)]: (a) Turn patient onto abdomen. (b) Assist patient to kneeling position arms and head should rest in pillow while upper chest rests on bed.	13. - - - (a) Facilitates positioning. (b) Complete positioning.
14. Positioning patient in lithotomy position [Fig. 12.7(G)]: (a) Request patient to slide buttocks to edge of examining table. (b) Lift both legs, have patient bend knees and place feet in stirrups. (c) Drape patient.	14. - - - (a) Facilitates positioning. (b) Position patient. (c) Provides privacy and prevents exposure.
15. Positioning patient in orthopneic position: (a) Elevate head of bed to 90°. (b) Place pillow between patients back and mattress. (c) Place pillow on over-head table and assist patient to learn over, placing head on pillow.	15. - - - (a) Facilitates positioning. (b) Provides back support. (c) Facilitates more-ease for breathing.
16. Positioning patient in semi-fowler's position [Fig. 12.7(J)]: (a) Slide patient and mattress to head of bed, and remove pillow. (b) Raise head of bed to about 30°. (c) Replace pillow. (d) Slightly raise foot of bed.	16. - - - (a) Helps ensure appropriate body alignment. (b) Position approximately. (c) Provides patient comfort. (d) Helps prevent patient from slipping in bed.
17. Positioning patient in semi-Fowler's position [Fig. 12.7(J)]: (a) Place patient head lower than the body with body and legs elevated and on an incline (bed may be elevated on blocks).	17. - - - (a) Used in performing abdominal surgery (not used if patient has head injury).
This position is not usually used to treat shock because of the pressure it causes on the diaphragm by the organs of the abdomen.	
18. Positioning patient in dorsal recumbent position [Fig. 12.7(C)]: (a) Slide the patient and mattress to head of bed, and remove pillow. (b) Lower head of the bed unless contraindicated. (c) Turn patient on the back. (d) Assist patient to raise legs, bend knees and allow legs to relax. (e) Replace pillow.	18. - - - (a) Helps to ensure appropriate body alignment. (b) Provides position safety. (c) Position patient. (d) Position patient comfort.
19. Wash hands.	19. Helps prevent cross infection.
20. Lower bed.	20. Provides for patient safety.
21. Observe body alignment position level of comfort and potential pressure points.	21. Determine effectiveness of positioning maintenance of body alignment and protection from pressure. Reduces risk of musculoskeletal injury related to improper positioning.
22. Records procedure in nurses notes including position assumed, frequency of turning, condition of skin, etc.	22. Documents effectiveness of nursing care. Provides for consistency among nursing staff.

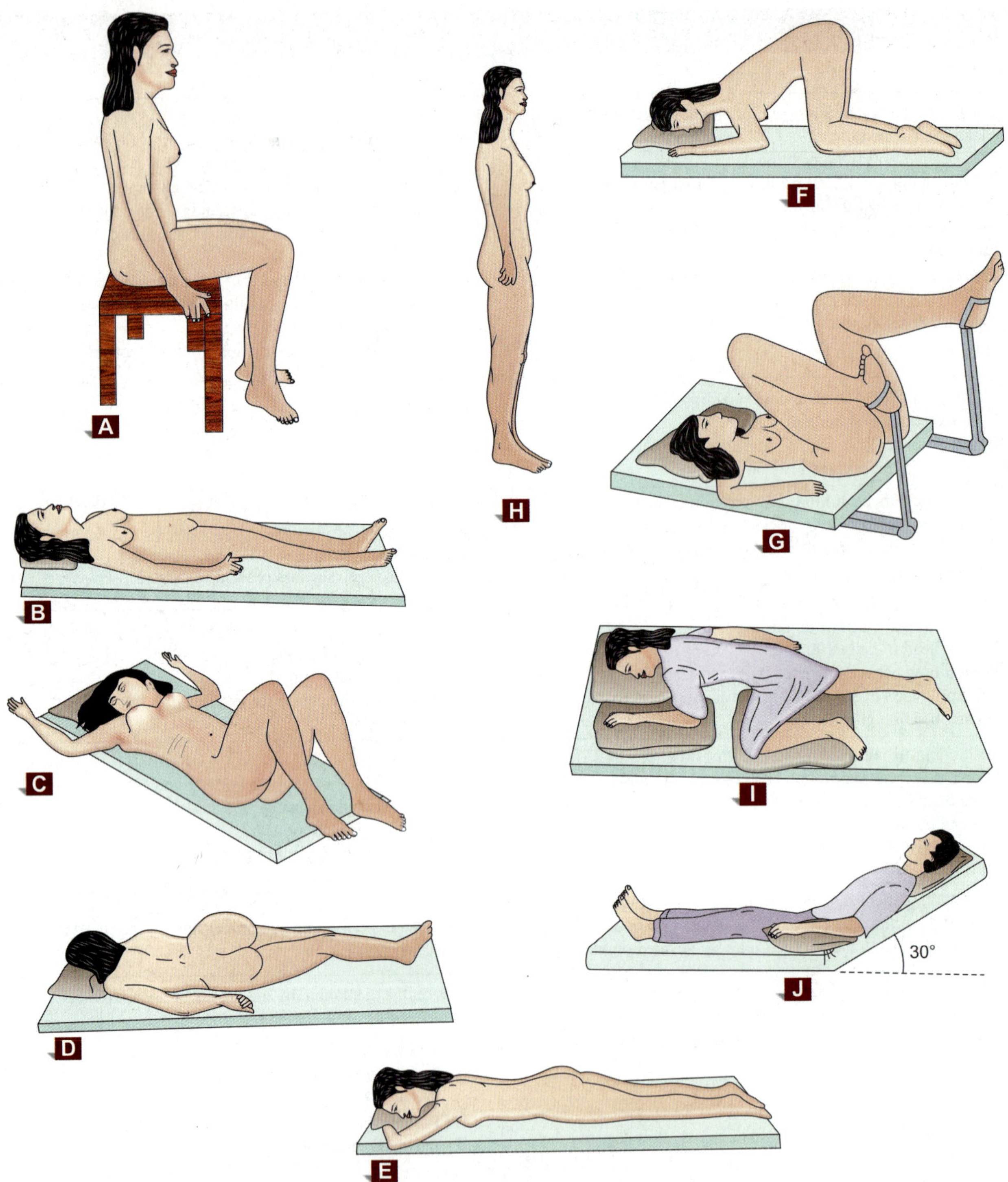

Figures 12.7A to J: Various client positions used during the nursing examinations: (A) Sitting position, (B) Supine position, (C) Doral recumbent position, (D) Sims' position, (E) Prone position, (F) Knee-chest position, (G) Lithotomy position, (H) Erect or standing position, (I) Lateral (side-lying) position (J) Semi-Fowler's position

for ambulation. Proper body mechanics enables the nurse to move, lift or transfer patients safely and also protects the nurse from injury to the musculorectal system.

There are certain guidelines the nurse should follow when moving and lifting patients. These are as follows:

- Know your patient diagnosis, capabilities and any movement not allowed. Place braces or any device the patient wears before helping from bed.
- Plan carefully what you will do before moving or lifting each client. Assess mobility attached equipment. You may injure the client or yourself if you have not planned well. If necessary, enlist the support of another nurse. This reduces strain on all involved.
- Explain to the patient what you plan to do. Then use what abilities the patient has to assist you. This technique often decrease work and possible injury to yourself.
- If the patient is in pain, administer the prescribed analgesics sufficiently in advance of the transfer to allow the client to participate in the move comfortably.
- Remove obstacle, if any that makes moving and lifting inconvenient.
- Elevate the bed as necessary, so that you are working at a height that is comfortable and safe for you.
- Lock the wheels of the bed, wheelchair or stretcher, so that they do not slide about while you are moving the client.
- Observe principles of body mechanics while you work to prevent injuring yourself.
- Be sure that patient is good body alignment while being moved and lifted to protect the patient from strain and muscle injury.

- Supporting the patients body well. Avoid grabbing and holding an extremity by its muscles.
- Avoid causing friction on the patients kin during moving. Friction can be reduced by sprinkling power of constretch on bedlines on the patients skin.
- Move your body and the patient in a smooth, rhythmic motion. Jerky movements tend to put extra strain on muscles and joints and are uncomfortable to the patient.
- Use mechanical devices such Hoyer lift or turning board, when they are available for moving patients. Be sure that you understand how the device operates and that patient is properly secured and informed of what will occur. Patient do not understand or are afraid may be unable to cooperate and may suffer injury as a result.
- Be a realistic about how much you can safely do without injury. Two small people cannot lift or move an obese patient without risking muscle strain and injury.

Principles and Techniques of Moving and Lifting

1. More force is required to lift an object than to pull or push it.
   - Use roller boards to pull patients on to another surface (roller boards have circular roles that revolve under a cover of material. The roller board is positioned partly under the patient, bridging the gap between a card and bed or any two flat surfaces. The patient is pulled across the board on to the bed. This board and the tubes revolve to move the patient with minimal friction and force needed)

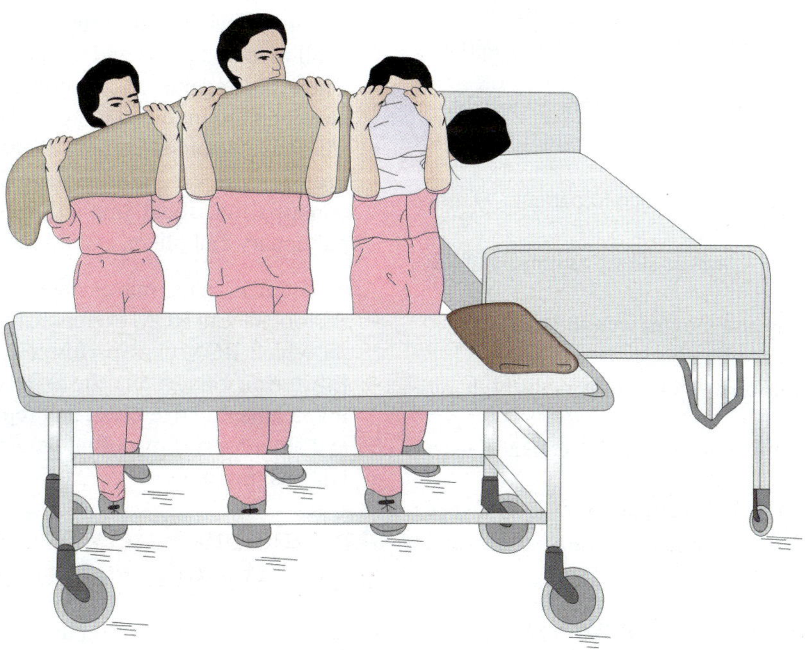

Figure 12.8: Lifting patient from stretcher to bed

- Use transfer board to slide the patient from bed to chair, bed to bed (transfer to wards are usually through flat pieces of solid material, often plastic, which bridge the gap between two surfaces, allowing the patient to slide into the new position gradually rather than being lifting which requires more work)
- Creation of friction on patients skin may cause damage.

2. Object is close to the lifters center of gravity require less force to it.
   - Patient moved does not nurse before lifting
   - Nurse's arms flexed rather than extended when lifting
   - Reaching while lifting is avoided
   - Kneel, seqat and wide basic supports to bring load closer to center of gravity

3. A wide base support giving stability to body
   - Feet apart approximately 1.5 feet
   - Feet flat on floor (parallel foot position with one foot forward and the one back pulls nurse up on to toes and ball of one foot as weight is shifted, leading to instability)
   - Angled foot position of approximately 60 to 90 degrees, with one foot forward and one back keeps both feet on floor improving stability

4. If the center of gravity moves outside the base of support; the body becomes unstable.
   - Position feet so center of gravity in pelvis is over feet
   - Bend knees to move down to lift load rather than bending over at waist
   - Knees behind, not back

5. A twisting motion when moving or lifting load places strain on the back muscle.
   - Back kept straight
   - Weight shifted from front foot to back foot to move load
   - Face direction opposite to movements

6. When load exceeds the force, no movement will occur
   - Get other lifters to help move heavy or immobile patient
   - Use mechanical lifters
   - Have the patient lift as much as own weight as possible
   - Provide patients bed with trapeze bar as appropriate to reduce nurses' load
   - Use body weight as a counter balance to patients weight to reduce force needed to move load

7. Muscles of the thighs are ten times as strong as muscle of the back.
   - Use the thighs in lifting and moving; not the back
   - Flex knees rather than bending back
   - Tighten abdominal muscles when lifting with thigh for maximum force

8. Healthy, active muscles are stronger than infrequently used muscle.
   - Keep abdominal, thigh, and biceps muscles in good shapes
   - Perform regular exercise to strengthen lifting muscles and reduce injury.

Moving the Patient up in Bed (One Nurse)

Children are light weight, adults are relatively easy to slide toward this head of the bed without assistance of second person.

The techniques used to move a patient up in bed when the client is able to assist are given in Tables 12.6 and 12.7

Performing Passive Range-of-Motion (ROM) Exercises

Passive range-of-motion (ROM or PROM) exercises seek to maintain or improve the current level of functional mobility of a client's extremities. The nurse provides, assists with, and teaches the client functional movements in all available planes and directions of involved joints. ROM exercises prevent contractures and shortening of muscles and tendons, increase circulation to extremities, decrease vascular complications of immobility, and facilitate comfort for the client. Methods for performing ROM exercises are shown in Figures 12.9A to E.

Before performing passive ROM exercise nurses should:

1. Be aware of the client's medical diagnosis. Understand the expected functional limit of a client with this diagnosis.
2. Familiarize yourself with the client's current range of motion. Note any joint pain, stiffness, or inflammation that might limit the client's motion. Understanding the client's current ROM will help you assess the functional limits of movement of each joint.
3. Assess client consciousness and cognitive function. Client should be encouraged to participate in ROM as actively as possible.

Equipment Needed

1. No special equipment is needed, except gloves when contact with body fluids is possible.

After procedure nurse should see than:
- Client has maintained or improved current functional mobility in all involved joints and extremities.
- Client has regained or improved strength and/or voluntary movement in involved joints and extremities.
- Client has avoided complications of immobility, including pressure ulcers, contractures, decreased peristalsis, constipation, fecal impaction, orthostatic hypotension, pulmonary embolism, and thrombophlebitis.

And document in the nurses notes:
- Performance of ROM exercises. Include joints and extremities on which ROM was performed, the types and degrees of limitation observed, the extend of the client's active involvement in exercises, any reports of pain or discomfort, and any observations of intolerance to exercise.
- Unusual findings.

Ambulation Safety and Assisting from Bed to Walking (Table 12.7)

Client ambulation (assisted or unassisted walking) is encouraged soon after the onset of illness or surgery to prevent the complications of immobility. First, assess the strength,

Table 12.6: Performing Passive ROM Exercises

	Nursing action		*Rationale*
	Check clients identification band Explain procedure before beginning		To identity right patient To get cooperation and reduce anxiety
1.	Cleanse hands, wear gloves if contact with body fluids is possible.	1.	Reduces the transmission of microorganisms.
2.	Provide for privacy, including exposing only the extremity to be exercised.	2.	Decreases embarrassment.
3.	Adjust bed to comfortable height for performing ROM.	3.	Prevents muscle strain and discomfort for nurse.
4.	Lower bed rail only on the side you are working.	4.	Prevents falls.
5.	Describe the passive ROM exercises you are performing, or verbally cue client to perform ROM exercises with your assistance.	5.	Exercises all joint areas.
6.	Start at the client's head and perform ROM exercises down each side of the body.	6.	Provides a systematic method to ensure that all body parts are exercised.
7.	Repeat each ROM exercise as the client tolerates, to a maximum of 5 times. Perform each motion is a slow, firm manner. Encourage full joint movement, but do not go beyond the point of pain, resistance, or fatigue.	7.	Provides exercise to the client's tolerance or to a level that will maintain the joint function.
8.	Head Perform these movements with the client in a sitting position, if possible. • Rotation: Turn the head from side to • side. • Flexion and extension: Tilt the head • toward the chest and then tilt slightly • upward. • Lateral flexion: Tilt the head on each side so as to almost touch the ear to the shoulder.	8.	Optimizes the performance of the movements, to preserve muscle tone and joint flexibility.
9.	Neck Perform these movements with the client in a sitting position, if possible. • Rotation: Rotate the neck in a semicircle while supporting the head.	9.	Optimizes the performance of the movements, to preserve muscle tone and joint flexibility.
10.	Trunk Perform these movements with the client in a sitting position. If possible. • Flexion and extension: Bend the trunk forward, straighten the trunk, and then extend slightly backward. • Rotation: Turn the shoulder forward and return to normal position. • Lateral flexion: tip trunk to the left side, straighten trunk, tip to the right side.	10.	Optimizes the performance of the movements, to preserve muscle tone and joint flexibility.
11.	Arm • Flexion and extension: Extend the arm in a straight position upward above the head, then downward along the side and back. • Adduction and abduction: Extend the arm in a straight position toward the midline (adduction) and away from the midline (abduction).	11.	Optimizes the performance of the movements, to preserve muscle tone and joint flexibility.

Contd...

	Table 12.6: *Contd...*		
	Nursing action		*Rationale*
12.	**Shoulder** • Internal and external rotation: Bend the elbow at a 90-degree angle with the upper arm parallel to the shoulder; rotate the shoulder by moving the lower arm upward and downward.	12.	Optimizes the performance of the movements, to preserve muscle tone and joint flexibility.
13.	**Elbow** • Flexion and extension: Supporting the arm, flex and extend the elbow. • Pronation and supination: Flex elbow, move the hand in palm-up and palm-down position.	13.	Optimizes the performance of the movements, to preserve muscle tone and joint flexibility.
14.	**Wrist** • Flexion and extension: Supporting the wrist, flex and extend the wrist (Fig 12.9A). • Adduction and abduction: Supporting the lower arm, turn wrist right to left, left to right, then rotate the wrist in a circular motion.	14.	Optimizes the performance of the movements, to preserve muscle tone and joint flexibility.
15.	**Hand** • Flexion and extension: Supporting the wrist, flex and extend the fingers (Fig. 12.9B). • Adduction and abduction: Supporting the wrist, spread fingers apart and then bring them close together. • Opposition: Supporting the wrist, touch each finger with the tip of the thumb. • Thumb rotation: supporting the wrist, rotate the thumb in a circular manner.	15.	Optimizes the performance of the movements, to preserve muscle tone and joint flexibility.
16.	**Hip and leg** Perform these movements with the client in a supine position, if possible. • Flexion and extension: Supporting the lower leg, flex the leg toward the chest and then extend the leg. • Internal and external rotation: Supporting the lower leg, angle the foot inward and outward. • Adduction and abduction: Slide the leg away from the client's midline and then back to the midline (Fig. 12.9C).	16.	Optimizes the performance of the movements, to preserve muscle tone and joint flexibility.
17.	**Knee** • Flexion and extension: Supporting the lower leg, flex the leg toward the knee (Fig. 12.9D).	17.	Optimizes the performance of the movements, to preserve muscle tone and joint flexibility.
18.	**Ankle** • Flexion and extension: Supporting the lower leg, flex and extend the ankle.	18.	Optimizes the performance of the movements, to preserve muscle tone and joint flexibility.
19.	**Foot** • Adduction and abduction: Supporting the ankle, spread the toes apart and then bring them close together. • Flexion and extension: Supporting the ankle, extend the toes upward and then flex the toes downward.	19.	Optimizes the performance of the movements, to preserve muscle tone and joint flexibility.
20.	Observe client's joints and face for signs of exertion, pain, or fatigue during movement.	20.	Alerts nurse to discontinue exercise.
21.	Replace covers and position client in proper body alignment.	21.	Promotes comfort.
22.	Place side rails in original position.	22.	Prevents falls.
23.	Place call light within reach.	23.	Facilitates communication.
24.	Cleanse hands.	24.	Reduces the transmission of microorganisms.

Neck
(to be done in sitting or standing position)

Flexion
Client instruction: "Bow your head forward with your chin toward your chest."

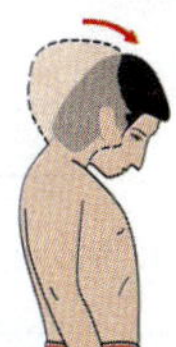

Extension
Client instruction: "Straighten your head back up."

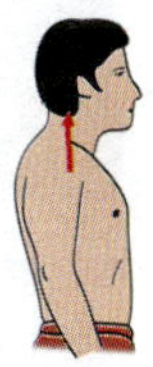

Hyperextension
Client instruction: "Bend your head back and look up toward the ceiling."

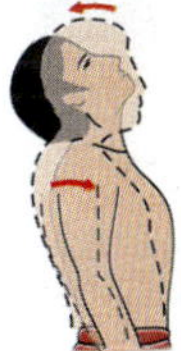

Lateral flexion
Client instruction: "Bend your head to the side with your ear toward your shoulder. Repeat this to the other side."

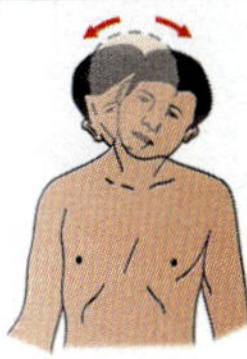

Rotation
Client instruction: "Trun your head to the side, chin toward shoulder, to look over your shoulder. Repeat this to the other side."

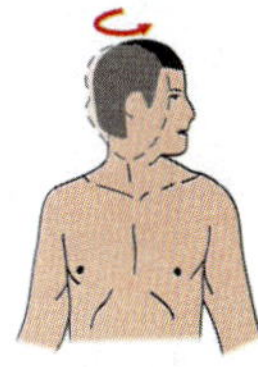

Vertebral column

Flexion
Client instruction: "Bend forward from the waist."

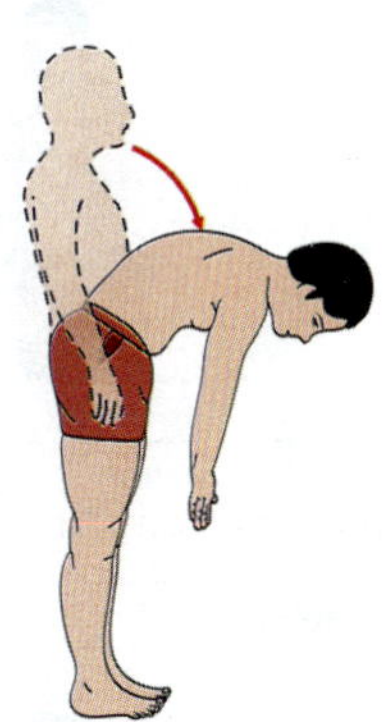

Extension
Client instruction: "Straighten back up."

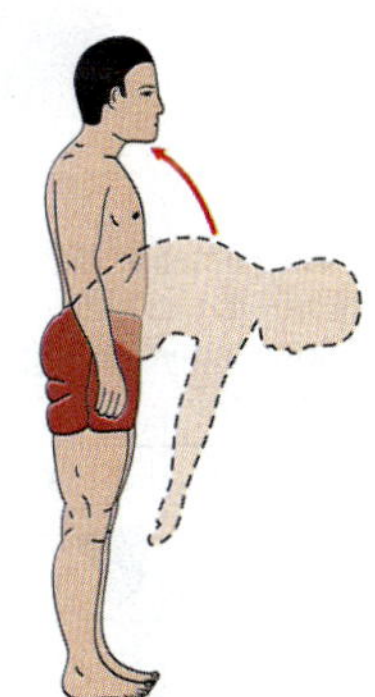

Hyperextension
Client instruction: "Keep your neck straight but bend backward from the waist while I stand beside you."

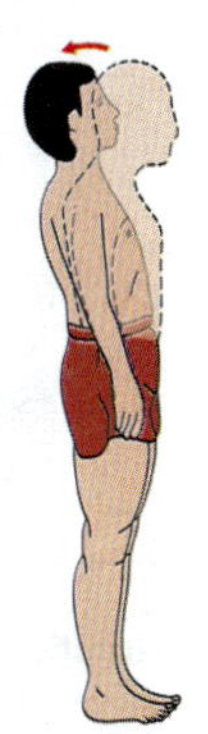

Lateral flexion
Client instruction: "Bend sideways from the waist while I stabilize your hips. Repeat this to the other side."

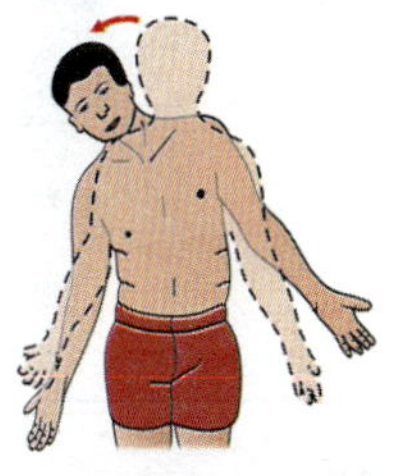

Rotation
Client instruction: "Without turning your head, turn from the waist to look behind you. Repeat to the opposite side."

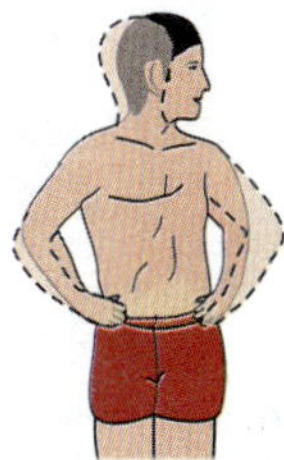

Figure 12.9A: Performing ROM exercises (contd...)

Shoulders
Flexion
Client instruction: "Reach both arms out in front of you and raise them straight up toward the ceiling."

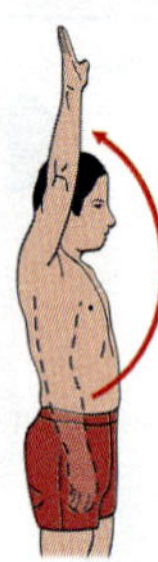

Extension
Client instruction: "Keeping them in front of you, bring them back down to your side.

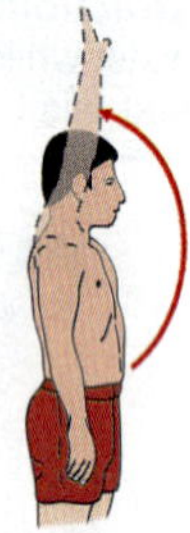

Hyperextension
Client instruction: "Continue moving them past your sides and back up behind you as far as you can reach."

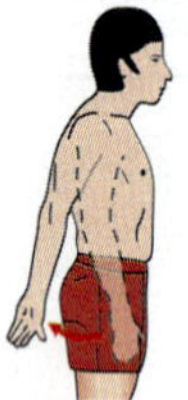

Abduction
Client instruction: "Raise your arms sideways until they point to the ceiling."

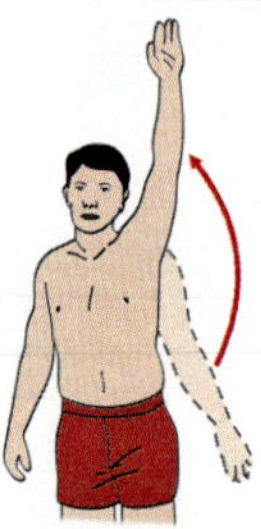

Adduction
Client instruction: "Moving them sideways, bring them back to your sides."

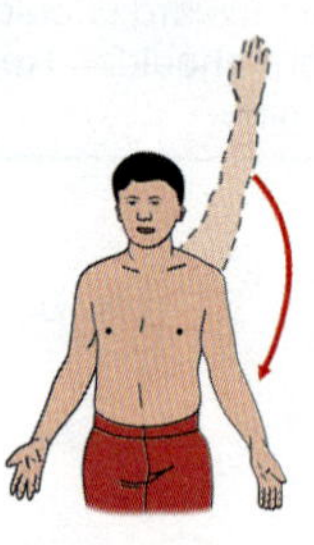

Horizontal adduction
Client instruction: "Lift your arms straight out to the side. Now, move them straight out in front of you and across your chest to your opposite side."

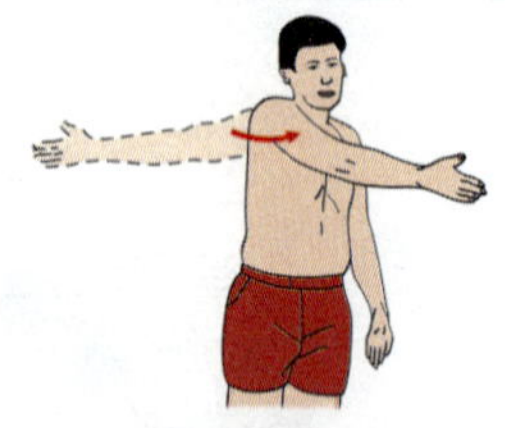

Horizontal abduction
Client instruction: "Bring them back to the beginning position, straight out to the side."

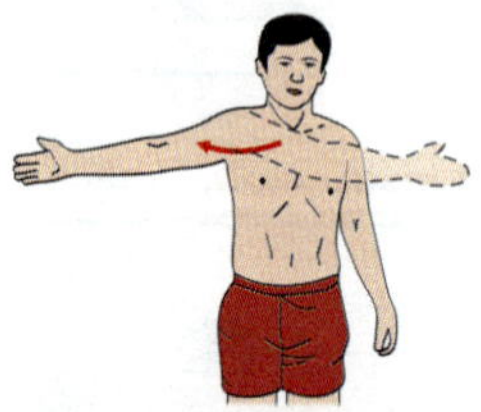

Internal rotation
Client instruction: "Bring your arms straight out to the sides and bend your elbows so your fingers point straight down."

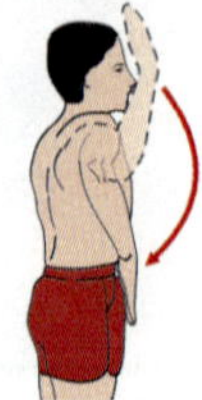

External rotation
Client instruction: "Now rotate your shoulders so your fingers point straight up."

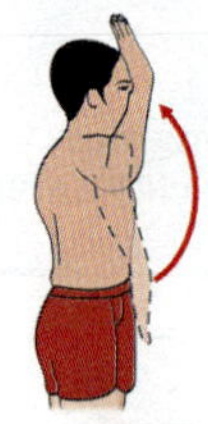

Circumduction
Client instruction: "Move each arm in a large circle."

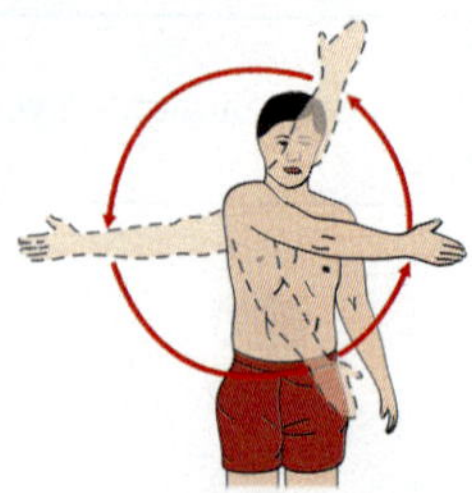

Elevation
Client instruction: "Shrug each shoulder."

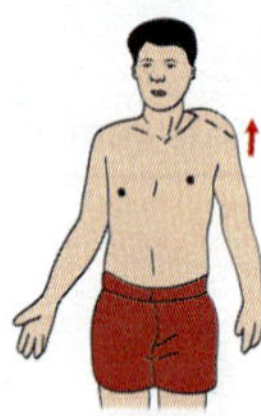

Depression
Client instruction: "Stretch your neck upward while pushing each shoulder down."

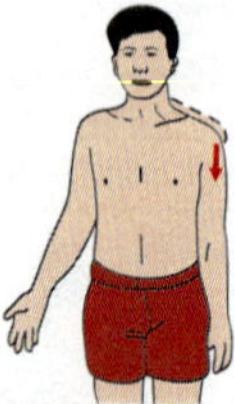

Figure 12.9B: Performing ROM exercises (contd…)

Protraction
Client instruction: "Put your arms out straight in front of you. Now stretch them farther forward from the shoulders."

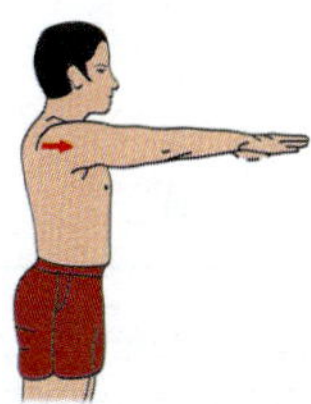

Retraction
Client instruction: "Keep your arms out, bring your shoulders back."

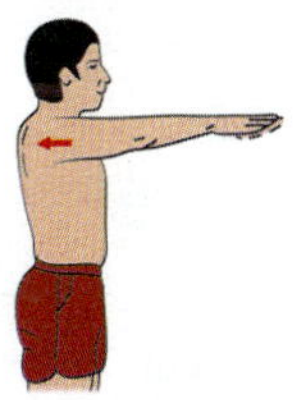

Elbows
Flexion
Client instruction: "With your arms at your sides and your palms facing forward, bring your palms up to touch your shoulders."

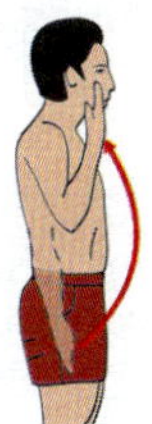

Extension
Client instruction: "Lower your palms to the beginning position."

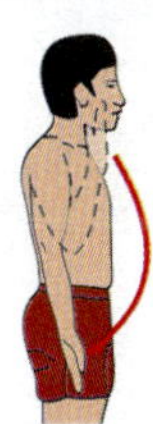

Forearms
Pronation
Client instruction: "With your arms out in front of you, rotate your forearms to turn your palms downward."

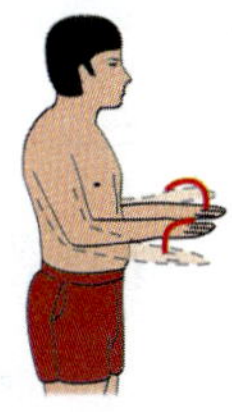

Supination
Client instruction: "Turn your palms back upward again."

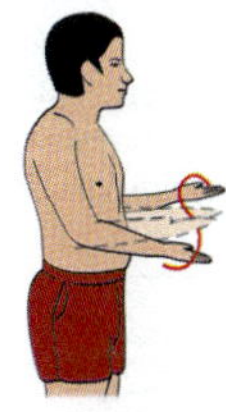

Wrists
Flexion (palmar flexion)
Client instruction: "Turn your palms down and bend your wrists so your fingers point toward the floor."

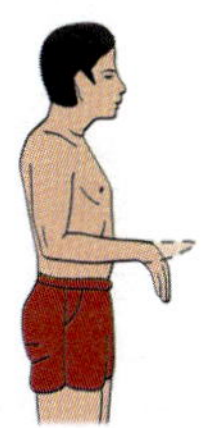

Extension
Client instruction: "Straighten your wrists back out again."

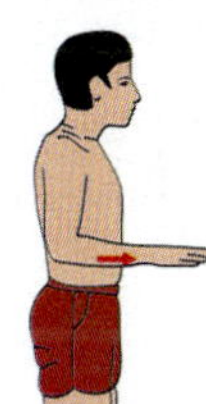

Hyperextension (dorsiflexion)
Client instruction: "Bend your wrists so your fingertips point toward the ceiling."

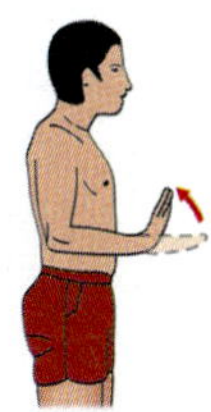

Radial flexion
Client instruction: "Bend your wrists sideways, toward your thumbs."

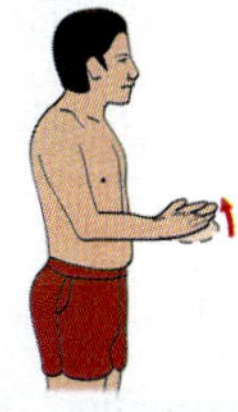

Ulnar flexion
Client instruction: "Bend your wrists in the opposite direction, toward your little fingers."

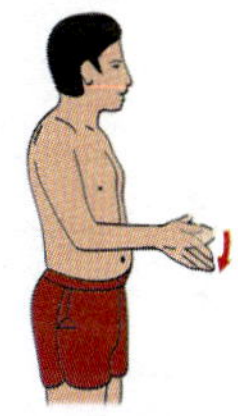

Fingers
Flexion
Client instruction: "Make tight fists."

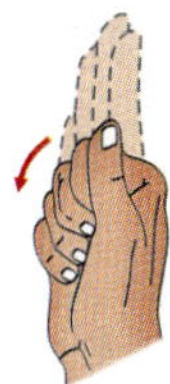

Figure 12.9C: Performing ROM exercises (contd…)

Extension
Client instruction: "Open your hands and straighten your fingers completely."

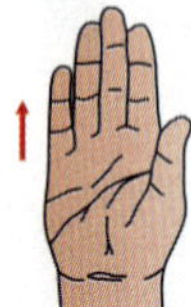

Abduction
Client instruction: "Spread your fingers and thumbs out sideways."

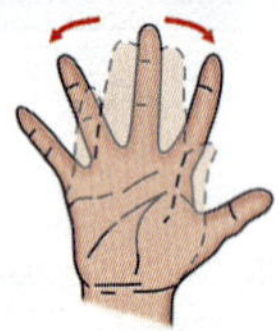

Adduction
Client instruction: "Bring them back together again so that the sides touch."

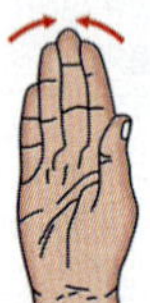

Thumbs
Flexion
Client instruction: "Try to touch the middle of each palm with your thumb tips."

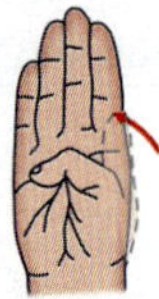

Extension
Client instruction: "Bring your thumbs back to their normal positions."

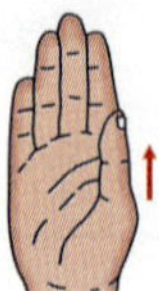

Abduction   (Tested with fingers)

Adduction   (Tested with fingers)

Opposition
Client instruction: "One at a time, touch the tip of your thumb to the tip of each of your other fingers on the same hand."

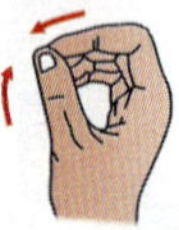

**Hips
(remainder of examination to be done in bed or on examination table. Being in supine position)**
Flexion
Client instruction: "Slowly lift one leg up as high as you can toward your chest. Bring it back down on the bed and rest 5 seconds. Repeat with the opposite leg."

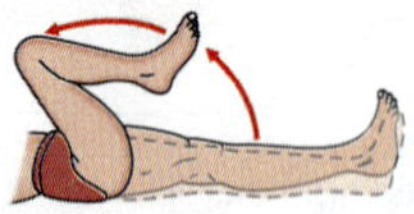

Extension
Client instruction: "Return both legs to a straightened position."

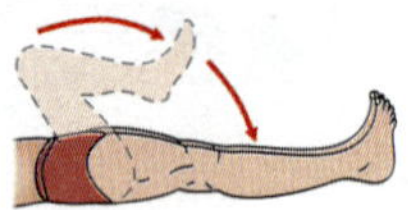

Abduction
Client instruction: "One leg at a time, move your leg out to the side as far as you can."

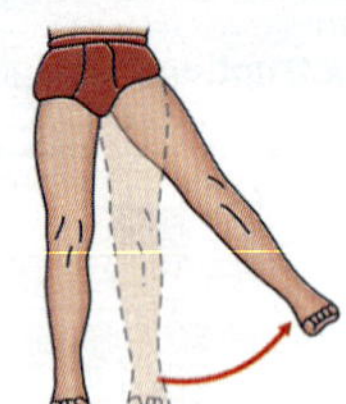

Adduction
Client instruction: "Bring the leg back in place."

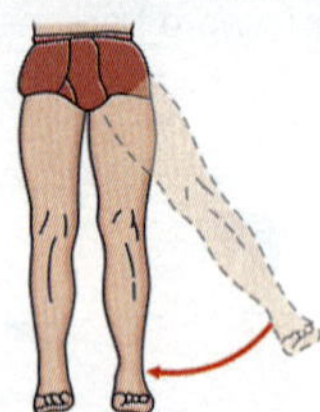

Cross-adduction
Client instruction: "Continue to carry the leg across the body to the opposite side."

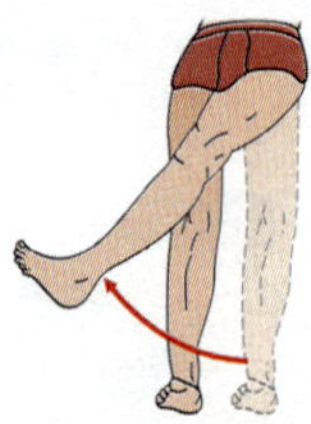

Internal rotation
Client instruction: "With your legs slightly apart, turn your toes inward, toward each other, as far as you can so that your legs roll inward."

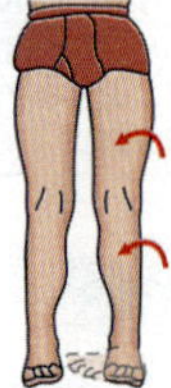

External rotation
Client instruction: "Now turn your toes in the opposite direction as far as you can so your legs roll outward."

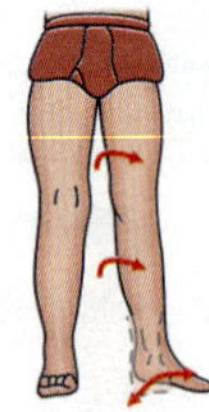

Figure 12.9D: Performing ROM exercises (contd...)

Circumduction
Client instruction: "One leg at a time, move your leg in the largest circle you can."

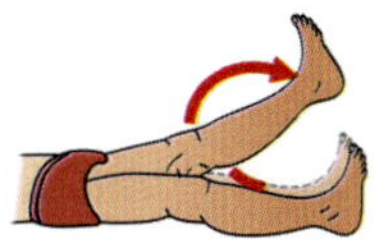

Ankles
Flexion (plantar flexion)
Client instruction: "Point your toes straight down."

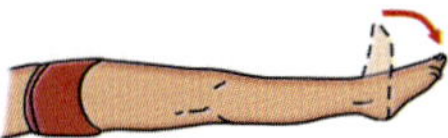

Extension
Client instruction: "Bring your feet back to your normal position."

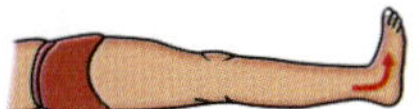

Hyperextension (dorsiflexion)
Client instruction: "Pull your toes up and backward so they point more toward your head."

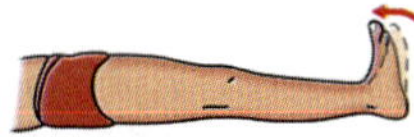

Inversion
Client instruction: "Relax your feet and ankles so the toes point upward. Then, with your feet about 6 inches apart, turn your ankles so each sole faces the other."

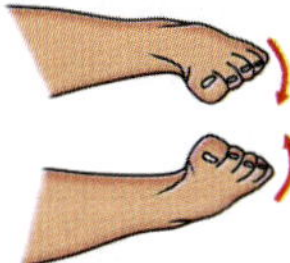

Eversion
Client instruction: "Move your ankles to the opposite side by turning your soles outward, away from each other."

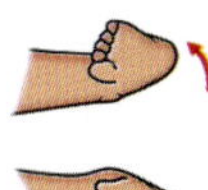

Matatarsals
Inversion
Client instruction: "While I hold your ankles still, try to turn as much of each of your soles toward the other as you can. The toe end of each foot should turn inward."

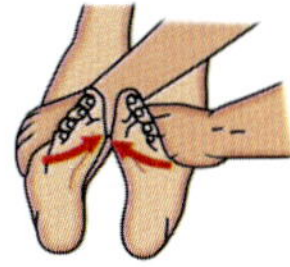

Eversion
Client instruction: "While I hold your ankles still, try to turn as much of each of your soles away from each other as you can. The toe end of each foot should turn outward."

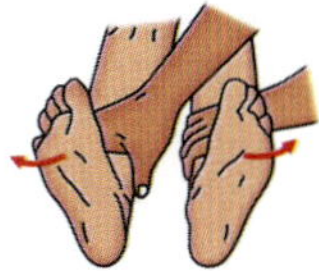

Toes
Flexion
Client instruction: "Make your toes curl up tightly."

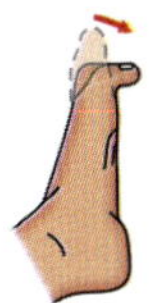

Extension
Client instruction: "Straighten them out."

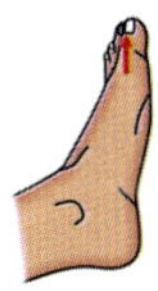

Hyperextension
Client instruction: "Bend them back and toward your head. Straighten them again."

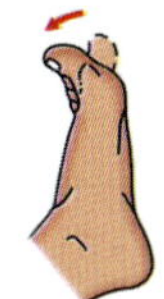

Abduction
Client instruction: "Spread them out."

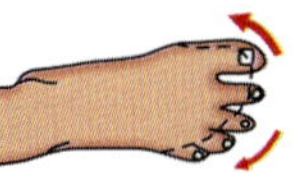

Adduction
Client instruction: "Let them come back together again."

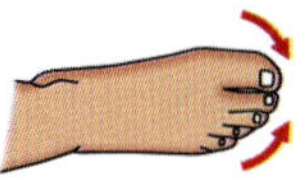

Hips and knees
(turn client to prone position for this assessment)
Hips
Hyperextension
Client instruction: "Lift one leg up off the bed as high as you can. Rest it on the bed for 5 seconds and repeat with the other leg."

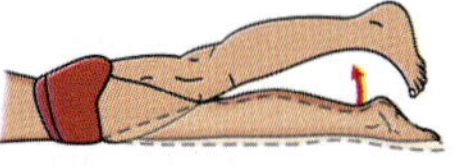

Knees

Flexion
Client instruction: "Bring your heels up toward your buttocks."

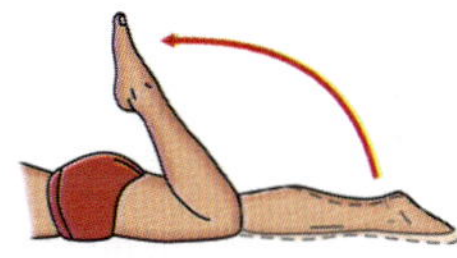

Extension
Client instruction: "Return them to the bed."

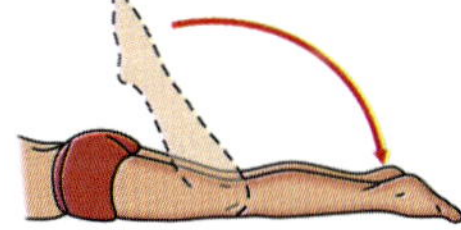

Figure 12.9E: Performing ROM exercises

endurance, mobility, and orientation of the client. Assist with client ambulation, especially if equipment (IV infusions, urinary catheters, closed chest drainage systems, drainage tubes) is present. Evaluate client ambulation to plan the progression of activity.

Clients at high risk for falls include those with prolonged hospitalization, those taking sedatives or tranquilizers, confused clients, or those with a history of physical restraint use. A great majority of falls:

- Occurs in the evening
- Occur in the client's room
- Involve wheelchairs
- Involve confused clients
- Involve clients with poor footwear
- Occur with poor lighting
- Involve clients with poor vision
- Occur with clients experiencing neuromuscular impairment

Awareness of risk factors for falls allows many client injuries to be prevented. When the client is comfortably able to tolerate sitting on the side of the bed and then standing at the side of the bed, progressive ambulation activities can be initiated. Disturbances in balance, coordination, proprioception, as well as weakness, low endurance, and deconditioning often occur as consequences of medical/surgical procedures. These clients need assistance with ambulation.

Continually evaluate the client's strength and endurance during the entire ambulation process.

Before the procedure nurse should:

1. Determine the client's most recent activity level and tolerance to evaluate the client's current ambulatory ability.
2. Assess the client's current status, including vital signs, fatigue, pain, and medications to identify conditions that might adversely affect ambulation.
3. To evaluate the client's environment for safety: Check for handrails to help the client stand and to hold onto while walking. Check that the floor is level, clean, and not slippery or wet. Make sure there is adequate lighting so the client can see where he or she is going.
4. Assess the client's ambulation equipment, including the use of a walker, cane, or other assistive device to determine whether the equipment is in safe condition.
5. Check the client's clothing to determine that the client's shoes or slippers are safe to walk in and that he or she has adequate covering for warmth and privacy.
6. While the client is ambulating, assess his or her gait and bearing. Determines how well he or she is tolerating the activity and allows detection of hypotension, diaphoresis, breathlessness, or weakness.
7. After ambulation, assess the client's ability to recover from the activity, including exhaustion, energy, and recovery times. Determine if modifications need to be made in the distance, type of assistance, or length of time the client is ambulating.

Equipment Needed

- Gait belt (transfer) as needed (PRN)
- Assistive devices
- Shoes or nonslip footwear.

After procedure nurse should see that:

- The client was able to walk a predetermined distance, with assistance as needed, and return to the starting point.
- While walking, the client did not suffer any injury.
- The client was able to increase the distance walked and/or required less assistance to accomplish the distance on a regular basis.

And document in the Nurses Notes as given below:

- Distance the client was able to ambulate and how the client tolerated the ambulation
- Assistive devices the client required and teaching done regarding using the device
- Special concerns or unusual findings observed while ambulating the client

Turning and Positioning a Client (Table 12.8)

Clients are not always able to independently move and position themselves in bed. Proper turning and positioning allows the health care provider to make clients as comfortable as possible, prevent contractures and pressure sores, make portions of the client's body available for treatment or procedures, and allows clients greater access to their environment. There are three key concepts to remember when positioning a client: pressure friction, and skin shear.

Any area that contacts the surface the client is lying on is a pressure site. Because of circulatory compromise, the pressure sites over bony prominences are at the highest risk of skin breakdown and ulceration. Always assess the blood flow to skin and tissue areas put under increased pressure when placing a client in a given position. When repositioning a client, be sure the sheets under the client are smooth. This helps prevent areas of increased pressure that could contribute to pressure sores.

Skin shear is caused when the skin is dragged across a hard surface. The deep layers of skin are torn by the resistance of being dragged. This damage to the skin can lead to skin breakdown and ulceration. To prevent skin shear; or friction burn from the sheets, do not drag a client across the bed. Lift the client into proper position or use a turning sheet.

Friction is caused when the skin is dragged across a rough surface, thereby causing heat and damaging the skin's surface. Any damage to the skin's integrity can lead to infection and skin breakdown.

Clients who cannot reposition themselves must be repositioned at least every two hours and more frequently if they are uncomfortable, incontinent, or have poor circulation, fragile skin, decreased cognition, decreased sensation, or poor nutritional status. When repositioning a client, assess the skin for redness and integrity. Area of redness should be resolved

Table 12.7: Ambulation Safety and Assist Bed to Walking

	Nursing action		*Rationale*
	Cleanse hands Check clients identification band Explain procedure before beginning		To prevent cross infection To identity right patient To get cooperation and reduce anxiety
1.	When assisting a client with an intravenous (IV) infusion, place the IV pole with wheels at the head of the bed before having the client dangle the legs, so there is room to swing the legs from the bed to the floor. If orders allow, place a saline lock on the IV.	1.	Prevents the client's legs from becoming tangled in the IV pole or tubing, causing a fall or causing the tubing to become dislodged. Provides more freedom of movement.
2.	Transfer the IV infusion from the bed IV pole to the portable IV pole. The client or the nurse can guide the portable IV pole ahead during ambulation.	2.	Supports the IV while the client ambulates.
3.	When assisting the client with a urinary drainage bag, empty the drainage bag before ambulation. Have the client sit on the side of the bed with legs dangling. Remove the urinary drainage bag from the bed. The nurse or client can hold the urinary drainage bag during ambulation. Make sure the drainage bag remains below the level of the bladder.	3.	Emptying the bag reduces the weight of the bag. An empty bag kept below the level of the bladder reduces the risk of urine flowing back into the bladder, and, hence, reduces risk of contamination. Having the nurse hold the drainage bag allows the client to concentrate on safe ambulation.
4.	When the client has a drainage tube such as a T-tube, hemovac, or Jackson-Pratt drainage system, be sure to secure the drainage tube and bag before ambulation. Place a rubber band around the drainage tube near the drainage bag. Secure the drainage tube and bag with a safety pin through the rubber band. Allow slack. The safety pin can be secured to the client's gown or robe.	4.	Prevents the tubing from becoming dislodged or tangled in clothing or other tubes.
5.	Ambulating the client with a closed chest tube drainage system often requires two nurses, one assisting the client and one nurse managing the closed chest tube drainage system. While the client is sitting on the edge of the bed with feet dangling, remove the hangers from the drainage system. Hold the closed chest tube drainage system upright at all times to maintain the water seal. Do not pull or tug on the chest tubes; they may not be sutured into place.	5.	Two nurses allow one to focus on the client's safety and ambulation while the other focuses on maintaining the chest drainage system and keeping tubes from becoming dislodged.
6.	Use a transfer belt or gait belt when ambulating a client who is weak. For additional safety, a wheelchair can be pushed alongside the client for ready access if the client feels weak, tired, or faint.	6.	The transfer belt is a 2-inch-wide webbed belt worn by the client for stabilization during transfers and ambulation. It provides more support for the client by having the nurse hold the back of the belt.
7.	If a client feels faint or dizzy during dangling, return the client to a supine position in bed and lower the head of the bed. Monitor the client's blood pressure and pulse.	7.	Keeps the client from falling from the bed. Lowering the head of the bed will allow gravity to support blood flow to the brain in the hypotensive client.
8.	If the client feels faint or dizzy during ambulation, allow the client to sit in a chair. Stay with the client for safety. Request another nurse to secure a wheelchair if not already available to return the client to bed.	8.	May stop the client from progressing to full syncope.
9.	If the client feels faint or dizzy during ambulation and starts to fall, ease the client to the floor while supporting and protecting the client's head. Position yourself next to and slightly behind the ambulating client, thus being able to step behind the client and safely ease the client to the floor. Ask other personnel to assist you in returning the client to bed. Assess orthostatic blood pressures.	9.	Easing the client to the floor prevents injury to the client.

Contd...

Table 12.7: *Contd...*

	Nursing action		Rationale
10.	Encourage the client to void before ambulating, especially with elderly clients.	10.	Prevents need to interrupt ambulation. Restroom may not be readily available.

Bed to walking

	Nursing action		Rationale
1.	Inform client of the purposes and distance of the walking exercise.	1.	Reduces client anxiety and increases cooperation.
2.	Elevate the head of the bed and wait several minutes.	2.	Prevents orthostatic hypotension.
3.	Lower the bed height.	3.	Reduces distance client has to step down, thus decreasing risk of injury.
4.	Encourage client to actively move legs, or this may be done passively.	4.	Stimulates flow of blood, especially elevation of systolic blood pressure to prevent possible orthostatic hypotension.
5.	With one arm on the client's back and one arm under the client' upper legs, move the client into the dangling position.	5.	Provides client support and reduces risk of falling.
6.	Encourage client to dangle at side of bed for several minutes.	6.	Prevents orthostatic hypotension. Allows for assessing tolerance for the sitting position.
7.	Place gait belt around client's waist; secure the buckle in front. Place ambulation device such as a walker within reach of the client, if necessary. Assist client into standing position. Make sure bed is locked and floor is not slippery. Client shoes should have nonslip soles.	7.	Provides handholds for the caregiver to support the client. Provides for client and caregiver safety.
8.	Stand in front of client with your knees touching client's knees.	8.	Prevents client from sliding forward if dizziness or faintness occurs.
9.	Place arms under client's axilla.	9.	Supports client's trunk.
10.	Assist client to a standing position, allowing client time to balance.	10.	Reduces risk of fall.
11.	If client is able to proceed with ambulating, assume a position beside the client and assist the client as necessary using the gait belt. Place yourself in a guarding position so as to assist client quickly and safely, if necessary. Use additional assistance, as necessary.	11.	Provides for client and caregiver safety.
12.	Following ambulation, return client to bed, remove gait belt, and monitor vital signs, as necessary. Make the client comfortable, and make sure all lines and tubes are secure.	12.	Promotes safety and comfort.
13.	Place the call light within reach of the client.	13.	Provides for client safety.
14.	Move the bedside table close to the bed and place items of frequent use within reach of the client.	14.	Provides for client safety.
15	Cleanse hands.	15	Reduces the transmission of microorganisms.

before the client is repositioned on that area. Areas of redness that do not resolve within 30 minutes after pressure relief should be documented. A plan to reposition the client more frequently may need to be instituted. Area of prolonged redness are more likely to sustain tissue damage, as are tissue areas covering bony prominences. Hip, back, neck, or head conditions may require that a client be turned keeping the body in alignment, turning as one unit, as a log. This is called log rolling. Remember that proper body mechanics are essential to protect the caregiver's back and to ensure client safety.

Prior to the procedure nurse should:

1. Assess the client's ability to move independently. Determine if the client can assist with turning and repositioning.
2. Assess the client's flexibility. If clients have contractures or other flexibility limitations, their positions may need to be modified to allow for the restrictions.
3. Assess the client's age, medical diagnosis, cognitive status, skin integrity, nutritional status, continence, altered sensation, as well as the overall condition of the musculoskeletal system. Helps determine the client's potential for pressure sore development.
4. Assess the physician's or qualified practitioner's orders for specific restrictions regarding client positioning to ensure the correct positioning is implemented.

Equipment Needed

- Pillows
- Rolled blankets or towels
- Footboard
- Heel protectors
- Hand rolls
- Gloves (if chance of exposure to body fluids).

Table 12.8: Turning and Positioning a Client			
	Nursing action		*Rationale*
	Check clients identification band Explain procedure before beginning		To identity right patient To get cooperation and reduce anxiety
1.	Cleanse hands.	1.	Reduces the transmission of microorganisms.
2.	Gather all necessary equipment. Provide for client privacy.	2.	Ensure client dignity and allows for a smooth procedure.
3.	Secure adequate assistance to safely complete task.	3.	Prevents caregiver back and muscle strain as well as provides for client safety.
4.	Adjust bed to comfortable working height. Lower side rail on side of bed from which you are assisting client.	4.	Prevents caregiver back and muscle strain.
5.	Follow proper body mechanics guidelines: When moving a client in bed, position the bed so that your legs are slightly bent at the knees and hips. Maintain the natural curves in your back while lifting. Position one foot slightly in front of the other and spreads feet apart to create a wide base for balance. When your arms are placed under the client, slowly lean backward onto your back leg using your body weight to help you lift the client to one side of the bed. Do not extend or rotate your back to move a client in bed. If you cannot move the client easily, always ask for and obtain assistance for both your and the client's safety. Be sure the floor is not slippery and that the bed is locked. Always use a turning sheet when rolling a client because this gives you better support and control of the client.	5.	Prevents caregiver back injury and muscle strain and promotes client safety. Spreading feet to create a wide base helps prevent loss of balance.
6.	Position drains, tubes and IVs to accommodate for new client position.	6.	Prevents accidental dislodgment and/or discomfort from movement by reduced mechanical tension.
7.	Place or assist client into appropriate starting position. Monitor client status, and provide adequate rest breaks or support as necessary.	7.	Prevents client injury.

Contd...

Table 12.8: *Contd...*

	Nursing action		Rationale
Moving from Supine to Side-Lying Position			
8.	Slide your hands underneath the client. Move the client to one side of the bed by lifting the client's body toward you in stages-first the upper trunk, then the lower trunk, and finally the legs. Lift the client's body; do not drag the client across the sheets. Move to other side of bed. Roll the client to side-lying position by placing the client's inside arm next to the client's body with the palm of the hand against the hip. Cross the client's outside arm and leg toward midline and log roll the client toward you using the client's outside shoulder and hip for leverage while maintaining stability and control of top arm and leg.	8.	Prevents shearing of skin tissue. Maintains client body alignment. Protects caregiver's back and prevents muscle strain. Prevents client injury and shearing of skin tissue.
Maintaining Side-Lying Position			
9.	Repeat Action 1-8.	9.	See Rationales 1-8.
10.	Pillows may be placed to support the client's head and arms. An additional pillow may be used to support the topside leg, and fully and equally support the thigh, knee, ankle, and foot. Move the lower arm forward slightly at the shoulder and bend the elbow for comfort. If the client is unstable, a pillow placed against the back will provide additional support and keep the client from rolling supine.	10.	Provides support and comfort.
Moving from Side-Lying to Prone Position			
11.	Repeat Actions 1-8.	11.	See Rationales 1-8.
12.	Remove positioning towels, pillows, or other support devices. Assess whether the client's position in bed needs to be adjusted to accommodate the continued movement into prone. Move the client's inside arm next to the client's body with palm against hip. Roll the client onto the stomach using the shoulder and hip as key points of control. The head must be placed in a comfortable position to one side without excessive pressure to sensitive areas. Pillows under the trunk are placed as needed to relieve pressure and increase comfort. The client's arms are placed comfortably at the client's side and the legs are uncrossed with the feet approximately a foot apart.	12.	Ensures comfort and safety in movement.
Maintaining Prone Position			
13.	A shallow pillow or a folded towel may be used to support the client's head comfortably as well as a pillow placed under the abdomen to support the back. An additional pillow may be placed under the lower leg to reduce the pressure of the toes and forefoot against the bed.	13.	Provides support and comfort.
Moving from Prone to Supine Position			
14.	Repeat Actions 1-8.	14.	See Rationales 1-8.

Contd...

Table 12.8: *Contd...*	
Nursing action	*Rationale*
15. Remove positioning towels, pillows, or other supporting devices. Slide your hands underneath the client. Move the client segmentally to one side of the bed to accommodate the new position. Position the inside arm next to the client's body with the client's palm next to the hip. Roll the client to supine by log rolling the client toward you using the client's outside shoulder and hip for leverage. Have the client's face positioned away from the direction of the roll to prevent undue pressure to the face or neck. When the client reaches supine, uncross the client's arms and legs and place them comfortably into anatomic positions.	15. Provides support and comfort.
Maintaining Supine Position	
16. A footboard may be used to support the foot as well as heel protectors or a pillow placed between the heel and gastrocnemius muscle to reduce the pressure on the heels. Assess and compare warmth, sensation, color, and movement of feet. To prevent excessive external rotation of the lower extremity, a trochanter roll may be used. For comfort, additional pillows may be used to support the client's head, arms, or lower back.	16. Provides support and comfort. Heel protectors and routine assessment of the feet help to prevent pressure sores. Trochanter rolls and pillows help to prevent displacement of the acetabulum (hip joint).
Log Rolling	
17. Repeat Actions 1-8.	17. See Rationales 1-8.
18. Use three nurses. Place a turning/draw sheet under client's head, back, and buttocks (if not already present).	18. Provides for client safety. Reduces shearing force.
19. Place pillow between client's legs.	19. Keeps legs in alignment with body.
20. Have client fold arms across chest.	20. Prevents getting the client's arms trapped or injured.
21. Roll up draw sheet on the far side until it is next to the client.	21. Provides support under the heavy parts of the client and places the nurses hands close to the weight to be turned.
22. One nurse places hands under the client's far leg, another holds rolled draw sheet at client's buttocks, and third nurse holds rolled draw sheet at chest and shoulder level.	22. Ensures client is turned like a log, as a unit.
23. Nurse nearest the client's head gives the signal to turn; 1-2-3 turn.	23. Ensures a smooth, coordinated turn.
24. Tuck pillows at client's back and abdomen.	24. Helps maintain side-lying position.
25. Assess the client for comfort and proper alignment.	25. Comfort is subjective. Ensure alignment.
26. Procedure can be reversed to reposition client on back or opposite side.	26. Reduces pressure ulcer development.
27. Be sure to replace side rails to upright position as well as to lower bed to beginning position.	27. Provides for client safety.
28. Place call light within reach of the client.	28. Provides for client safety.
29. Move bedside table close to bed and place items of frequent use within reach of the client.	29. Provides for client safety.
30. Cleanse hands.	30. Reduces the transmission of microorganisms.

After procedure nurse should observe the following:
- Safe and proper body alignment and movement were achieved for both client and caregiver.
- The client is comfortable in the new position as evident by verbal and nonverbal cues.
- The client's skin and underlying organs and tissues were protected from pressure, friction, and shear.

And document in the Nurses' notes:
- Client's new position and time of the position change
- Report or observation of pain, discomfort, or dyspnea
- Integumentary assessment, including color and integrity of skin and length of time redness persists over bony prominences.

Moving a Client in Bed (Table 12.9)

Prolonged immobility is uncomfortable and presents an increased risk of many complications. Muscle wasting, clot formation, and skin breakdown are the most common risks associated with immobility. Clients who are unable to move themselves in bed or are only able to assist with moving in bed are at risk for discomfort and complications related to immobility. Often, clients' restlessness in bed will cause them to slide down toward the foot of the bed. This is especially true in beds where the head raises up to a Fowler's or semi-Fowler's position. If the client slides down toward the foot of the bed while the beds where the head raises up to a Fowler's or semi-Fowler's position. If the client slides down toward the foot of the bed while the head is elevated, it can lead to reduced respiratory effort, reduced lung capacity, and skin breakdown, thus impairing the client's recovery.

The Nurse is often called on to move a client to a more comfortable position. Repositioning a client can sometimes be done by a single staff member, but often it requires two or more people to do this procedure safely.

Before the procedure nurse should:
1. Assess the client's ability to assist with repositioning. Determine if the client can move with the aid of an overhead trapeze or the side rail. Judge how much assistance will be needed. Determines safety for the client and the nurse and good body mechanics for the nurse.
2. Assess the client's ability to understand and follow directions and assist and cooperate with the move. Affects how the procedure will be carried out. Affects client teaching.
3. Assess the client's environment. Check the bed for cleanliness. Has the client been restless, sweaty, or incontinent? Check to see if the sheets have been turned or twisted. Tubes, lines, wires, traction, casts, or splints must be moved carefully. Affects how the procedure will be carried out. Affects what additional procedures will be performed. Prepares the caregivers to keep tubes and equipment from becoming dislodged or tipping or pulling.

Equipment Needed

- Hospital bed with side rails
- Trapeze if required
- Turn sheet or draw sheet.

After the procedure nurse should see that:
- The client was moved without injury to self or staff.
- The client reported an increase in comfort following the move.
- All tubes, lines, and drains remained intact.

And document in the Nurses' notes:
- Time and position the client was moved
- Unusual findings.

Transferring from Bed to Wheelchair, Commode, or Chair (Table 12.10)

Client activity is an important part of the healing process. Activity improves muscle tone, increases venous return to the heart and stimulates peristalsis. Moving a client from the bed to a chair is an important part of client activity.

Moving a client from the bed to a chair, wheelchair commode, or stretcher is called a transfer. Transferring a client requires good planning to avoid injury to the client and the nurse. When transferring a client, consider the client's ability to assist with the transfer. If the client is unable to provide any assistance or is large, on or more staff members may be needed to help perform the transfer safely.

The most frequent complication in transferring a client is falling during the transfer. If a client does start to fall while being transferred, lower him or her gently to the floor, making sure the head does not strike anything. If a client does fall, obtain assistance and perform a thorough assessment of the client before moving him or her.

Another possible hazard in client transfers is pulling on or dislodging indwelling tubes or catheters. Think ahead about ways tubes will move with the transfer and try to avoid snagging them. Take care to appropriately anchor all tubes and catheters before transferring a client.

Clients are also at risk of damage to the skin during a transfer sliding across the sheets, side rails, and wheelchair armrest can bruise or injure the client. Use a transfer board or pad any sharp exposed areas to help prevent injury to the client.

Be sure the client is wearing should sappers with firm, non slip soles when transferring a client. Even if the client will be standing only briefly, the feet need to protected from potential injury and contamination from the floor and the client from slipping.

When transferring a client with slides on one side of the body, use the "Good to go" maxim. This means that the client needs to lead off with the "good" one side of the body. Perform the transfer in the direction of the good side, so the client pivots and supports the weight on the body inside. This allows maximum strength and stability on the client's part.

Table 12.9: Moving a Client in Bed

	Nursing action		Rationale
	Check clients identification band Explain procedure before beginning		To identity right patient To get cooperation and reduce anxiety
1.	Cleanse hands.	1.	Reduces the transmission of microorganisms.
2.	Elevate bed to just below waist height. Lower head of bed if tolerated by client. Lower side rails on the side where you are standing.	2.	Lessens strain on nurse's back muscles.
3.	Remove the pillow and place it against the headboard.	3.	Prevents having to move against the pillow. Provides padding of the headboard if the client should be moved too high in the bed.
4.	Have client hold on to the overhead trapeze, if available.	4.	Promotes client autonomy by allowing the client to assist with the move.
5.	Have the client bend the knees and place the feet flat on the bed if available.	5.	Allows the client to assist in the move; promotes client autonomy.
6.	Stand at an angle to the head of the bed, feet apart, knees bent, feet toward the head of the bed.	6.	Promotes good body mechanics.
7.	Slide one hand and arm under the client's shoulder, the other under the client's thigh.	7.	Distributes the client's weight more evenly. Promotes good lifting technique.
8.	Rock forward toward the head of the bed, lifting the client with you. Simultaneously have the client push with the legs.	8.	Allows a smooth motion to lift the client. Client assistance lessens strain on nurse's back muscles; promotes client autonomy.
9.	If the client has a trapeze, have the client pull up holding onto the trapeze as you move the client upward in bed.	9.	Client assistance lessens strain on nurse's back muscles; promotes client autonomy.
10.	Repeat these steps until the client is moved up high enough in bed.	10.	Large or very immobile clients are often not moved far enough in one step.
11.	Return the client's pillow under the head.	11.	Promotes client comfort.
12.	Elevate head of bed, if tolerated by client.	12.	Promotes comfort; facilitates eating and drinking; facilitates communication.
13.	Assess client for comfort.	13.	Comfort is subjective.
14.	Adjust the client's bedclothes as needed for comfort.	14.	Promotes comfort.
15.	Lower bed and elevate side rails.	15.	Promotes client safety.
16.	Cleanse hands.	16.	Reduces the transmission of microorganisms.

Contd...

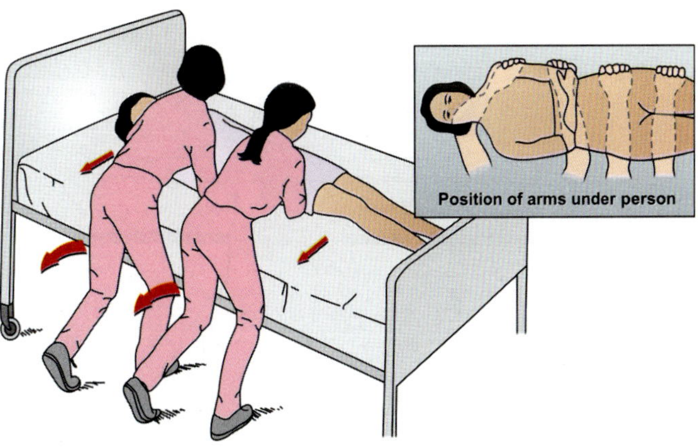

Figure 12.10: Two nurses moving helpless patient in bed

<table>
<tr><td colspan="2" align="center">Table 12.9: Contd...</td></tr>
<tr><td>Nursing action</td><td>Rationale</td></tr>
</table>

Moving a client up in bed with two or more nurses (Fig. 12.10)

#	Nursing action	#	Rationale
17.	Cleanse hands and apply gloves if needed.	17.	Reduces the transmission of microorganisms.
18.	Elevate bed to just below waist height. Lower head of bed if tolerated by client. Lower side rails.	18.	Lessens strain on nurses' back muscles.
19.	With two nurses, place turn/draw sheet under client's back and head.	19.	Reduces shearing force, which can precipitate skin breakdown.
20.	Roll up the draw sheet on each side until it is next to the client	20.	Provides support under the heavy parts of the body and places the nurse's hands close to the weight to be moved.
21.	Follow Actions 3-5.	21.	See Rationales 3-5.
22.	The nurses stand on either side of the bed, at an angle to the head of the bed, with knees flexed, feet apart in a wide stance.	22.	Promotes good body mechanics.
23.	The nurses hold their elbows as close as possible to their bodies.	23.	Allows the muscle of the torso to assist the arm muscles in bearing and moving the weight of the client.
24.	The lead nurse gives the signal to move; 1-2-3 go. The nurses will lift up (off the bed) on the turn/draw sheet and forward (toward the head of the bed) in one smooth motion (Fig. 12.11). The move is coordinated to transfer the client toward the head of the bed. Simultaneously, have the client push with the legs or pull using the trapeze.	24.	Allows a smooth motion to lift the client. Client assistance lessens strain on the nurses' back muscles; promotes client autonomy.
25.	Repeat until the client is moved up high enough in bed to be comfortable.	25.	Large or very immobile clients are often not moved far enough in one step.
26.	Return the client's pillow under the head.	26.	Promotes client comfort.
27.	Elevate head of bed, if tolerated by client.	27.	Promotes comfort; facilitates eating and drinking; facilitates communication.
28.	Assess client for comfort.	28.	Promotes comfort.
29.	Adjust the client's bedclothes for comfort.	29.	Promotes comfort.
30.	Lower bed and elevate side rails.	30.	Promotes client safety.
31.	Cleanse hands.	31.	Reduces the transmission of microorganisms.

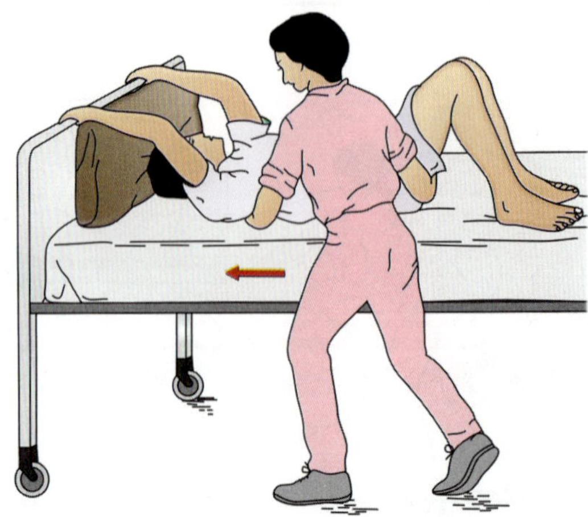

Figure 12.11: One nurse moving client in bed

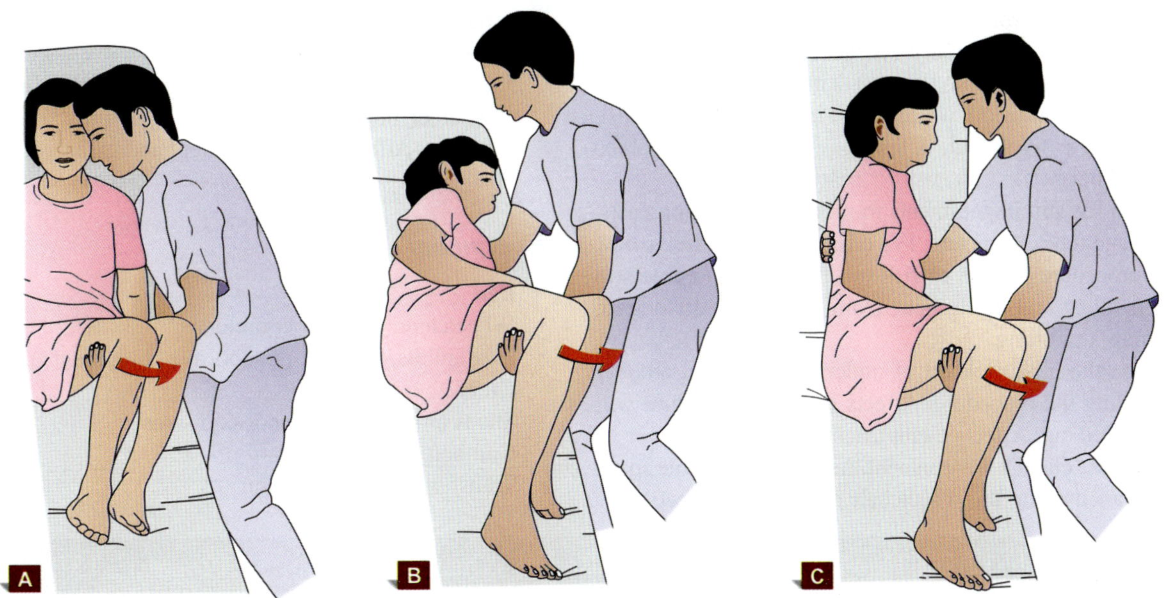

Figure 12.12: Transferring client from bed to wheel chair

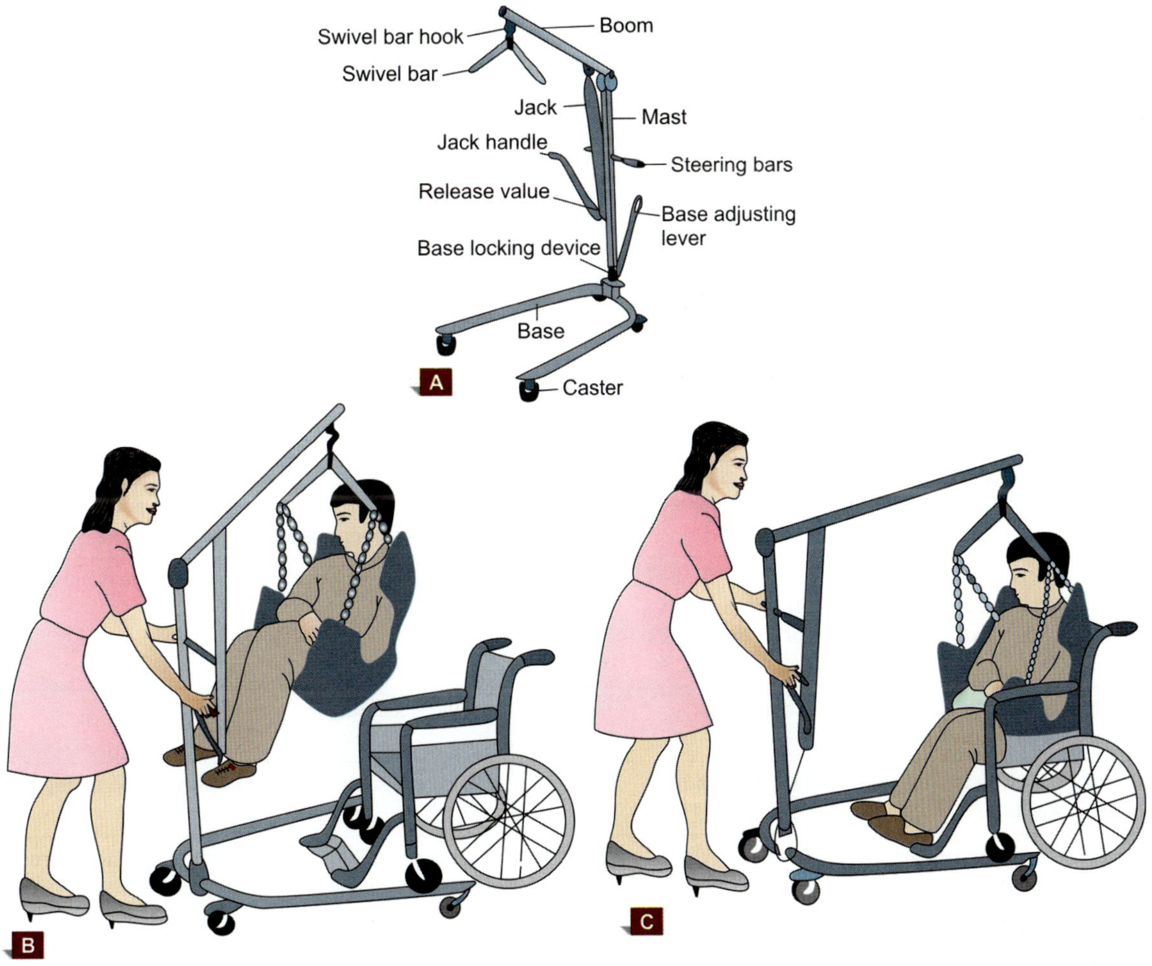

Figure 12.13: Transferring client to a wheel chair using a mechanical patient lift

Before the procedure nurse should:
1. Assess the client's current level of mobility. Determine how much the client is able to assist with the transfer. Assess for pain or confusion, which might impair ability to assist. Check for a "weak" side Affects how the procedure will be carried out.
2. Assess for any impediments to mobility, including casts, drainage tubes, catheters, IVs or intubations. Affects how the procedure will be carried out. Prepares caregivers to keep tubes and equipment from becoming dislodged, tipping, or pulling.
3. Assess the client's level of under standing and anxiety regarding the procedure. Affects how the procedure will be carried out. Affects client teaching.
4. Assess the client's environment. Assess the available space for maneuvering the wheelchair to the bed. Affects how the procedure will be carried out. Affects safety and good body, mechanics for caregivers.
5. Assess the equipment. Check the bed and chair height. See whether they are adjustable for footings and wheelchair brakes. Affects safety for client and caregivers.

Equipment Needed

- Bed
- Wheelchair, chair, or commode
- Any splints, braces, or supportive equipment specific to the client
- Shoes or slippers with nonskid soles
- Gait belt
- Transfer board (if necessary).

Table 12.10: Transferring Client from Bed to Wheel Chair (Figs 12.12 and 12.13)

	Nursing action		*Rationale*
	Check clients identification band Explain procedure before beginning		To identity right patient To get cooperation and reduce anxiety
1.	Cleanse hands.	1.	Reduces the transmission of microorganisms.
2.	Assess client for ability to assist with the transfer and for presence of cognitive sensory deficits.	2.	Allows planning regarding the amount of assistance and cooperation to expect from the client.
3.	Lock the bed in position.	3.	Prevents the bed from rolling during the procedure.
4.	Place any splints, braces, or other devices on the client.	4.	Provides support and prevents injury to the client.
5.	Place the client's shoes or slippers on the client's feet.	5.	Provides a nonslip surface for stability.
6.	Lower the height of the bed to lowest possible position.	6.	Reduces distance client has to step down, thus decreasing risk of injury.
7.	Slowly raise the head of the bed if this is not contraindicated by the client's condition.	7.	Minimizes lifting.
8.	Place one arm under the client's legs and one arm behind the client's back. Slowly pivot the client so the client's legs are dangling over the edge of the bed and the client is in a sitting position on the edge of the bed.	8.	Supports the client while sitting him or her upright.
9.	Allow client to dangle for 2 to 5 minutes. Help support client if necessary.	9.	Allows time for assessing client's response to sitting; reduces possibility of orthostatic hypotension.
10.	Bring the chair or wheelchair close to the side of the bed. Place it at a 45-degree angle to the bed. If the client has a weaker side, place the chair or wheelchair on the client's strong side.	10.	Minimizes transfer distance. Allows the client to pivot on the stronger leg.
11.	Lock wheelchair brakes and elevate the foot pedals. For chairs, lock brakes if available.	11.	Provides stability.
12.	If using a gait belt to assist the client, place it around the client's waist.	12.	Provides a secure handhold for the nurse during the transfer.
13.	Assist client to side of bed until feet are firmly on the floor and slightly apart.	13.	Moves client into proper position for transfer. Provides stable footing for client.
14.	Grasp the sides of the gait belt or place your hands just below the client's axilla. Using a wide stance, bend your knees and assist the client to a standing position.	14.	Wide stances increases nurse stability and minimizes strain on the back. Avoids putting pressure directly on the axilla, and risking never damage or shoulder subluxation.

Contd...

<table>
<tr><td colspan="4" align="center">**Table 12.10:** *Contd...*</td></tr>
<tr><td colspan="2">*Nursing action*</td><td colspan="2">*Rationale*</td></tr>
<tr><td>15.</td><td>Standing close to the client, pivot until the client's back is toward the chair.</td><td>15.</td><td>Moves client into proper position to be seated.</td></tr>
<tr><td>16.</td><td>Instruct the client to place hands on the arm supports, or place the client's hands on the arm supports of the chair.</td><td>16.</td><td>Allows client to gain balance and judge distance to seat.</td></tr>
<tr><td>17.</td><td>Bend at the knees and ease the client into a sitting position.</td><td>17.</td><td>Increases stability ands minimizes strain on back.</td></tr>
<tr><td>18.</td><td>Assist client to maintain proper posture. Support weak side with pillow if needed.</td><td>18.</td><td>Increases client comfort.</td></tr>
<tr><td>19.</td><td>Secure the safety belt, place client's feet on feet pedals, and release brakes if you will be moving the client immediately. Make sure tubes and lines, arms, and hands are not pinched or caught between the client and the chair. If the client is sitting in a chair, offer a footstool if available.</td><td>19.</td><td>Ensures client safety; prepares client for movement.</td></tr>
<tr><td>20.</td><td>Cleanse hands.</td><td>20.</td><td>Reduces the transmission of microorganisms.</td></tr>
</table>

After the procedure nurse should see that:

- Client was transferred from the bed to the wheelchair without pain or injury.
- Drainage tubes, IVs, or other devices remain intact.
- Client's skin is intact and undamaged.

And document in the Nurses' notes

- Client's tolerance of the activity, any aids that were required, how much assistance was required, and the client's ability to assist
- Unusual events during the transfer

Transferring from Bed to Stretcher (Fig. 12.14 and Table 12.11)

Some clients are not strong enough to sit erect in a wheelchair or have some injury that prevents them from sitting, so they must be moved while lying flat. The most commonly used equipment for transferring a client is a stretcher (gurney). A stretcher is a narrow, cart like bed that rolls on wheels on a stretchers are equipped with side rails or safety straps to prevent accidental falls during transport. The wheels on a stretcher lock to prevent accidental movement during client transfers.

Before the procedure nurse should:

1. Assess the client's current level of mobility. Knowing whether a client is able to assist with the transfer will affect how the transfer is performed.
2. Assess for injury. Caregivers may need to keep the client in the same alignment as much as possible.
3. Assess for any impediments to mobility such as a cast, drainage tubes, IVs, or intubation. This will affect how the transfer is performed.
4. Assess the client's level of understanding of the procedure. This will affect client comfort, anxiety, and cooperation.
5. Assess the client's environment. Assess how close the stretcher will move to the bed. Assess the height of the bed. This allows for a safe transfer. Plan for good body mechanics.
6. Make sure the stretcher is safe to use. Check for working brakes, side rails, safety straps that are intact and usable, and an IV pole attachment if needed. This allows for a safe transfer. Plan for good body mechanics.

Equipment Needed

Transferring a Client with Minimum Assistance
- Bed
- Stretcher.

Transferring a Client with Maximum Assistance
- Bed
- Stretcher
- Pillows
- Transfer/slider boards
- Lift sheet
- Other qualified personnel to assist.

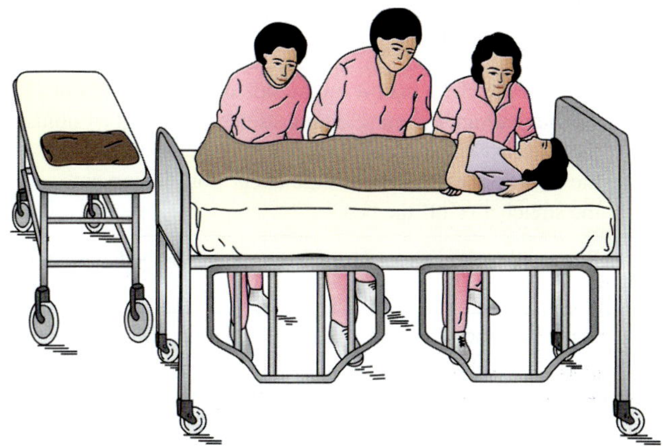

Figure 12.14: Transferring client from bed to stretcher

Table 12.11: Transferring Client from Bed to Stretcher (Fig. 12.15)

	Nursing action		*Rationale*
	Check clients identification band		To identity right patient
	Explain procedure before beginning		To get cooperation and reduce anxiety

Minimum Assistance

	Nursing action		Rationale
1.	Cleanse hands.	1.	Reduces the transmission of microorganisms.
2.	Raise the height of bed to 1 inch higher than the stretcher and lock brakes of bed.	2.	Reduces distance nurse must bend, thus preventing back strain; prevents bed from moving.
3.	Instruct client to move to side of bed close to stretcher. Lower side rails of bed an stretcher. Leave side rails on opposite side up.	3.	Decreases risk of client falling.
4.	Stand at outer side of stretcher and push it toward bed.	4.	Diminishes the gap between bed and stretcher; secures the stretcher position.
5.	Instruct client to move onto stretcher with assistance as needed.	5.	Promotes client independence.
6.	Cover client to move onto stretcher with assistance as needed.	6.	Promotes comfort; protects privacy.
7.	Cover client with sheet or bath blanket.	7.	Prevents falls.
8.	Elevate side rails on stretcher and secure safety belts about client. Release brakes of stretcher.	8.	Pushing, not pulling, ensures proper body mechanics.
9.	Cleanse hands.	9.	Reduces the transmission of microorganisms.

Maximum Assistance

	Nursing action		Rationale
10.	Repeat Actions 1 and 2.	10.	See Rationales 1 and 2.
11.	Assess amount of assistance required for transfer. Usually 2 to 4 staff members are required for the maximum-assisted transfer.	11.	Promotes client independence; ensures that enough staff are present before beginning transfer.
12.	Lock wheels of bed and stretcher.	12.	Prevents falls.
13.	Have one nurse stand close to client's head.	13.	Supports client's head during the move.
14.	Log roll the client (keep in straight alignment) and place a lift sheet under the client's back, trunk, and upper legs. The lift sheet can extend under the head if client lacks head control abilities.	14.	Prevents flexion and rotation of client's hips and spine; maintains correct body alignment.
15.	Empty all drainage bags (e.g. T-tube, Hemo Vac, Jackson-Pratt). Record amounts. Secure drainage system to client's gown before transfer.	15.	Decreases possibility og spills; prevents dislodging of tubes.
16.	Move client to edge of bed near stretcher. Lift up and over to avoid dragging.	16.	Prevents dragging, which causes shearing force.
17.	Because the client is now on the side of the bed, without the side rail up, the nurse on nonstretcher side of bed holds the stretcher side of the lift sheet up (by reaching across the client's chest) to prevent the client from falling onto the stretcher or off the bed.	17.	Protects the client from falling.
18.	Place pillow and slider board overlapping the bed and stretcher.	18.	Protects head from injury. Slider board eases movement of the client.
19.	Have staff members grasp edges of lift sheet. Be sure to use good body mechanics.	19.	Provides surface for client to slide on. Prevents dragging and shearing.

Contd...

Table 12.11: Contd...

	Nursing action		*Rationale*
20.	On the count of three, have staff members pull lift sheet and the client onto the stretcher.	20.	Working in unison makes the overall job easier and prevents staff injury.
21.	Position client on stretcher, place pillow under head, and cover with a sheet or bath blanket.	21.	Promotes comfort and provides for privacy.
22.	Secure safety belts and elevate side rails of stretcher.	22.	Prevents falls.
23.	If IV is present, move it from bed IV pole to stretcher IV pole after client transfer.	23.	Prevents tubing from being pulled and IV from being dislodged.
24.	Cleanse hands.	24.	Reduces the transmission of microorganisms.

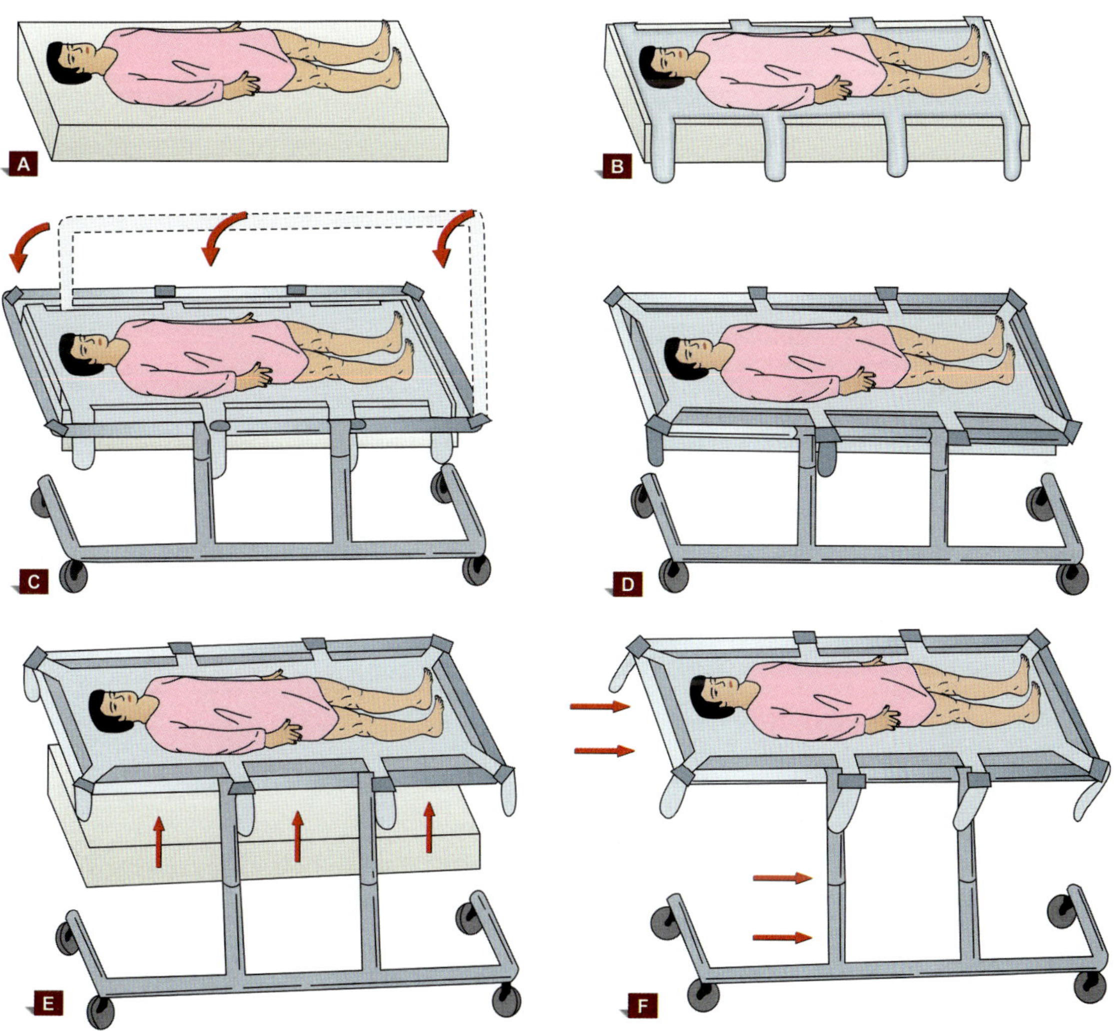

Figure 12.15: Transferring helpless client from the bed

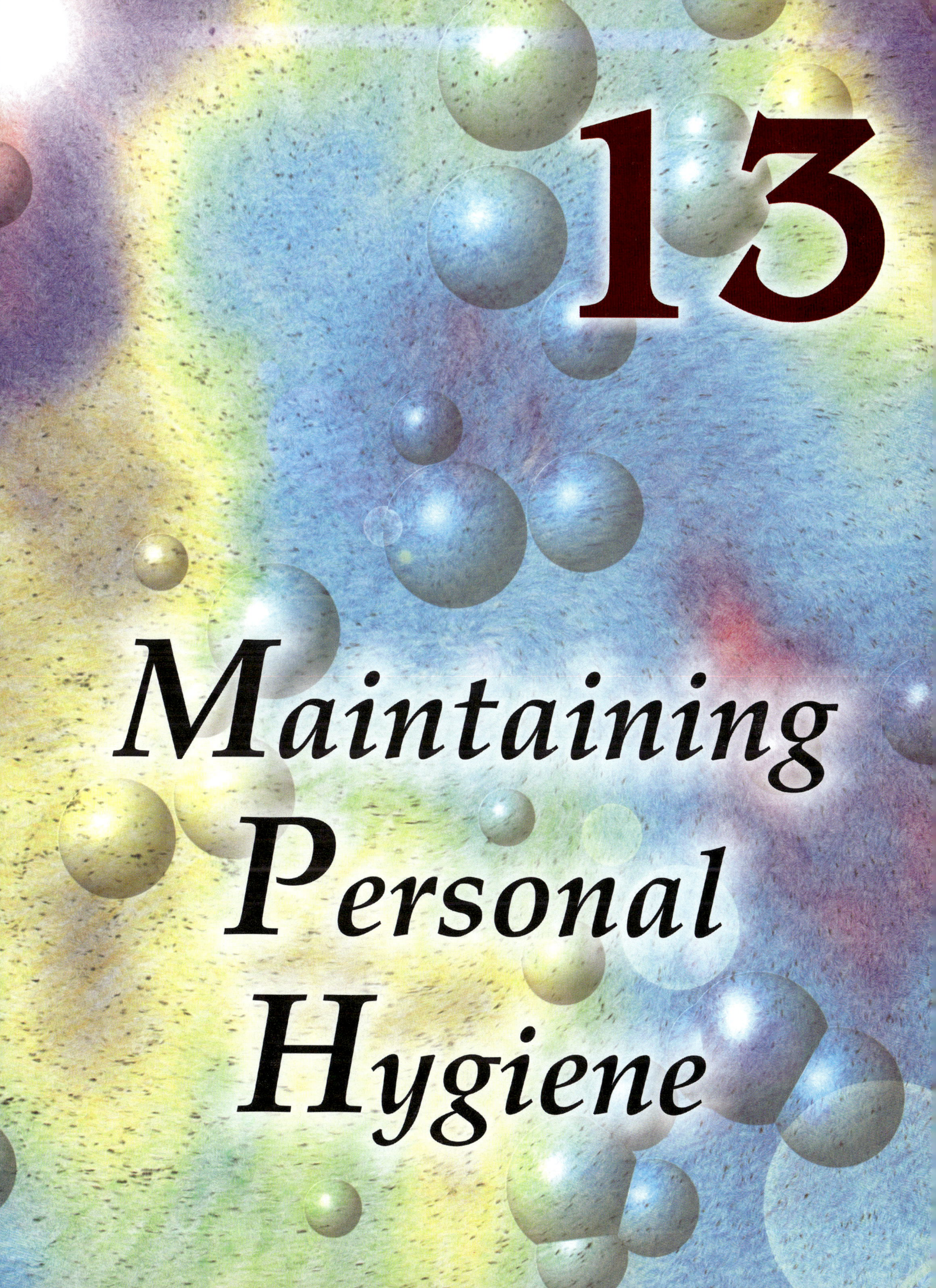

13
Maintaining Personal Hygiene

Introduction

Hygiene is the science of health. The self care measures people use to maintain their health are personal hygiene. Personal hygiene deals with matters, which are personal responsibility of every person. It is concern itself with the adjustments, which the individual must make to preserve and improve the health of his or her body and mind.

Personal hygiene may be defined as "the measures for personal cleanliness and grooming that promote physical and psychological wellbeing". Maintenance of personal hygiene is necessary for an individual comfort, safety, and well-being. Thus, personal hygiene is the health care of own self for which a person himself is responsible. It deals with the personal care of health so that man is able to enjoy healthy life and should get satisfaction about his health. As for the quality of life, health enables the individual to live most and serve best.

Maintenance of personal hygiene is necessary for an individuals comfort, safety as well-being. Healthy persons are capable of meeting their own hygiene needs, whereas ill or physically handicapped persons may require the nurse's assistance to carry out routine hygiene practices illness, hospitalization and industrialization may demand modifications in hygiene practices. In addition personal and sociocultural factors (i.e. body image, social practices, socioeconomic status, knowledge, cultural variables, personal preferences, physical condition) influence the client's hygiene practices. The nurse determines a client's ability to perform self care and provides hygienic care according to the client needs and preferences. In these situations the nurse helps the client to continue sound hygienic practices and has an opportunity to teach the client and family members regarding hygiene.

The main objective of personal hygiene is to maintain high standard of health. Healthy living depends upon the practice of a few principles of health and hygiene. Ill health results mostly from harmful habits. Man is a creature of environment, his health is the state in which his psychological, physical, physiological and sociological activities of the body and mind are adjusted satisfactorily to the environments. Personal hygiene is not only concerned with matters pertaining to health of a person but also includes certain personal factors conducive to good health. These are habits, constitution, hereditary, idiosyncrasy, temperament, cleanliness, sleep, clothing, exercise, sex, etc.

Habit

Habit plays an important part in the preservation of health. Habit grows into practice and it is said to be the second nature of human being because once it is formed, it is very difficult to get rid of. To keep one fit and ready for actions, the habits decent. Habits influence should necessarily be the physical, physiological and psychosocial condition of the individual. Man by birth desires to be socially well-being when he becomes major he wants to ear; when married his families added up. He works

more and should keep good habits. Temperament should remain under the control of will and he should not tilt towards bad habits (e.g. smoking, alcohol, substance abuse, gambling, prostitution, etc.) as they affect the health. Health of the community also depends a great deal on the habits of each member of that community.

The development of good habits which influence in the child is right action and right thinking. Proper healthy habits constitute the only sound foundation upon which permanent physical and mental health should be built at expected level.

(i) *Eating Habits*

It is essential to create a regular habit of taking food including water. Only wholesome food should be taken for the preservation of health. Eating time is not fixed by watch in Indian families, but in India the habit of taking food is more or less fixed pattern. Meals should be taken after due intervals at fixed hours and quantities compatible with one's work. In a few families and only 10 percent of Indian population believe in taking regular nutritious diet at the fixed hours of the day. Food should be taken slowly after desire comes for it, i.e. when the appetite particularly craves for and mind should be calm and clear. It should be properly masticated and eaten slowly. Every morsel should be bitten 32 times. Bolting of unchewed morsels should not be done. Reading should be avoided while taking meals. Excessive eating is not a good habit.

Food should not be taken more than actual requirements of the body since gluttony or over-eating results in obesity, apart from digestive and other disorders. And too much of food should not be taken at simple sitting, but the meals should be spread out over the course of the day. It is desirable that there should be agreeable society at the time of taking meals. Water should be sparingly taken along with meals, but should be taken freely between principal meals. It is good to take a glass of cold water early in the morning on rise from the bed.

Alcohol should never be encouraged with food, since it is harmful to health. Adverse effects of faulty food habits results in indigestion, constipation, obesity.

Indigestion: It occurs when the food fails to get digested properly. The causes for indigestion are as follows:
- Unbalanced diet
- Eating between meals
- Rapid eating
- Too little chewing of the food
- Constipation
- Unpleasing surroundings while eating
- Eating during anger, worried or fatigue
- Disease condition such as gallstone, ulcers or chronic illness.

When indigestion occurs from any of these causes, do not eat any food and if hungry take liquid foods for the next 24 hours.

Constipation: It is the failure to evacuate the waste matters from the bowel in sufficient quantity. Sedentary habits and lack of regular exercise often lead to weakening of intestinal and abdominal muscle, which results in constipation. If prolonged, it may lead to piles. As a matter of fact, the residue of the meal should be expelled out within 48 hours and if this does not take place there is stagnation in the bowel. It is reasonable to eliminate waste matter for alimentary tract as soon as possible. It has been physiologically accepted that one good motion a day is sufficient, provided adequate quantity of fecal matter is expelled out. It is healthful and ideally practical also.

Usual causes of constipation are as follows:
- Habits of using drugs to relieve constipation upset the intestinal system
- Ignoring the call to evacuate the bowel / rectum
- Lack of exercises
- Insufficient intake of fluids and roughage in the diet
- Eating too much fats
- Hurried eating habits and too little rest
- Poor posture leads to bending of the body forward and crowding of abdominal organs lead to weakening muscles

To prevent constipation the following measures may be helpful:
- Adoption of correct position and regularly attending to the nature call is most essential
- Drinking plenty of water between principal meals, especially a glass of water early in the morning
- Since the habit of using medicine in any form to relieve constipation is harmful and should be avoided unless it is prescribed, e.g., purgatives
- Faulty diet must be corrected by modification in diet and habits
- Diet must contain simple fibrous material in order to give sufficient bulk of stool
- Sufficient roughage in the diet is necessary in old age
- Whole wheat bread, grams, vegetables, pulses and fruits in place of meat and egg should encouraged in the diet
- Yeast is very valuable as it contains enough of vitamin 'B' complex which tones the nerves of the intestine and improve its power of contraction and movement of the bowel
- Eating some course bulky foods, e.g. green vegetables, bran, whole grain cereals, fruits with their skin
- Taking regularly outdoor exercise
- Constipation is often associated with the weakness of abdomen and pelvic muscles. In order to strengthen these muscle remedial exercise should be taken (see exercise)

Obesity or overweight: It is an abnormal and dangerous condition in which there is stored a large surplus of fat within the body. Its accumulation beyond the normal limit, may be due to endocrine dysfunction, i.e. hypothyroidism causing an abnormally low metabolic rate but in large majority of cases, it is due to either excessive intake of food or to a deficient utilization of the food than the produce energy. Obesity may be defined as an abnormal growth of adipose tissue due to an enlargement of fatcell size (hyper tropic obesity) increase in fat cell number (hyperplastic obesity) or increases in fat cell number (hyperplastic obesity) or a combination of both obesity expressed in terms of body mass index (BMI). Overweight is usually due to obesity but can arise from other causes such as abnormal muscle development or fluid retentions. However obese individual differ not only in the amount of excess fat that they store, but also in the regional distribution of this fat within the body

Fat in food is the most common cause of overweight, which at first may cause merely discomfort and later on menace in life. It increases susceptibility to diabetes, renal diseases, cardiac failure, diseases of the arteries, lever and gallbladder diseases. Cerebral hemorrhage and number of other ailments. Excessive weight of 10 percent above the normal increases the mortality toll, about 20 percent and the greater the amount of surplus weight, the higher the death toll.

Table 13.1 deals with the ideal height and weight chart for men and women of 25 years and above. The principle underlying in that weight should not be restricted by interfering with the normal development of bones and muscles. Obesity can be prevented in those taking too rich food, by increased exercise, or in those taking too little exercise or by food restriction.

To control increased weight needs a selection of food and by restriction of its amount, which includes non-fatty diet which may provide proteins liberally, but should restrict fats and carbohydrates.

Table 13.1: Ideal Height and Weight for Men and Women (25 years and above)			
Men		*Women*	
Height in cm with shoes	*Weight in kg*	*Height in kg with shoes*	*Weight in cm*
157	56.2-60.3	152	50.8-54.5
160	57.6-61.7	155	51.7-55.3
163	59.0-63.5	157	53.1-56.1
175	60.8-65.3	160	54.5-58.1
168	62.1-66.7	163	56.2-59.9
170	64.0-68.5	165	57.6-61.2
173	65.8-70.8	168	59.0-63.5
175	67.6-72.6	170	60.8-65.3
180	71.2-76.2	173	62.1-66.7
183	73.0-78.5	175	64.0-68.5
185	75.3-80.7	178	65.8-70.3
188	77.6-83.5	180	67.1-71.7
191	79.8-85.7	183	68.5-73.9

- Bulk which satisfies hunger, is achieved by the use of foods rich in water, poor carbohydrates and fats, with considerable proportion of material which cannot be absorbed, e.g. fruits and leafy vegetables
- Protein food should not be reduced in amount unless the individual happens to use them in excess
- Starchy food should not be entirely eliminated, as the stored fat is oxidized much more readily and safely in the presence of carbohydrates
- It is very dangerous to reduce weight rapidly, it should not be more than 0.5 pound or 226.5 gm per day. Rapid reduction leads to the production of fatty acids in excessive amounts.

These acids cannot be neutralized and lead to low alkaline reserves in the body which in turn lead to acidosis
- Food restrictions to become slim should never be encouraged
- Weight reducing drugs should not be encouraged.

Underweight: Individuals should have normal weight according to their age, sex and height. Underweight also leads to many problems. The common causes of underweight are as follows:
- Insufficient intake of food
- An unbalanced diet
- Too little sleep
- Chronic infections
- Worry.

If the individual is undernourished, he may look pale, have poor posture, flabby muscles, dark circles under his eyes, decreased appetite and he often shows irritation.

(ii) *Drinking Habit*

Drinking water is very essential and good habit for all purposes. Nowadays there are so many drinks are available to people for drinking purposes, e.g. soft drinks, hot drinks, which may provide some amount of stimulation but some are not nutritious which include coffee, tea, coca cola, alcohol, etc.

Use of Coffee and Tea: Coffee or tea is an ideal stimulant of body tissue when properly used but its abuse constitutes a problem. In moderate doses, it lessens the feeling of fatigue and is of value during hard mental and physical work and in cases of shock.

Coffee contains caffeine which speeds up burning of food in the tissues and increases the functional activities. It whips the brain and makes the mental process keener. As a result of its intake the heart works faster and special sense become more acute, the body thus becomes highly active and vital. The habitual use of coffee repeatedly leads to the tissue response becomes dull and exhaustion results and the uses go on increasing their dose to get stimulation which is harmful to health.

The users of coffee admit that they drink coffee for the pick-up and feeling of increased strength and freshness. They get help from coffee in getting through days of stress and strain. These people with a rapid pace of life get a temporary sense of fitness and efficiency but actually the habit increases the underlying exhaustion of their body tissues leading to breakdown. It masks the underlying fatigue and under its influence the users perform more work than their system and, by cutting down sleep and upsetting relaxation. This combination of overwork and lack of rest gradually leads to physical and mental break down.

The heart has to work harder and blood pressure may be raised. So it has been suggested the use of coffee should be prohibited among persons with impaired health. Healthy persons may use coffee in moderation during cold season as it gives feeling of comfort and mental alertness.

Tea is freely used as a stimulant due to the presence of tannin, caffeine. Average black tea contain cellulose (40 %), albumin (17.9 %), tannic acid (16.4 %), water (8.2 %), ash (8.6 %), resin (4.6 %), caffeine (3.2 %) and others (1.1 %). Among these, caffeine is most important constituent and then comes tannic acid. Preparation of tea is important. When water begins to boil, it should be poured in a separate pot which is warm and contains the tea leaves. Tea is infused for five minutes after which it should be poured off and stained. Prolonged boiling should be avoided, because the longer the tea is infused, the more tannic acid is dissolved out. Tannic acid produces constipation and the taste of the tea becomes bitter. Addition of milk renders some of the tannic acid insoluble. Increase use of tea causes constipation, dyspepsia, insomnia and nervousness. Light and hard tea may be taken up to 2-3 cups a day by a healthy person.

Use of coca and chocolates: they contain an alkaloid, closely related to caffeine, called the obromine. Its stimulating effects are mainly exerted on the brain and central nervous system. Tea and coffee, if taken without milk and sugar, have no food value but coca and chocolate are nutritious.

Use of alcohol: Alcohol acts as a sedative. It is a food and a narcotic but its food value is very limited. In certain occasions, if used in small doses it may help digestion, or induce sleep, but it has a devitalizing action upon the tissues, the symptoms of which range from some impairment of functions to gross degenerative poisons. The feeling of exhilaration that follows after taking a mild dose of alcohol is due to paralysis of higher nerve centers that normally provide inhibition. It bottles up the disagreeable thoughts and sensations and produces a feeling of well-being and happiness. It kills the sense of fatigue and mental unrest. But excess of alcohol or its misuse acts a slow poison.

Now it has become a social evil, it may cause gastrointestinal disorders, fatty degeneration of heart and liver, arteriosclerosis, peripheral neuritis, etc. in its passage through different tissues, alcohol has different effects:

1. On the casual nervous system, alcohol acts as a narcotic which may begin with the production of pleasant state or euphoria, i.e. the facing out of disturbing and unpleasant facts of life, progress to stupor, then coma and even death in rare cases. The first higher centers of the brain to be affected are those which control memory, attention, thought, judgement of self control and subsequently muscular and sensory functions are interfered with. They loose the power of concentration and memory, and may develop dullness and may commit some breaches of the law bringing trouble on himself and on his family.
2. Alcohol increases the rate of contraction causing rapid heartbeat through the nerve tissue covering the heart.
3. By dilating the blood vessel, at the surface of the body alcohol interferes with the heart regulating mechanism producing a sense of warmth in the skin and actual loss of internal body heat. The loss can be serious in cold weather, by the body is not well wrapped.
4. By acting on the nerve tissue which is the special sensory organs, it can produce error and delay in observing through eye and ear. It has very dangerous effect on persons driving a vehicle or an aeroplane. In view of its slow rate of elimination from the body, these effects of alcohol usually remain for some hours after alcohol has been taken.

5. As regards to respiratory process moderate amounts of alcohol produce little effect but large amounts may cause paralysis of the respiratory centers and lead to even death.

6. In the cases of digestive process, peristaltic action may be lessened and flow of saliva increased as also of gastric juice with the difference that this is lower in pepsin contents but higher in hydrochloric acid contents than normal – a change liable to be harmful to persons suffering from peptic ulcer. Persons addicted to alcohol loss their appetite. They get nausea and vomiting in the morning, which is an expression of resentment by the outraged stomach. They suffer from gastric catarrh, windy spasms and heart burns. Alcohol, which absorbed, passes through the liver and damages; it leads to liver disorder.

7. Usually excessive intake of alcohol is that normal restraint in conduct may be lost, involving the risk of promiscuity, and of contracting such diseases in STD, gonorrhea and syphilis.

Alcoholism is a social evil; its economic and social costs are heavy. It affects the personality of the man as well as his social status and family relationship. Family discards his security and happiness of home is shattered. Alcohol develops unusual cunningness to cover up one's use of alcohol and want to maintain normal behavior with friends and family members. Alcoholism can easily found out by relatives and friends. The following signs may serve as guidelines:

- Drinking alone
- Constantly drinking and thinking
- Getting drunk without really intending to
- Drinking frequently
- Needing drinks at odd hours
- Making excuses for drinking.

Consumption of alcohol does not remove fatigue but makes one unconscious of it and blunts one's recollections of the difficulties and worries of the day. The real danger of its use is its habit formation nature and for persons having weak self control, it very quickly ceases to be under control but becomes their master. It is responsible for many crimes, accidents and so many physical, physiological and psychological injuries and diseases. Therefore, use of alcohol and other such liquids should be avoided.

Use of tobacco: Tobacco is the most common form of substance abuse which leads to social addiction. It is used mostly in smoking, chewing and snuffing.

1. *Smoking:* It is a habit which comes from indisciplined society. The children start smoking at a very young age in case their father is chain smoker. Smoking is injurious to health and it should not be encouraged.

It is noticed that smoking in any form is injurious to health but nobody pay least importance to it. It has been proved that cigarette smoking, has been important factor in the development of cancer of lungs and cancer of larynx. Many cases of lung carcinoma and lip cancer are due to the use of lip tobacco and smoking cigarette or beedi. Smokers have higher death rate from coronary heart disease and it is also one of the major causes of chronic bronchitis. The smoke of tobacco consists of a mixture of gasses and various vaporized chemicals including vaporized nicotine, which is a toxic substance. A smoker gets more nicotine and tar if he smokes cigarette to the end. When smoker inhales nicotine, which increases stimulation it further intensifies the habit of smoking. Smoking is used as a means of relaxation, specially during tension in an individual smoking tends to have 20 percent more illness. Smoking pipe and cigar are less dangerous while smoking beedi/biri which is being used extensively throughout India is more harmful. In beedi, burning of leaf in which tobacco is wrapped for making beedi irritates the throat. Hookah-smoking is a better method of smoking tobacco. When the smoke of tobacco passed through water in the hookah, nicotine is dissolved in water to a great extent, and hookah fumes pass through water reservoir and most of the alkaloids of the tobacco are precipitated in this way.

2. *Tobacco-chewing:* Here the tobacco leaf is powdered and little lime is mixed and then it is kept between the lower lip and teeth and chewed. This habit is the worst habit; on this operation, a large quantity of salivary juice and even the particles of tobacco are swallowed, causing chronic sore throat, disorders of digestion, impaired vision and nervous tremor. This is associated with high prevalence of oral cancer; cancer of the lip and tongue.

3. *Snuffing:* It is another form of tobacco which is used widely. The habitual snuff users suffer from hypertrophy and later atrophy of nasal mucosa. This is more risky than smoking and chewing of tobacco.

Once the people addicted to use of tobacco, it is very difficult to give up the habit. To give up smoking do not use any drugs or medicine which has no value. Success in dropping smoking depends upon desire and will power to quit it. It requires motivation which leads to positive action in the act of stopping smoking. It may begin with gradual withdrawal but it usually fails. But to stop it suddenly becomes uncomfortable physically and emotionally. Most smokers crave for smoking after each meal and some during office break. In order to quit smoking change in the living pattern is required.

Cleanliness or Maintaining of Personal Hygiene

Cultivating the habit of maintaining cleanliness is very essential for the upkeep of health and for the normal growth of our body. Cleanliness is next to godliness. Dirt is not only harmful but it is antagonistic even to our very existence. Therefore, special emphasis should be paid on cleanliness with regard to the food we eat, the air we breath in and the water we drink. While taking care of the body in relation to cleanliness, emphasis should be made to take care of skin, hairs, mouth, teeth, hands, feet, nails, eyes, ear, external genitals, etc.

1. Care of the Skin

The skin is an active organ with the function of protection, secretion, sensation, respiration, temperature regulation and excretion. Skin has around two millions sweat glands, which has at least three functions, i.e. to keep body temperature normal, to keep the skin permeable and to get rid the body of the waste material and dirt. Skin is of immense value as a lot of perspiration and excretion of solids take place through its innumerable minute pores. As a matter of fact, a great deal of work of lungs and kidneys is performed by the skin. The amounts of sweat varies from person to person. Emotional stress, worry, fear or excitement can also cause excessive sweating. Certain parts of the body, like armpits give out an unpleasant odors from the secretion of sweat.

The skin exchanges oxygen, nutrients and fluid with underlying blood vessels, synthesizes new cells and eliminated dead, nonfunctioning cells. The cells of the integument requires adequate nutrition and hydration to resist injury and disease. Adequate circulation is essential to maintain cell life. The skin often reflects a change in physical condition by alteration in color, thickness, texture, turgor, temperature and hydration. As long as the skin remains intact and healthy, its physiological function remains optional.

Skin cleanliness is desirable from the aesthetic as well as hygienic standpoint. It makes bodily comfort and self respect. Hence, it is most necessary to keep the skin clean from dirt, so that the sweat glands may function properly. The best way to maintain cleanliness is the removal of sebaceous secretions of the skin which is best affected by taking bath regularly by using soap and water, which should be followed by liberal application of some toilet powder containing a deodorant.

Baths

Baths are not only very necessary for cleanliness but also for their beneficial action on the skin and internal organs. The purposes of bathing are as follows:

(i) *Cleansing the skin* Cleansing removes perspiration, some bacteria, sebum and dead skin cells, which minimizes skin irritation and reduces the chance of infection.

(ii) *Stimulation of circulation* Good circulation is promoted through the use of warm water and gentle stroking of the extremities.

(iii) *Improved self image* Bathing promotes relaxation and feeling of being refreshed and comfortable.

(iv) *Reduction of body odors* Excessive secretion of sweat from apocrine glands located in the axillae and pubic areas causes unpleasant body odors. Bathing and use of antiperspiratants minimized odors.

(v) *Promotion of range of motions (ROM)* Movement of the extremities during bathing maintains joint function.

A bath should be taken early in the morning or in the middle of the day, before taking meals. It should not be taken immediately after meals or after exhaustion due to fatigue. A good quality soap should be used while taking bath, since the function of soap is to wash away the sweat and dirt and to emulsify the sebaceous secretions of the skin or the skin oils, thus rendering the cleansing of skin easier and quicker. Cheap toilet avoided. Baths may be classified as under:

- Cold bath 33° to 65° F (0.5°C to 18.3°C)
- Tepid bath 80° to 90° F (26.6°C to 32.2°C)
- Warm bath 90° to 98° F (32.2°C to 36.6°C)
- Hot bath 98° to 100° F (36.6°C to 37.7°C).

Cold bath: Cold bath acts as a stimulant to heart and it contracts the peripheral blood vessels. Young healthy persons should use cold water for a bath as it is invigorating, more refreshing and acts very simulative to improve the texture, tone, firmness and color of the skin and stimulates the circulation of the blood throughout the body. It stimulates the skin and increases the power of the body to react to variations in the temperature. Cold bath should be taken as quickly as possible and body covered immediately afterwards. The first effect produced by taking a cold bath is to chill the surface of the body and that of a shock followed by constriction of superficial blood vessels, but vessels dilate very soon giving feeling of warmth and pleasure to the individual. Some people taking plunge bath by immersing their whole body in the water (e.g. river, lake or stream) such baths are beneficial and are invigorating.

Bathing in cool water can relieve tension or lower body temperature. Water temperature should be tepid (37°C / 98.6°F) rather than cold to avoid chilling and to promote slow cooling; this avoids temperature fluctuations. This type of bath is especially effective in reducing the body temperature of a small child with a fever.

Warm bath: Bathing in warm water relieves muscle tension. Water temperature should be 43°C (109.4°F). In warm bath the temperature is approximately that of the body. It is of value chiefly to clean the skin, particularly when soap is used. It does not have much stimulating effect on skin or the circulation. It soothes the nervous system and may be used to induce sleep, if taken just before retiring.

Hot bath: This bath has a temperature above that of the body. It raises the temperature of the surface of the body and dilates the superficial blood vessels and stimulates the sweat glands. It thus causes hyperemia through the skin by with drawing a large quantity of blood from the interior organs. There is a danger of chilling of the body due to dilated skin vessels and so it is not advisable to go out in the cold after taking a hot bath. If hot bath is continued for long it becomes depressing. Hot bath is not desirable for persons with heart disease. It is also not desirable to take hot bath soon after meal. Frequent hot bath in a day is not desired as an undue heat is lost. It lowers the blood pressure. It relaxes the body and removes fatigue and also means of combating insomnia. Vigorous rubbing of the body with rough and dry towel, after taking a bath is very beneficial, as it act as a massage to the skin and provides a certain amount of bodily exercise and excites circulation of the blood in the skin. It gives splendid feeling of glow and well-being.

A good bath influences the structure of the skin, heart, blood pressure and respiration, muscle tone, fibrous tissues and joints. There are several type of therapeutic baths such as soak, sitz baths, bran bath, electric bath, mud bath, and mineral bath.

(i) Soak: Local application of water or a medicated solution can remove dead tissue or soften encrusted secretions. An aseptic technique is necessary when cleansing open or abraded areas of the skin. Soaks are also useful in reducing pain and swelling of inflamed or irritated skin surfaces.

(ii) Sitz bath: A sitz bath cleanses and reduces inflammation of the perineal areas and of a client who has undergone rectal or vaginal surgery or childbirth or who has local rectal irritation from hemorrhoids or tissues water temperature depends on the clients condition but should be 43-45°C to 90-98°C. Cold sitz bath are more effective and relieving pain in the postpartum period.

(iii) Bran bath: A bran bath is used for removing the irritation of certain types of skin diseases and for soothing effects. This type of bath is prepared by adding one pound of fresh bran in the five gallons of water at 103°F and the affected parts are bathed for 40 to 50 minutes keeping the temperature at about 103°F by adding hot water.

(iv) Electric bath: It is suitable for parts with impaired circulation and also in chronic rheumatism, weak muscle, and flat foot, etc.

(v) Mud bath: It is useful in chronic irritation of the skin and in constipation. Mud contains mineral matters and some of the mud may contain radioactive substances useful to the system.

(vi) Mineral bath Hot mineral bath in the warm space, i.e. hot springs (e.g. Rajgir in Bihar) is suitable for helping in cure of certain types of ailments. Water of such springs contains usually calcium, sulphur and radioactive substances. By taking such bath regularly for a few days in these springs, patients ailments such as gout, chronic rheumatism of muscles, joints and ligaments, arthritis of septic origin and osteoarthritis, etc. are generally benefited. Regular bath is not advisable to hypertensive and weak persons.

Bathing a Client

Bathing a client is a part of total hygienic care. Bath can be categorized as cleansing or therapeutic. A physician's order is necessary for bath designed for therapeutic purposes (e.g. tepid sponging), the order designates bath temperature, the body part being treated (soak) and any medicated solution used (i.e. saline, sodium bicarbonate, potassium permanganate). The complete bed bath, needed for clients who are totally depended and required total hygienic care (Tables 13.2 to 13.6). Bathing serves a variety of purposes, including the following:

- It cleanses the skin
- It act as a skin conditioner
- It helps relax a restless person
- It promotes circulation by stimulating the skin peripheral nerve endings and underlying tissues
- It serves as a musculoskeletal exercises through activity involved with bathing and thus improves joint mobility and muscle tone

Table 13.2: Procedures for Giving a Bedbath

	Nursing actions		Rationales
1.	Discuss procedure with the client and assess the client's ability to assist in the bathing process as well as process as well as personal hygiene preferences. Review the client's chart for any limitations in physical activity.	1.	This discussion promotes reassurance and provides knowledge about the procedure. Dialogue also encourages client participation and allows for individualized nursing care.
2.	Bring necessary equipment to the bedside stand or over bed table. Remove sequential compression devices and antiembolism stockings from lower extremities according to agency protocol.	2.	Bringing everything to the bedside conserves time and energy. Arranging items nearby is convenient, saves time, and helps prevent unnecessary stretching and twisting of muscles on the part of the nurse. Most manufacturers and agencies recommend removal of these devices during the bath to allow for assessment.
3.	Close the curtains around the bed and close the door to the room if possible.	3.	This ensures the client's privacy and lessens the possibility of loss of body heat during the bath.
4.	Offer the client the bedpan or urinal.	4.	Voiding or defecating before the bath lessens the likelihood that the bath will be interrupted, because warm bath water may stimulate the urge to void.
5.	Wash your hands.	5.	Handwashing deters the spread of microorganisms.
6.	Raise the client's bed to the high position.	6.	Having the bed in a high position prevents strain on the nurse's back.

Contd...

Table 13.2: *Contd...*

	Nursing actions		Rationales
7.	Lower the side rail nearer to you and assist the client to the side of the bed where you will work. Have the client lie on his or her back.	7.	Having the client positioned near the nurse and lowering the side rail help prevent unnecessary stretching and twisting of muscles on the part of the nurse.
8.	Loosen top covers and remove all except the top sheet. Place bath blanket over the client and then remove the top sheet while the client holds the bath blanket in place. If linen is to be reused, fold it over a chair. Place soiled linen in the laundry bag.	8.	The client is not exposed unnecessarily and warmth is maintained. If a bath blanket is unavailable, the top sheet may be used in place of the bath blanket.
9.	Assist the client with oral hygiene, as necessary.	9.	This helps maintain teeth and gums in good condition, alleviates unpleasant odor and taste, and may improve appetite. Some clients may prefer oral care after the bath is completed.
10.	Remove the client's gown and keep the bath blanket in place. If client has an intravenous line, remove the gown from the other arm first. Lower the intravenous container and pass the gown over the tubing and the container. Rehang the container and check the drip rate.	10.	This provides uncluttered access during the bath and maintains warmth of the client. Intravenous fluids must be maintained at the prescribed rate.
11.	Raise the side rail. Fill the basin with a sufficient amount of comfortably warm water (between 43° and 46°C, 110° to 115°F). Change as necessary throughout the bath. Lower the side rail closer to you when you return to the bedside to being the bath.	11.	Warm water is comfortable and relaxing for the client. It also stimulates circulation and provides for more effective cleansing. Side rails maintain client safety.
12.	Fold the washcloth like a mitter on your hand so there are no loose ends, as illustrated in Figure 13.1.	12.	Having loose ends of cloth drag across the client's skin is uncomfortable. Loose ends cool quickly and will feel cold to the client.
13.	Lay a towel across the client's chest and on top of the bath blanket.	13.	This prevents chilling the keeps the bath blanket dry.
14.	With no soap on the washcloth, wipe one eye from the inner part of the eye, near the nose, to the outer part. Rinse or turn the cloth before washing the other eye (Fig. 13.2).	14.	Rinsing, returning the washcloth, prevents spreading organisms from one eye to the other. Soap is irritating to the eyes. Moving from the inner to the outer aspect of the eye prevents carrying debris toward the naso-lacrimal duct.
15.	Bathe the client's face, neck, and ears, avoiding soap on the face if the client prefers.	15.	Soap can be drying and may be avoided as a matter of personal preference.
16.	Expose the fore arm of the client and place the towel lengthwise under it. Using firm strokes, wash and the arm and axilla, rinse, and dry.	16.	The towel helps to keep the bed dry. Washing the far side first eliminates contaminating a clean area once it is washed. Gentle friction stimulates circulation and muscles and helps remove dirt, oil, and organisms. Long, firm strokes are relaxing and more comfortable than short, uneven strokes.
17.	Place a folded towel on the bed next to the client's hand and put the basin on it. Soak the client's hand in the basin. Wash, rinse, and dry and hand.	17.	Placing the hands in the basin of water is comfortable and relaxing for the client, allows for a thorough washing of the hands and between the fingers, and facilitates removal of debris from under the nails.
18.	Repeat actions 16 and 17 for the arm nearer to you (an option for the shorter nurse or one prone to back strain might be to bathe one side of the client and move to the other side of the bed to complete the bath).	18.	—

Contd...

<table>
<tr><td colspan="2" align="center">Table 13.2: Contd...</td></tr>
<tr><td align="center">Nursing actions</td><td align="center">Rationales</td></tr>
<tr><td>19. Spread a towel across the client's chest. Lower the bath blanket to the client's umbilical area. Wash, rinse, and dry the client's chest. Keep the client's chest covered with the towel between the wash and rinse. Pay special attention to skin folds under the breasts of clients.</td><td>19. Exposing, washing, rinsing, and drying one part of the body at a time avoids unnecessary exposure and chilling. Skin fold areas may be sources of odor and skin breakdown if not cleansed and dried properly.</td></tr>
<tr><td>20. Lower the bath blanket to the client's perineal area. Place a towel over the client's chest. Perform normal perineal care (Figs 13.3A and B and 13.4A to C).</td><td>20. Keeping the bath blanket and towel in place avoids exposure and chilling.</td></tr>
<tr><td>21. Wash, rinse, and dry the client's abdomen. Carefully inspect and cleanse the umbilical area and any abdominal folds or creases.</td><td>21. Skin-fold areas may be sources of odor and skin breakdown if not cleansed and dried properly.</td></tr>
<tr><td>22. Return the bath blanket to its original position and expose the far leg of the client. Place the towel under the far leg. Using firm strokes, wash, rinse, and dry the client's leg from ankle to knee and knee to groin.</td><td>22. The towel protects linens and prevents the client from feeling uncomfortable from a damp or wet bed. Washing from ankle to groin with firm strokes promotes venous return.</td></tr>
<tr><td>23. Fold a towel near the client's foot area and place the basin on it. Place the client's foot in the basin while supporting the client's ankle and heel in your hand and the leg on your arm. Wash, rinse, and dry, paying particular attention to the area between the toes (Fig. 13.5).</td><td>23. Supporting the client's foot and leg helps reduce strain and discomfort for the client. Placing the feet in a basin of water is comfortable and relaxing and allows for a thorough cleaning of the feet and the areas between the toes and under the nails.</td></tr>
<tr><td>24. Repeat actions 22 and 23 for the other leg and foot.</td><td>24. —</td></tr>
<tr><td>25. Make sure that the client is covered with the bath blanket. Change water at this point or earlier if necessary. Assist the client onto his or her side.</td><td>25. The bath blanket maintains warmth and privacy. Clean, warm water prevents chilling and maintains the client's comfort.</td></tr>
<tr><td>26. Assist the client to a prone or side-lying position. Position the bath blanket and towel to expose only the back and buttocks (Fig. 13.6).</td><td>26. Positioning of the towel and bath blanket protects the client's privacy and provides warmth.</td></tr>
<tr><td>27. Wash, rinse, and dry the client's back and buttocks area. Pay particular attention to cleansing between gluteal folds and observe for any indication of redness or skin breakdown in the sacral area.</td><td>27. Fecal material near the anus may be a source of microorganisms. Prolonged pressure on the sacral area or other body prominences may compromise circulation and lead to development of decubitus ulcer.</td></tr>
<tr><td>28. If not contraindicated, give the client a backrub, as described in Table 13.24. Back massage may be given also after perineal care.</td><td>28. A backrub improves circulation to the tissues and is an aid to relaxation. A backrub may be contraindicated in clients with cardiovascular disease or musculoskeletal injuries.</td></tr>
<tr><td>29. Refill basin with clean water. Discard washcloth and towel.</td><td>29. The washcloth, towel, and water are contaminated after washing the client's gluteal area. Changing to clean supplies decreases the spread of organisms from the anal area to the genitals.</td></tr>
<tr><td>30. Clean the client's perineal area or set up the client so he or she has complete perineal self-care.</td><td>30. Providing perineal self-care decrease embarrassment for the client. Effective perineal care reduces odor and decreases the chance of infection through contamination.</td></tr>
<tr><td>31. Help the client put on a clean gown and attend to personal hygiene needs.</td><td>31. This provides for the client's warmth and comfort.</td></tr>
<tr><td>32. Protect the pillow with a towel, and groom the client's hair, as described in the text.</td><td>32. —</td></tr>
<tr><td>33. Change bed linens, as described in respective procedures.</td><td>33. —</td></tr>
<tr><td>34. Record any significant observation and communication on the client's chart.</td><td>34. A careful record is important for planning and individualizing the client's care.</td></tr>
</table>

- It stimulates the rate and depth of respiration.
- It promotes comfort through muscle relaxation and skin stimulation
- It provides the performance with sensory input
- It helps improve self image
- It gives the nurse an excellent opportunity to strengthen the nurse-patient relationship, to observe the physiologic and emotional status

Equipment

- Wash basin
- Soap and dish
- Wash cloths
- Bath blanket
- Gown or pajamas
- Bed linen
- Towels (2)
- Disposable gloves for anal and perineal care (optional for remainder of bath)
- Personal hygiene supplies deodorant, lotion, and others
- Bedpan or urinal
- Laundry bag or cart

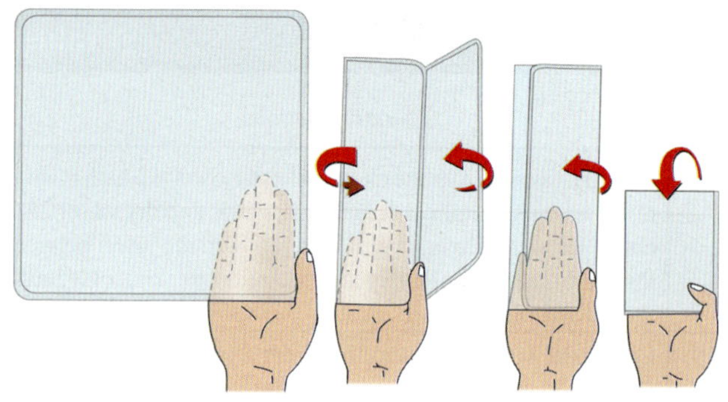

Figure 13.1: Forming a mitten with bath cloth around hands

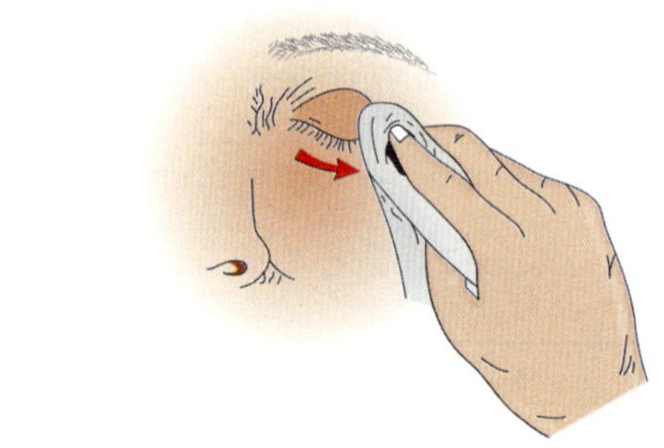

Figure 13.2: Washing around patient's eye

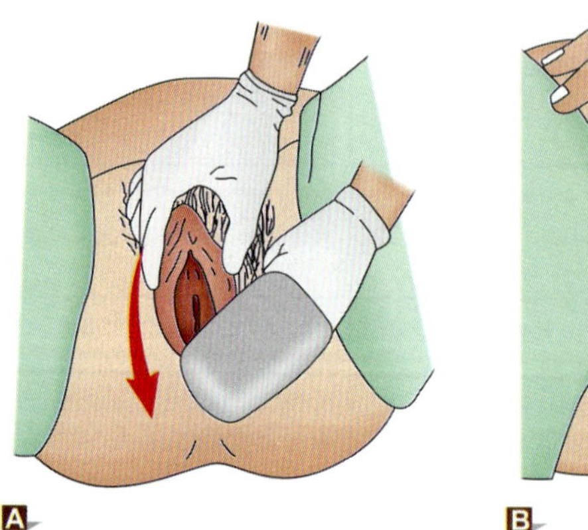
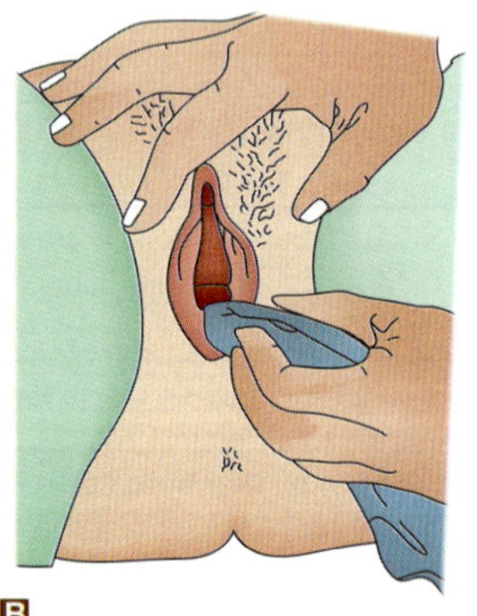

Figures 13.3A and B: Performing normal perineal care (female): (A) Separate labia to expose urinary meatus, (B) Cleaning urinary meatus

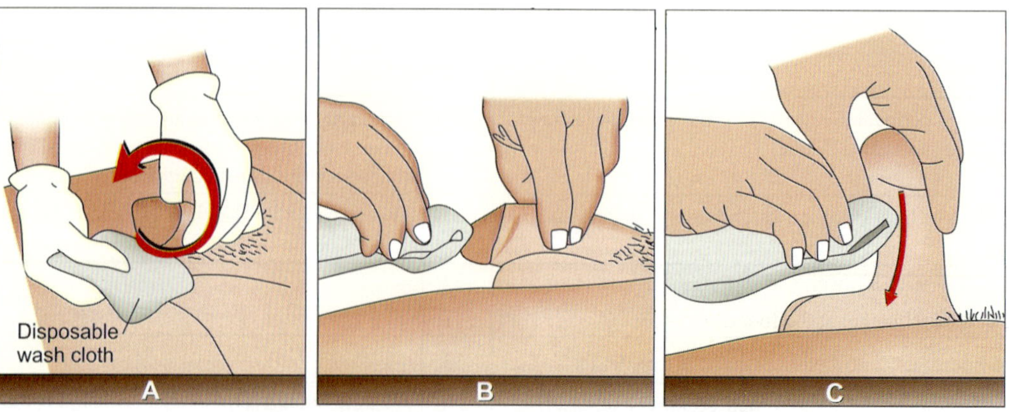

Figures 13.4A to C: Performing normal perineal care: Cleaning penis with disposable

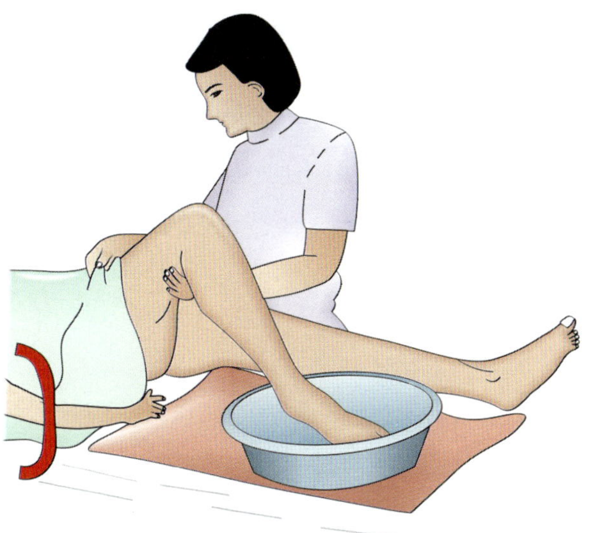

Fig. 13.5: Placing foot in basin

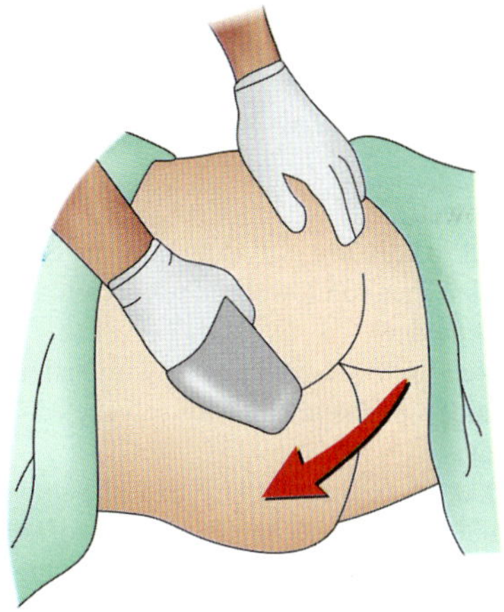

Figure 13.6: Side lying position

Closely, to teach the client and indicator, to demonstrate than the nurse care for the client and is interested in the client's general welfare.

	Table 13.3: Procedures for Administering a Towel Bath		
	Nursing actions		*Rationales*
1.	Check physician's order. Confer with charge nurse to determine need for towel bath.	1.	Ensures accuracy of procedure.
2.	Explain procedure.	2.	Reduces anxiety
3.	Adjust room temperature, and provide privacy.	3.	Prevents chilling, and encourages relaxation.
4.	Obtain supplies: • Concentrate/solution (e.g. septi-soft) • Measuring device, such as plastic medication cup of liter-calibrated container • Towel-bath towel (31 ft × 7½ ft) • Large plastic bag • Bath towel • Wash cloths (2) • Bath blankets (2 or 3) • Disposable gloves • Linens for bedmaking • Articles for personal hygiene – comb, toothbrush lotion, toothpaste and mouthwash.	4.	Promotes orderly procedure.
5. (a) (b) (c) (d)	Prepare patient. Remove patient's clothing and excess bedding (top linens, bedspread). Place patient on bath blanket, and cover patient with bath blanket. Cover with plastic any surgical dressings, casts, or areas that should not be wet. Fan fold a clean bath blanket at the foot of the bed. Position patient supine (lying on back with legs partially separated and arms loosely at sides).	5. (a) (b)	Preparing patient ensures bath towel will be warm enough for patient's comfort, as well as for effective towel bath. Prevents contamination of dressing or cast.

Contd...

Table 13.3: *Contd...*	
Nursing actions	*Rationales*
6. Prepare towel: (a) Fold towel in half, top to bottom, now half again, procedure. (b) side to side. Then roll towel and wash cloth inside, beginning with folded edge. (c) Place rolled-up towel-bath towel (with bath towel and wash cloths inside) in plastic bag with solvage edges toward open end of bag. (d) Draw 2000 mL of water at 115° to 120°F into plastic pitcher. Measure 30 mL of concentrate or 90 mL of solution. If using dispenser with a pump, single stroke measures (30 mL) mix 2000 mL of water and septi-soft. (e) Pour mixture over towel in plastic bag. (f) Knead the solution quickly into towel, position plastic bag with open end in sink, and squeeze out excess water, giving added wringing twist to solvage edges of towel.	6. Preparing towel prevents unnecessary clean-ups and promotes effective.
7. Bathe patient: (a) Fold bath blanket down to waist. Remove warm, moist towel from plastic bag and place on patient's right or left chest with open edges up and outward (Unroll towel across chest). (b) Open towel to cover entire body while removing top bath blanket. Tuck towel-bath towel in and around body (Leave bath towel and wash clothes in plastic bag to keep warm). (c) Begin bathing at feet, using gentle, massaging motion. Employ clean section of towel for each part of body as nurse moves towards patient's head. (d) Fold lower part of towel upward away from feet as bathing continues. (e) Put clean bath blanket up over patient as nurse moves upward. Leave in or exposed skin between towel and bath blanket. Skin will dry in 2 or 3 sec. (f) Wash face, neck and ears with one of prepared wash cloths. (g) Turn patient onto side. (h) Use bath towel for back care. (i) Use second wash cloth for perineal care (don disposable gloves). (j) When bath is completed, remove towel and place with soiled linens in plastic laundry bag. (k) If top bath blanket is not	7. Bathing patient following these steps promotes effective towel bath, provides warmth, and keeps bed dry, avoiding causing the patient to chill.

Age considerations When bathing an infant or young child, have supplies within easy reach and support or hold the child securely at all times to ensure safety. Never leave the child along.

Check temperature of water, particularly before bathing an older client because sensitivity to temperature may be impaired.

An older client who is not incontinent may not require a full bed bath with soap and water everyday. If dry skin is a problem, water and skin lotion or bath oil may be used on alternate days.

Special considerations Removal of gown if client has an intravenous line necessitates taking the gown off, uninvolved arm first, and then threading the intravenous tubing and bottle or bag through the arm of the gown after the affected arm has been removed from the gown. To replace the gown. Place the clean gown on the unaffected arm first and thread intravenous tubing and bottle or bag from inside the arm of the gown on the involved side. Never disconnect intravenous tubing to change a gown because this causes a break in a sterile system and introduces the potential for infection.

Lying flat in bed during the bed bath may be contraindicated for certain clients. Position may have to be modified to accommodate their needs.

Perineal care for a client with an indwelling catheter may vary based on agency protocol.

Change water as often as necessary to maintain at a comfortable temperature. Always change the water after performing perineal care or when the water is foiled.

Table 13.4: Procedures for Assisting the Patient to Take a Tub or Shower Bath

	Nursing actions		*Rationales*
1.	Determine if activity is allowed, consult with RN in charge, and check physician's order.	1.	Provides a basis for patient care.
2.	Make certain tub or shower appliance is clean. See agency's policy. Place nonskid mat on tub or shower floor and disposable mat outside of tub or shower.	2.	Promotes patient safety.
3.	Gather all items necessary for bathing. • Towel • Washcloth • Soap • Deodorant • Lotion • Clean gown.	3.	Prevents unnecessary interruptions.
4.	Assist patient to tub or shower. Be certain patient wears robe and slippers.	4.	Promotes patient safety. Prevents patient from chilling.
5.	Instruct patient on how to use call signal and place "in use" sign on tub or shower door if private bath is not being used.	5.	Provides for patient safety and privacy.
6.	If a tub is used, fill with warm water; temperature 109°F (43°C) have patient test water, and adjust. Instruct patient on use of faucets – which is hot and which is cold. If shower is used, turn water on and adjust temperature.	6.	Prevents accidental burns and promotes safety.
7.	Caution patient to use safety bars, and discourage use of bath oil in water. Check on patient q 5 min. do not allow patient to remain in tub more than 20 min.	7.	Maintains patient safety. Prevents vertigo and syncope.
8.	Return to room which patient signals, to assist from tub. Knock before entering.	8.	Provides privacy.
9.	Assist patient out of tub and with drying. If patient complains of weakness, vertigo or syncope, drain tub before patient gets out and place towel over patient's shoulder.	9.	Prevents falls.
10.	Assist patient into clean gown, robe, and slippers. Accompany to room, and position for comfort, in either chair or bed.	10.	Maintains warmth.
11.	Make unoccupied bed if patient can tolerate sitting in chair. Perform back, hair, nail and skin care.	11.	Maintains clean environment. Promotes positive self-image and promotes medical asepsis.
12.	Return to shower or tub. Clean according to agency policy. Place all soiled linens in laundry bag and return all articles to patient's bedside.	12.	Promotes orderly environment.
13.	Wash hands.	13.	Reduces spread of microorganisms.

• Evaluate the safety of the bathing area in the home. Tub mats, adhesive stips, grab bars, and shower stools are helpful accessories to prevent falls.

Tepid Sponge Bath

A tepid sponge bath is administered to reduce an elevated temperature. This procedure is commonly used for patients who are febrile (Table 13.5).

A medicated bath may be ordered. This bath may include agents such as oatmeal, cornstarch, Burow's solution, and sodium bicarbonate (alkaline bath) (Table 13.6). The medicated bath is ordered to reduce tension and relax the patient and to relieve pruritus or certain skin disorders.

Purposes: The nurse provides or facilitates a patient's bath for the following reasons:
• To cleanse the skin
• To apply medication
• To stimulate circulation
• To improve self-image
• To reduce body odors
• To promote range of motion
• To demonstrate caring – an important aspect of the nurse/patient relationship.

Table 13.5: Procedures for Administering a Tepid Sponge Bath for Temperature Reduction

	Nursing actions		Rationales
1.	Observe patient for elevated temperature. Review physician's orders.	1.	Provides basis for care.
2.	Explain to patient; outline steps of the procedure.	2.	Reduces anxiety.
3.	Prepare equipment: • Bath basin • Tepid water (37°C or 98.6°F) • Wash cloths (4) • Bath thermometer • Bath blanket • Patient thermometer.	3.	Promotes organization
4.	Provide privacy, and wash hands.	4.	Promotes relaxation. Prevents spread of microorganisms.
5.	Cover patient with bath blanket, remove gown, and close windows and doors.	5.	Prevents chilling.
6.	Test water temperature. Place wash cloths in water, and then apply wet cloths to each axilla and groin. If patient is in tub, allow to stay in water for 20 to 30 min.	6.	Promotes cooler temperature. Allows for more effective heat loss because blood vessels are close to the surface of the body in the axilla and groin.
7.	Gently sponge an extremity for about 5 min. if patient in tub, gently sponge water over upper torso, chest, and back.	7.	Prevents sudden drop in body temperature.
8.	Continue sponge bath to other extremities, back, and buttocks for 3 to 5 min each. Determine temperature q 15 min.	8.	Minimizes risk of patient chilling.
9.	Change water, and reapply freshly moistened was cloths to axilla and groin as necessary.	9.	Maintain tepid water temperature.
10.	Continue with sponge bath until body temperature falls to slightly above normal. Discontinue procedure according to agency's policy.	10.	Prevents body temperature from falling below normal.
11.	Dry patient thoroughly, and cover with light blanket or sheet.	11.	Prevents patient from chilling.
12.	Return equipment to storage, clean area, and change bed linens as necessary. Wash hands.	12.	Prevents spread of microorganisms.
13.	Record time procedure was started, when ended, vital signs and patient's response.	13.	Temperature and pulse indicate patient's response to treatment.

Table 13.6: Procedures for Administering a Medicated Bath

	Nursing actions		Rationales
1.	Prepare tub bath (see skill).	1.	Promotes an orderly procedure.
2.	Add appropriate agent as ordered by physician.	2.	Follows physician's orders.
3.	Assist patient to tub.	3.	Maintains patient safety.
4.	Allow patient to remain in tub for required time.	4.	Promotes effective procedure.
5.	Assist patient out of tub.	5.	Maintains patients safety.
6.	Gently pat dry.	6.	Allows medication to remain on patient's skin.
7.	Assist patient into gown or pajamas.	7.	Prevents patient from chilling.
8.	Assist patient to return to bed, and position for comfort.	8.	Allows patient to rest and relax
9.	Wash hands.	9.	Prevents spread of microorganisms.

Documentation

• Record procedure.	Proves performance. Communicates patient care.

Sample charting		
Date	12/4/99	Notes
Time	0830	Alkaline bath with sodium bicarbonate 1:5 solution administered as tub bath for 3 minutes. Patted dry gently. Assisted to bed and positioned for comforts. States "the itching is not quite as bad." Edematous / erythematous patches over lower extremities are as prominent as yesterday. Reported to Lalitha RN. (Nurse's signature)

Patient Teaching

• Teach patient not to scratch the lesions to avoid further irritation and to prevent infection.

2. *Care of Hair*

Hair Care

Proper hair care is important to the patient's self image. Combing, brushing, and shampooing are basic hygiene measures for all patients. Illness or disability may prevent patients from performing their own daily hair care. A bedfast patient's hair may soon become tangled. It is important for the nurse to remember that most patients are aware of their appearance at all times. Therefore, good hair care must be performed routinely, at least daily to meet the hygiene needs of the patient. If the patient cannot carry out this part of his personal hygiene, the nurse will be required to give assistance. If the patient can take a shower or tub bath, the hair can be shampooed easily. A portable chair may be used in the shower, or a chair may be placed in front of a sink.

For the helpless, bedfast patient, the shampoo must be done in bed. A physician's instruction may or may not be necessary. Most facilities have portable blow dryers and curling irons available, as well as shampoo boards (Table 13.7).

Hair should be kept thoroughly clean and should always be kept combed and dressed. Proper and thorough cleansing is required both by men and women. The scalp needs a good blood supply and massaging for a few minutes daily is of great benefit. Fresh air is stimulating and to go without a heat (except in great heat) is good. If the hair is not properly looked after, disease like ring worm and dandruff may arise. Lice may appear if hair is kept untidy. A dry scalp, seborrhea sicca, is a condition of 'dandruff', i.e. epithelial scales are shed in excess. Only soft soap shampoos should be used. A good home made shampoo consists of 50 parts of soft soap, 15 parts of water, 33 parts of alcohol and 2 parts of oil of lavender. An oily sclap, seborrhea oleosa, is a condition of overactive sebaceous glands. Shampoos should be readily drying, and so spirit is added to them. It is necessary to wash the hair once in a week with soap and water or soap nut solution, prepared by steeping podered soap nuts for a few hours, in water (preferably hot water). Oil should not be used too frequently. It may however, be used once a week after washing the hair with soap to restore and natural grease. One should always practice to have ownself and as far as possible, avoid going to barber's shop for the purpose to avoid getting danger of infection.

Care of the Mouth/ Oral Care

Oral Hygiene

Oral hygiene helps to maintain a healthy state of the mouth, teeth gums and lips. Brushing the teeth removes food particles, plaque, and bacteria, massages the gums, and relieves discomfort resulting from unpleasant odors and tastes. Complete oral hygiene gives a sense of well-being and thus can stimulate appetite.

Certain patients are at risk for oral disorders because of: (i) lack of knowledge about oral hygiene, (ii) an inability to perform oral care, or (iii) an alteration in the integrity of teeth and mucosa resulting from disease or treatments.

Patients who are particularly at risk are those who are (i) paralyzed, (ii) seriously ill, (iii) have upper extremity activity limitations, (iv) unconscious, (v) confused, (vi) diabetic, or (vii) NPO status. Patients who are undergoing radiation therapy, receiving chemotherapeutic drugs or undergoing oral surgery also are at risk.

The nurse will allow the patient to brush his own teeth whenever possible. When the patient is unable to do so, the nurse will need to perform this procedure for him (Tables 13.8 and 13.9).

Denture Care

• Patients should be encouraged to care for their own dentures as often as for natural teeth to prevent infection and irritation.
• If the patient becomes disabled, incapacitated, or confused, the nurse must assist with denture care (Tables 13.8 and 13.10).
• Dentures are expensive and easily broken and are the patient's personal property; therefore they must be handled with care.
• Dentures should be stored in an enclosed and labelled cup during soaking or when not worn; patients should be

Table 13.7: Procedures for Administering a Bed Shampoo

	Nursing actions		*Rationales*
1.	Review physician's order instruction.	1.	Special shampoos may be ordered.
2.	Explain procedure.	2.	Patient may be anxious.
3.	Prepare equipment: • Bath towels (2) • Was cloth or hand towel • Water pitcher • Shampoo • Shampoo board • Wash basin • Bath blanket • Comb and brush, hair dryer and curling iron, if needed.	3.	Promotes an orderly procedure.
4.	Wash hands.	4.	Prevents spread of microorganism.
5.	Arrange equipment conveniently.	5.	Prevents interruptions during procedure.
6.	Position the patient close to one side of the bed. Place shampoo board under patient's head and wash basin at end of spout. Make sure spout extends over edge of mattress.	6.	Prevents getting bed linen wet.
7.	Position rolled-up bath towel under patient's neck.	7.	Minimizes discomfort.
8.	Brush and comb patient's hair.	8.	Removes tangles and loosens dried secretions.
9.	Obtain water in pitcher about 110°F (43°C).	9.	Prevents burns.
10.	If patient is able, instruct patient to hold washcloth over eyes. Completely wet hair and apply small amount of shampoo.	10.	Prevents water and shampoo from getting into eyes.
11.	Massage scalp with fingertips, not nails. Shampoo hair-line, back of neck (lift head slightly) and sides of hair.	11.	Ensures thorough cleansing and increases scalp circulation.
12.	Rinse thoroughly and apply more shampoo, repeating steps 10 and 11. Rinse, and repeat rinsing until hair is free of shampoo.	12.	Prevents scalp irritation.
13.	Wrap dry towel around patient's head. Dry patient's face, neck and shoulders. Dry hair and scalp using second towel if necessary.	13.	Prevents patient from chilling.
14.	Comb hair and/or dry with blow dryer as quickly as possible.	14.	Prevents patients from chilling.
15.	Complete styling hair, and position patient for comfort.	15.	Promotes sense of well-being.
16.	Place soiled linens in hamper. Clean and store equipment. Wash hands.	16.	Prevents spread of microorganisms.

discouraged from wrapping them in tissue or placing them on meal trays, since the dentures may be accidentally discarded.

In mouth, there are many species of bacteria always present as a rule a healthy mouth is capable of dealing with these. Under conditions of sepsis, however, such as caries teeth, septic tonsils, unhealthy mucous membrane or infected sinuses, the stream of bacteria are constantly pouring into the mouth, find these ideal conditions of growth, helped by remnants of food. The tongue becomes coated and sordes collect around teeth and lips. Such a mouth may give rise to parotitis, otitismedia, infected of respiratory passages and via general circulation, rheumatic conditions and remote septic foci. The tongue should be cleaned every morning by a tongue cleanser.

Mouth should be well rinsed with some pleasant antiseptic mouthwash, such as glycerine of thymol and little of it should be used for gargling in the morning and at night after taking the last meal or drink.

The oral cavity functions in mastication, secretion of mucus to moisten and lubricate the digestive system, secretion of digestive enzymes, and absorption of essential nutrients. Common problems occurring in the oral cavity include the following:

• Bad breath (halitosis)

- Dental cavities (caries)
- Plaque
- Periodontal disease
- Inflammation of the gums (gingivitis)
- Inflammation of the oral mucosa (stomatitis)

Poor oral hygiene and loss of teeth may affect a client's social interaction and body image as well as nutritional intake. Daily oral care is essential to maintain the integrity of the mucous membranes, teeth, gums, and lips. Through preventive measures, the oral cavity and teeth can be preserved. Preventive oral care consists of fluoride rinsing, flossing, and brushing.

Fluoride: Fluoride can prevent dental caries. Fluoride is a common component of many mouthwashes and toothpastes; however, people with excessive dryness or irritated mucous membranes should avoid commercial mouthwashes because of the alcohol content, which causes drying of mucous membranes. Educate clients about fluoride being an excellent preventive measure against dental caries, but excessive fluoride exposure can affect the color of tooth enamel.

Flossing: Floss daily in conjunction with brushing of teeth. Flossing prevents the formation of plaque, removes plaque between the teeth, and removes food debris. Dental caries and periodontal disease can be prevented by regular flossing. Many floss holders are available to facilitate flossing.

Brushing: Teeth should be brushed after each meal. Brushing should be performed using a dentifrice (toothpaste) that contains fluoride to aid in preventing dental caries. An effective homemade dentifrice is the combination of two parts salt with one part baking soda. Brushing removes plaque and food debris and promotes blood circulation of the gums. Dentures should be brushed using the same brushing motion as that used for brushing teeth.

Before the procedure the nurse should
- Assess whether the client is able to assist with oral care and to what extent. Promotes independence where possible.
- Evaluate whether the client has an understanding of proper oral hygiene. Promotes self-care and teaching.
- Check whether the client has dentures. Determines how oral care will be performed.
- Assess the condition of the client's mouth. Determines how oral care will be performed.
- Assess whether inflammation, bleeding, infection, or ulceration is present. Determines how oral care will be performed. Determines the need for additional assessment and intervention.
- Assess what cultural practices must be taken into consideration. Determines how oral care will be performed.
- Assess whether there are any appliances or devices present in the client's mouth such as braces, **endotracheal tube, or bridgework. Determines how oral care will be performed.**
- Check that the proper equipment is available to perform oral care. Ensures a smooth procedure.

Equipment Needed

Brushing and Flossing
- Toothbrush
- Toothpaste with fluoride
- Emesis basin
- Towel
- Cup of water
- Nonsterile gloves
- Dental floss, floss holder
- Mirror
- Lip moisturizer

Denture Care
- Denture brush
- Denture cleaner
- Emesis basin
- Towel
- Cup of water
- Nonsterile gloves
- Tissue
- Denture cup

Special Care Items for Clients with Impaired Physical Mobility or Who Are Unconscious (comatose)
- Soft toothbrush or toothette
- Tongue blade
- 3×3 gauze sponges
- cotton-tip applicators
- prescribed solution
- plastic Asepto syringe
- suction machine and catheter

After procedure nurse should see that:
- The client's mouth, teeth, gums, and lips are clean and free of food particles.
- Inflammation, bleeding, infection, or ulceration are noted and cared for.
- The oral mucosa is clean, intact, and well hydrated.
- The oral care was performed with a minimum of trauma to the client.

And document in the Nurses' Notes
- Unusual findings

Care of Teeth

A tooth is a hard structure composed of dentine and the enamel covering the dentine although it resembles bone, yet it is much harder. The enamel of teeth is the hardest tissue in the body. Once the enamel of teeth is completely formed, the cells that produced, it, disappear. Thus it can then no longer receive nourishment from the body, the enamel is therefore incapable of repair. It covers only the exposed surface of the tooth, as within the jaw bone the dentine of the tooth, as within the jaw bone the dentine of the tooth is covered with a cement like material, called cementum.

Table 13.8: Oral Care

	Nursing actions		Rationales
	Check clients identification band		To identity right patient
	Explain procedure before beginning		To get cooperation and reduce anxiety

Self-Care Client: Flossing and Brushing

	Nursing actions		Rationales
1.	Assemble articles for flossing and brushing.	1.	Promotes efficiency.
2.	Provide privacy.	2.	Relaxes the client.
3.	Place client in a high Fowler's position.	3.	Decreases risk of aspiration.
4.	Cleanse hands and apply gloves.	4.	Reduces the transmission of microorganisms.
5.	Arrange articles within client's reach.	5.	Facilitates self-care.
6.	Assist client with flossing and brushing as necessary. Position mirror, emesis basin, water with straw near the client, and a towel across the chest.	6.	Flossing and brushing decrease microorganism growth in the mouth. Use of mirror permits cleaning back and sides of teeth.
7.	Assist client with rinsing mouth.	7.	Removes toothpaste and oral secretions.
8.	Reposition client, raise side rails, and place call button within reach.	8.	Promotes comfort, safety, and communication.
9.	Rinse, dry, and return articles to proper place.	9.	Promotes a clean environment.
10.	Remove gloves, cleanse hands, and document care.	10.	Reduces the transmission of microorganisms and documents nursing care.

Self-Care Client: Denture Care

	Nursing actions		Rationales
11.	Assemble articles for denture cleaning.	11.	Promotes efficiency.
12.	Provide privacy.	12.	Relaxes the client.
13.	Assist client to a high Fowler's position.	13.	Facilitates removal of dentures.
14.	Cleanse hands and apply gloves.	14.	Reduces the transmission of microorganisms and exposure to body fluids.
15.	Assist client with denture removal: (a) Top denture: • With tissue, grasp the denture with thumb and forefinger and pull downward. • Place in denture cup. (b) Bottom denture: • Place thumbs on the gums and release the denture. Grasp denture with thumb and forefinger and pull upward. • Place in denture cup.	15.	Breaks seal created with dentures without causing pressure and injury to oral membranes. Prevents breaking of dentures.
16.	Apply toothpaste to brush, and brush dentures either with cool water in the emesis basin or under running water in the sink. Pad sink with towel to protect dentures in case they are dropped (Fig. 13.11).	16.	Facilitates removal of microorganisms.
17.	Rinse thoroughly.	17.	Removes toothpaste.
18.	Assist client with rinsing mouth and replacing dentures.	18.	Freshens mouth and facilitates intake of solid food.
19.	Reposition client, with side rails up and call button within reach.	19.	Promotes comfort, safety, and communication.
20.	Rinse, dry, and return articles to proper place.	20.	Maintains a clean environment.
21.	Remove gloves and cleanse hands.	21.	Reduces the transmission of microorganisms.

Contd...

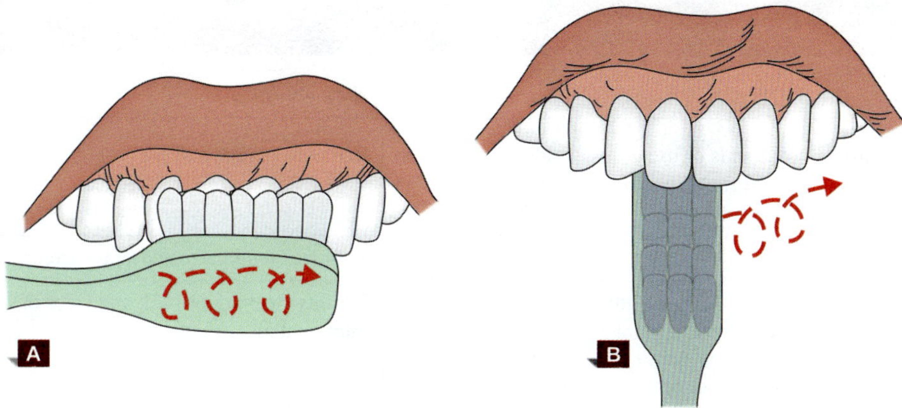

Figures 13.7A and B: A. Brushing outer surface of upper teeth, B. Clean inside surface of teeth with end of toothbrush, using vibratory motion. Hold brush at 45° angle to the teeth.

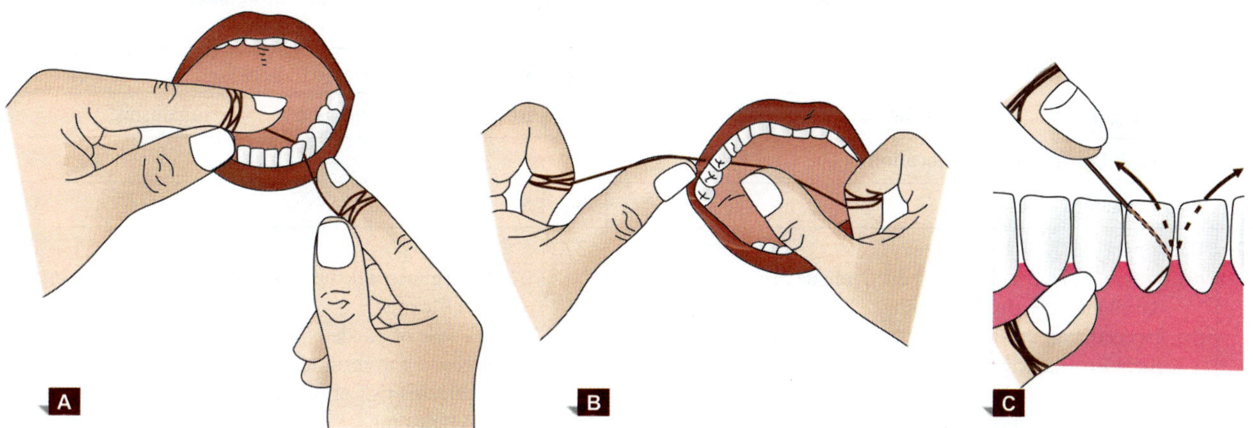

Figures 13.8A and B: Flossing technique A. Flossing bottom teeth, B. Flossing top teeth, C. Directions of flossing. Floss should wrap around side of tooth and go between bottom of tooth and gum tissue

<table>
<tr><td colspan="4" align="center">Table 13.8: Contd...</td></tr>
<tr><td colspan="2">Nursing actions</td><td colspan="2">Rationales</td></tr>
<tr><td colspan="4">Full-Care Client: Brushing and Flossing (Figs 13.7 and 13.8)</td></tr>
<tr><td>22.</td><td>Assemble articles for flossing and brushing.</td><td>22.</td><td>Promotes efficiency.</td></tr>
<tr><td>23.</td><td>Provide privacy.</td><td>23.</td><td>Relaxes client.</td></tr>
<tr><td>24.</td><td>Cleanse hands and apply gloves.</td><td>24.</td><td>Reduces the transmission of microorganisms and exposure to body fluids.</td></tr>
<tr><td>25.</td><td>Position client as condition allows: high Fowler's, semi-Fowler's or lateral position, head turned toward side (Fig. 13.9).</td><td>25.</td><td>Decreases risk of aspiration.</td></tr>
<tr><td>26.</td><td>Place towel across client's chest or under face and mouth if head is turned to one side.</td><td>26.</td><td>Catches secretions.</td></tr>
<tr><td>27.</td><td>Moisten toothbrush or toothette, apply small amount of toothpaste, and brush teeth and gums.</td><td>27.</td><td>Moistens mouth and facilitates plaque removal.</td></tr>
</table>

Contd...

Table 13.8: *Contd...*

	Nursing actions		Rationales
28.	Grasp the dental floss in both hands or use a floss holder and floss between all teeth: hold floss against tooth while moving floss up and down sides of teeth.	28.	Removes plaque and prevents gum disease.
29.	Assist the client in rinsing mouth.	29.	Removes toothpaste and oral secretions.
30.	Reapply toothpaste and brush the teeth and gums using friction in a vertical or circular motion. On inner and outer surfaces of teeth, hold brush at 45-degree angle against teeth and brush from sulcus to crowns of teeth. On bit	30.	Permits cleaning of back and sides of teeth and decreases microorganism growth in mouth.
31.	Assist the client in rinsing and drying mouth.	31.	Removes toothpaste and oral secretions
32.	Apply lip moisturizer, if appropriate.	32.	Maintains skin integrity of lips.
33.	Reposition client, raise side rails, and place call button within reach.	33.	Promotes comfort, safety, and communication.
34.	Rinse, dry, and return articles to proper place.	34.	Provides an orderly environment.
35.	Remove gloves and cleanse hands.	35.	Reduces the transmission of microorganisms.
Clients at Risk for or with an Alteration of the Oral Cavity			
36.	Follow Actions 22-24.	36.	See Rationales 22-24.
37.	Bleeding: (a) Assess oral cavity with a padded tongue blade and flashlight for signs of bleeding. (b) Proceed with the actions for oral care for a full-care client except: • Do not floss. • Use a soft toothbrush, toothette, or a tongue blade padded with 3 × 3 gauze sponges to gently swab teeth and gums. • Rinse with tepid water.	37.	(a) Determines whether bleeding is present, amount, and specific area. • Dispose of padded tongue blade into a biohazard bag according to institutional policy. • Decreases risk of bleeding and trauma to gums. • Promotes proper disposal of contaminated waste. • Cleanses mouth.
38.	Infection: (a) Assess oral cavity with a tongue blade and flash-light for signs of infection. (b) Culture lesions as ordered. (c) Proceed with the actions for oral care for a full-care client except: • Do not floss. • Use prescribed antiseptic solution. • Use a tongue blade padded with 3 × 3 gauze sponges to gently swab the teeth and gums. • Dispose of padded tongue blade into a biohazard bag according to institutional policy. • Rinse mouth with tepid water. • Apply additional solution as prescribed.	38.	(a) Determines appearance, integrity, and general condition. • Identifies growth of specific microorganisms. • Prevents irritation, pain, and bleeding. • Antiseptic solutions decrease growth of microorganisms. • Promotes proper disposal of contaminated materials. • Cleanses mouth. • Provides a coating that promotes healing of the tissue.
39.	Ulceration: (a) Assess oral cavity with a tongue blade and flash-light for signs of ulceration. (b) Culture lesions as ordered. (c) Proceed with actions for oral care for a full-care client except: • Do not floss. • Use prescribed antiseptic solution.	39.	(a) Determines appearance, integrity, and general condition. (b) Identifies growth of specific microorganisms. • Prevents irritation, pain, and bleeding, • Antiseptic solutions decrease growth of microorganisms. • Promotes proper disposal of contaminated materials. • Cleanses mouth.

Contd...

Table 13.8: *Contd...*

	Nursing actions		Rationales
	• Use a tongue blade padded with 3 × 3 gauze sponges to gently swab the teeth and gums. • Dispose of padded tongue blade into a biohazard bag according to institutional policy. • Rinse mouth with tepid water. • Apply additional solution as prescribed.		• Provides a coating that promotes healing of the tissue.
40.	Follow Actions 22-24.	40.	See Rationales 22-24.
41.	Place the client in a lateral position, with the head turned toward the side.	41.	Prevents aspiration.
42.	Use a floss holder and floss between all teeth.	42.	Prevents transfer of microorganisms from a client bite.
43.	Moisten toothbrush or toothette, and brush the teeth and gums using friction in a vertical or circular motion. Do not use toothpaste. On inner and outer surfaces of teeth, hold brush at 45-degree angle against teeth and brush from sulcus to crowns of teeth. On biting surfaces, move brush back and forth in short strokes. All surfaces of teeth should be brushed from every angle.	43.	Permits cleaning of back and sides of teeth and decreases microorganism growth in mouth. Toothpaste may foam and cause aspiration.
44.	After flossing and brushing, rinse mouth with an asepto syringe (do not force water into the mouth) and perform oral suction.	44.	Promotes cleansing and removal of secretions and prevents aspiration.
45.	Dry the client's mouth.	45.	Prevents skin irritation.
46.	Apply lip moisturizer.	46.	Maintains skin integrity of lips.
47.	Leave the client in a lateral position with head turned toward side for 30 to 60 minutes after oral hygiene care. Suction one more time. Remove the towel from under the client's mouthy and face.	47.	Prevents pooling of secretions and aspiration.
48.	Dispose of any contaminated items in a biohazard bag and clean, dry, and return all articles to the appropriate place.	48.	Promotes proper disposal of contaminated materials.
49.	Remove gloves and cleanse hands.	49.	Reduces the transmission of microorganisms.

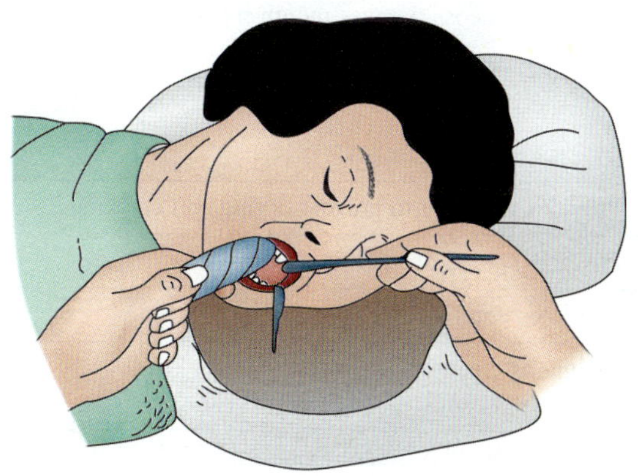

Figure 13.9: Giving mouth care to a comatose or helpless person unconscious (Comatose) client

A proper wholesome diet is necessary not only for building of strong teeth, but also to ward off dental diseases. Milk, eggs, tomatoes, guavas, amlas and other citrus fruits including green leafy vegetables rich in vitamin C content should be included in our daily diet. If the diet happens to be lacking in minerals and vitamin C, children may suffer from structural defects of teeth, gums and bones. Full grown teeth also require balanced nourishment for their maintenance.

A set of sound teeth is a valuable asset because it contributes to personal appearance, in addition to providing an efficient chewing apparatus. Defective teeth make difficult or impossible the proper mastication of food and when teeth are infected, health of the body may become seriously impaired. So it is very essential that the teeth should be regularly and thoroughly cleaned to ensure good digestion. They should be scrupulously cleaned at least twice a day. The first thing in the morning and last thing at night should be with a brush of moderate stiffness. Any place between the teeth where food gets lodged habitually and hence it is not removed promptly and regularly is quite sure to decay sooner or later. The teeth rarely decay on a fully exposed surface. If there are cavities in the teeth they should be promptly got filled up. If they are altogether decayed and carious they should be removed at once so that near by teeth will not be decayed. Deposit of tartar upon the teeth should receive due attention and in this case the teeth require scaling or else the roots will become exposed which will eventually make the teeth loose. Children often suffer from caries either on account of deficiency of vitamin D or due to acid forming bacteria formed on account of fermentation of carbohydrates. Especially amongst children, eating of sweets, chocolates, toffees and chewing gums, etc. are the promoting causes of dental caries or decay of teeth, because starch and sugar undergo fermentation of the mouth and are converted into acids. Acid acts on the enamel of the teeth, exerting a corroding action, destroying it and exposing underlying dentine. The microorganisms, which are teeming in our mouths subsequently, attach the exposed dentine. Therefore natural fruits in the form of dry fruits such as figs, dates, apricots, plums, etc. may be given to children, which act as nourishing substitutes for candles.

Table 13.9: Administering Oral Hygiene (Patient without Denture)

	Nursing actions		*Rationales*
1.	Position patient's head to side toward nurse (dependent side if possible) as close to nurse as possible.	1.	Prevents aspiration.
2.	Explain procedure even to unconscious patient.	2.	Unconscious patients may be able to hear.
3.	Prepare equipment: • Cleansing solution, such as diluted hydrogen peroxide, toothpaste, normal saline, soda solution, or mouthwash • Toothed comb, toothbrush, or tongue blade wrapped with gauze • Towel • Emesis basin • Disposable wash cloths • Water glass filled with cool water • Water-soluble lubricant • Disposable gloves • Flashlight.	3.	Organizes procedure.
4.	Wash hands, and don gloves.	4.	Prevents spread of microorganisms.
5.	Provide privacy, and arrange equipment.	5.	Promotes an orderly procedure.
6.	Raise bed to working level, and lower side rail.	6.	Enables good body mechanics.
7.	Place towel under patient's face and emesis basin under patient's chin.	7.	Facilitates procedure. Prevents soiling bed.
8.	Carefully separate patient's jaws.	8.	Protect nurse's fingers.
9.	Cleanse teeth using brush (Fig. 13.10), tongue blade, or toothette moistened with cleansing agent. Clean inner and outer teeth surfaces. Swab roof of mouth and inside cheeks. Use flashlight for better visualization of oral cavity. Gently swab tongue. Rinse several times.	9.	Removes food particles, secretions, and dried exudes and moistens mucosa. Leaves mouth fresh.
10.	Apply lubricant on lips.	10.	Provides moisture to prevent drying and cracking.
11.	Remove gloves, and dispose of properly.	11.	Prevents spread of microorganisms.
12.	Position patient for comfort, raise side rail, and lower bed.	12.	Promotes comfort and safety.
13.	Clean and return equipment to storage. Place soiled linen in laundry bag.	13.	Maintains clean environment.
14.	Wash hands.	14.	Prevents spread of microorganisms.
15.	Record procedure. Include any pertinent observations, such as gum bleeding or ulcerations.	15.	Documents patient response – any unusual findings may indicate more serious problems.

In tropics, one has to be very careful about the occurrence of pyorrhea, alveolaris among adults which is perhaps form the scurvy due to deficiency of vitamin C. Pyorrhea is essentially a disease, which is characterized by the formation of pus pockets between the teeth surfaces and gums, where germs freely thrive and become a source of danger to the body. Since germs from the pyorrhea may threaten the danger of poisoning even the whole body, these germs from the pyorrhea pockets can reach any part of the body and give rise to conditions like digestive disorders, pain in joints, eye trouble, heart and kidneys diseases. Moreover, apart from these ailments, pyorrhea has its social aspects too. Pockets of pus and germs give rise to foul breath which may lead to avoidance of social relations and loss of friends.

The movement of the brush should not only be from side to side but also from above downwards and inside the teeth. While brushing the teeth, sufficient pressure should be exercised so that bristles of the brush may be forced between the teeth. All the inner, outer and biting surfaces should be brushed alike at least 5 times. Upper and lower teeth should be brushed downwards and upwards respectively. The chewing and biting surfaces should, however be particularly at night followed by a hot and tepid water gargles will go along way to prevent caries and pyorrhea. The gum tissues may be benefited by massaging them with a finger tip smeared with tooth paste.

The use of tooth brush is not very sanitary because there is always the difficulty of keeping clean and the same brush is generally used for a considerably long period. If the toothbrush is to be used, it should be kept in boiling water for sometime after use. It should be frequently changed.

In India a green neem or kiker twig, *datun* is used for cleansing teeth, which is very good from hygienic point of view, since it requires chewing and provides massage to the gums.

The tongue should be cleaned by a tongue cleanser every morning.

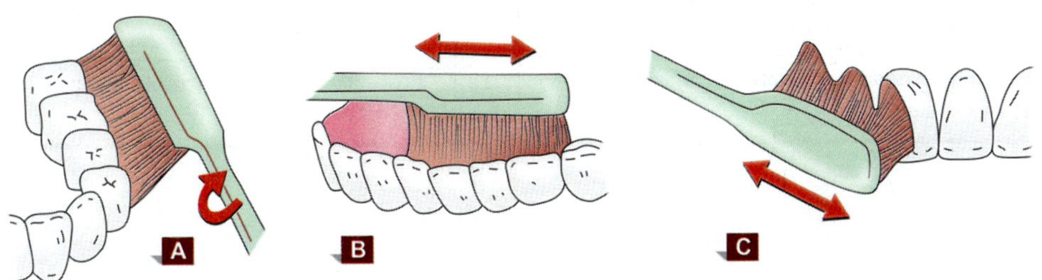

Figure 13.10: Cleaning teeth using brush

		Table 13.10: Administering Oral Hygiene (Patients with Denture)		
	Nursing actions			*Rationales*
1.	Explain procedure patient.		1.	Promotes cooperation.
2.	Prepare equipment: • Soft-bristled toothbrush • Denture brush • Emesis basin or sink • Cleansing agent • Water glass • Wash cloth • 4 × 4 gauze • denture cup • Disposable gloves.		2.	Promotes orderly procedure.
3.	Wash hands.		3.	Prevents spread of microorganisms.
4.	Arrange supplies close by		4.	Promotes organized procedure
5.	Fill emesis basin ½ full of tepid water		5.	Acts as a cushion for the dentures if accidentally dropped, preventing damage to dentures.
6.	Don gloves.		6.	Prevents spread of microorganisms.

Contd...

Table 13.10: Contd...

	Nursing actions		*Rationales*
7.	Ask patient to remove dentures and place in emesis basin. If patient is unable to remove own dentures, break suction that holds upper denture in place by using thumb and finger. With gauze apply gentle downward tug and carefully remove from patient's mouth. Next remove lower denture by carefully lifting up and turning sideways. Remove and place in emesis basin.	7.	Prevents slipping while handling dentures.
8.	Cleanse biting surfaces. Cleanse outer and inner teeth surfaces. Be certain to cleanse under surface of dentures (Fig. 13.11).	8.	Cleansing prevents food, bacteria, odor, and stain formation.
9.	Rinse dentures thoroughly with tepid water.	9.	Warm water is more effective than cold water.
10.	Replace dentures either in patient's mouth or in container of solution placed in safe place	10.	Dentures may become brittle and warped if not kept mlist.
11.	Before replacing dentures in patient's mouth or after storing dentures properly, gently brush patient's gums, tongue, and inside of check, and rinse thoroughly.	11.	Oral cavity needs cleansing also to promote healthy gums and mucosa.
12.	Remove gloves, and discard appropriately. Clean and store equipment. Wash hands.	12.	Prevents spread of microorganisms.

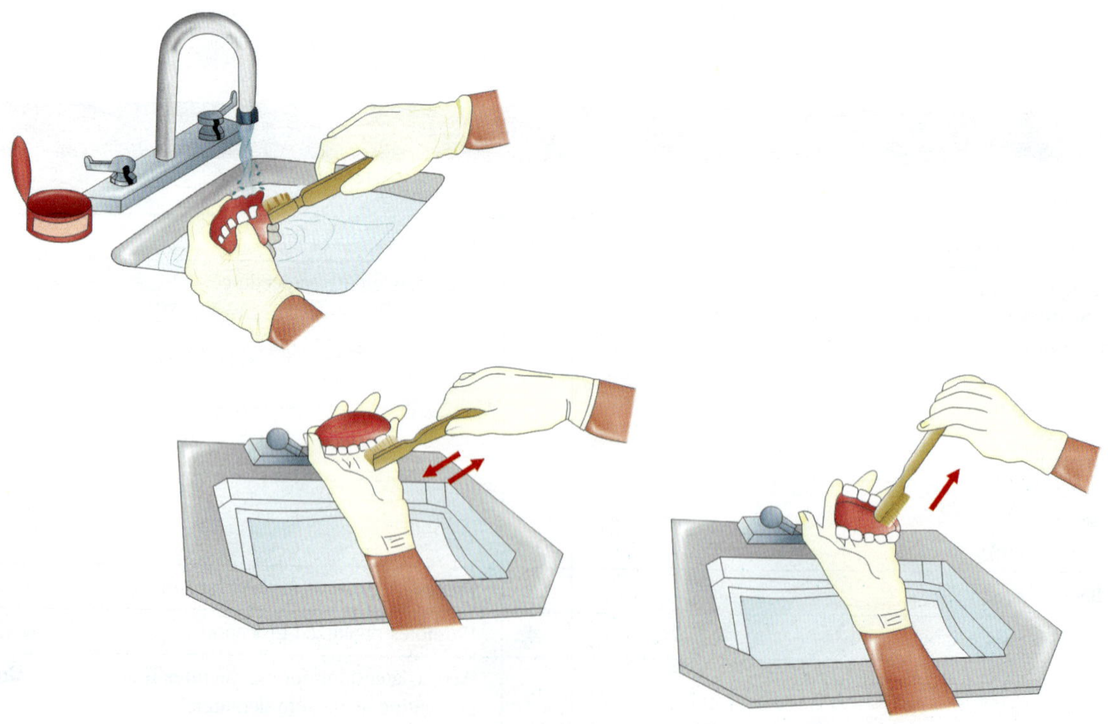

Figure 13.11: Cleaning dentures

4. *Care of the Hands*

Hands and Feet Care

Hands and feet often require special attention to prevent infection, odors, and injury. Problems arise from abuse or poor care of the hands and feet, for example, biting nails or wearing ill-fitting shoes.

Assessment of the feet involves a thorough examination of all skin surfaces. The area between the toes should be carefully checked. Patients with diabetes mellitus or peripheral vascular disease should be observed for adequate circulation to the feet. The elderly are also at the risk for foot disorders, because of poor vision or decreased mobility.

Care of the hands and feet can be administered during the morning bath or at another time (Table 13.11).

Hands should be kept free from the cracks and roughness due to cold wind or constant use of antiseptic solutions. Glycerine (diluted) in account of its action of drawing fluid to it or some skin cream which will prevent evaporation should be used until cracks heal. Scrupulous cleansing of hands with soap and water is very essential to prevent spread of infectious diseases like cholera, typhoid, dysentery, etc. they should invariably be washed before taking meals and during handling or preparing food.

5. *Care of the Feet*

Next to hands, the feet carry the greatest load of any part of the body, so obviously they have a tremendous effect on the rest of the body. These must be kept scrupulously clean by daily washing and carefully drying between the toes.

The feet contain many sweat glands, and excessive sweating or hyperhidrosis necessitates frequent washing and change of soacks. Bromidrosis is excessive sweating with offensive odors and soreness of feet. The odor is due to decomposition of sweat. For this condition the feet should be washed several times a day in boric acid solution, dried, dabbed with methylated spirit mixed with starch and boric powder. Sock and shoes must be changed each time after use; used sockings washing and shoes be aired. Shoes with cork heels are good and should be washed with a spirit lotion.

Corns: These are caused by pressure of badly fitting shoes. The epidermis thickens and becomes horny and grows inward to a point. If they occur between the toes, they are kept moist and are called 'softcorns.'

Callosities: These are formed as a result of pointed shoes. The great toe becomes bent in producing an angle at the junction of metatarsophalangeal joint. The head of the metatarsal is thus a projecting point on the inner border of the foot and is exposed to pressure. A callosity forms on this point of pressure and the bursa underneath becomes chronically inflamed.

These conditions may be avoided by wearing suitable shoes.

Arch of the foot: The inner bony arch should be 1 to 1½ inches (25.4-38.1 mm) from the ground. Dropped arch is very painful and is caused for want of tone in the leg muscles with stretching of the supporting tendons and ligaments under the arch. The chief remedies are massage of leg muscles, a built up sole, raised ¼ to ½ inch (6.1-12.2 mm) on the inner side and provision of arch supports.

6. *Care of the Nails*

Nails require to be kept clean and should be cut short periodically otherwise dirts will get lodged under them and may carry infection. The cuticle surrounding the nails should be pressed back periodically, say once or twice a week, with a wooden stick. If necessary, the cuticle may be softened to bed by applying the dilute glycerine or liquid paraffin at night before retiring. As a majority of Indians eat their meals with their hands and do not use spoon and forks, they should be very careful about regular cleansing of their nails. The fingers should never be put in the mouth of the nose. Biting of nails with the teeth is also an unclean habit and is particularly dangerous in tropics, as intestinal infections are very likely to be carried in this way to the human system. The nails should be cut horizontally, because if curved, the skin around them will be pressed over the nails and the pressure of the nails on this enfolding skin will cause symptoms usually attributed to 'ingrowing toe nails'.

Hypertrophied nails: These are hard, horny, thickened growths of nails and are of a yellowish or blakish color. They should be treated as soon as the symptoms start, by soaking in a solution of sodium bicarbonate and careful filing.

7. *Care of the Eyes/ Eyes Care*

Eye, Ear and Nose Care

Special attention is paid to the cleaning of the eyes, ears, and nose during the patient's bath. The nurse often has the responsibility of assisting patients in the care of eye glasses, contact lenses, or artificial eyes. For patients who wear eye glasses, contact lenses, artificial eyes, or hearing aids, the nurse will assess the patient's knowledge and methods used to care for the aids, as well as any problems caused by the aids. Patients who cannot grasp small objects, have limited mobility in the upper extremities, have reduced, or are seriously fatigued will require assistance from the nurse.

The eyes, ears and nose are sensitive, and therefore extracare should be taken to avoid injury to these tissues.

Care of the Eyes

Cleansing of the circumorbital (circular area around the eye) area of the eyes is usually performed during the bath and involves washing with a clean wash cloth moistened with clear water. The use of soap is generally omitted because it may cause burning and irritation. The eye is cleansed from the inner to outer canthus. A separate section of the wash cloth is used each time to prevents spread of infection. If he patient has dried exudate that is not removed easily with gentle cleansing, the nurse may first place a damp cotton ball or gauze on the lid margins to loosen secretions. Never apply direct pressure over the eyeball, because this may cause serious injury. Exudates from the eyes should be

Table 13.11: Procedures for Caring the Hands and Feet

	Nursing actions		*Rationales*
1.	Obtain physician's order if necessary.	1.	The patient's physical condition may place him at risk for infection.
2.	Explain procedure.	2.	Patient may be anxious or fatigued.
3.	Prepare equipment: • Wash basin • Emesis basin • Wash cloth • Hand towel • Nail clippers, emory board, and orange wood stick • Lotion • Disposable bath mat • Disposable gloves (optionals).	3.	Prevents interruptions during procedure.
4.	Wash hands. Arrange supplies within easy reach.	4.	Prevents spread of microorganisms.
5.	Provide privacy. Position patient in chair. If possible place disposable mat under patient's feet.	5.	Protects patient's bare feet from floor.
6.	Fill basin with water at 100° to 110°F (43° to 44°C). Place basin on disposable mat, and assist patient to place feet into basin. Allow to soak 10 to 20 min. Rewarm water as necessary.	6.	Soaking in warm water will soften nails and ensures easy manipulation of cuticles.
7.	Place over bed table, in low position in front of patient. Fill emesis basin with water at 100° to 110°F (43° to 44°C). Place basin on table, and place patient's fingers in basin. Allow fingernails to soak 10 to 20 min. Rewarm water as necessary.	7.	Soaking loosens foreign particles under nails and ensures easy manipulation of cuticles.
8.	Using orange stick, gently clean under fingernails. With clippers, trim nails straight across and even with tip of fingers. With emory board shape fingernails. Push cuticles back gently with wash cloth or orange wood stick.	8.	Prevents injury to delicate nailbeds.
9.	Don gloves, and with a wash cloth scrub area of feet that are calloused.	9.	Prevents spread of microorganisms.
10.	Trim and clean toenails following step 8.	10.	Prevents injury, infection.
11.	Apply lotion or cream to hands and feet. Return patient to bed, and position for comfort.	11.	Creams and lotions lubricate dry skin.
12.	Remove and dispose of gloves in proper container. Clean and store equipment. Place soiled linen in laundry bag. Wash hands.	12.	Prevents spread of microorganisms.

removed carefully and as often as necessary to keep the eye clean.

The eyes are well-protected with eyelashes, tearing, and a split second blink reflex and usually do not require special care. Secretions may collect along the margins of the lid and inner cantus when the blink reflex is absent or when the eyes do not completely close. Lubricating eye drops may be ordered by the physicians. Sometimes the eyes may be medicated and covered to prevent corneal drying and irritation.

Many patients wear eyeglasses. This represents a large financial investment for them. Therefore, the nurse will use car

when cleaning glasses and should protect them from breakage or other damage when not worn.

Eye glasses should be stored in the case and placed in the drawer of the bedside stand when not in use to avoid accidental damage. Glasses are made of hardened glass or plastic that is impact resistant to prevent shattering but can be easily scratched. Plastic lenses require special cleansing solutions and drying tissues. Warm water is adequate to clean glass lenses, and the use of a soft cloth to dry is best to prevent of the lenses.

Most patients prefer caring for their own contact lenses. A contact lens is a small, round, sometimes colored disk that fits on the cornea of the eye over the pupil. If the patient's condition does not permit him to remove the lenses, the nurse should seek assistance from someone who is familiar with the procedure. The lenses need not be reinserted until the patient is more capable of caring for the lenses himself. It is important that the nurse protect those patients who are unable to care for their lenses properly, because prolonged wearing of contact lenses may cause serious damage to the cornea. There is a large variety of products available for lens care. Each type of lens (hard, soft or rigid gas-permeable) requires a different cleansing technique. Each set of lenses is stored in a case with solution according to manufacturer's directions.

It is highly specialized receptor of the optic nerve. Its mechanism enables the light waves to reach the optic nerve endings producing sight.

Eyes of the school children should be periodically examined and defects corrected and treated. Children with such defects as myopia and those whose vision is liable to deteriorate should be kept under constant supervision and suitable work chosen for them.

Tears have considerably bactericidal power and are less injurious to conjunctiva than any other lotion. They are brought about by some emotional crisis, by frustration, anger, sorrow or even by the sudden lifting of some frightening crisis, as for example, when a mother finds her lost child who has not been drowned or kidnapped. Frequent bathing of eyes should not be encouraged. Disinfectant lotions should be used only when prescribed.

School children should be taught the importance of looking after their eyes. They should be asked to hold the printed page about a foot and a half (0.45 meters) from the eyes and at an angle of 45 to 70 degrees from horizontal surface. The light in the class room should be satisfactory and the print of the books should be large enough to prevent eye strain. An inflammation or accident to the eyes should receive immediate attention.

Sore eye is an infective disease and fairly widespread in villages all over the country. The infection is present in the discharge of the eyes and is transmitted to the healthy persons through handkerchiefs or towels soiled with discharge by direct contact with the eyes of an infected person. Indirectly the infection is spread through flies. When the germs of sore eye infect an individual, then transparent covering of the eye called conjunctiva is damaged or it may get hurt by particles of foreign bodies such as dust particles and the eyes may therefore get red and watery. In due course of time a discharge secretes from the eyes, which is infective and is disease producing.

Prevention

The following measures should be adopted:
1. One should avoid open cases of sore eye as the disease is highly infectious.
2. Children with sore eye should never be allowed to mix up with the others.
3. Mothers should not use the end of *dhotis* or *sarees* to wipe away the eye discharge of their children.

4. Flies should not be allowed to sit on the sore eye.
5. Persons infected with sore eye should be asked to use separate handkerchiefs, towels, etc.

Generally, the eye needs little daily care. Normally, eyes are continually cleansed by the production of tears and movement of eyelids over the eyes. Some clients, however, do have special eye care needs.

Contact Lenses: Self-care is the best method of care for a client with contact lenses; however, accidents or illness may render a client unable to remove or care for the lenses. Some lenses may be left on the cornea for up to a week without damage. Most must be removed daily for cleaning and to prevent hypoxia of the cornea. It is a nursing responsibility to determine whether the client is wearing contact lenses and to properly care for the lenses and the client's eyes. In acute care situations, encourage the client to wear glasses if possible and send the contact lenses home with a family member.

Prosthetic Eyes: Some clients have an artificial eye (ocular prosthesis) in place. Artificial eyes are created to look identical to the client's biologic eye. They are generally made from glass or plastic. Some artificial eyes are permanently implanted in the eye socket, but others must be removed daily for cleaning. The eye socket should also be gently cleansed to remove crusts and mucus, and the prosthesis replaced in the eye socket.

For procedure of eye, ear care please see Table 13.12.

Before the procedure the nurse should
1. Determine if the client is wearing contact lenses or has an ocular prosthesis. If the client is unable to answer questions, you will need to find out another way. Does it indicate in the client's chart if the client wears contact lenses or has a prosthesis? Are there family members present to ask? This will affect how eye care is given.
2. Are the eye care supplies needed available? If the client can tell you what kind of eye care products he or she normally uses, ask or have a family member bring these products from home. This will affect how eye care is given.
3. Assess whether the client can do his or her own eye care. If not, evaluate what kind of assistance the client will need. This promotes maximum independence in the client.

Equipment Needed

Artificial Eye
- Storage container
- Mild soap
- 3 × 3 gauze sponges
- Cotton balls
- Towel
- Emesis basins
- Eye irrigation syringe (optional)
- Running water
- Sterile gloves
- Biohazard bag
- Saline solution
- Protector pad

	Table 13.12: Eye Ears with Artificial Eye		
	Nursing actions		*Rationales*
	Check clients identification band Explain procedure before beginning		To identity right patient To get cooperation and reduce anxiety
1.	Inquire about client's care regimen and gather equipment accordingly.	1.	Promotes continuity of care.
2.	Provide privacy.	2.	Relaxes the client.
3.	Cleanse hands; apply gloves.	3.	Reduces the transmission of microorganisms.
4.	Place client in a semi- Fowler's position.	4.	Facilitates procedure and client participation.
5.	Place the cotton balls in an emesis basin filled halfway with warm tap water.	5.	Dry cotton balls could cause irritation.
6.	Place 3 × 3 gauze sponges in bottom of second emesis basin and fill halfway with mild soap and tepid water.	6.	Gauze serves as padding to prevent breakage of the prosthesis.
7.	Grasp and squeeze excess water from a cotton ball. Cleanse the eyelid with the moistened cotton ball, starting at the inner canthus and moving outward toward the outer canthus. After each use, dispose of cotton ball in biohazard bag. Repeat procedure until eyelid is clean (without dried secretions).	7.	Eliminating the excess water prevents water from running down the client's face. Cleansing the eyelid prevents contamination of the lacrimal system (inner canthus area). Disposal of cotton balls reduces transmission of microorganisms to other health care workers.
8. (a) (b) (c)	Remove the artificial eye: Using dominant hand, raise the client's upper eyelid with index finger and depress the lower eyelid with thumb. Cup nondominant hand under the client's lower eyelid. Apply slight pressure with index finger between the brow and the artificial eye and remove it. Place it in an emesis basin filled with warm, soapy water.	8. (a) (b) (c)	Cleanses the artificial eye. Promotes removal of artificial eye. Cupping reduces dropping and possible breaking of the eye. Applying pressure will help the prosthesis to slip out.
9.	Grasp a moistened cotton ball and cleanse around the edge of the eye socket. Dispose of the soiled cotton ball into biohazard bag.	9.	Cleanses the eye socket. Disposal of cotton ball reduces transmission of microorganisms to other health care workers.
10.	Inspect the eye socket for any signs of irritation, drainage, or crusting. *Note:* If the client's usual care regimen or physician order requires irrigation of the socket, proceed with Action 11; otherwise, go to Action 12.	10.	Indicates an infection.
11. (a) (b) (c) (d) (e) (f) (g) (h) (i)	Eye socket irrigation: Lower the head of the bed and place the client in a supine position. Place protector pad on bed; turn head toward socket side and slightly extend neck. Fill the irrigation syringe with the prescribed amount and type of irrigating solution (warm tap water or normal saline). With nondominant hand, separate the eyelids with your forefinger and thumb while resting fingers on the brow and cheekbone. Hold the irrigating syringe in dominant hand several inches above the inner canthus; with thumb, gently apply pressure on the plunger, directing the flow of solution from the inner canthus along the conjunctival sac. Irrigate until the prescribed amount of solution has been used. Wipe the eyelids with a moistened cotton ball after irrigating. Dispose of soiled cotton ball in biohazard bag. Pat the skin dry with the towel. Return the client to a semi-Fowler's position. Remove gloves, cleanse hands, and apply clean gloves.	11. (a) (b) (c) (d) (e) (f) (g) (h) (i)	Cleanses the eye socket and removes secretions. Positioning of client facilitates ease in performing the procedure and client comfort. Ensures compliance with client's regimen or prescribed orders. Keeps the eyelid open and the socket visible. Prevents injury to the client. Ensures compliance with client's regimen of prescribed orders. Reduces the transmission of microorganisms to prosthesis. Prevents maceration of the skin. Promotes client comfort. Reduces the transmission of microorganisms.

Contd...

Table 13.12: *Contd...*

	Nursing actions		Rationales
12.	Rub the artificial eye between index finger and thumb in the basin of warm, soapy water.	12.	Creates cleaning with friction and prevents breakage of the prosthesis.
13.	Rinse the prosthesis under running water or place in the clean basin of tepid water. Do not dry the prosthesis. *Note:* Either reinsert the prosthesis (Action 14) or store in a container (Action 15).	13.	Removes soap and secretions. Keeping the artificial eye wet prevents irritation from lint or other particles that night adhere to it and facilitates reinsertion.
14. (a) (b) (c) (d)	Reinsert the prosthesis: With the thumb of the nondominant hand, raise and hold the upper eyelid open. With the dominant hand, grasp the artificial eye so that the indented part is facing toward the client's nose and slide it under the upper eyelid as far as possible. Depress the lower lid. Pull the lower lid forwards to cover the edge of the prosthesis.	14. (a) (b) (c) (d)	Allows for client comfort. Facilitates reinsertion of the prosthesis without discomfort to the client. Positions the prosthesis for insertion. Allows the prosthesis to slide into place. Holds the prosthesis in place.
15.	Place the cleaned artificial eye in a labeled container with saline or tap water solution.	15.	Protects the prosthesis from scratches and keeps it clean.
16.	Grasp a moistened cotton ball and squeeze out excessive moisture. Wipe the eyelid from the inner to the outer canthus. Dispose of the soiled cotton ball in a biohazard bag.	16.	Squeezing the cotton ball removes moisture. Cleansing the eyelid prevents contamination of lacrimal system. Disposal of cotton ball reduces the transmission of microorganisms to other health care workers.
17.	Clean, dry, and replace equipment.	17.	Promotes a clean environment.
18.	Reposition the client, raise side rails, and place call light in reach.	18.	Promotes client's comfort, safety, and communication.
19.	Dispose of biohazard bag according to institutional policy.	19.	Reduces the transmission of microorganisms to other health care workers.
20.	Remove gloves and cleanse hands.	20.	Same as Rationale 19.
Contact Lens Removal			
21.	Assess level of assistance needed and provide privacy.	21.	Level of assistance determines level of intervention. Privacy reduces anxiety.
22.	Cleanse hands.	22.	Reduces the transmission of microorganisms.
23.	Assist the client to a semi-Fowler's position if needed.	23.	Facilitates removal of lens.
24.	Drape a clean towel over the client's chest.	24.	Provides a clean surface and facilitates the location of a lens if it falls during removal.
25.	Prepare the lens storage case with the prescribed solution.	25.	Hard lenses can be stored dry or in a special soaking solution. Soft lenses are stored in sterile normal saline without a preservative.
26.	Instruct the client to look straight ahead. Assess the location of the lens. If it is not on the cornea, either you or the client should gently move the lens toward the cornea with pad of index finger	26.	Client's position promotes easy removal of lens. Positioning lens on the cornea aids removal. Use of the finger pad of the index finger prevents damage to cornea and lens.

Contd...

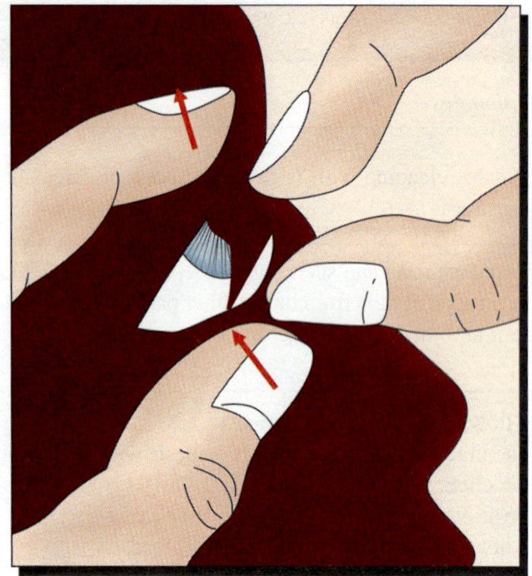

Figure 13.12: Removal of hard lens

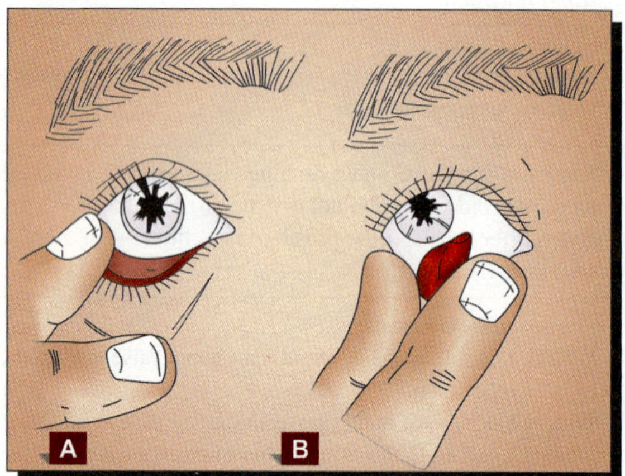

Figure 13.13: Removal of soft lens

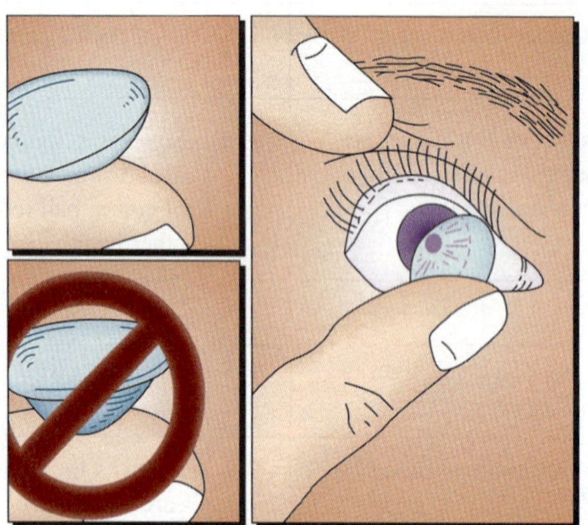

Figure 13.14: Removal of soft contact lens

Table 13.12: *Contd...*

Nursing actions		Rationales	
27. (a)	Remove the lens (Figs 13.12 to 13.14) Hard lens: • Cup nondominant hand under the eye. • Gently place index finger on the outside corner of the eye and pull toward the temple and ask client to blink. Catch the lens in your nondominant hand.	27. (a)	Provides for cleaning and storage of the lens. • Cupping the hand under eye helps catch the lens and prevent breakage. • Pulling the corner of the eye tightens the eyelid against the eyeball. Pressure on the upper edge of lens causes the lens to tip forward.
(b)	Soft lens: • With nondominant hand, separate the eyelid with your thumb and middle finger. • With the index finger of the dominant hand gently placed on the lower edge of the lens, slide the lens downward onto the sclera and gently squeeze the lens. • Release the top eyelid (continue holding the lower lid down) and remove the lens with your index finger and thumb *Note:* If action 27 is unsuccessful, secure a suction cup to remove the contact lens. If you are unable to remove the lens, notify the physician or qualified practitioner.	(b)	• Separating the eyelid exposes the lower edge of lens. • Positions lens for easy grasping with the pad of the index finger, which prevents injury to the cornea and lens. Squeezing the lens allows air to enter and release the suction. • Ensures control of the lens. • Suction cup is used to remove a lens from an unconscious or dependent client.

Contd...

Table 13.12: *Contd....*

	Nursing actions		Rationales
28.	Store the lens in the correct compartment of the case ("right" or "left"). Label with the client's name.	28.	Storage prevents damage to the lenses and ensures that each lens will be reinserted into the correct eye.
29.	Remove and store the other lens by repeating Actions 27 and 28.	29.	Refer to Rationales 27 and 28.
30.	Assess eyes for irritation or redness.	30.	Signs of corneal irritation.
31.	Store the lens case in a safe place.	31.	Prevents damage or loss.
32.	Dispose of soiled articles and clean and return reusable articles to proper location.	32.	Reduces the transmission of infection.
33.	Reposition the client, raise side rails, and place call light in reach.	33.	Promotes client comfort, safety, and communication.
34.	Remove gloves and cleanse hands.	34.	Reduces the transmission of infection.

Contact Lenses

- Lens container
- Soaking solution—type used by client
- Towel
- Suction cup (optional)
- Scotch tape (optional)
- Nonsterile gloves

After procedure nurse should see that:
- The client's contact lenses were safely removed and stored.
- The client's ocular prosthesis was safely removed, cleaned, and either stored or returned to the client's eye socket.
- The client's contacts or prosthesis were cared for with a minimum of trauma to the client's eyes.
- The client's eyes are free of crusts and exudates.
- The client is comfortable.

And document in the Nurses' Notes
- Whether the client wears contact lenses
- Location and condition of the lenses
- Whether the client requires assistance to place and remove the contact lenses
- Whether the client has an ocular prosthesis and which eye.
- Condition of the prosthesis and the condition of the eye socket
- Care performed on the prosthesis and the socket and how the client tolerated the activity
- Client teaching

8. *Care of the Ears*

The ears require proper care and attention. The child with running ears is in constant danger of deafness or mastoiditis. Wax in ears, sometimes gives rise to partial deafness, so it should be removed by syringing. If dirt is allowed to collect for sometime, it may develop into a large hard plug causing earache, boils and even deafness. No attempt should be made to remove wax by prodding any sharp pencil, hairpin or any pointed instrument. Similarly, do not let inexperienced people remove wax by unsterilized instruments or forcibly syringe the ear. The best way is to put a drop of warm oil like olive, mustard, coconut oil or glycerine (if available) for a few days. It will soften the hard wax and bring it to the surface, which can be conveniently removed by a lean cotton swab wrapped on the point of a match stick or through syringing. The child with a running ear, or perforation is drum should plug in his ear with cotton wool before entering a swimming pool for a bath. The infliction of casement by 'boxing' a person's ears should be heavily punished.

The ears are cleansed by the nurse during the bedbath. A clean corner of a moistened wash cloth rotated gently into the ear canal works best for cleaning. Also, a cotton-tipped applicator is useful for cleansing the pinna. The nurse should teach patients never to use bobby pins, toothpicks or cotton-tipped applicators to clean the external auditory canal. These objects may damage the tympanic membrane (eardrum) or cause wax (cerumen) impacted within the canal.

Hearing aids: Hearing loss is a common health problem. The ability to hear enables patients to communicate and react appropriately within their environment. There are several types of hearing aids available. The care of the hearing aid involves routine cleanings, battery care, and proper insertion technique. The nurse will assess the patient's knowledge and routines for cleaning and caring for the hearing aid. The nurse will determine whether the patient can hear clearly with the use of the aid by taking slowly and clearly in a normal voice tone. The nurse should have suggested the patient any additional tips for care of the hearing aid. When not in use, the hearing aid should be stored where it will not be damaged. The hearing aid should be turned off when not in use to prolong the life of the battery. The outside of the hearing aid should be cleaned with a dry, soft cloth.

9. *Care of the Nose*

The patient can usually remove secretions from the nose by gently blowing into a soft tissue. This could be the only daily hygiene necessary. The nurse should teach the patient that harsh blowing causes pressure capable of injuring the eardrum, nasal mucosa, and even sensitive eye structures. If the patient is not able to clean his nose, the nurse will assist using a saline-moistened wash cloth or cotton-tipped applicator. The applicator should not be inserted beyond the cotton tip. If nasal secretions are excessive, suctioning may be necessary. When patients receive oxygen per nasal cannula or have a nasogastric tube, the nurse should cleanse the nares every 8 hours with a cotton-tipped applicator moistened with saline. Because secretions are more likely to collect and dry around the tube, the nurse will also need to gently cleanse the tube with soap and water.

10. *Care of External Genitalia*

The sexual organs require cleansing even more than other parts of the body. In the case of uncircumcised male penis, the foreskin should be retracted in the bath and the secretion washing away. If this is not regularly done smegma collects and undergoes bacterial decomposition, with consequent irritation, which may lead to excitement and unclean habits, e.g. masturbation, etc. (Please See Perineal care Page no. 432)

In case of females, the vulva should be washed in the bath. Commencement of menstruation is not a reason for stopping baths but rather calls for their greater frequency. Girls in their childhood should be taught to wipe the anus backward and not in the reverse direction so as to avoid introducing fecal organisms into vulva or the genital passage. Hygiene of menstruation is also important in girls.

11. *Maintaining Posture*

By posture is meant the characteristic form in which the body is maintained during its various activities. There is no single good posture known. Goodness of a posture consists in alignment of parts in relaxation rather than tension and readiness for action. It may be added that the postures often recommended are stiff, awkward and undesirable. The posture of the soldier on parade is generally taken as an ideal one, but it is a mistaken concept. Correct mechanical use of body permits the internal organs to function efficiently. Good posture is desirable social asset because of its aesthetic value. The vital body functions, i.e. respiration, circulation, excretion, digestion and coordination of body are in perfect physiological balance. The human body makes a poor show when a part of its anatomy is out of alignment.

The causes of faulty posture are:
1. Inherited structural irregularities.

2. Malnutrition, which brings with it, insufficient muscular power to balance the body properly against the force of gravity.
3. Tight or constricting garments worn during pre-adolescent and adolescent ages.
4. Incorrect foot wear especially shoes with high heels.
5. Insufficient physical activity which results in muscular insufficiency, and lack of wholesome mental attitude towards life.
6. Occupation which confines the body in an improper posture for many hours a day.

Incorrect posture may interfere with the functioning of the diaphragm, causing it to sage down wards, thus seriously limiting the amplitude of movements, limiting the action of the diaphragm affects the flow of blood in the large veins because the diaphragm does not produce the necessary pumping action to cause rapid return of blood. The sagging of diaphragm displaces the heart and abdominal organs by forcing them downward and forward. This may cause circulatory and digestive disturbances and in women may cause displacement of uterus, ovaries and other pelvic organs.

A common and troublesome fault of postures is an increase of lumbar curvature. This condition, known as 'lordosis' or 'sway-back' is accompanied by a forward and downward till of pelvic organs and protrusion of the abdomen. In this position the last lumbar vertebra rests at too sharp an angle on the sacrum, producing a weak joint at this place. This results in a general strain on the muscles and ligaments of the lumbar region, producing pain; faulty posture is a frequent cause of low back pain which is a common ailment of modern mankind.

A common structural change in the spinal column is 'kyphosis' or 'round back' which may result from a stopping posture habitually maintained. In this condition thoracic curve is increased, the shoulders and head are bent forward and the chest is flat. Lateran curvature of spine, known as 'scoliosis' is a condition in which the spine deviates sideways. It usually starts as a simple functional lateral deviation. If untreated it usually progresses to a double curve and finally the vertebrae and ribs become permanently altered in shape. An individual may have both 'kyphosis' and 'lordosis' at the same time.

12. *Performing Exercise*

Exercise is very essential for the normal growth and development of the body and perfect maintenance of health. It is also required to excite the demand for oxygen required for utilization of food and to promote the repair of worn out tissues. Attainment of bodily strength is essential to achieve success in life. A strong man can work with great vigor and zeal and withstand cares and snares of life better than another, who is comparatively weak in constitution.

Effects of exercise: The effects of exercise on various systems are as follows:

1. ***Respiratory system:*** During exercise the number of respiration is increased and breathing becomes deeper. The pulmonary circulation is quickened and brings into use all the air sacs of the lungs. There is a considerable increase in the amount of oxygen inhaled and carbon dioxide and water vapors exhaled. Outdoor exercise plays an important role in prevention of tuberculosis.

2. ***Circulatory system:*** Active exercise increases the force and frequency of the heart. Blood and lymph circulate more freely through the whole body. Oxygenation of the blood is very much increased. Lack of muscular activity tends the blood to stagnate in the abdominal viscera. Exercise is beneficial to the normal heart; for it keeps it well nourished, in good tone and prolongs its usefulness.

3. ***Muscular system:*** The nutrition of the muscles is improved, which contributes to their growth and energy. Without exercise, muscles become pale and flabby and begin to waste and wither away.

4. ***Cutaneous system:*** There is a marked increase of perspiration owing to the increased action of the skin.

5. ***Alimentary system:*** Exercise brings about an increased assimilation of food and thus creates a demand for food. The appetite is improved and the action of bowels is stimulated it plays an important role in the prevention of constipation.

6. ***Urinary system:*** Quantity of urine is diminished, though the amount of urea remains unaltered. The excretion of uric acid is slightly increased.

7. ***Nervous system:*** The mind is refreshed and the powers of observation, precision and tolerance are developed.

Effects of excessive exercise: It causes either nervous or muscular fatigue or even both. It causes breathlessness, palpitation and hypertrophy of left ventricle and renders pulse small, frequent and irregular. The voluntary muscles become exhausted due to over exertion, suffer in nutrition and gradually begin to wither away.

Exercise should never be carried on up to a stage when the body becomes entirely exhausted. This fact is of paramount importance, especially when the person taking exercise happens to be raw of untrained. It should not be too strenuous for the age, physical development and the training of a person. After the age of 40 years, intense exercise may do harm to persons not accustomed to vigorous physical activity. For middle age and old persons, walking is one of the best forms of exercise.

Exercise should be done in early hours of the morning or in the evening. It should not be taken within two hours of heavy meal. One should not eat too soon either before or after exercise. Games should be encouraged since they combine recreation with exercise.

The risk of getting chill, however, increases after exercise and therefore the surface of the body, which is exposed during exercise, requires to be covered and protected from undue loss of heat.

13. Clothing

Unlike animals man has not developed natural means of protection from heat, cold and atmospheric phenomena. He has neither fur or feathers nor a thick layer of fat under the skin. Thus, he has to provide himself with clothing and shelter. Clothing serves as a protective covering. In modern life, in the case of a civilized man only about 20 percent of body surface is normally exposed to air.

The kind and the extend of clothing worn have a direct bearing on the human well-being:

1. To afford protection to the body against effects of heat and cold and to protect the body from external injuries.
2. To assist in the maintenance of body heat.
3. For decency and personal decoration.
4. Clothing influences metabolic change. If sufficient clothing is used.

Maintenance of Skin Integrity

When a person's physical condition changes, the skin often reflects this by alterations in color, thickness, texture, turgor, temperature and hydration. As long as the skin remains intact and healthy, the physiological function remains optimal. Intact, without abrasions, warm, localized changes in texture across surface, good turgor (elastic and firm) and generally smooth and soft, color variations from body part to body part.

The nursing diagnosis of impairment of skin integrity, either actual or potential, applies to every patient with whom the nurse has contact. Prevention and treatment of skin impairment are often responsibilities of the nurse. Prevention is the ultimate goal, but when this is not possible, good nursing interventions can result in: (i) optimal healing of the impaired skin without complications, (ii) a decrease in the patient's discomfort, (iii) a decrease in length of hospitalization, and (iv) a decrease in the cost of ongoing care.

A major manifestation of impairment of skin integrity is decubitus ulcers (pressure sores). A patient who stays in one position without relief of pressure, especially over bony prominences, can develop a decubitus ulcer. Patients especially at risk are those who are chronically ill, debilitated, elderly, or disabled or who have a spinal cord injury. Decubitus ulcers occur when there is sufficient pressure on the skin to cause the blood vessels in an area to collapse. The flow of blood and fluid to the cells is impaired, resulting in ischemia, or lack of oxygen and nutrients, to the cells. If the pressure continues without relief for more than 2 hours, cell necrosis may occur in the layers of skin involved. Pressure is usually most severe over bony prominences; for example, the sacrum, ischial tuberosities, trochanteric area of the hips, heels, and malleoli of the ankles. The most common pressure points are supine, side lying and prone positions as shown in Figure 13.15.

In addition to unrelieved pressure, two mechanical factors can result in decubitus ulcers. The first is "shearing force". This occurs when the tissue layers of skin slide on each other, resulting

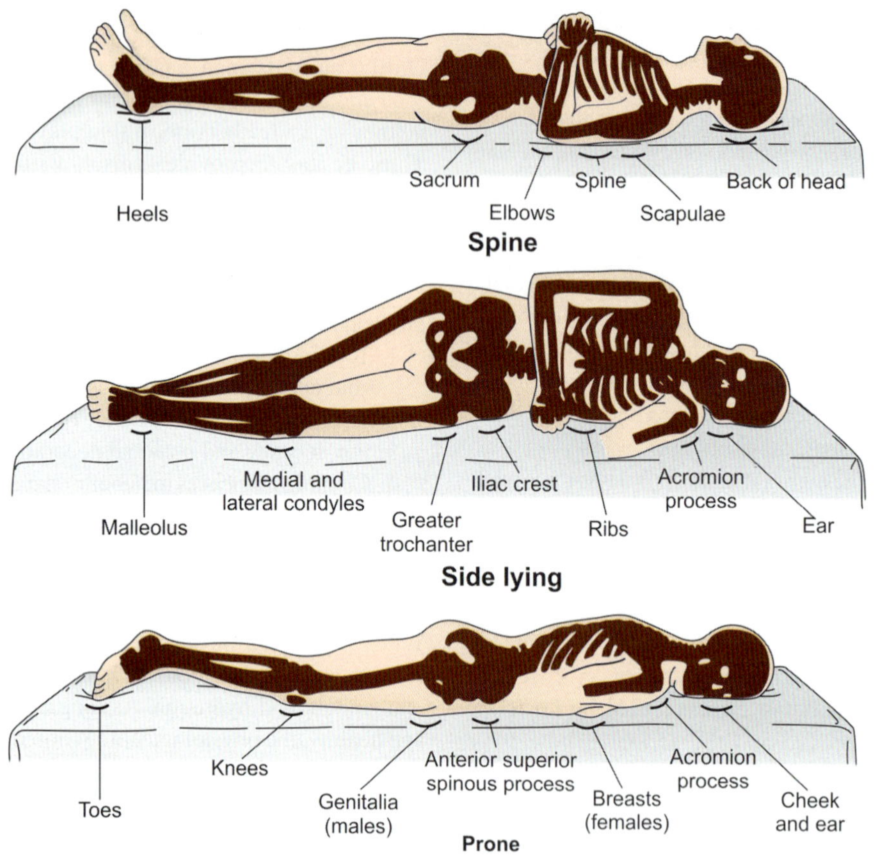

Figure 13.15: Most common pressure points in supine, side lying and prone positions

in kinking or stretching of subcutaneous blood vessels, which results in an interruption of blood flow to the skin.

The second mechanical factor is "friction". The rubbing of skin over a surface produces friction, which may remove layers of tissue. Examples of when this might occur are: (i) moving the patient in bed by sliding him over the linen, (ii) improper lifting of the patient, or (iii) improper placement of the bedpan.

The first goal in the care of the patient's skin is to prevent skin impairment. A critical factor in achieving this goal is careful observation of each patient to determine who is at increased risk for impairment in skin integrity. The six areas to include in the data collection are as follows:

1. General physical condition.
2. Level of consciousness.
3. Level of activity.
4. Mobility.
5. Presence of continence of incontinence.
6. Nutritional state.

The patients at highest risk are those who are confined to a bed or chair, who have limited mobility, who are incontinent, or who have poor overall nutrition. Those who are incontinent are at risk because continual contact of the skin with urine and feces may cause chemical irritation, resulting in skin impairment. Nutritional factors are pertinent for those who are overweight and those who are underweight. Obesity increases the risk

because fat decreased vascularity and resistance, and increases weight and pressure on bony prominences. Underweight increases the risk because of a lack of cushion over the bones and muscles. In addition, any condition that results in a decrease in oxygen and nutrients to the cells, such as anemia, atherosclerosis, or edema, increases the risk of skin impairment, because the cells are not adequately nourished.

Patients who are at increased risk for any reason will need careful, ongoing observation and a plan of care aimed at the prevention of skin impairment. To prevent, perform the following (Tables 13.14 and 13.15).

If the patient has a skin impairment, it is necessary to assess the severity of the decubitus ulcer. A commonly accepted system of classifying decubitus ulcers divides them into five stages (Table 13.13).

Nursing interventions for these patients include ongoing assessment for evaluating whether improvement is occurring. Assessment data include the size and depth of the ulcer, the amount and color of any exudates, the presence of pain or odor, and the color of the exposed tissue. Healing is a long-term process; therefore, the plan of care should be consistent over time and evaluated for effectiveness.

Nursing interventions are aimed at preventing, as well as healing the ulcers. Specific interventions are determined by the stage of the ulcer.

Table 13.13: Five Stages of Decubitus Ulcers	
Stage I :	Transient circulatory disturbances: erythema or blanching with pressure that disappears when pressure is removed. The signs are the result of a compensatory mechanism. When pressure is released, circulation is restored to the area. With prolonged pressure, estimated to be more than 2 hours, this compensatory mechanism may not be able to respond and the skin at the site suffers ischemia and necrosis.
Stage II :	Erythematous or blanched area with no impairment of skin integrity. Patient may complain of pain at the site.
Stage III :	Erythema and edema with vesicle and/or impairment of skin integrity.
Stage IV :	Full-thickness lesion extending to subcutaneous fat with or without serosanguineous exudates (drainage).
Stage V : and beyond	Full thickness lesion extending to deep fascia, muscle and bone.

Table 13.14 : Prevention of Skin Impairment	
Nursing diagnosis	*Nursing interventions*
• Potential impaired skin integrity related immobilization	• Inspect skin for to presence of pressure points at least tid • Provide daily baths • Provide perineal care after each voiding and defecation • Apply skin lotion to areas of skin that becomes easily erythematous (coccyx, heels, scapulae, and greater trochanteric regions) • Keep bed linen clean, dry, neat and wrinkle-free as possible • Encourage adequate fluid intake • Perform range-of-motion exercises • Use mechanical means, such as sheep skin pads, eggerate mattress, heel and elbow protectors, and foam-or water-filled chair cushions. Turn q 2 hr.

Table 13.15: Preventing Infection and Healing of Ulcers	
Nursing diagnosis	*Nursing interventions*

• Impaired skin integrity, related to pressure ulcer (stages I, II and III)	• Assess skin and identify stage of ulcer development
	• Eliminate causative factors, and initiate appropriate ulcer care
	• Cleanse area at least q 4 hr with mild soap and water and pat dry
	• Massage area gently to increase circulation; avoid vigorous rubbing. If possible, expose are to sunlight and air q 2 to 4 hr or to heat lamp every day for 15 minutes; observe area frequently to prevent burning. Position patient on unaffected areas.
	• Protect skin surface and affected area with one or combination of the following:
	  - Apply talcum powder lightly: dust off excess
	  - Apply skin prep or skin gel
	  - Cover area with moisture permeable adhesive or water barrier
	  - Apply Granulex spray q 8 hr or commercial fat pad, according to manufacturer's directions
	  - Continue one type of application or combination for 48 to 72 hr; if improvement is apparent, continue applications; if no improvement is noted, begin another type of treatment

• Impairment of skin integrity, related to pressure ulcer (stages IV and V)	• Assess ulcer for size, color, odor and amount and type of drainage. • Monitor temperature for elevation. Culture ulcer as needed. Continue applications to promote healing. If healing is not evident, prepare for debridement as ordered. • After debridement, change dressings as ordered. If available, consult enterostomal therapist.

Many kinds of tropical agents are available for application to the wound and edges of the wound to facilitate healing. Care should be taken to evaluate the effectiveness of any produce used on the ulcer. Products that might damage fragile skin and prevent epithelialization, such as hydrogen peroxide or alcohol, should be used with caution.

Shaving a Client

Many patients prefer to shave at the time of bathing. The nurse should remember that those patients who have a bleeding disorder or are taking anticoagulants (medications that increase the tendency to bleed) should use electric razors. The nurse will not allow a confused or depressed patient to use a razor with a blade, to prevent accidental or self-inflicted injury. Patient's beard, moustache, or sideburns are never removed without written consent, except for emergency purpose.

Shaving the male client is done to remove facial hair if the client is unable to complete this self-care. It is usually done after a bath or shower and as often as required to remove unwanted facial hair. Most men shave every day, although the facial hair of older clients does not grow as rapidly. If a beard or moustache is present, it should be groomed daily and trimmed as appropriate. Do not shave off beards or moustaches without the client's permission.

For procedures refer Tables 13.16 and 13.17).

Before the procedure the nurse should
- Assess whether the client is able to perform self-care. Promote independence when possible.
- Assess the client's skin for areas of redness, skin break down, moles, or skin lesions. Shaving could irritate the skin further.

Table 13.16: Shaving a Client

	Nursing actions		*Rationales*
	Check clients identification band Explain procedure before beginning		To identity right patient To get cooperation and reduce anxiety
1.	Cleanse hands and apply gloves.	1.	Reduces the transmission of microorganisms.
2.	Assist the client to a comfortable position. If the client can shave himself, set up the equipment and supplies, including warm water, and watch the client for safety. Adjust lighting as needed.	2.	Facilitates comfort and ease of shaving. Encourages sense of self-control and independence.
3.	Place a towel over the client's chest and shoulder.	3.	Protects the client and gown from soil.
4.	Raise the bed to a comfortable height.	4.	Facilitates comfort of staff.
5.	Fill a washbasin with water at approximately 44°C (110°F). Check temperature for comfort.	5.	Warm water helps soften the skin and bread. Warmth can be relaxing.
6.	Place the washcloth in the basin and wring out thoroughly. Apply the cloth over the client's entire face.	6.	Warm water helps soften the skin and bread. Warmth can be relaxing.
7.	Apply shaving cream.	7.	Helps soften the whiskers.
8.	Take the razor in the dominant hand and hold it at a 45-degree angle to the client's skin. Start having across one side of the client's face. Use the nondominant hand to gently pull the skin taut while shaving. Use short, firm strokes in the direction hair grows. Use short, downward strokes over the upper lip area.	8.	Holding the skin taut prevents razor cuts and discomfort during shaving.
9.	Rinse the razor in water as cream accumulates.	9.	Keeps the cutting edge of the razor clean.
10.	Check the face to see if all the facial hair is removed.	10.	Ensures a neat appearance.
11.	After all the facial hair is removed, rinse the face thoroughly with a moistened washcloth	11.	Promotes comfort and cleanliness.
12.	Dry the face thoroughly and apply aftershave lotion if desired.	12.	Stimulates and lubricates the skin.
13.	Assist the client to a comfortable position and allow him to inspect the results of the shave.	13.	Facilitates comfort and a sense of control.
14.	Dispose of equipment in proper receptacle.	14.	Equipment should not be shared between clients in accordance with Standard Precautions because disruption of skin and bleeding may occur. The client may, however, keep his own razor. Clean and store it at the bedside.
15.	Cleanse hands.	15.	Reduces the transmission of microorganisms.

- Assess whether the client has a bleeding tendency or is on anticoagulants. If there is an increased risk of bleeding, an electric razor should be used.
- If the client prefers to shave himself, assess the client's ability to manipulate the razor. The client must be able to shave safely.
- Assess the client's preference for the type of shaving, type of equipment, and type of lotion (if there are options). This promotes independence.

Equipment Needed

- Electric razor or disposable razor
- Shaving cream or soap
- Warm water
- Washcloth and bath towel
- Washbasin
- Aftershave lotion (if the client has no skin irritation and prefers lotion)

- Mirror
- Sharp scissors and comb if moustache care required
- Gloves

After procedure nurse should see that:
- The client is neat and well-groomed.
- The client's skin integrity remained intact.
- If the client was able to shave or able to assist, the client attained a sense of independence.
- The client is comfortable following the procedure.

And document in the Nurses' Notes
- Procedure, if the client was able to assist, and how the client tolerated the activity
- Unusual findings or injury that may have occurred

The nurse will need to shave the patient when he is unable, e.g. because he is too ill or an arm is immobilized in traction or a cast (Table 13.17).

	Table 13.17: Shaving the Patients		
	Nursing actions		*Rationales*
1.	Determine patient's usual shaving method. Explain procedures.	1.	Attempts to follow patient's pattern as much as possible.
2.	Wash hands.	2.	Prevents spread of microorganisms.
3.	Assemble equipment: • Razor with sharp blade • Shaving cream/soap/brush • Bath towel • Face towel • Bath blanket • Basin with hot water (46ºC/115ºF) or as patient prefers • After-shave lotion/powder • Mirror	3.	Organizes procedures. Choose equipment with safety in mind.
4.	Assist patient to sitting position if patient is able. Provide privacy. Drape patient with bath blanket.	4.	Similar to normal position. Some patients prefer privacy. Keeps patient warm.
5.	Observe face and neck for lesions moles, or birthmarks.	5.	Cutting could cause infection, bleeding, or irritation.
6.	Use shaving cream or soap.	6.	Lathering will soften beard and facilitate shave.
7.	Shave in direction half grows. Use short strokes. Start with upper face and lip, and then extend to neck. If patient is able, it will help if he will hyperextend his head to help shave curved areas.	7.	Provides for closer shave without irritation.
8.	Pull skin taut with nondominant hand below the area being shaved.	8.	Promotes uniform shaving.
9.	Rinse razor after each stroke.	9.	Keeps cutting edge clean.
10.	Rinse and dry face.	10.	Removes remnants of lather and shaved hair.
11.	If patient desires, apply lotion or cologne.	11.	This will cause cooling sensation that feels refreshing.
12.	Clean and store equipment. Dispose of used blades in safety container.	12.	Protects others from accidental injury.
13.	Wash hands.	13.	Prevents spread of microorganisms.

Perineal Care

Perineal care (pericare) is part of the complete bedbath. The patients most in need of scrupulous pericare are those at risk for acquiring an infection, for example, patients with indwelling catheters, patients recovering from rectal or genital surgery, or postpartum patients. If patients are able to do their own pericare, they should be allowed to do so. Embarrassment should never cause the nurse to overlook this nursing intervention. A professional dignified attitude can diminish embarrassment and put patients at ease. And nurses should know the anatomy of perineal area (Fig. 13.16).

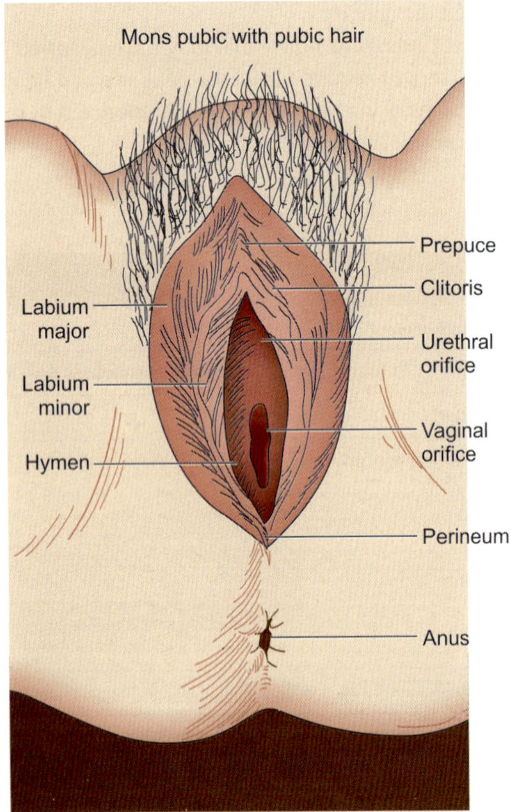

Figure 13.16: Female perineal area

The perineum is the external structure of the pelvic floor. It is composed of the skin and muscle surrounding the genitalia: it is the area between the scrotum and anus in the male and between the vulva and anus in the female. Care of the perineum and genitalia is directed toward maintaining a hygienic perineal environment. Perineal and genital care is usually self-care: however, alterations in the client's ability to perform self-care or alterations in the perineum and genitalia are reasons for nurses or other care providers to perform this skill. Perineal and genital care is an emotionally and culturally difficult subject. Many cultures have specific beliefs and taboos regarding the perineal/genital area. Many people are embarrassed by the idea of anyone else seeing or touching their genitals, particularly a stranger. Be aware of these possibilities when approaching genital/perineal care. In general, a professional, nonjudgmental approach will put the client more at ease with the procedure. Ask the client or the client's caregiver, if possible, about any preferences the client may have in this area.

For procedures of perineal care please see Table 13.18.

Before the procedure the nurse should

- Evaluate client status: level of consciousness, ability to ambulate, ability to perform self-care, frequency of urination and defecation, skin condition. This allows the nurse to decide who, where, how, and when to perform perineal care.
- Identify cultural preferences for perineal care. Perineal care is strongly associated with cultural practices, for example, who may touch the perineal area and how, and the proper way to "wipe." To the extent possible, these preferences should be identified and incorporated into the client's care.
- Assess the client's perineal health. Ask the male client if he has any perineal/genital itching or discomfort. Ask the female client if she has any urethral, vaginal, or anal discharge. Determines the presence of signs and symptoms that may need additional assessment and intervention.
- Determine if the client is incontinent of urine or stool. Affects how the procedure may be necessary.
- Assess whether the client has recently had perineal/genital surgery. Affects how the procedure will be done and what additional procedures may be necessary.

Equipment Needed

- Personal protective equipment (gloves, gown)
- Toilet paper/washcloths
- Waterproof pads
- Cleansing solution if needed
- Perineal wash bottle (fill with plain, warm water).
- Water receptacle (bedpan or toilet if client is ambulatory)
- Dry towels
- Perineal treatment (i.e., ointment or lotions) if necessary
- Linen receptacle
- Room deodorizer

After procedure nurse should see than
- The perineum and genitalia are dry, clean, and free of secretions and unpleasant odors.
- The client reports feeling comfortable and clean in the perineal area.
- The client did not experience discomfort or undue embarrassment during the procedure.

And document in the Nurses' Notes
- Time and type of perineal care provided
- Unusual findings such as skin breakdown, infection, or unusual drainage
- Client special preferences or cultural considerations

Routine Catheter Care

An indwelling catheter is used to provide continuous drainage of urine from the bladder. The catheter, which is attached to a drainage bag, may be used for episodic or long-term urinary drainage. Because the catheter is in the bladder through the

Table 13.18: Perineal Care

	Nursing actions		Rationales
	Check clients identification band Explain procedure before beginning		To identity right patient To get cooperation and reduce anxiety
1.	Cleanse hands and wear gloves. If appropriate and splashing is likely, wear gown, mask, and goggles.	1.	Reduces the transmission of microorganisms.
2.	Close privacy curtain or door.	2.	Provides privacy.
3.	Position client.	3.	If client is ambulatory, perineal care may be done either with client on or standing at the toilet. If perineal care is to be performed in the bed, place the client on the side or over a deep bedpan.
4.	Place waterproof pads under the client in the bed or under bedpan if used.	4.	Protects bed linen.
5.	Remove fecal debris with toilet paper and dispose in toilet.	5.	May require several attempts. If performing at the bedside, may collect paper in disposable pad or linens until end of procedure.
6.	Spray perineum with washing solution if indicated. Alternatively, plain water may be used.	6.	Several perineal solutions are available, which may or may not require rinsing. Carefully evaluate this requirement. Solutions that require rinsing may cause skin breakdown if left on the skin.
7.	Cleanse perineum with wet washcloths (front to back on females), changing to clean area on washcloth with each wipe. Cleanse the penis on the male (Figs 13.17 and 13.18)	7.	Maximizes cleaning; prevents spread of rectal flora to vagina.
8.	Carefully examine gluteal folds and scrotal folds for debris. Gently visualize vulva for debris.	8.	Fecal material causes irritation and skin breakdown rapidly when left in contact with skin.
9.	If soap is used, spray area with clean water from the peri-bottle.	9.	Rinses soap, which can irritate the skin, from the area.
10.	Change gloves.	10.	Reduces the transmission of microorganisms.
11.	Dry perineum carefully with towel.	11.	Residual moisture provides an ideal environment for the growth of microorganisms.
12.	If indicated, apply barrier lotion or ointment. folds tend to harbor moisture.	12.	Barrier ointments may be used if client is incontinent or skin
13.	Reposition or dress client as appropriate.	13.	Promotes client comfort.
14.	Dispose of linens and garbage according to hospital policy.	14.	Prevents spread of disease or bacteria.
15.	Cleanse hands.	15.	Reduces the transmission of microorganisms.
16.	Deodorize room if appropriate.	16.	Promotes client comfort. This may also be done at the beginning of the procedure.

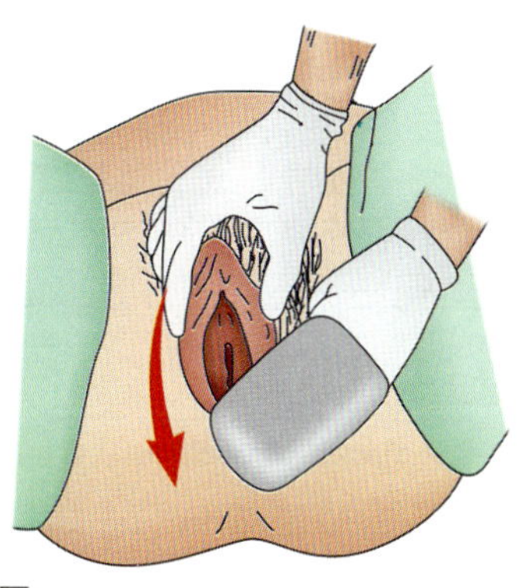
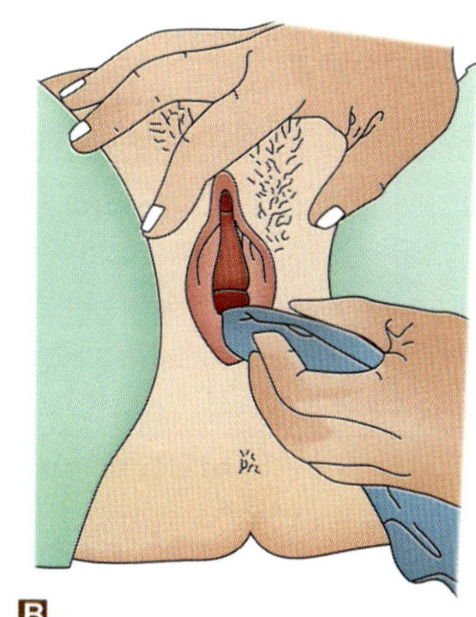

Figures 13.17A and B: Performing normal perineal care (female): (A) Separate labia to expose urinary meatus (B) Cleaning urinary meatus

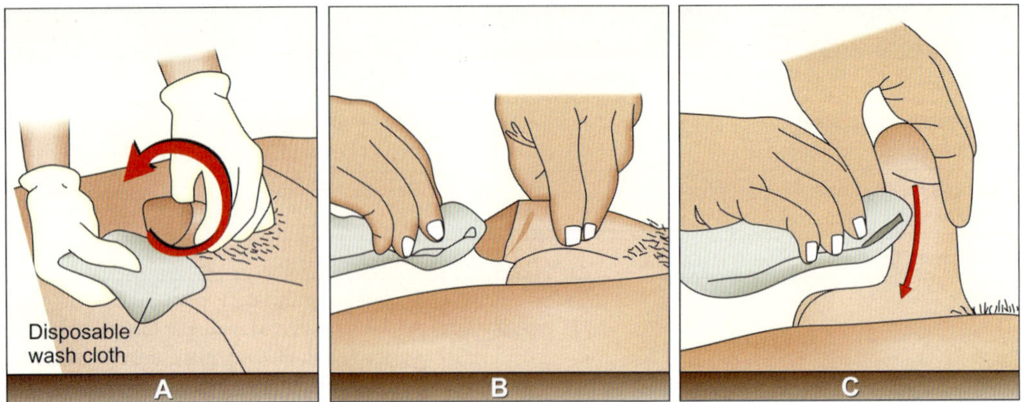

Figures 13.18A to C: Performing normal perineal care: Cleaning penis with disposable

urethra, bacteria may enter the urinary system; therefore, care must be taken to ensure that the surrounding area is clean to decrease contamination of the catheter by bacterial flora. Clients may be embarrassed or frightened by the catheter and related care and, therefore, require emotional support.

For procedure of routine catheter care please refer Table 13.19.

Before procedure the nurse should
- Assess catheter patency and urine color, consistency, and amount while performing the care to determine if catheter and drainage system are functioning correctly.

- Determine the condition of the urinary meatus and perineal area to monitor for redness, swelling, or drainage, stool, or vaginal discharge, as indicators of infection. External infections may migrate up the catheter and lead to urinary tract infection.
- Determine the clients emotional reaction and feelings related to the catheter. This may prevent untoward reactions to the care and allow the nurse to help the client deal with some deeper emotional issues.

	Table 13.19: Routine Catheter Care			
	Nursing actions			*Rationales*
	Check clients identification band Explain procedure before beginning			To identity right patient To get cooperation and reduce anxiety
1.	Cleanse hands.		1.	Reduces the transmission of microorganisms.
2.	Check institutional protocol or care plan.		2.	Ensures proper procedure.
3.	Provide privacy.		3.	Protects client dignity.
4.	Place client in supine position and expose perineal area and catheter.		4.	Allows for visualization of field. If unable to visualize the perineal area with the client supine, try placing the client in a side-lying position.
5.	Place waterproof pad under client.		5.	Protects bed linens.
6.	Put on clean gloves.		6.	Reduces transmission of microorganisms.
7.	After performing perineal care (Procedure 26-18), cleanse meatus if there is excessive purulent drainage with nonirritating antiseptic solutions on cotton balls.		7.	Moving from the most clean area out decreases risk of recontamination.
8.	Cleanse catheter from meatus out to end of catheter, taking care not to pull on catheter.		8.	Moving from most clean area out does not traumatize urethra or bladder.
9.	Be sure to repeat catheter care any time it becomes soiled with stool or other drainage.		9.	Reduces chance of infection.
10.	Place linen or cotton balls in proper receptacle for laundry or disposal.		10.	Reduces transmission of infection to other clients.
11.	Cleanse hands.		11.	Reduces transmission of microorganisms.

Equipment Needed

- Clean latex-free gloves
- Washcloth, soap, and water
- Waterproof pad
- Antiseptic solution
- Sterile swabs

After procedure nurse should see that:
- The client is free of signs and symptoms of urinary tract infection.

- The client understands the reason for the catheter and related care.
- The meatus and surrounding area are clean, intact, and free of drainage.

And document in the Nurses' Notes
- Time the procedure was performed and condition of area surrounding the catheter

The nurse should be alert for signs of vaginal or urethral discharge, skin impairment, unpleasant odors, complaints of burning urination, or localized tenderness or pain of the perineum.

Table 13.20: Procedures for Administering Perineal Care for Male and Female Patients

	Nursing actions		*Rationales*
1.	Explain procedure.	1.	Minimizes anxiety.
2.	Prepare equipment: • Soap dish/soap • Wash basin • Wash cloths (2) • Bath towel • Bath blanket • Bedpan • Toilet tissue • Disposable gloves. When perineal care is given other than routinely during the bath, the nurse will need perineal bottle (peribottle) filled with cleansing solution.	2.	Promotes organization.
3.	Provide privacy. Arrange supplies within easy reach.	3.	Reduces anxiety. Ensures orderliness.
4.	Raise bed height to working position and lower the side rail. Assist patient to the dorsal recumbent position for females or supine position for males.	4.	Enables good body mechanics.

Contd...

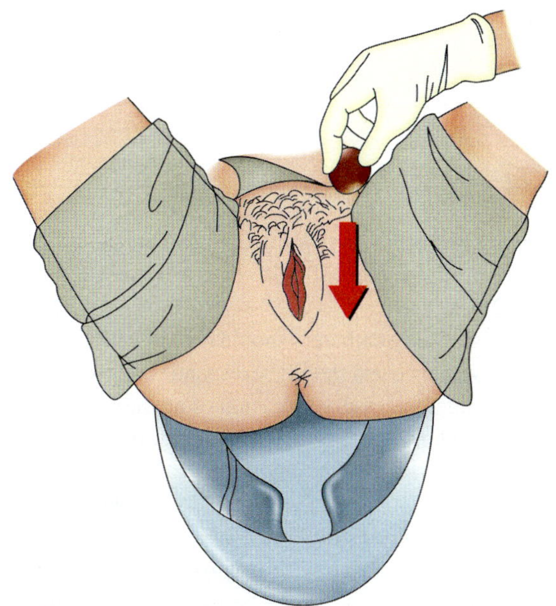

Figure 13.19: Female perineal care

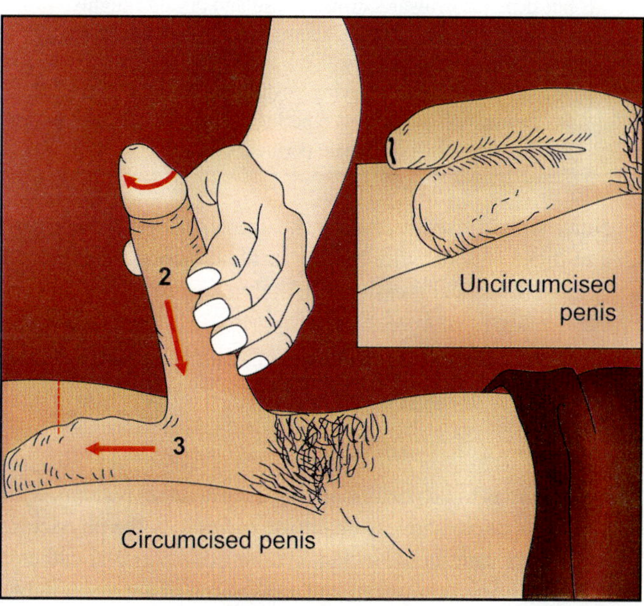

Figure 13.20: Male perineal care

Table 13.20: *Contd....*			
Nursing actions		*Rationales*	
5.	Female perineal care (Figs 13.17 and 13.19)	5.	
(a)	Drape patient with bath blanket.	(a)	Prevents unnecessary exposure.
(b)	Raise side rail, and fill basin 2/3 full with water at 105° to 109°F (41248 to 43°C).	(b)	Promotes patient safety.
(c)	Wash hands, and don gloves.	(c)	Prevents spread of microorganisms.
(d)	Wash and dry patient's upper thighs.	(d)	Surrounding skin surfaces need cleansing also.
(e)	Wash both labia majora and labia minora. Wash carefully in skin folds. Cleanse in direction anterior to posterior.	(e)	Use separate corner of wash cloth for each skin folds.
(f)	Separate labia to expose the urinary meatus and vaginal orifice. Wash downward toward rectum with smooth strokes.	(f)	Prevents spread of microorganisms.
(g)	Cleanse, rinse, and dry thoroughly (If patient is on bedpan and peribottle is used, direct flow of cleansing solution down over perineal area and dry thoroughly).	(g)	Use separate corner of wash cloth for each smooth stroke. Prevents spread of microorganisms.
(h)	Assist patient to side-lying position, and cleanse rectal area with toilet tissue if necessary. Wash area by cleansing from perineal area toward anus (Several wash cloths may be needed). Wash, rinse, and dry thoroughly.	(h)	Retained moisture harbors microorganisms.
(i)	Remove and discard gloves properly.	(i)	Prevents spread of microorganisms, prevents skin impairment.
(j)	Position patient for comfort, and provide warmth.	(j)	Prevents spread of microorganisms.
(k)	Clean and store equipment. Place soiled linen in laundry bag.	(k)	Promotes patient's comfort.
(l)	Wash hands.	(l)	Promotes an orderly environment.
		(m)	Prevents spread of microorganisms.
6	Male perineal care (Figs 13.18 and 13.20)	6	—
(a)	Female perineal care.	(a)	Facilitates procedure.
(b)	Raise bed to working height.	(b)	Enables good body mechanics
(c)	Drape patient.	(c)	Provides privacy.
(d)	Raise side rail, fill basin 2/3 full with water 105° to 110°F (41° to 43°C).	(d)	Provides for patient safety.
(e)	Wash hands, and don gloves.	(e)	Prevent spread of microorganisms
(f)	Gently grasp shaft of penis. Retract foreskin of uncircumcised patient.	(f)	Secretions collect under foreskin.
(g)	Wash tip of penis with circular motion. Cleanse from meatus outward. Two wash cloths may be necessary. Wash, rinse and dry gently.	(g)	Prevents microorganisms from entering urethra.
(h)	Replace foreskin, and wash shaft of penis with a firm but gentle downward stroke. Rinse and dry thoroughly.	(h)	Retained moisture harbors microorganisms.
(i)	Cleanse serotum gently. Cleanse carefully in underlying skin folds. Rinse and dry.	(i)	Pressure on scrotal tissue can be very painful.
(j)	Assist patient to a side-lying position. Cleanse anal area following step 5h of female perineal care.	(j)	Facilitates procedure.
(k)	Follow steps 5 i-l of female perineal care.	(k)	–

Nurse should also observe for skin impairment in the perineal area in those patients with urinary or fecal incontinence, rectal and perineal surgical dressings and indwelling urinary catheters (Table 13.20).

Perineal Care for the Patient with an Indwelling Catheter

Catheter care is to be performed twice daily on all patients with indwelling catheters unless otherwise ordered by the physician. Daily catheter care should include cleaning of the meatal-catheter junction with soap and water and application of a water soluble microbicidal ointment (Betadine) unless other ointment or cream is ordered by physician. If possible, the patient should perform the procedure, but the nurse should observe for proper technique (Table 13.21).

Indwelling urinary catheters should never be used solely as a matter of convenience and should be discontinued promptly when they are no longer necessary. Insertion of an indwelling urinary catheter should be done only by adequately trained personnel using sterile technique, including gloves, catheter, microbicidal antiseptic solution (Betadine) and a water-soluble microbicidal ointment (Betadine) or as ordered.

A sterile, closed-drainage system with disposable, clear plastic bag and connecting tubes should be used. The system should provide for removal of urine without break in sterile continuity

Table 13.21: Procedures for Administering Perineal Care for the Patients with an Indwelling Catheter

	Nursing actions		*Rationales*
1.	Check physician's instruction.	1.	Provides basis for care.
2.	Introduce self and explain procedure.	2.	Promotes cooperation.
3.	Provide privacy.	3.	Encourages relaxation.
4.	Obtain supplies: • Betadine (or ointment of physician's choice) • Soft wash cloth • Soap and water • Sterile cotton-tipped applicator and gloves	4.	Promotes orderly procedure.
5.	Wash hands, and don gloves.	5.	Prevents cross-contamination.
6.	Position patient for comfort.	6.	Promotes ease of procedure.
7.	Cleanse around urethral meatus and adjacent catheter. Cleanse entire catheter with soap and water.	7.	Prevents urinary tract infections.
8.	Repeat cleansing to remove all exudates from meatus and catheter.	8.	Exudates can be irritating and serve as good medium for infectious organisms.
9.	Open package of sterile cotton-tipped applicators. Do not touch cotton tip. Apply Betadine ointment to applicator. Do not touch wrapper to cotton tip.	9.	Maintains sterility.
10.	Apply ointment to junction of catheter and urethral meatus.	10.	Reduces irritation and prevents spread of microorganisms.
11.	Remove gloves. Clean and store equipment. Dispose of contaminated supplies in proper receptacle.	11.	Prevents spread of microorganisms.
12.	Wash hands.	12.	Prevents spread of microorganisms.
13.	Position patient for comfort.	13.	Promotes relaxation.

and should be changed if sterility is compromised by a break in tubing or technique. Drainage bags should never be inverted or elevated to or above the level of the patient's bladder.

Giving a Back Rub

Giving a back rub is a basic nursing skill. Back massage can be an effective means of building a sense of trust and increased rapport between the nurse and client. Clients are often touch-deprived in the busy health care industry of today. The small amount of time that it takes to do a simple back massage can often soothe and relax a "difficult" client and increase the effectiveness of the nurse – client relationship.

The backrub is usually administered after the patient's bath. It should be offered to the patient because it promotes relaxation, relieves muscular tension, and stimulates circulation. During the backrub, the nurse is able to observe the patient's

Massage can be performed in many different ways, from light strokes to heavy kneading. Various forms include effleurage, deep or gentle stroking, and petrissage, a kneading performed with the tips of the fingers and thumbs or palm of the hand. Massage stimulates circulation and promotes lymphatic drainage, thereby helping to rid the body of metabolic wastes, speed healing, and provide gentle relaxation. Massage can open lines of communication and improve the therapeutic relationship between a nurse and client.

Before the procedure the nurse should
• Assess the client's willingness to have a massage. The client may not want a massage or may not enjoy the tactile experience of a massage.
• Assess the client for contraindications of a back rub. Conditions include open sores or lesions, vertebral fractures, burns, and signs of pressure ulcers. To prevent injuring the client.
• Assess any limitations the client has in positioning to determine if the client has any conditions that prohibit a side-lying or prone position.
• Assess the client for fatigue, stiffness, or soreness in the back and shoulders. Knowing areas of particular concern allows you to focus your energies toward "trouble area."
• Assess the client for anxiety or emotional disturbances. Massage can help reduce anxiety and calm people in distress.
• If possible, have the client quantify the degree of discomfort using a 1 to 10 rating scale. Quantifying the results can provide more validity to the intervention.

<table>
<tr><td colspan="2" align="center">Table 13.22: Giving Back Rub</td></tr>
<tr><td>Nursing actions</td><td>Rationales</td></tr>
<tr><td>Check clients identification band
Explain procedure before beginning</td><td>To identity right patient
To get cooperation and reduce anxiety</td></tr>
<tr><td>1. Cleanse hands and apply gloves if necessary.</td><td>1. Reduces the transmission of microorganisms.</td></tr>
<tr><td>2. Help client to a prone or side-lying position (Figs 13.21 to 13.23).</td><td>2. Allows exposure of back and shoulder area.</td></tr>
<tr><td>3. Drape the bath blanket, and undo the client's gown, exposing the back, shoulder, and sacral area, but keeping the remainder of the body covered.</td><td>3. Prevents chilling and excess exposure.</td></tr>
<tr><td>4. Pour a small amount of lotion in your hand and warm between your palms for a few moments. The lotion bottle can also be submerged in a bowl of warm water for a few minutes to warm the lotion. Baby powder may be substituted for oils or lotions</td><td>4. Prevents the shock of cold lotion being applied to the body. Some clients may be sensitive to oils or lotions.</td></tr>
<tr><td>5. Begin in the sacral area with smooth, circular strokes, moving upward toward the shoulders. Gradually lengthen the strokes to the upper back, scapulae, and upper arms. Apply firm, continuous pressure without breaking contact with the client</td><td>5. Applying firm, continuous pressure increases circulation and relaxation.</td></tr>
<tr><td>6. Assess client's back as you are massaging for areas of redness and signs of decreased circulation.</td><td>6. Monitors for signs of early skin breakdown.</td></tr>
<tr><td>7. Provide a firm, kneading massage to areas of increased tension if desired, in areas such as the shoulders and gluteal muscles.</td><td>7. Firm, kneading strokes can decrease muscle tension, reducing pain and increasing relaxation.</td></tr>
<tr><td>8. Complete the massage with long, very light brush strokes, using the tips of the finger</td><td>8. This is a very relaxing stroke and signals an end to the massage.</td></tr>
<tr><td>9. Gently pat or wipe excess lubricant off the client and cover the client.</td><td>9. Prevents soiling of the bed with excess lotions and keeps the client warm.</td></tr>
<tr><td>10. Cleanse hands.</td><td>10. Reduces the transmission of microorganisms.</td></tr>
</table>

Equipment Needed

- Quiet environment, free of interruptions, with a comfortable room temperature
- Comfortable bed or massage table that allows a client to lie in a side-lying or prone position
- Bath blanket
- Bath towel, to absorb excess moisture, oils
- Lotion, baby powder, or massage oil
- Gloves if necessary

After procedure nurse should see that:
- The client experienced a reduction in tension, anxiety, pain, and fatigue.
- The nurse established better rapport with the client.

And document in the Nurses' Notes
- Time and date the back rub was performed
- Client's response to the back rub
- Complaints of pain or tension the client reported
- Unusual findings

To give an effective backrub, the nurse will massage the back for 3 to 5 minutes (Tables 13.22 and 13.23).

The nurse provides a verities of hygienic measures. Hygienic measures cover a variety of basic physical needs that clients are often unable to meet themselves promoting independence and participation in personal hygiene which is a part of the nurses' role. A nurse should be resourceful when delivering hygienic measure. The nurse takes time for therapeutic communication, teaching and provision of emotional support. When client needs assistance, the nurse can conduct of portion of physical examination.

Applying Antiembolic Stockings

Antiembolic hose, also called TED hose or elastic stockings, are used to promote circulation by compression and are useful to prevent thrombophlebitis. They are used on the legs of a client after surgery, on clients who are immobile, and on clients who have vascular disorders such as thrombophlebitis, varicose veins, and other conditions of impaired circulation of the lower extremities.

Table 13.23: Procedures for Administering the Back Rub

	Nursing actions		*Rationales*
1.	Explain procedure.	1.	Promotes relaxation.
2.	Prepare equipment: • Bath blanket (optional) • Bath towel • Skin lotion, alcohol, or powder	2.	Lotion lubricates skin, whereas alcohol has drying effect.
3.	Adjust bed height to working level.	3.	Ensures proper body mechanics.
4.	Provide privacy and quieten environment.	4.	Promotes relaxation.
5.	Lower side rail. Position patient with back toward nurse. Cover patient so that only parts to massage or exposed.	5.	Prevents unnecessary exposure.
6.	Wash hands, and warm if necessary. Warm lotion by holding some in hands. Explain that the lotion may feel cool	6.	Enhances relaxation.
7.	Begin massage by starting in sacral area using circular motions stroke upwards to shoulders. Use firm, smooth strokes to massage age over scapulae. Continue to upper arms with one smooth stroke and down along side of back to iliac crests. Do not break contact with patient's skin. Complete massage in 3 to 5 minutes (Fig. 13.21).	7.	Firm, gentle pressure provides relaxation. Using firm pressure prevents tickling sensation. Continuous contact with skin surface is soothing and stimulates circulation.
8.	Gently but firmly knead skin by grasping area between thumb and fingers. Work across each shoulder and around nape of neck. Continue downward along each side to sacrum.	8.	Increases circulation. Is soothing and relaxing.
9.	With long, smooth strokes, and massage. Remove excess lubricant from patient's back with towel, and retic gown. Position for comfort. Lower bed, and raise side rail as needed.	9.	Most soothing of all massage movements. Promotes patient safety.
10.	Place soiled laundry in proper receptacle. Wash hands.	10.	Prevents spread of microorganisms

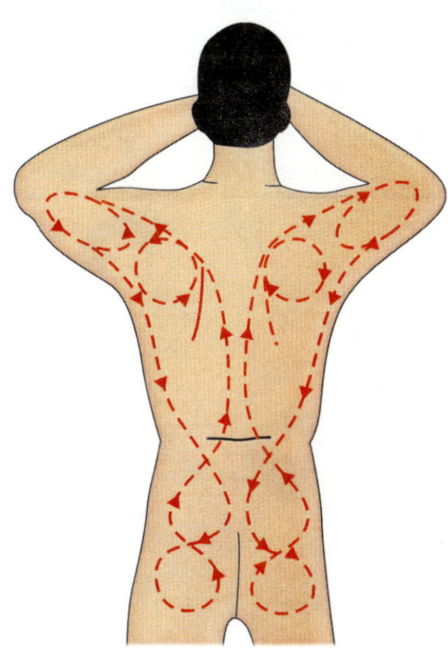

Figure 13.21: Back rub

Table 13.24: Procedures for Giving a Back Massage

Equipment	
• Massage lubricant or lotion • Powder	• Bath blanket • Towel

	Nursing actions		Rationales
1.	Explain the procedures and offer back massage to the client.	1.	Back massage can facilitate circulation and promote relaxation.
2.	Wash your hands.	2.	Hand washing deters the spread of microorganisms.
3.	Close the curtain or door.	3.	Privacy increases relaxation.
4.	Assist the client to the prone position or side-lying position with the back exposed from the shoulders to the sacral area. Use the bath blanket to drape the client. Raise the bed to the high position and lower the side rail closest to you.	4.	This position exposes an adequate area for massage with privacy and warmth maintained. Having the bed in the high position reduces back strain for the nurse.
5.	Warm the lubricant or lotion in the palm of your hand or place the container in warm water.	5.	Cold lotion causes chilling and uncomfortable sensation.
6.	Using light gliding strokes (effcurage apply lotion to client's shoulders, back, and sacral area (Fig. 13.22).	6.	Encourage relaxes the client and lessens tension.
7.	Place your hands beside each other at the base of the client's spine and stroke upward to the shoulders and back downward to the buttocks in show continuous strokes. Continue for several minutes.	7.	Continuous contact is soothing and simulates circulation and muscle relaxation.
8.	Massage the client's shoulders, entire back, area over iliac crests, and sacrum with circular stroking motion. Keep your hands in contact with the client's skin. Continue for several minutes applying additional lotion as necessary.	8.	A firmer stroke with continuous contact promotes relaxation.
9.	Knead the client's skin by gently alternating grasping and compression motions	9.	Kneading increases blood circulation to areas.
10.	Complete the massage with additional long stroking movements.	10.	Long stroking motion is soothing and promotes relaxation.
11.	During massage, observe the client's skin for reddened or open areas. Pay particular attention to the skin over bony prominences.	11.	Pressure may interfere with circulation and lead to development of decubitus ulcer. Back rub stimulates circulation to these areas.

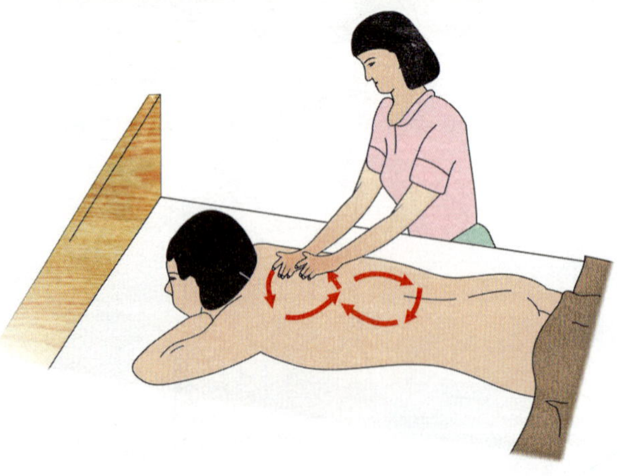

Figure 13.22: Back massage

Table 13.24: *Contd...*

	Nursing actions		Rationales
12.	Use the towel to pat the client dry and to remove excess lotion. Apply powder if the client requests it.	12.	This provides additional comfort for the client.
13.	Wash your hands.	13.	Handwashing deters the spread of microorganisms.
14.	Assess the client's response and record your observations on the client's chart.	14.	This provides accurate documentation of the procedure and condition of the client's skin.

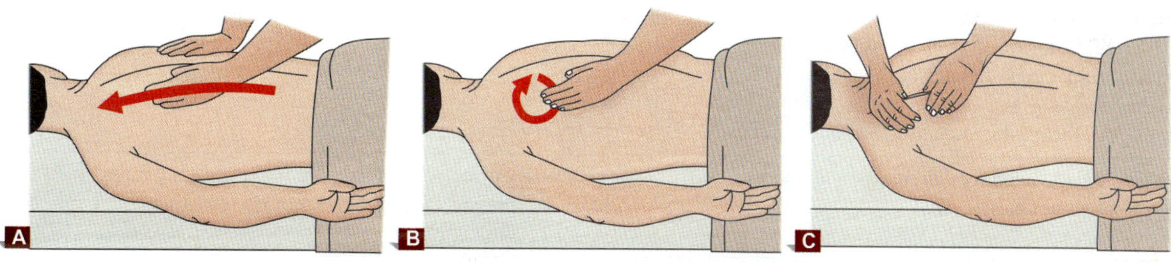

**Figures 13.23A to C: Three basic types of massage. A. Straight and deep, firm sticking (effieurage),
B. Light, circular friction, C. Kneading of muscles with a lifting motion**

For procedure of applying antiembolic stockings, please see Table 13.25.

Before the procedure the nurse should

1. Assess the condition of the client's lower extremities, noting edema, color, temperature, intact skin, ulcers, or infections. Establishes a baseline for comparison.
2. Assess the quality and equality of peripheral pulses in the legs (either dorsalis pedis or posterior tibial pulses) to determine circulatory status.
3. Assess the client's understanding of the reasons for, and the use of, the antiembolic stockings to determine the amount of client teaching required.
4. Assess the client for signs and symptoms of deep vein thrombosis, such as increased calf size or color change, to determine the appropriateness of the TED hose placement.

Please see Figure 13.24 for method of apply of antiembolic stockings.

Equipment Needed

- Antiembolic stockings and package directions (latex-free, if necessary)
- Tape measure

After procedure nurse should see that:

- The client has not experienced any signs or symptoms of deep venous thrombosis or thrombophlebitis.
- The client's venous return is improved.
- The client's popliteal, posterior tibial, and dorsalis pedis pulses remain intact while stockings are in place.
- The client has good circulation while stockings are in place, as evident by warm skin temperature, capillary return within normal limits, sensation within normal limits, and no edema in either extremities.

And document in the Nurses' Notes

- Use of stockings
- Skin integrity, any presence of venous problems, and circulatory status of extremities
- Equality of pedal pulses
- Size and length of stockings

Assisting with a Bedpan or Urinal (Table 13.26)

Voiding and bowel elimination for the client confined to bed require a bedpan and/or a urinal. Reduced mobility, pain, privacy issues, the need for assistance, delays in getting assistance when needed, and the fear of interruption can all alter normal elimination patterns. Fear of creating embarrassing noises, sights, or odors may compel the client to reduce fluid intake or avoid the urge to eliminate while in the hospital. This can lead to an increased risk of urinary tract infection. Sensitivity and proper technique by caregivers support the client on bed rest.

Before the procedure the nurse should

- Assess your equipment. Do you have the necessary items within reach? Prevents having to stop the procedure and leave the client's bedside.
- Assess how much the client can assist in positioning and removing the bedpan. Determines how the procedure will be done and whether assistance will be required.

Table 13.25: Applying Antiembolic Stockings

	Nursing actions		*Rationales*
	Check clients identification band Explain procedure before beginning		To identity right patient To get cooperation and reduce anxiety
1.	Cleanse hands.	1.	Reduces the transmission of microorganisms.
2.	Review the orders with the client, including the reason for the stockings and the type of stockings ordered (e.g., knee or thigh high).	2.	Facilitates compliance.
3.	With the client in a supine position in bed, measure the client's leg for the correct size: • Thigh-high stockings: from Achilles tendon to the gluteal fold, circumference of the midthigh • Below-the-knee stockings: from the Achilles tendon to the popliteal fold, circumference of the midcalf	3.	Supine position encourages venous return and decreases swelling, thereby allowing accurate measurement for size of stockings.
4.	Compare the obtained measurements with the package insert to ascertain proper size.	4.	Correct size is essential for stockings to apply the appropriate pressure for adequate venous return without compromise to circulation.
5.	Apply stockings. The best time to apply stockings is early in the morning, before the client in supine position until stockings are applied.	5.	Feet are less swollen in the morning because the feet have been in a nondependent position during the night and most venous return has occurred. This, of course, is not the case in a client who has been up frequently during the night.
6.	Open the package and turn stockings inside out over hand and arm. Place hand deep enough inside a stocking to grasp the stocking toe.	6.	Because stockings contain strong elastic, application can be difficult if not initiated from the bottom up and if stockings are not turned inside out. Wrinkles in stockings can also occur if a systematic approach is not used for application.
7.	Using the hand inside the stocking, hold onto the client's toes. Invert the stocking with the other hand and pull it over the hand and the client's toes. Release toes.	7.	See Rationale 6.
8.	Hold each side of the stocking and pull it from the client's toes to the heel in one motion	8.	See Rationale 6.
9.	Continuing to hold each side of the stockings, firmly pull the stocking up by using the thumbs to guide the stockings upward over the ankles and up the client's leg.	9.	See Rationale 6.
10.	Repeat with the other leg, if necessary.	10.	See Rationale 6.
11.	Smooth and remove any wrinkles in the stockings.	11.	Wrinkles can create skin breakdown and can cause a tourniquet effect on the leg.
12.	Assess circulatory and neurostatus of feet. (CMS: circulatory, movement, sensation)	12.	Establishes baseline assessment.
13.	Cleanse hands.	13.	Reduces the transmission of microorganisms.

• Check whether the client is confused, combative, in traction, or immobile. Determines how the procedure will be done and whether assistance will be required.
• Check for casts, braces, or dressings, which need to be protected from accidental contamination with waste products. Determines how much preparation will need to be done before toileting.
• Check for privacy and unexpected interruptions. Determines if extra steps need to be taken to ensure privacy before toileting.

• Assess if client has orders to record intake and output. Determines need to take steps for measurement and may require containers with measurement markings.

Equipment needed for assessing Bedpan and Urinal are
• Bedpan (regular or fracture) or urinal
• Disposable gloves
• Bedpan cover
• Toilet paper
• Washcloth and towel

Note the style. Hose may be knee length, midthigh length, or groin length with opening over ball of foot or over tops of toes.

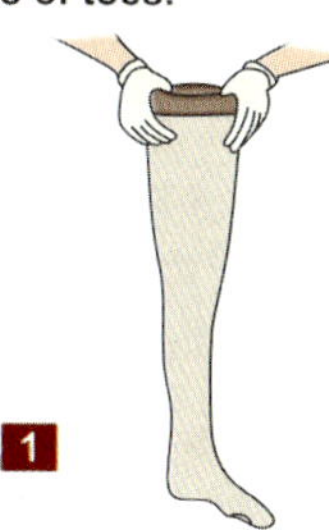

Invert the upper half of the stocking down so stocking is dobbled and covers almost all of the foot. Leave enough of the foot visible to be able to identify toe and heel

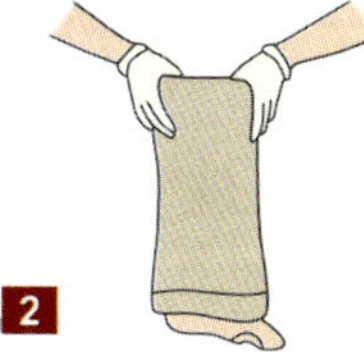

Gather the doubled stocking down to approximately the level of the ankle.

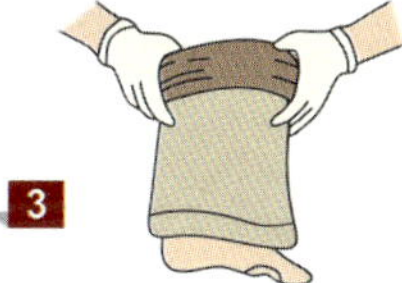

Work gathered stocking over the client's ankle

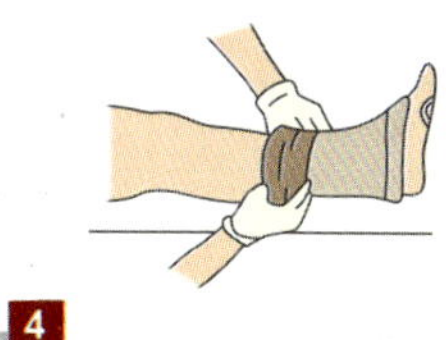

Pull the doubled stocking up firmly, smoothing all wrinkles in the process

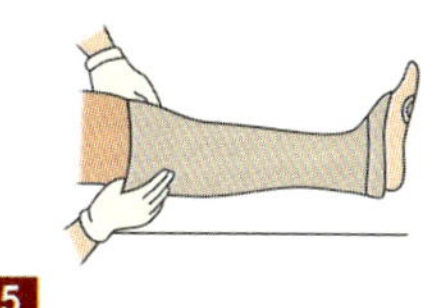

Pull the remaining stocking up to its full length, smoothing all remaining wrinkles from the stocking

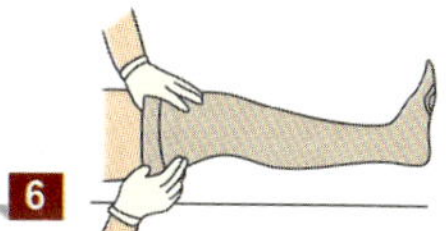

Figure 13.24: Method of applying antimobilism hosiery

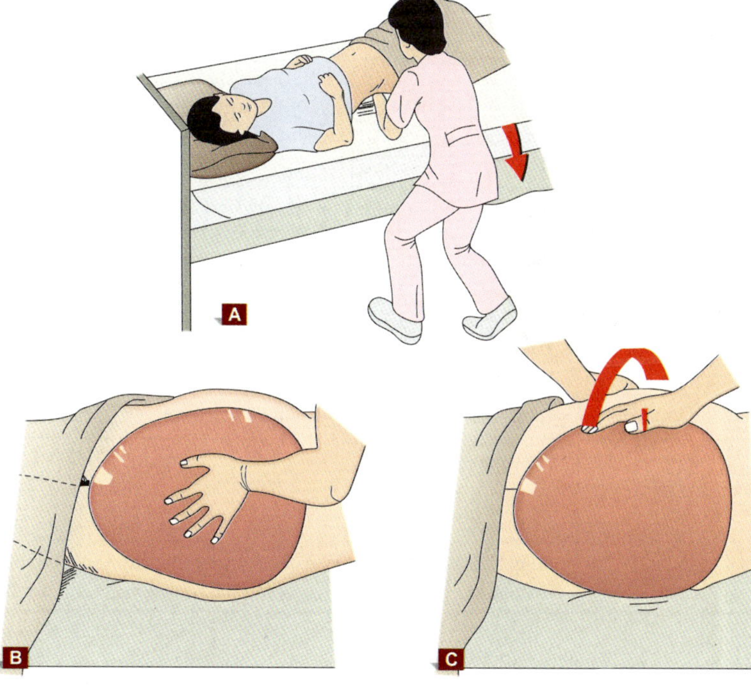

Figures 13.25A to C: Two methods of giving a bed pan to a person who can assist with lifting self. A. With person on back, B. With person on side, C. Nurse places hand on person's hip and gently while rolling person onto back

Table 13.26: Assessing with a Bedpan and Urinal

	Nursing actions		*Rationales*
	Check clients identification band Explain procedure before beginning		To identity right patient To get cooperation and reduce anxiety
1.	Close curtain or door.	1.	Provides for privacy.
2.	Cleanse hands; apply gloves.	2.	Reduces the transmission of microorganisms.
3.	Lower head of bed so client is in supine position (Fig. 13.25A)	3.	The supine position will increase ability of client to move to side-lying position.
4.	Elevate bed.	4.	Ensure proper body mechanics.
5.	Assist client to side-lying position using side rail for support (Fig. 13.25B).	5.	Provides for best position for proper placement of bedpan.
6.	Warm bedpan under warm water if needed; powder bedpan if necessary.	6.	For comfort; prevents bedpan from sticking to the skin.
7.	While holding the bedpan with one hand, help the client roll onto his or her back, while pushing against the bedpan (toward the center of the bed) to hold it in place.	7.	Prevents dislocation or alignment of bedpan.
8.	Alternate: Help the client raise the hips using the over bed trapeze, and slide the pan in place (Fig. 13.25C). Alternate: If the client is unable to turn or raise hips, use a fracture pan instead of a bedpan. With a fracture pan, the flat side is placed toward the client's head.	8.	Provides an alternate way to position the pan. Fracture pan reduces the amount of movement and lift required to place the pan.
9.	Check placement of bedpan by looking between client's legs.	9.	May prevent spillage from misalignment of bedpan.
10.	If indicated; elevate head of bed to 45-degree angle or higher for comfort.	10.	Check order of physician or qualified practitioner; bed remains flat if client has a spinal cord injury or spinal surgery. Elevating the head of bed creates a more normal elimination position.
11.	Place call light within reach of client; place side rails in upright position, lower bed, and provide privacy.	11.	Privacy allows for a more comfortable elimination environment; elevated side rails provide for safety.
12.	Remove gloves; cleanse hands.	12.	Reduces the transmission of microorganisms.
Positioning a Urinal			
13.	Repeat Actions 1 and 2.	13.	See Rationales 1 and 2.
14.	Lift the covers and place the urinal so the client may grasp the handle and position it. If the client cannot do this, you must position the urinal and place the penis into the opening	14.	Ensures proper placement of the urinal and reduces the risk of spillage.
15.	Remove gloves; cleanse hands.	15.	Reduces the transmission of microorganisms.
Removing a Bedpan			
16.	Cleanse hands; apply gloves.	16.	Reduces the transmission of microorganisms.
17.	Gather toilet paper and washing supplies.	17.	Having supplies at the bedside allows smooth and safe completion
18.	Lower head of bed to supine position.	18.	Increases client's ability to move to side-lying position.
19.	While holding bedpan with one hand, roll client to side and remove the pan, being careful not to pull or shear skin sticking to the pan and being careful not to spill contents.	19.	Prevents possible spillage of bedpan contents.
20.	Assist with cleaning or wiping; always wipe from front to back.	20.	Client may not be able to clean self; wiping from front to back decreases chances of cross-contamination from anus to urethra.

Contd...

Table 13.26: *Contd...*

	Nursing actions		Rationales
21.	Empty bedpan (observe and measure urine output and check for occult blood if ordered), clean bedpan, and store it in proper place; if bedpan is to be emptied outside client's room, cover it during transport.	21.	Promotes privacy and decreases the chance of spilling contents. Assessment of types of stool evaluates for constipation and diarrhea.
22.	Remove soiled gloves. Cleanse hands.	22.	Reduces the transmission of microorganisms.
23.	Allow client to cleanse hands.	23.	Provides for physical hygiene and comfort.
24.	Place call light within reach; recheck that side rails are in the upright position.	24.	Ensures client safety and comfort.
25.	Cleanse hands.	25.	Reduces the transmission of microorganisms.
Removing a Urinal			
26.	Cleanse hands and apply gloves.	26.	Reduces the transmission of microorganisms.
27.	Empty the urinal, measuring urine output if ordered, rinse the urinal and replace it within the client's reach. Observe odor and color of urine before discarding.	27.	Provides a way to measure the client's output. Keeping the urinal within reach promotes client autonomy. Helps evaluate for concentrated urine, infection, and renal problems.
28.	Remove soiled gloves. Cleanse hands.	28.	Reduces the transmission of microorganisms.
29.	Allow client to cleanse hands.	29.	Provides for physical hygiene and comfort.
30.	Place call light within reach; rechecks that side rails are in the upright position.	30.	Ensures client safety and comfort.
31.	Cleanse hands.	31.	Reduces the transmission of microorganisms.

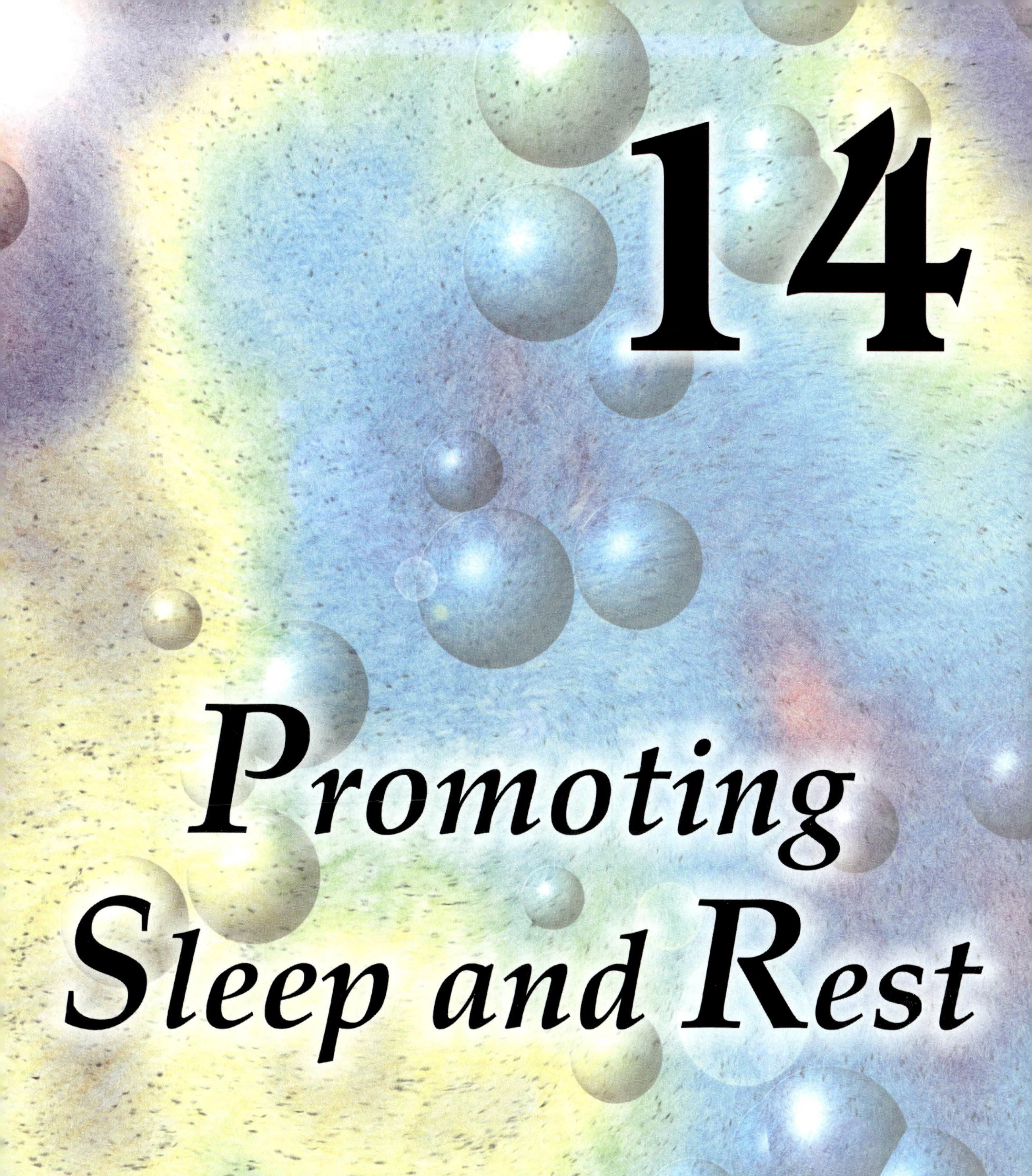

14
Promoting
Sleep and Rest

Introduction

Sleep means a state of altered consciousness, through out which varying degrees of stimuli produce wakefulness. It is a recurrent, altered state of consciousness that occurs for sustained periods, restoring energy and wellbeing. Sleep is an active and complex rhythmic state involving a progression of repeated cycles, each representing different phases of body and brain activity.

Sleep is a cyclically occurring state of decreased motor activity and perception. Body functions slow, and metabolism falls by 20 to 30%, so the body conserves energy. Sleep is characterized by altered consciousness: a sleeping person is unaware of the environment and responds selectively to external stimuli. For example, an alarm clock, bright light, or other "meaningful" stimuli usually will awaken a sleeper, but everyday background noises and soft light will not.

Rest refers to a condition in which the body is in a decreased state of activity with the consequent feeling of being refreshed. People at rest feel mentally relaxed free from anxiety, and physically calm. Persons at rest are in a state of decreased mental and physical activity that leaves them feeling refreshed, rejuvenated, and ready to resume the activities of the day.

Rest is a condition in which the body is inactive or engaging in mild activity, after which the person feels refreshed. A person at rest is calm, at ease, relaxed, and free of anxiety and stress. People rest by doing things that they find calming and relaxing, for example reading, listening to music, watching television, doing needlework, praying or meditating, gardening, baking, playing golf, walking, and camping.

Although necessary and beneficial, rest without sleep is inadequate. At rest, the body is disturbed by all exterior stimuli, whereas in sleep it is screened from them by altered consciousness. Thus, as we discuss next, sleep restores the body; rest alone cannot do this.

The need for sleep and rest is important in quality of life for all people. All individuals need and receive different amounts and qualities of sleep and rest, physical and emotional health depend on the ability to fulfill this basic human need, without rest and sleep, the ability to concentrate, make judgments and participate to activities decrease and irritability increase. It has been relieved then sleep restores wellbeing; relieves stress an anxiety; and restores ability to cope and to concentrate on activities of daily living.

Sleep problems may cause clients to seek healthcare or problem may go unnoticed period. Nurses care for clients who often have pre-existing sleep disturbance and for clients who develop sleep problems as a result of illness or hospitalization. Ill persons often require more sleep and rest than healthy ones. The environment of a hospital or long-term care facility and activities of healthcare personnel may also make sleep difficult. Identifying and treated sleep disturbances is an important goal of a nurse. Nurse must understand the nature of sleep, the factors influencing the client's sleep habits.

We spend more time sleeping than engaging in any other single activity: about 8 hours a day, or 2688 hours a year–nearly one-third of our lives! So why is sleep so important? Before you try to answer, think back to the last time you had a poor night's sleep. Remember the mental fogginess, the physical fatigue, the feeling of slight nausea? Missing even one night of sleep can reduce mental performance, and long periods of sleep deprivation can result in stress-related illnesses and injuries (e.g. from an automobile accident). The reason is that sleep and rest are essential for physical, mental, and spiritual well-being.

Theorists do not agree on all of the functions of sleep, but studies have shown that adequate sleep restores energy. Despite the fact that some regions of the brain are more active during sleep than when we are awake, our total energy output is reduced while we sleep, giving the body time for restoration and repair. Research also indicates that sleep strengthens the immune system: Animals deprived of sleep are more vulnerable to infection. Sleep may also improve learning and adaptation, giving the individual a chance to mentally repeat and rehearse facts and situations before they are encountered in wakeful life. Some evidence suggests that sleep and dreaming may facilitate the storage of long-term memory, perhaps by assisting the brain in reorganizing and storing information. Sleep also appears to reduce stress and anxiety, improving our ability to cope and concentrate on activities of daily living.

Sleep/rest and illness are interrelated (Fig. 14.1). Illness and injury increase the need to sleep and at the same time make it difficult to sleep. In turn, lack of sleep increases the susceptibility to illness by compromising the immune system. People who are ill or injured need more sleep than usual to restore energy needed for tissue repair and healing. However, they often have difficulty resting because of pain and other symptoms of their illness. Lack of sleep and rest increases our susceptibility to illness, and the pain of illness and injury increases our susceptibility to disturbed sleep.

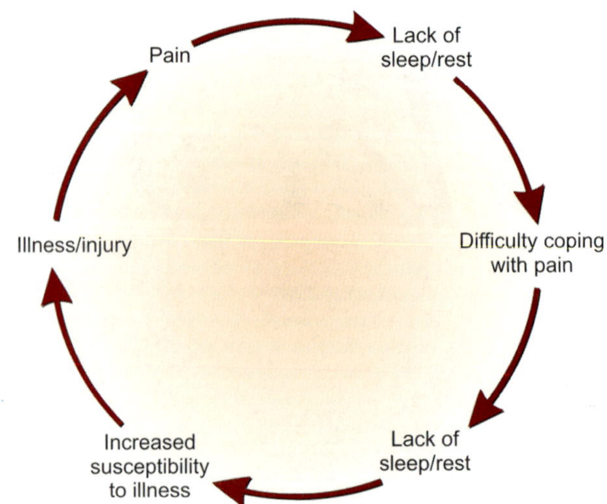

Figure 14.1: Relationship between sleep/rest and illness

Because sleep enhances wellness and speeds recovery from illness, promoting sleep is an important independent nursing intervention. In this chapter, you'll learn how to recognize signs of sleep disturbance, as well as factors that interfere with patients' sleep, and specific measures to facilitate sleep for each client.

Sleep Requirements

Sleep needs vary widely among individuals. Average sleep requirements based on age are shown in Table 14.1. Even though the accepted standard has been 8 hours per night for adults, there is really no "correct" amount or pattern of sleep that maintains well-being in all people. In spite of individual variations, however, different sleep patterns are characteristic of different age groups.

Infants have an overall greater total sleep time than any other age group. Newborns sleep as much as 16 to 20 hours a day, in periods ranging from one to several hours. Sleep time gradually decreases over the next few months, but throughout the first year of life, a minimum of 14 hours of sleep per day is recommended. Most infants sleep several hours during one overnight period, with a morning and afternoon nap each day.

After the first year of life, sleep duration gradually decreases. In most adults, sleep of 7 to 8 hours is fully restorative; however, there are wide individual variations. In some cultures, total sleep time is divided into an overnight sleep period and a midafternoon nap.

Older adults spend significantly less time sleeping but need more rest than younger adults. Usually older adults rest or nap during the day, go to bed early, and get up early. They take longer falling asleep, and their arousal periods during sleep are longer and more frequent. Frequent waking is commonly due to physical discomfort, anxiety, and nocturia. If the sleep is interrupted, the person will need to sleep longer to feel restored. If the older adult does not increase the total time in bed, she may experience fatigue, irritability, and impaired cognition.

Table 14.1: Average Sleep Requirements to Age	
Age Group	*Hours per Day*
Newborns (birth to 4 weeks)	16-20
Infants (4 weeks to 1 year)	14-16
Toddlers (1-3 years)	12-14
Preschoolers (3-6 years)	11-13
Middle and late childhood (6-12 years)	10-11
Adolescents (12-18 years)	8-9
Young adults (18-40 years)	7-8
Middle-age adults (40-65 years)	7
Older adults (65 years and older)	5-7

Physiology of Sleep

Sleep is a set of complete physiological processes. It involves a sequence of state maintained by highly integrated central nervous system, endocrine, cardiovascular, respiratory, and muscular system. Each sequence can be identified by specific behavior, physiologic responses, and pattern of brain activity.

The timing of the sleep-wake cycle and other circadian rhythms such as body temperature, is controlled, atleast in part, by the superchiasmatic nucleus in the anterior hypothalamus. Located above the optic chiasm, his area receives input from the retina, which provide information about darkness and light. The superchiasmatic nucleus control the production of melatonin, which is believed to be a potent sleep induced. Sleep is a rationally occurring readily reversible altered state of arousal characterized by a decreased responsiveness to the environment. The mediator of arousal and of sensory stimulation is the reticular activity system (RAS). The RAS is located in the brains tern and contains projections to the thalamus and cortex. The diffuse network of neurons in the RAS is in a strategic position to monitor ascending and descending stimuli through feedback loop.

Although the RAS provides the anatomic framework for arousal it in the neurotransmitters than serve on the chemical messengers. The onset of sleep and each subsequent sleep stage is an active process involving delicate shifts in the balance of several of these transmitters.

The transition from the awake state to non-rapid eye movement (NREM). Sleep is marked by decreases in the concentration of serotonin, nor-epineprine and acetylcholine. The later transition to rapid eye movements (REM) sleep is marked by a dramatic increases in acetylcholine and further drop in serotonin, nor-epinephrine. As REM sleep continues the concentration of serotonin and nor-epinephrine increases eventually stopping REM sleep. Cholinergic activation with the release of acetylcholine seems to reestablish REM sleep the continuous interaction of these two system thought to produce the normal alterations between NREM and REM sleep. Other neurotransmitters such as gamma aminobutyric acid (GABA) and dopamine, are also relieved to have part in the reciprocal process involved in shifts in sleep state.

All of these neurotransmitters are actively involved and waking processes as well. For example, neurons that produce serotonin and nor-epinephrine playa role in the modulation of sensory input, mood, energy, and information processing including attention, learning, and memory. Thus it can be seen that imbalances in these neurotransmitters induced through sleep pattern disturbances, medications, or diseases may reciprocally affect not only sleep but also aspect of sensory processing mood and cognition. REM sleep may be especially important for maintaining mental activities such as learning, reasoning and emotional adjustments sleep also serves as an energy-conserving measure for most of the body parts except the brain.

Sleep can be defined behaviorally, functionally and electrophysiologically. Electrophysiologic monitoring of sleep, which is called polysomnography, can divide sleep into REM and NREM sleep. NREM further divided into stages 1 through 4. These stages vary in depth but are characterized by lack of eye movements, low and fragmented cognitive activity, maintenance of moderate muscle tone, and slower but generally rhythmic respirations, and pulse rate. As individual progress from stage 1 to stage 4 sleep, the wave form recorded by EEG becomes more synchronized, slower and greater amplitude.

Stage 1: NREM sleep is very light. Respiration begins to slow, and muscle relax. At sleep onset, some erratic breathing may occur as well as sudden myoclonic jerks (sleep starts) as the body shifts from as awake to a sleep state. Stage 1 is such a light stage of sleep than persons wakened from it will often claim that they were not asleep at all.

Stage 2: NREM is still light sleep. The brain waves are frequently mixed and low voltage in pattern, with bursts of activities called sleep spindles and large-amplitude waves called "K" complexes. More than 50% of sleep occur as stage 2 sleep.

Stages 3 and 4: NREM are known as slow-wave sleep, named for the characteristics high-voltage, low frequency delta waves. Respirations become slow and ever. The pulse and blood pressure fall. Oxygen consumption by muscle tissue and urine formation are decreased.

Dreams occur during the NREM stages of sleep, are generally thought like ruminations of recent events and current concerns with little story line.

REM sleep: It is characterized by low voltage random fast waves as in stage 1. NREM clients in REM sleep have been characterized by rapid eye movement, erratic respirations charges in heart rate and very low muscle tone. During REM sleep, ventilation primarily depends on the movement of the diaphragm, because intercostal and accessory muscle tone is markedly diminished, and all postural and non-respiratory muscles are essentially paralyzed. Dreams in REM sleep are vivid, story like emotional and bizarre.

Biorhythms are "biological clocks" that are controlled within the body and synchronized with environmental factors (e.g. gravity, electromagnetic forces, light, and darkness). Biorhythms influence many physical and mental functions. For example, body temperature is typically lowest when the person wakes up in the morning, and female menstruation follows an approximately 28-day cycle, like the lunar cycle on which our calendar months are based. A **circadian rhythm** is a biorhythm based on the day-night pattern in a 24-hour cycle. The term comes from the Latin words *circa,* meaning "about" and *dies,* meaning "day"–once a day. A person's circadian rhythm is regulated by a cluster of cells in the hypothalamus of the brain stem that respond to changing levels of light. Circadian rhythm affects our overall level of functioning; most people have a higher energy level in the daytime and less energy at night. However, some people are more alert and active in the morning, whereas others function at a higher level in the afternoon or evening.

Do you find yourself feeling sleepy at about the same time each night? Do you often awaken before the alarm clock goes off? If so, that's because the timing of sleep and waking is also influenced by your circadian biorhythm. Sleep quality is best when the time at which you go to sleep and wake up is in synchrony with your circadian rhythm. For this reason, people who work evening and night shifts (e.g. healthcare workers, police officers, and so on) can suffer significant sleep deprivation until their bodies adjust to the new pattern. Changing time zones can also disrupt sleep-wake cycles and can thus be troublesome for people who travel frequently on business. Hospitalization can also interfere with a patient's circadian rhythm. Noises, lights, waking the patient for assessment's or medications, absence of normal bedtime rituals, absence or presence of family members, recent losses, or fear of the unknown may hinder the patient's ability to sleep at his usual time.

Regulation of Sleep and Wakefulness

Major factor in regulating sleep is the amount of light received through the eyes. The increasing light of a dawning sky signals the hypothalamus (Fig. 14.2) to induce gradual arousal from sleep. Another collection of nerve cell bodies within the brain stem, called the reticular formation, is responsible for maintaining wakefulness. The reticular formation is activated by stimuli from the cerebral cortex. Together, these reticular and cortical neurons are called the reticular activating system (RAS). Neurotransmitters associated with excitatory and inhibitory sleep mechanisms include catecholamines, acetylcholine, serotonin, histamine, and prostaglandins. L-tryptophan and adenosine promote feelings of sleepiness.

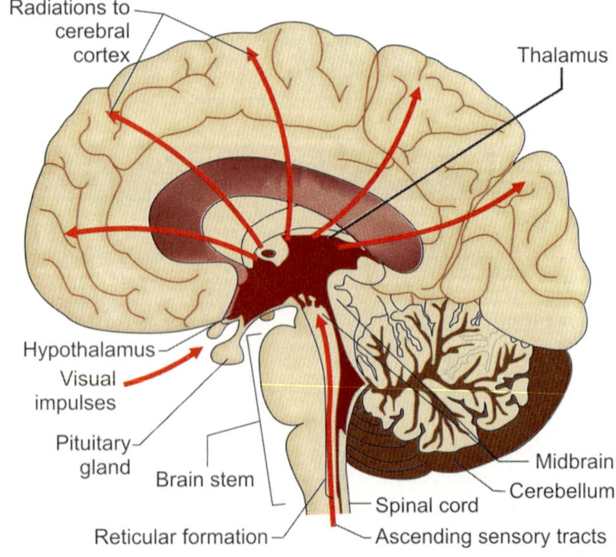

Figure 14.2: Regulation of sleep and wakefulness by RAS

An electroencephalogram (EEG) is a machine that is used to record the electrical activity of the neurons in the brain. Electrical impulses are transmitted from the brain to the machine through electrodes attached to the scalp. These impulses create wave patterns commonly known as *brain waves.* Any of four different types of brain waves may be recorded (Fig. 14.3):

Alpha waves are high-frequency, medium-amplitude, irregular waves.

Beta waves are high-frequency, low-amplitude, irregular waves.

Theta waves are high-amplitude waves that are common in children but rare in adults.

Delta waves are low-frequency, high-amplitude, regular waves common in deep sleep.

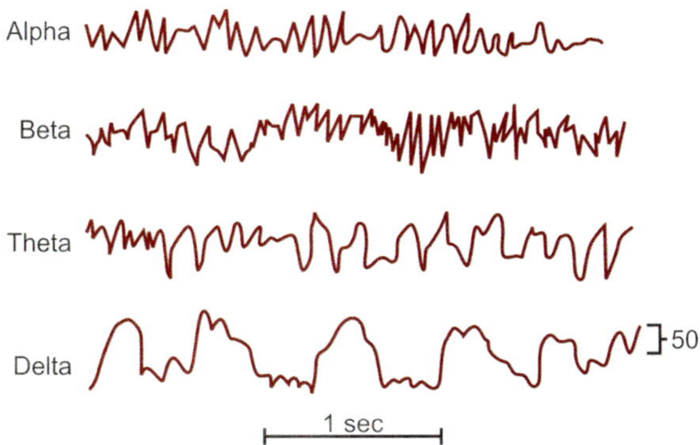

Figure 14.3: Four different types of brain waves

The EEG of a waking person differs greatly from that of a sleeping person. In general, the greater the brain activity, the more rapid the brain waves on the EEG. While the person is awake, brain waves are very rapid, irregular, and low in amplitude, mostly alpha and beta waves. Many neurons are firing at different intervals, at different times, and with different strengths. When a person is relaxed (e.g. sitting on the couch watching TV without any mental arousal), the EEG records mostly alpha activity. During sleep, alpha waves disappear. They are replaced by slower, higher amplitude delta waves.

Stages of Sleep

There are two distinct types of sleep:

1. **NREM** (non-rapid eye movement) sleep is produced by withdrawal of neurotransmitters from the reticular formation and inhibition of arousal mechanisms in the cerebral cortex.
2. In **REM** (rapid eye movement) sleep, the brain is highly active with rapid, low-amplitude waves similar to those that occur when a person is awake and alert. REM sleep is primarily initiated by the reticular formation.

Five stages of sleep (four NREM stages and the REM stage) have been identified, based on brain activity and other physiological characteristics. See Table 14.2 for characteristics of each stage of sleep.

1. NREM Sleep Stages

NREM sleep is also called *slow-wave sleep (SWS)* because it is characterized by the presence of delta waves. NREM is divided into four stages, each deeper than the one preceding it. The parasympathetic branch of the autonomic nervous system becomes progressively more dominant during each stage *of*

NREM sleep, so the metabolic rate and all vital signs progressively decrease.

- **Stage I** is a light sleep from which the sleeper can easily be awakened. The person is relaxed; breathing is regular and deep; the eyelids slowly open and close, and the eyes roll from side to side. The person feels groggy, the eyelids feel heavy, and suddenly without notice the person falls asleep. Within 5 to 10 minutes, sleep progresses to stage II. Stage I accounts for about 5% *of* our total sleep during the night. Brain activity consists *of* alpha waves, with occasional low-frequency theta waves.
- **Stage II** is also light sleep. Brain activity slows. The eyes are still, and body processes begin to slow down (e.g. temperature, pulse, and BP decrease). The sleeper is easily roused. Stage II, which usually lasts for 10 to 15 minutes, helps us disconnect from the outside world.
- **Stage III** is a deeper sleep. Slow-wave activity begins to occur in this stage. The person is difficult to rouse, slow eye movement stops, skeletal muscles are very relaxed, and snoring may occur. This stage may last 5 to 15 minutes. A young adult spends about 8% of sleep time in stage III.
- **Stage IV** is the deepest sleep. In this stage, the delta waves are highest in amplitude, slowest in frequency, and highly synchronized. The body, mind, and muscles are very relaxed. The heart rate is about 25% lower than when awake. It is difficult to awaken someone in stage IV slow wave sleep, and if she is awakened, the person may appear confused and react slowly. Some dreaming may occur in stage IV, but dreams are less vivid than those that occur in REM sleep. A young adult spends about 11 % of sleep time in stage IV.

Stage IV sleep appears to be especially important for restorative processes such as protein synthesis, cell division, and tissue renewal. During this stage, the body releases human growth hormone, which is essential for repair and renewal of brain and other cells.

2. REM Sleep (Stage V)

About 90 minutes after the onset of sleep and following the deep sleep of stage IV, the brain becomes highly active, and the brain waves resemble those of a person who is fully awake. This is REM sleep, so called because of its characteristic rapid eye movements, which can often be detected even though the sleeper's eyelids are closed. Metabolism, temperature, pulse, heart rate, and blood pressure increase, but muscle activity and deep tendon reflexes are depressed. Because most people awakened during REM sleep report that they have been dreaming, this loss of muscle tone is thought to be a protective response that prevents the person from acting out the dreams. People are more difficult to rouse during REM sleep than during any other stage of sleep; however, more spontaneous awakenings occur during this stage than any other. For this reason, REM sleep is also called *paradoxical sleep*. When sleepers are successfully awakened during this stage, they are usually alert and can react normally; in contrast, sleepers who are awakened during stages III or IV of slow-wave (NREM) sleep take a few moments to wake up and react.

Table 14.2: Characteristics of Stages of Sleep

Stage	Typical Duration	Characteristics
I	5–10 minutes	• Transition between wakefulness and sleep • Light sleep; can be awakened easily • Relaxed but aware of surroundings • Groggy, heavy lidded • Regular, deep breathing; eyelids open and close slowly • Accounts for about 5% of total sleep • Dreams usually not remembered
II	10–15 minutes	• Light sleep • Easily roused • Temperature, heart rate, and blood pressure decrease slightly • Accounts for about 50% of total sleep
III	5–15 minutes	• Deep sleep • Difficult to rouse • Parasympathetic nervous system predominates: temperature, pulse, respirations, and blood pressure slow even more • Skeletal muscles very relaxed • Snoring may occur • Accounts for about 8% of total sleep
IV	20–50 minutes	• The deepest sleep • Difficult to awaken • Body, mind, and muscles very relaxed • Parasympathetic nervous system still predominates; heart rate and respirations are slow and regular; temperature and BP are low • If roused, may be confused • Accounts for about 11 % of total sleep
REM (V)	5–30 minutes (usually at least 20–30)	• Paradoxical sleep • Less restful than NREM sleep • Eyes move rapidly • Small muscles twitch • Metabolism, temperature, pulse, and BP increase • Pulse may be rapid and irregular • Apnea may occur • Gastric secretions increase • Large muscle activity and deep-tendon reflexes are depressed • Dreaming occurs • If awakened, will react normally • Accounts for about 25% of total sleep

REM sleep is essential for mental and emotional restoration. Loss of REM sleep impairs memory and learning. A person who is deprived of REM sleep for several nights will usually experience *REM rebound;* that is, the person will spend a greater amount of time in REM sleep on successive nights, keeping the total amount of REM sleep constant over time.

Sleep Cycles

Sleep is cyclic. Not only do we sleep for several hours each day, but also a sleeper progresses back and forth through lighter and deeper stages of sleep about six times during an 8-hour sleep. After falling asleep in stage I, a person progresses through successively deeper stages of NREM sleep to stage IV. Then the sequence reverses, and the person progresses through successively lighter stages to stage II. Instead of proceeding to stage I, however, the person enters 'the REM stage. After REM sleep, the person cycles back through NREM stages II, III, and IV, and back again from IV to II to REM. If awakened at any time, however, the sleeper starts the cycle again at stage I. Figure 14.4 illustrates the normal sleep cycle of young adults.

All but NREM stage I are repeated four or more times a night. The *NREM/REM* sleep cycle repeats four to six times throughout the night, depending on the total amount of time spent sleeping. Each cycle lasts approximately 90 to 100 minutes. The first REM period may last only about 20 minutes, but with each cycle, the REM period lengthens until, in the last cycle of an 8-hours sleep period, REM may last as long as 60 minutes. The amount of time spent in each sleep stage varies over the life span.

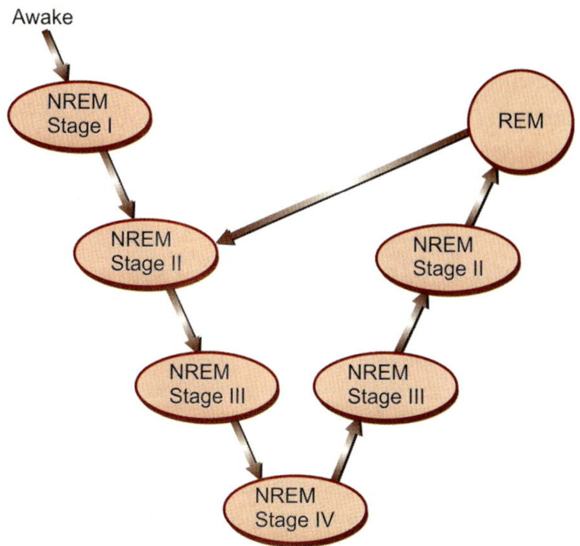

Figure 14.4: The normal adult sleep cycle

Factors Affecting Sleep

People vary not only in the amount of sleep they need, but also in their sleep patterns. Some people are refreshed after napping for 15 or 20 minutes; others feel groggy after napping; still others cannot nap at all. Many people routinely waken several times a night and do not report being tired, whereas others report fatigue and loss of mental clarity if their sleep is even minimally interrupted. In short, sleep quality has both subjective and objective components. It is related to (1) the total amount of sleep, (2) how well the person slept, and (3) whether the person obtained the needed amounts of NREM and REM. Several factors affect the amount and quality of sleep.

(i) Age

Age is an important factor affecting the duration of sleep. But sleep *patterns* are also affected by age. For example, newborns and young children experience prolonged REM sleep periods; young adults spend about 25% of their sleep in REM sleep; and older adults experience significantly less REM sleep.

Children and Adolescents: Young children experience sleep-related problems a few times a week. The problems included trouble falling asleep, frequent awakenings, nightmares, and heavy snoring. Environmental stimuli, such as the sounds and lights of older family members' activities, may make it difficult for a young child to sleep, or the child may have difficulty "winding down" after hectic activities in the late afternoon and early evening hours. Toddlers and preschoolers are often frightened to go to bed because of imagined monsters or intruders, or they may waken frequently at night because of bad dreams, the need to use the bathroom, illness, heavy snoring, tossing off the bedclothes, or falling out of bed. School-age children may suffer sleep disturbances because they are anxious about meeting new classmates or having a new schedule, or they may be excited about an upcoming competition or other activity.

The growth spurt that occurs during adolescence increases the need for sleep. At the same time, teenagers may not sleep well because of increased demands at school; staying up late to watch television, surf the Internet, or study; dating or staying out late with friends; or the effect of alcohol or drugs. Some teens consume large amounts of caffeinated colas and other beverages that can delay or disturb sleep.

Young Adults: College students may pull "all-nighters" to cram for exams or experience insomnia because of worries about grades or future career choices. Young adults may drive themselves too hard to succeed, prompting late nights at work or sleep loss due to hectic travel schedules or work-related stress.

Parents of young children often sleep poorly. Breastfeeding mothers typically need to feed their infants one or more times each night until the infant begins solid foods. Parents of toddlers often wake to care for a child who is having a nightmare, is ill, or needs to use the bathroom. Studies found that some parents lose as many as 200 hours of sleep a year because of their children's poor sleeping patterns.

Middle-Aged and Older Adults: Middle-aged adults may experience insomnia because of the stress of career demands, the need to care for a parent, or marital or financial problems. Menopausal women may be awakened by hot flashes. Older adults may feel displaced in the workforce and worry about their impending retirement. Older adults also suffer sleep disturbances because of nocturia, the side effects of medications, and discomfort or pain.

(ii) Lifestyle Factors

Lifestyle factors influencing sleep include work, exercise, nutrition, and use of medications and drugs. As noted earlier, a person who changes work shifts frequently may find it difficult to sleep at the right time. Moreover, people who cross time zones frequently because of business travel may experience difficulty falling asleep, early wakening, or day time fatigue.

- *Exercise* promotes sleep if it occurs at least 2 hours prior to bedtime. Fatigue from a normal physically active day is thought to promote a restful night's sleep. However, the more tired a person is, the shorter the first period of REM sleep.
- *Foods* can either promote or interfere with sleep. A meal high in saturated fat near bedtime may interfere with sleep. Dietary L-tryptophan, an amino acid found in milk and cheese, may help to induce sleep, although some studies indicate that the protein in these foods actually increases alertness and concentration. Carbohydrates seem to promote relaxation through their effects on brain serotonin levels. In general, satiation induces sleep, whereas many people, especially infants and children, have difficulty falling asleep when they are hungry.
- *Nicotine and caffeine,* both central nervous system stimulants, interfere with sleep. Smokers tend to have more difficulty

falling asleep and are more easily roused than nonsmokers. People who stop smoking often experience temporary sleep disturbances during the withdrawal period. Caffeine blocks adenosine and thereby inhibits sleep. However, individuals vary greatly in their sensitivity to caffeine. Some people can consume coffee throughout the day and evening and suffer no loss of sleep, whereas others cannot consume even small amounts of caffeine past noon without suffering insomnia.

- *Alcohol consumption,* if heavy, may hasten the onset of sleep; however, it disrupts REM and slow wave sleep and may cause spontaneous awakenings with difficulty returning to sleep. In addition, in some people heavy alcohol can prompt nightmares during REM sleep. Because alcohol is a diuretic, it can interrupt sleep by inducing nocturia.

- *Medications* can also affect sleep. Medications to induce sleep (i.e., *hypnotics)* tend to increase the amount of sleep while decreasing the quality. Ambien (zolpidem tartrate) promotes normal REM sleep and appears to influence sleep quality less than do other hypnotics. Amphetamines, tranquilizers, and antidepressants reduce the amount of REM sleep; barbiturates, in addition, interfere with NREM sleep. Opioids such as morphine suppress REM sleep and cause frequent awakening. Beta-blockers are reported to cause insomnia and nightmares.

(iii) Illness

As we noted earlier, illness increases the need for sleep and rest. At the same time, its associated mental and physical distress can cause sleep problems. Fear of the unknown outcome of an illness and role changes associated with hospitalization can cause anxiety. Disease symptoms such as fever, pain, nausea, and respiratory conditions (e.g. shortness of breath, dyspnea, sinus congestion) can also interfere with sleep.

Anxiety increases gastric secretions, intestinal motility, heart rate, and respirations. All of these factors contribute to a restless night. Anxiety also stimulates the sympathetic nervous system, increasing the level of norepinephrine. This decreases stage IV and REM sleep and leads to more awakenings. Depression may be associated either with almost constant sleeping or with insomnia.

(iv) Environmental Factors

Environmental factors can promote or inhibit sleep. Some people need a cool room, whereas others need warmth. Some prefer heavy bedclothes, and others like to sleep with just a light sheet. Noise can also inhibit sleep, but a person can become habituated to noise over time and be less affected by it. Some people routinely fall asleep to music or while listening to a radio or television. Usually loud noises are needed to awaken a person in NREM stages III and IV and REM sleep.

Any change in the usual environmental stimuli can affect sleep. For example, when people who are accustomed to sleeping in a dark room are hospitalized, they may have trouble falling asleep because of light outside their window or filtering into the room from the hallway. A patient used to falling asleep next to his wife may have trouble sleeping alone in a hospital bed. Equipment noise, the muffled sounds of a busy med-surg unit, or the labored breathing or snoring of a roommate also can interfere with the patient's ability to sleep.

Common Sleep Disorders

Sleep disorders are classified by their signs and symptoms. The more common disorders fall into two groups: (1) Dyssomnias–sleep disorders characterized by insomnia or excessive sleepiness. They include insomnia, sleep-wake schedule (circadian) disorders, sleep apnea, restless leg syndrome, hypersomnia, and narcolepsy and (2) Parasomnias– patterns of waking behavior that appear during sleep (e.g. sleepwalking).

1. Dyssomnias

- **Insomnia:** Insomnia is the inability to fall asleep, remain asleep, or go back to sleep. Insomnia may be *transient/short term* (less than a month) or *chronic* (longer than a month). People with insomnia usually report an insufficient quantity and quality of sleep, although people complaining of insomnia are often observed to fall asleep more quickly and sleep more than they perceive that they do. Most people are very distressed by this condition, which includes symptoms of excessive daytime sleepiness, inability to concentrate, fatigue, lethargy, and irritability.

Insomnia is the most common sleep disorder. It affects up to 30% of the adult population and rivals the common cold, stomach disorders, and headaches as a reason to seek medical assistance. It is more prevalent in women and in adults older than 60 years. Insomnia may occur as a result of illness, depression, anxiety disorders, acute stress, substance abuse, the side effects of medications (e.g. steroids, central adrenergic blockers, bronchodilating agents), or inadequate sleep hygiene (e.g. watching TV in bed, drinking caffeine-containing beverages before bedtime). It may also be the presenting symptom of other primary sleep disorders, such as restless leg syndrome.

Primary care providers can diagnose and manage most cases of insomnia. Once underlying medical or psychiatric conditions have been identified and treated, a combination of behavioral and pharmacological therapy may be effective. The use of sleeping medications is controversial because they are habit-forming, become less effective when taken continuously, and can have serious side effects. However, sedative-hypnotic treatment is justified in short-term insomnia to avoid the negative effects of insomnia on mood and performance. Short-term aggressive treatment may prevent the development of chronic insomnia.

- **Sleep-wake Schedule (Circadian) Disorders:** Abnormalities in sleep-wake schedules may be caused by rapid time-zone changes (jet lag), shift work, or a change in total sleep time from day to day. Symptoms include decreased vigilance, decreased ability to perform psychomotor tasks, and short sleep episodes *(microsleeps)* that the person is not aware of. People suffering jet lag need several days to adjust their sleep-wake schedule.

- **Restless Leg Syndrome (RLS):** Restless leg syndrome is a disorder of the central nervous system characterized by an uncontrollable movement of the legs while resting or prior to sleep onset. Children and young adults experience this condition, but it is especially common in older adults, in whom it is associated with low levels of iron (Earley, Hecklev, & Allen, 2004; Sun et al. 1998). Symptoms include unpleasant creeping, crawling, itching, or tingling sensations in the legs. Symptoms are relieved only by moving the legs, which prevents the person from relaxing and falling asleep. RLS may also keep the bed partner awake. If RLS is severe, treatment may include sedatives and avoidance of stimulants (e.g. caffeine).

- **Sleep Deprivation:** Sleep deprivation is a NANDA nursing diagnosis. It is not actually a sleep disorder, but rather a result of prolonged sleep disturbances (e.g. insomnia and parasomnias). It can result from NREM or REM deprivation, or both. Signs and symptoms of sleep deprivation include daytime sleepiness, disorientation, slurred speech, impaired cognitive functioning, irritability, many somatic (body) complaints, and a general feeling of malaise. If sleep deprivation is severe and prolonged, delusions, paranoia, and other psychotic behavior may occur. Illness and hospital care are common causes of sleep deprivation, especially for patients in critical care units (CCUs). In the CCU, lights are on most of the time, and equipment noise, frequent treatments, and assessments all combine with the client's fragile physical condition to create sleep deprivation.

- **Hypersomnia:** Hypersomnia is excessive sleeping, especially in the daytime. People with excessive daytime sleepiness doze, nap, or fall asleep at times and in situations when they need or wish to be awake and alert. The sleep disorders that commonly cause hypersomnia are obstructive sleep apnea and narcolepsy. Hypersomnia may also be caused by disorders of the central nervous system, kidney, or liver or by metabolic disorders (e.g. diabetic acidosis and hypothyroidism).

- **Sleep Apnea:** Sleep apnea is a periodic lack of breathing during sleep-an absence of air flow through the nose or mouth for at least 10 seconds at a time. Episodes may occur several or even hundreds of times a night and may last for as long as 1 minute or more. During periods of apnea, the oxygen level in the blood drops, and the carbon dioxide level rises, causing the person to wake up. This may result in cardiac dysrhythmias (irregularities) and increases in pulse and blood pressure. Many people with sleep apnea complain of fatigue and morning headache; however, some may experience mild sleep apnea without any symptoms.

To diagnose sleep apnea, a sleep study consisting of an EEG, monitoring of arterial oxygen saturation, and an electrocardiogram (ECG) is recommended. Treatment depends on the type of apnea involved. Untreated sleep apnea is associated with polycythemia, hypertension, angina, coronary artery disease, right-sided heart failure, stroke, impotence, depression, personality changes, and mood swings.

The three types of sleep apnea have different etiologies:
- **(i) Obstructive sleep apnea (OSA)** is caused by airway occlusion (usually by the tongue or palate) during sleep, but the person continues to try to breathe. The person is not aware of waking. Sleeping partners often report that the person snores, snorts, or thrashes about during sleep. Airway occlusion may be due to a collapse of the hypopharynx or from other structural abnormalities (e.g. enlarged tonsils, adenoids, a deviated nasal septum, or thyroid enlargement). Treatment of OSA is surgical removal of the obstruction or CPAP (continuous positive airway pressure) treatment by means of a device that delivers oxygen and keeps the airways open when apnea occurs. Patients with OSA should avoid alcohol and smoking and lose excess weight.
- **(ii) Central sleep apnea (CSA)** is a complete suspension of breathing resulting from a dysfunction in central respiratory control. Only about 10% of sleep apnea is central in origin. People with CSA tend to awaken during sleep and, therefore, experience daytime sleepiness.
- **(iii) Mixed apnea** is a combination of both OSA and CSA.

- **Snoring:** Snoring is a hallmark sign of obstructive sleep apnea, but it does not necessarily indicate OSA. Even so, snoring can significantly reduce the quality of sleep for the bed partner. Snoring results when the muscles at the back of the mouth relax during sleep, obstruct the airway, and vibrate with each breath. Obstruction is usually more pronounced when the person sleeps on his back. Many treatments have been invented to open the air passages, such as nose tapes or even surgery. Saline sprays, nose drops, and cortisone sprays are also used–all with mixed success.

- **Narcolepsy:** Narcolepsy is a chronic disorder that causes sudden, uncontrollable episodes of sleep during the day, even though the person sleeps well at night. The person cannot avoid the "sleep attacks" but awakens easily. Narcolepsy is characterized by sleepiness, slurred speech, slackening of the facial muscles, a feeling of impending weakness of the knees, paralysis, and hallucinations. Because sleep attacks can come on suddenly, even while the person is standing up or working, they can be dangerous. Some people have symptoms only during sedentary activities such as reading, working at a computer, or driving a motor vehicle. Some have other symptoms, such as cataplexy, a sudden loss of muscle tone usually triggered by an emotional event (e.g. laughter, surprise, or anger), but most only have hypersomnia.

Narcolepsy affects up to 1 in every 1000 individuals, making it as common as Parkinson's disease and multiple sclerosis. It is thought to be caused by a genetic defect of the central nervous system in which REM sleep cannot be controlled. Each sleep attack *begins* in the REM stage instead of progressing through the NREM stages first. People with narcolepsy do not tolerate irregular wake-sleep patterns, such as shift work. The condition is controlled by central nervous system stimulants, such as methylphenidate (Ritalin), with little evidence of tolerance, dependence, or abuse.

2. Parasomnias

The parasomnias include sleepwalking, sleeptalking, bruxism, night terrors, REM sleep behavior disorders, and enuresis.

- **Sleepwalking (somnambulism)** occurs during stages III and IV of NREM sleep, usually 1 to 2 hours after the person falls asleep. The sleeper leaves the bed and walks about, with little awareness of surroundings. He may perform what appear to be conscious motor activities (e.g. brush his teeth, make coffee), but he does not wake up. The person is not aware of sleepwalking and has no memory of the event on awakening. The event may last 3 to 4 minutes or longer. Children sleepwalk more than adults. If the child does not outgrow the condition or serious safety risks exist, drugs may be given to suppress stage IV sleep. Stress, fatigue, and some drugs can cause sleepwalking.

- **Sleep talking** occurs during NREM sleep, just before the REM stage. It does not usually interfere with the person's rest but may be disturbing to a bed partner.

- **Bruxism,** grinding and clenching of the teeth, usually occurs during stage II NREM sleep. It can eventually erode tooth enamel and loosen the teeth. The noise can also disturb the bed partner's sleep.

- **Night terrors** are sudden arousals in which the person (usually a child) is physically active, often hallucinatory, and expresses a strong emotion such as terror. Children experiencing night terrors typically cry or scream in fear, thrash about, and resist all attempts by their parents or other caregivers to hold or console them. The child appears to be fully awake, but she is not; in fact, children in the midst of night terrors are extremely difficult to awaken. Episodes may last from 10 to 30 minutes and are quite distressing to witness. However, the child typically returns to sleep without awakening, and in the morning has no memory of the event. Unlike *nightmares* (unpleasant, frightening dreams), which occur during REM sleep, night terrors occur during stage IV (deep NREM) sleep.

- **REM sleep behavior disorders** are associated with REM (or dreaming period) sleep, in which the sleeper violently acts out the dream. People have actually injured themselves or others without waking.

- **Enuresis** (bedwetting) is night time incontinence past the stage at which toilet training has been well established. It has incorrectly been associated with dreaming; however, most incidents occur during NREM sleep, during the first third of the night when the child is difficult to rouse. It is distressing because of the importance society places on continence, the inconvenience of keeping bed linens clean, and the misconception that the child is bedwetting to act out against parents. Because the great majority of children outgrow enuresis, the best strategy is patience. If the problem persists, the child should have a full medical evaluation.

- **Secondary Sleep Disorders**

Secondary sleep disorders occur when a disease causes alterations in sleep stages or in quantity and quality of sleep. The following are the most common causes:

- *Depression:* Depressed people may spend a great deal of time in bed. However, in general, they have difficulty falling asleep, experience less slow-wave (deep) sleep, spend less time in REM sleep, awaken early, and have less total sleep time.
- *Hyperthyroidism* or *hypothyroidism:* An increase in thyroid secretion causes an increase in stage III and IV sleep; hypothyroidism causes a decrease in those stages. Hyperthyroidism increases metabolic rate, making it difficult for the person to fall asleep.
- *Pain:* Both acute and chronic pain interfere with sleep. Chronic pain affects both the quality and quantity of sleep. It inhibits sleep, increases arousals during sleep, and causes longer waking intervals during the night.
- *Airway passage obstruction* or *CNS dysfunction, which cause sleep apnea.*

- **Sleep Provoking Disorders**

Sleep-provoked disorders are those that occur when signs and symptoms of the disease appear or become worse during sleep. Diseases affected by sleep include the following:

- *Coronary artery disease:* During REM sleep, dreams may increase heart rate and provoke angina and ECG changes.
- *Bronchial asthma:* People with asthma may experience bronchospasm during REM sleep. In adults, asthma attacks may occur at any time during the night. In children, they occur mostly during the final two-thirds of the night, when there is less stage IV sleep.
- *Chronic obstructive pulmonary disease (COPD):* Persons with COPD experience lowered oxygen tension and increased carbon dioxide retention during sleep, especially during REM sleep, when neuromuscular control is normally depressed. This can result in pulmonary spasm and transient pulmonary hypertension.
- *Diabetes:* Blood glucose levels vary during sleep. When diabetes is uncontrolled, it may profoundly affect the blood sugar during sleep, when the person is not alert enough to deal with it. Therefore, patients with uncontrolled diabetes may need to have blood glucose levels monitored during sleep.
- *Duodenal ulcers:* During REM sleep, people with duodenal ulcers secrete up to 20 times more gastric acid than do people who do not have duodenal ulcers. This increased acid often produces nocturnal epigastric pain and sleep loss.

Nursing Management

It is important to assess usual sleep patterns and rituals for all patients who are being admitted to the hospital or seeking help for a sleep problem. A brief assessment for all patients should include questions about the following:

- Usual sleeping pattern
- Sleeping environment
- Bedtime routines/rituals
- Sleep aids
- Sleep changes or problems

If the person reports experiencing satisfactory sleep, that is an adequate assessment, and nurse merely need to support her usual sleep patterns and rituals. When nurse suspect a sleep problem, nurse will perform a more in-depth assessment, such as a detailed sleep history or sleep diary. A **sleep history** includes in-depth questions about the person's usual times for sleep, any preparation, preferences and routines, quality of sleep, napping habits (if any), and whether she wakes early and cannot return to sleep. A **sleep diary** provides very specific information on their patient's patterns of sleep. Nurse will usually tell the patient to keep the diary for 14 days; remind him that it is important to be diligent in maintaining it.

It is important to determine whether lack of sleep is a problem, is a symptom of a problem, or is contributing to (etiology of) a different problem. For health promotion applications, use the diagnosis "Readiness for Enhanced Sleep" when a client has no particular sleep problem but wishes to move to a higher level of functioning in the area of sleep. To focus on interventions to promote sleep, use the diagnoses Disturbed Sleep Pattern or Sleep Deprivation on the problem side of the nursing diagnosis.

Use *sleep deprivation* as the nursing diagnosis when the patient's amount, consistency, or quality of sleep is decreased over prolonged periods of time. Defining characteristics of Sleep Deprivation are more severe than those for Disturbed Sleep Pattern, so nursing activities may focus as much on relieving symptoms (e.g. confusion, paranoia) as on sleep promotion.

Use *disturbed sleep pattern* as the diagnosis when assessment data points to a time-limited sleep problem that can be treated by nursing therapy (e.g. inability to sleep in the unfamiliar hospital environment). Add modifying words to specify the type of sleep problem, as in the examples. This will help you to focus goals appropriately.

- Disturbed Sleep Pattern (insomnia: difficulty falling asleep) related to worries about family
- Disturbed Sleep Pattern (insomnia: difficulty falling and remaining asleep) related to noise of hospital environment and need for scheduled treatments
- Disturbed Sleep Pattern (insomnia: premature awakening) related to sleeping aid dependence and lack of knowledge of nonpharmacological aids for insomnia
- Disturbed Sleep Pattern (excessive daytime sleeping) related to effects of biological aging and depression
- Disturbed Sleep Pattern (altered sleep-wake patterns) related to frequent rotations of shift and overtime

Nurse carefully describe the etiologies for sleep problems, because they determine nursing interventions to avoid interrupting sleep use nursing judgment to decide when a procedure must be done and when it is more important for your patient to sleep. Healthcare routines usually allow time for rest periods. In addition, you may consider the following:

- Some patients need to rest after a procedure or after meals.
- If the person looks sleepy, give a prescribed sleeping pill early to avoid waking him later in the evening.
- You can often alter routines; for example, you can allow the patient to sleep as long as he can in the morning and bring his breakfast later.
- Unless the patient is critically ill, do not wake him for morning vital signs if he is sleeping.
- Keep the noise level down. Be aware that activities, conversation, and equipment, even outside the patient's room, can disrupt sleep.

Many people find it difficult to sleep in a strange bed, even a comfortable one. Hospital beds are not noted for their luxury, but you can help make them more comfortable. To create a restful environment following measures will be helpful:

- Be sure the bed linens are tight on the bottom and loose on top to allow movement.
- Keep linens clean, dry, and free of irritants. Perspiration on the hospital gown or linens can lead to chill.
- Good body alignment also facilitates relaxation. Use extra pillows, a blanket from home, or any other item which may help the patient rest.
- Keep the room dark and quiet, unless the patient prefers a light.
- As much as possible, control the temperature of the room and provide good ventilation.

In addition following measures are helpful to promote sleep:

- **Promote Comfort:** Pain, itching, and nausea may all be deterrents to rest and sleep in an ill person. Be sure to offer pain medications at their scheduled times, and before the patient's sleep time. Other comfort measures include providing a restful environment (see the preceding intervention) and offering fluids, cool cloths, or a massage or back rub.

- **Support Bedtime Rituals and Routines:** Most people have some kind of a routine before bed, be it reading, watching TV, drinking warm milk, or praying or meditating, to allow them to prepare for sleep. For children, a favorite doll, blanket, bedtime story, as well as brushing their teeth and hair, may enhance sleepiness. Be sure to include any routines or rituals in the nursing plan of care to ensure continuity. Advise patients who smoke not to smoke after the evening meal.

- **Offer Appropriate Bedtime Snacks or Beverages:** Carbohydrates (e.g. a juice drink, crackers) seem to help most people sleep. Newer information suggests that protein (e.g. milk, cheese) may increase alertness and concentration, although in the past it was believed the dietary amino acid L-tryptophan promotes sleep. Advise the client to avoid alcohol. Although it may induce sleepiness at first, alcohol is contraindicated because it interferes with the deep sleep cycle. The client should also avoid taking caffeine-containing foods and beverages (e.g. tea, coffee, chocolate, colas) after the evening meal. Advise the client to drink plenty of fluids during the day but to restrict fluids close to bedtime.

- **Promote Relaxation:** You will base your choice of relaxation strategies on your repertoire of techniques and on patient preference. Relaxation strategies may include a massage, a warm bath, or one of the following:
  - *Guided imagery* can be used to help your patient move in his mind to a safe place, where relaxation is possible. You may ask the patient what type of place will soothe him and "guide" him there through visualization.
  - *Progressive muscle relaxation,* relaxing each muscle independently and progressing from head to toe, may help to promote sleep.
  - *Music therapy* has been shown to be effective in promoting relaxation. Some patients respond well and can put away their troubles while listening to music, whereas others may find music irritating. Slow, quiet music, or a recording of forest or ocean sounds may be soothing.

- **Maintain Patient Safety:** A person who sleepwalks needs protection from injury, because the risk of falling is great. A sleep walker tends not to notice dangers (e.g. stairs). Intravenous infusions, catheters, and nasogastric tubes can produce injury if they are pulled out of the body when the person gets out of bed. Guide sleepwalkers back to bed, and remember that they startle easily, so be gentle and quiet.

- **Teach About Sleep Hygiene:** Most people with sleep problems manage them at home. Teaching clients self-care regarding sleep as given below:
  - Follow a regular routine for bedtime and morning awakenings.
  - Go to bed each night at the same time, even on days you are off work.
  - If you cannot fall asleep in 15 minutes, get up and do something monotonous. When you feel sleepy, go back to bed.
  - Use relaxation methods to promote sleep: Read a book, pray, or meditate.
  - Avoid going to bed angry.
  - Don't depend on sleeping aids. Be aware of the potential dangers of sleeping medications.
  - Use your bedroom only for sleep; do not turn your bedroom into the family room.
  - Avoid caffeine, alcohol, smoking, and heavy meals before retiring.
  - Eat a small amount of carbohydrates (e.g. crackers, cereal, or bread) before bed; they aid in sleeping.
  - If you take prescription drugs, ask your physician or pharmacist about the side effects.
  - Use earplugs to block out noise.
  - Walk or exercise in the early evening. Doing so will raise your body temperature and tire your muscles.

- Take a warm bath just before retiring. This will raise your body temperature, and when your body starts to cool off, you will fall asleep more easily.
- Don't try to "catch up" on sleep. Rise at your regular time, even if you went to bed later than usual.

Medications to Produce Sleep

When considering sleep medications, it is important for the patient to understand the options, be aware of potential side effects, and know what questions to ask. Some medications are habit-forming; others may have unpleasant side effects. As a general rule, they are not recommended for long-term use. The most common side effects of sleep medicines include dizziness, lightheadedness, daytime drowsiness, diarrhea, and difficulty with coordination.

Prescription sleep medications includes:

- *Non-benzodiazepines.* This is the newest class of sedative/hypnotics (sleep medicines). These have a short half-life, which means that they are eliminated from the body quickly and do not cause "hangover" (daytime sleepiness). They are also selective, which means that they target specific receptors that are thought to be associated with sleep rather than depressing the entire central nervous system. Examples are zolpidem tartrate (Ambien) and zaleplon (Sonata). Long-term effects of these medications are not yet known.
- *Benzodiazepines.* This class of sedative/hypnotics includes both long-acting and short-acting drugs. Long-acting medications linger in the body and potentially cause daytime drowsiness. Many benzodiazepines were originally formulated to treat anxiety. Examples are diazepam (Valium), alprazolam (Xanax), flurazepam (Dalmane), lorazepam (Ativan), and triazolam (Halcion).
- *Barbiturates.* These sedative/hypnotics and anticonvulsants are rarely prescribed for insomnia because of the risk of addiction, abuse, and overdose. Examples are amobarbital (Amytal), pentobarbital (Nembutal), and secobarbital (Seconal).
- *Tricyclic antidepressants.* At times, primary care providers prescribe antidepressants to promote sleep, although none of these medicines is specifically approved for this purpose. Examples are amitriptyline (Elavil), doxepin (Sinequan), imipramine (Tofranil), and nortriptyline (Aventyl, Pamelor).

Nonprescription Sleep Medications includes:

Nonprescription sleep medications usually contain an antihistamine, which may induce drowsiness that lasts into the next day. It is important to check the ingredient label of any over-the-counter (OTC) medication to see whether it contains an antihistamine. Advise clients that OTC sleep medications can interact with other medicines they may be taking, so they should consult their doctor or pharmacist before using them. An example is diphenhydramine hydrochloride (Benadryl). Other nonprescription sleep aids include the following:

- *Melatonin:* This is widely sold as a sleep aid but remains controversial in medical circles. Melatonin is a hormone produced by the pineal gland.
- *Herbal sleep aids:* Herbal remedies for sleep problems include chamomile tea, valerian root, hops, lavender, and passionflower. Like melatonin, these herbal remedies have not undergone extensive testing for benefits and safety. Factors affecting sleep should be assessed as given below:
- *Physical illness:* For example, respiratory disease, (asthma, cold), hypertension and cardiac disease (chest pain).
- *Drugs and substances:* For example, hypotonics, diuretics, antidepressant and stimulant alcohol, caffeine, diagoxin, beta-blockers, narcotics (morphine).
- *Lifestyle:* Night duties, late night, etc.
- *Sleep pattern:* Day time sleepness or sleep.
- *Emotional stress:* Worries.
- *Environment:* Lack of ventilation, noise.
- *Exercise fatigue*
- *Calorie intake:* Weight loss or gain influence sleep, i.e. less calories and excess calories intake.

And keep in mind the sleep requirement of individuals that is generally 8 hours sleep every night has been accepted giving no reasons. There is not rigid formula for normal periodicity and duration of sleep. It is important, however, that each person follow a pattern of rest that maintains wellbeing. Usually, on the average, infants sleep from 14 to 20 hours each day. Growing children require from 10 hours to 14 hours of sleep. Adults average 7 to 9 hours; although 4 hours of range observed in many normal adults.

As already stated the following common sleep disorders while promoting sleep includes:

- *Insomnia:* It is characterized by difficulty in falling asleep, intermittent sleep or early awakening from sleep.
- *Hypersomnia:* It is characterized by excessive sleep, particularly during day.
- *Narcolepsy:* It is a condition characterized by uncontrollable desire to sleep (force while conversation or while driving, etc).
- *Sleep apnea:* It refers to periods of no breathing between snoring intervals. The person may not breath for periods of 10 to 20 seconds to as long as 2 minutes. Long periods of interval drop oxygen level in blood.
- *Sleep deprivation:* It refers to a decrease in the amount consistency and quality of sleep. The symptoms of sleep deprivation are enlisted in Table 14.3.
- *Somnambulism:* Sleep waling, night terrors, nightmares.
- *Nocturnal enuresis:* Bedwetting.
- *Bruxism:* Tooth grindly.

And take measures to induce sleep.

Table 14.3: Symptoms of Sleep Deprivation

Physiological symptoms	*Psychological symptoms*
• Hand tremors • Decreased reflexes • Slowed response time • Reduction in word memory • Decreased reasoning, judgment • Cardiac dysrhythmias • Decreased auditory and visual alertness	• Moods • Disorientation • Irritability • Decreased motivation • Fatigue association • Sleepiness • Hyperactivity

Nursing Measures to Induce Sleep

All ailments require a sleeping environment with a comfortable room temperature and proper ventilation, minimal sources of noise, a comfortable bed and proper lighting. In a hospital the nurse can control noise in several ways, 'which include the following:

- Close doors to a clients room
- Reduce volume of nearly telephone and paying equipment
- Wear rubber, soled shoes, avoid wearing clogs
- Turn off bedside equipment that is not in use, e.g. oxygen and suction
- Avoid abrupt loud noise such as flushing a toilet or moving a bed
- Keep necessary conversation as low levels, particularly at night
- Conduct discussion or nursing reports in a private separate room away from client
- Turn off the TV or radio unless client prefers soft music.

And nurse can apply following comfort measures to promote sleep:

- Administer analgesic or sedatives about 30 minutes before bed time
- Encourage clients, to wear loose-fitting night wear
- Remove any irritant against the clients skin such as moist or wrinkled or drainage tubing
- Position and support body parts to protect pressure points and aid muscle relaxation
- Offer a massage just before bed time
- Provide caps and shock for older clients and those from the cold
- Administer necessary hygienic measures
- Keep bed linen clean and dry
- Provide comfortable mattresses
- Encourage client to void before going to sleep.

15

Meeting Nutritional Needs/Nutrition in Nursing

Introduction

Nutrition is a basic human need that changes throughout life cycle and along the health-illness continuum. The body requires food to provide energy for organ functions, body movement and work maintain body temperature; and to provide raw materials for enzymes function, growth replacement of cells and repair. Food provides nutrition for both the body and the mind. Eating has evolved from being simply a necessity; it may be a source of pleasure for past time, a social happening, a political statement, a religious symbol, a cultural emblem or an integral component of medical treatment.

The science of nutrition encompasses the study of nutrients and how they are handled by the body, as well as the impact of human behavior and environment on the process of nourishment. Nutrients are specific historical substances used by the body for growth and development activity, reproduction, lactation, health maintenance and recovery from illness or injury.

Nurses must understand the functions of the basic nutrients and metabolism. An understanding of the guidelines for adequate diet is essential so that nurses can teach about nutrients and answer questions related to diet. Nurses must be able to assist the nutrients of the diet. They must also recognize that many divergent factors influence food intake and considering the factors when attempting to modifying food intake. The factors that influence nutrient requirements are developmental consideration, i.e. age, sex, health, status, culture, and religion, socioeconomic status, personal preference, medications, alcohol and drugs, etc. Nurse also must be able to identify clients at risk for nutritional problems and be aware of common nutritional conditions.

Good nutrition is a basic component of health, growth, and development for maintaining health throughout life. Proper nutrition of the nation is necessary for the nation's growth and economic development.

Meaning of Food and Nutrition

The term 'food' refers to anything, which nourishes the body. It would obviously include solids, semisolids, and liquids which can be consumed and which help to sustain the body and keep it healthy. The terms 'food' and 'nutrition' are sometimes used synonymously; but it is not strictly correct. Food is defined as what one feeds on and is a composite mixture of many substances ranging from a fraction of a gram in some cases to hundred of grams in others. The foodstuff if defined as anything which can be used for food. Therefore, the word 'nutrition' is derived from the word *nutricus*, which means "to suckle at the breast". Nutrition is defined as combination of dynamic process by which the consumed food is utilized for nourishment and structural and functional efficiency of every cell of the body.

The body requires food to provide energy for organ function, body movement, and work; to maintain body temperature, and provide raw materials for enzyme function, growth, replacement of cells and repair. Metabolism refers to all biochemical reactions within body. It consists of anabolic reactions that build substances and body tissues and catabolic reactions that breakdown substances. Food is ingested, digested, and absorbed to produce the energy needed for these reactions. The energy requirement of an awake person at rest is called the basal metabolic rate (BMR). BMR is the energy needed at a person's lowest level of cellular functions. Age, body size, body temperature, growth, sex, nutritional status, emotional status, and good intake affect individual energy requirements beyond the BMR.

When energy requirements are completely met by caloric intake in food, people maintain that activity levels without weight change. If the number of calories ingested exceeds energy needs, people gain weight. When the calories ingested fail to meet energy requirements, people loss weight.

Nutrition encompasses all of the processes involved in consuming and utilizing food for energy, maintenance, and growth. These processes are ingestion, digestion, absorption, metabolism, and excretion. Much of the discussion throughout this chapter focuses on ingestion. Because this is the process that the individual can control and with which the nurse can be of assistance to the client. Basic information is presented about proper nutrition and the role of the nurse in assisting clients to meet their nutritional needs. Topics covered include specific nutrients and their functions in the body; phytochemicals; promoting proper nutrition; factors influencing nutrition; nutritional needs during the life cycle: nutrition and health; weight management; food labeling, quality, and safety; food allergies; and nutrition and the nursing process,

Physiology of Nutrition

Five processes are involved in the body's use of nutrients: ingestion, digestion, absorption, metabolism, and excretion.

Ingestion: Nutrition begins with ingestion, taking food into the digestive tract, generally through the mouth. In special circumstances, ingestion occurs directly into the stomach, through a feeding tube.

Digestion: Digestion refers to the mechanical and chemical processes that convert nutrients into a physically absorbable state mechanical digestion includes mastication (chewing), breaking food into fine particles and mixing it with enzymes in saliva, and deglutition (swallowing food), the peristaltic waves and mucus secretions that move the food down the esophagus. Chemical digestion juices change food into the individual nutrients that can be used by the body.

Digestion begins in the stomach (except in the case of some starches. for which digestion begins in the mouth) and is completed in the intestines. *Peristalsis* (rhythmic, coordinated, serial contractions of the smooth muscles of the GI tract) forces *chyme* (an acidic, semifluid paste) through the small and large intestines. Only carbohydrates, proteins, and fats require chemical digestion to make the nutrients available for absorption.

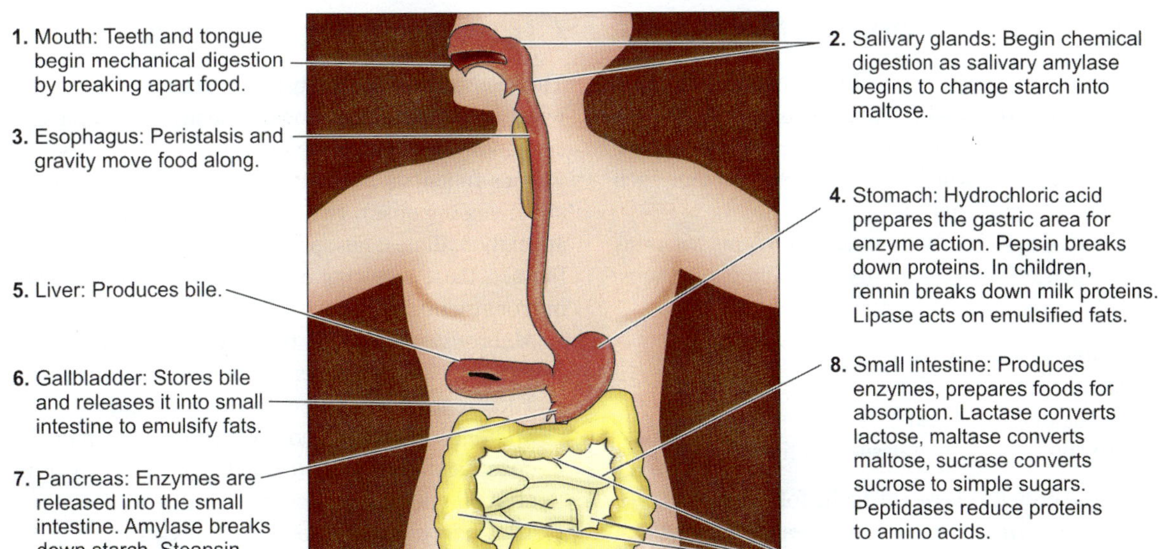

Figure 15.1: Functions of the digestive system

Figure 15.1 illustrates the basic elements and functions of the digestive system.

Absorption: Absorption is the process whereby the end products of digestion (i.e., individual nutrients) pass through the epithelial membranes in the small and large intestines and into the blood or lymph systems, The nutrients are absorbed and taken to the parts of the body that need them. Most nutrients are water soluble and can be absorbed directly through the *villi* (fingerlike projections that line the small intestine) and into the blood. Fats, which are not water soluble, are absorbed first into the lymph system and eventually enter the circulatory system.

Metabolism: The conversion of nutrients into energy by the body is called *metabolism;* this process is the sum total of all the biological and chemical processes in the body as they relate to the use of nutrients in every body cell. Metabolism involves two processes: anabolism and catabolism. *Anabolism* is the constructive process of metabolism, wherein new molecules are synthesized and new tissues are formed, as in growth and repair. This process requires energy. *Catabolism* is the destructive process of metabolism, wherein tissues or substances are broken into their component parts. This process releases energy. During metabolism, energy is also produced by the process of *oxidation,* which is the chemical process of combining nutrients with oxygen. The energy produced by the body is used in a number of ways: electrical energy for brain and nerve activities, chemical energy for metabolism, mechanical energy for muscle contractions, and thermal energy to keep the body warm.

Metabolic rate is the rate of energy utilization in the body; it is expressed in units called calories. One *calorie* is the amount of heat required to raise the temperature of one gram of water by $1°$ celsius. Because of the large quantity of energy released during metabolism, the energy is expressed in *kilocalories* (kcal), each of which is equal to 1,000 calories.

Basal metabolism is the amount of energy needed to maintain essential physiologic functions, when a person is at *complete* rest. It is the lowest level of energy expenditure.

The major factor affecting basal metabolism is body composition. Lean muscle tissue has a higher metabolic rate and thus produces more energy than does fatly tissue. Generally, women have a lower metabolism than men because they have a higher percentage of fat tissue; however, metabolism increases during menstruation, pregnancy, and lactation. Age is also an influence, because growth periods increase metabolism. Glandular activity, especially of the thyroid gland, affects metabolism. The rate of metabolism is governed primarily by the hormones triiodothyronine (T_1) and thyroxine (T_4). Hypothyroid activity, a decrease in the secretion of thyroid hormones, causes a lower rate of metabolism, whereas hyperthyroid activity, an increase in the secretion of thyroid hormones, causes a higher rate of metabolism.

Excretion: Excretion is the process of eliminating or removing waste products from the body. Dietary fiber and other indigestible materials, salts, and other products such as bile and water are formed into feces and excreted from the body as solid waste. Other excretory organs that aid the digestive system in the elimination of wastes include the kidneys, bladder, sweat glands, skin, and lungs. Most liquid waste is sent through the kidneys and bladder to be excreted as urine. Some liquid waste is removed through the sweat glands of the skin as perspiration. Gaseous waste is eliminated through the lungs.

Classification of Foodstuffs

Food is classified on the basis of their functions:
- *Energy yielding foods*—in which foods are rich in carbohydrates and fats such as cereals, sugar, roots and tubers.
- *Body building foods*—in which foods are rich in protein, such as meat, liver, fish, milk, pulses.
- *Protective foods*—in which food are rich in proteins, vitamins and minerals such as fruits, green leafy, vegetables, liver, eggs, milk and fish.

The main functions of food are:
- The provision of energy.
- Tissue building and repair, and
- Maintenance and regulation of tissue functions.

Foodstuffs may be broadly classified as the following:
- Cereals, e.g. rice, *ragi,* wheat, maize, *jowar,* etc., which produce carbohydrate.
- Pulses, which give proteins.
- Nuts and oilseed, e.g. groundnut, almond, cashewnut, mustard seed, soyabean, etc. provide protein and fat.
- Vegetables, e.g.
  - Green leafy vegetables (spinach, amaranth which provide carotene)
  - Root vegetables, e.g. tapioca, potato, sweet potato, etc. provide carbohydrate
  - Other vegetable (brinjal, lady finger, french beans) which provide vitamins.
- Fruits, e.g. guavas, amla, citrus fruits, etc., provide vitamins. Mangoes, orange, papaya, etc., provide carotene. Dried fruits like dates and raisins provide iron.
- Milk and milk products, e.g. milk, curds, cheese, which provide proteins.
- Flesh foods, e.g. fish, poultry, meat provide class proteins.

Nutrients

The body must have six types of nutrients to function efficiently and effectively. These are water, carbohydrates, fats, proteins, vitamins, and minerals. If a person eats a well-balanced diet, all the nutrients the body requires are provided by the food.

Nutrients are classified as energy nutrients, organic nutrients, and inorganic nutrients.

Energy nutrients release energy for use by the body. Organic nutrients build and maintain body tissues and regulate body processes. Inorganic nutrients provide a medium for the body's chemical reactions, transport materials, maintain body temperature, promote bone formation, and conduct nerve impulses.

The functions of the nutrients are interrelated. Intake changes in one nutrient may lead to functional changes in another. Some examples of interrelated functions include: (1) Iron is better absorbed when vitamin C is present, and (2) Calcium absorption depends on the presence of vitamin D.

Classification of Nutrients

The foodstuff contains substances known as 'nutrients' some of which have been already mentioned in these examples. Nutrients are foods that contain the elements, necessary which perform various functions in the body that food is consumed daily by any living organism. There are six categories of nutrients. They are carbohydrates, fats, proteins, vitamins, minerals, and water. Further, these nutrients can be groups as macronutrients and micronutrients.
- *Macronutrients*—are those which the body requires in relatively large amounts, e.g. protein, fat, carbohydrate, water. Their requirements are measured in gram.
- *Micronutrients*—are those which the body requires in small quantities. These requirements are measures in milligrams (1/1000 gm) and micrograms (1/10,00,000 gm).

The energy value of food is expressed in terms of calories. The calories refer to the amount of heat required to raise one gram (1 gm) of water to one degree celsius (1°C) at atmosphere. A kilocalorie or large calorie used to represent energy values of food, is 1000 times as large as small calorie, the unit used in physics to describe energy exchange in the body.

1 gram of fat yields 9.3 calories.

1 gram of carbohydrate yields 4.1 calories.

1 gram of protein yields 4.1 calories.

Now we shall examine the classification of nutrients for details as given in Figure 15.2.

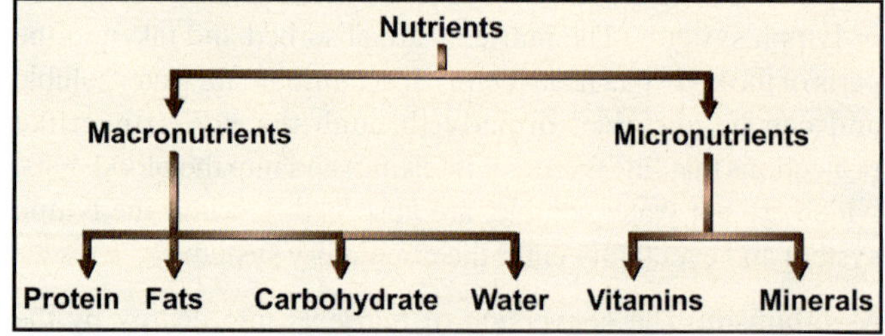

Figure 15.2: Classification of nutrients

Proteins

Proteins comes from the word *protos* meaning 'to take first place.' Proteins are the chief substances in the cells of the body. They are composed of hydrogen, oxygen, carbon, and nitrogen. Some proteins also contain sulfur, phosphorous and iron and occasionally other elements. A human adult contains about 10 kg of proteins. The proteins are made up of simpler substances called amino acids. Further they are categorized into essential and nonessential amino acids follows (Fig. 15.3).

Amino acids are the most important nutrients of proteins. They are essential for synthesis (building) of body tissues in growth, maintenance and repair. Proteins can also be used as a source of energy. Certain amino acids when present in excessive amounts have been found to affect the health and growth.

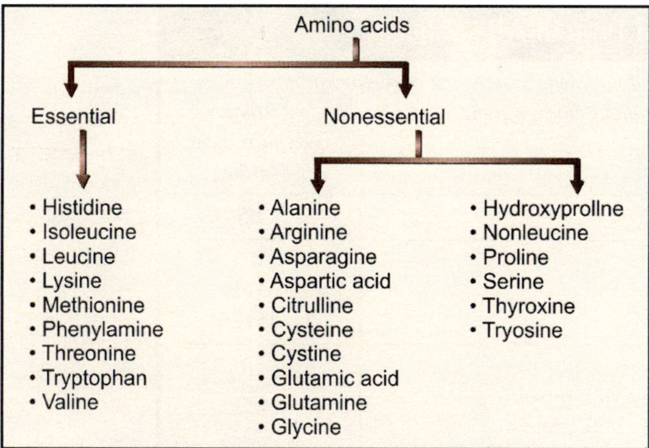

Figure 15.3: Types of amino acids

Functions of Proteins

- It helps in growth and development.
- It helps in wear and tear of the tissue repair and maintenance.
- It helps in the formation of immune bodies, enzymes, and hormones.
- It acts as a source of energy when consumed in excess of body need.

Sources of Proteins

- Animal sources, e.g. cheese, milk, liver, fish, meat, eggs.
- Plant sources, e.g. pulses, nuts, beans, and soybeans.
- Conventional sources, e.g. oil seeds, cakes, sea weeds, leaf, protein and yeast.

Animal proteins are called first class proteins or superior proteins as they are more easily digestible and contain more and several types of amino acids. Human beings are able to synthesize about 12 nonessential amino acids. The essential amino acids are to be derived from the food we eat. So the animal protein contains all amino acids. Pulses contain about 25 percent proteins and they are cheap. By proper continuation of two or more vegetables food (cereals, pulses and vegetables) it is possible to produce a mixture containing all the essential amino acids cheaper than animal proteins. This is the reason that vegetarian mixing of 3-4 types of pulses is essential.

Protein Requirement

The protein requirement will depend upon the age, sex, physical, physiological and psychological factors and other factors.

ICMR (1981) recommended one gram of protein per kilogram of body weight per day. Far an Indian adult, assuming a net protein utilization of 65 gm for the dietary pattern. The recommended daily protein allowance by ICMR is enlisted in Table 15.1.

An extra-amount is to be provided for heavy workers and also should be provided in ailments involving either loss, destruction or degeneration of body tissue, e.g. blood loss, surgery etc.

Deficiencies of Proteins/Protein-Energy Malnutrition

Our Indian diet is mostly composed of carbohydrates. Protein is inadequate, especially protein of animal origin, which leads to protein deficiency, which is called as condition of protein-energy malnutrition or protein caloric malnutrition (PEM/PCM). The PEM is an important cause of infant and young child's morbidity, mortality, stunted physical growth, impaired mental growth, low work output, premature ageing and reduced lifespan in the developing countries. The wide occurrence of PEM especially among infants, preschool children, expectant and lactating mothers in many developing nations poses a great danger. It is widely prevalent among the poor class of Indian population. The rice eating belts in South India, Orissa, West Bengal, etc. are affected.

Causes

These are as follows:
- Sociocultural patterns of Indians leads to poor environmental conditions, large family size, poor maternal health, failure in lactation, premature termination of breastfeeding, faulty child rearing practices, etc.
- Population explosion in India is responsible for wide gap between per capita demand and availability of proteins.
- Infections and infestations have precipitating roles, e.g. ARI, measles, diarrhea, worm infestation, etc.
- Inadequacy of food supplies, poverty, ignorance and food prejudice.

Forms of PEM, their preventive measures: The most serious forms of PEM are kwashiorkor and marasmus and also anemia, particularly during pregnancy. The first indicator of PEM is underweight. The most practical method to detect the PEM is maintenance of road to health chart by any health workers in the field, including Nursing Personnel of peripheri. These charts indicate whether children are gaining weight or losing weight at a glance.

The main features of kwashiorkor and marasmus are given in Table 15.2.

PEM is the nutritional disorder due to deficiency of proteins in the diet. This condition will spread among the children in the tropical countries where diets of the children lack in adequate and good quantity of protein. This condition is rarely during period of breastfeeding. It appears generally during the weaning period of the child when starchy food is introduced to child in place of milk.

The preventive measures of PEM in the community, adopted from the FAO/WHO (1971) are as follow:

(a) Health promotion
- Measures directed to pregnant and lactating women (education, distribution of supplements)
- Promotion of breastfeeding
- Development of low cost weaning foods, the child should be made to eat more food at frequent intervals

Table 15.1: Recommended Protein Allowances

	Age (Years)	Daily allowance in terms of dietary pattern Gram/kg body weight	Total Requirement (Gram)
1.	Man (55 kg)	1.0	55
2.	Women (45 kg) Women pregnancy (1st and 2nd trimester) Women lactation (0-6 months)	1.0	45 45+14 45+25
3.	Infants 0 to 3 months 3 to 6 months 6 to 9 months 9 to 12 months	 2.3 (Milk protein) 1.8 (Milk protein) 1.8 (Partly vegetable proteins) 1.5 (Partly vegetable proteins)	
4.	Children 1 to 3 years 4 to 6 years 7 to 9 years	 1.83 1.56 1.35	 22 29 36
5.	Males 10 to 12 years 13 to 15 years 16 to 18 years	 1.24 1.10 0.94	 43 52 53
6.	Females 10 to 12 years 13 to 15 years 16 to 18 years	 1.17 0.95 0.88	 43 43 44

Table 15.2: Main Features of PEM in Children

Features	Marasmus	Kwashiorkor
Essential features		
1. Edema	None	Lower legs, sometimes face or generalized
2. Wasting	Marked, all skin and bone	Less obvious, sometimes fat, blubbery
3. Muscle wasting	Severe	Sometimes
4. Growth retardation (In terms of body weight)	Severe	Less than marasmus
5. Mental changes	Usually good	Usually present
Variable features		
1. Appetite	Usually good	Usually poor
2. Diarrhea	Often (past or present)	Often (past or present)
3. Skin changes	Usually none	Often, diffuse, dyspigmentation often sparse
4. Hair changes	Texture may be modified	Straight and silky, dyspigmentation, grayish, or reddish
5. Moonface	None	Often
6. Hepatitic enlargement	None	Frequent

- Measures to improve family diets
- Nutritional education-promotion of correct feeding practices
- Home economics
- Family planning and spacing of birth
- Family environment.

(b) Specific protection
- The child's diet must contain proteins and energy-rich foods e.g. milk, eggs, etc.
- Immunization
- Food fortification.

(c) Early diagnosis and treatment
- Periodic surveillance
- Early diagnosis of any lag in growth
- Early diagnosis and treatment of infections and diarrhea
- Development of program for early dehydration of children with diarrhea
- Development of supplementary feeding programs during epidemic
- Deworming of heavily infested children.

(d) Rehabilitation
- Nutritional rehabilitation services
- Hospital treatment
- Follow-up care.

By keeping these above preventive points in mind, the community health nurse has to take certain measures to make:

- Provision of sufficient whole or skimmed milk to expectant and nursing mothers; eggs and fish, etc. with the help of team members
- Supply of animal proteins to be increased by development of milk producing livestock and fishery in coordination with related sectors
- Provision and intake of mixtures of adequate vegetable protein especially such as pulses, nuts, beans, and green vegetables, through nutrition education, and counseling
- Supplementary feeding of infants and young children with good quality of proteins as *Balahar* and groundnut flour, a cheap food proteins. Blackgram flour should be mixed with wheat four
- Provision to treat malnutrition with Hyderabad mixture that is formulated by National Institute of Nutritions, Hyderabad:

Whole wheat (roasted)	—	40 gm
Bengal gram	—	16 gm
Groundnut	—	10 gm
Jaggery	—	20 gm
Total	**—**	**86 gm**

Which yields energy of 330 Kcal and has 11.3 grams of protein. Many children with PEM have been treated with this mixture; they were cured of PEM within 3 months.

Fats

Fats are concentrated resources of energy. The term 'lipid' is also used for fats. Lipid is a comprehensive term applied to compounds that are insoluble in water but soluble in organic solvents (for example, ethanol, ether, benzene and acetone). Lipids include fats that are solid at room temperature and oils that are liquid at room temperature. Lipids are composed of carbon, hydrogen, and oxygen, but the proportion of each element differs from that of carbohydrate.

Lipids are classified as simple, compound and derived:
1. *Simple lipids*—such as monoglycerides, diglycerides, and triglycerides are combination of glycerol and fatty acids. Monoglyceride contains one fatty acid, diglycerides contain two, and a triglycerids contains three.
2. *Compound lipids*—are simple lipids combined with a non-lipid substance, such as carbohydrate in glycolipids, phosphorous in phospholipids, and proteins in lipoproteins.
3. *Derived lipids*—such as cholesterol, steroid hormones and fat soluble vitamins, are produced during the crackdown of simple of compound lipids.

Functions

1. Fat is a concentrated source of energy.
2. It is vehicle of fat soluble vitamins such as A, D, E, K, etc.
3. Fats are sources of essential fatty acids.
4. Excess fat is stored as fat depot in the body. Fat not used by the body is stored by adipose tissue.

Fat is a concentrated source of energy and it supplied per unit weight more than double the energy furnished by either protein or carbohydrate. One gram of fat yields 9.3 calories of energy (and as such it reduces the bulk of diet). Fats and oils are changed to fatty acids and glycerol in the digestive tract. These simpler substances pass through the interstitial wall to be used as fuel to be stored in body fat or to be changed into carbohydrate and stored as glycogen. Stored fat has value in addition to its availability in fuel. It is stored just below the skin and serves as insulation against cold as well as contributing to the smoothness of the skin itself. It also helps to round off the angular contours of the body. Some of the stored fat is packed around the vital organs such as the kidney and heart. The fat layer around the skin prevents excessive heat loss and keeps the body warm. The padding around the vital organs protects them from the damage or injury.

As already stated, the fats are the sources of fatty acids. Fatty acids can be saturated, unsaturated or polysaturated. A saturated fatty acid contains as much hydrogen as it can hold. An unsaturated fatty acid can take up another hydrogen atom, and a polyunsaturated fatty acid can take up many more hydrogen atoms. Unsaturated and polyunsaturated fatty acids are oils. They have a low melting point and are liquid at room temperature. Hydrogenation is the process by which these oils are made solid by the addition of hydrogen. The addition of hydrogen also makes them more saturated. Ingestion of saturated fatty acids appears to increase blood cholesterol levels. Ingestion of unsaturated fatty acids has a minimal effect on blood cholesterol and poly-unsaturated fatty acids appear to lower blood cholesterol levels.

Fatty acids are usually not purely saturated, unsaturated or polyunsaturated. Most animal fats have high proportions of saturated fatty acids. Most vegetable fats have higher amounts of unsaturated and polyunsaturated fatty acids, that are called as "essential fatty acids (EFA), e.g. linoleic, linolenic and arachidonic acids. Usually essential fatty acids found in vegetable oils such as soybean, corn, cottonseed, and peanut, groundnut oils.

Sources of Fats:

Animal source: It includes butter, ghee, cheese, lard (pigs fat) and fish oils. Animal fats are poor sources of EFA with exceptions of marine fish oil such as cod liver oil and sardine oil but they are good sources of retinol and cholicalciferol, which all lack in vegetable oils.

Vegetable source: They include various edible oils, such as ground nut, gingerly, mustard, sesame (til), palm oil, sunflower oil, rapeseed oil and coconut oil, etc. Mostly all vegetable oils (except coconut oil) are rich sources of essential fatty acids.

Deficiency Diseases of Fat: The deficiency of essential fatty acids leads to phrynoderma. Excessive fatty acids in the body leads to increased blood cholesterol levels which are associated with atherosclerosis, cardiovascular accident (stroke) or coronary occlusion.

Daily requirement: It is suggested that 10 to 20 gram of fat per day, depending upon the level of calories consumed, i.e. 20 percent of the total energy (ICMR 1976).

Carbohydrates

Carbohydrates are the main sources of energy composed of carbon, hydrogen and oxygen. The ratio of hydrogen to oxygen is the same as in water, i.e. two hydrogen ions for every oxygen ion. One gram of carbohydrate yields energy of 4.1 calories. Ninety percent of calorie requirement is supplied by carbohydrates. In balanced diet, not more than 60 percent or less than 50 percent of the total calorie requirements should be obtained from carbohydrated food.

Functions of Carbohydrates

- It is the chief and cheap source of energy.
- It is essential for combustion of fat as fat burns in the flame of carbohydrate.

Sources of Carbohydrate

Starches These are present in abundance in cereals and millets, e.g. wheat, rice, millet, soji, maize, etc.

Sugars

There are following types of sugars:
1. Monosaccharides, e.g. glucose, galactose, and fructose and found in grapes, sugar, honey and fruits.
2. Disaccharides, e.g. sucrose, lactose and maltose are found in starches, dextrin, and cellulose.

Daily Requirement

The optimum quantity of carbohydrate in balanced diet is placed between 50 to 70 percent of total energy intake. Most Indian diets contain excessive amount of carbohydrate, providing as much as 90 percent of total energy intake. The carbohydrate reserve of a human adult is only about 500 gm, when man is fasting, this reserve is rapidly exhausted.

Deficiency of Carbohydrate

Carbohydrates are necessary to prevent excessive breakdown of fats and proteins. If there is not much enough carbohydrates available, incompletely oxidized ketonecides will collect in the blood resulting in ketosis. A wide range of diseased conditions are now being thought to be related to fiber deficiency such as constipation, colonic cancer, atherosclerosis, coronary artery disease, appendicitis and gallstones.

Water

Water is the most important nutrient because the function of cells depend on a fluid environment. Water composes 60 percent to 70 percent of total body weight. Lean people's body contains more water than obese people's bodies. Infants have the greatest percentage of total body weight as water and older people have the least. As a result, they are most vulnerable to water deprivation or loss. Yet, no one when deprived of water, can survive more than a few hours in a desert or few days in the most protective environment. The ranges of *daily fluid requirements* for different ages (Behrman *et al* 1987)* is enlisted in Table 15.3.

Fluid needs are met by consumption of liquids and solid foods such as fresh fruits and vegetables, and water is produced when foot is oxidized during digestion. In healthy individual the fluid intake from all sources equals the fluid output through elimination, respiration, and sweating. An ill person can have an increased need for fluid (e.g. fever). An ill person can also have a decreased need for fluid (e.g. cardio-pulmonary or renal disease).

Vitamins

Vitamins are complex chemical substances required by the body in very small quantities. They are present in minute amounts in food, that are essential to normal metabolism. They do not yield energy and act as a catalyst in various body processes. Since it cannot be manufactured in the body insufficient quantity they have to be supplemented by diet. Although they are contained in many foods vitamins are affected by processing, storage and preparation. Usually vitamin content is highest in fresh foods that are used quickly after minimal exposure to heat air or water.

<table>
<tr><td colspan="2">Table 15.3: Daily Fluid Requirements According to Age</td></tr>
<tr><td>Age</td><td>Fluid requirement (ml/kg/day)</td></tr>
<tr><td>3 days</td><td>80-100</td></tr>
<tr><td>10 days</td><td>125-150</td></tr>
<tr><td>3 months</td><td>140-160</td></tr>
<tr><td>6 months</td><td>130-155</td></tr>
<tr><td>9 months</td><td>125-145</td></tr>
<tr><td>1 year</td><td>120-135</td></tr>
<tr><td>2 years</td><td>115-125</td></tr>
<tr><td>4 years</td><td>100-110</td></tr>
<tr><td>6 years</td><td>100-110</td></tr>
<tr><td>10 years</td><td>90-100</td></tr>
<tr><td>14 years</td><td>50-60</td></tr>
<tr><td>18 years</td><td>40-50</td></tr>
<tr><td>10 to 50 years</td><td>50</td></tr>
</table>

Classification of Vitamins

Vitamins are classified as water soluble vitamins and fat soluble vitamins (Fig. 15.4).

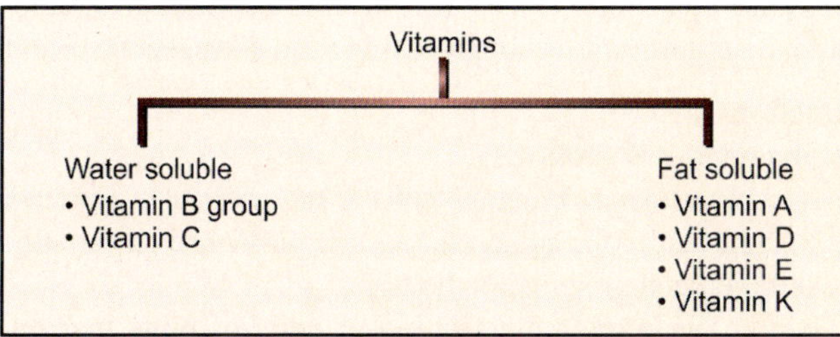

Figure 15.4: Classification of vitamins

As each vitamin has a specific function in the body, minimum intake of many vitamins has been determined but optimum remain speculative.

Water soluble vitamins: The water soluble vitamins are vitamin C and vitamin B complex, which consist of eight different vitamins. Water soluble vitamins cannot be stored in the body and must be provided in the daily food intake. These vitamins are chemically used as catalysts in biochemical reactions. When there is enough of any specific vitamin to meet the catalytic demands, the rest of the vitamin supply acts as a free chemical and may be toxic to the body.

1. Vitamin C ($H_6H_8O_6$)

Vitamin C is an antiscorbutic factor also called ascorbic acid, which is a white crystalline substance, a highly soluble in water but rapidly destroyed in oxidation and high temperature such as those involved in cooking.

Functions

Its functions are as follows:

- It aids utilization of iron, forms cement that holds cells together, strengthens the blood vessels promotes healing, increases resistance to infection.
- It helps in production of collagen; integrity of capillary walls; formations of red blood cells; metabolism of amino acids, reduction of iron salts; protection of other vitamins from oxidations.
- To sum up, vitamin C has enzymatic act, so it is a metabolite of connective tissue. It assists in wound healing, it mitigates infection and stress and arrests bleeding. It acts as a cementing material between endothelial cells of the blood vessels and maintains cohesion and integrity.

Sources: Amla, rose, roots and tubers, citrus fruits like lemon and orange, guava, papaya and green leafy vegetable, straw berries, potatoes, cabbages, tomatoes, cantaloupe, green peppers, broccoli.

Daily requirements: The daily requirement of an Indian is as follows:

1. Adults   –   50 mg daily
2. Pregnancy –   50 mg daily
3. Lactation –   50 + 30 mg daily
4. Infants   –   30 mg daily

Deficiency of vitamin C: It leads to scurvy, poor wound healing, bleeding gums and mucus membrane, minor hemorrhage, bruising loose teeth and the effects of excessive intake may lead to kidney stones, scurvy on withdrawal, and urinary tract infections.

2. Vitamin B Complex

(i) Vitamin B_1 or Thiamine ($C_{12}H_{18}N_4O_2Cl_2$)

Thiamine is relatively stable to heat in the dry form but it is otherwise liable to oxidation and is rapidly destroyed in neutral or alkaline solution.

Functions

Its functions are as follows:

- It acts as a coenzyme in carbohydrate metabolism, promotes normal appetite, functions of heart, nerves and muscles.
- As a component of enzyme helps in carbohydrate oxidation; oxidation conversion of pyruvic acid and citric acid cycle. Its deficiency leads to pyruvic acid or lactic acid accumulation in blood.

So, vitamin B_1 is essential for proper functioning of nervous system and also helps in maintaining good appetite and normal digestion.

Sources: Whole grains, unmilled cereal, wheat germ, pulses, milk, nuts, meat, lentils, potatoes, pork, fish, eggs, poultry, dried beans, green peas and beans, green leafy vegetables.

Daily requirement: The daily requirement of vitamin B_1 is 5 mg for 1000 calories.

Deficiencies: Thiamine deficiency leads to beriberi, mental confusion, muscular weakness, calf tenderness, loss of deep jerks, ataxia, muscle pain, heart disorders, cardiac rhythmic disturbances, cardiac enlargement, depression, irritability, Wrenick-Karskoffs syndrome, etc. The excessive thiamine may lead to rapid pulse, headaches, weakness, irritability, insomnia.

(ii) Vitamin B_2 ($C_{17}H_{20}N_4O_6$)

It is also called as riboflavin or lactoflavin. It is a yellow crystalline substance.

Functions

It acts as a coenzyme in proteins and energy metabolism; promotes healthy skin and eyes.

In brief it helps the metabolism of nutrients; essential for growth; and involving in oxidation and reduction of fats, carbohydrate, and proteins.

Sources: Whole grain, eggs, milk and milk products, liver, fish, eggs, cereals, green leafy vegetables.

Daily requirement: The recommended daily allowance is 0.6 mg/1000 Kcal.

Deficiency of riboflavin: It includes, eye symptoms, redness and burning sensation of eye, frontal headache, sore dry skin, i.e., ariboflavinosis–cracks at mouth corners, scaly desquamation of skin around mouth, eye irritation, glossitis, (shiny red and sore tongue), photophobia (light sensibility) soreness of lips, cheilosis, greasy skin around angle of nose, scrotal dermatitis.

The effects of excessive riboflavin includes ulcer, elevated blood glucose level, increased uric acid levels in blood.

(iii) Niacin ($C_6H_6O_2N$)

It is also called nicotinic acid, required by body for utilization of carbohydrates. It is necessary to normal cell respiration and to maintain health of epithelial and nervous tissue. Amino acid, tryptophan, is converted into niacin in the body. Sixty milligram of tryptophan yields 1 gram of niacin.

Functions

Niacin's functions are as follow:
- Niacin acts as coenzyme in energy productions, promotes healthy skin, gastro-intestinal and nervous system functions
- It helps in protein utilization, glycolysis, fat synthesis and tissue repair.

Sources: Meats, liver, fish, eggs. Whole grains, legumes, dairy products cereals, tuna. Maize is low in tryptophane. Jowar contains excessive leucine.

Daily requirement: The recommended daily allowance is 6.6 mgm/1000 calories.

Deficiency: Its deficiency leads to pellagra, soreness of tongue, loss of appetite, lethargy and diarrhea, dementia, depression.

Those who are on isoniazid drugs (TB) leads to deficiency of niacin.

The effects of excess of niacin leads to ulcer, liver: dysfunction, elevated blood glucose level, increased blood, uric acid levels, diarrhea, nausea, flushing.

(iv) Vitamin B_6

Vitamin B_6 occurs in three forms. Pyridoxine, pyridoxal, and pyridoxamine.

Functions

Its functions are as follows:
- It is important as protein metabolism, hemoglobin synthesis, integrity of central nervous system.
- In metabolism, it helps in synthesis of nonessential amino acids and conversion of tryptophan to niacin, and helps to proper function of blood and central nervous system.

Sources: Meat, seeds, whole grain, potatoes, bananas, green leafy vegetables, liver, fish, poultry, green beans, nuts.

Daily requirements: The recommended daily allowance of vitamin B_6 is 0.2 to 0.3 mg daily.

Deficiency of vitamin: B_6 Its deficiency leads to cheilosis, anemia, irritability, skin lesions, crack at corner of mouth, CNS disturbances.

The effects of excessive vitamin B_6 leads to bloating, depressions, fatigue, headache, nerve damage, irritability.

(v) Vitamin B_{12}

Vitamin B_{12} is also called as cyanocobalamine, is a red crystalline substance containing cobalt. It is synthesized in human colon but in bound form. It is not present in food of vegetable origin.

Functions

Its functions are as follows:
- It manufactures enzymes essential to metabolism of nutrients. Nucleic acid, folic acid, has got some influence on carbohydrate, fat and protein metabolism.
- It helps in proper functioning of cells of bone marrow, essential for red blood cell and maturation.
- It is important for function of all body cells which include gastrointestinal and nervous system.
- It helps in formation of purines and thus RNA and DNA. It is essential for synthesis of DNA.

Sources: Milk, egg, cheese, meat, fish, poultry, foods of animal origin. Plant food contains no vitamin B_{12}.

Daily requirements: The recommended daily allowance of vitamin B_{12} is as follows:
- Adult—2 micrograms daily
- Pregnancy—2 micrograms daily
- Lactation—2.5 micrograms daily.

Deficiency of vitamin B_{12}: Its deficiency leads to the following:
- Megaloblastic anemia, infertility, and sterility
- Pernicious anemia
- Neurological disorder, i.e. demyelinating neurologicalleisons.

(vi) Folates

Folic acid occurs in food in two forms, i.e. (a) free folates, and (b) the bound folates and also called as folacin, folic acid, folate.

Functions: All these helps in metabolism of some amino acids, maturation of red blood cells and synthesis of purines and pyrimidines, which are necessary for RNA and DNA.

Sources: Liver, green leafy vegetables, meat, fish, poultry, whole grains.

Daily requirement: Recommended daily allowance of folates is as follows:

- Healthy adults—100 micrograms daily
- Pregnancy—300 micrograms daily
- Lactation—150 micrograms daily
- Children—100 micrograms daily

Deficiency of folates: It leads to macrocytic anemia. The excess or folates also leads to diarrhea, insomnia, irritability, masking of vitamin B_{12} deficiency.

(vii) Pantothenic acid

Pantothenic acid is member of vitamin B complex group. It helps in metabolism of nutrients, synthesis of cholesterol and steroid hormones, activity of adrenal cortex.

Sources: It is widely distributed in animal and vegetable foods, i.e. meats, whole grains, cereals, legumes.

Daily requirements: It is considered 10 mgm will satisfy the daily need.

Deficiency: No deficiency symptoms have been reported in human beings.

The effect of excessive pantothenic acid leads to increased need to thiamine, occasionally diarrhea and water retention.

(viii) Biotin

Biotin also considered a B complex groups. It helps in synthesis of fatty acids, utilization of glucose, metabolism of proteins, and utilization of vitamin B_{12} and folic acid.

Its effects of deficiency and effects of excess if not yet known.

Sources: Liver, kidneys, dark green vegetables, egg yolk, green beans.

Fat Soluble Vitamins

The fat soluble vitamins, e.g. A, D, E, K can be stored in the body, and therefore, their daily intake is not needed. However, with the exception of vitamin D, these vitamins should be provided through dietary intake. Some fat soluble vitamins lead to toxicity. Toxicity usually is the result of megadoses of synthetic vitamins and large intake of fish liver. The processing, storage and preparation of food have less effect on fat soluble vitamins.

Now we will examine the fat soluble vitamin.

(i) Vitamin A ($C_{20}H_{20}OH$)

Vitamin A is a fat soluble vitamin and has little loss during cooking but presence of acid it becomes rancid. No loss during canning and processing. The vitamin is also referred as retinol, retinal and retinoic acid.

Functions

It helps in the following:

- Growth and maintenance of epithelial tissue – assists formation and maintenance of skin and mucus membrane, thus increasing resistance to infections
- Maintenance of visual acuity (in dim light), formations of visual purple and promotes health of eye tissue and eye adaptation of dim light
- Promotion of bone growth
- It has got immune function especially antigen recognition.

Sources: Whole milk, whole milk product, eggs, green leafy vegetables, yellow fruits, and vegetables, i.e. spinach, cabbage, carrot, amaranth, fish liver oils, (codliver oil), liver, halibut liver oil, synthetic from Indian lemon grass.

Daily requirement: 500 units of carotene daily for adult. 3000 IU or 1 mgm of vitamin A is needed daily.

Deficiency of vitamin A: It deficiency leads to night blindness, xerophthalmia, Bitot's spots, (triangular, foamy, rough and raised patches seen on the bulbar conjunctiva), keratomalacia (softening of entire thickness of cornea), rough scaly skin, dry mucus membrane, decreased resistance to infection, faulty tooth and bone development.

The effects of excessive of vitamin A leads to nausea, vomiting, abdominal pain and growth failure in children, weight loss in adults. Megadoses of vitamin A leads to hair loss, bone swelling and tenderness, joint pain, hepatomegaly, splenomegaly, headache.

(ii) Vitamin D ($C_{28}H_{44}C_4$) (Inviosterol)

Vitamin D is not a single substance. They are closely related compounds. For human nutrition point of view, cholecalciferol and ergosterol are important. Calcifer is a antirachitic factor. Cholecalciferol naturally occurs in vitamin called vitamin D_3. It occurs in animal fat and fish liver oil. Ergocalciferol does not occur in nature. it is vegetable sterol, ultraviolet rays.

Functions

- It promotes absorption and utilization of calcium and phosphorous in bone and tooth development.
- It has direct action on mineralizations of bones and teeth.

Sources: Exposure to sunlight, fortified milk, fistofortified margarines, fish liver oils.

Daily requirement: The recommended daily allowance is 100 IU (2.5 microgram) for adults and 400 IU during pregnancy.

Deficiency of vitamin D: Its deficiency leads to the following:

- Rickets and delayed dentition in children.
- Osteomalacia (softening of bones) in adults.
- The deficiency is more common in pregnant and lactating mothers.

The megadoses of vitamin D leads to loss of appetite, vomiting, growth failure, weight loss, increased calcium deposit in soft tissue, blood vessels, and kidneys, polyurea drowsiness.

(iii) Vitamin E (Tocopherol)

Vitamin E is an anti sterility factor, and antioxidance, chemically identified as tocopherol.

Functions

- It acts as an antioxidant, and protects vitamin A and unsaturated fatty acids, integrity of normal cell membrane from oxidation and synthesis.
- It is important for wound healing and immune system of health.

Sources: Vegetable oils, green leafy vegetables, milk, eggs, meats, cereals, nuts, wheatgerm oil.

Daily requirement: A current estimate of vitamin E requirement is 15 IU per day for normal adult.

Deficiency of vitamin E: It deficiency is associated with habitual abortions and testicular degeneration in laboratory animals. The effects of deficiency also leads to increased hemolysis of red blood cells and macrocytic anemia in premature infants.

The effects of excessive of vitamin E doses leads to interference with utilization of vitamins A and K prolonged prothrombin time, intestinal irritability, headache, fatigue, dizziness.

(iv) Vitamin K

It is also a fat soluble vitamin.

Function

The main function of vitamin K is prothrombin formation in the liver during coagulation of blood or clotting.

Sources: Vitamin K is found in fresh green leafy vegetables, (liver synthesis in gastrointestinal tract) lettuce, cabbage, egg yolk soybean oil, liver.

Daily requirements: The adult requirement is unknown. For premature baby, 0.5 to 1 mgm intramusculary or 1-2 morally.

Deficiency of vitamin K: Its deficiency leads to generalized bleeding, hemorrhagic diseases of the newborn, prolonged clotting time in adults.

The excessive doses, of vitamin K leads to hyperbilirubinemia in infants, vomiting in adults.

Minerals

Minerals are inorganic elements, essential to the body because of their role as catalysts in biochemical reaction.

- The body contains more than 19 minerals all of which must be derived from foods. A well-balanced diet will supply a sufficient quantity of minerals. Human beings needs mineral because: They maintain osmotic pressure.
- They supply necessary electrolytes for the action of muscles and nerves.
- They are present in all enzymic systems.

- They have specific action such as iron for blood formation, etc.
- They are required in small quantities.

Classification of Mineral

Minerals are classified as macrominerals when the daily requirement' is 100 mg or more and micro minerals, when less then 100 mg is needed daily (Fig. 15.5).

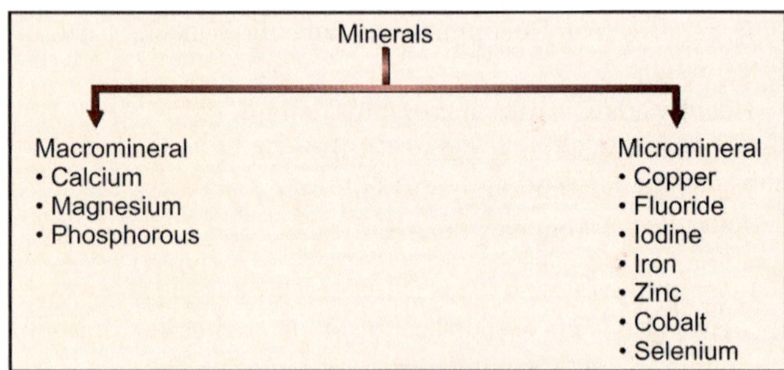

Figure 15.5: Classification of minerals

1. Calcium

Calcium is a major mineral element in the body. The body of a men contains two percent of calcium. At birth, child contains about 25 to 35 gm of calcium, whereas in adults it may come to about 850 to 1400 gram. Ninety percent of the calcium is found in bone and 10-11 mg of calcium found in 100 cc of blood.

Functions

It with other minerals (Phosphorous) within protein framework to give strength and structure to bones and teeth. It helps in formation of teeth and bones. It helps also in the following:

- Contractions of muscles and rigidity to skeletal structures
- Transmission of nerve impulses
- Activation of enzymes
- Permeability of cell membrane
- Coagulation of blood
- Cardiac functions.

Sources: Calcium is found in milk, milk products, leafy vegetables, fish with bones, vegetable greens, small edible bones.

Daily requirement: The recommended daily allowance for adults 600 to 800 mg/ day, 1500 mg/ day for pregnant and lactating mothers, 100 mg/ day for children.

Deficiency of calcium: Its deficiency includes tingling of fingers, and area around mouth, muscle cramps, carpopedas (thumb or toe) spasm, tetany, convulsions, pathological fractures, stunted growth in children, bone loss in adults, hypertension, tremors.

The excessive effects of calcium include relaxed skeletal muscles, cardiac irregularities and hypercalcemia.

2. Phosphorous

Phosphorous is also an important mineral required for the body. It is widely distributed in food.

Function

It helps in the following:
- Formation of bone and teeth
- Activation of 'B' vitamins
- Transfer of energy in cells
- Promotion of muscles and nerve activity
- Metabolism of carbohydrates
- Regulation of acid-base balance
- Transmission of hereditary traits.

Sources: It is found in pork, beef, dried peas and beans, milk and milk products.

Daily requirements: The recommended daily allowance of phosphorous is 1-2 grams daily. *Deficiency of phosphorous.* Its deficiency includes hemolytic anemia, defective white blood cell function, delayed clotting, bone pain, pathological fractures.

The excessive dose of phosphorous will lead to erosion of jaw and calcium loss.

3. Magnesium

Magnesium is the macro mineral, which supports the function of the 'B' vitamins.

Function

It helps in utilization of calcium, potassium, protein and maintenance of electrical activity in nerves and muscles.

Sources: Whole grains, nuts, legumes, green vegetables.

Daily requirement: It is estimated to be 200-300 mg/ day for adults.

Deficiency of magnesium: It will lead to neuromuscular irritability, confusion, hallucinations, and growth failure. The excessive dose of magnesium leads to lethargy and diarrhea.

4. Copper

It is a trace element and helps in the following:
- Formation of hemoglobin
- Synthesis of phospholipids
- Formation and activity of some enzymes, etc.
- Synthesis of prostaglandin.

Sources: Liver, kidney, shellfish, nuts, raisins.

Deficiency of copper: It leads to abnormal blood cell development in infants, bone demineralization. The effects of excessive consumption of copper leads to headache, dizziness, heartburn, weakness, nausea, vomiting, diarrhea, Wilson's disease.

5. Iron

An average man contains about 4.5 gram of iron. Blood contains 40-50 mg per 100 cc. It is absorbed in ferrous form, passes through intestinal mucosa cells, delivered to transferrin in the plasma. This transferrin transfers it to all body sites especially bone marrow.

Function

It helps in the following processes:
- Formation of hemoglobin, combines with protein to form hemoglobin, which carries oxygen in blood, increases resistance to infection, functions as a part of enzymes involved in tissue respiration
- Synthesis of vitamins, purines, and antibodies.

Sources: Iron is found in liver, lean meats, meat, whole grains, enriched breads, and cereals, dried beans, and peas, dark green leafy vegetables.

Daily requirements: The recommended daily allowance for men is 0.20 mg per day and women due to menses, pregnancy and lactation, require double of this dose approximately.

Deficiency of iron: It leads to lowered resistance to infection, anaemia, fatigue, weakness, lethargy.

The excessive intake of iron may lead to hemosiderosis, hemochromatosis, (Bronze coloration), liver damage, cramps, abdominal pain, nausea, vomiting, black stools, cirrhosis.

6. Iodine

Iodine exists in thyroxine in thyroid gland which helps in oxidation process of the body, i.e. it is a basic component of thyroid hormone.

Sources: We can get iodine from iodized salt, seafood, food additives, dough oxidizers, dairy disinfectants, coloring agents and national food and water. Richest sources are crude common salt prepared from sea water, seafish and codliver oil.

Daily requirement of iodine: It will be 0.2 gram daily.

Deficiency of iodine: It leads to cretinism in infants, depressed thyroid activity. The excessive dose of iodine leads to toxic goiter.

7. Fluorine

Fluorine is one of the most active element of the halogen group. It is never found in nature. About 96 percent of fluorine is found in bones and teeth. It is essential for normal mineralization of bones and formation of dental enamel.

Function

It helps in formation of teeth and prevention of dental caries. The mottling of teeth occurs in fluorine contents in food and drink in about 2 PPM (part per million). It is called dental fluorosis. If content is below 0.2 PPM caries occurs. Defluoridation is done by adding lime and alum in well water. Dental caries is prevented by fluoridation of community water supply.

8. Chlorine

Chlorine is necessary to maintain the composition of blood and formation of hydrochloric acid. The sources of chlorine are tomatoes, bananas, and green leafy vegetables.

9. Zinc

Zinc is a constituent of crystalline insulin found in pancreas. It is required for the following:

- Connective tissue integrity
- Immune response
- Formation of enzymes and insulin
- Protein synthesis.

The sources of zinc includes oysters, liver, meats, poultry, legumes, nuts, etc.

Deficiency of zinc: It leads to impaired wound healing, decreased sensation of taste and smell, skin lesions, delayed growth. The excessive dose of zinc leads to anemia, fever, nausea, vomiting, diarrhea, muscle pain and weakness, decreased calcium absorption.

10. Cobalt

Cobalt is an essential molecule of vitamin B_{12}. It is suggested that it is necessary for the first stage of hormone production, i.e. capture of iodine by the gland. Cobalt may interact with iodine and affects its utilization.

11. Selenium

Selenium when given to child suffering from kwashiorkor increases the weight of the child. Studies indicate that human selenium deficiency may occur in PEM.

12. Potassium

Potassium occurs widely in foodstuffs. The adult human body consists of about 250 gram of potassium. It exerts an influence on the excitation of nerve tissue and contractibility of all types of muscles. The sources of potassium are brain, cereal, milk, fish, and meat. The daily requirement will be 3-4 grams. The deficiency of potassium leads to disorders of kidney.

13. Sodium

Sodium is found in all body fluids. The adult human body contains about 100 grams of sodium ion. It is mainly used in food as salt (NaCl). It is also present in the bile and gastric juice.

It is essential for maintenance of pH concentration and osmotic pressure of blood and other tissue maintenance. The daily requirement is 10 to 15 gm.

Deficiency of sodium leads to marked general weakness, cramps, dyspnea in exertion and heat exhaustion.

14. Chromium

It plays a role in relation to carbohydrate and insulin function.

15. Molybdenum

Excess of molybdenum leads to bony deformities and deficiency associated with mouth and esophagus cancer.

Malnutrition

Malnutrition implies the result of imperfect assimilation nutrition or both. It has been defined as a pathological state resulting from a relative or absolute deficiency or excess of one or more essential nutrients.

Malnutrition may be in the following forms:

Undernutrition: It is due to insufficient food eaten over an extended period of time due to poverty or ignorance.

Overnutrition: It is due to consumption of excessive quantity of food over an extended period of time leads to high sickness rate mortality rate.

Imbalance: It is due to imbalance such as quantitative imbalance of calcium, phosphorus and vitamin D.

Specific deficiency: It is due to specific deficiency such as goiter in iodine deficiency.

Malnutrition is a condition that is most prevalent in our country. It is more common among children, pregnant ladies and nursing mothers. Its effects are kwashiorkor, marasmus, xerophthalmia, beriberi, pellagra, goiter, rickets, etc. This malnutrition condition predisposes to diseases like tuberculosis, diarrhea, parasitic infestation, leads to high sickness rate and increased infant mortality rate.

Causes for Malnutrition

Population growth: The rapid growth of population leads to gap between food consumption which causes malnutrition.

Agriculture and food production: In India food production depends upon nature. There is no proper adequate source of timely irrigation. Farmers have to depend on natural rainfall, which is unpredictable. At one time unprecedented drought is followed by flood at another time. Fragmentation of land and bad socioeconomic conditions are also responsible.

Prevalence of parasitic and infectious diseases: These diseases responsible for decreased intestinal absorption and lack of proper work which is important for poor and inadequate diet.

Religious and cultural food fads: These prevent the people from using the locally available nutritious food. Cooking methods also differ according to tradition.

General illiteracy and ignorance: About the importance of balanced diet and poverty.

Economic barrier: It is also resulted in malnutrition among the children of the nation.

Preventive Measures of Malnutrition

1. Increased food production by scientific cultivation.
2. Vulnerable group, i.e., infants, preschool children, expectant and lactating mothers should be protected by best utilization of locally available food substitution, midday meal, cheap supplementary food, etc.
3. Fortification of *atta* (flour) with protein and calcium or milk should be fortified with vitamin A and vitamin D.
4. Improvement of environmental sanitation is necessary to prevent the parasitic infections.

5. Projects and programs in the field of food and nutrition including nutrition education should receive high priority.
6. Applied nutrition program should be extended to all the affected areas and it should run sincerely and should be beneficial to vulnerable groups.
7. Prevention of unnecessary loss of food in the fields, store, transport and cooking is necessary.
8. Education of public on fundamentals of diet and nutrition and help from voluntary and international organization are necessary.

Malnutrition is a disease of society, poverty and ignorance. In this, everyone, i.e. teacher, nurse, physician, farmer and all organizations have to contribute much to combat this malnutrition. The steps have already taken by the government of India to tackle the problem.

Role or Nurses in Nutritional Assessment and Nutrition Education

Nurses are concerned about the nutritional status of all their clients. All people eat to stay alive, and what is eaten affects health from conception to old age. Throughout the world, chronic malnutrition affects physical and mental development. In industrialized societies, diet-related conditions are among the leading causes of disease and death. Many diet-related diseases result from nutritional excess rather than undernourishment. For example, coronary heart disease is linked with excessive intake of saturated fats and cholesterol; cancer is linked to high-fat, low fiber diet, and alcohol consumption; hypertension, a risk factor for strokes is associated with intakes of excessive calories and salt; liver diseases is associated with heavy alcohol consumption; and diabetes mellitus is associated with excessive calorie intake and subsequent obesity.

Community health nurses are often the contact community residents have with the health care system. Because of frequent and extended contact with clients in the community, nurses have excellent opportunities to provide information and counseling about the role of nutrition in health promotion and prevention of illness.

The role of the nurse has changed with the current preventive health care focus and emphasis upon wellness and with the expanding responsibilities that nurses are assuming in their care of clients in hospital as well as in primary health care facilities. The nurse must assume an epidemiologic approach when taking nutritional histories and developing care plans for clients with nutritional inadequacies. Nutritional problems are usually the result of multiple factors. All clients (hosts) have a genetic care and this together with the influence of past life experiences, may make them more susceptible to problems. The environment made up of social, physical and biological factors, in influenced by the host and likewise contribute to nutritional problems. To sum up the factors influencing on nutrition, i.e. biological, psychological sociocultural, and environment factors were discussed briefly as follows:

Biological Factors

The human body requires certain nutrients to maintain health. The nutrients are needed for growth, development and repair of body structures, and maintenance of body processes. Level of activity and stress, age and rate of growth, genetics and variety of factors such as temperature, taste, and smell affect intake of food. In addition, medications, tobacco, alcohol and caffeine affect absorption of vitamins and minerals.

Sociocultural Factors

The cultural and ethnic background of clients plays a major role in food selection and eating behaviors. Many cultural practices have evolved because they are healthful recognition of and respect for these food preferences are important for nurses counseling clients in the community.

Psychological Factor

Eating behavior is affected both by positive emotions, such as enjoyment and tranquility, and negative feelings like anger and insecurity. Food may represent rewards, comforts, and security. Some eating habits, self-esteem and knowledge about nutrition are also affecting the foods as person selects.

Environmental Factor

Food selection is influenced by many factors like cost, accessibility, convenience, and safety. When counseling the clients on nutritional aspect, the nurse should consider the all these environmental factors. That is, which food contains necessary nutrients which cost low and yield more nutrients; advising to take locally available foodstuffs, which reach the clients easily and which food stuffs, that reach the clients easily and which food stuffs are safe and so on.

With the changing responsibilities, the nurse has to come to assume a major role in health education. Formal nutrition classes and individualized nutritional counseling require the nurse to be skilled in teaching and learning principles as well as to have a strong knowledge of nutrition. The nurse needs to know if the community resources for financial assistance, meal preparation assistance and nutrition classes.

The nurse within any health care setting should assume responsibility for provision of optimal nutrition and nutrition counseling for the clients. Preventive health teaching should be initiated during first visit to clients or client's first visit to the agency. Referral to appropriate community resources helps the client maintain a preventive approach to health care.

Table 15.4: Clinical Signs of Nutritional Status

	Body area	Signs of good nutrition	Signs of poor nutrition
1	General appearance	Alert, responsible	Listless, apathetic, cachetic appearance
2	Weight	Weight normal for height age body build	Obesity or underweight appearance (spl. concern for underweight)
3	Posture	Erect posture, straight arms and legs	Sagging shoulders, sunken chest, humped back
4	Muscles	Well developed firm muscles; good tone; some fat under the skin wasted appearance, inability to walk	Flaccid appearance, poor tone; underdeveloped tone tenderness, edema, properly
5	Skeleton	Lack of malformations	Bowlegs; knock knees; chest deformity; at diaphragm; beaded ribs; prominent scupulac
6	Legs and feet	Lack of tenderness. Weakness of selling good color	Edema, tender calf; tingling, weakness
7	Nerve control	Good attention span; lack of irritability or restlessness; normal reflexes; psychological stability	In attention; irritability; confusion; burning and tingling of hand and feet; (paresthesia); loss of position and vibratory sense, weakness and tenderness of muscles (may result in inability to walk); decrease or loss of ankle and knee reflexes; absent vibratory sense
8	GI function	Good appetite and digestion; normal regular elimination; no palpable organs or mass	Anorexia; indigestion; constipation or diarrhea liver or spleen enlargement
9	Cardiovascular functions	Normal heart rate and rhythm; lack of murmurs; normal blood pressure for age	Rapid heart rate, enlarged heart, abnormal rhythm; elevated blood pressure
10	General vitality	Endurance; energy; good sleep habits vigorous appearance	Ability to be easily fatigued; lack of energy; falling asleep easily, tired and apathetic appearance
11	Hair	Shiny, lustrous appearance; firmness; strands not easily plucked, healthy scalp	Stringy, dull, brittle, dry, thin, and sparse, depigmented appearance, strands that can be easily plucked
12	Nails	Firm, pink appearance	Spoon shape (kiolonychia), brittleness, ridges
13	Face and neck	Uniform color; smooth, pink, healthy appearance, lack of selling	Greasy, discolored, scaly, swollen appearance; dark skin over cheeks and under eyes, lumpiness or flakiness of skin around nose and mouth
14	Neck glands	Lack of enlargement	Thyroid enlargement
15	Legs	Smoothness; good color; moist (not chaffed or swollen appearance)	Dry, scaly, swollen appearance redness and selling (cheilosis) angular lesions at corners of mouth; fissures or scars (stomatitis)
16	Mouth, oral membrane	Reddish, pink mucus membrane in oral cavity	Swollen, boggy, oral mucus membrane
17	Gums	Good pink color; healthy and red appearance; lack of swelling or bleeding	Spongy gums that bleed easily; marginal redness; inflammation; receding gums
18	Tongue	Good pink or deep reddish color; lack of swelling; smoothness, presence of surface paillae; lack of lesions	Swelling; scarlet and raw appearance; magenta color beefiness (glossitis) hyperemic or hypertrophic papillae, atrophic papillae
19	Teeth	Lack of cavities and pain; bright, straight appearance; lack of crowning well-shaped jaw; clean appearance with no discoloration	Unfilled caries; absent teeth; worm surfaces; mottled (fluorosis) malpositioned appearance
20	Eyes	Bright, clear, shiny appearance; lack of sores, at corner of membranes; eyelids; moist and healthy pink color; prominent blood vessels; or lack of mourid of tissue or sclera; lack of fatigue circles beneath eyes	Pale eye membranes, redness of membrane, dryness sign of infection; Bitot's spots; redness and fissuring of eyelid corners (angular palpebritis) dryness of eyes dull appearance of cornea; soft cornea

Nutritional Assessment

Nurses are in an excellent position to recognize signs of poor nutrition and to take effective step to initiate charge. The nutritional assessment consists of nursing and diet history observation (physical anthropometry, and laboratory data). In addition, the assessment is individualized to determine clients at risk for nutritional alteration. The diet history focuses on the clients habitual intake of food and liquids, as well as preferences, allergies, problems and other relevant areas and nurses also should assess the factors influencing on dietary pattern of the client which includes health status, cultural background, religion, socioeconomic status, personal preference, psychological factors, use of alcohol, or drugs and misinformation of beliefs about food values. In addition the community heal the nurses also observes the client for signs of actual or potential nutritional need. The physical examination can enable the nurse to document signs and symptoms of inadequate nutrition as follows (Williams 1989) (Table 15.4).

Anthropometry

Anthropometry is a system of measurement of the body size, and make up of the body and specific body parts. Anthropometric measurements that aid in identifying nutritional problems include weight, height, wrist circumference, mid-upper arm circumference (MUAC) and triceps skin fold (TSF).

Weight: The weight should be taken with minimum clothing and recorded to the nearest quarter kilogram. For taking correct weight, liver balance is good than spring balance.

Height: The height should be taken in a standing position without foot-wear, and is recorded to the nearest half-contractor. For correct measuring by height, steel measuring tape is good.

It is equally important to record the age of the individual correctly for proper interpretation of height and weights. The clients height and weight can be compared to the usual measurement and to standards for normal height-weight relationship.

Wrist circumference: The wrist circumference was used to estimate the client's bodyframe. A tape measure is used to measure the wrist distal to the styloid process. The nurses calculates the frame size (r-value) by dividing wrist circumference into the client's height (cm) wrist circumference. The result is the calculated r-value. Bodyframe normal values include greater than 10.4 to 10.9 cm (small), 10.4 to 9.6 cm (medium), and less than 9.6 cm (large).

Mid-upper arm circumference (MUAC): The MUAC determines muscle wasting. It is a useful indicator of nutritional status of individuals and communities. Accuracy in measuring this is improved by use of an insertion tape. This measurement of mid upper arm circumference is useful for the following:

- Evaluating nutrition status in community health programs
- Nurses with a device for detecting severe under nutrition

- Supplying community leaders and parents with a measure for monitoring the extents of undernutrition in their communities and children. They raises their "level of consciousness" concerning the problem.
- Preparing baseline surveys and periodic surveys of nutritional status of the population served by community health projects
- Selecting malnourished children for feeding program
- Selecting villages which deserve priority for feeding in time of food scarcity
- Monitoring the effect of feeding and nutrition education schemes on individuals and communities.

Technique of Insertion Tape

1. Push up the clothing. Put the tape round the middle of the left arm.
2. Put the end of the tape through the small slot on the wide end of the tape.
3. Pull the tape firmly but not so tightly that it pinches or pulls the skin.
4. Now read the result in centimeters in the windows between the arrows.

Interpretation of MUAC

Arm circumference includes bone, fat the muscle. Muscle and fat, which are the body's protein and energy reserves, are reduced by the body does not absorb or take in enough food, as in PEM.

Arm circumference increases with age, but from the first of fifth birth days, it does not change much. At this time fat is gradually replaced by muscle. Thus when using the tape with this age group, we do not need to know the exact age of the child in order to know the nutritional status.

Triceps Skin Fold (TSF)

Skin fold measurements are used to determine fat content of subcutaneous tissue. TSF is the most common and easiest measure. With the thumb and forefinger, pinch lengthwise a double fold of fat about 1 cm above middle of the MUAC. With the other hand, place the teeth of calipers (skin calipers) on either side of the fat-fold. The average measurement is taken from three readings. Normal values include 12.5 cm (men) and 18.0 cm (women). The other anatomical areas for skin fold measurements include the biceps, scapula and abdominal. The mid -arm muscle circumference (MAMC) is an estimation of skeletal mass. It is calculated from the MUAC and TSF anthropometric measures. The formula is MAMC = MUAC – (TSF × 3.14). The normal values include 25.3 cm (men) or 23.2 cm (women).

A primary nutritional disease occurs when nutrition is the cause of the disease. Usually, there is an inadequate intake of one or more nutrients. Some examples of such diseases are scurvy, from inadequate intake of vitamin C; rickets, from insufficient intake of vitamin D; and anemia, from a deficiency of iron in the diet.

Excesses of nutrients can also cause illness. These, however, occur when nutrient supplements are taken in excess, rather than from food intake. For instance, excess vitamin D may cause nausea, diarrhea, weight loss, and calcification of the renal tubules, blood vessels, and bronchi. Excess niacin may cause flushing, itching, and hypotension.

Most nutritional diseases are secondary diseases; that is, they are a complication of another disease or condition. The original disease or condition interferes with digestion or absorption, or there is an increased need for one or more nutrients. For instance, in pregnancy, the body's need for iron increases. Not receiving the increased amount may cause anemia in the mother. In malabsorption disorders, the body is unable to absorb sufficient amounts of certain nutrients. The amount ingested may be adequate, but the body is unable to use it. Rapid excretion from the body, as in diarrhea, docs not allow the nutrients to be absorbed and utilized. Uncontrolled diarrhea can lead to dehydration along with electrolyte and acid-base imbalance.

Weight Management

Maintaining weight at a desired level can be very difficult for some people. Weight management is based on the relationship between the intake and use of kcal. When these two elements are balanced, weight is maintained at a steady level. A range of 10% over or under the desired weight is considered appropriate.

Determining Caloric Needs: The number of kcal needed to achieve or maintain a desired weight is based on two factors: basal energy needs and total energy requirements.

Basal Energy Needs

Basal energy need refers to the number of kcal required to keep an individual alive when at rest. There are two ways to determine basal energy (kcal) needs. One is based on the person's desired weight (Table 15.5), the other on the person's actual weight.

Table 15.5: Determining Desired Weight		
Build	*Women*	*Men*
Medium	100 Ib for 5 ft of height, plus 5 Ib for each additional inch	106 Ib for 5 ft of height, plus 6 Ib for each additional inch
Small	Subtract 10%	Subtract 10%
Large	Add 10%	Add 10%

Calculation using desired weight is as follows:
Basal energy needs = desired weight × 10

Examples
Female:
    5 ft 5 in tall
    5 ft = 100 Ib

5 in= 25 Ib
        125 Ib desired weight
125 × 10 = 1.250
Basal energy needs = 1,250 kcal

Male:
    5 ft 9 in tall
    5 ft = 106 Ib
    9 in =54 Ib
        160 Ib desired weight
    160 × 10 = 1,600
    Basal energy needs = 1.600 kcal

Calculation using actual weight is as follows:
    Female weight in kg × 0.9 × 24 = basal kcal
    Male weight in kg × 1 × 24 = basal kcal
    (Weight in Ib ÷ 2.2 = weight in kg)

Examples
    Female weighs 130 Ib
    130 ÷ 2.2 = 59.1 kg
    59.1 kg × 0.9 × 24 = 1.276.6
    Basal energy needs = 1,276.6 kcal
    Male weighs 170 Ib
    170 ÷ 2.2 = 77.3 kg
    77.3 kg × 1 × 24 = 1,855.2
    Basal energy needs = 1,855.2 kcal

Total Energy Requirements

People do not live their lives at rest. They are active! Kilocalories must be added to the basal metabolic requirement in order to meet the needs of activity. All activity is not equal in kcal needed, however. A person's overall activity level can be divided into sedentary (light, such as watching television), moderate (such as playing tennis), or strenuous (such as running a marathon). The following formulas can be used to determine the number of kcal to add given the activity level:
Sedimentary: basal kcal × 1.3 = total kcal
Moderate: basal kcal × 1.5 = total kcal
Strenuous: basal kcal × 2.0 = total kcal

Example: The 125-lb woman in the preceding example who is planning on running a marathon would need the following:

    1,250 (basal kcal) × 2 = 2,500 kcal

Factors in addition to activity that have an effect on the total kcal need are state of health and climate. A person who is ill needs more kcal to repair tissue. A cold climate requires a person to take in more kcal to provide more thermal energy to maintain body temperature.

Overweight

A person is considered to be overweight when 11% to 19% above the desired weight. Obesity is considered present in a person who is 20% or more above the desired weight. Overweight conditions can become serious health hazards by placing increased strain on the heart, lungs, muscles, bones, and joints. Overweight and obese people are more susceptible to diabetes and hypertension and tend to have a shorter life span.

Study indicated that obesity is rising in the States. Among children between the ages of 6 and 11 years, 13.7% are overweight; among adolescents ages 12 to 17. 11.5% are overweight. Among adults, 36.4% of men and 33.3% of women are overweight.

Causes: There is no single cause of obesity. Genetic, physiologic, biochemical, and psychological factors may all contribute to overweight conditions. Most often, the cause of being overweight or obese is an energy imbalance. That is, more kcal are being taken in than are being used. When this occurs, the body stores the excess kcal as adipose tissue. Hypothyroidism is a possible, but rare, cause of obesity. In this condition. Basal metabolism is low, thereby reducing the number of kcal needed for energy. Unless corrected, this condition can result in excess weight.

Treatment: Treatment for an overweight person involves two parts: revised eating habits and exercise. Revised eating habits include reducing daily kcal intake at mealtime, limiting between-meal snacks to fresh fruits or vegetables, and restricting or eliminating empty calories.

One pound of body weight equals 3.500 kcal. Therefore, to lose 1 pound per week, a person must reduce kcal intake by 500 kcal each day. Weight loss should be limited to 1 to 2 pounds per week, unless the client is under strict medical supervision. Diets should be planned according to the minimum servings of the food guide pyramid and should not be reduced to below 1,200 kcal/day in order for the dieter to receive adequate nutrients to sustain health.

Attention should also be given to food preparation. Frying adds many kcal from fat to a food item. Broiling, grilling, baking, roasting, boiling, and poaching are healthy ways to prepare foods. Vegetables should be eaten raw or steamed; the addition of butter, margarine, or sauces should be avoided. Eating habits may be adopted to decrease the amount eaten, and yet provide satisfaction: place food on a smaller plate; cut food into smaller bites; chew each bite at least 12 times; and place the fork on the plate between bites.

Exercise, particularly aerobic exercise, is an excellent adjunct to any weight-loss program. Aerobic exercise uses energy from the body's fat reserves, as it increases the amount of oxygen the body takes in. Examples of aerobic exercise are dancing, jogging, bicycling, skiing, rowing, and power walking. Such exercise helps tone the muscles, burns kcal, increases the basal metabolism so that food is burned faster, and is fun for the participant. Any exercise program must begin slowly and increase over time so that no physical damage occurs.

Exercise alone can only rarely replace the need to be mindful of diet, however. The dieter should be made aware of the number of kcal burned by specific exercises to avoid overeating after the workout.

Underweight

Persons are considered to be underweight when their weight is 10% to 15% below the desired weight. An underweight person is more likely to have nutritional deficiencies because of the decreased intake of food. For women, this can cause complications during pregnancy. Being underweight may lower a person's resistance to infection. Being severely underweight may even cause death.

Causes: There are several possible causes of being underweight, such as an inadequate intake of food, excessive exercise, poor absorption of nutrients, or severe infection. Occasionally, hyperthyroidism may be the cause. After the adequacy of food intake and the appropriate activity level are ascertained, specific diagnostic tests must be done to determine whether poor absorption, infection, or hyperthyroidism are present.

Treatment: Dietary treatment for an inadequate intake of food is to gradually increase the amount of food eaten. Also, higher-kcal foods can be eaten. Between-meal snacks and a bedtime snack can help increase the intake of food.

If the individual is to gain 1 pound per week, 3.500 kcal in addition to the individual's basic normal weekly kcal requirement are prescribed. This means an extra 500 kcal must be taken in each day. If a weight gain of 2 pounds per week is required, an additional 7,000 kcal each week, or an additional 1,000 kcal per day, are necessary. This diet cannot be immediately accepted at full kcal value. Time will be needed to gradually increase the daily kcal value by increasing intake of foods rich in carbohydrates, some fats, and protein. Vitamins and minerals are supplied in adequate amounts. If there are deficiencies of some vitamins and minerals, supplements are prescribed.

Nursing Process

Collection of subjective and objective data regarding the client's nutrition serves as the basis for determining the type of nutritional care the client requires.

Assessment

Proper assessment allows the health care team to determine the degree to which the client's nutritional needs are being met. Assessment must be performed logically and should include a nutritional history, physical examination, and the results of laboratory tests.

Age and pregnancy determine some specific items to be included in the nutritional assessment.

Nutritional assessment for an infant should include:
- Height and weight
- Sleeping habits
- Type of feeding (breast- or bottle-fed)
- If breastfeeding, the mother's nutritional status and use of alcohol, tobacco, caffeine, and drugs; infant's feeding schedule (how often fed and for how long)

- If formula feeding, type, frequency, and method of preparation and storage; feeding schedule; amount taken at each feeding
- Use of vitamin/mineral supplements
- If on solid foods, age at introduction, and any reactions or allergies
- Family attitudes about eating, food and weight.

The basic nutritional assessment for everyone over 1 year old should include:

- Nutritional status
- Height and weight
- Meal and snack pattern (food record or 24-hour recall)
- Adequacy of intake based on the food guide pyramid
- Food allergies
- Physical activity
- Cultural, ethnic, and family influences
- Use of vitamin/mineral supplements.

In addition to the basic nutritional assessment, during childhood dental health should also be assessed.

In addition to the basic nutritional assessment, the following should be assessed for the adolescent client:

- Use of alcohol, tobacco, caffeine, and drugs
- Use of fad diets
- Family attitude toward thinness and the adolescent's weight.

In addition to the basic nutritional assessment, the following should be assessed for the adult client:

- Use of alcohol, tobacco, caffeine, and drugs
- Use of fad diets
- Prescribed restricted diet.

In addition to the basic nutritional assessment, the following should be assessed for elderly clients.

- Undesirable change in weight
- Dentition and swallowing
- Appetite
- Vision
- Hand-eye coordination
- Adequacy of daily intake of food
- Ability to self-feed
- Prescribed restricted diet
- Use of alcohol, tobacco, caffeine, and drugs.

In addition to the basic nutritional assessment, the following should be assessed for the pregnant client:

- Weight and rate of weight gain
- Diet changes in response to pregnancy
- Cravings for foods or nonfoods (pica)
- Intake of supplemental vitamins/minerals
- Feeding plans (breast or formula)
- Use of alcohol, caffeine, tobacco, or drugs.

Subjective Data

Subjective data can be obtained through a nutritional history by asking clients questions. Several methods can be used in collecting these subjective data: 24-hour recall, food-frequency questionnaire, food record, and diet history. Although the history data may indicate adequate nutrition, clients must be reassessed periodically to prevent nutritional problems,

24-Hour Recall: The 24-hour recall requires client identification of everything consumed in the previous 24 hours. It is performed easily and quickly by asking pertinent questions: however, clients may be unable to accurately recall their intake or anything atypical in the diet. Family members can often assist with these data, if necessary.

Food-Frequency Questionnaire: The food-frequency method gathers data relative to the number of times per day, week, or month that the client eats particular foods. The nurse can tailor the questions to particular nutrients, such as cholesterol and saturated fat. This method helps to validate the accuracy of the 24-hour recall and provides a more complete picture of foods consumed.

Food Record: The food record provides quantitative information regarding all foods consumed, with portions weighed and measured for three consecutive days. This method requires full client or family member cooperation.

Diet History: The diet history elicits detailed information regarding the client's nutritional status, general health pattern, socioeconomic status, and cultural factors. This method incorporates information similar to that collected by the 24-hour recall and food-frequency questionnaire. The history may require more than one interview because of the amount of data to be collected.

Objective Data

A physical examination may elicit findings that suggest nutritional imbalance. Table 15.6 lists physical indicators of nutritional status.

The measurement of a client's intake and output and daily weight are critical assessments, especially for hospitalized clients.

Anthropometric measurements (Measurement of the size, weight, and proportions of the body) are indicative of the client's caloric-energy expenditure balance, muscle mass, body fat, and protein reserves. The measurements used are body mass index (calculated using weight and height), skinfolds, and limb and girth circumferences.

Body Mass Index (BMI) is a measurement used to determine whether a person's weight (in kilograms) is appropriate for height (in meters). It is calculated using a simple formula:

$$BMI = \frac{weight\ (kg)}{[height\ (m)]^2}$$

A BMI of 27 or greater indicates obesity. For example, a person who weighs 65 kilograms and is 1.6 meters tall would have a BMI of $65\ kg/(1.6)^2$, or 25.4. Go to the CDC's website for a body mass index calculator at www.cdc.gov.

Skinfold Measurement: Skinfold measurement indicates the amount of body fat. The skinfold is measured by grasping the subcutaneous tissue and taking a reading using a special caliper. Measurements can be taken of the tricep, subscapular, bicep, and supra iliac skinfolds.

Table 15.6: Physical Indicators of Nutritional Status

Body area	Good nutrition	Inadequate nutrition
General	Alert, responsive, sleeps well, energetic, seldom ill	Apathetic, easily fatigued, looks tired, often ill
Weight	Appropriate for age, height, body build	Overweight, underweight
Skeleton	Good posture, no malformations	Poor posture
Skin	Good color, no rashes or swelling, smooth, moist, good turgor	Rough, dry, pale, poor turgor
Muscles	Firm, good tone	Flaccid, poor tone
Nails	Pink, firm	Pale, brittle
Eyes	Clear, bright, moist	Dull, pale, dry
Hair	Shiny, smooth	Dull, dry, brittle
Elimination	Regular, soft	Diarrhea or constipation

Other Measurements: Mid-upper-arm circumference serves as an index of skeletal muscle mass and protein reserve. Abdominal-girth measurement serves as an index as to whether the abdomen is increasing, decreasing, or remaining the same. Both of these measurements should be made repeatedly over a span of time, for best assessment.

Laboratory Tests: Several laboratory tests provide information about a client's nutritional status. These include the protein indices of serum albumin, pre-albumin, and serum transferring; hemoglobin; total lymphocyte count; blood urea nitrogen (BUN); and urine creatinine. The serum albumin blood test is used to measure prolonged protein depletion that occurs in chronic malnutrition, liver disease, and nephrosis. The pre-albumin test indicates protein depletion in acute conditions such as trauma and inflammation. Serum transferrin also measures the protein level as indicated by iron stores. Hemoglobin is a measurement of the oxygen- and iron-carrying capacity of the blood. Total lymphocyte count may reflect protein-caloric malnutrition, which inhibits lymphocyte synthesis. Blood urea nitrogen is a nitrogen balance study that indicates the degree to which protein is being depleted or replaced, and urine creatinine excretion indicates the amount of creatinine eliminated by the kidneys.

Nursing Diagnosis

Nursing diagnoses related specifically *to* nutrition include:
> *Imbalanced Nutrition: Less than Body Requirements*
> *Imbalanced Nutrition: More than Body Requirements*
> *Risk for Imbalanced Nutrition: More than Body Requirements*

Other possible nursing diagnoses related to nutritional problems include the following:
> *Disturbed Body Image*
> *Ineffective Breastfeeding*
> *Impaired Dentition*
> *Deficient Knowledge (specify)*
> *Impaired Oral Mucous Membrane*
> *Acute Pain, Chronic Pain*
> *Feeding Self-Care Deficit*
> *Chronic Low Self-Esteem*
> *Risk for Impaired Skin Integrity*

Planning

A plan should be formulated by the nurse and client to achieve mutually agreed-upon goals. The plan is individualized to meet the client's specific needs. These needs may include achieving desired weight, correcting nutritional deficiencies, maintaining a special diet. Preventing nutritional disorders secondary to a particular therapy, or improving nutrition to promote health and prevent disease.

Goals for clients with nutritional alterations might be as follows:
- Client will maintain intake and output balance.
- Client will comply with diet therapy, avoiding high sodium foods.
- Client will gain 2 pounds in 4 weeks.

Implementation

The nurse and client actually carry out the plan through specific actions. Interventions to accomplish the goals may include diet therapy, assistance with meals, weight and intake monitoring, and nutritional support.

Diet Therapy

Diet therapy is the treatment of a disease or disorder with a special diet. A dietary prescription/order is an order written by the physician for food, including liquids. This is similar to a medication prescription written for medications a client receives. A client must not be given anything to eat or drink without an order. The dietary prescription is written for one or more of the following purposes:
- Provide the client with nutrients needed for maintenance or growth.

- Prepare a client for diagnostic tests.
- Treat the client with a disease or condition.

When the dietary prescription has been received, the dietary department must be noticed so the proper food will be sent to the client.

Many times a client needs some help in understanding changes in the diet and the reasons the changes are necessary. A basic knowledge of nutrition and diet therapy contributes to the nurse's ability to competently answer the client's questions about nutrition and diet. It is important, however, for the nurse to recognize when to refer questions to the dietitian.

The dietary prescription may be for nothing by mouth, a standard diet, or a special diet.

Nothing by Mouth: Nothing by mouth (nil per os, NPO) status is a type of diet modification as well as a fluid restriction. This is often prescribed before surgery and certain diagnostic procedures, to rest the GI tract, or when the client's nutritional problem has not been identified.

Standard Diets: Each health care agency has standard or house diets. The standard diets include general (sometimes called regular), soft, clear liquid, full liquid, mechanical soft, and pureed.

General or Regular Diet: The general or regular diet is planned according to the food guide pyramid. There are no restrictions of any kind. It is an adequate diet providing approximately 2,000 kcal a day.

Soft Diet: A soft diet provides foods that are easy to chew and swallow, thus promoting mechanical digestion of foods. Foods to be avoided include nuts, seeds (tomatoes and berries with seeds), raw fruits and vegetables, fried foods, and whole grains. The food guide pyramid is the basis for this diet, although fewer kcal, usually approximately 1,800, are provided.

Clear-Liquid Diet: The clear-liquid diet, also called the surgical liquid diet, is ordered as preparation for diagnostic tests or as the first meal or two after surgery. It consists mostly of water and carbohydrates, providing approximately 500 kcal/day. This is a very nutritionally inadequate diet but does relieve thirst, aids in hydration, and mildly stimulates peristalsis. Liquids included are water; clear, fat-free broth; tea; coffee; clear and strained fruit juices; jello; popsicles; and carbonated drinks such as lemon-lime soda.

Full-Liquid Diet: A full-liquid diet provides approximately 800 to 1,000 kcal per day. It includes all foods that are liquid at room temperature. In addition to the liquids on a clear-liquid diet, milk: milk drinks; cream soups; strained, cooked cereals; ice cream: puddings; all fruit and vegetable juices; and custard are included.

Mechanical Soft or Edentulous Diet: A mechanical soft or edentulous diet consists of food fixed especially for a person who has no teeth or has difficulty chewing. The food is either ground or chopped into very small pieces and cooked very soft, to ease the work of chewing.

Pureed Diet: A pureed did uses foods that has been blended to a smooth consistency. It is prescribed for clients who have difficulty swallowing.

Special Diets: A special diet restores or maintains a client's nutritional status. These diets are variations of the general diet; however, they still must provide all the nutrients of the general diets. Special diets may provide specific amounts of nutrients or may increase or restrict certain foods. Low-residue, high-fiber, liberal bland, fat-controlled, and sodium-restricted are types of special diets.

Low-Residue Diet: The low-residue diet of fiber a day reduces the normal work of the intestines by reducing food residue. Some low-residue diets limit tough or coarse meats, milk, and milk products. The low residue diet is prescribed to decrease GI mucosal irritation in clients with diverticulitis, ulcerative colitis, and Crohn's disease. Foods to be avoided include raw fruits (except bananas), vegetables, seeds, plant fiber, and whole grains. Dairy products are limited to two servings per day.

High-Fiber Diet: A high-fiber diet contains 25 to 35 g or more of dietary fiber. A high-fiber diet is an integral part of the treatment regimen for diverticulosis because it increases the forward motion of the indigestible wastes through the colon. This diet is believed to help prevent constipation, hemorrhoids, and colon cancer, along with helping to treat diabetes mellitus and atherosclerosis.

The recommended foods for this diet include coarse and whole-grain breads and cereals, bran, all fruits, vegetables (especially raw), and legumes. This nutritionally adequate diet must be introduced gradually to prevent the formation of gas and the discomfort that accompanies it. Fight 8-oz glasses of water also must be consumed along with the increased fiber.

Liberal Bland Diet: A liberal bland diet eliminates chemical and mechanical food irritants such as fried foods, alcohol, and caffeine. This diet is prescribed for clients with gastritis and ulcers because it reduces GI irritation.

Fat-Controlled Diet: The fat-controlled diet reduces the total fat ingested by replacing saturated fats with monounsaturated and polyunsaturated fats and restricting cholesterol. This diet is prescribed for clients with atherosclerosis, heart disease, and obesity. Saturated-fat foods to be avoided include animal fats, gravies, sauces, chocolate, and whole-milk products.

Sodium-Restricted Diet: Sodium-restricted diets tailor the level of sodium to mild (2 to 3 g); moderate (1,000 mg); strict (500 mg); or severe (250 mg). This diet is prescribed for clients with fluid volume excess, hypertension, heart failure, myocardial infarction, or renal failure.

Assistance with Meals

Assisting with meals consists of preparing the client preparing the environment, serving the tray, and assisting with eating.

Preparing the Client: Before taking a meal tray into a client's room, the nurse must ensure that the client is ready to eat; face and hands are washed, oral hygiene completed, and if necessary, the bladder emptied. The nurse should help the client into a comfortable eating position; this must be individualized to each client, as not everyone is allowed or able to sit up to eat a meal.

Preparing the Environment: The nurse should make every effort to see that the physical environment is as conducive to a pleasant mealtime atmosphere as possible. This may necessitate cleaning and clearing the overbed table so the tray can be placed on it, tidying the room to remove offensive sights and smells, and brightening the room.

Serving the Tray: The nurse should check that the tray contains the diet ordered, that everything on the tray is appropriate for the diet, and that nothing has spilled. For example, if a low-sodium did tray has a salt packet, the packet should be removed. The nurse should then check the client's ID band against the name on the tray: it is very important that the correct meal is served to each client. The nurse should prepare the food by opening cartons or cutting food, if necessary.

Assisting with Eating: The client who needs assistance in eating should be served last. This way, the nurse will have ample time and not have to hurry the client through the meal.

Weight and Intake Monitoring

Measuring weight daily or weekly and measuring the amount of food and fluid intake monitors therapy effectiveness.

Recording and Reporting

After the client has finished eating, the tray should be promptly removed. The amount of food eaten should be recorded, usually as the percentage of the meal eaten. When a client with diabetes does not eat all the food on the tray, both the charge nurse and the dietitian must be noticed so that a supplemental feeding can be sent later. If the client is on intake and output (I & O), the amount of fluids consumed during the meal must be recorded. Any problems or difficulty in eating as well as likes and dislikes should be reported and documented on the client's medical record.

Nutritional Support

There are two ways nutritional support for adult clients are delivered: enteral nutrition and parenteral nutrition. *Enteral nutrition* includes both the ingestion of food orally and the delivery of nutrients through a GI tube, but is generally used to mean the latter. *Parenteral nutrition* refers to nutrients bypassing the GI system and entering the blood directly.

Enteral Nutrition: When clients cannot or will not take food by mouth, but their GI tracts are working, they are given tube feedings (TF). Sometimes, this may be necessary because of

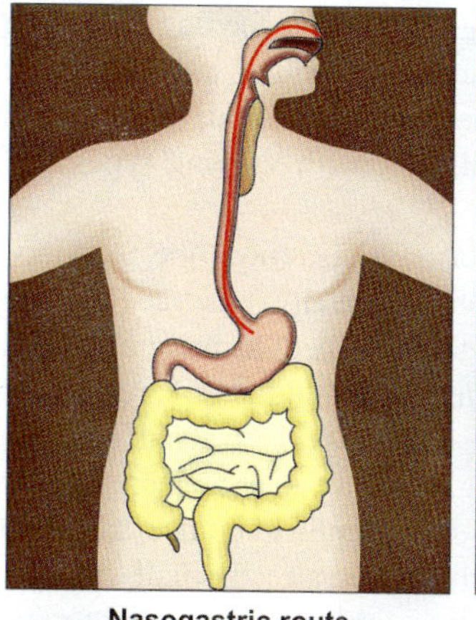

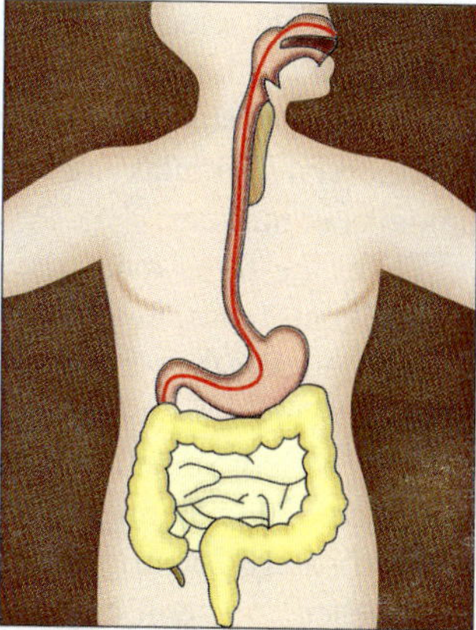

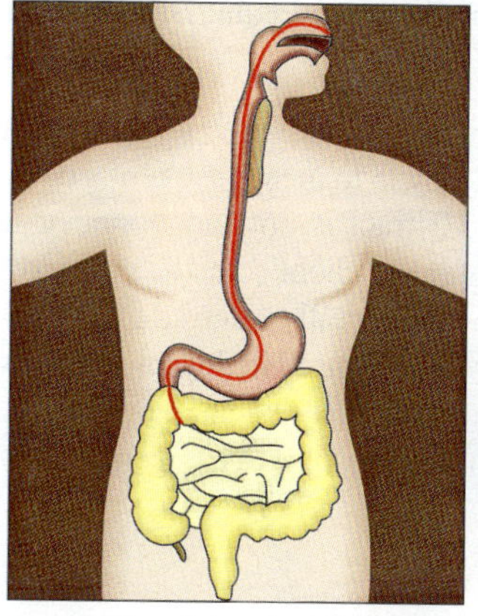

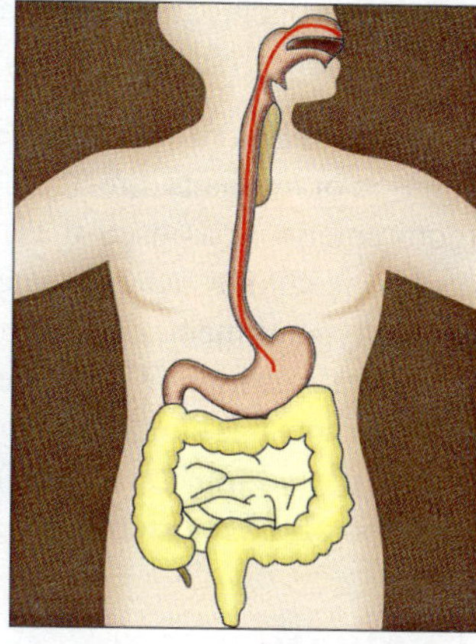

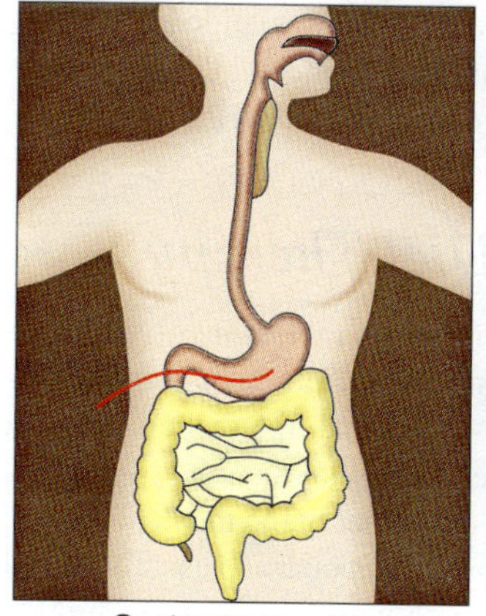

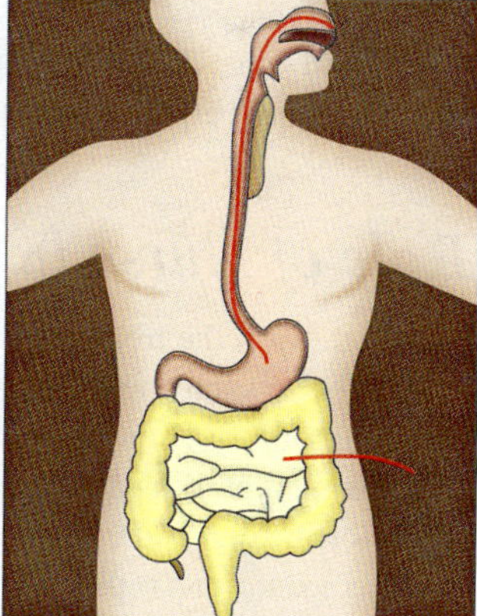

Figure 15.6: Enteral feeding routes

unconsciousness, surgery, stroke, severe malnutrition, or extensive burns. Tube feedings maintain the structural and functional integrity of the GI tract, enhance the utilization of nutrients, and are a safe, economical way to provide nutrients.

Usually, for periods that do not exceed 6 weeks, tube feeding is administered through a nasogastric (NG) tube inserted through the nose and into the stomach or small intestine. When the tube cannot be placed in the nose or when tube feedings will be required for more than 6 weeks, an opening called an ostomy is surgically created into the esophagus (esophagostomy), the stomach (gastrostomy), or the intestine (jejunostomy) (Fig. 15.6).

The physician selects the route and type of feeding tube. The tubes used for these feedings are soft, flexible, and as small as they can be and still allow the feeding to pass through. Numerous commercial formulas are available, with varying types and amounts of nutrients.

There are three methods for administering tube feedings: intermittent, bolus, and continuous. Usually, tube feedings are administered by the continuous infusion method, preferably with a pump. This means the feeding is continuous over a 16- to 24-hour period. Sometimes, the formula is given at half strength at a rate of 30 to 50 ml per hour. This rate may be increased by approximately 25 ml every 4 hours until tolerance has been established. As soon as the client tolerates the half-strength formula, a full-strength formula is initiated at the appropriate rate. When clients are ready to return to oral feedings, the transfer must be done gradually.

Parenteral Nutrition: Parenteral nutrition is the infusion of a solution or nutrients directly into a win to meet the client's daily requirements. It is used if the GI tract is not functional or if normal feeding is not adequate for the client's needs. Formerly called hyperalimentation, it is now generally referred to as total parenteral nutrition (TPN). The solution used in this intravenous infusion contains dextrose, amino acids, fats, essential fatty acids, vitamins, and minerals. Administration of TPN is generally a function of the registered nurse.

Evaluation

The effectiveness of the plan is evaluated in relation to attaining the desired goals. The nurse must assess whether the goals were met. The plan is continued, or modified based on the evaluation.

Role of Nurse in Diet Therapy

Diet therapy is the treatment of disease diet. It involves modifying diets in such a way as to meet the requirements created by disease or injury. A diet used as a medical treatment is called a therapeutic diet. If a patient needs a special diet, the physicians prescribe the diet and write the diet order in the medical record. The therapeutic diet is planned by the dietician and usually served and monitored by the nurse. Nurses and other health professionals should consult with the physician when conditions may necessitate a change in diet order.

Hospital food service must accommodate a wide range of patients from varying backgrounds. Many different therapeutic diets must be planned, and the number and type of meals to be served changes daily. It is no wonder hospital food does not always measure up to "home cooking. Nevertheless, hospital menus are planned to be nutritionally adequate and well balanced. Efforts are made to accommodate each individual patient. Patients sometimes have a negative perception of hospital food. If they are on a restricted diet, they may have even less of a desire to eat.

The nurse can make an impact on the patients nutritional therapy in a number of ways. First, it is imperative for the nursing and dietary department to have a working communication link. For example, if a patient who has a food allergy is admitted, the nurse should inform the dietary department promptly so as to avoid having that particular food sent to the patient, or, if a diagnostic test is being performed that requires the patient omit breakfast, the nurse could alert dietary the night before and ask them to withhold breakfast but send a snack at the time the patient will be back from the test. Also the nurse works closely with the patient on a daily basis and may notice whether inappropriate foods are served or whether the patient has an inadequate intake or manifest clinical signs of malnutrition. It is essential for the nurse to report these findings to the dietician and physician so that proper nutrition intervention can be made.

Second, meal trays should be served in a positive manner. Nurses should avoid making negative statements about the food. Meal trays should be served promptly while foods are at the correct temperature. Some patients may need assistance opening milk cartons, cutting meats, or sitting up to eat. The nurse must be sensitive to these needs, for many patients will leave the food uneaten rather than ask for help.

Therapeutic Diets

Most hospitals have standard diets based on consistency, specially, liquid, soft and regular diets.

Liquid Diets

The two types of liquid diets are clear liquid and full liquid. The clear liquid diet is a nonirritating diet consisting of liquid that are easily digested and absorbed and leave little residue in the gastrointestinal (GI) tract. This diet may be used before diagnostic tests, particularly tests on the GI tract, or before surgery. It is commonly used postoperatively until the bowel resumes activity any may also be used during times of vomiting or diarrhea. The clear liquid diet is low in kilocalories, protein, and most nutrients. It should be used temporarily and for less than one week (Table 15.7).

Table 15.7: Foods Included in Liquid Diets

Clear Liquids	Full Liquids
Bouillon	All clear liquids
Fat-free broth	Strained cereals
Grape, apple, cranberry juice	Strained soups
Fruit drinks	Fruit and vegetable juices
Popsicles	Milk, milkshakes
Gelatin	Ice-cream, sherbet
Tea, coffee	Custard
Ginger, lemon-lime soda	Puddings

The full liquid diet is used as a transition diet after a clear liquid diet. It may be used until the patient is ready for solid foods. A full liquid diet is more nutritionally complete than clear liquid one but is still lacking in some nutrients, such as iron and zinc and fiber. This diet too, should only be used temporarily.

Soft Diets

Soft diets can be used as an intermediate diet when the patient is progressing from a liquid to a regular diet. Soft diets may also be used on a long-term basis for those with conditions affecting the GI tract. A soft diet is sometime called a low-fiber diet. It can include foods from all four food groups including meats, fish, poultry, eggs, milk, grains, and fruits and vegetables. Foods excluded are whole grains and cereals; nuts; seeds; bran; fried meats, fish or poultry; fried eggs, fried breads and pastries; legumes, peas, corn, and gas-producing vegetables such as cabbage, raw fruits (except bananas); and raw vegetables. Foods with strong spices may also be limited.

The low-residue diet is a variation of the soft diet. Its restrictions are similar to the soft or low-fiber diet, but the diet may also exclude milk and milk products because they leave ore residue in the colon. If milk is omitted, care should be taken that the patient receives adequate calcium from other sources.

Both soft and low-residue diets are used in the treatment of diverticulitis, particularly during periods of exacerbation. Other GI conditions for which diets are prescribed include inflammatory bowel disease, gastritis and periods of diarrhea or indigestion.

The mechanical soft diet is specifically for those with chewing or swallowing difficulties. The diet eliminates foods that are difficult to chew or swallow. Other foods may be chopped, pureed or liquefied. This diet must be individualized depending on the extent of chewing or swallowing difficulties.

Bland Diet

Bland diet of the past was a restrictive diet prescribed most often for patients with peptic ulcer (erosion of the tissue lining the stomach or duodenum). Spices and fiber were avoided, and milk and cream were consumed in excess. A liberalized bland diet is now the preferred dietary treatment. Patients with peptic ulcers are instructed to individualize their diet, omitting foods that tend to bother them. In addition, all patients are to (i) eat smaller meals more often and eat in a relaxed environment; (ii) avoid caffeinated beverages, such as coffee, tea, and colas (decaffeinated coffee is also restricted); (iii) avoid pepper, chili powder and coca; and (iv) avoid alcohol. Adequate protein is necessary for the ulcer to heal. Treatment for peptic ulcer includes a combination of diet, medication and rest.

High Fiber Diet

The high fiber diet is a variation of the regular diet and may be used therapeutically. It may be used as a treatment for some GI disorders and may include a preventive effect against some diseases. High-fiber diets are used in the treatment of constipation. With adequate fluids, fiber can reduce constipation in the young, as well as the elderly. This diet is recommended for those with diverticulosis during the latent stages of the disease. Fiber seems to lessen the occurrence of diverticulitis. It may also help prevent diverticulitis in susceptible individuals. High fiber diets are often used in treating diabetes, with other dietary controls to help regulate blood sugar. Complex carbohydrates and fiber seen to moderate the rise in postprandial blood glucose levels. High-fiber diets may also be used in the treatment of atherosclerosis.

The high fiber diet uses foods with high fiber content in place of similar foods with little, if any, fiber. For example, whole grain products, rather than refined are used. Fresh cooked or raw fruits and vegetables including peelings where possible, should be used, rather than canned or processed fruits and vegetables. Nurses should advise patients who are just beginning a high fiber diet to increase intake gradually so the body can become accustomed to larger amounts of fiber.

Meal Frequency Modifications

Meal frequency modifications often, especially in GI related disorders, small frequent meals will be used rather than three larger meals. Perhaps as many as six to eight small meals or snacks may be consumed daily. By eating smaller meals, the work load placed on the GI tract and cardiovascular system is less than that with a large meal.

Small frequent meals may be used for GI disorders, such as hiatal hernia and epigastric distress, during periods of nausea or indigestion, for esophageal reflux and in pancreatitis. They may also be prescribed after myocardial infarction (MI) and in congestive heart failure.

Kilocalorie Modifications

The body requires a specific amount of energy each day to carry out its tasks. Energy intake includes foods and beverages consumed daily. Energy output includes energy used for (i) basal metabolic rate (BMR), (ii) physical activity, and (iii) digestion of food. Energy balance is achieved when energy intake equals output. During energy balance, weight should remain constant if energy intake is greater than output, positive energy balance results, causing weight gain. On the other hand if intake is less than output, negative energy balance occurs leading to weight loss.

High Kilocalorie and High Protein Diets

During times of physiological stress, such as after surgery, bone fractures, sepsis, burns, cancer and some other disease states, the body's energy and protein needs are increased. Medical trauma can greatly increase the BMR, so that if energy needs are not met by diet, negative energy balance will result. The patient will lose protein stores and weight.

Many trauma and cancer patients suffer from anorexia, or lack of appetite, and may also have difficulty with the eating process. This further complicates the problem of nutritional inadequacies. Dietary treatment should aim at restoring energy balance in the normal weight patient or creating a positive energy balance in the under weight patient. High-kilocalorie and high-protein diets should provide increased amounts of kilocalories and protein in a small volume. Commercially prepared liquid supplements may be used.

Suggestions to Increase Kilocalories and Protein

- Add extra-powdered milk to milkshakes, beverages, soups, puddings and cooked cereals
- Spread peanut butter on crackers, fruit or celery
- Add cheese to casseroles, soups, and sauces
- Use extra-meat, chicken or fish in casseroles an soups
- Add sugar to foods where reasonable (this only adds kilocalories)
- Use generous amounts of kilocalorie-dense foods such as butter, margarine, mayonnaise, cream cheese, sour cream, and cream in recipes, as spreads or as dips
- Have snacks available at all times
- Encourage the patient to eat high-kilocalorie foods first and eat the lower kilocalorie foods if still hungry.

Of course, the diet should still provide a balance of foods from all the food groups. It should be kept in mind that the appearance of the food and how it is served may determine whether or not it is eaten. Those serving foods should do so with a positive attitude and encouragement. The meals should be as attractive as possible. Beverages, especially liquid supplements should be served in glasses, not cans. Foods should be served at the correct temperature; meals should be served promptly, and snacks and supplements should be refrigerated, it necessary.

If a patient is not able to consume adequate kilocalories or refuses to eat, nutritional support in the form of tube feedings or intravenous (IV) feedings may be considered.

Kilocalorie Controlled and Low Kilocalorie Diets

Obesity is the condition of having an abnormally large amount of fat on the body.

Ideally obesity should be determined using measures of body composition. Methods of measuring body composition include hydrostatic weighting (submerging the body in a tank of water and measuring displacement), fat-fold thickness measures (measuring pinch of skin using skinfold calipers), and electrical impedance tests (a small electrical current is transmitted through the body and its resistance measured). These methods measure percent of body fat and are better suited for determining obesity; however, they are not always available nor are they as simple as using a weight scale.

The cause of obesity is at best difficult to explain. Many factors may contribute to the positive energy balance that leads to obesity. Most experts agree that both heredity and lifestyle contribute to obesity. Regardless of cause, obesity is a major heath problem particularly in well developed countries. Obese people have a higher incidence of non insulin-dependent diabetes mellitus (NIDDM), high blood lipid levels, hypertension, coronary heart disease, postsurgical complications, gynecological irregularities, pregnancy induced hypertension and gout. Excess weight exacerbates arthritis and some respiratory problems. It can lead to varicose veins and abdominal hernia.

Obesity is resistant to treatment. Some studies have shown that if "cure" from obesity is defined as reduction to ideal weight and maintenance of that weight for 5 years, a person is more likely to recover from many forms of cancer than from obesity. Treatment of obesity has ranged from diets, medications, and psychotherapy to surgery. The goal of any treatment is to cause a negative energy balance resulting weight loss. By far, the most common treatment and probably the safest is a low kilocalorie diet and exercise. Low kilocalorie diet must be based on the exchange lists for meal planning discussed later on under the heading of diabetes mellitus. A successful weight reduction program should incorporate three major components:

1. A lower-kilocalorie diet.
2. Exercise and physical activity, and
3. Behavior modification and other lifestyle changes.

The program should help and prepare patients to control weight throughout life and not just on a temporary basis. Diet should be not less than 1200 kcal/day, and weight loss should occur at the rate of approximately 1 to 2 lb/week. Diets that require the purchase of specially prepared foods, supplements or "magic" diet aides should be avoided. Persons trying to loss weight must learn to take charge of their own life and not rely on expensive products for weight control. Individuals consuming less than 1500 kcal/day may need to take a multivitamin/minor supplement providing approximately 100 percent of the recommended dietary allowance (RDA).

Very Low Calorie Diet (VLCD)

Very low calorie diet programs, sometimes called liquid fasts, are being used increasingly in many hospital outpatient clinics and doctors' offices. These diets consists of a low-kilocalorie and nutritionally balanced. Liquid diet providing 300 to 500 kcal/day. Throughout the liquid fast, patients are monitored by their physician and other health professionals. They should receive dietary and behavioral counseling and should be involved in an exercise program. The patient continues on the liquid fast for a given period, eating the other foods, and then begins a gradual refeeding program and is instructed on a diet for weight maintenance.

Long-term results of VLCDs prove disappointing, showing a higher percentage of dieters regaining over half of the weight lost on the program. With VLCDs as with any weight reduction regimen, the principles of weight management still apply. Unless exercise continues, food intake is controlled and dietary habits are changed, weight loss will be only temporary.

Carbohydrate Modified Diets

Diabetes Mellitus

Probably the most common type of carbohydrate modified diet is the diabetic diet used for those with diabetes mellitus. In diabetes mellitus beta cells in the pancreas do not produce enough insulin or cannot use it properly. Insulin is the hormone necessary to move glucose from the blood stream into the cells where it is used for energy. Without insulin, glucose builds up in the blood stream, leading to hyperglyceme (elevated blood glucose). Diabetes also may affect fat metabolism and increase levels of blood lipids (cholesterol and triglycerides) over time, elevated blood glucose and lipid levels may cause serious long-term complications.

Perhaps not enough emphasis has been placed on the role of diet in the management of diabetes. Proper diet is essential for blood glucose control and may help reduce insulin needs if strictly followed. By keeping blood glucose levels relatively constant and in an appropriate range the risk of diabetic complications may be lessened. Persons with diabetes should continually be encouraged to follow their individualized meal plan. Dietary goals differ somewhat depending on the type of diabetes being treated.

Insulin-dependent diabetes mellitus(IDDM): It occurs most often in children and adolescents. Those with IDDM do not produce insulin their body cannot use glucose for energy and begins to bum fat. When fat is burned for energy in the absence of glucose, and wastes called ketones are formed. Ketone build up in the blood and lead to a life-threatening condition called ketoacidosis. People with IDDM must take insulin to avoid this condition.

The most important principle for those with IDDM is consistency. Meals and snacks should be eaten at about the same time each day. The types and amounts of foods eaten should be similar from day to day. This is necessary because the carbohydrate eaten must balance the insulin administered each day. Carbohydrate intake should be distributed evenly throughout the day to provide adequate amounts of glucose for the available insulin to move from the blood stream to the cells. This is called carbohydrate distribution.

The patient should be given a meal plan to follow that specified the number of food choices (exchanges) to be consumed at each meal and snack. Carbohydrate is distributed among the meals to correspond with insulin dosage.

If a person taking insulin fails to consume adequate carbohydrate, blood glucose levels may drop, causing hypoglycemia (low blood glucose). Symptoms of hypoglycemia may include headache, confusion, weakness, perspiration, shallow breathing, nervousness, visual disturbances, and vertigo and may lead to unconsciousness. Sometime the person experiencing hypoglycemia may be mistakenly judged to be intoxicated. Proper medical identification should be worked to prevent such a mistake. Hypoglycemia should be treated with immediate administration of glucose in a readily available form, such as orange juice, followed by food containing both carbohydrate and protein. If juice is not available, sugar or hard candy may be eaten. In the event of unconsciousness, glucose should be administered intravenously.

In times of illness, the patient with diabetes may not want to eat the usual foods on the meal plan. In such cases, it is essential to provide carbohydrates in the diet to correspond with insulin dosage. Carbohydrate-containing beverages, such as juices and punch, should be offered. Popsicles, flavored gelatin, crackers, puddings, and ice milk provide carbohydrate and may be better accepted during illness.

Noninsulin-dependent diabetes mellitus (NIDDM) it usually occurs in adults, many of whom are overweight. People with NIDDM produce insulin but either there is not enough insulin or the body is unable to use it properly. This type of diabetes often may be controlled by diet and exercise. Some people with NIDDM use oral hypoglycemic agents, medications that stimulate insulin production and use. In some instances insulin injections may be needed to help regulate blood glucose levels. Whenever insulin is administered, the dietary principles for IDDM should be used.

Many people with NIDDM are overweight, and one of the major dietary goals with this type of diabetes is weight control. For the obese person with NIDDM, weight reduction can help control blood glucose and reduce the need for medication. Kilocalorie control is more important than carbohydrate distribution in this type of diabetes. A diet using the exchange lists is an ideal method of weight control. As with IDDM, simple sugar should be restricted and adequate fiber intake emphasized.

Exercise reduces blood glucose levels. This is helpful in the control of blood glucose and is also important for weight control. People with either type of the diabetes may be able to reduce insulin or medication needs with regular exercise. Diet can also be adjusted to compensate for exercise. If a patient with IDDM is to be involved in a physical activity that he is not accustomed to, some carbohydrate-containing food (milk, fruits, vegetables, or starches) may be added to the meal just before engaging in the activity. In this way, the extra-carbohydrate will provide more glucose to satisfy the demands of exercise.

Dumping Syndrome

Dumping syndrome may occur after surgery where a portion of all of the stomach is removed (partial or total gastrectomy). After partial of total gastrectomy, the stomach contents may empty too rapidly into the jejunum. The body reacts by sending water to the intestinal tract, thus blood pressure is reduced. The load on the intestinal tract increases peristalsis (contractions that move food through the GI tract), leading to diarrhea. Symptoms occur 15 to 30 minutes after meals and include cramping, weakness, diaphoresis, vertigo, nausea, and possibly vomiting.

Diet therapy involves giving small, frequent meals that are higher in protein and fat and lower in carbohydrates. Concentrated sweets should be avoided, and fluids should be taken 30 to 60 minutes before or after a meal. The dumping syndrome diet may be needed only temporarily until the body adjusts to the changes caused by surgery.

Lactose Intolerance

Lactose intolerance occurs as a result of lack of the digestive enzyme, lactase. Because of this, the GI tract is unable to breakdown lactose, the milk sugar. Symptoms occur after ingestion of milk products and include nausea, cramps, a bloated feeling flatulence, and diarrhea.

Diet for lactose intolerance excludes milk and milk products, such as icecream, puddings, cheese, powdered milk. Food wit milk added, such as biscuit or muffin mixes, some soups, and other prepared foods, may need to be avoided.

Some individuals have a deficiency rather than a total absence of lactase. These individuals may be able to tolerate small amount of milk products. Yogurt and cheese are often well tolerated. Lactase enzyme-containing preparations are available and can be added to milk before drinking.

Fat Modified Diets

Dietary fat intake may also be modified in the treatment of disease.

Fat-Controlled Diets

A fat-controlled diet is desirable for the treatment of atherosclerosis, heart disease, and hyperlipidemias. Diabetic diets also incorporate fat control. A fat-controlled diet limits both total fat and saturated fat intake. Usually when saturated fat intake is reduced, cholesterol intake also drops, since it is often found in foods containing saturated fat. The individual who is reducing saturated fat in the diet should choose low-fat dairy products, lean meats, skinless poultry, and fish. Eggs should be limited to three per week and organ meats, such as liver, limited to one serving per week or less. Visible fats, such as butter, margarine, mayonnaise, cream, sour cream, nuts, and rich desserts, should be limited. Cooking methods may need to be altered as well. Patients should be encouraged to bake, boil or poach food, rather than to fry and add breading or butter to it. Foods should be eaten without the addition of sauces, gravies, or dips that are high in fat.

When fat is necessary in food preparation, unsaturated fats (monounsaturated and polyunsaturated) should be used in place of saturated fats.

Low Fat Diets

Other medical conditions warrant the use of a low fat diet. Low fat diets differ from fat-controlled diets in that all fats are limited, regardless of saturation. Any time fat malabsorption occurs, dietary fat should be limited. GI diseases that involve malabsorption of fat include cystic fibrosis, inflammatory bowel disease, pancreatitis, and short-bowel syndrome secondary to bowel resection). Gallbladder disease often requires a low fat diet. The gallbladder stores bile and contracts whenever fat is present in the intestinal tract. If gallstones are present or inflammation of the gallbladder exists, contraction may be painful. A low fat diet may alleviate some discomfort. After the gallbladder is removed (cholecystectomy), as low fat diet is no longer required. Some patients with gallbladder disease may be overweight or obese. Weight reduction is indicated for these individuals and may reduce symptoms of gallbladder disease.

Protein, Electrolyte and Fluid Modified Diets

Protein Restricted Diets

In disease states, increased protein needs are often considered to facilitate healing. However, in the presence of defects in protein metabolism or excretion, protein intake should be reduced or controlled. One such case is during renal failure, or may progress slowly (end-stage renal disease). Acute renal failure if often temporary, whereas end-stage renal disease is irreversible.

The kidney normally functions to excrete wastes, concentrate urine and conserve needed electrolytes. During renal failure, the nephrons (working units of the kidney) fail to maintain normal function. Oliguria (decreased urine output) or anuria (no urine output) may result. Urea and other nitrogenous wastes, the end products of protein metabolism, build up in the blood steam, leading to a condition known as azotemia. Many electrolytes, particularly potassium, sodium and phosphorous, are retained and increased blood levels of these nutrients may occur.

Because of the build up of protein waste products, dietary protein should be restricted. A therapeutic diet for renal failure limits the amount of protein consumed; the degree of limitation depends on the extend of renal failure. Patients are encouraged to consume moderate amounts of only high-quality, or complete, proteins found in milk, meat, fish, poultry, and eggs. Incomplete proteins, those found in plant products, contribute to uremia and should be restricted. Other dietary modification in renal failure include the restriction of potassium, sodium, phosphorous and fluids. Vitamin-mineral supplements are generally prescribed.

Cirrhosis is a chronic, degenerative disease of the liver. It is most often seen secondary to alcoholism but may also be seen as a result of hepatitis A and B or other infection. Scar tissue develops in the liver, hampering its effectiveness in removing waste products from the blood stream. In this case ammonia, a waste product of protein metabolism, builds up in the blood stream. If not controlled, high ammonia levels may contribute to hepatic coma (coma secondary to liver disease), brain damage and death. Ascites, a condition characterized by accumulation of fluid in the abdominal cavity, may occur. If the liver is unable to produce bile, fat malabsorption also may take place.

In the presence of cirrhosis, protein intake should initially be at or above the RDA to facilitate healing and tissue regeneration. However, if blood ammonia levels become elevated and signs of impending coma are present, such as confusion, apathy, and drowsiness, a strict low-protein diet should be followed. The low-protein diets for cirrhosis restrict milk and milk products, meats, fish, poultry, cheese, eggs, legumes and nuts. Special nutritional support formulates with modified protein content have also been developed for hepatic coma.

The veins at the lower end of the esophagus may become enlarged and tortuous during cirrhosis, a condition called esophageal varices. Esophageal varices are painful and the use of a soft or liquid diet may be beneficial in this case. Other dietary modifications for cirrhosis include total abstinence from alcohol and may require restriction if malabsorption is present. Vitamin-mineral supplements are also given.

Sodium Restricted Diets

Sodium restrictions may be used to treat a number of medical conditions. Hypertension is often responsive to a lowered sodium intake. It is estimated that 20 percent of the population is "sodium sensitive", that is, they have a genetic sensitivity to sodium that leads to hypertension. In such individuals sodium reduction appears beneficial in controlling blood pressure.

Sodium is also restricted when water retention or edema is present. In the presence of congestive heart failure sodium intake should be decreased to alleviate pulmonary and peripheral edema. Directly after a myocardial infarction, sodium fluid, kilocalorie, and fat restrictions may be implemented. These restrictions are to minimize the work load on the heart. As recovery progresses, the diet will be liberalized as individual condition permits. It cirrhosis is accompanied by ascites, sodium intake should be reduced, and in renal failure, if anuria or oliguria exists, sodium should be restricted.

Sodium restricted diets vary in degree of restriction. The no-add-salt (NAS) diet is the least restrictive, allowing 2000 to 3000 mg of sodium/ day. This diet allows the use of most foods with the exception of highly salted snack foods and prepared foods. Patients following this diet should read nutrition labels to assess the sodium content of food products and determine which would be appropriate for their diet. No salt should be added in cooking or at the table. Other sodium restricted diets range from 2000 mg (2 g) sodium to as little as 250 mg of sodium/day.

In the presence of cystic fibrosis, the sweat glands produce excessive amounts of sodium and chloride. In this special condition sodium intake is not restricted, but generous amounts of sodium and salt are encouraged to compensate for the large losses of sodium.

Potassium Modified Diets

Potassium is considered to playa role in blood pressure control. Evidence indicates that populations with higher potassium intakes have less incidence of hypertension. Increased potassium intake from foods may be beneficial for blood pressure control. Many patients with hypertension or other conditions that cause water retention may take potassium-wasting diuretics. An increased intake of potassium is needed to counteract the loss of potassium caused by the diuretic.

In end-stage renal disease and other kidney diseases, potassium intake may need to be restricted to as little as 1500 to 2000 mg/day.

Fluid Modified Diets

Fluid is found in the diet in a number of forms. Of course, all beverages, milk, juices, coffee and tea add fluid to the diet. Other dietary fluid sources include gelatins, icecream, sherbet, puddings, popsicles, fruit ices, and soups.

During end-stage renal disease and other kidney disease with oliguria and anuria fluid is restricted to 400 to 500 mL/day plus an amount equal to daily urine output, if any. Fluid restrictions may also be implemented during congestive heart failure, directly after an MI, or in hepatic coma or ascites.

During fluid restrictions, patients may experience excessive thirst. Some suggestions to help alleviate thirst include rinsing the mouth with cold mouthwash, putting lemon into cold water to make it more refreshing, freezing fluid so it takes longer to consume, eating cold fruits and raw vegetables, chewing gum sucking on breath mints or hard candies (in moderation), and brushing teeth often.

Increased fluid intake is a common dietary treatment for renal calculi (kidney stones) an urinary tract infection. Additional fluid helps to dilute the urine and increase urinary output. Fluid needs are also increased during periods of diarrhea, vomiting, or malabsorption such as in inflammatory bowel disease. Care should be taken to replace fluids that are lost, to prevent dehydration.

The burn victim loses a large volume of fluids from the wounds, immediately after a severe burn, fluids, electrolytes, and protein are given intravenously rather than orally, because burn patients experience a temporary loss of bowel function. Once bowel activity resumes, adequate fluids should be a part of dietary treatment.

Most conditions requiring diet therapy involve combinations of therapeutic diets. A summary of diet modifications are given in Table 15.8.

Nutrition Support

Occasionally a patient may not be able to consume an oral diet. For whatever reason alternative feeding methods are available in the form of tube feedings or intravenous feedings.

Tube Feedings

A tube feeding is often referred to as 'enteral nutrition support'. Tube feedings may be indicated when a patient is unable to chew or swallow, such as after oral surgery or facial trauma; when a person has no appetite or refuses to eat; in times of great nutritional needs, such as in the burn or trauma patient; in the comatose patient or during periods of moderate malabsorption or diarrhea.

Indications for the use of enteral nutrition support (tube feeding)

- Protein kilocalorie malnutrition with inadequate intake for past five days

Table 15.8: Summary of Diet Modifications

Conditions	Possible diet modifications
Acquired immune deficiency syndrome (AIDS)	High kilocalorie and protein, increased fluid intake mechanical soft; possible tube feeding or TPN
A therosclerosis	Fat controlled; high fiber; when necessary kilocaloric and/or sodium-restricted diet
Burns	High kilocalorie and protein; increased fluid intake; vitamin-mineral therapy
Cancer	High kilocalorie and protein; dietary adjustments made based on symptoms; possible tube feeding or TPN
Cirrhosis/hepatic coma	Protein restricted; possible sodium and fluid restriction
Congestive heart failure	Sodium-restricted; fluid-restricted, small, frequent feedings; soft diet, possible kilocalorie restriction
Constipation	High fiber, increased fluid intake
Cystic fibrosis	High kilocalorie and protein; low fat; generous sodium; vitamin and mineral supplementation
Diabetes mellitus IDDM	Carbohydrate controlled; no concentrated sweets fat controlled; high fiber
NIDDM	Kilocalorie restricted; no concentrated sweets; fat controlled; high fiber
Diverticulitis	Soft, low residue
Diverticulosis	High fiber
Dumping syndrome	Carbohydrate restricted; no concentrated sweets; small, frequent feedings; fluids before or after meals; when necessary, fluid and electrolyte replacement
Gallbladder disease	Low fat, kilocalorie restricted
Gastritis	Low residue, liberalized bland
Hepatitis	High kilocalorie and protein
Hiatal hernia	Small, frequent feelings; low fat; bland; when necessary, kilocalorie restricted
Hyperlipidemia	Fat controlled; when necessary, kilocalorie restricted; carbohydrate controlled
Hypertension	Sodium restricted; high potassium; fat controlled; when necessary, kilocalorie restricted
Hypoglycemia	No concentrated sweets; small, frequent feedings
Inflammatory bowel disease	Low residue; low fat, high kilocalorie and protein fluid and electrolyte replacement; vitamin-mineral supplementation; possible lactose restriction, tube feeding, or TPN
Lactose intolerance	Lactose restricted
Malabsorption	Low fat, high kilocalorie and protein, fluid and electrolyte replacement
Mouth, conditions affecting broken jaw/oral surgery	Mechanical soft; possible tube feeding
Dental caries/peridontal disease/ ill fitting dentures/missing teeth	Mechanical soft
Dry mouth	Mechanical soft; increased fluid intake
Dysphagia (difficulty in swallowing)	Mechanical soft; possible tube feeding
Ulcers of mouth or gums	Mechanical soft; bland
Myocardial infarction	Low sodium, kilocalorie restricted, soft, bland small, frequent feedings; fat controlled; fluid restricted (temporary); moderate temperature food
Nausea	Soft; bland; small; frequent feedings
Obesity	Kilocalorie restricted; fat controlled, high fiber
Pancreatitis	Low fat, small, frequent feedings, possible tube feedings or TPN
Peptic ulcer	Liberalized bland diet
Reflux esophagus	Small frequent feedings; low fat; bland
Renal calculi (kidney stones)	Increased fluid intake; possible calcium controlled
Acute renal failure	Protein restricted, high kilocalorie; fluid, sodium, and potassium controlled
Chronic renal failure	Protein restricted, low sodium; potassium, fluid and phosphorous restricted; vitamin-mineral supplement
Underweight	High kilocalorie and protein
Vomiting	Fluid and electrolyte replacement

- Hospitalized patient consuming less than 50 percent of nutritional needs for past 7 to 10 days
- Severe dysphagia (difficulty swallowing)
- Major burns
- Sustained major trauma wounds
- Liver failure
- Renal dysfunction
- Radiation therapy
- Mild chemotherapy
- As adjunctive therapy with TPN for small bowel regeneration
- Low output enterocutaneous fistulas (abnormal passage from the intestine to the body surface) that can be successfully bypassed with a tube.

Tube feedings should be used only when all or at least part of the GI tract is functioning. Tube feedings are most commonly administered by way of a nasogastric tube, that is, a tube that is passed through the nose and into the stomach. If regurgitation is common or gastric-residual is high, a nasojejunal tube (a tube that is passed through the nose and into the jejunum) may be used to reduce the risk of aspiration (Tables 15.9 to 15.12).

Table 15.9: Procedures for Inserting a Nasogastric Tube

Equipment

• Nasogastric tube of appropriate size (8 to 18 French)	• Stethoscope	• Suction apparatus (if ordered)
• Small basin filled with ice or warm water (optional)	• Normal saline solution for (irrigation only)	• Bath towel or disposable pad
• Water-soluble lubricant	• Aseptobulb syringe or	• Safety pin and rubber band
• Tongue blade	• Toomey syringe (20 to 50 mL)	• Clamp
• Flashlight	• Nonallergenic tape (1 inch wide)	• Emesis basin
• Topical analgesic (optional)	• Tissues	• Disposable gloves
	• Glass of water with straw	• Tincture or benzoin

	Nursing actions	*Rationales*
1.	Check physician's order for insertion of naso-gastric tube.	This clarifies procedure and type of equipment required.
2.	Explain procedure to client.	Explanation facilitates client cooperation.
3.	Gather equipment.	This provides for organized approach to task.
4.	If nasogastric tube is rubber place it is a basin with ice for 5 to 10 minutes or place a plastic tube in a basin of warm water.	Cold stiffens the rubber tube, making it easier to insert. Plastic tube may be placed in warm water to make it more flexible.
5.	Assess client's abdomen.	Assessment determines presence of bowel sounds and amount of abdominal distention.
6.	Wash your hands. Don disposable gloves.	Handwashing deters the spread of microorganisms. Gloves protect from exposure to body fluids.
7.	Assist the client to high Fowler's position, or 45°, if unable to maintain upright position, and drape chest with bath towel or disposable pad. Have emesis basin and tissues handy.	Upright position is more natural for swallowing and protects against aspiration, if the client should vomit. Passage of tube may stimulate gagging and tearing of eyes.
8.	Check the nares for patency by asking the client to occlude one nostril and breathe normally through the other. Select the nostril through which air passes more easily.	Tube passes more easily through the nostril with the largest opening.
9.	Measure the distance to insert the tube by placing tip of tube.	Measurement ensures that the tube will be long enough to enter the client's stomach at client's nostril and extending to tip of earlobe and then to tip of xiphoid process. Mark tube with a piece of tape.
10.	Lubricate the tip of the tube (at least 1-2 in) with a water-soluble lubricant. Apply topical analgesic to nostril and oropharynx or ask client to hold ice chips in mouth for several minutes (according to physician's preference).	Lubrication reduces friction and facilitates passage of the tube into the stomach. Water soluble lubricant will not cause pneumonia if tube accidentally enters the lungs. Topical analgesic or ice acts as a local anesthetic, reducing discomfort.
11.	Ask the client to lift the head, and insert the tube into the nostril while directing the tube downward and backward. The client may gag when the tube reaches the pharynx.	Following the normal contour of the nasal passage while inserting the tube reduces irritation and the likelihood of mucosal injury. The gag reflex is readily stimulated by the tube.

Contd...

Table 15.9: *Contd...*

	Nursing actions	Rationales
12.	Instruct the client to keep head in upright or normal eating position. Encourage him or her to swallow even if no fluids are permitted. Advance the tube in a downward and backward direction when the client swallows. Stop when the client breathes. Provide tissues for tearing or watering of eyes. If gagging and coughing persist, check placement of tube with a tongue blade and flashlight. Keep advancing the tube until the tape marking is reached. Do not use force. Rotate the tube if it meets resistance.	Bringing the head forward helps close the trachea and open the esophagus. Swallowing helps advance the tube, causes the epiglotis to cover the opening of the trachea, and helps to eliminate gagging and coughing. Tears are a natural response as the tube passes into the nasopharynx. Excessive coughing and gagging may occur is the tube has curled in the back of throat. Forcing the tube may injure mucous membranes.
13.	Discontinue the procedure and remove the tube if there are signs of distress, such as gasping, coughing, cyanosis, and the inability to speak or hum.	The tube is not in the esophagus if the client shows signs of distress and is unable to speak or hum.
14.	Determine that the tube is in the client's stomach (these methods are appropriate for large-bore tubes but may be ineffective to check placement of small-bores, pliable tubes):	
	(a) Attach the syringe to the end of the tube and aspirate 10 to 30 mL of stomach contents.	The tube is in the stomach if its contents can be aspirated; pH of aspirate can then be treated to determine gastric placement.
	(b) Measure the pH of aspirated fluid using pH paper or a meter.	The pH of gastric contents is acidic (4 or less), compared with an average pH of 7.0 or greater for respiratory fluid. Because pH of intestinal fluid also is slightly basic, this method will not effectively differentiate between intestinal fluid and pleural fluid.
	(c) Obtain X-ray of placement of tube (as directed by physician).	X-ray visualization is the most definitive measure to determine tube placement.
15.	Apply tincture of benzoin to tip of nose. Secure the tube with tape to the client's nose. Be careful not to pull the tube too tightly against the nose. (a) Cut a 4-inch piece of tape and split bottom 2 inches or use packaged nose tape for NG tubes. (b) Place unsplit and over bridge of client's nose. (c) Wrap split ends under the tubing and up and over onto the nose.	Tincture of benzoin facilitates attachment of tape. Constant pressure of the tube against the skin and mucous membranes causes tissue injury.
16.	Attach tube to suction or clamp the tube and cap it according to the physician's directions. (Fig. 15.7)	Suction provides for decompression of stomach and drainage of gastric contents.
17.	Secure tube to the client's gown by using a rubber band or tape and a safety pin. If double-lumen tube is used, secure vent above stomach level. Attach at shoulder level.	This prevents tension and tugging on the tube. Securing and double-lumen tube above stomach level prevents seepage of gastric contents and keeps the lumen clear for venting air.
18.	Assist with or provide client with oral hygiene at regular intervals.	Oral hygiene keeps mouth clean and moist and promotes comfort.
19.	Wash hands. Remove all equipment and make client comfortable.	Handwashing deters the spread of microorganisms.
20.	Record the insertion procedure type and size of tube, description of gastric contents, and client's response.	This facilitates documentation and provides for comprehensive care.

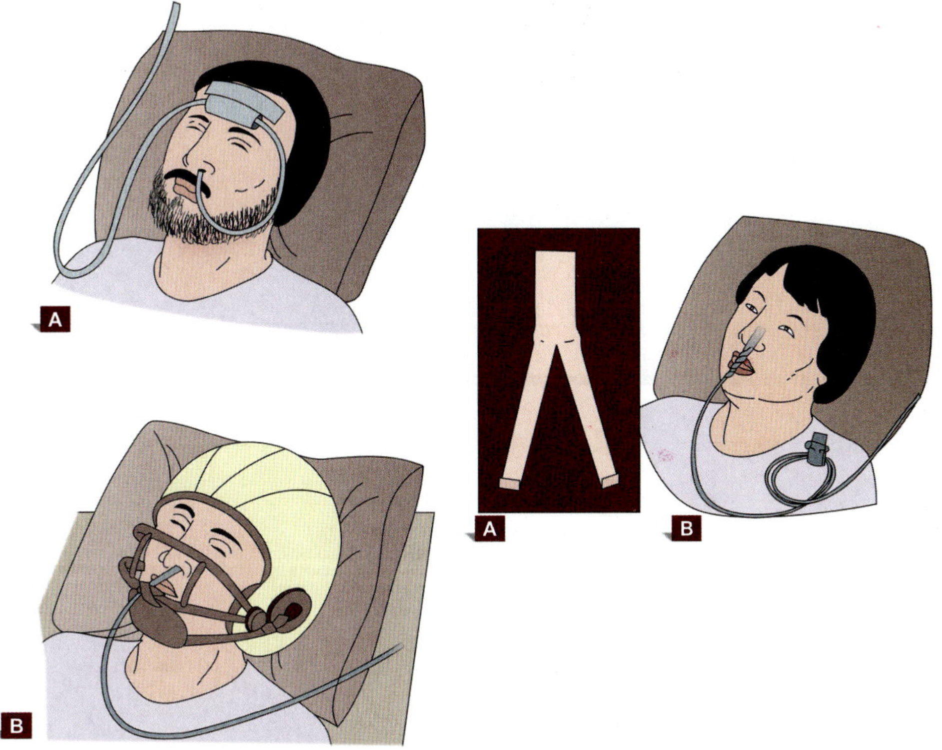

Figure 15.7: Inserted Nasogastric Tube

Table 15.10: Procedures for Administering a Tube Feeding

Equipment

• Tube feeding at room temperature	• Clamp (Hoffman or butterfly)	• Rubber band
• Stethoscope	• Disposable pad or towel	• Enteral feeding pump (if ordered)
• Feeding bag or prefilled tube feeding set	• Sterile water for irrigation	• IV pole
• Alcohol preps	• Asepto or Toomey syringe	• Disposable gloves

	Nursing actions	*Rationales*
1.	Explain procedure to client. Use stethoscope to assess bowel sounds.	This facilitates cooperation and provides reassurance for client. Presence of bowel sounds indicates functional GI tract.
2.	Assemble equipment. Check amount, concentration, type, and frequency of tube feeding on client's chart. Check expiration date of formula.	This provides for organized approach to task. Ensures that correct feeding will be administered. Outdated formula may be contaminated.
3.	Wash your hands. Don disposable gloves.	Handwashing deters the spread of microorganisms. Gloves protect from exposure to blood or body fluids.
4.	Position client with head of bed elevated at least 30° or as near normal position for eating as possible.	This position minimizes possibility of aspiration into trachea.
5.	Unpin tube from client's gown and check to see that the nasogastric tube is properly located in the stomach, as described in Table 15.9, Action 14.	Even when initially positioned correctly, a nasogastric tube left in place can become dislodged between feedings. The instillation of water or nourishment could lead to serious respiratory problems if a gastric tube is in the trachea or a bronchus, rather than in the stomach.
6.	Aspirate all gastric contents with a syringe and measure. Return immediately through tube, flush tube with 30 mL of sterile water for irrigation. Proceed with feeding if amount of residual does not exceed policy of agency of physician's guideline. Disconnect syringe from tubing. (Fig. 15.8)	This indicates gastric emptying time. A residual more then 100 mL or more than 10 or 20 percent the hourly feeding rate must be reported to physician. Fluid should be returned to stomach so as not to cause any fluid or electrolyte losses.

Contd...

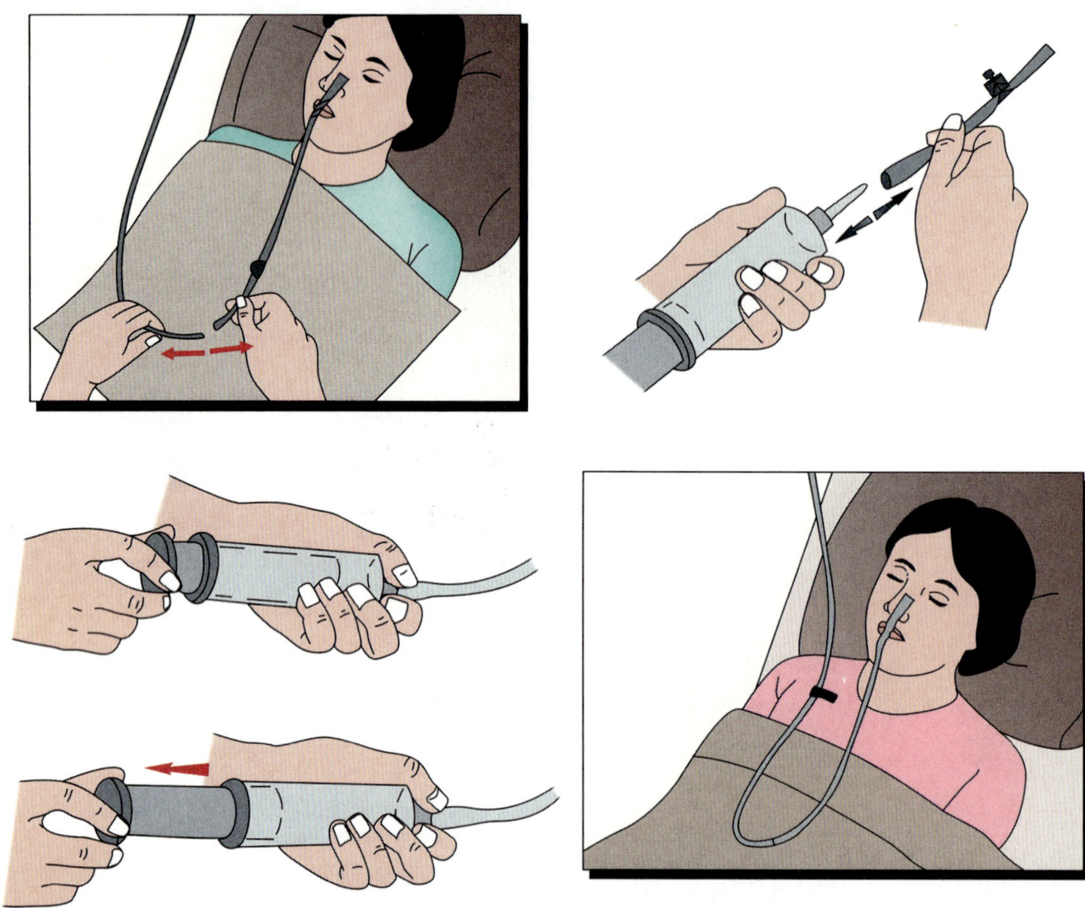

Figure 15.8: Administering a Tube Feeding

Table 15.10: *Contd...*		

	Nursing actions	Rationales
For intermittent feedings		
7.	When using a feeding bas (open system);	Formula displaces air in the tubing. Cleansing container top with alcohol minimizes risk or contaminants entering feeding bag. Formula displaces air in tubing.
(a)	Hang bag on IV pole and adjust to about 12 inches above the stomach. Clamp tubing.	
(b)	Cleanse top of feeding container with alcohol before opening it. Pour formula into feeding bag and allow solution to run through tubing. Close clamp.	
(c)	Attach feeding set-up to feeding tube, open clamp, and regulate drip according to physician's order or allow feeding to run in over 30 minutes.	Introducing the formula at a show, regular rate allows the stomach to accommodate to the feeding and decreases gastrointestinal distress.
(d)	Add 30 to 60 mL (1-2 oz) of sterile water for irrigation to feeding bag when feeding is almost completed and allow it to run through tube.	Water rinses the feeding from the tube and helps to keep it patient.
(e)	Clamp the tubing immediately after water has been instilled. Disconnect from tube. Clamp tube and cover end with sterile gauze secured with a rubber band or apply cap.	Clamping the tube prevents air from entering the stomach. Cover on end of tube deters entry of microorganisms and protects client and linens from fluid leakage from tube.

Contd...

Table 15.10: *Contd....*

	Nursing actions	Rationales
8. (a)	When using prefilled tube feeding set-up (closed system): Remove screw-on cap and attach administration set-up with drip chamber and tubing. Hang set on IV pole and adjust to about 12 inches above the stomach. Clamp tubing and squeeze drip chamber to fill one-third to one-half of capacity. Release clamp and run formula through tubing. Close clamp.	Formula displaces air in tubing.
(b)	Follow Actions 7c, 7d, and 7e. Feeding pump may be used with tube feeding set-up to regulate drip.	
9.	When using a feeding pump:	
(a)	Close flow regulator clamp on tubing and fill feeding bag with prescribed formula. The amount used depends on agency policy. Place label on container.	Feeding intolerance is less likely to occur with smaller volumes. Hanging smaller amount of feeding also reduces risk of bacteria growth and contamination of feeding at room temperature.
(b)	Hang feeding container on IV pole and allow solution to flow through tubing.	This prevents air from being forced into the stomach or intestines.
(c)	Connect to feeding pump following manufacturer's directions. Set rate.	Smaller volume of feeding is infused continuously and is more easily tolerated by client.
(d)	Check residual every 4 to 8 hours.	Checking verifies placement of the tube and proper absorption of the feeding.
10.	Observe client's response during and after tube feeding.	Pain may indicate stomach distention which may lead to vomiting.
11.	Have client remain in upright position for at least 30 minutes to 1 hour after feeding.	This position minimizes risk of backflow and discourages aspiration, if any vomiting should occur.
12.	Wash and clean equipment or replace according to agency policy. Remove gloves and wash your hands.	This prevents contamination and deters spread of microorganisms.
13.	Record type and amount of feeding and client's response. Monitor blood glucose, if ordered by physician.	This provides accurate documentation of procedure. Many feedings contain high amounts of carbohydrates.

Table 15.11: Procedures for Removing a Nasogastric Tube

Equipment

- Tissues
- Bath towel or disposable pad
- Disposable plastic bag
- 50 mL syringe (optional)
- Normal saline solution for irrigation (optional)
- Disposable gloves

	Nursing actions	Rationales
1.	Check physician's direction for removal of nasogastric tube.	This ensures correct implementation of physician's direction.
2.	Explain procedure to client and assist to semi-Flowler's position.	Explanation facilitates client cooperation. Sitting position decreases risk of aspiration, if vomiting should occur.
3.	Gather equipment.	This provides for organized approach to task.
4.	Wash your hands. Don clean disposable gloves.	Handwashing deters the spread of microorganisms. Gloves protect hands from contact with abdominal secretions.
5.	Place towel or disposable pad across client's chest. Give tissues to client.	Precautions protect client from contact with gastric secretions. Tissues are necessary if client wants to blow his or her nose when tube is removed.

Contd...

Table 15.11: *Contd...*

	Nursing actions	Rationales
6.	Discontinue suction and separate tube from suction. Unpin tube from client's gown and carefully remove adhesive tape from client's nose.	Disconnecting tube allows for its unrestricted removal.
7.	Attach syringe and flush with 10 mL normal saline solution or clear with 30 to 50 cc of air (optional).	Air or saline solution clears the tube of feeding or debris.
8.	Instruct client to take a deep breath and hold it.	This prevents accidental aspiration of gastric secretions in tube.
9.	Clamp tube with fingers by doubling tube on itself. Quickly and carefully remove tube while client holds breath.	Carefully removal minimizes trauma and discomfort for client. Clamping prevents drainage of gastric contents in tube.
10.	Place tube in disposable plastic bag. Remove gloves and place in bag.	This prevents contamination with microorganisms.
11.	Offer mouth care to client and make client comfortable.	Provides for comfort.
12.	Measure nasogastric drainage. Remove all equipments and dispose according to agency policy. Wash your hands.	Measuring nasogastric drainage provides for accurate recording of output. Proper disposal deters spread of microorganisms.
13.	Record renewal of tube, client's response, and measurement of drainage.	Facilitates documentation and provides for comprehensive care.

Table 15.12: Procedures for Irrigating a Nasogastric Tube Connected to Suction

Equipment

- Nasogastric tube connected to continuous or intermittent suction
- Irrigation set (Asepto or Toomey syringe and container for irrigating solution)
- Normal saline solution (0.9% sodium chloride solution) for irrigation
- Stethoscope
- Disposable pad or bath towel clamp
- Disposable gloves

	Nursing actions	Rationales
1.	Check physician's direction for irrigation. Explain procedure to client.	This clarifies schedule and irrigating solution. An explanation encourages client cooperation and reduces apprehension.
2.	Gather necessary equipment. Check expiration dates on irrigating saline solution and irrigation set.	This provides for organized approach to task. Agency policy dictates safe interval for reuse of equipment.
3.	Wash your hands.	Handwashing deters the spread of microorganisms.
4.	Assist client to semi-Fowler's position, unless this is contraindicated.	This position minimizes risk of aspiration.
5.	Check placement of nasogastric tube.	
6.	Clamp suction tubing near connection site. Disconnect tube from suction apparatus and lay on disposable pad or towel.	This protects client from leakage of nasogastric drainage.
7.	Pour irrigating solution into container. Draw up 30 mL of saline solution (or amount directed by physician) into syringe.	This delivers measured amount of irrigant through tube. Saline solution compensates for electrolytes lost through nasogastric drainage.
8.	Place tip of syringe in tube. If Salem sump or double-lumen tube is used, make sure that syringe tip is placed in drainage port and not in air bent. Hold syringe upright and gently insert the irrigant for allow solution to flow in by gravity if agency or physician indicates. Do not force solution into tube.	Position of syringe prevents entry of air into stomach. Gentle insertion of saline solution (for gravity insertion) is less traumatic to gastric mucosa.
9.	If unable to irrigate tube, reposition client and attempt irrigation again. Check with physician if repeated attempts to irrigate tube fail.	Tube may be positioned against gastric mucosa, making it difficult to irrigate.

Table 15.12: *Contd...*	
Nursing actions	*Rationales*
10. Withdraw or aspirate fluid into syringe. If not return, inject 20 cc of air and aspirate again.	Injection of air may reposition the end of tube.
11. Reconnect tube to suction. Observe movement of solution or drainage.	Observation determines patency of tube and correct operation of suction apparatus.
12. Measure and record amount and description of irrigant and returned solution.	Irrigant placed in tube is considered intake, solution returned is recorded as output.
13. Rinse equipment if it will be reused.	This promotes cleanliness and prepares equipment for next irrigation.
14. Wash your hands.	Handwashing deters the spread of microorganisms.
15. Record irrigation procedure, description of drainage, and client's response.	This facilitates documentation of procedure and provides for comprehensive care.

In case where long-term tube feedings are necessary such as in a patient with a gastrectomy or intestinal resection, or in a patient with an upper GI obstruction, feeding ostomies may be employed. Ostomies are surgical openings through which a feeding tube may pass. Ostomies may be made into the pharynx (pharyngostomy), esophagus (esophagostomy), stomach (gastronomy), or the jejunum Oejunostomy). Ostomy feeding need not be continuous, but can be given intermittently, permitting more freedom of movement.

Formulas vary in composition. If the tube feeding is the sole source of nutrition, a complete formula that provides adequate kilocalories, protein, carbohydrate, fat, vitamins, and minerals to meet RDAs should be used. Intact formulas are formulas containing proteins, carbohydrates, and fats in whole forms, as found in foods. These formulas are available with or without fiber. Elemental or hydrolyzed formulas are available for individuals experiencing malabsorption, such as in inflammatory bowel disease, or for those who experience diarrhea and malabsorption with intact formulas. Elemental formula are predigested, that is, the nutrients are already broken down into smaller units. Therefore, they require little digestive action before being absorbed.

In the hospital, tube feedings can be fed on a continuous basis, using a continuous drip pump that administers the formula slowly over 16 to 24 hours. Feedings may also be given intermittently. This involves giving a specific volume of formula over a short time, about 20 to 30 minutes. This may be done to six times daily. Intermittent feeding is preferred by many long-term tubefed patients. Bolus fee dings (giving a 4 to 6 hour volume of formula in a matter of minutes) may be given but are poorly tolerated in most patients.

Tube feedings should always be started slowly and most formulas should be diluted to one-third to one-half of regular strength. The strength and the amount of formula can then be increased at different intervals until the full prescription is given. Distention, diarrhea and nausea may indicate that the formula strength and/ or volume is too great. Dumping syndrome may also occur with rapid and concentrated formula delivery.

Tube feeling is considered to be aggressive nutritional therapy. Complications may arise, including diarrhea, contamination of formula, infection, aspiration; overhydration or dehydration; abnormalities of blood concentrations of electrolytes, glucose, and other nutrients; and development of liver abnormalities.

Parenteral Nutrition Support

Parenteral nutritional is the term used to describe intravenous feedings. Parenteral nutrition may be administered through peripheral veins, such as those in the arms or legs. The administration route is called 'peripheral parenteral nutrition' (TPN). The term 'total parenteral nutrition' (TPN) usually refers to administration into a large central vein (most often the superior vena cava), by way of the subclavian vein, or by way of the internal jugular vein. TPN and PPN formulas are composed of glucose, amino acids, vitamins, minerals, and electrolytes. Fat, in the form of triglycerides, is also given as a supplement to the main formula. It is administered separately through a Y-connector tube.

Parenteral nutrition support is indicated for the patient with a nonfunctioning or dysfunctioning GI tract. Many patients with nonfunctioning GI tracts can be maintained on saline solutions for 5 to 7 days, but if the digestive tract is still nonfunctioning after that time, PPN or TPN should be initiated.

When intravenous nutrition is necessary, PPN should be the first choice of administration where possible. PPN carries less risk of complications, requires less monitoring, and costs less than the central venous route. Candidates for PPN are those needing 3000 or fewer kilocalories/ day, those needing supplementation to oral diet, or those requiring short-term therapy (less than 3 weeks).

Total parenteral nutrition is indicated for patients needing a highly concentrated formula, such as those who need more kilocalories than can be administered peripherally or those requiring a third restriction-a concentrated formula delivers more kilocalories and nutrients in a smaller volume. Other candidates for TPN include those who must be on IV feedings for more than 3 weeks and those with unsuitable or unavailable peripheral veins.

Possible indications for the use of total parenteral nutrition are:
- Bone marrow transplantation
- Chronic intractable vomiting (such as hyperemesis gravidarum, the severe nausea and vomiting of pregnancy)
- Severe malabsorption and diarrhea
- Inflammatory bowel disease
- Enterocutaneous fistulas (abnormal passage from the intestine to the body surface)
- Small bowel obstruction or surgical resection
- Moderate to acute pancreatitis
- High-dose chemotherapy
- High-dose radiation therapy affecting the GI tract
- Preoperative therapy when intensive medical or surgical intervention is used in the malnourished
- Severe malnutrition in the face of a nonfunctioning GI tract

Table 15.13: Procedures for Monitoring the Blood Glucose Level		
Equipment		
• Blood glucose meter • Testing strips	• Sterile lancet • Cotton balls	• Alcohol swab or soap and water • Disposable gloves

	Nursing actions	*Rationales*
1.	Check physician's direction for monitoring schedule.	This confirms times for checking blood glucose.
2.	Gather equipment.	This provides an organized approach to the task.
3.	Explain procedure to client.	Explanation encourages client cooperation.
4.	Wash, hands, not disposable gloves. from exposure to blood or body fluids.	Handwashing deters the spread of microorganisms. Gloves protect
5.	Prepare lancet.	Aseptic technique maintains sterility.
6.	Remove test strip and recap container immediately. Turn monitor on and check that code number on strip matches the code number on the monitor screen.	Immediate recapping protects strips from exposure to light and discoloration. Matching code numbers on the strip and glucose monitor ensure that machine is calibrated correctly.
7.	Massage side of finger for adults (or heel for child) toward puncture site.	Massage encourages blood flow to the area.
8.	Have client wash hands with soap and warm water or cleanse area with alcohol. Dry thoroughly.	Washing with soap and water or alcohol cleanses the puncture site. Warm water also help to cause vasodilation.
9.	With finger in dependent position, hold lancet perpendicular to skin and prick site with the lancet.	Dependent position increases blood flow to the site. Holding lancet in proper position facilitates proper skin penetration.
10.	Wipe away first drop of blood with cotton ball if recommended by manufacturer of monitor.	Some feel first drop of blood may be contaminated by serum or cleansing product and produce an inaccurate reading.
11.	Lightly squeeze or milk the puncture site until a hanging drop of blood has formed (check instructions for monitor).	Large droplet facilitates accurate test results.
12.	Gently touch drop of blood to pad on test strip without smearing it.	Smearing blood on strip may result in inaccurate test results.
13.	Insert strip into the meter according to directions for that specific device.	Correctly inserted strip allows meter to read blood glucose level accurately.
14.	Apply pressure to puncture site.	Pressure causes hemostasis.
15.	Read blood glucose results and document appropriately at bedside. Inform client of test result.	Timing when awaiting results depends on type of meter.
16.	Turn meter off, dispose of supplies appropriately, and place lancet in sharps container.	Proper disposal prevents exposure to blood and accidental needle sticks.
17.	Remove gloves and wash hands.	Handwashing prevents the spread of microorganisms.
18.	Record blood glucose on chart or medication record.	This facilitates documentation of procedure and provides for comprehensive care.

- Hospitalization, when adequate enteral nutrition cannot be established within 7 to 10 days.

In any condition, TPN should not be used for those patients whose dependence on parenteral nutritional support is expected to be shorter than 5 days.

TPN requires constant medical care. Central venous administration requires surgical placement of a catheter in one of the central veins. This imposes significant risks on the patient, including sepsis (major infection), pneumothorax (air in the pleural cavity), homothorax (blood in the pleural cavity), phlebitis 'inflammation of the vein), or thrombosis (blood clots).

The catheter site must be kept aseptic, and feeding solutions must be sterile. Biochemical and clinical status of the patient must be constantly monitored.

The patient receiving TPN may experience fluid and electrolytic imbalances, hyperglycemia or hypoglycemia, metabolic disturbances, and bone disorders, such as osteomalacia (softening of the bones). For this reason blood chemistries should be monitored frequently. Blood glucose should be checked several times each day. Regular insulin may be administered in a sliding scale to maintain blood glucose levels below 200 mg/dL (Table 15.13).

16

Management of Bowel Elimination

Introduction

Bowel elimination is a natural process critical to human functioning in which body excretes waste products of digestion. It is essential component of the healthy body functioning. Alterations in bowel elimination can cause problems with gastrointestinal and other body systems. Because bowel function depends on the balance of several factors, elimination patterns and habits vary among individuals. Patients often need assistance from the nurse to maintain normal bowel elimination habits, because certain illnesses prevent normal bowel habits. To manage patients' elimination problems, the nurse must understand normal eliminations and factors that promote or impede elimination. Supportive nursing care respects patients' privacy and emotional needs. Measures designed to promote normal elimination should also minimize discomfort. The nurse provides therapies that promote or minimize factors affecting peristalsis and or the absorption and secretion of intestinal contents. Care usually involves educating clients about daily activities or habits that affect defecation.

Many factors influence the process of bowel elimination, which include growth and development, dietary patterns, food and fluid intake, activity and muscle tone, lifestyles variables, psychologic variables, pathologic conditions, medications, diagnostic tests, surgery and anesthesia. The specific factors which promote and impair bowel elimination are as follows:

(i) *Factors promoting elimination*

- Stress-free environment
- Ability to follow personal bowel habits, privacy
- High-fiber diet
- Normal fluid intake (fruit juices, warm liquids)
- Exercise (walking)
- Ability to assume squatting position
- Properly-administered laxatives and cathartics

(ii)   *Factors impairing elimination*

- Emotional stress (anxiety or depression)
- Failure to heed defecation reflex, lack of time or privacy
- High carbohydrate, high fat diet
- Reduced fluid intake
- Immobility or inactivity
- Inability to squat because of immobility, advanced age, pain, advanced pregnancy, pain during defecation
- Use of narcotics, antibiotics, and general anesthesia
- Use of excessive cathartics

Physiology of Elimination

Reabsorbtion of water from chime in the large intestine produces a semisolid mass known as **feces.** Feces is a mixture of fiber and undigested food, shed epithelial cells, inorganic material (e.g., calcium and phosphates), bacteria, and water. Small amounts of fat may be present. Gas, or **flatus,** which is produced during digestion, may also be present.

• The Process of Defecation

The process by which the bowel eliminates waste is called **defecation.** When fecal material reaches the rectum, distention stimulates stretch receptors to initiate contraction of the sigmoid colon and rectal muscles, along with relaxation of the internal anal sphincter. At the same time, sensory impulses transmitted to the central nervous system (CNS) produce a conscious urge to defecate. We respond to this signal by voluntarily contracting our diaphragmatic and abdominal muscles to increase downward pressure, while at the same time relaxing the external anal sphincter. These actions allow feces to be propelled through the anus. If we ignore the signal to defecate, the reflexive contractions ease for a few minutes, until mass peristalsis occurs again. A person can increase the pressure to expel feces by contracting the abdominal muscles while maintaining a closed airway. This is called the **Valsalva maneuver.** Although it assists with the passage of stool, clients with heart disease, glaucoma, increased intracranial pressure, or a new surgical wound should be cautioned to avoid the Valsalva maneuver because it raises blood pressure, increases pressure within the abdominal cavity, and is associated with an increased risk for cardiac arrhythmias.

• Normal Defecation Patterns

Many grocery stores, pharmacies, and even convenience stores have half an aisle or more of products devoted to bowel function. Some products promote bowel movements (BMs), and others treat diarrhea. All claim to return the consumer to "regularity." The sheer volume of products suggests that bowel function problems are common. Nevertheless, many people avoid the topic of bowel elimination – it is not typically something they chat about with their neighbors. As a result, many patients have unanswered questions about their bowel function and may turn to you for information. Part of the confusion about bowel function is that there is a wide range of "normal." The frequency of BMs may range from several times per day to once a week. As long as the person passes stools without excessive urgency (needing to rush to the toilet), with minimal effort and no straining, without blood loss, and without the use of laxatives, you can regard bowel function as normal.

Normally stool is approximately 75 % water and 25% solid when expelled. This combination yields a soft, formed semisolid. If passage through the colon is slowed, more water is reabsorbed from the feces. The result is the formation of dry, hard stool that requires more effort to pass. If transit time through the colon is faster than normal, less water is reabsorbed, and stools are watery. Feces is usually brown in color because **bile salts,** which aid in the digestion of fat, are excreted in the feces. Bile is normally golden yellow, but the action of bacteria in the GI tract change the color to brown. Bacteria are also responsible for the odor of feces. Flatus, or gas, is formed in the digestive process. Some is swallowed air that accompanies the intake of food. A small portion diffuses from blood into the GI tract. However, most of the gas is created by bacterial fermentation in the colon. Flatus is a mixture of nitrogen, carbon dioxide, hydrogen, methane, and hydrogen sulphide.

Factors Affect Bowel Elimination

There is a wide range of acceptable frequency for BMs. Each person develops a pattern that is based on several factors.

Developmental Stage: Bowel elimination patterns change throughout the life span. During the first 2 days of life, the newborn passes meconium through the anus. **Meconium** is green-black in color, tarry, and sticky and results from swallowed amniotic fluid. Stools transition to a yellow-green color over the next few days. After that, the appearance of the feces depends largely on the type of feeding the infant receives. Breastfed babies pass golden yellow stools, whereas formula-fed babies pass tan stools. Initially babies defecate frequently, usually after each feeding. The stools tend to be watery while the large intestine is still immature. Gradually normal flora develops in the colon, and stools become firmer and less frequent.

The ability to control defecation typically develops at about 2 to 3 years of age. Toilet training requires neural and muscular control as well as conscious effort. The child must be aware of the urge to defecate, be able to maintain closure of the external anal sphincter while getting to the toilet, and be able to remove clothing. When toddlers become engrossed in play, they sometimes ignore the need to move their bowels, and soiling is common. As children mature, they gradually learn to gain more control over defecation. In fact, school-age children and adolescents often delay defecation until they have come home or have completed an activity.

The bowel pattern set in childhood normally continues into late adulthood if the client consumes adequate fiber and fluid and engages in regular physical activity. However, peristalsis, intestinal smooth muscle tone, perineal muscle tone, and sphincter control normally decrease with aging. These physiological processes can contribute to bowel elimination problems among older adults, especially if they decrease their activity and fiber intake.

Personal and Sociocultural Factors: Privacy is important to most people, as is sufficient time to have a bowel movement without feeling the need to hurry. Clients working in fast-paced jobs may have difficulty even consciously recognizing the need to defecate, and some habitually ignore the need, promoting bowel dysfunction. Parents and caregivers of infants and toddlers may postpone their own toileting needs because of fear of leaving the children alone. Some clients are acutely embarrassed by the thought that anyone might realize they are having a bowel movement and will wait until they are entirely alone before even entering the bathroom.

Stress has a major influence on motility of the GI tract. It may cause diarrhea or constipation, and it is a primary risk factor in the development of *irritable bowel syndrome,* a disorder associated with bloating, pain, and altered bowel function.

Nutrition, Hydration, and Activity Level: Nutrition, hydration, and activity all relate to bowel function.
- *Fiber:* As noted earlier, regular intake of food promotes peristalsis. People who eat on a regular schedule are likely to develop a regular pattern of defecation. Irregular eating creates irregular bowel elimination. The type of food eaten is also important. High-fiber foods promote peristalsis and defecation by increasing bulk certain high-fiber foods are given below:
  - Apples with skin
  - Bran cereal
  - Broccoli, cauliflower, and other cruciferous vegetables
  - Cabbage
  - Carrots
  - Cherries
  - Corn
  - Dried beans, peas, and legumes
  - Dried fruits
  - Flaxseed
  - Greens such as chard,
  - Kale, collards, and turnip greens
  - Oatmeal
  - Oranges
  - Pears with skin
  - Plums with skin
  - Popcorn
  - Potato with skin
  - Prunes
  - Raisins
  - Strawberries
  - Whole-grain cereal products

  Bulky foods absorb fluids and increase stool mass. The increased mass stretches bowel walls, initiating peristalsis and the defecation reflex. Other foods have specific effects in the bowel. For example, the active bacteria in yogurt stimulate peristalsis, while at the same time promoting healing of intestinal infections. Low-fiber foods, such as pasta and other simple carbohydrates and lean meats, slow peristalsis. Foods like broccoli, onions, and beans lead to excess gas in many people. Spicy foods may also cause gas, as well as more frequent bowel movements.

  Dietary supplements can also affect bowel function. For example, calcium supplements cause constipation in many clients, whereas magnesium loosens stools. Supplemental vitamin C softens stools and, in high doses, may cause diarrhea in sensitive clients.
- *Fluids:* A minimum of 6 to 8 glasses (1400 to 2000 mL) of fluid per day is required to promote healthful bowel function. Inadequate fluid intake or excessive fluid loss, as in diarrhea or vomiting, slows peristalsis and leads to dry, hard stools that are difficult to pass. Excessive fluid intake (especially beverages with high sugar content) may lead to rapid passage through the colon and soft or watery stools. Different types of fluids have varying effects on sensitive individuals. For instance, consuming large amounts of milk may cause constipation in some people. Coffee promotes peristalsis in many clients and may even cause loose stools in sensitive clients.
- *Activity:* Physical activity seems to stimulate peristalsis and bowel elimination. In addition, sedentary people are likely to have weaker abdominal muscles. Clients with health concerns that limit activity (e.g., such as shortness of breath, pain, or required bed rest) often experience constipation.

Medications and Procedures: Many medications may affect peristalsis. All oral medicines have the potential to affect the function of the GI tract. Examples include the following:
- *Antacids,* often used for heartburn, neutralize stomach acid but may slow peristalsis.

- *Aspirin and other nonsteroidal anti-inflammatory drugs (NSAIDs),* such as ibuprofen, irritate the stomach. Repeated use can lead to ulceration of the stomach or duodenum.
- *Antibiotics* given to combat infection decrease the normal flora in the colon. The result is often diarrhea. Bacterial populations can be maintained with supplements of probiotics (e.g., acidophilus) or daily consumption of yogurt.
- *Iron,* a common mineral supplement, is available as an over-the-counter (OTC) medication and is often prescribed for the treatment of anemia. Iron has an astringent effect on the bowel and is notorious for causing constipation.
- *Pain medications,* particularly opioids (narcotics), slow peristalsis and are associated with a high incidence of constipation.
- *Antimotility drugs,* such as diphenoxylate (Lomotil) may be used to treat diarrhea. They work by slowing peristalsis.
- *Laxatives* are used to treat constipation. In general, laxatives work by stimulating peristalsis. They come in many forms and are frequently abused by people who self-medicate with OTC drugs.

Clients undergoing anesthesia and surgery often experience sluggish bowel elimination. The delay in bowel elimination may be caused by a variety of circumstances:

- *Anesthesia:* General anesthesia (which renders the patient unconscious) and analgesics (administered preoperatively and postoperatively for pain) slow bowel motility. Spinal anesthesia and epidural anesthesia are less likely to cause this effect.
- *Stress:* Regardless of the type of anesthesia, most clients find surgery a stressful event. If stress activates the general adaptation syndrome (GAS), autonomic nervous system and endocrine responses ensue. Among those responses is a slowing of peristalsis.
- *Manipulation of the bowel during surgery:* Abdominal or pelvic surgery in which the bowel is manipulated may result in a **paralytic ileus,** a cessation of bowel peristalsis. Although peristalsis halts, the bowel continues to produce secretions. Without peristalsis, secretions remain stagnant, causing distention and discomfort. To decrease the complications of paralytic ileus, patients who have had bowel surgery typically have a nasogastric (NG) tube with low constant or intermittent suction. The NG tube removes secretions until peristalsis returns.
- *Decreased mobility:* After surgery, patients often experience discomfort that affects mobility. This further hinders GI motility and increases the risk for constipation.
- *Perineal surgery:* Patients who have had surgical interventions involving the perineal region may fear pain or that their sutures will "tear" or "break" during bowel elimination, and therefore they resist the urge to evacuate their bowel.
- *Anal sphincter surgery:* Patients who have had surgery that disrupts the anal sphincter may experience uncontrolled drainage after surgery.

Pregnancy: In early pregnancy, many women experience fluid loss due to "morning sickness" – periods of nausea and vomiting – which, despite the name, may occur at any time of day. As the pregnancy progresses, the growing uterus crowds and displaces the intestines, and the increased level of progesterone slows intestinal motility. As a result, pregnant women often experience constipation, decreased appetite, and irregular food intake. In addition, the increasing pressure of the uterus and the increased blood volume of normal pregnancy increase the woman's risk for hemorrhoids.

Pathological Conditions: Several disorders affect bowel function. Among them are neurological disorders that affect innervation of the lower GI tract, cognitive conditions that limit the ability to sense the urge to defecate, pain or immobility that leads to sluggish peristalsis, and pathological conditions of the GI tract. Constipation and diarrhea are discussed in the "Nursing Diagnosis" section of the chapter. Other common disorders are food allergies, food intolerances, and diverticulosis.

- *Food allergies:* Food allergy is a true immune system reaction prompted by the presence in the body of an allergenic food. Some common food allergens include dairy products, egg whites, shellfish, wheat, peanuts, citrus fruits, and soy. Immune responses to foods manifest as a variety of symptoms ranging from a mild rash to anaphylactic shock. Common GI symptoms suggesting food allergy include constipation, diarrhea, a burn like rash around the anus, abdominal discomfort, bloating, excessive gas, and intestinal bleeding.
- *Food intolerances:* In contrast to a food allergy, a **food intolerance** is specifically linked to the GI system. It produces such symptoms as GI discomfort, pain, gas, bloating, diarrhea, or constipation after the person consumes the food. An example is *lactose intolerance,* a deficiency of the enzyme lactase, which is responsible for the breakdown of milk sugar (lactose). Such symptoms can mimic those of a food allergy, but food intolerances are not caused by immune responses.
- *Diverticulosis:* When the colon must repeatedly move highly compacted fecal material, over time the longitudinal and circular muscles enlarge. This increases force on the mucosal tissues, causing them to "balloon" out between the muscles and to form pouches in which fecal matter becomes trapped. The development of these saclike outpouchings of mucosa through the muscle layers of the colon wall is a condition called **diverticulosis.** In some cases, the pouches become infected, a condition called **diverticulitis,** and antibiotics or surgery is required. People whose diets are low in fiber or consist mainly of refined foods are especially at risk for diverticulosis.

Bowel Diversions: A bowel diversion is a surgically created opening for elimination of digestive waste products. The procedure is performed for clients with a variety of conditions, including cancer, ulcerations, trauma, or inadequate blood supply. A client with a bowel diversion does not eliminate via the anus. Instead, the **effluent** (output) is expelled through a surgically created opening in the abdominal wall, called a **stoma** or **ostomy.** The effluent may range from liquid to solid, depending on the part of the bowel that is being diverted. A bowel diversion close to the ileocecal valve (between the small

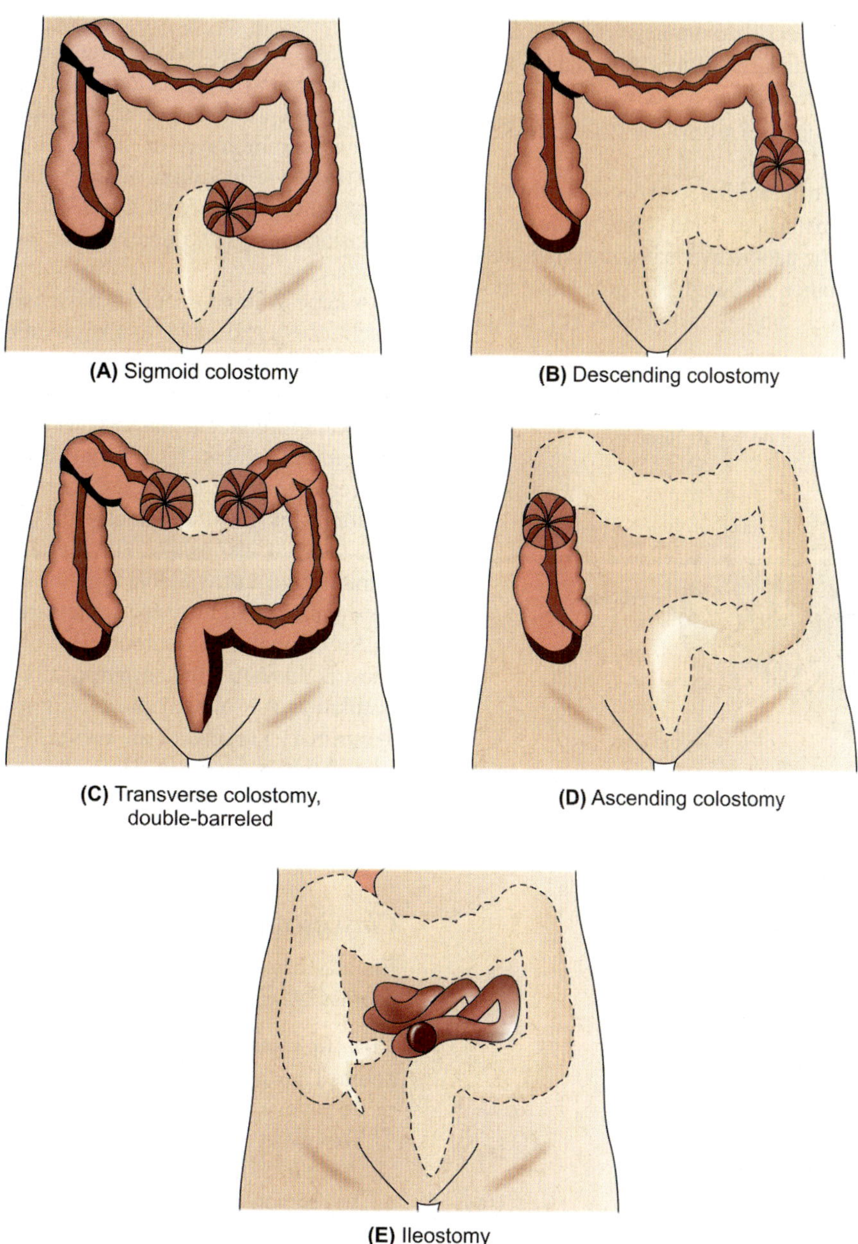

Figure 16.1: Location of various bowel diversion ostomies

and large intestine) will have a constant flow of liquid effluent. In contrast, a bowel diversion close to the rectum will have effluent that resembles feces (Fig. 16.1).

Bowel diversions may be temporary or permanent. *Temporary bowel diversions* are common after surgical interventions for being conditions of the bowel. They allow healing of the distal portion of the bowel. Once adequate healing has occurred, surgical **reanastomosis** (reconnection) of the bowel is performed, and the patient once again has BMs from the anus. *Permanent bowel diversions* are performed if the bowel is necrotic (Dead) or cannot be salvaged because of severe disease or trauma. An **ileostomy** brings a portion of the ileum through a

surgical opening in the abdomen, bypassing the large intestine entirely. Drainage at this level is liquid and continuous. The patient must wear an ostomy appliance at all times to collect the drainage. Two variations of an ileostomy are designed to control drainage more effectively and to cause less body image disturbance. However, many clients are not candidates for these procedures because of their underlying disease

(a) Sigmoid colostomy

(b) Descending colostomy

(c) Transverse colostomy double-barrelled

(d) Ascending colostomy

(e) Ileostomy

- A **Kock pouch,** or continent ileostomy, creates an internal pouch, or reservoir, to collect ileal drainage (Fig. 16.2A). to drain the pouch, the patient inserts a tube through the external stoma into the pouch several times per day. This alternative avoids continuous drainage and allows the patient to be free of an ostomy appliance.

A **total colectomy with ileaoanal reservoir** removes the colon, creates a pouch from the ileum, and connects the ileum to the rectum (Fig. 16.2B). The patient evacuates the bowel on the commode in the usual manner. Although this procedure should result in continence of bowel elimination, the feces will be liquid.

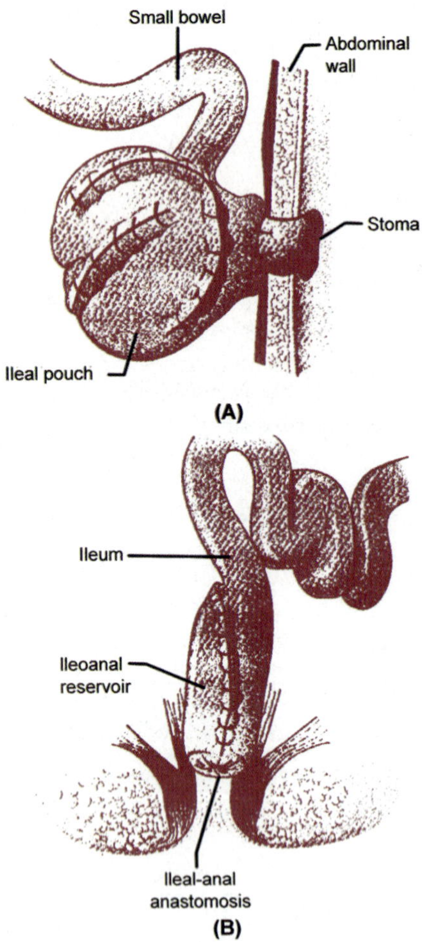

Figures 16.2A and B: Ileostomy variations. A. Continent ileostomy (Kock pouch) B. Ileoanal reservoir

A **colostomy** brings a portion of the colon through a surgical opening in the abdomen. The location of the colostomy determines the consistency of the feces eliminated, as well as the need to wear an ostomy appliance. The closer the colostomy is to the ascending colon, the more liquid and continuous the drainage will be. In contrast, a colostomy close to the sigmoid colon will produce solid feces. Colostomies near the rectum, such as sigmoid colostomies, can often be controlled by diet and irrigation. As a result, the client may not need to wear an ostomy appliance to collect drainage.

Enemas

An enema is a solution inserted into the rectum and sigmoid colon to remove feces and/or flatus. Enemas can also be used to instill medications or nutrition. A cleansing enema is probably the most common type of enema. This type of enema stimulates peristalsis via irritation of the colon/rectum and by causing intestinal distention with fluid. There are two general types of cleansing enemas; the large-volume enema and the small-volume enema.

A large-volume enema is designed to clean the colon of as much feces as possible. In a large-volume enema, between 500 and 1,000 cc of fluid are instilled into the rectum/colon, and the client is asked to retain the fluid as long as possible.

Small-volume enemas are designed to clear the rectum and the sigmoid colon of fecal matter. Small-volume enemas can be delivered with the traditional enema kit using 50 to 200 cc of solution, but most frequently they are administered using a prepackaged disposable kit. Prepackaged enemas are easily administered and available over-the-counter in most drugstores. This makes them ideal for home care use.

An enema is the introduction of a solution into the large intestine, usually for the purpose of removing feces. It is the instillation of a solution into the sigmoid colon. As stated earlier, the primary purpose of an enema is to promote defecation by stimulating peristalsis. Here the instilled solution distends intestine, may irritate intestinal mucosa, and then increases peristalsis. The volume of fluid instilled breaks up the fecal mass, stretches the rectal wall and initiates the defecation reflex.

Classification of Enemas

Enemas are classified as cleansing, retention or return flow enemas. A brief description of enemas are as follows.

Cleansing enemas: These are given to remove feces from the colon. They are used for following purposes:
- To relieve constipation or fecal impaction
- To prevent involuntary escape of fecal material during surgical procedures
- To promote visualization of the intestinal tract by X-ray film or instrument examination
- To help establish regular bowel function during a bowel training program

The most frequent types of solution used for cleansing enemas are tap water (hyptonic), normal saline solution (isotonic), soapsuds solution, and low volume hypertonic solution. The suggested maximum volume according to age groups of clients are as follows:
- Infant   150 to 250 mL
- Toddler   250 to 350 mL
- Schoolage   300 to 500 mL
- Adolescent   500 to 750 mL
- Adult   750 to 1000 mL

The large volumes of solution may present a danger to clients with weakened intestinal walls. These solutions often require special preparation and equipment.

Hypertonic solution preparations are available commercially and are administered in smaller volume (adult 70 to 130 mL). These solutions draw water into the colon, which stimulates the defecation relax. They may be contraindicated in clients for whom sodium retention is a protcem, and clients who dehydrated and young infants.

Soapsuds may be added to tap water or saline to create the effect the intestinal irrigation. Only pure castile soap is safe. Harsh soaps or detergents can cause serious bowels inflammation. The recommended ratio of soap solution is 5 mL (1 teaspoon) of castile soap to 1000 mL of warm water or saline.

A doctor may prescribe a high or low cleansing enema. The term high or low refers to the height from which and hence the pressure with which the fluid is delivered. High enemas are given to cleanse the entire colon. Fluid is delivered at a high pressure by raising the enema container to a high level. During administration of a regular enema, the enema can or bag is held 30 inches (12 cm) above the client hips. With a high enema the bag or can will be raised 5 to 45 cm (125 to 18 inches) or slightly higher. The client is asked to turn from the left lateral to the dorsal recumbent, over to the right lateral position. The position change ensures that fluid reaches the large bowel. With a low enema the nurse holds the can 7.5 cm or 3 inches or less above the clients hips. Low enema cleans only the rectum and sigmoid colon.

Retention enemas: These are retained in the bowel for a prolonged period for different reasons as given below:
- *Oil retention enemas*—lubricate the blood and intestinal mucosa, making defecation easier. About 150 to 200 mL of solution is administered to adults
- *Carminative enemas*—help to expel flatus from the rectum and provide relief from gaseous distention. Common solution includes milk and molasses enema (equal parts) and the MCW enema (30 mL of magnesium sulphate, 60 mL of glycerin and 90 mL of warm water)
- *Medicated enema*—used to administer medication that are absorbed through rectal mucosa (e.g. dexamethosone and ulcerative colitis, neomycin solution, before bowel surgery)
- *Antihelminthic enema*—administered to destroy intestinal parasites
- *Nutritive enema*—administered fluids and nutrition rectally.

Return-flow enemas or Harris flush enemas: These are occasionally presented to expel flatus. For an adult, 100 to 200 ml of a solution is instilled into the rectum and sigmoid colon and then the solution container is lowered so that the solution flows back into the container. This process is repeated five or six times, and the alternating flow of solution stimulates peristalsis and helps on the expelling flatus. The procedure is terminated when abdominal distention is released. If the return solution becomes thick with feces, it is replaced by fresh solution.

An oil retention enema is a small-volume enema that instills oil into the rectum, retained for up to an hour to soften very hard stool. It is often followed by a large-volume cleansing enema. A small-volume enema can deliver a medicated solution directly to the rectal mucosa. This method is useful when the rectum is the area to be medicated, if the client is unable to take oral medications, or if rapid absorption of the medication is required. The return-flow enema, used to remove flatus and stimulate peristalsis, is frequently given following abdominal surgery to reduce intestinal distention and to stimulate the resumption of bowel function.

Many different solutions are used for enemas, including tap water, normal saline, hypertonic solutions, soap solutions, oil, and carminative solutions. Tap water is a hypotonic solution. Because it is a less concentrated solution than the body's cell, it is drawn into the body and may cause water toxicity, electrolyte imbalance, or circulatory overload. Normal saline is an isotonic solution. It is the same concentration as the body's own fluids and is considered a safe enema solution. It is important that children and infants be given only normal saline enemas because their small size predisposes them to fluid imbalances. Prepackaged small-volume enemas use hypertonic solutions to draw fluid from the body to lubricate the stool and distend the rectum. Hypertonic solutions are contraindicated in dehydrated clients and small children. Carminative solutions are used to prevent gas from forming.

Enemas are contraindicated in clients with bowel obstruction, inflammation, or infection of the abdomen or if the client has had recent rectal or anal surgery. If there is any question regarding the advisability of administering an enema, consult the client's health care provider.

Administration of Enema (Table 16.1)

Prior to procedure the nurse should
1. Identify the type of enema ordered as well as the rationale for the enema. Allows the nurse to verify the appropriateness of the type of enema ordered.
2. Assess the physical condition of the client. Determine if the client has bowel sounds. Assess for a history of constipation, hemorrhoids, or diverticulitis. Determine if the client will be able to hold a side-lying or knee-chest position or be able to retain the enema solution. Allows the nurse to plan the procedure with the client's limitations in mind.
3. Assess the client's mental state, including ability to understand and cooperate with the procedure, the client's knowledge level regarding the procedure, and any preexisting fears the client may have regarding the procedure, knowing if the client can comprehend and cooperate with the procedure will help the nurse plan ahead. Many clients have preexisting fears and beliefs regarding enemas and their administration.

Equipment Needed For Giving Enema includes

Large-Volume Cleansing Enema
- Absorbent pad for the bed
- Disposable gloves
- Bedside commode or bedpan if client will not be able to ambulate to bathroom

- Lubricant
- Enema container
- Tubing with clamp and nozzle
- Thermometer for enema solution
- Toilet tissue
- IV pole
- Washcloth, towel, and basin

Small-Volume Prepackaged Enema
- Prescribed prepackaged enema
- Lubricant if the tip is not prelubricated

- Toilet tissue
- Bedpan or commode if the client cannot use the bathroom
- Absorbent pad for bed
- Gloves

Return-Flow Enema
- Absorbent pad for the bed
- Disposable gloves
- Bedside commode or bedpan if client will not be able to ambulate to bathroom
- Prescribed solution

Table 16.1: Administration of Enema			
	Nursing actions		*Rationales*
	Check clients identification band Explain procedure before beginning		To identity right patient To get cooperation and reduce anxiety
1.	Cleanse hands.	1.	Reduces the transmission of microorganisms.
2.	Assess client's understanding of procedure and provide privacy.	2.	Prepares client for procedure.
3.	Apply gloves.	3.	Prevents contact with feces.
4.	Prepare equipment	4.	Ensures a smooth procedure.
5.	Place absorbent pad on bed under client. Assist client in attaining left lateral position with right leg flexed as sharply as possible. If there is a question regarding the client's ability to hold the solution, place a bedpan on the bed nearby	5.	Facilitates flow of solution into the rectum and colon. The flexed leg provides the best exposure of the anus.
6.	If specified, heat solution to desired temperature using thermometer to measure. Enemas administered to adults are usually given at 105° to 110°F(40.5° to 43°C), and those administered to children are usually administered at 100°F (37.7°C). Solution should be at least body temperature to prevent cramping and discomfort.	6.	Enemas work best when solution is warm. If enemas are too hot, damage can be done to the bowel mucosa. If enemas are too cold, spasms may occur.
7.	Pour solution into the bag or bucket; add water if needed. Open clamp and allow solution to prime tubing. Clamp tubing when primed.	7.	Expels air from the tubing, which could cause intestinal distention and discomfort.
8.	Lubricate 5 cm (2 inches) of the rectal tube unless the tube is part of prelubricated enema set.	8.	Minimizes trauma to the anal sphincter during insertion of the rectal tube.
9.	Hold the enema container level with the rectum. Ask the client to take a deep breath. Simultaneously, slowly and smoothly insert rectal tube into rectum approximately 7 to 10 cm in an adult. The rectum of an adult is usually 10 to 20 cm (4 to 6 inches). The tube should be inserted beyond the internal sphincter. Aim the rectal tube toward the client's umbilicus.	9.	A deep breath helps relax the sphincter. Insertion of rectal tube toward the umbilicus guides tube along rectum.
10.	Raise the solution container and open clamp. (If using an enema set, squeeze the container holding solution). The solution should be 30 to 45 cm (12 to 18 inches) above the rectum for an adult and 7.5 cm (3 inches) above the rectum for an infant. The solution may be placed on an IV pole at the proper height (Fig. 16.3)	10.	Solution should be at a height above rectum that allows gravity flow of solution into the rectum, but does not cause damage to the rectal lining because of a too-rapid increase in rectal pressure.
11.	Slowly administer the fluid.	11.	Decreases the incidence of intestinal spasms and cramps.

Contd...

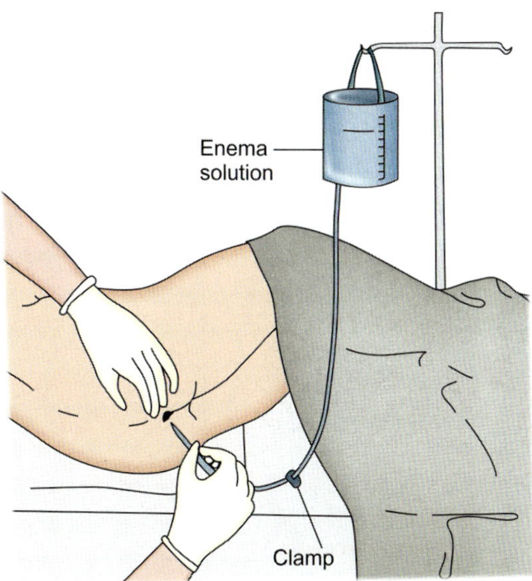

Figure 16.3: Enema administration

	Table 16.1: *Contd....*			
	Nursing actions			*Rationales*
12.	When solution has been completely administered or when the client cannot hold any more fluid, clamp the tubing, remove the rectal tube, and dispose of it properly.		12.	The urge to defecate indicates that a sufficient amount of fluid has been administered.
13.	Clean lubricant, any solution, and any feces from the anus with toilet tissue.		13.	Minimizes skin irritation.
14.	Have the client continue to lie on the left side for the prescribed length of time.		14.	Certain types of enemas are more effective when retained for a specified amount of time. It is easier for the client to retain the enema in a lying position, where gravity can be resisted.
15.	When the client has retained the enema for the prescribed amount of time, assist to the bedside commode or toilet or onto the bedpan. If the client is using the bathroom, instruct not to flush the toilet when finished.		15.	Client will be prepared to expel fluid and feces. Caregiver can see results of the enema.
16.	When the client is finished expelling the enema, assist to clean the perineal area if needed.		16.	Prevents skin breakdown and excoriation.
17.	Return the client to a comfortable position. Place a clean, dry protective pad under the client to catch any solution or feces that may continue to be expelled.		17.	Provides comfort for the client and protects the linen from potential soiling.
18.	Remove gloves and cleanse hands.		18.	Reduces transmission of microorganisms.
Small-Volume Prepackaged Enema				
19.	Cleanse hands.		19.	Reduces transmission of microorganisms.
20.	Remove prepackaged enema from packaging. Be familiar with any special instructions included with the enema. The packaged enema may be stood in a basin of warm the fluid before use.		20.	Prepares the enema for use.
21.	Apply gloves.		21.	Protects hands from exposure to feces.

Contd...

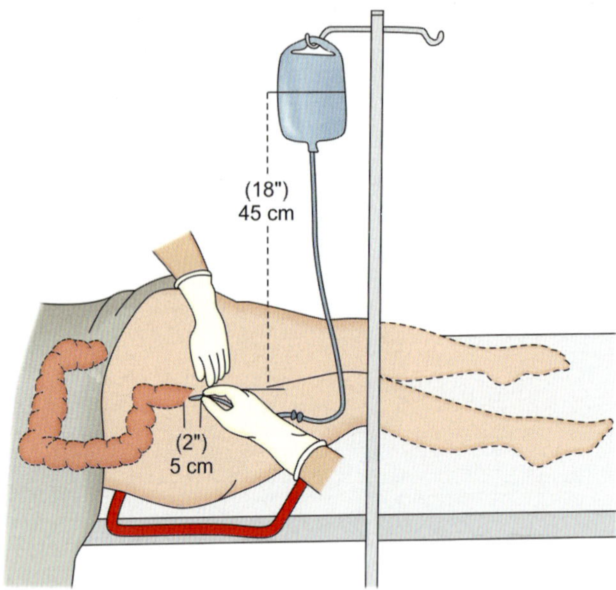

Figure 16.4: Placing the patient in left lateral position while administering enema

		Table 16.1: *Contd....*		
	Nursing actions			*Rationales*
22.	Place absorbent pad on bed under client. Assist client in attaining left lateral position with right leg flexed as sharply as possible, or you may use the knee-chest position (Fig. 16.4). If there is a question regarding the client's ability to hold the solution, place a bedpan on the bed nearby.		22.	Facilitates flow of solution into the rectum and colon. The flexed leg provides the best exposure of the anus. The knee-chest position provides good exposure and allows gravity to aid in retention of the enema.
23.	Remove the protective cap from the nozzle for lubrication. If the lubrication is not adequate, add more.		23.	Prevents trauma to the rectal mucosa.
24.	Squeeze the container gently to remove any air and prime the nozzle.		24.	Reduces introduction of air into the rectum.
25.	Have the client take a deep breath. Simultaneously, gently insert the enema nozzle into the anus, pointing the nozzle toward the umbilicus.		25.	Relaxes the rectal sphincter. Pointing the nozzle toward the umbilicus positions the nozzle away from the rectal walls.
26.	Squeeze the container until all the solution is instilled.		26.	Allows the client to get the full benefit of the solution.
27.	Remove the nozzle from the anus and dispose of the empty container in a trash receptacle.		27.	Prevents the spread of microorganisms.
28.	Clean lubricant, any solution, and any feces from the anus with toilet tissue.		28.	Minimizes skin irritation.
29.	Have the client continue to lie on the left side for the prescribed length of time.		29.	Certain types of enemas are more effective when retained for a specified amount of time. It is easier for the client to retain the enema in a lying position, where gravity can be resisted.
30.	When the client has retained the enema for the prescribed amount of time, assist to the bedside commode or toilet or onto the bedpan. If the client is using the bathroom, instruct not to flush the toilet when finished.		30.	Client will be prepared to expel fluid and feces.
31.	When the client is finished expelling the enema, assist to clean the perineal area if needed.		31.	Prevents skin breakdown and excoriation.

Contd...

Table 16.1: *Contd....*

	Nursing Actions		Rationales
32.	Return the client to a comfortable position. Place a clean, dry protective pad under the client to catch any solution or feces that may continue to be expelled.	32.	Provides comfort for the client and protects the linen from potential soiling.
33.	Remove gloves and cleanse hands.	33.	Reduces transmission of microorganisms.
Return-Flow Enema			
34.	Follow Actions 1–9	34.	See Rationales 1–9.
35.	Raise the solution container and open clamp. The solution should be 30 to 45 cm (12 to 18 inches) above the rectum for an adult and 7.5 cm (3 inches) above the rectum for an infant.	35.	Solution should be at a height that allows gravity flow of solution into the rectum, but does not cause damage to the rectal lining because of a too rapid increase in rectal pressure.
36.	Slowly administer approximately 200 cc of solution.	36.	Momentary pauses decrease the incidence of intestinal spasms and cramps.
37.	Clamp the tubing and lower the enema container 12 to 18 inches below the client's rectum. Open the clamp.	37.	Allows the solution to flow back out of the rectum.
38.	Observe the solution container for air bubbles as the solution returns. Not any fecal particles that may be returned.	38.	Assesses the effectiveness of the procedure. Air bubbles in the container indicate flatus being passed from the rectum.
39.	When no further solution is returned to the container, clamp the tubing and raise the enema container 12 to 18 inches above the client's rectum. Open the clamp and instill approximately 200 cc of fluid.	39.	Continues to stimulate peristalsis and remove flatus.
40.	Repeat raising and lowering the solution container until no further flatus is seen. Most institutions have guidelines regarding the number of returns to perform. A good rule of thumb is not more than 3 times.	40.	Limiting the number of returns prevents unduly tiring or stressing the client.
41.	After the final return of fluid, clamp the tubing and gently remove it from the client's anus. Clean the anus with tissue to remove any lubricant or solution.	41.	Prevents skin irritation.
42.	If the client feels the need to empty his or her rectum, assist onto the bedpan or up to the bathroom or commode.	42.	Allows any retained solution to be expelled. Stimulates peristalsis.
43.	When the client is finished expelling any retained solution, assist to clean the perineal area if needed.	43.	Prevents skin breakdown and excoriation.
44.	Return the client to a comfortable position. Place a clean, dry protective pad under the client to catch any solution or feces that may continues to be expelled.	44.	Provides comfort for the client and protects the linen from potential soiling.
45.	Remove gloves and cleanse hands.	45.	Reduces transmission of microorganisms.

- Lubricant
- Enema container
- Tubing with clamp and nozzle
- Thermometer
- Toilet tissue

After Procedure the Nurse should see that
- The client's rectum is free of feces or flatus.
- The client experienced a minimum of trauma and embarrassment from the procedure.

And Document the Procedure in Nurses' Notes
- Time and date of the procedure
- Type of enema given, amount of fluid infused and returned, and amount and description of the feces expelled
- Client's tolerance for the procedure and any complaints or unusual findings

Medication Administration Record (MAR)
- If this is a medicated enema, be sure to note it on the MAR

And Maintain Intake and Output Record
- If the amount of fluid returned is significantly less than the amount infused, note this on the I&O record.

Administering a Cleansing Enema (Table 16.2)

Equipment: Commercially-prepared enema kits include a flexible bottle containing hypertonic solution with an attaches prelubricated firm tip about 5 to 7.5 cm (2 to 3 inches) in length. Its easy use makes it particularly convenient in the home setting; client can readily administer their own enema in many instances.

For the hypotonic, isotonic or soapsuds enema, a container, rubber or plastic tubing with side openings near its distal end, a tubing clamp, lubricant and the solution are necessary. Although the commercially-prepared equipment is sterile, and any reusable equipment is sterile, and any reusable equipment is sterilized between clients in a hospital, the procedure of administering an enema requires clean or medical asepsis technique, not sterile technique. Disposable gloves protect the caregiver from exposure to blood, body substances and microorganism. In brief, the following equipments are needed:
- Disposable enema set or enema can with accessories
- Water soluble lubricant
- Solution as ordered by physicians
- Temperature: For adults: 105°-110°F (40°-43°C)
                            For children: 100°F (37.7°C)
- Amount will vary, depending on type of solution, age of the person, and the client's ability to return the solution (see suggested volume)
- Necessary additives (soap, salt and so forth)
- Bath thermometer
- Waterproof pad
- Bath blanket
- Bed pan and toilet tissue
- IV pole
- Disposable gloves
- Paper towel
- Wash cloth, soap and towel or handwipes.

Table 16.2: Procedures for Administering Cleansing Enema (Home Setting)

	Nursing actions		*Rationales*
1.	Assemble the necessary equipment. Warm solutions in amount ordered, and check temperature with a bath thermometer if available. If tap water is used, adjust temperature as it flows from faucet.	1.	Organization facilitates performance of task; if bath thermometer is not available, warm to room temperature or slightly higher and test on inner wrist.
2.	Explain this procedure to the client and plan where he or she will defecate. Have a bedpan commode, or nearly bathroom ready for his or her use.	2.	The client is better able to relax and cooperate if he or she is familiarized with the procedure and knows every thing is in readiness when the urge to defecate is felt.
3.	Wash your hands.	3.	It deters spread of microorganism.
4.	Add enema solution to container. Release the clamp and allow fluid to progress through tube before reclamping.	4.	This may cause air to be expelled from the tubing. Although allowing air to enter the intestine is not harmful, it may further distend the intestine.
5.	Position waterproof pad under the client.	5.	This protects bed linen.
6.	Provide for client's privacy, position and drape the client on the left side (Sims' position) with anus exposed or on the back, as dictated by client comfort and condition.	6.	The client's comfort and warmth help him or her to relax. The exact position of the relining person has not been found to alter results of an enema significantly.
7.	Put on disposable gloves.	7.	This protects the nurse from microorganisms in the feces.
8.	Elevate the solution so that it is 45 cm (18 inches) above the level of the client's anus. Plan to give the solution slowly over a period of 5 to 10 minutes. The container may be hung on a IV pole or held in the nurse's hands at the proper height.	8.	Gravity forces the solution to enter the intestine. The amount of pressure determines the rate of flow and pressure exerted on the intestinal wall. Giving the solution too quickly causes rapid distention and pressure in the intestine, resulting in too rapid expulsion of the solution, poor defecation, or damage to the mucous membrane.
9.	Generally lubricate the end of the rectal tube for 5 to 7 cm (2-3 inches). A disposable enema set may have a prelubricated rectal tube.	9.	This facilitates passage of the rectal tube through the anal sphincter and prevents injury to the mucosa.
10.	Lift the buttock to expose the anus. Slowly and gently insert the rectal tube 7 to 10 cm (3-4 inches). Direct it at an angle pointing toward the umbilicus.	10.	Good visualization of the anus helps prevent injury to tissues. The anal canal is about 2.5 to 5 cm in length. The tube should be inserted past the internal sphincter. Further insertion may damage intestinal mucosa membrane. The suggested angle follows the normal intestinal contour. Slow insertion of the tube minimizes spasms of the intestinal wall and sphincters.

Contd...

Table 16.2: *Contd...*

	Nursing actions		Rationales
11.	If the tube meets resistance while inserting it, permit a small amount of solution to enter, withdraw the tube slightly and then continue to insert it. Do not force entry of the tube. Ask the client to take several deep breaths.	11.	Resistance may be due to spasms of the intestine of failure of the internal sphincter to open. The solution may help reduce spasms are relax the sphincter, thus making continued insertion of the tube safe. Facing a tube may injure the intestinal wall. Taking deep breath helps relax the anal sphincter.
12.	Introduce the solution slowly over a period of 5 to 10 minutes. Hold tubing all the time that solution is being instilled. Commercial preparations may be administered by compressing container with hands, according to package directions.	12.	Introducing solution slowly helps prevent rapid distention of the intestine and a desire to defecate.
13.	Clamp the tubing or lower the container if the client has the desire to defecate or clamping occurs. Client also may be instructed to take small, fast breaths or to part.	13.	These techniques help relax muscles and prevent the expulsion of the solution prematurely.
14.	After solution has been given, clamp the tubing and remove the tube, have paper towel ready to receive tube as it is withdrawn. Have the client retain the solution until the urge to defect becomes strong, usually in about 5 to 15 minutes.	14.	This amount of time usually allows muscle contraction to become sufficient to produce good results.
15.	Remove disposable gloves from inside out and discard.	15.	This protects the nurse from contact with any microorganism.
16.	When the client has a strong urge to defecate, place him or her in a sitting position on a bedpan or assist to a commode or to the toilet.	16.	The sitting position is most natural and facilitates the act of defecation.
17.	Record the character of the stool, and the client's reaction to enema. Remind the client not to flush commode before nurse inspects result of enema.	17.	The nurse needs to observe and record the results. Additional enema may be necessary if physician may order enemas 'until clear.'
18.	Assist client if necessary with cleaning of anal area. After wash cloth, soap, and water to wash clients hands.	18.	Deters spread of microorganism.
19.	Leave the client clean and comfortable, care for equipment properly.	19.	There is abundant growth of bacteria in the intestines which can spread to others, when equipment is improper.
20.	Wash your hands.	20.	It deters spread of microorganism.

Special consideration: Many different types of appliances are available, the nurse should always read manufacturer's instructions or check with the enterostomal therapist before handling unfamiliar equipment. Flatus may cause a pouch to balloon out. This requires immediate attention because if flatus is not released, the pouch may separate from the skin barrier causing seepage of fecal contents or release of fecal odor. Open the clamp and release the flatus. Never puncture a hole in the appliance.

Age considerations: A one-piece appliance makes application easier for an older client, particularly if impaired vision or compromised mobility from arthritis is present.

Home care: Written directions should always be sent home with the client.

Considerations: Encourage client to participate in a support group.

Changing a Stone Appliance on Ileal Conduit

Refer to Tables 16.3 and 16.4.

Table 16.3: Procedures for Changing a Stoma Appliance on Ileal Conduit

Equipment

- Basin with warm water, soap, towel, washcloth or cotton ball
- Graduated container
- Skin protectant or barrier
- Sterile 2 × 2 gauze squares
- Ostomy bag cut to the correct stomal size (with adhesive backed faceplate, if available)
- Ostomy belt (optional)
- Adhesive cement (optional for reusable pouches)
- Disposable gloves

	Nursing actions		*Rationales*
1.	Explain the procedure and encourage the client to observe or participate if possible. Provide for privacy.	1.	Observing or assisting with procedure encourages self-acceptance.
2.	Assemble the equipment.	2.	Organization facilitates performance of task.
3.	Wash your hands and don disposable gloves. Gloves protect the nurse from blood, body substances, and microorganisms.	3.	Handwashing deters the spread of microorganisms.
4.	Have the client sit or stand if able to assist with procedure or assume supine position on the bed.	4.	These positions result in less abdominal folds and facilitate removal and application of the device.
5.	Empty the pouch being warm into the graduated container (before removing, if it is reusable and not attached to straight drainage).	5.	Having the pouch empty before handling it reduces the likelihood of spilling the excretions. The physician may have ordered recording of intake and output.
6.	Gently remove the pouch face plate from the skin.	6.	The seal between the surface of the faceplate can be removed. Harsh handling of the appliance can damage the skin and impair the development of a secure seal in the future.
7.	Discard the pouch appropriately if disposable, or wash reusable pouch in lukewarm soap and water and allow to air dry.	7.	Thorough cleaning and airing of the appliance reduce odor and deterioration. For aesthetic and infection control purposes, used appliances should be discarded appropriately.
8.	Clean the skin around the stoma with soap and water or a commercial cleaner using washcloth or cotton balls. Make sure you remove all of old adhesive from the skin.	8.	Cleaning the skin removes excretions and old adhesive and skin protectant. Excretions or a build-up of other substances can irritate and damage the skin.
9.	Gently pat dry. Make sure the skin around the stoma is thoroughly dry. Assess the stoma and the condition of the surrounding skin.	9.	Careful drying prevents trauma to the skin and stoma. An intact, properly applied urinary collection device protects skin integrity. Any change in the color and size of the stoma may indicate circulatory problems.
10.	Place a gauze square or two over the stoma opening.	10.	Continuous drainage must be absorbed to keep the skin dry during the appliance change.
11.	Apply a skin protectant to a 5 cm (2 inches) radius around the stoma, and allow it to dry completely, which takes about 30 seconds.	11.	The skin needs protection from the excoriating effect of the excretion and appliance adhesive. Allowing the protectant to dry completely enhances its effectiveness.
12.	If necessary, enlarge the size of the faceplate opening to fit the stoma.	12.	The appliance should fit snugly around the stoma, with only 1/16 to 1/8 inch of skin visible around the opening. A faceplate opening that is too small can cause trauma to the stoma. Exposed skin will be irritated by urine if the opening is too large.
13.	Apply adhesive to the faceplate or remove the protective covering from the disposable faceplate, carefully position the appliance, and press it in place, moving from the center outward. Remove the gauze squares from the stoma before applying the pouch.	13.	The appliance is effective only if it is properly positioned and securely adhered. Commercial deodorants may be used if odor is a problem.
14.	Secure the optional belt to the appliance and around the client.	14.	An elasticized belt helps support the appliance for some people.
15.	Remove or discard the equipment and assess the client's response to the procedure. Wash your hands and remove gloves.	15.	The client's response may indicate acceptance of the ostomy as well as the need for health teaching. Handwashing deters the spread of microorganisms.
16.	Record the appearance of the stoma and the surrounding skin as well as the client's reaction to the procedure.	16.	A careful record is important for planning the client's care.

Table 16.4: Procedures for Changing or Emptying an Ostomy Appliance

Equipment

- Clean ostomy appliance
- Closure clamp
- Stoma measuring guide
- Scissors
- Toilet tissue
- Cleansing products (warm water, mild soap (optional), washcloth, and towel)

- Adhesive solvent (optional)
- Plastic bag
- Toilet or bedpan
- Water or special solution to clean pouch

- Gauze pad
- Disposable gloves
- Disposable pad (optional)
- Skin barrier (optional)
- Deodorant for pouch (optional)

	Nursing actions		*Rationales*
1.	Assemble the necessary equipment.	1.	Organization facilitates performance of the task.
2.	Explain the procedure to the client.	2.	The client is better able to cooperate and learn the technique when he or she is aware of the procedures.
3.	Wash your hands and don disposable gloves.	3.	Handwashing deters the spread of microorganisms. Gloves protect the nurse from exposure to blood or microorganisms in the feces.
4.	Provide for client's privacy. Assist to a comfortable sitting or lying position in bed or a standing or sitting position in the bathroom.	4.	Either position should allow the client to view the procedure in preparation for learning to apply it independently. Lying flat or sitting upright facilitates smooth application of the appliance.
5.	Empty the partially filled appliance into a bedpan if it is a drainable pouch.	5.	Emptying the contents before removal of the pouch prevents accidental spillage of fecal that material. Poches are too full can detach or leak.

To change the pouch

6.	Slowly remove the appliance beginning at the top while keeping the abdominal skin taut. If any resistance is felt, use warm water or the adhesive solvent to facilitate removal. Discard the disposable pouch in the plastic bag.	6.	Careful removal protects the underlying skin from damage and minimizes discomfort for the client. Solvent is rarely necessary to ease removal of the pouch.
7.	Use toilet tissue to remove any excess stool from the stoma. Cover stoma with a gauze pad. Gently wash and pat dry the peristomal skin. Mild soap or a cleansing agent may be used according to agency.	7.	Soap may not be recommended because it may be irritating to the peristomal skin. Toilet tissue, used gently, will not damage the stoma. The gauze absorbs any drainage from the stoma while the skin is being prepared.
8.	Assess the appearance of the peristomal skin and stoma. A moist, reddish-pink stoma is considered normal.	8.	Any change in normal appearance may indicate either anemia (pale stoma) or altered circulation (bluish-purple color) and the physician should be notified.
9.	Apply the skin barrier and appliance together (water or disc style): • Select size for stoma opening by using the measurement guide • Trace same size circle on the back and center of the skin barrier • Use scissors to cut an opening 1/7 to 1/8 inch larger than stoma • Remove the backing to expose sticky side • Remove gauze pad covering stoma • Ease barrier and pouch over the stoma and gently press onto skin while smoothing out creases or wrinkles. Hold the pouch in place for five minutes.	9.	Placing both the skin barrier disc and the appliance together over the stoma makes application easier for the client. The opening is cut slightly larger to prevent irritation to the stoma as peristalsis occurs. Smooth application of the pouch prevents escape of odor and feces. The warmth from the nurse's hands facilitates a tight seal.
10.	Close the pouch if it is drainable by folding the end upward and using a clamp or clip (see manufacturer's directions).	10.	A tightly sealed appliance will not leak and cause embarrassment and discomfort for the client.

Contd...

Table 16.4: *Contd...*

	Nursing actions		Rationales
	To empty the pouch		
11.	Plan to drain the pouch when it is 1/3 to 1/2 full. Remove clamp and fold the end of the pouch upward like a cuff.	11.	Allowing the pouch to fill more than half-way increases its weight and makes it more likely to separate of loosen from the skin. Creating a cuff before emptying prevents additional soilage and odor.
12.	Empty contents into bedpan or toilet. Rinse pouch with tepid water or water mixed with a drop of mouthwash administered via a squeeze bottle.	12.	Rinsing the inside of the pouch provides a cleaner appearance and minimizes odor.
13.	Wipe the lower 2 inches of the pouch with toilet tissue.	13.	Drying the lower section of the pouch removes any additional fecal material.
14.	Uncuff the edge of the pouch and apply the clip or clamp.	14.	The edge of the pouch should remain clean. The clamp secures closure of the appliance.
15.	Dispose the used equipment according to agency policy. Remove gloves and wash hands.	15.	Proper disposal of equipment and hand-washing prevents contamination from microorganisms.
16.	Document appearance of stoma, condition of peristomal skin, characteristics of drainage (amount, color, consistency, unusual odor), and client's reaction to the procedure.	16.	Careful documentation facilitates continuity of care.

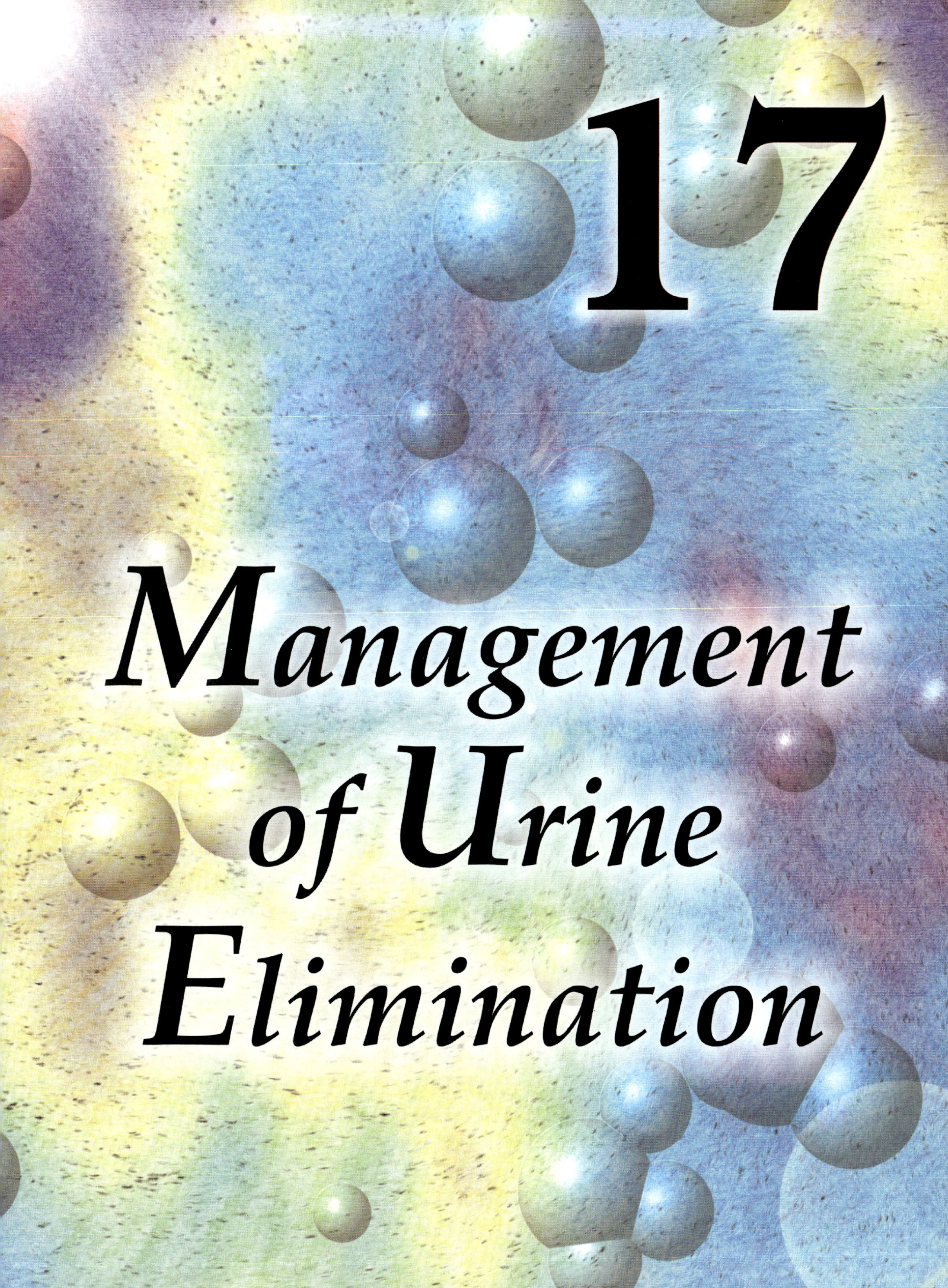
17
Management
of Urine
Elimination

Urinary Elimination

The kidneys filter metabolic wastes, drains excess ions, and water from the bloodstream and excrete their urine. When the bladder is empty, it shrivels and its elastic was becomes heavily folded. As it receives newly formed urine, it expands and the wall becomes smooth. An average, normal bladder can store 500 mL (one pint) of urine, but it may distend when needed to a capacity twice that amount. We cannot palpate an empty bladder, but a full or distended bladder, but a full or distended bladder extends upward to form a pear shape that you can feel in the suprapubic region.

Urinary elimination, a natural process in which the body excretes waste products and materials that exceeded bodily needs, usually is taken for granted. When the urinary system fails to function properly, virtually organ systems can be affected. Persons with alterations in urinary elimination may also suffer emotionally from body image changes. The proper functioning of the urinary system is vital to the body's physical well being, to life itself, and a person's general sense of well being. Nursing therapies promote or minimize factors that influence urinary elimination. Each client has a different pattern of elimination. The nurse must assess this pattern and design therapies to promote normal urinary elimination when necessary. The nurse uses devices such as a condom or an indwelling catheter to assist the client with urinary elimination. The nurse assisting a client with urination or intervening to resolve health problems related to urinary needs may have specialized abilities.

The urethra transports urine from the bladder to the body exterior. In females, the urethra is about 3 to 4 cm (1.5 in) long and is anchored to the anterior wall of the vagina by connective tissue; it opens at the **urinary meatus** between the clitoris and vaginal opening. In males the urethra extends about 20 cm (8 in) from the bladder to the urinary meatus at the distal end of the penis. As it leaves the bladder, the male urethra passes through a surrounding gland known as the **prostate.** In addition to urine, the male urethra also carries semen.

Because the female urethra is so short, women are especially prone to urinary tract infection from microorganisms residing in the vagina and rectum. The mucous membrane of the urethra (in both men and women) is continuous with the bladder and the ureters. Therefore, infection in the urethra can easily spread through the bladder and up into the kidneys.

Physiology of Urinary Elimination

Urinary elimination depends on the function of the kidneys, ureters, bladder, and urethra. Kidneys remove waste from the blood to form urine. Ureters transport urine from the kidneys to the bladder. The bladder holds urine until the urge to urinate develops. Urine leaves the body through the urethra. All organs of the urinary system must be intact and functional for successful removal of urinary wastes.

The process of emptying the bladder is known as micturition or voiding or urination. The bladder normally holds as much as 600 mL of urine. However, the desire to urinate can be sensed when the bladder contains only a small amount of urine (150 to 200 mL in adults and 50 to 200 mL in a child). As the volume increases, the bladder walls stretch, sending sensory impulses to micturition center in the sacral spinal cord. Parasympathetic impulses from the micturition center stimulate the detrusor muscle to contract rhythmically. The internal sphincter also relaxes so that urine may enter the urethra, although voiding does not yet occur. As the bladder contracts, nerve impulses travel up the spinal cord to the midbrain and cerebral cortex. A person is thus conscious of the need to urinate. If the person chooses not to void, the external urinary sphincter remains contracted, and the micturition reflex is inhibited. However, when a person is ready to void, the external sphincter relaxes, the micturition reflex stimulates the detrusor muscle to contract and urination occurs. The act of micturition normally is painless.

Where the bladder connects to the urethra is a thickening of smooth muscle called the **internal urethral sphincter.** When closed, the internal sphincter keeps urine in the bladder from entering the urethra. When the bladder contains 200 to 450 mL of urine (50 to 200 mL in children), the distention activates stretch receptors in the bladder wall. The stretch receptors send sensory impulses to the *voiding reflex center* in the spinal cord, triggering motor impulses that cause the detrusor muscle to contract and the internal sphincter to relax. The internal urethral sphincter is not under voluntary control. **Voiding** (also called **urination** or **micturition**) occurs when contraction of the detrusor muscle pushes stored urine through the relaxed internal urethral sphincter into the urethra. This triggers the conscious urge to void. However, voiding may be voluntarily delayed by inhibiting release of a second, **external urethral sphincter.** When the person is ready to urinate, the brain signals the external sphincter to relax, and urine flows through the urethra. Further contraction of the detrusor muscle normally forces out any urine remaining in the bladder. After the detrusor muscle relaxes, the bladder begins to fill with urine again.

Voiding and control of urination require that, in addition to normal functioning of the bladder and urethra, the brain, spinal cord, and nerves supplying the bladder and urethra be intact. The person must be aware of the need to urinate and able to respond by either inhibiting the reflex or by going to the toilet. The kidneys produce urine at a rate of about 60 mL per hour, or 1500 mL per day. However, output may fluctuate by 1000 mL to 2000 mL depending on various factors discussed in the next section. Most people void about five or six times per day – normally on awakening, after each meal, and just prior to bedtime. **Specific gravity** is a measure of dissolved solutes in a solution. As the concentration of solutes increases, specific gravity increases. The specific gravity of distilled water is 1.000 because there are no dissolved solutes. The normal specific gravity range for urine is 1.002 to 1.028. As fluid intake increases, urine becomes dilute and lighter in color and may even become almost colorless as specific gravity approaches 1.000. In contrast, if fluid intake is low or there have been fluid losses, as with diarrhea or vomiting, the urine darkens and the specific gravity rises.

Factors Affect Urinary Elimination

Given the complex structure and physiology of the urinary organs, it isn't surprising that many variables effect their function.

(i) Developmental Factors

Developmental factors affect urine volume and frequency and control of voiding.

- *Infants and Children:* A newborn's kidneys produce 15 to 60 mL of urine per kilogram of body weight per day. Newborns do not concentrate urine well and, therefore, may void up to 25 times during the first 24 hours of life. Normal specific gravity of their urine is 1.008. over the first weeks of life, the urine gradually becomes more concentrated, and the well-hydrated infant produces eight to ten wet diapers a day (Polan & Taylor, 2003). Infants do not have voluntary control of voiding because neuromuscular functioning is immature.

The timing of toilet training is highly variable and is influenced by family and culture, as well as the presence of older children who can act as role models. In the United States, most parents begin toilet training when their child is between 18 and 24 months of age. This timing can vary widely among cultures. For example, it is not unusual for Chinese children to be completely toilet-trained by their first birthday. Before toilet training can occur, toddlers must be able to control the external urethral sphincter, sense the urge to void, communicate their need to use the toilet, and remove their clothing. Full control over urination is usually established by age 3 but may occur as late as age 5. Daytime dryness usually occurs before toddlers can go without a diaper all night.

Occasional wetting (**enuresis**) is entirely normal in children, even in the early school years, especially when the child is intensely involved in a game, test, or other absorbing activity. Such events should be accepted calmly and not punished. **Nocturnal enuresis,** or bed-wetting, is considered normal until well after toilet training has been firmly established and should not be considered a problem until age 6.

- *Older Adults:* The size and functioning of the kidneys begin to decrease at about age 50, and by age 80 only about two-thirds of the functioning nephrons remain. This results in a decline in filtration rate, which affects the ability to dilute and concentrate urine, but does not normally create problems unless an illness alters fluid balance. For example, when older adults lose fluids and electrolytes through vomiting and diarrhea, it is difficult for their kidneys to maintain acid-base and electrolyte balances. Chronic diseases such as arteriosclerosis, common in older adults, can reduce blood flow and impair renal function. Decreased kidney function places older adults at risk for drug toxicity, as well.

(ii) Personal, Sociocultural, and Environmental Factors

Many people put off voiding while they are working, watching TV, or busy with other tasks. Delaying urination promotes urinary stasis and can lead to bladder infections. Other situations can inhibit voiding, as well. A person who is anxious and tense cannot relax the abdominal and perineal muscles and the external urethral sphincter. It is then difficult to void, as in the following situations:

- *Lack of time:* Most people find it difficult to void when they feel rushed; therefore, when helping patients to void, make sure you have scheduled enough time for them to relax fully.
- *Lack of privacy:* Many people require privacy for voiding and if they are in a restaurant or other unfamiliar environment, they may be embarrassed even to ask for directions to a bathroom. Some hospitalized clients may also avoid asking for assistance to the bathroom.
- *Loss of dignity:* In chapter 10, we talked about the loss of dignity that hospitalized patient's experience. Patients who need assistance with toileting may be especially vulnerable to such feelings, especially if they require catheterization or a bedpan. It is important, therefore, to acknowledge such feelings and encourage the patient to participate in other aspects of self-care, such as bathing and dressing.
- *Cultural influences:* Some patients will state personal, cultural, or religious requirements for toileting assistance to be provided by a person of the same gender, or they will wait until a visit from a family member before acknowledging their need for help with voiding.

(iii) Nutrition, Hydration, and Activity Level

Substances that contain caffeine, such as coffee, tea, cola, and chocolate, act as diuretics and increase urine production. Consuming large amounts of alcohol impairs the release of antidiuretic hormone (ADH), resulting in increased production of urine. In contrast, a diet high in salt causes water retention and decreases urine production.

The kidneys also "spare" water when a person is dehydrated, such as after heavy exercise or simply when fluid intake is inadequate. This causes the urine to be concentrated and low in volume. During lengthy sessions of physical activity, especially in hot weather, the body loses sodium and other electrolytes rapidly through sweat; for this reason, a nutrient-balanced sports beverage may be more beneficial than plain water in helping to prevent dehydration. For most adults, plate to clear urine indicates adequate hydration.

(iv) Medications

Various medications affect urination. *Phenazopyridine hydrochloride (Pyridium),* a bladder analgesic, turns the urine a deep orange-red color. *Diuretics,* sometimes called "water pills," treat blood pressure, fluid retention, and edema by increasing elimination of urine. Diuretics are classified as thiazide, potassium-sparing, or loop-acting diuretics. In contrast, a number of medications have a side effect of urinary retention. They inhibit the free flow of urine due to *anticholinergic effects* (e.g., medications given to relieve bladder spasms). The most common medications associated with urinary retention as given below.

Medications Associated with Urinary Retention

Class	Examples
Antihistamines	Chlorpheniramine (Chlortrimeton), loratadine (Claritin)
Tricyclic antidepressants	Amitriptyline (Elavil), desipramine (Norpramin)
MAO inhibitors	Phenelzine (Nardil), tranylcypromine (Parnate)
Antispasmodics	Dicyclomine (Bentyl)
Antiparkinsonism medications	Benztropine mesylate (Cogentin), levodopa
Beta-adrenergic blockers	Propranolol (Inderal), naldolol (Corgard)

Medications associated with urine elimination, see Table 17.1.

Still other medications are **nephrotoxic** (damaging to the kidneys). These include some antibiotics, such as gentamicin (Garamycin) and amphotericin B (Amphotex, a fungicide), and high doses or long-term use of aspirin and ibuprofen (Motrin).

(v) Surgery and Anesthesia

Reproductive and urinary tract surgeries can affect urine solutes, normal urine characteristics, and the ability to pass urine normally. Manipulation of the urinary tract frequently leads to trauma, bleeding, or the introduction of bacteria into a normally sterile tract. Swelling after diagnostic or invasive procedures and childbirth may cause urinary retention.

Surgery in the pubic area, vagina, or rectum is associated with a high incidence of trauma to the urinary organs, lower abdominal swelling, loss of pelvic muscle control, and increased pressure on the kidneys, ureters, or bladder. Surgery on the reproductive organs, such as hysterectomy in women or

Table 17.1: Medications Associated with Urine Elimination

Diuretics	• Midamore (amiloride) • Novospiroton (spironolactone)
Thiazide Diuretics	**Loop-Acting Diuretics**
Thiazide diuretics are used to treat high blood pressure by reducing the amount of sodium and water in the body. They also dilate blood vessels, thereby lowering blood pressure. In the United States, numerous thiazide diuretics are available. Below are several that are widely used: • Aquatensen (methyclothiazie) • Diulo, mykrox (metolazone) • Diuril (chlorothiazide) • Esidrix (hydrochlorothiazide) • Hygroton or Thalitone (chlorthalidone) • Naturetin (bendroflumethiazide)	Loop-acting diuretics cause the kidneys to excrete more urine by reabsorbing less water. This reduces the amount of water in the body and lowers blood pressure. Commonly used brand names in the United States include the following: • Bumex (bumetanide) • Demadex (torsemide) • Edecrin (ethacrynic acid) • Lasix (furosemide)
In Cananda, numerous thiazide diuretics are available. Below are several that are widely used: • Apo-Chlorthalidone, Hygroton, Nove-Thalidone, Uridon (chlorthalidone) • Apo-Hydro, Diuchlor H, Hydro diuril, Neo-Codema, Novo-Hydrazide (hydrochlorothiazide) • Diuretic (methyclothiazide), • Naturetin (bendroflumethiazide)	Commonly used brand names in Canada include the following: • Apo-Furosemide (furosemide) • Edecrine (ethacrynic acid) • Furoside, lasix, Novosemide, or Uritol (furosemide) **Medications that have Significant Interactions with Diuretics** • Digoxin • Certain antidepressants, especially when taking thiazide or loop-acting diuretics • Other medicines for high blood pressure • Lithium • Cyclosporin (an immunosuppressant), especially when the patient is taking a potassium-sparing diuretic
Potassium-Sparing Diuretics Potassium-sparing diuretics reduce the amount of water in the body. Unlike other diuretic medicines, these medicines do not cause potassium loss. Commonly used brand names in the United States include the following: • Aldactone (spironolactone) • Dyrenium (traimterene) • Midamor (amiloride) Commonly used brand names in Canada include the following: • Aldactone (spironolactone) • Dyrenium (triamterene)	**Common Side Effects of Diuretics** • Weakness • Muscle cramps • Skin rash • Increased sensitivity to sunlight (with thiazide diuretics) • Dizziness or lightheadedness • Joint pain

transurethral resection of the prostate in men, usually requires the use of an indwelling catheter (tube) for draining the bladder postoperatively. The urine may be red or pinkinged after any invasive urinary tract surgery or procedure.

Anesthetic agents can decrease blood pressure and glomerular filtration, thus decreasing urine formation. Spinal anesthesia decreases the patient's awareness of the need to void, which may lead to bladder distention.

(vi) Pathological Conditions

Disorders of the urinary system that affect urinary elimination include the following:

- Infection or inflammation of the bladder, ureters, or kidneys
- **Renal calculi** (kidney stones) or tumors, which obstruct the normal flow of urine
- In older men **hypertrophy** (excessive growth) of the prostate gland due to benign or cancerous lesions, which interferes with flow of urine from the bladder into the urethra

Diseases involving other systems can indirectly affect urinary function. For example:

- Cardiovascular and metabolic disorders decrease blood flow through the glomeruli and thus impair filtration and urine production
- Any condition that affects the nervous system controlling the urinary system organs will impair urinary elimination. After a stroke or spinal cord injury, for example, some patients may lose bladder control
- **Neurogenic bladder** occurs as a result of impaired neurological function. The person cannot perceive bladder fullness nor control the urinary sphincters. The bladder becomes flaccid or spastic, causing frequent involuntary loss of urine.
- Systemic infection, especially when accompanied by a high fever, causes the kidneys to reabsorb and retain water
- Mobility and communication problems may cause inability to get to the bathroom in time or inability to communicate the need for assistance. This may result in urination in inappropriate settings or at inappropriate times
- Cognitive changes that alter perception of the urge to void or severe psychiatric concerns that alter perception or ability to manage activities of daily living may lead to "accidents".

To sum up numerous factors which affect the amount and quality of urine produced by the body and manner which it is excreted. These are as follows.

Growth and development of individual: It influences urination. Usually infants or children with 6 to 8 kg excrete 400 to 500 mL per day and child cannot withhold urination. The adult normally voids 1500 to 1600 mL per day and has normal urine color; also has control over urination. Aging impairs urination, e.g. elder adults.

Food and fluid: Foods high in water content increased urine production. Certain foods affect the color and odor of urine. Certain fluid needed when person is dehydrated to maintain fluids and electrolyte balance.

Lifestyles: Some sociocultural variables influence a person's normal voiding habits. Privacy and adequate time to urinate are usually important for most people; they think voiding is private act. The nurse approach in or to a client's elimination must consider cultural and social habits.

Psychologic variable: Anxiety and stress do not change the characteristics of urine, but may cause a sense of urgency and increase frequency of urination.

Activity and muscle tone: Regular exercise increases the metabolism and helps in optimal urine production and elimination. Weak abdominal and pelvic floor muscles impair bladder contraction and control of external urethral sphincter.

Pathologic condition: Several diseases can affect the ability to micturate. Any lesion of peripheral nerves leading to the bladder causes loss of bladder tone, reduced sensation of bladder-fullness and difficulty in controlling urination (e.g. diabetis mellitus).

Medications: These have numerous effects on urine production and elimination. Diuretics prevent reabsorption of water and certain electrolytes to increase urine output. Urinary retention may be caused by use of anticholenergics, antihistamines, antihypertensives and beta-adrenergic blockers. Certain drugs also change the color of urine. For example, diuretics lead to pale yellow, B complex preparations lead to green or blue-green. Iron tablets lead to brown or black color urine.

Diagnostic Examination

Diagnostic examination of the urinary system can also influence micturition, for example, IVP.

Conditions which Alter Urinary Elimination

The most common conditions which alter urine elimination encountered by the nurse, involve disturbance in the act of micturition. These disturbances result from impaired bladder function, obstruction to urine outflow, or inability of voluntary control of micturition. The common renal conditions causing alteration in urinary elimination are as follows:

(i) *Prerenal conditions*

- Decreased intravascular volume, dehydration, hemorrhage, burns shock
- Altered peripheral vascular resistance; sepsis, anaphylactic shock and reactions
- Cardiac pump failure; congestive heart failure, myocardial infarction, hypertensive heart disease, valvular disease, pericardial tamponade.

(ii) *Renal conditions*

- Use of nephrotoxic agents (e.g. gentamycin)
- Transfusion reactions
- Diseases of the glomeruli (e.g. nephritis)
- Neoplasms
- Systemic diseases (e.g. diabetes)

- Hereditary diseases (e.g. polycystic kidney)
- Infections.

(iii) *Postrenal conditions*
- Ureteral, bladder or urethral obstructions, due to calculi, blood clot, tumors, strictures
- Prostatic hypertrophy
- Neurogenic bladder
- Pelvic tumor
- Retroperitoneal fibrosis.

Role of Nurse in Urinary Elimination

The role and responsibilities of nurse, when managing the urinary elimination in their clients include the following:
- Taking nursing history pertaining to client with partial emphasis on urinary elimination
- Conducting or assessing physical assessment of kidneys, bladder, urethral orifice, skin integrity and hydration and urine
- In addition, carrying out the following assessment measures like measuring urine output, collecting urine specimens, determining the presence of abnormal constituents, assisting with diagnostic procedure.

Nursing procedures related to urinary elimination shown in Tables 17.2 to 17.8.

Common Urinary Problems

Anuria: Technically, no urine is voided or 24-hour urine output is less than 100 mL.

Dysuria: Difficulty in voiding, may or may not be associated with pain, a feeling of warm local irritation occurring during voiding is called 'burning'.

Enuresis: Most often used to refer to the child who involuntarily urinates during night, i.e. bedwetting.

Frequency: Increased incidence of voiding.

Glycosuria: Presence of sugar in the urine. It may be due to an unusually large intake of sugar or to marked emotional disturbance and is temporary.

Hematuria: Presence of blood in the urine.

Hesitancy: Delay or difficulty in initiating voiding.

Incontinence: Inability to voluntarily control the discharge of urine.

Nocturia: Frequency of urination during the nights.

Oligurea: Scanty or greatly diminished amount of urine voided in a given time (24 hours urine output is 100 to 400 mL).

Table 17.2: Procedures for Offering and Removing a Bedpan or Urinal		
Equipment		
• Bedpan or urinal Graduated container • Toilet tissue	• Handwashing supplies • Disposable gloves	• Cover for bedpan or urinal (Use chux or disposable cover if other are not available)

	Nursing actions		Rationales
1.	Bring the bedpan or urinal and equipment to bedside. Don disposable gloves.	1.	Having equipment on hand saves time by avoiding unnecessary trips to the storage area. Gloves protect against exposure to blood and body substances.
2.	Warm the bedpan, if it is made of metal, by rinsing it with warm water.	2.	A cold bedpan feels uncomfortable and may make it difficult for the client to void. Plastic bedpans do not require warming.
3.	Place an adjustable bed in the high position.	3.	Keeping the bed in the high position reduces strain on the nurse's back while assisting the client onto the bedpan.
4.	Place the bedpan or urinal on the chair next to the bed or on the foot of the bed. Fold the top linen back just enough to allow for placement of bedpan or urinal.	4.	Folding back the linen in this manner prevents unnecessary exposure while still allowing the nurse to place the bedpan or urinal.
5.	If the client needs assistance to move onto the bedpan, have him or her bend the knees and rest some of his or her weight on the heels. Lift the client by placing one hand under the lower back, and slip the bedpan into place with the other hand.	5.	The client uses less energy as the nurse assists by lifting him or her onto the bedpan. The nurse uses less energy when the client can assist by placing some of his or her weight on the heels.
6.	If the client is helpless, two people may be required to lift him or her onto the bedpan. Or, the client may be placed on his or her side, the bedpan is placed against the buttocks, and the client is rolled back onto the bedpan.	6.	Having two people lift a helpless client causes less strain on the nurse's back. Rolling the client takes less energy than lifting the client onto a bedpan.

Contd...

Table 17.2: *Contd...*	
Nursing actions	*Rationales*
7. When the bedpan is in the proper place, the client's buttocks rest on the rounded shelf of the bedpan. For male clients, the urinal is properly placed between slightly spread legs with the penis positioned in it and with the urinal resting on the bed.	7. Having the bedpan or urinal in the proper place prevents spilling contents onto the bed and prevents injury to the skin from a misplaced bedpan.
8. If permitted, raise the head of the bed as near to the sitting position as tolerated.	8. This position makes it easier for the client to void or defecate, avoids strain on the client's back, and allows gravity to aid in elimination.
9. Place cell device and toilet tissue within easy reach. Leave the client if it is safe to do so. Use siderails appropriately.	9. Falls can be prevented when the client does not have to reach for items he or she needs. Siderail is an additional safety precaution. Leaving client alone, if possible, promotes self-esteem and respects privacy.
10. Remove the bedpan in the same manner in which it was offered, being careful to hold it steady. If necessary to assist the client, don disposable gloves, wrap tissue around the hand several times, and wipe the client clean, using one stroke from the public area toward the anal area. Discard tissue, and use more until the client is clean. Place the client on his or her side, and spread the buttocks to clean the anal area. Cover bedpan.	10. Holding the pan steady prevents spilling its contents. Cleaning an area from front to back minimizes focal contamination of the vagina and urinary meatus. Cleaning the client after he or she has used the bedpan prevents offensive odors and irritation to the skin.
11. Do not place toilet tissue in the bedpan if a specimen is required or if measurement of elimination is required. Have a receptacle handy for discarding the tissue.	11. Toilet tissue mixed with a specimen makes laboratory examination more difficult and interferes with accurate output measurement.
12. Offer the client supplies to wash and dry his or her hands, assisting as necessary.	12. Washing hands after using the bedpan or urinal helps prevent the spread of organisms.
13. Empty and clean the bedpan and urinal. Wash your hands. Record according to agency procedure	13. Provides adequate documentation. Hand washing helps prevent the spread of organisms.

Orthostatic albuminuria: Presence of albumin in urine that is voided after periods of standing, walking or running. It is the phenomenon of circulatory systems.

Pneumaturia: Passage of urine containing gas.

Polyuria: Excessive output of urine (diuresis).

Proteinuria: Presence of protein, usually albumin, in the urine.

Pyuria: Pus in the urine. Urine appears cloudy.

Nursing considerations: A fracture bedpan may be substituted when it is difficult or uncomfortable to use a regular bedpan. If it is difficult to slide client onto the bedpan, powder may be used on the resting surfaces of the pan to eliminate friction. Powder should not be used if a specimen is required because contamination could result.

Different catheter configuration are as shown in Figure 17.1.

Age considerations: If the client is a child, the size of the catheter must be adapted accordingly. Elderly women may be uncomfortable in the lithotomy position, and require variable positions for catheterization. If the client is able to remain on her back, another nurse can assist her to flex her knees and hips, this is bringing the knees closer to the abdomen and allowing visualization of the urinary meatus. Catheterization also is possible with the client on her side in a modified Sims' position as discussed and shown in Figures 17.2A and B.

Home care considerations: If self-catheterization must be performed in the home, clean technique is appropriate. The bladder's natural resistance to microorganisms normally found in the home makes sterile technique unnecessary. Rubber catheters must be washed thoroughly before boiling for 20 minutes. Dry and store properly for next usage. A shower rather than a tub bath is recommended for clients with an indwelling catheter. Sitting in the bath tub may allow for easier access of bacteria into the urinary tract.

Special considerations: If there is not an immediate flow of urine after the catheter has been inserted, several measures may prove helpful:
- Have the client take a deep breath, which helps to relax the perineal and abdominal muscles

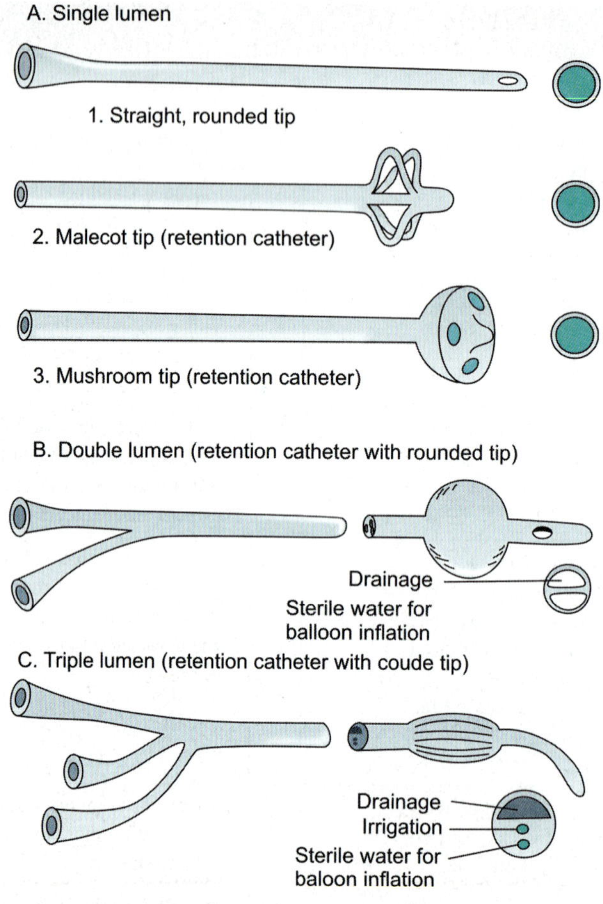

Figure 17.1: Catheter configuration

Table 17.3: Procedures for Catheterizing the Female Urinary Bladder (Straight and Indwelling)

Equipment

• Sterile catheterization kit	• Forceps	• Urine collection bag and drainage
• Sterile gloves	• Straight or indwelling catheter	• tubing (may be connected to sterile
• Sterile drapes (one of is fenestrated)	(Size must be appropriate for client)	indwelling catheter if a closed drainage
• Antiseptic solution	• Prefilled syringe	system is used)
• Lubricant	• Basin (base of kit usually serves as this)	• Velcro leg strap or tape
• Cotton balls or gauze squares	• Specimen container	• Waterproof pad or chux
	• Flashlight or lamp	

	Nursing actions		*Rationales*
1.	Assemble equipment. Wash your hands. Explain the procedure and its purpose to the client.	1.	Organization facilitates performance of the task. Hand washing deters spread of microorganisms. An explanation encourages client cooperation and reduces apprehension.
2.	Provide for good light. Artificial light is recommended (Use of a flash light requires an assistant to hold and position it).	2.	Good lighting is necessary to see the meatus clearly.
3.	Provide for privacy by closing the curtains or door.	3.	The procedure may be embarrassing for the client.
4.	Assist the client to the dorsal recumbent position with the kness flexed and the legs about 2 feet apart and drape the client. Or, if preferable, the client can be placed in the side-lying position (refer Figs 12.7C and I in chapter 12), slide the waterproof drape under the client.	4.	Good visualization of the meatus is important. Embarrassment, chillness, and feeling tense can interfere with introducing the catheter. The client's comfort will promote relaxation. The drape will protect bed linens from moisture.

Contd...

Table 17.3: *Contd...*

	Nursing actions		Rationales
5.	Clean the genital and perineal area with warm soap and water. Rinse and dry. Wash your hands again.	5.	Clean technique decreases the possibility of introducing organisms into the bladder.
6.	Prepare urine drainage set-up if indwelling catheter is to be inserted and separate urine collection system is used. Secure to bedframe according to manufacturer's directions.	6.	This facilitates connection of the catheter to the drainage system and provides for easy access.
7.	Open the sterile catheterization tray on over-bed table using sterile technique.	7.	Placement of equipment near the work site increases efficiency. Sterile technique protects the client and prevents and spread of microorganisms.
8.	Put on sterile gloves. Grasp the upper corners of the drape and unfold the drape without touching unsterile areas. Fold back a cuff over gloved hands. Ask the client to lift her buttocks and slide the sterile drape under her with gloves protected by cuff.	8.	The drape provides sterile field close to the meatus. Covering the gloved hands will help keep the gloves sterile while placing the drape.
9.	A fenestrated sterile drape may be placed over the perineal area, exposing the labia.	9.	The drape expands the sterile field and protects against contamination. Use of a fenestrated drape may limit visualization and is considered optional by some practitioners.
10.	Place the sterile tray on the drape between the client's thighs.	10.	This provides easy access to supplies.
11. (a) (b) (c)	Open all supplies: If the catheter is to be indwelling, test the catheter balloon. Remove the protective cap on the tip of the syringe and attach the syringe prefilled with sterile water to injection port. Inject appropriate amount of fluid. If the balloon inflates properly, withdraw build and leave the syringe attached the port. Pour antiseptic solution over cotton balls or gauze. Open the specimen container if specimen is to be obtained. Lubricate 1 to 2 inches of the catheter tip.	11. (a) (b) (c)	— A balloon that does not inflate or that leaks needs to be replaced before insertion in the client. It is necessary to open all supplies and prepare for the procedure while both hands are sterile. Lubrication facilitates the insertion of the catheter and reduces trauma to the issues.

Contd...

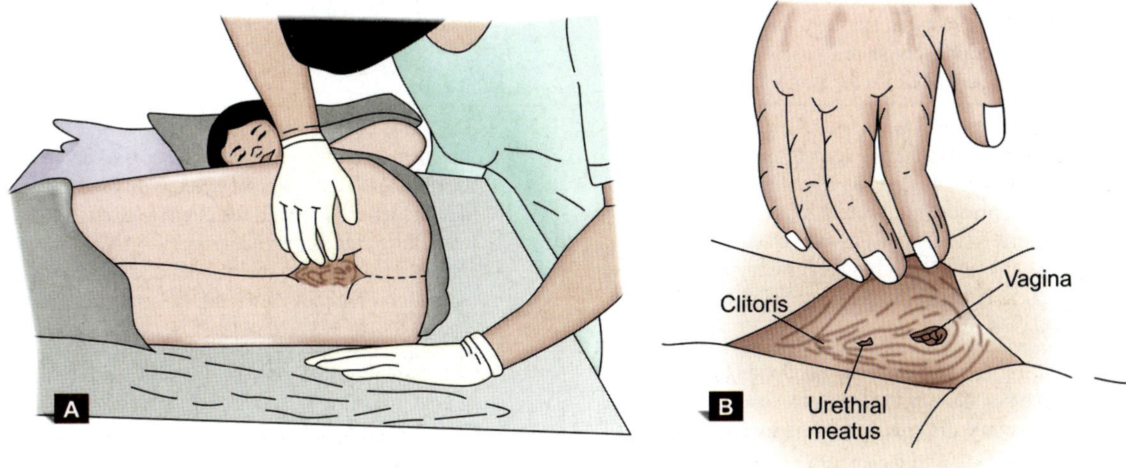

Figure 17.2: Placing the patient in modified sim's position to identify the urethral meatus

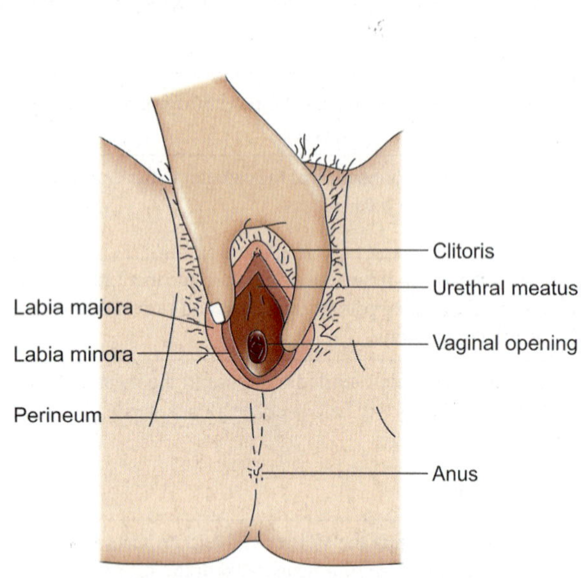

Figure 17.3: Identifying the urethral meatus

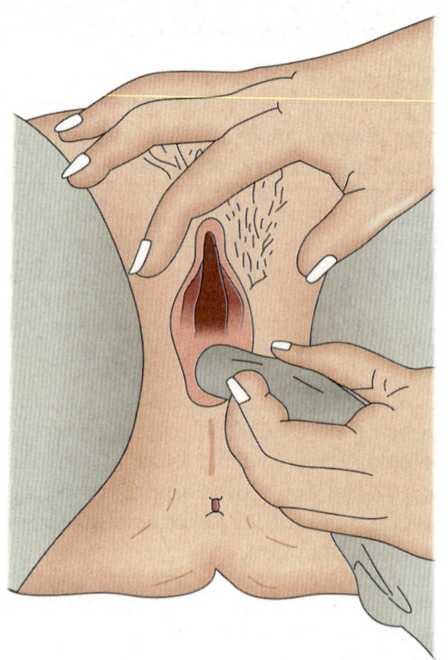

Figure 17.4: Cleaning the labia and meatus

		Table 17.3: *Contd...*	
	Nursing actions		*Rationales*
12.	With the thumb and one finger of your nondominant hand, spread the labia and identify the meatus as shown in Figs 17.3 and 17.5 be prepared to maintain separation of the labia with one hand until urine is flowing well and continuously.	12.	Smoothing the area immediately surrounding the meatus helps to make it visible. Allowing the labia to drop back into position may contaminate the area around the meatus, as well as the catheter. Your nondominant hand is now contaminated.
13.	Using cotton balls held with forceps, clean both labial folds and then directly over the meatus. Move the cotton ball from above the meatus downward the rectum. Discard each cotton ball after one downward stroke (Fig. 17.4).	13.	Moving from an area where there is likely to be less contamination to an area where there is more contamination helps prevent the spread of organisms. Cleaning the meatus last helps reduce the possibility of introducing organisms into the bladder.
14.	With the uncontaminated gloved hand, place the drainage end of the catheter in the receptacle. For insertion of an indwelling catheter that is preattached to sterile tubing and drainage container (closed drainage system), position the catheter and set up within easy reach on the sterile field.	14.	This facilitates drainage of urine and minimizes risk of contaminating sterile equipment.
15.	Insert the catheter tip into the meatus 5 to 7.5 cm (2-3 inches) or until urine flows. Do not use force to push the catheter through the urethra into the bladder. Ask the client to breathe deeply, and rotate the catheter gently if slight resistance is met as the catheter reaches the external sphincter. For an indwelling catheter, once urine drains, advance the catheter another 2.5 to 5 cm (1-2 inches).	15.	The female urethra is about 3.7 to 6.2 cm (1 ½ - 2 ½ inches) long. Applying force on the catheter is likely to injure mucous membranes. The sphincter relaxes and the catheter can enter the bladder easily when the client relaxes. Advancing an indwelling catheter an additional 1.3 to 2.5 cm (1/2-1 inches) ensures placement in the bladder and facilitates inflation of the balloon without damaging the urethra.
16.	Hold the catheter securely with the nondominant hand while the bladder empties. Collect a specimen if required. Continue drainage according to agency policy.	16.	Withdrawing and reinserting the catheter increases the chances of contaminating it. In general, no more than 750 ml of urine should be removed at one time. Pelvic floor blood vessels may become engorged from the sudden release of pressure leading to possible hypotensive episode.

Contd...

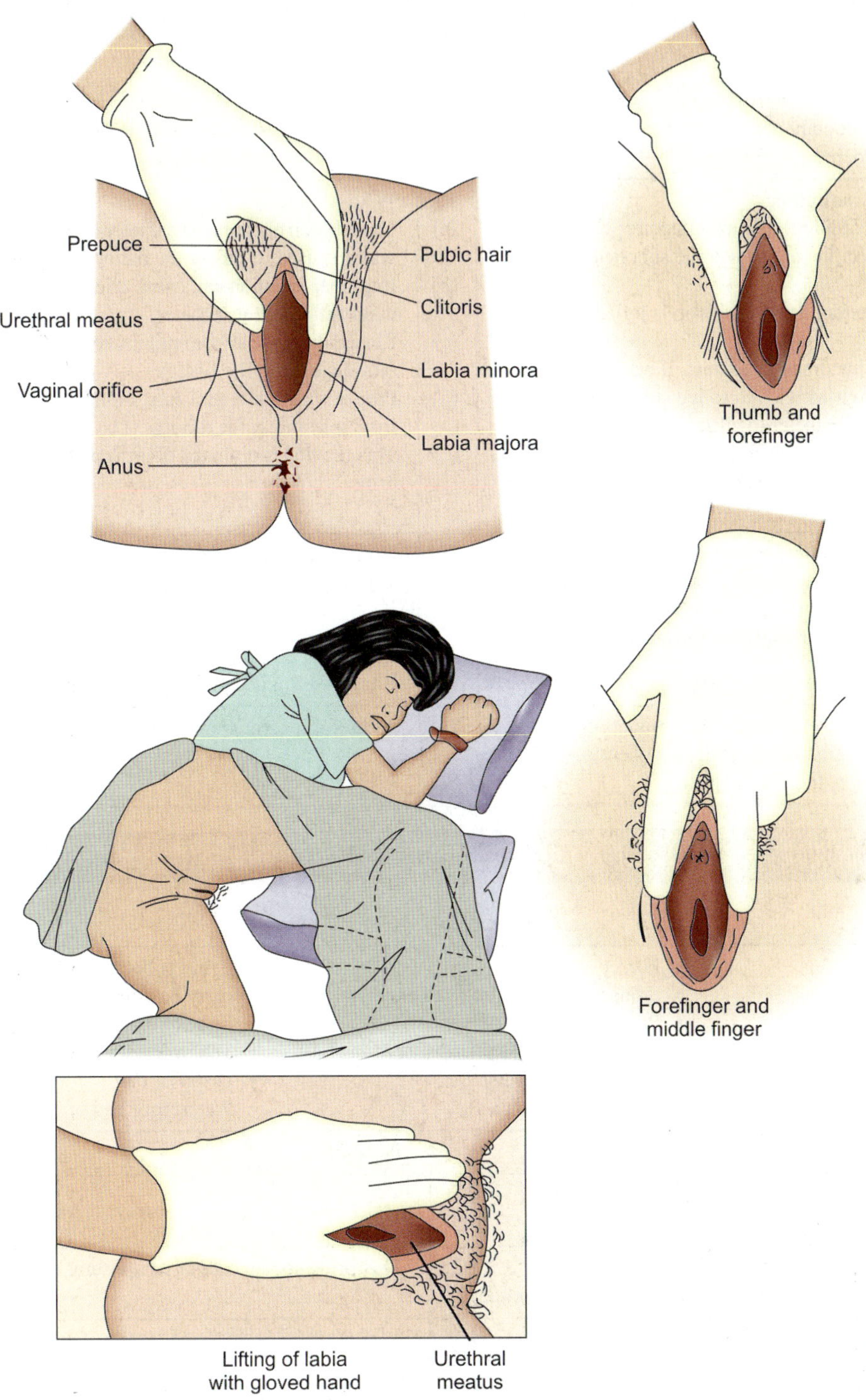

Figure 17.5: Steps for catheterizing the female patient

Table 17.3: *Contd...*

	Nursing actions		Rationales
17.	Remove the catheter smoothly and slowly if a straight catheterization was ordered.	17.	This causes less discomfort to the client.
18. (a) (b) (c) (d) (e)	If the catheter is to be indwelling: Inflate the balloon according to the manufacturer's recommendations. Inject the entire volume supplied in the prefilled syringe Tug gently on the catheter after the balloon is inflated to feel resistance Attach the catheter to the drainage system, if necessary. Secure to the upper thigh with a Velcro leg strap or tape. Leave some slack in the catheter to allow for leg movement Check that the drainage tubing is not kinked and that movement of siderails does not interfere with catheter or drainage bag	18. (a) (b) (c) (d) (e)	— The balloon anchors the catheter in place in the bladder. Sterile water is used to inflate the balloon as a precaution Improper inflation can cause client discomfort and malpositioning of catheter Closed drainage system minimizes the risk of organisms being introduced into the bladder Proper attachment prevents trauma to the urethra and meatus from tension on the tubing This facilitates drainage of urine and prevents the backflow of urine
19.	Remove the equipment and make the client comfortable in bed. Clean and dry the perineal area, if necessary. Care for the equipment according to agency policy. Send the urine specimen to the laboratory promptly or refrigerate it.	19.	Urine kept at room temperature may cause organisms, if present, to grow and distort laboratory findings.
20.	Wash your hands.	20.	Handwashing deters the spread of microorganisms
21.	Record the time of the catheterization, the amount of urine removed, a description of the urine, the client's reaction to the procedure, and your name.	21.	A careful record is important for planning the client's care.

Table 17.4: Procedures for Catheterizing the Male Urinary Bladder (Straight and Indwelling)

Equipment

- Sterile catheterization kit
- Sterile gloves
- Sterile drapes (one of is fenestrated)
- Antiseptic solution
- Lubricant
- Cotton balls or gauze
- Forceps
- Straight or indwelling catheter
- Prefilled syringe
- Basin (base of kit usually serves as this)
- Specimen container
- Flashlight or lamp
- Urine collection bag and drainage tubing (may be connected to sterile indwelling catheter if a closed drainage system is used)
- Velcro leg strap or tape
- Disposal bag
- Waterproof pad or chux

	Nursing actions		Rationales
1.	Assemble the equipment and follow actions 1 to 3 for female catheterization procedures of Table 17.3.	1.	—
2.	Position the client on his back with the thighs slightly apart. Drape the client so that only the area around the penis is exposed.	2.	This prevents unnecessary exposure.
3.	Follow actions 5 to 7 for female catheterization procedures of Table 17.3.	3.	—
4.	Put on sterile gloves. Open the sterile drape and place on the client's thigh. Place the fenestrated drape with the opening over the penis.	4.	This maintains a sterile working area.
5.	Place the catheter set on or next to the client's left on nurse's the sterile drape.	5.	The sterile set-up should be arranged so that the back is not turned to it, nor should it be out of the nurse's range of vision.
6. (a)	Open all supplies: If the catheter is to be indwelling, test the catheter balloon. Remove the cap on the tip of the syringe and attach the syringe	6. (a)	— A balloon that does not inflate or that leaks must be replaced before insertion in the client.

Contd...

<table>
<tr><td colspan="2" align="center">Table 17.4: Contd...</td></tr>
<tr><td colspan="2">Nursing actions</td><td colspan="2">Rationales</td></tr>
</table>

	Nursing actions		Rationales
(b)	prefilled with sterile water to the injection port. Inject appropriate amount of fluid. If balloon inflates properly, withdraw fluid and leave syringe attached to port. Pour antiseptic solution over cotton balls or gauze. Open the specimen container if specimen is to be obtained.	(b)	It is necessary to open all supplies and prepare for the procedure while both hands are sterile.
7.	Generously lubricate the catheter for about 15 to 18 cm (6 to 7 inches).	7.	Generous lubrication is especially important because of the length and tortuousness of the male urethra. The lubricant decreases friction
8.	Lift the penis with your nondominant hand, which is then considered contaminated. Retract the foreskin in the uncircumcised penis. Clean the area at the meatus with a cotton ball held with a forceps. Use a circular motion, moving from the meatus toward the based of the penis for three cleansings.	8.	The hand touching of the penis can be contaminated. Cleansing the area around the meatus and under the foreskin of the uncircumcised penis helps prevent infection. Moving from the meatus towards the based of the penis prevents bringing organisms to the meatus
9.	Hold the penis with slight upward tension and perpendicular to the client's body. Ask the client to bear down as if voiding. With your dominant hand, place the drainage at the end of the catheter in the receptacle. For insertion of an indwelling catheter that is preattached to sterile tubing and a drainage container (closed drainage system) (Fig. 17.6), position the catheter and set up within easy reach on the sterile field.	9.	Holding the penis up with slight traction helps straighten the urethra.
10.	Insert the tip into the meatus. Advance the catheter 15 to 20 cm (6-8 inches) or until urine flows. Do not use force to introduce the catheter. If the catheter resists entry, ask the client to breathe deeply and rotate the catheter slightly. For an indwelling catheter, once drains advance the catheter to the bifurcation of the catheter. Once the balloon is inflated, the catheter may be gently pulled back into place. The catheter can be taped laterally to the thigh (Fig. 17.7) Lower the penis.	10.	The male urethra is about 20 cm long. Deep breaths or slight twisting of the catheter may ease the catheter past resistance at the sphincters. Advancing an indwelling catheter to the bifurcation ensures its placement in the bladder and facilitates inflation of the balloon without damaging the urethra.
11.	Follow actions 16 to 21 for female catheterization procedure of Table 17.3, except that the catheter may be secured to the upper thigh or lower abdomen with the penis directed toward the client's chest (Figs 17.9A and B). Slack should be left in the catheter to prevent tension.	11.	This is done to prevent irritation at the angle of the penis and scrotum. Slack left in the catheter allows for penile erection, which can occur naturally during sleep.

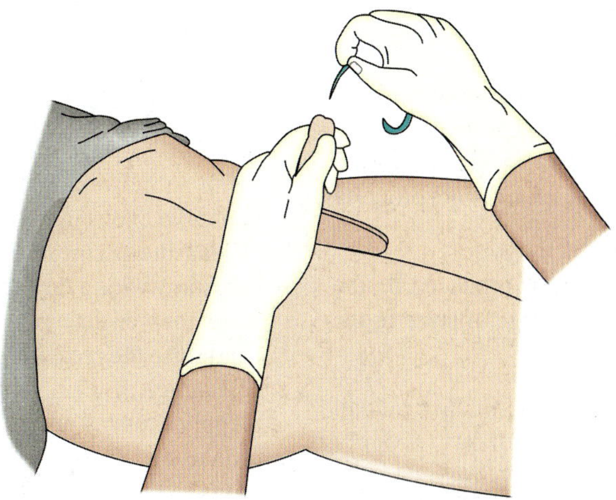

Figure 17.6: Position of the penis for catheterization

- Rotate the catheter slightly because a drainage hole may be resting against the bladder wall
- Raise the head of the client's bed to increase pressure in the bladder area
- Place a gloved finger in the vagina to feel digitally for the position of the catheter through the anterior vaginal wall
- Temporarily leave a catheter that has inadvertently been placed in the vagina in place as a guide while the nurse regloves and inserts another sterile catheter directly above it into the urinary meatus.

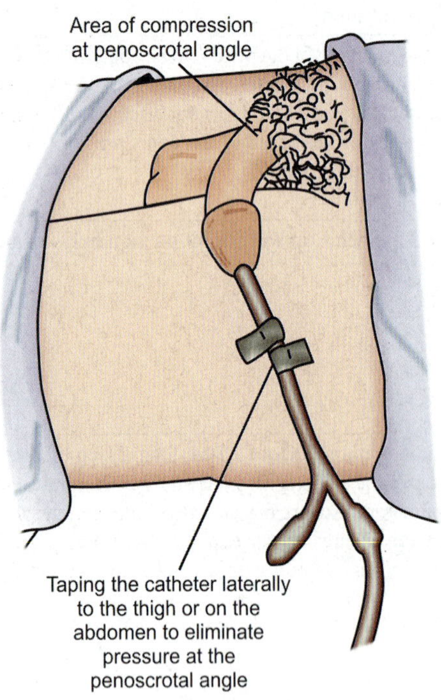

Figure 17.7: Catheterizing the male patient

Age considerations: If the client is a child, the size of the catheter must be adapted accordingly.

Home care: If self-catheterization must be performed in the home, cleanse technique

Considerations is appropriate. The bladder's natural resistance to microorganisms normally found in the home makes sterile technique unnecessary. Rubber catheters must be washed thoroughly before boiling for 20 minutes. Dry and store properly for next usage.

Retention: Inability to void although urine is produced by the kidney and enter the bladder. Excessive storage of urine in the bladder.

Suppression: Stoppage of urine production; normally the adult kidneys produce urine continuously at the rate of 60 to 120 mL/hour.

Urgency: Strong desire to void.

In addition to taking care of client with urinary problem, the nurses also have got responsibility to perform certain procedures related to urinary elimination which are as follows:
- Offering and removing bedpan or urinal (Table 17.2)
- Catheterizing the client's urinary bladder (Table 17.3 and 17.4)

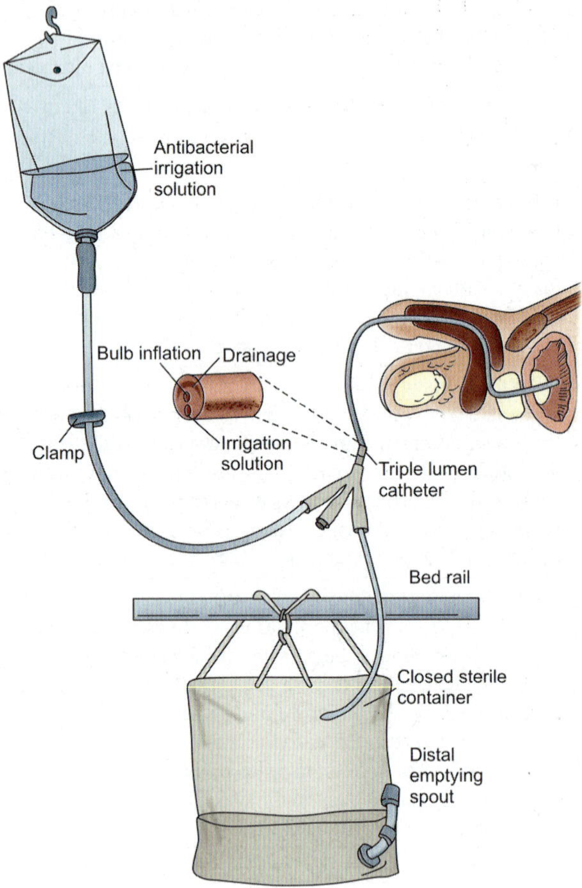

Figure 17.8: Position of drainage bag and tubing for an indwelling catheter

Instructions

While taking care of the patient with indwelling catheter, the nurse must keep following points which include the following:
- Be sure to wash hands before and after caring for a client with an indwelling catheter. Wear gloves to protect against possible exposure to blood and body substances
- Clean the perineal area thoroughly, especially around the meatus, twice a day and after each bowel movement
- Use soap or detergent and water to clean the perineal area, and rinse the area well. Do not use powders and lotions after cleaning
- Apply a topical antibiotic ointment at the meatus, as ordered
- Make sure that the client maintains a generous fluid intake. This helps prevent infection and irrigates the catheter naturally by increasing urine output

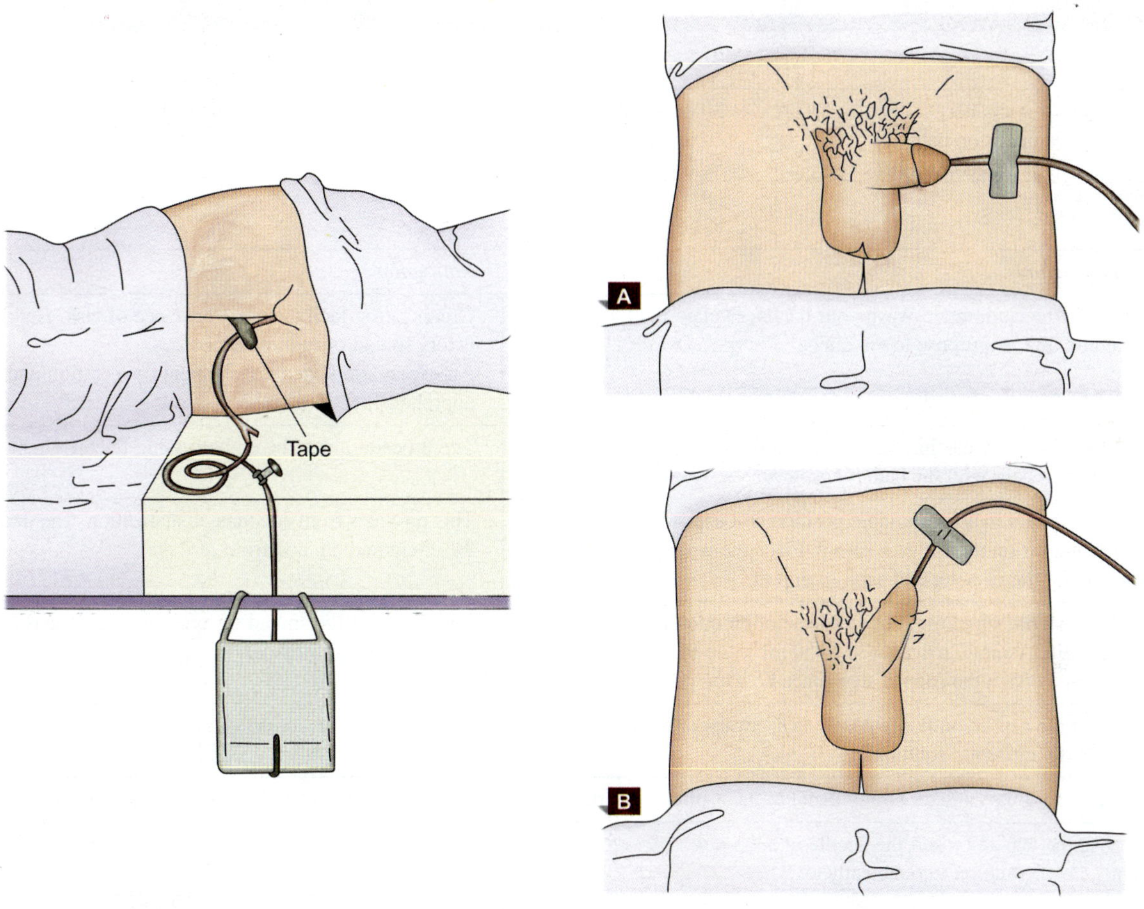

Figures 17.9A and B: Stabilization of the catheter in a male by taping it to A. The thigh, B. The abdomen

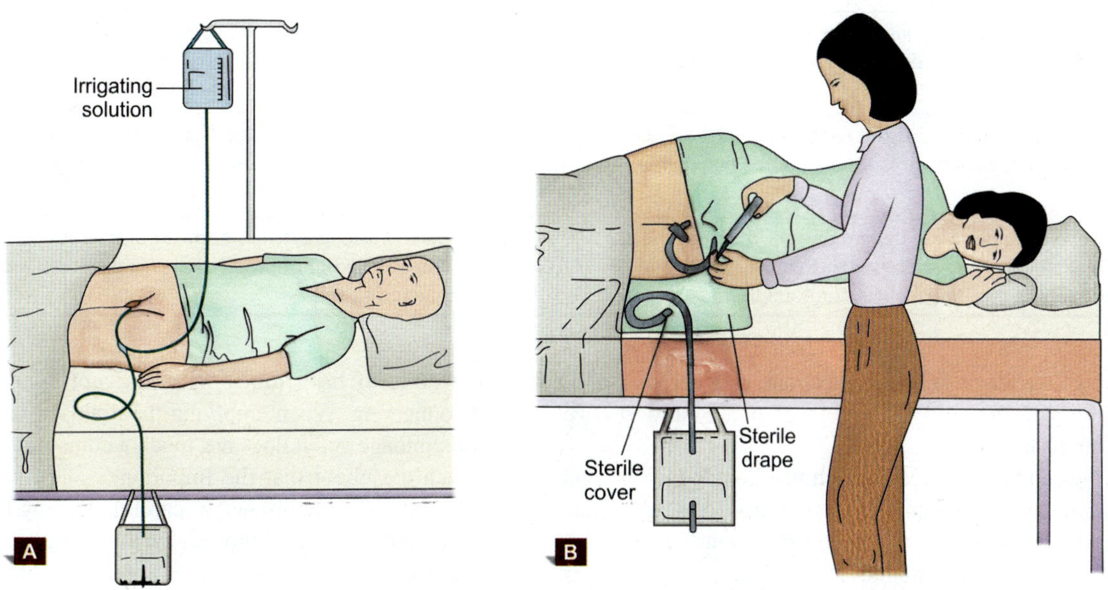

Figures 17.10A and B: A. Closed system for catheter of bladder irrigation of bladder instillation B. Open method of catheter irrigation

Table 17.5: Procedures for Irrigating the Catheter Using the Closed System

Equipment

- Sterile basin or container
- Gauze squares or cotton balls with disinfectant or alcohol swabs
- Waterproof drape
- 30 to 60 mL syringe with 19 or 19 gauge needle
- Sterile irrigating solution (at room temperature or warmed to body temperature)
- Bath blanket
- Disposable gloves

	Nursing actions		*Rationales*
1.	Assemble the equipment. Wash your hands. Explain the procedure and its purpose to the client.	1.	Organization facilitates performance of task. Handwashing deters spread of microorganisms. An explanation encourages client cooperation and reduces apprehension.
2.	Provide privacy by closing the curtains or door and draping the client with the bath blanket.	2.	The procedure may be embarrassing for the client.
3.	Assist the client to a comfortable position and expose the aspiration port on the catheter set-up. Place the waterproof drape under the catheter and aspiration port.	3.	This provides from adequate visualization. The drape protects the client and the bed from leakage.
4.	Open the sterile supplies. Pour sterile solution into the sterile basin. Aspirate irrigant (30 to 50 mL) into the sterile syringe and attach the capped sterile needle. Don gloves.	4.	This prevents the spread of microorganisms and contact with blood o body substances.
5.	Disinfect the aspiration port with alcohol. Swabs or gauze square with antiseptic solution.	5.	This prevents the spread of microorganisms.
6.	Clamp or fold the catheter tubing distal to the aspiration port.	6.	This directs the irrigating solution into the bladder.
7.	Remove the cap and insert the needle into the port. Gently instill solution into the catheter.	7.	Gentle irrigation prevents damage to the lining of the bladder.
8.	Remove the needle from the port. Unclamp the tubing and allow irrigant and urine to drain. Repeat the procedure as necessary (Figs 17.10A and B).	8.	Gravity aids drainage of urine and irrigant from the bladder.
9.	Assess the client's response to the procedure and the quality and amount of drainage. Document on the client's chart.	9.	This provides accurate documentation of the procedures.
10.	Record the amount of irrigant used on the intake and output record. Subtract this from the urine output when totalled.	10.	Subtracting irrigant total from drainage in urine collection bag provides accurate recording of urine output.
11.	Remove equipment and discard uncapped needle and syringe in appropriate receptacle. Remove gloves and wash your hands. Make client comfortable.	11.	Hand-washing deters the spread of microorganisms. Proper disposal of needle prevents the nurse accidentally puncturing self.

- Encourage the client to be up and about, as ordered
- Note the volume and character of urine, and record observations carefully
- The urine can be observed through the drainage tubing and in the collecting container. The usual procedure is to note and record the amount of urine on the client's intake and output record every 8 hours. The collecting container is calibrated, but the volume markings are only approximations. The urine should be emptied into a graduated container that is accurately calibrated for correct determination of output
- Do not open the drainage system to obtain urine specimens or to measure urine. If the tubing becomes disconnected, wipe the ends of both tubes with antiseptic solution before reconnecting. When emptying the drainage bag, make sure the drainage spout does not touch a contaminated surface
- Teach the client that the importance of personal hygiene, especially the importance of careful cleaning after having a bowel movement and thorough washing of hands frequently
- Promptly report any signs of infection. These include a burning sensation and irritation at the meatus, cloudy urine, a strong odor to the urine, an elevated temperature, and chills
- Help keep the urine acid in character, since acidity retards bacterial growth. Plain water in increased amounts, cranberry

Table 17.6: Procedures for Giving Continuous Bladder Irrigation

Equipment

- Sterile irrigating solution (at room temperature or warmed to body temperature), usually 2000 ml bags
- Sterile tubing with drip chamber and clamp for connection to irrigating solution
- IV pole
- Three-way Foley catheter in place in client's bladder
- Flossy drainage set-up (tubing and collection bag)
- Bath blanket
- Disposable gloves (optional)

	Nursing actions		*Rationales*
1.	Explain the procedure and its purpose to the client.	1.	An explanation encourages client cooperation and reduces apprehension.
2.	Assemble the equipment.	2.	Organization facilitates performance of tasks.
3.	Wash your hands.	3.	Handwashing deters the spread of microorganisms.
4.	Provide for privacy by closing the curtains or door and draping the client with the bath blanket.	4.	The procedure may be embarrassing for the client.
5.	Prepare the sterile irrigation bag for use as directed by the manufacturer. Secure the clamp and attach the sterile tubing with drip chamber to the container. Hang the bag on IV pole 2½ to 3 feet above the level of the client's bladder. Release the clamp and remove the protective cover on the end of the tubing without contaminating it. Allow the solution to flush the tubing and remove air. Reclamp (Fig. 17.8).	5.	Irrigating solution continuously bathes the lining of the bladder and keeps the catheter patent. Flushing the tubing before irrigation clears air from the tubing that might cause bladder distention.
6.	Using sterile technique, attach the irrigation tubing to the irrigation port of the three-way Foley catheter. If a closed system is used, tubing may already be connected to the irrigation port on the catheter.	6.	Sterile technique prevents the spread of microorganisms into the bladder.
7.	Release the clamp on the irrigation tubing and regulate the flow according to the physician's order.	7.	This allows for continual gentle irrigation without causing discomfort to the client.
8.	As irrigation is completed, clamp the tubing. Do not allow the drip chamber to empty. Disconnect the empty bag and attach a full irrigation bag. Continue as ordered by the physician.	8.	This eliminates the need to separate tubing from the catheter and clear air from the tubing. Opening the drainage system provides access for introduction of microorganisms.
9.	Assess the client's response to the procedure and the quality and amount of drainage. Document on the client's chart.	9.	This provides accurate documentation of the procedures.
10.	Record the amount of irrigant used on the intake and output record. Don gloves and empty the drainage collection bag as each new container is hung and record.	10.	This ensures accurate recording of urine output. Gloves protect against exposure to blood, body substances, and microorganisms.
11.	Wash your hands.	11.	Handwashing deters the spread of microorganisms

juice, prune juice, and ascorbic acid are helpful in acidifying urine. Regular use of cranberry juice cocktail reduced the bacterial and white blood cell count in a population of older women.

- Help the client take a tub or shower bath when permitted. The catheter should be clamped temporarily if the collecting container is higher than the bladder at any time. In a tub, with the catheter clamped, the container can be hung over the side of the tub. Care should be taken so that the catheter does not remain clamped after the bath. In a shower, the container can be attached to the client's leg, in which case clamping the tube usually is unnecessary

- Plan to change indwelling catheters only as necessary. If rolling the drainage tubing between the hands frees the tubing of sandy particles, it is time to change the catheter. The usual interval between catheter changes varies from five days to two weeks. The lesser often a catheter is changed, the less likehood that an infection will develop.

Table 17.7: Procedures for Applying a Condom Catheter

Equipment

• Condom sheath in appropriate size • Basin of warm water and soap • Wash cloth and towel	• Bath blanket • Disposable gloves (optional) • Elastic strip or Velcro strap (optional)	• Reusable leg bag with drainage tubing or urinary drainage set-up

	Nursing actions		*Rationales*
1.	Explain the procedure to the client. Ask if the client is aware of any allergy to latex.	1.	This provides reassurance and promotes client cooperation. If the client is allergic to latex, a latex-free condom catheter must be used.
2.	Assemble the equipment. Prepare urinary drainage set-up or reusable leg bag for attachment to the condom sheath.	2.	This provides for an organized approach to the task.
3.	Wash your hands.	3.	Handwashing deters the spread of microorganisms
4.	Assist the client to assume the supine position. Close the curtain or door. Use the bath blanket and sheet to expose only the client's genital area.	4.	This provides privacy for the client.
5.	Don disposable gloves. Wash the genital area with soap and water, rinse, and dry thoroughly.	5.	Washing removes urine, secretions, and microorganisms. The penis must be clean and dry to minimize skin irritation.
6.	Roll the condom sheath outward onto itself. Grasp the penis firmly with your nondominant hand. Apply the condom sheath by rolling it into the penis with your dominant hand. Leave 2.5 to 5 cm (1 to 2 inches) space between the tip of the penis and the end of the condom sheath.	6.	Rolling the condom sheath outward allows for easier application. The space prevents irritation to the tip of the penis and allows for free drainage of urine.
7.	Apply the elastic or Velcro strap in a snug but not tight manner. Do not allow the elastic or Velcro to come in contact with the skin.	7.	The elastic or Velcro strap should secure the condom sheath but not interfere with blood circulation to the penis.
8.	Connect the condom sheath to the drainage set-up. Avoid kinking or twisting of the drainage tubing.	8.	The collection device keeps the client dry. Kinked tubing encourages back-flow of urine.
9.	Remove the equipment. Place the client in a comfortable, safe position. Wash your hands.	9.	This provides a safe, comfortable setting for the client. Handwashing deters the spread of microorganisms.
10.	Assess the client's response and record observations on the client's chart.	10.	This provides accurate documentation and observation of urine output.

Applying a Condom Catheter

The condom catheter is an external drainage system to collect urine from male clients who have incontinence. It is less invasive than a retention catheter and allows less contact of the skin with urine than a diaper or blue pad. Condom catheters require an order from an appropriate health care provider. Before applying condom catheter nurse has to do the following

- Assess skin integrity around the penis and perineal are to look for signs of irritation and skin breakdown
- Assess the client for ability to cooperate with the application and retention of the condom catheter to determine what type of teaching will be necessary
- Assess the amount and pattern of urinary incontinence to determine if the condom catheter is the best continence method for the client
- Assess for latex allergy.

Equipment Needed

- Condom catheter kit with adhesive strip
- Urinary drainage bag
- Clean gloves
- Basin with warm water and soap
- Towel and washcloth.

After procedure evaluate that:

- The client's condom catheter is in place without leakage or discomfort.
- The client does not have any skin irritation from the condom catheter.
- The client understands the reason for, and cooperates with, the placement and retention of the condom catheter.

And document the same in nurses' notes:

- Time the procedure was performed

Table 17.8: Applying Condom Catheter

	Nursing actions		*Rationales*
	Check clients identification band Explain procedure before beginning		To identity right patient To get cooperation and reduce anxiety
1.	Cleanse hands.	1.	Reduces transmission of microorganisms.
2.	Protect the client's privacy by closing the door and pulling curtains around the bed.	2.	Allows privacy for the client.
3.	Position the client in a comfortable position, preferably a supine position, if tolerated by the client. Raise the bed to a comfortable height for the nurse.	3.	Facilitates the cleaning and application of the catheter. Raising the bed to a comfortable height promotes good body mechanics.
4.	Apply latex-free gloves.	4.	Prevents possible transmission of microorganisms.
5.	Fold the client's gown across the abdomen and the sheet just below pubic area.	5.	Provides minimal exposure of the client, thereby reducing the client's embarrassment.
6.	Assess the client's penis for any signs of redness, irritation, or skin breakdown.	6.	A significant amount of skin breakdown may require an indwelling catheter. Provides baseline data for comparison with future assessments.
7.	Clean the client's penis with warm soapy water. Retract the foreskin on the uncircumcised male and clean thoroughly in folds.	7.	Removes microorganisms that could enter the urinary meatus and cause a urinary tract infection. Avoids trapping microorganisms in folds around the meatus.
8.	Return the client's foreskin to its normal position.	8.	Failure to return the foreskin to a normal position can lead to swelling of the penis and possible constriction.
9.	Shave any excess hair around the base of penis if required by institutional policy.	9.	Prevents discomfort from the adhesive strip when the condom catheter is removed.
10.	Rinse and dry the area.	10.	Moist warm environment can lead to the growth of microorganisms.
11.	If a condom kit used, open the package containing the skin preparation. Wipe and apply skin preparation solution to the shaft of the penis. If the client has an erection, wait for termination of erection before applying the catheter.	11.	Preparation solution protects the client's skin from irritation. An erection may occur from manipulation of the penis while cleaning the area. This is a normal reaction and will terminate in a few minutes.
12.	Apply the double-sided adhesive trip around the base of the client's penis in a spiral fashion. The strip is applied 1 inch from the proximal end of the penis. Do not completely encircle the penis or tightly encompass penis.	12.	Applying the adhesive in a spiral fashion does not compromise circulation of the penis. Encircling the penis can constrict the penis, impair circulation, and cause edema.
13.	Position the rolled condom at the distal portion of the penis and unroll it, covering the penis and the double-sided strip of adhesive. Leave a 1- to 2-inch space between the tip of the penis and the end of the condom.	13.	The condom sticks to the adhesive and remains in place. The extra spacing prevents pressure and erosion of the tip of the penis.
14.	Gently press the condom to the adhesive strip.	14.	Enables the condom to adhere evenly to the adhesive strip.
15.	Attach the drainage bag tubing to the catheter tubing. Make sure the tubing lays over the client's legs, not under. Secure the drainage bag to the side of the bed below the level of the client's bladder or to the drainage bag attached to the leg.	15.	Promotes urine flow away from the client. Constant exposure to urine and moisture can irritate the penis. Prevents reflux of the urine onto the penis and microorganisms from entering the penis.
16.	Determine that the condom and tubing are not twisted.	16.	If the condom or tubing is twisted, the urine cannot flow out and the condom will leak or fall off.
17.	Cover the client.	17.	Maintains privacy of the client.
18.	Dispose of the used equipment in appropriate receptacle.	18.	Reduces transmission of microorganisms.

Contd...

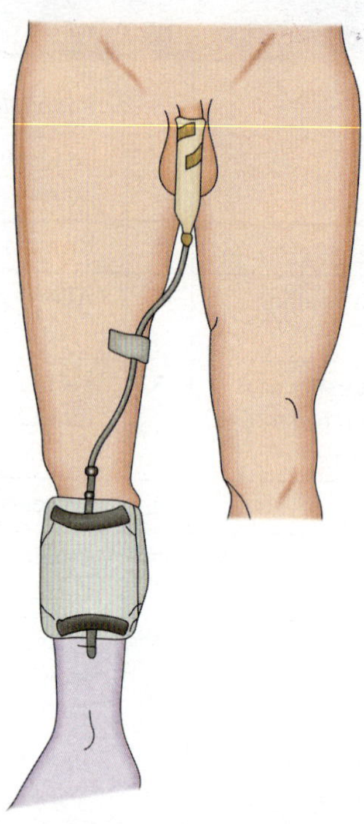

Figure 17.11: Condom catheter with drainage bag in place

	Table 17.8: *Contd...*			
	Nursing actions			*Rationales*
19.	Empty the bag, measure the client's urinary output, and record every 4 hours. Remove gloves and cleanse hands after procedure.		19.	Records output and prevents bag from becoming overly full and/or too heavy. Reduces transmission of microorganisms.
20	Return the client's bed to the lowest position and reposition client to comfortable or appropriate position.		20	Reduces potential injury from falls.
21.	Remove the condom once a day to clean the area and assess the skin for signs of impaired skin integrity.		21.	Promotes hygiene and reduces the possibility of skin breakdown.

- Condition of the client's skin, recording any irritation, rashes, or open area
- Client teaching performed
- Amount of urine emptied from the urine drainage bag

Measuring Intake and Output

One of the most basic methods of monitoring a client's health is measuring intake and output, commonly called "I&O." By monitoring the amount of fluids a client takes in and comparing this to the amount of fluid a client puts out, the health care team gains valuable insights into the client's general health as well as monitors specific disease conditions.

To maintain good health, fluid intake should approximately equal fluid output. Intake that exceeds output can indicate medical conditions ranging from renal failure to congestive heart failure. Output that exceeds intake can be caused by things as serious as life-threatening diarrhea or as benign as diuretic medications. An accurate record of a client's fluid balance is an important nursing function.

I&O monitoring is often ordered by the health care provider but can also be initiated by the nurse. Ideally, I&O should be monitored over several days to obtain an accurate record of the client's status. In critical situations, however, this may not be possible, and the client's I&O may be monitored and reported on an hourly basis. A urine output of less than 30 cc per hour should be reported.

A daily weight is often done in conjunction with I&O because it can indicate fluid retention or loss. One gallon of water weights 8 pounds. An 8 pound weight gain over a 24- to 48-hour period could indicate a life-threatening condition for the client. A significant change in a client's weight or a significant difference in a client's total I&O should be reported to the client's health care provider.

Intake is considered to be any fluid consumed or infused. This includes water, juice, coffee, milk, ice cream, soup broth, and Jell-O. Be sure to calculate the amount of water the client has consumed from the bedside water pitcher. Any fluids infused through IV lines, central lines, feeding tubes, or irrigant that is not returned is considered intake. Blood and blood products as well as the saline used to flush IV lines before and after the transfusion are also included in this count. IV piggybacks, fluids used to measure cardiac output, central line flushes, and *TKO* (to keep open) fluids are also considered in the intake total.

Urine is the largest component of output fluid volume, but several other fluid loss avenues must be considered. Diarrhea, diaphoresis, wound drainage, gastric or other fluids removed by suction, and bleeding are all fluid losses as well. These losses should be measured or estimated and recorded in the total output.

Client who are able to understand and cooperate with the I&O measurement should be encouraged to keep track of their fluid balance. Particularly in clients who are on a fluid restriction, client understanding and participation can greatly increase cooperation.

Table 17.9: Measuring Intake and Output (I & O)

	Nursing actions		*Rationales*
	Check clients identification band Explain procedure before beginning		To identity right patient To get cooperation and reduce anxiety
1.	Cleanse hands.	1.	Reduces the transmission of microorganisms.
2.	Explain the rules of I&O record. All fluids taken orally must be recorded on the client's intake and output form (sometimes called a fluid balance flow sheet). • Client must void into bedpan, urinal, or "hat" in toilet for collecting urine, not into toilet. • Toilet tissue should be disposed of in plastic-lined container, not in bedpan.	2.	Elicits client support. • Fluid voided into the toilet cannot be measured. • Liquids absorbed into toilet tissue cannot be measured by volume.
Intake			
3.	Measure all oral fluids in accord with agency policy (e.g., cup = 150 mL, glass = 240 mL).	3.	Provides for consistency of measurement.
4.	Record time and amount of all fluid intake in the designated space on bedside form (e.g., oral, tube feedings, IV fluids).	4.	Documents fluids.
5.	Transfer 8-hour total fluid intake from bedside I&O record to graphic sheet or 24-hour I&O record on client's chart.	5.	Provides for data analysis of the client's fluid status.
6.	Record all fluid intake in the appropriate column of the 24-hour record.	6.	Documents intake by type and amount.
7.	Complete 24-hour intake record by adding all 8-hour totals.	7.	Provides consistent data for analysis of the client's fluid status over a 24-hour period.
Output			
8.	Cleanse hands and apply nonsterile gloves.	8.	Reduces potential for transmission of pathogens.
9.	Empty urinal, bedpan, or Foley drainage bag (Fig. 17.11) into graduated container or commode "hat".	9.	Provides accurate measurement of urine.
10.	Remove gloves and cleanse hands.	10.	Prevents cross-contamination.
11.	Record time and amount of output (e.g., urine, drainage from nasogastric tube, drainage tube) on I&O record.	11.	Documents output.
12.	Transfer 8-hour output totals to graphic sheet or 24-hour I&O record on the client's chart.	12.	Provides for data analysis of the client's fluid status.
13.	Complete 24-hour output record by totaling all 8-hour totals. over a 24-hour period.	13.	Provides consistent data for analysis of the client's fluid status
14.	Cleanse hands.	14.	Reduces transmission of microorganisms.

Before measuring intake and output the nurse should:
- Assess the client's risk factors for fluid overload, such as congestive heart failure, renal failure, or ascites because edema can result from excess volume in extracellular fluid spaces and transferring of fluid into tissues
- Determine if the client is receiving fluids or medications that would predispose to fluid overload, such as large amounts of IV fluids or steroid therapy, because steroids cause sodium and water retention and excretion of potassium
- Assess the client's risk factors for fluid loss, such as diaphoresis, rapid respirations, diarrhea, gastric suction, blood loss, or wound drainage, because dehydration can result from reduction of fluid within the tissues and circulatory system
- Determine if the client's urine output is in excess of fluid intake because the kidneys excrete excess fluid during periods of overhydration and conserve body water during periods of dehydration
- Assess the client's ability to understand and cooperate with intake and output measurement because cooperation in these measurements will help ensure accuracy.

Equipment Needed

- I&O form at bedside
- I&O graphic record in chart
- Glass or cup
- Bedpan, urinal, or bedside commode
- Graduated container for output
- Nonsterile gloves
- Sign at bedside stating client is on I&O.
  Procedure of intake and output measuring, see Table 17.9.

After measuring I&O the nurse should see that:
- The client's fluid intake and output was accurately measured and recorded
- Note if the client was able to participate in the recording of fluid intake and output to the best of his or her ability
- Note and report any abnormal findings to the client's health care provider.

And document the following intake and output record:
- All fluid I&O
- Totals at the end of every shift
- Totals for 24 hours.

After it should be documented in the Nurses' Notes as given below:
- Unusual findings, excessive intake, excessive output, or serious imbalance of intake and output and report to the client's health care provider.

18

Management of Fluid, Electrolyte and Acid-base Balance

Introduction of Body Fluids

A fluid medium is essential for normal body function. It is the most vital and at the same time the most abundant component of the human body. Life depends upon a constant source and regulation of fluid in the body. Without fluid there would be no form of life.

Electrolyte balance is closely related to fluid balance. The fluid disturbance or electrolyte disturbance leads to fatality. Fluid deprivation brings about death more early than food deprivation.

The cells that make up body tissues exist chemically in constant but physiologically in dynamic internal environment. Physiologic processes function to regulate this environment so that responses to stimuli minimally affect the body. The chemical consistency is achieved through fluid, electrolyte and acid-base balance. Physiologic homeostasis and life itself, depend on normal fluid and electrolyte balance and acid-base balance. It is essential to maintain homeostasis. Homeostasis is the term used to describe the ability to maintain internal balance in the presence of external stressors.

The homeostatic mechanism that regulates fluid and electrolyte balance represents interaction between chemical and physiologic processes. Promoting balance in either a wellness or an illness state can prevent fluid and electrolyte imbalances that may be life-threatening. Nurses have primary professional contact for most clients. In any setting it is natural for them to play an action role in the prevention, early detection and treatment of fluid and electrolyte imbalances. Now nurses not only have the opportunity, but also they have broad base of knowledge of normal physiology and pathology, to assist in the identification of clients at risk and recognizing early manifestations of imbalance and taking measures to correct imbalance through nursing process.

The external environment within which we live undergoes continual changes, both small and large. For example, the daily and seasonal temperatures may fluctuate over a wide range. The light intensity is bright on sunny days and less so on cloudy days. The humidity may be either high or low. These are just a few of the many factors that constantly change in the external environment. Our bodies must continually adjust to such changes in the external environment. In order for life to continue, however, our internal environment-the one inside our bodies must remain relatively constant, varying only slightly within narrow ranges. This internal environment consists of the various body fluids such as the fluid inside cells, the blood, tissue fluids that bathe the cells, and other fluids. Maintenance of the internal environment within very narrow limits is termed homeostasis (equilibrium).

Homeostasis

Homeostasis is an ongoing process; that is, the body simply does not reach a state of equilibrium and remain there. Small changes constantly occur in response to physiologic processes. The body must therefore continuously make subtle adjustments to maintain the constancy of the internal environment within a normal range.

- Homeostasis is accomplished by various physiologic processes and the coordinated activities of the organ systems. Some examples are as follows:
- The gastrointestinal (GI) system changes large, complex molecules of ingested food to simpler, less-complex molecules that can be utilized by the cells of the body to produce the energy necessary for life.
- The respiratory system supplies the cells with the constant source of oxygen required to release the energy from the products of digestion. It also eliminates carbon dioxide, the waste product produced by the cells as a result of energy production.
- The blood acts as a transport mechanism, carrying the products of digestion along with hormones and oxygen to the cells, where these substances are utilized.
- It also transports carbon dioxide from the energy-releasing processes of the cells to the lungs, where it will be eliminated.
- All of the activities of the various organ systems are integrated and coordinated through the nervous system and the endocrine system.

When the body loses the ability to maintain homeostasis and the internal environment changes, the physiologic processes can be interrupted or changed, leading to disease, disorder, or death. In essence, then, maintaining homeostasis is essential to life. Because the processes of homeostasis involve many chemical and physical processes, it is necessary to examine some of these before studying homeostasis in more detail.

Distribution of Fluid

The fluid is distributed in the body in three compartments that are separated by semipermeable membrane. This is roughly distributed as follows:

Intracellular fluid is within the cell and interstitial fluid surrounds all living cells and allows for diffusion of nutrients, electrolytes, water, hormones, oxygen and waste products. Intravascular fluid is within the blood vessels.

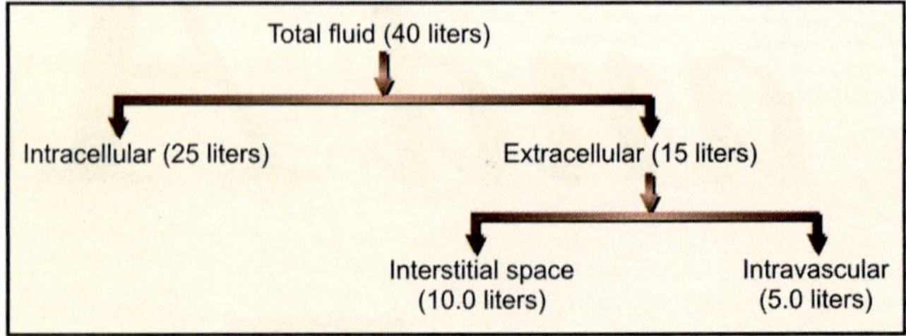

Normal control of body fluid:
Fluid intake
The body receives water from two sources:
(a) Exogenous - as drinks or with solid foods.
(b) Endogenous - released during the metabolic oxidation.

The total fluid intake per day:

Water intake	300 c.c.
Water from solid food	1000 c.c.
Water produced from internal metabolic oxidation	300 c.c.
Total	2600 c.c. per 24 hours

Fluid Loss: Daily fluid loss of an average adult taking normal amount of fluid is usually through various sources as follows:

(1) Lung	400 c.c.
(2) Kidney	1500 c.c.
(3) Skin	600 c.c. (may be 1000 c.c. in hot
(4) Bowel	100 c.c. climate)
(5) Negligible amount along saliva and tears	________
	2600 c.c. per 24 hours

The fluid loss in babies and growing children are proportionately greater than that of an adult. Kidneys of an infant do not conserve water as effectively as the kidneys of adults. In older child and adult if the body needs water, the pituitary antidiuretic hormone promotes its reabsorption from the renal tubules and excessive fluid intake is eliminated through the kidneys. If large quantity of fluid is taken rapid absorption of fluid into the plasma compartment takes place. Blood volume may be temporarily increased as well as an increase in cardiac output. There is rapid adjustment to the increased fluid.

The normal daily replacement of water equals the normal daily loss. Since daily turnover of water of a baby is more than half of his extracellular fluid volume, it is essential that his fluid losses be replaced at once.

Body Electrolyte Component

All body fluids contain chemical compounds. Chemical compounds in solution may be classified as electrolytes or non-electrolytes. An electrolyte is a substance which when dissolves in water splits into separate electrically charged particles known as ions. Positively charged ions are called cations and negatively charged ions are called anions.

They are as follows:

CATIONS	ANIONS
Sodium (Na^+)	Chloride (Cl^-)
Potassium (K^+)	Bicarbonate (HCO_3^-)
Calcium (Ca^{++})	Phosphates (HPO_4, $H_2PO_4^-$)
Magnesium (Mg_2^{++})	Sulphates (SO_4^-)

They are important in maintenance of acid base balance and help to control body water volume. Identical electrolytes are in three fluid compartments but the concentration of the various electrolytes in each compartment varies markedly.

In general higher the concentration of the ions the more active is the solution. Some electrolytes ionize freely and provide high concentration of ions and are known as strong electrolytes. Some others maintain a reserve of neutral molecules in the solution. These are known as weak electrolytes.

In health the ratio of cations to anions in each of the body fluids and concentration of the various ions in these fluids is relatively constant. Electrolytes move more readily between interstitial and intravascular fluid than between the intracellular and interstitial fluids.

Electrolyte loss is mainly through the kidneys. Besides this, smaller amount of loss is through the skin, lungs and bowel. The kidneys selectively excrete electrolytes, retaining those needed for normal body fluid composition. Hormones influence the selective function of kidney.

A well balanced diet contains all the substances need to maintain electrolyte balance. Any excess of electrolytes ingested will be excreted by the kidneys.

Chemical Organization

The human body is highly organized. This organization exists in increasing levels of complexity. Most basic is the chemical level. To understand the higher levels of organization. it is necessary to know something about basic chemical and physical principles.

Elements

The cell consists of living matter. *Matter* is anything that occupies space and possesses mass. All matter has certain physical properties such as color, odor, hardness, and density. Matter also has extensive properties such as size, shape, and weight. Matter is composed of basic substances called *elements*. Elements are made of tiny units called atoms. Atoms of each element are alike. Different elements have different kinds of atoms. Presently, 108 elements are recognized. Some examples are iron, gold, carbon, hydrogen, oxygen, nitrogen, and copper. Many of the elements occur in the human body in varying amounts. Some are present in large amounts, and others are found in only trace amounts. The time elements oxygen, carbon, hydrogen, and nitrogen constitute more than 95% of the total body weight of the elements. Some of the elements and their function in the body are presented in Table 18.1.

Atoms

An atom is the smallest unit of chemical structure, and no chemical change can alter it. Atoms are made up of three basic particles: protons, neutrons, and electrons. Protons and neutrons are similar in size, but whereas protons have a positive electrical charge, neutrons have no charge. Together, they form the nucleus of the atom. Because the protons have a positive charge and the neutrons are neutral, the nucleus of an atom has a positive charge. The electrons have a negative charge and move in an orbit around the nucleus. There are as many electrons as protons, rendering

Table 18.1: Elements Occurring in the Human Body

Element	Approximate % of body weight	Function
Major Elements		
Oxygen (O)	65.0	Found in both organic and inorganic compounds; as a gas, is necessary in metabolizing glucose and other chemical compounds into energy
Carbon (C)	18.5	Found in all organic compounds such as carbohydrates, protein, lipids, and nucleic acids; necessary for cellular respiration
Hydrogen (H)	9.5	Found in many organic and inorganic compounds; in ionic form, involved in pH; component of water; necessary for life
Nitrogen (N)	3.2	Important in proteins, which are the body's building blocks, an energy source, and a component of hormones
Calcium (Ca)	1.5	Important element in bone and tooth composition; involved in nerve conduction, muscle contraction, and blood clotting
Phosphorus (P)	1.0	Found in bones, teeth, the high-energy carrying compound adenosine triphosphatase (ATP), some proteins, and nucleic acid
Potassium (K)	0.4	Major electrolyte in intracellular fluid; important in muscle contraction and transmission of nerve impulses; activates enzymes; influences cellular osmotic pressure; involved in kidney function and acid-base balance
Sulfur (5)	0.3	Found in some proteins, nucleic acids, and some vitamins and hormones
Sodium (Na)	0.2	Constitutes major electrolyte in extracellular fluid; important in osmoregulation and acid-base balance; necessary for nerve transmission and muscle contraction
Chlorine (CI)	0.2	Found in extracellular fluid; important in water balance, acid-base balance, and production of hydrochloric acid in the stomach
Magnesium (Mg)	0.1	Important to muscle and nerve function and bone formation and in some coenzymes
Essential Trace Elements		
Present in the human body in minimal amounts, constituting approximately 0.1 % of body weight; have known functions		
Cobalt (Co)		Important component of vitamin B_{12}
Copper (Cu)		Necessary for formation of hemoglobin and for bone development
Chromium (Cr)		A cofactor involved with enzymes for fat, cholesterol, and glucose metabolism
Fluorine (F)		Gives hardness to teeth and bones
Iodine (I)		Necessary for synthesis of thyroid hormone
Iron (Fe)		Necessary for transportation of oxygen by hemoglobin
Manganese (Mn)		Necessary in activating some enzymes
Selenium (Se)		Acts with vitamin E as an antioxidant; component of teeth
Zinc (Zn)		Found in some enzymes; needed for protein metabolism and carbon dioxide transport
Other Trace Elements		
Have probable, but as yet undetected, functions		
Aluminum (AI), Nickel (Ni), Arsenic (As), Tin (Sn), Boron (B), Silicon (Si), Cadmium (Cd), Vanadium (V)		

the overall atom neutral. The number of protons in an atom is called its atomic number. The simplest element is hydrogen. It has an atomic number of 1. One proton with a positive charge forms the nucleus, and one electron moves in an orbit around the nucleus. Hydrogen atoms may or may not have a neutron. A hydrogen atom is illustrated in Figure 18.1 shows positively charged proton in the nucleus and negatively charged electron in orbit.

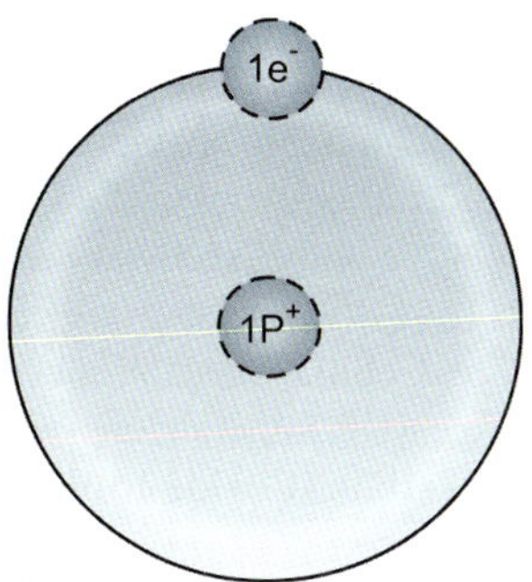

Figure 18.1: Hydrogen atom

Depending on the element, other atoms may have more than one proton and one electron and may have neutrons. The number of protons and neutrons in the nucleus is approximately equal to the atomic weight. Thus hydrogen has an atomic weight of 1.

Isotopes

The number of protons in the nucleus is the same for all atoms of a given element, but the number of neutrons may vary in atoms of the same element. For instance, all hydrogen atoms have one proton and one electron; however, some hydrogen atoms have one neutron in the nucleus, while others have two (Fig. 18.2). Atoms of the same element that have different atomic weights (i.e., have a different number of neutrons) are called isotopes. All of the isotopes of a given element react the same way chemically. A. Deuteridium has one positively charged proton and one neutron in the nucleus and one electron in orbit; B. Tritium has one positively charged proton and two neutrons in the nucleus and one electron in orbit.

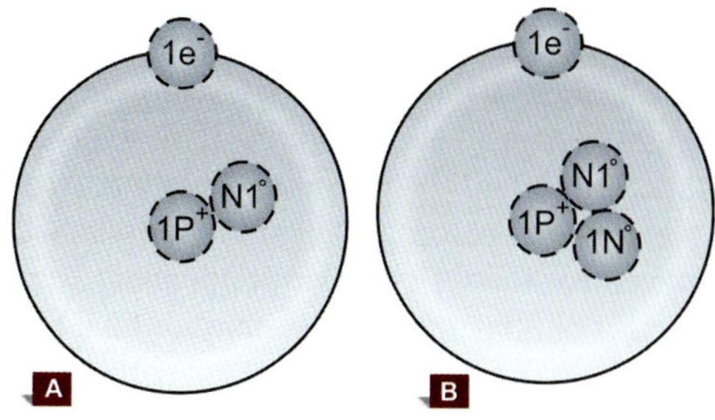

Figure 18.2: Isotopes of hydrogen

Some isotopes, called radioactive isotopes, have an unstable nucleus, which decomposes and gives off energy in the form of radiation. This radiation can be in the form of alpha, beta, or gamma rays. All are damaging to cells. Alpha radiation is the least harmful, and gamma radiation is the most harmful. Iodine, oxygen, and cobalt are examples of elements having radioactive isotopes. Some of the radioactive isotopes are useful as biological markers and can be used *to* track metabolic pathways of food. Others such as iodine can be injected into the body and used to track the circulation of blood. Still others such as cobalt are used in cancer treatment.

Molecules and Compounds

Atoms of the same element can unite with each other to form a molecule. For example, atoms of hydrogen unite to form a hydrogen molecule. This can be expressed in a chemical equation using the chemical symbol for hydrogen:

$$H + H \rightarrow H_2$$

In this reaction, the atoms on the left are the reactants; the arrow is read as "yield"; and the last symbol is the product–a molecule of hydrogen. A chemical equation uses the chemical symbols of elements and shows the ratios by which they combine. Because atoms of elements always combine in the same ratio under similar conditions, it is possible to predict the nature of a chemical change.

When atoms of two or more different elements combine (react), they form a compound. For example, if one atom of sodium (Na) and one atom of chlorine (Cl) react, they form a molecule of the compound called sodium chloride. This is expressed in the following equation:

$$Na + Cl \rightarrow NaCl$$

Compounds can be divided into two groups. Those without carbon are inorganic compounds, and those with carbon are organic compounds. By using chemical equations, chemical changes, called reactions, can be shown. Sometimes, different substances are combined in no specific way, and the components do not have a definite ratio every time. For instance, water, sugar, and table salt mixed without being measured will yield different results depending on the ratio of each substance. Such a combination is called a mixture. Its composition may vary each time the components are mixed.

Chemical reactions occur whenever atoms join together or separate. They join together by forming bonds, and they separate by breaking bonds. Either way, new combinations result. When two or more atoms (reactants) bond and form a more complex molecular product, the reaction is called synthesis. A sample equation would be as follows:

$$2H \quad + \quad O \quad \rightarrow \quad H_2O$$
hydrogen and oxygen yields water

When the bonding between the atoms in a molecule is broken and simpler products are formed, the reaction is called decomposition. If a molecule of sodium chloride is decomposed, it forms sodium and chlorine. This can be expressed as follows:

NaCI ?   →   Na   +   Cl
sodium chloride   yields sodium   and   chloride
(decomposition)

It is important to understand that when synthesis occurs, energy is tied up in the bonds formed during the reaction. When decomposition occurs, energy is released. In the cells of the body, these kinds of chemical reactions are repeatedly occurring: Molecules form and decompose. Body cells can utilize these reactions to form energy sources and to free energy to drive the various metabolic processes of the cells.

Ions

When some compounds are placed in water, they decompose, or ionize. The result is an ion, an atom bearing an electrical charge. An ion with a positive charge is called a cation; an ion with a negative charge is termed an anion. For example, sodium chloride in water dissociates to form sodium ions bearing a positive charge and chloride ions bearing a negative charge (Fig. 18.3). Because the atoms in this combination are charged, they will conduct electricity. The reaction can be shown as follows:

NaCI ?   →   Na⁺   +   Cl
sodium chloride   yields sodium   and   chloride
(cation)   (anion)

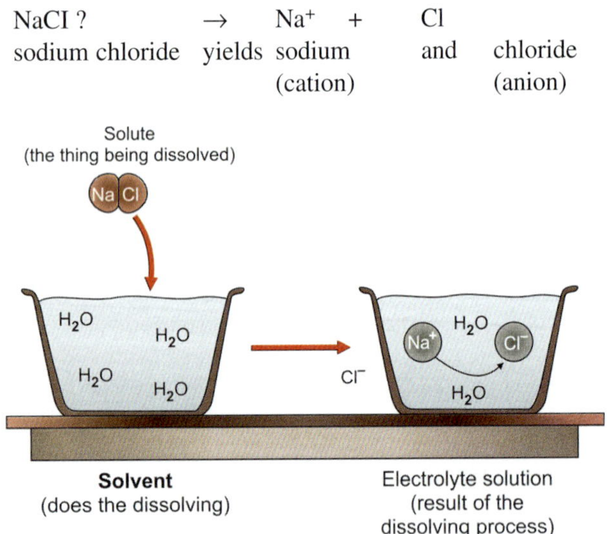

Figure 18.3: Dissociation of electrolytes

A compound that dissociates into ions in water is called an electrolyte. Many electrolytes are extremely important in body chemistry.

Water

Water constitutes approximately 60% of the total body weight of all adult and is involved in many of the physical and physiological processes of the body. Because water is so integral to the body's processes, fluctuations in the amount of water in the body can have harmful or even fatal consequences.

Body Water and Body Size

The amount of body water is inversely proportional to body size. The smaller the body, the higher the water content:

Embryo: 97%
Infant: 77%
Child: 60% to 77%
Adult: 60%
Elders: 45% to 50%

Body water diminishment in elderly persons is related to tissue loss.

Water is the major component of blood. Approximately 92% of the body's organic and inorganic compounds dissolve in this water into less-complex molecules and atoms and then are transported throughout the body. Necessary substances such as oxygen and nutrients from the GI system are carried to the cells, where they are utilized. Cellular waste products such as carbon dioxide, urea, and excessive minerals are carried by water to sites of elimination: carbon dioxide to the lungs, urea and minerals to the kidneys.

Water also absorbs heat resulting from muscle contractions and distributes this heat over the body. Water in the form of perspiration released from sweat glands in the skin can cool the body by evaporation. Water also can break apart the bonds in large molecules such as starches to form smaller molecules in the digestive process. This type of reaction is called hydration.

Water is the primary component of all body fluids. It is the solvent used to transport nutrients to cells and to remove waste products produced by the cellular metabolism. Temperature regulation is assisted by evaporation of water on the body surface. Approximately 60 percent of weight in a typical adult is composed of fluids, i.e. water and electrolytes. Factors that influence the amount of body fluids are age, gender, and body content. As a general rule, younger people have a higher percentage of body fluid than older people and men have proportionately more body fluid than women. Obese people have less fluid than thin people because fat cells contain little water. Adipose tissue contains less water than an equivalent amount of muscle tissue. In the older adult, body water contents averages 45 to 55 percent of the body weight. In infant, water content averages 70 to 80 percent of body weight. Therefore, the young are at risk because they have less fluid reserves. Both the very young and the very old have a decreased ability to compensate for fluid loss.

Body fluid is located in the two compartments, viz. intracellular space (fluid in the cells) and the extracellular space (fluids outside the cells). Intracellular fluid (ICF) is located (primarily in the skeletal muscle mass) and constitutes 40 percent of body weight or 70 percent or two-third of the total body fluids/water. Extracellular fluid (ECF) constitutes about 20 percent of the body weight or 30 percent or one-third of total body fluids/water. Extracellular fluid (ECF) constitutes about 20 percent of the body weight or 30 percent or one-third of total body water. ECF consists of interstitial (between cells and lymph) intravascular (fluid within the cell is plasma), cerebrospinal, and intraocular fluid, as well as secretions of the gastrointestinal (GI) tract. Sometimes, the term 'transcellular', i.e., a product of secretion and diffusion from cells is used to refer to cerebrospinal, pericardial, synovial, intraocular and pleural fluids, sweat and digestive secretions.

ECF transports nutrients, electrolytes and oxygen to cells, carries waste products for excretion, regulates heat, lubricates and cushions, joints and membranes, hydrolizes food for digestion and maintains vascular volume by passing easily through the capillary walls. ICF provides the cell with the internal aqueous medium necessary for its chemical functions. Normally, the fluid volume inside and outside of the cells maintains a steady state due to compensatory responses.

Fluid Spacing

Fluid spacing is a term used to classify the distribution of body water. The term 'fluid' is used because more water is found in these ICF and ECF compartments such as glucose, sodium and potassium.

First spacing: It is a normal distribution of fluid in both the ECF and ICF components.

Second spacing: It refers to an excess accumulation of interstitial fluid (edema).

Third spacing: It occurs when fluids accumulate in areas that normally have no fluid or only a minimum amount of fluid (e.g., ascitis, sequestration of fluid in the bowel in peritonitis and edema associated with bums).

Water is not only responsible for the body's structure and functions but it is also necessary for the maintenance of equilibrium (homeostasis) and of life itself. Body fluids normally shift between the two major compartments or spaces in an effort to maintain the equilibrium between the spaces. Loss of fluid from the body can also disrupt the equilibrium. Sometimes fluid is not lost from the body, but it is unavailable for use by either ICF or ECF spaces. Loss of ECF into a space that does not contribute to equilibrium between ICF and ECF is referred to as *third space fluid shift*. Third spacing is a concern because it takes fluid away from the normal fluid compartments and may produce hypovolemia. An early clue of a third space fluid shift is a decrease in urinary output despite adequate fluid therapy. Urine output decreases because fluid shift out of the intravascular space; the kidneys that receive less blood flow and attempt to compensate by decreasing urine output. Other signs and symptoms of 'third spacing' that indicates an intravascular fluid volume deficit include increased heart rate, decreased blood pressure, decreased central venous pressure, edema, increased body weight and imbalance in fluid intake and output. For example, third space occurs in ascitis, burns, massive bleeding into a joint or body cavity.

Gases

Two important gases in the body are oxygen (O_2) and carbon dioxide (CO_2). Because these elements are gases, their molecules are free and can move swiftly in all directions. Oxygen enters the body through the lungs and is transported by the red blood cells throughout the body to the cells. The cells use oxygen in the release of energy from glucose and other molecules. This energy is needed by the cells to carry out their activities. As a result of the energy-releasing processes, carbon dioxide is produced by the cells and transported in the blood to the lungs, where it is eliminated.

Acids, Bases, Salts and pH

Other chemical substances important for life are acids, bases, and salts: pH is the measure of acid and base strength.

Acids: An acid is any substance that in solution yields hydrogen ions bearing a positive charge. As an example, hydrochloric acid (HCl) in water dissociates as shown following:

$$HCl \rightarrow H^+ + Cl$$

hydrochloric acid   yields   hydrogen   and   chlorine

The hydrogen ion characterizes this as an acid. Important acids in the body are hydrochloric acid, produced in the stomach, and carbonic acid, formed when the carbon dioxide released from cells reacts with some of the water in the extracellular fluid (all body fluids except for those contained within the cells).

Bases: A base is a substance that when dissociated produces ions that will combine with hydrogen ions. For example, when sodium hydroxide dissociates in water, it forms a sodium ion bearing a positive charge and a hydroxyl ion bearing a negative charge as shown following:

$$NaOH \rightarrow Na^+ + OH^-$$

sodium hydroxide   yields sodium   and   hydroxyl

The hydroxyl ion is capable of combining with a hydrogen ion to form water. Sodium bicarbonate is an example of a base found in the body.

Salts: A salt is formed when an acid and a base react with each other. Salts result from the neutralization of an acid by a base, as illustrated by the following reaction:

$$HCl + NaOH \rightarrow H_2O + NaCl$$

hydrochloric   and   sodium   yields   water and   sodium
acid   hydroxide   chloride

The hydrochloric acid reacts with the sodium hydroxide to form a molecule of water and a molecule of a salt–sodium chloride. When salts are placed in water, they dissociate into a cation and an anion. For instance, in water, the sodium chloride would dissociate into Na^+ and Cl^-. One reason salts are of great biological importance is that many of the compounds that dissociate into ions in living cells are salts. For example, sodium and chlorine ions are present in great amounts in body fluids. Many other salts occur in lesser amounts.

pH: Acid and bases are classified as either strong or weak by the number of hydrogen ions or hydroxyl ions they produce when they dissociate. Strong acids release many hydrogen ions; weak acids release relatively few. The same is true of hydroxyl ions in strong and weak bases. The acidity or alkalinity of a solution is determined by the concentration of hydrogen ions in the solution. Potential hydrogen (pH) indicates the hydrogen ion concentration in a solution, expressed as a number from 0 to 14. A solution with a pH of 7 is neutral (i.e. it is neither an acid or a base). A solution with a pH greater than 7 is a base or alkaline. A solution with a pH less than 7 is an acid. The higher above 7 the pH, the more alkaline the solution; the lower below 7 the pH, the more acid the solution. pH is of great biological importance. The human body can tolerate only very slight changes in pH. For example, the pH of human blood ranges from 7.35 to 7.45. Blood pH above or below this range can cause severe or even fatal physiological problems.

Although small amounts of acids may enter the body through food intake, the greatest source of acids–and thus H^+ ions–is cellular metabolism, resulting in products including lactic acid, phosphoric acid, pyruvic acid, and many fatty acids. When blood pH falls below 7.35 as a result of an elevated concentration of H^+ ions, *acidosis* occurs. Rarely does blood pH fall to 7 or become acidic, because death will usually occur first. As acidosis increases, the central nervous system (CNS) becomes involved, and the client may become unconscious. The heartbeat may become weak and irregular, and blood pressure may decrease or even disappear.

When blood pH increases above 7.45, *alkalosis* occurs. Alkalosis is a condition characterized by an excessive loss of hydrogen ions. This happens less often than does acidosis. Symptoms of alkalosis include a heightened state of nervous system activity, resulting in spasmodic muscle contractions, convulsions, and even death.

Buffers

Buffers are substances that attempt to maintain pH range, or H^+ ion concentration, in the presence of added acids or bases. Buffers usually occur in pairs in the body fluids. They act to keep the pH of body fluids within normal range. If body fluids become acidic, buffers in the body fluids combine with the excess hydrogen ions and restore normal pH. Likewise, if the body fluids become alkaline, other buffers in the blood combine with the strong bases, converting them to weak bases and restoring normal pH.

Three important buffer systems occur in body fluids: the bicarbonate buffer system, the phosphate buffer system, and the protein buffer system. Because a change in pH of one fluid may bring corresponding changes in the pH of other fluids, an interplay between buffer systems acts to maintain the body's pH. The buffer systems react quickly to prevent excessive changes in the hydrogen ion concentration.

Bicarbonate Buffer System: The bicarbonate buffer system is found in both the extracellular and intracellular fluids and is the body's primary buffer system. It has two components: carbonic

acid (H_2CO_3) and sodium bicarbonate ($NaHCO_3$). When a strong acid such as hydrochloric acid is added to this buffer system, the acid will react with the sodium bicarbonate and form a weaker acid (carbonic acid) and a salt (sodium chloride).

HCl	+	$NaHCO_3$	$\rightarrow$	H_2CO_3	+	NaCl
hydrochloric acid	and	sodium bicarbonate	yields	carbonic acid	and	sodium chloride

The strong acid is converted into a weak acid, and the pH is raised toward normal.

If a strong base such as sodium hydroxide is added to this buffer system, the carbonic acid will react with it to form a weak base (sodium bicarbonate) and water.

NaOH	+	H_2CO_3	$\rightarrow$	$NaHCO_3$	+	H_2O
sodium hydroxide	and	carbonic acid	yields	sodium bicarbonate	and	water

The strong base, which initially raised the pH, is converted to a weak base, which will lower the pH toward normal. It is vital to note that hydrochloric acid and sodium hydroxide are substances not normally added to the blood. They are used here only as good examples of the way buffers work. This buffer system normally buffers organic acids found in body fluids.

In the body, bicarbonate helps stabilize pH by combining reversibly with hydrogen ions. Most of the body's bicarbonate is produced in red blood cells, where the enzyme carbonic anhydrase accelerates the conversion of carbon dioxide to carbonic acid. The production of bicarbonate is illustrated in the following reversible equation:

CO_2	+	H_2O	$\rightarrow$	H_2CO_3	$\leftrightarrow$	H^+	+	HCO_3^-
carbon dioxide	water			carbonic acid		hydrogen chloride		bicarbonate

When the hydrogen ion concentration increases in the extracellular (outside of the cell) space, the reaction shifts toward the left. A decreased concentration of hydrogen ions drives the reaction to the right.

Phosphate Buffer System: The phosphate buffer system is involved in regulating the pH of intracellular fluid and the fluid of the kidney tubules. It has two phosphate compounds: sodium monohydrogen phosphate ($NaHPO_4$) and sodium dihydrogen phosphate (NaH_2PO_4). In the presence of a strong acid such as hydrochloric acid, the sodium monohydrogen phosphate reacts with the acid to form a weak acid (sodium dihydrogen phosphate) and a salt (sodium chloride), thus raising the pH.

HCl	+	$NaHPO_4$	$\rightarrow$	NaH_2PO_4	+	NaCl
hydrochloric acid	and	sodium mono hydrogen phosphate	yields	sodium dihydrogen phosphate	and	sodium chloride

When sodium dihydrogen phosphate encounters a strong base such as sodium hydroxide, a weak base (sodium monohydrogen phosphate) and water are formed.

NaOH	+	NaH_2PO_4	$\rightarrow$	$NaHPO_4$	+	H_2O
Sodium hydroxide	and	sodium dihydrogen phosphate	yields	sodium monohydrogen phosphate	and	sodium chloride

Protein Buffers: Proteins are complex substances formed when amino acids bond. Each amino acid contains a carboxyl group (COOH) and an amino group (NH_2). The carboxyl group can ionize and release hydrogen, thus acting as an acid. The amino group can accept hydrogen, thus acting as a base. This ability allows proteins to act as a buffer system. The protein buffer system is found inside cells, especially in the hemoglobin of red blood cells, where the proteins can act to maintain the pH inside the cell. They are also found in the plasma.

Movement of Substance

Substances must be able to both enter and leave cells. For example, oxygen and various end products of digestion must enter a cell through the cell membrane for use by the cell. Waste products from cellular processes must be eliminated from the cell. Various ions must also both enter and leave cells. Everything that enters and leaves the cell must pass through the cell membrane. Thus the cell membrane serves not only as an envelope around the cell, but also as a gatekeeper, regulating which substances can enter and leave the cell. The cell membrane is a very thin and delicate, but complex and living, elastic covering around each cell. It consists of an inner and outer layer of phospholipids in which protein molecules are embedded. Many small channels pass through the membrane. These channels allow some water molecules and some water-soluble substances to pass through the membrane. The ability of a membrane to permit substances to pass through it is called *permeability*. Because a cell membrane allows passage of only certain substances, it is called a selective permeable membrane, or *semipermeable membrane*.

Some substances can pass through the cell membrane without energy expenditure on the part of the cell. This is called passive transport. The passage of other substances requires an expenditure of energy by the cell. This is called active transport.

Passive Transport

There are several types of passive transport: diffusion, osmosis, and filtration.

Diffusion: Diffusion is the tendency of molecules of either gases, liquids, or solids to move from a region of higher molecular concentration to a region of lower molecular concentration until an equilibrium is reached. This movement is caused by the kinetic energy ill molecules. Kinetic energy causes the molecules to move constantly, colliding with one another and knocking each other about, thus causing them to move farther apart. An example is a drop of black ink placed in a glass of water: over time, the glass of water will turn a uniform black color because of diffusion, as shown in Figure 18.4 is the spreading of particles from an area of greater concentration to an area of lesser concentration. Dye put into a beaker of water gradually spreads throughout the water.

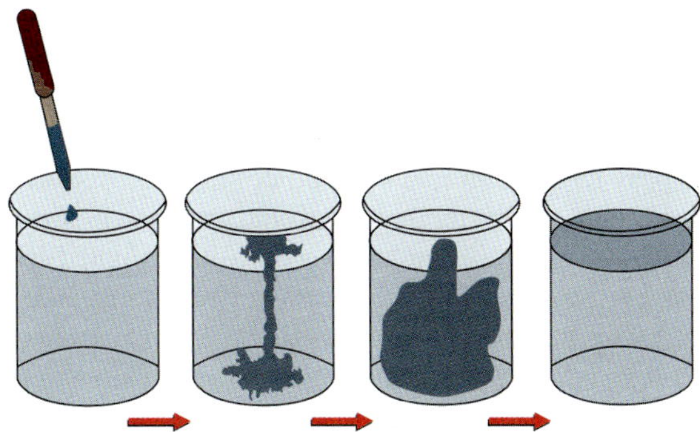

Figure 18.4: Diffusion

In the body, oxygen moves by diffusion from the lungs to the bloodstream because the oxygen concentration is higher in the lungs and lower in the blood. Carbon dioxide moves by diffusion from the bloodstream, where the concentration of carbon dioxide is higher, to the lungs, for elimination. The size of the channels in the cell membrane can prevent large molecules from passing through the membrane. Some substances, such as glucose molecules, combine with carrier molecules, which carry them into the interior of the cell, where they are released.

The term *dialysis* is used when diffusion is employed to separate molecules out of a solution by passing them through a semipermeable membrane. Dialysis is the process used in the artificial kidney. As blood from a client circulates through a machine, small, toxic waste molecules such as urea leave the blood and pass through the semipermeable membrane by diffusion and out into the surrounding fluid. The blood, thus cleaned, is then returned to the body.

Osmosis: Osmosis is the diffusion of water through a semipermeable membrane from a region of higher water concentration to a region of lower water concentration. In a solution undergoing osmosis, only the water (solvent) molecules move through the membrane; the dissolved molecules do not (Fig. 18.5).

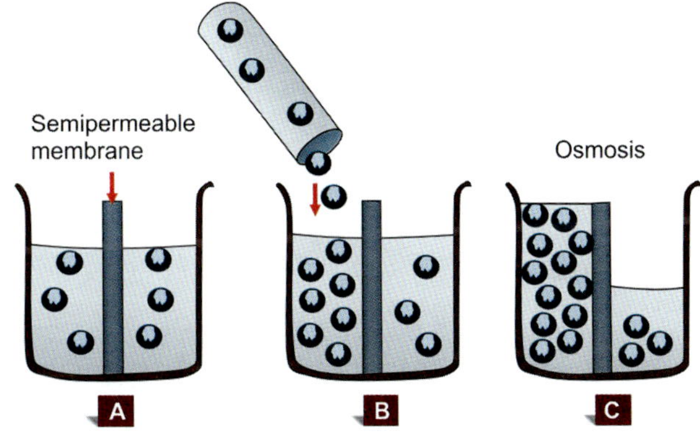

Figure 18.5: The process of osmosis

If a cell, having both a membrane that will not allow sodium chloride to pass through and a molecular concentration of 10%, sodium chloride, were placed in a container with a 5% sodium chloride solution, the cell would contain 10% sodium chloride and 90% water, and the 5% solution in which it was placed would contain 5% dissolved sodium chloride and 95% water. There would be more water outside than inside the cell: thus water would pass through the membrane into the cell. Because the cell membrane is elastic, the cell would increase in size as a result of the water accumulation within it facilitated by the process of osmosis. The pressure exerted against the cell membrane by the water inside the cell is called *osmotic pressure*.

A solution that bas the same molecular concentration as the cell is called an *isotonic solution*. It neither increases nor decreases the size of the cell. A solution that has a lower molecular concentration than the cell is called a *hypotonic solution*. Placing cells in a hypotonic solution causes them to swell, possibly to the point of eventual rupture. The rupture of red blood cells due to osmosis is called *hemolysis*. As red blood cells swell, the hemoglobin contained within passes to the outside of the cell and into the solution surrounding the cell, rendering the blood cells no longer capable of carrying oxygen. A solution that has a higher molecular concentration than the cell is called a *hypertonic solution*. When placed in such a solution, water leaves the cell, and the cell decreases in size. In the case of red blood cells, they shrivel and become wrinkled. This shrinkage, called *crenation*, leaves the cells incapable of functioning.

In persons who have lost large volumes of blood, it is sometimes necessary to administer additional fluids to maintain blood pressure. Generally, normal saline can be used. This 0.9% sodium chloride solution has approximately the same osmotic concentration as blood. Because it is isotonic, it will not damage the cells. Figure 18.6 shows osmosis in cells with different solution concentrations. A. In a hypotonic solution, the water moves into the cells, causing them to swell and burst. B. In an isotonic solution, cells are normal in size and shape because the same amount of water is entering and leaving the cells. C. In a hypertonic solution, cells are losing water because water moves from an area of lower concentration (inside the cell) to an area of higher concentration (outside the cell).

Filtration: In filtration, fluids and the substances dissolved in them are forced through cell membranes by *hydrostatic pressure–* the pressure the fluid exerts against the membrane. The molecules passing through the membrane are determined by the size of the pores in the membrane. Tissue fluids are formed by filtration. As blood passes through the capillaries, hydrostatic pressure exerted by the pumping action of the heart causes some of the liquid fraction of the blood (but not the cells) to pass out of the capillaries, resulting in formation of the tissue fluid (Fig. 18.7). (i) Pressure in the arteriole is greater then interstitial (between the cells) pressure, causing fluid with dissolved substances to move out of capillaries. (ii) Pressure in venules is less than interstitial fluid pressure, causing fluid and waste products to move back into the capillaries. As the blood circulates through the capillaries of the kidneys, the hydrostatic pressure of the blood causes many materials to leave the blood through the filtration process. These materials pass into the tubules of the kidneys, where the toxic waste products are removed to form urine. The urine is then eliminated from the body.

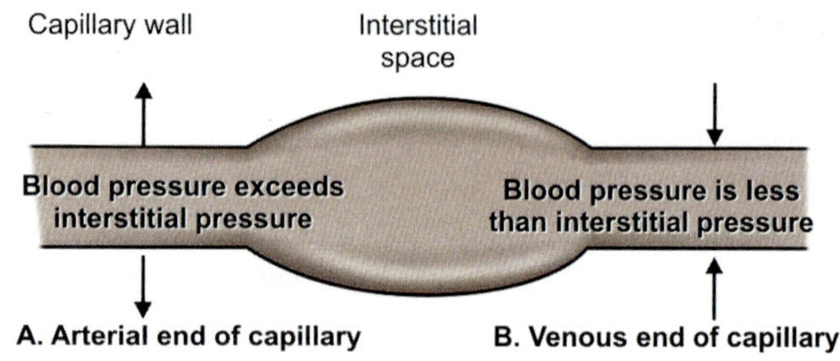

Figure 18.7: Filtration

Active Transport

In the processes discussed thus far, the movement of molecules depends on the concentration of molecules or on pressure. In other words, the cells do not have to expend energy to move the molecules in or out of the cell. In active transport, the cell must use energy to move the molecules. For instance, in the body, sodium ions are in higher concentration in the fluids surrounding the cell than inside the cell. Although some sodium ions can diffuse into the cell, the cell actively transports them through the membrane to the outside. Active transport is accomplished by means of carrier molecules, which can latch onto specific molecules and transport them in or out of the cell. This process requires an expenditure of cellular energy (Fig. 18.8). Examples of important ions transported by this process are calcium, sodium,

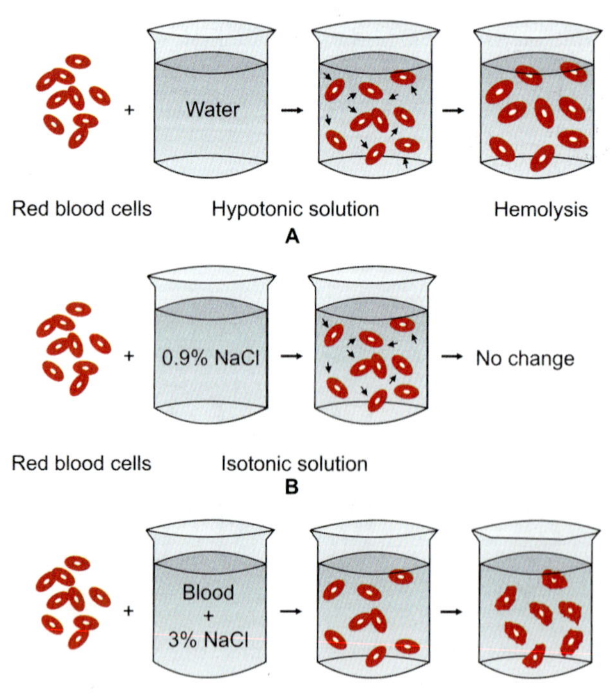

Figure 18.6: Osmosis is the movement of water through a membrane from an area of lower concentration to one of higher concentration

potassium, and magnesium. Active transport of molecules takes place from an area of lesser concentration to an area of greater concentration.

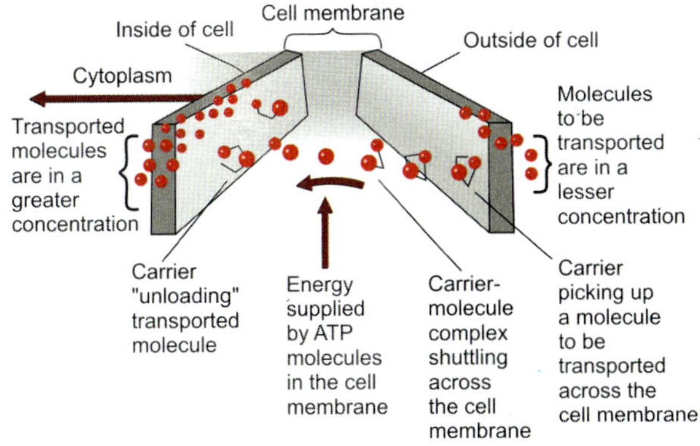

Figure 18.8: Active transport of molecules

Fluid and Electrolyte Balance

Human life is suspended in a saline solution having a salt concentration of 0.9%. This solution, which both surrounds the cells and is contained within them, constitutes the body fluids. The water and electrolytes composing these body fluids come from ingested water and nutrients, and from the water that results from metabolism.

For life to continue and the cells to function properly, the body fluids must remain fairly constant with regard to the amount *of* water and the specific electrolytes *of* which they are composed. Water is essential because it is the basic component of all the body fluids. Water is involved in many of the metabolic processes in the body and is a by-product of some of these reactions. The various electrolytes all have essential roles in cellular physiological processes. If some of either is lost, it must be replaced, and if either water or an electrolyte is in excess, it must be removed. Maintaining the consistency of this fluid environment is homeostasis.

For cells to survive and carry out their multitude of physiologic functions, they need both a continuing source of water, nutrients, and oxygen and a mechanism to remove cellular wastes. These physiologic processes affect the amount of water, the pH, and the ions both inside and outside the cells. A balance most be maintained between the components of the fluids inside and outside the cell. Because the ions are dissolved in water, these two components are tied together: Anything affecting the amount of water in the body will affect the ion concentration.

Body Fluids

Much of the body weight of an average adult is due to the water in the body fluids surrounding the cells and contained within them. The fluid around the cells cushions them and serves as the medium of exchange. Everything that enters or leaves the cells must pass through this fluid layer.

There are two kinds of body fluids. They can be thought of as being contained within two separate containers, called compartments. The *intracellular fluid* (ICF) compartment contains all of the water and ions inside the cells. By far the largest amount of water in the body, approximately 65% is found within this compartment.

The extracellular fluid compartment contains the remaining body fluids, called *extracellular fluid* (ECF), or fluid outside the cells. These can be further subdivided into interstitial, intravascular, and other fluids. *Interstitial fluid* is the fluid in the tissue spaces around each cell. The *intravascular fluid* is the plasma in the blood vessels and the lymph in the lymphatic system (Fig. 18.9). There are also small amounts of other specialized body fluids such as synovial fluid, cerebrospinal fluid, serous fluid, aqueous and vitreous humor, and the endolymph and perilymph. The proportions of extracellular fluid and intracellular fluid vary with age.

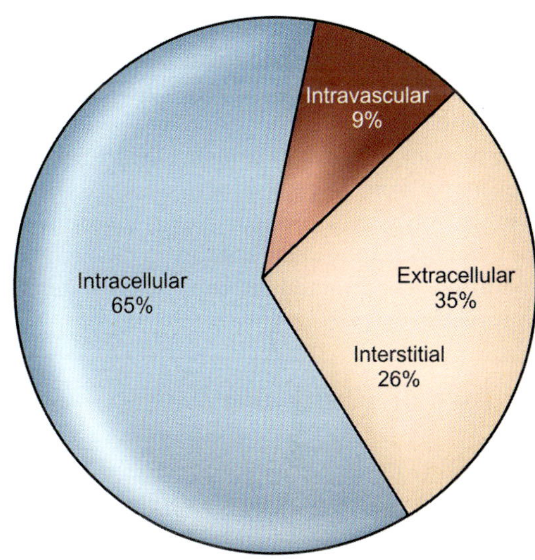

Figure 18.9: Body fluid compartments of an adult

Generally speaking, the major ions in the extracellular fluid are sodium (Na^+), chloride (Cl^-), and bicarbonate (HCO_3^-), although other ions do occur. In the intracellular fluid, the major ions are potassium (K^+), phosphate (PO_4^{--}), and magnesium (Mg^{++}), with lesser amounts of other ions present. There are also large numbers of protein molecules bearing a negative charge.

Exchange between the ECF and ICF

Water and ions moving between the extracellular and intracellular fluids must first pass through the selectively permeable cell membrane. This movement is governed primarily by osmosis. Diffusion and active transport also playa role.

The difference in the ion concentration inside the cell and outside the cell is primarily due to the cell's ability to pump some ions inside and pump others out. If the intracellular fluid becomes hypertonic to the extracellular fluid, water from the extracellular fluid will move by osmosis into the cell to restore the balance, and *vice versa*.

A fluid balance also occurs between the interstitial fluid and the plasma. This balance is regulated primarily by hydrostatic pressure (blood pressure) and osmotic pressure. When the circulating blood passes from the arterioles into the capillaries, the pressure in the capillaries is higher than that in the interstitial fluid. This forces some of the water from the plasma *out* of the capillaries and into the interstitial fluid. Because of osmotic pressure, some of the water in the interstitial fluid is forced back into the capillaries in the area where they join the venules. Some water is also returned to the bloodstream through the lymphatic system. If the amount of interstitial fluid returned to the circulatory system lessens and the fluid accumulates in the tissue spaces. the tissues become swollen. This condition is called edema. Several conditions can cause edema, including kidney or liver disease and heart disorders. Many of these conditions can have serious consequences.

When more water is lost from the body than is replaced, *dehydration* occurs. Among the various causes of dehydration are water deprivation, excessive urine production, profuse sweating, diarrhea, and extended periods of vomiting. As water is lost, the amount of water in the interstitial fluid decreases. Water then moves from the cells to the tissue spaces by osmosis, causing an electrolyte imbalance. Circulatory impairment occurs, which in turn affects the kidney's ability to function normally. This condition is corrected by supplying water and the appropriate electrolytes.

Regulators of Fluid and Electrolyte Balance

There must be a balance in the amounts of fluids and electrolytes consumed and lost daily. Under typical conditions, the average adult loses some water through the skin, lungs, and GI tract and loses the largest amount of water through urine production. This can amount to a per-day fluid loss of approximately 2,500 mL, depending on conditions.

- *Skin:* In the average adult, an estimated water loss of 300 to 400 mL per day occurs by diffusion through the skin. Because the person is not aware of this water loss, it is called *insensible loss.* Water is also lost through the skin by perspiration. The total amount of water lost through perspiration varies depending on environmental factors and body temperature.
- *Lungs:* In the average adult, an estimated insensible water loss of 300 to 400 mL per day occurs with expired air, which is saturated with water vapor. This varies with the rate and depth of respirations.
- *Gastrointestinal Tract:* Although a large amount of fluid– approximately 8,000 mL per day in the average adult–is secreted into the gastrointestinal tract, almost all of this fluid is reabsorbed by the body. In adults, approximately 200 mL of water is lost per day in feces. Severe diarrhea can cause a fluid and electrolyte deficit because the GI fluids contain a large amount of electrolytes.

- *Kidneys:* The kidneys playa major role in maintaining fluid balance by excreting 1.200 to 1,500 mL of water per day in the average adult. The excretion of water by healthy kidneys is proportional to the fluid ingested and the amount of waste or solutes excreted.

When an extracellular fluid volume deficit occurs, hormones playa key role in restoring the extracellular fluid volume. Release of the following hormones into circulation causes the kidneys to conserve water:

- *Antidiuretic hormone (ADH)*: Released by the posterior pituitary gland; acts on the distal tubules of the kidneys to reabsorb water
- *Aldosterone:* Produced in the adrenal cortex; causes the reabsorption of sodium from the renal tubules, leading to water retention in the extracellular fluid, thereby increasing its volume
- *Renin:* Released by the juxtaglomerular cells of the kidneys; promotes vasoconstriction and the release of aldosterone.

The interaction of these hormones with regard to renal functions serves as the body's compensatory mechanism to maintain homeostasis.

Sodium is the main electrolyte that promotes the retention of water. An intravascular water deficit causes the renal tubules to reabsorb mare sodium into circulation. Because water molecules go with the sodium ions, the intravascular water deficit is corrected by this action of the renal tubules.

Fluid and Food Intake

Fluids must be replaced in the amounts lost. The primary source of fluid replacement is water consumption. Approximately 60% may be obtained in this way, with an additional 30% being obtained from foods and 8% to 10% being a product of metabolism (metabolic water), for a total of 2,500 mL.

Thirst

Water consumption usually occurs in response to the sensation of thirst. This mechanism is poorly understood. It is generally believed to be brought about by the loss of body fluids, which in turn causes a dryness in the mouth and the thirst sensation. Replacing the lost fluids by water consumption causes the sensation to diminish. The thirst mechanism appears to be regarded by the hypothalamus in the brain.

Dehydration is one of the must common and most serious fluid imbalances that can result from poor monitoring of fluid intake. One nursing goal is to ensure that all clients understand both the role that water plays in health and the way to maintain adequate hydration.

The primary body fluid, i.e. water is the most important nutrient of life. Whereas life can be sustained for many days without food, but it can be sustained for only a few days without water. The primary functions of water in the body are as follows:

- Provides a medium for transporting nutrients to cells and wastes from cells and transporting substances such as

hormones, enzyme, blood platelets, and red and white blood cells
- Facilitates cellular metabolism and proper cellular chemical functioning
- Acts as a solvent for electrolytes and nonelectrolytes
- Helps to maintain normal body temperature
- Facilitates digestion and promotes elimination
- Acts as a tissue lubricant.

Regulation of Body Fluids

As water moves through all parts of the body it is constantly being lost. Fluid leaves the body through the kidneys, lungs, skin, and GI tract. To maintain homeostasis, the normal daily loss must be met by the normal daily intake. Homeostasis is a relatively constancy in the internal environments of the body, naturally maintained by adaptive responses and that promote healthy survival. An approximate daily water intake and output of an adult eating 2500 calories per day are given in Table 18.2.

Table 18.2: Daily Water Intake and Output of an Adult			
Intake		*Output*	
Route	*Gain (mL)*	*Route*	*Loss (mL)*
Water in food	1,000	Skin	500
Water from oxidation	300	Lungs	350
Water as liquid	1,200	Feces	150
		Kidney	1,500
Total	2,500	Total	2,500

There are many different processes which control the movement of fluid and electrolytes between the ICF and ECF spaces. These processes include simple diffusion, facilitated diffusion, active transport, osmosis, fluid presence (hydrostatic pressure and oncotic pressure).

Simple Diffusion: Diffusion is defined as the natural tendency of a substance or solutes to move from an area of higher concentration to that of lower concentration. It occurs through the random movement of ions and molecules. It occurs in liquids, gases, and solids. For example, exchange of oxygen and carbon dioxide between pulmonary capillaries and alveoli. Net movement of the molecules stops when the concentrations are equal in both areas. The membrane separating the two areas must be permeable to the diffusing substance for the process to occur.

These molecules move without external energy. Diffusion is an efficient mechanism for the movement of molecules in and out of cells. Diffusion does not require energy.

Facilitated Diffusion: Some molecules diffuse slowly into the cell because of the composition of cellular membrane. However, when they are combined with a specific carrier molecule, the rate of diffusion accelerates. Like simple diffusion, facilitated diffusion moves molecules from an area of high concentration to one of low concentration. Glucose transport into the cell is an example of facilitated diffusion. The hormone insulin increases the rate of facilitated diffusion of glucose in most tissues.

Active Transport: Active transport is a process in which molecules move in the absence of a favorable diffusion gradient. In which, the physiologic pump (Naik) that moves fluid from an area of lower concentration to one of higher concentration. External energy is required for this process because molecules are being moved against a concentration gradient. Active transport requires adenosine triphosphate (ATP) for energy. The energy production depends on oxygen and glucose availability. The concentration of sodium and potassium differs greatly, intracellularly and extracellularly. By active transport, sodium moves out of the cell and potassium moves into the cell. The energy source for the sodium-potassium pump is ATP which is produced in the mitochondria. By definition, active transport implies that energy expenditure must take place for the movement to occur against a concentration of gradient.

Osmosis: Osmosis, a special type of diffusion, is the flow of water between too compartments separated by a membrane permeable to water but not to solute. Here the movement of fluid across a semipermeable membrane from an area of low solute concentration to an area of high solute concentration. This process stops when the solute concentrations are equal on both sides of the membrane. In this, water moves from the compartments that is more dilute (has more water) to the side that is more concentrated (has less water). The semipermeable membrane prevents movement of solute particles. Osmosis requires no outside energy sources and stops when concentration differences disappear. In addition to diffusion, osmosis is very important for maintaining the chemical stability of body cells.

Osmotic Pressure or Force

Osmotic pressure is a term used to describe the movement of water by the process of osmosis. It can be described as a pulling of water. Osmotic pressure is an important factor in the movement of water between fluid compartments. 'Osmolarity' and 'osmolality' both are measurements of osmotic pressure.

Osmolality: It measures the osmotic force of solute per unit of weight of solvent. It reflects the concentration of fluid that affects the movement of water between fluid compartments by osmosis. It measures the solute concentration per kilogram in blood and urine. It is measured in milliosmole per kg of water (mosm/kg). The normal osmolality of body fluids is between 275 and 295 mmol/kg or mosm/kg. The major determinants of osmolality are sodium, glucose, and urea with sodium. Increased in the concentration of these substances in the plasma causes fluid movement into plasma because of its increased osmotic pressure.

Osmolarity: It measures the total milliosmole of solutes per unit of a total volume of solution. The number of osmoles, the standard unit of osmotic pressure per liter of solution. It is expressed as milliosmole per liter (mosm/L) used to describe the concentration of solutes or dissolved particles.

In clinical practice, osmolality is used most frequently. Serum osmolality may be measured directly through laboratory tests or estimated at the bedside by doubling the serum sodium level or by utilizing the following formula:

$$Na^+ \times 2 + \frac{glucose}{18} + \frac{BUN\ (Blood\ urea\ nitrogen)}{3} = \text{Approximate value of serum osmolality}$$

In osmotic movement of fluid, cells are affected by the osmolality of the fluid that surrounds them. Where fluids are added to the body those that have same osmolality as cell interior are "isotonic". Solutions that contain more water than the cell are "hypotonic" (hypoosmolar), those with less water than the cell are hypertonic (hyperosmolar).

Fluid Pressure: As a result of pressure, body fluids shift between the interstitial space and the vascular space within the capillary. The pressure in the body fluids are either hydrostatic or oncotic.

Hydrostatic Pressure

Hydrostatic pressure is the force exerted by a fluid against the walls of its container. The heart is a main component in generating pressure in blood vessels. Hydrostatic pressure in the vascular system gradually decreases as the blood moves through the arteries until it is about 40 mm Hg at the arterial end of a capillary. Because of the size of the capillary bed and fluid movement into the interstitial, the pressure decreases to about 10 mm Hg at the venous end of the vessel. Hydrostatic pressure in the capillaries tends to filter fluid out of the vascular compartment into the interstitial fluid.

Oncotic Pressure (Colloidal Osmotic Pressure)

Oncotic pressure is an osmotic pressure exerted by colloidal, in solution. In plasma, proteins and molecules attract water and contribute to the total osmotic pressure in the vascular system. Unlike electrolytes, the large molecular size prevents proteins from leaving the vascular space through pores in capillary walls. Plasma oncotic pressure is approximately 25 mm Hg. Some patients are found in the interstitial space, and they exert an oncotic pressure of approximately 1 mm Hg.

Filtration

The movement of the fluid through a capillary via the above stated two pressures (hydrostatic and oncotic) is called 'filtration'. An example of filtration is the passage of water and electrolytes from the arterial capillary bed to the interstitial fluid. In this instance, the hydrostatic pressure is furnished by the pumping action of the heart. Through filtration, absorption or reabsorption, and resorption will take place.

Absorption: It usually refers to the initial movement of substances such as end products of digestion or medications from organ such as GI tract or tissues such as the muscle, subcutaneous or dermal tissue, buccal or pharyngeal tissues, into the vascular system.

Reabsorption: It refers to movement of water, electrolytes, vitamins, amino acids, glucose, lactate or other essential substances from one compartment, such as the interstitial or renal tubules, back into vascular capillaries.

Resorption: It refers to the process of calcium salts leaving the bone and moving to the blood in an ionized form.

Homeostatic Mechanism

The body is equipped with remarkable homeostatic mechanisms to keep the composition and volume of body fluid within narrow limits of normal. Organs involved in the homeostatic mechanism or regulation of fluid and electrolytes include hypothalamus, pituitary gland, adrenal gland, kidney, GI tract, parathyroid gland, heart and blood vessels, lungs, etc. (Table 18.3).

Hypothalamus: Water ingestion in the conscious client is regulated by the thirst receptors located in the hypothalamus. The thirst mechanism is stimulated by the hypotension and increased serum osmolality. In addition thirst may result from polyuria, fluid volume depletion as small as 0.5 percent, excess sodium intake, hypertonic feedings, and hypertonic IV fluids. Although thirst can be reported and is an important clinical manifestation of fluid imbalances, it is not a true indicator of fluid balance in all persons. The thirst mechanism is depressed in the elderly. The desire to consume fluids is also affected by social and psychologic factors not related to fluid balance. A dry mouth will cause the client to drink, even when there is no measurable body water deficit. Water ingestion will equal water excretion in the individual who has free access to water, a normal thirst and ADH mechanism and normally-functioning kidneys.

Pituitary Gland: The hypothalamus manufactures a substance known as antidiuretic hormone (ADH) which is stored in vesicle in the posterior pituitary gland and released as needed. ADH regulates water retention by kidneys. The distal tubules and collecting ducts in the kidneys respond to the ADH by becoming more permeable in water so that water is absorbed into the blood and not excreted. When there is a normal plasma osmolality and normal circulating plasma volume, continued ADH secretion is called" syndrome inappropriate to antidiuretic hormone (SIADH)". ADH is released in response to many conditions–an increase in plasma osmolality, ECF volume depletion, pain, stress, and use of certain medications such as narcotics, barbiturates, and anesthetics–stress may be physiologic or psychologic. The factors which suppressing ADH include

Table 18.3: Organs that Maintain Homeostasis

Kidneys
- Regulate ECF volume and osmolality by selective retention and excretion of body fluids
- Regulate electrolytic levels in the ECF by selective retention of needed substances and excretion of unneeded substances
- Regulate pH of ECF by excretion or retention of hydrogen ions
- Excrete metabolic wastes (primarily acids) and toxic substances

Heart and blood vessels
- Circulate blood through the kidneys under sufficient pressure of urine to form (pumping action of the heart)
- React to hypovolemia by stimulating fluid retention (stretch receptors in the atria and blood vessels)

Lungs
- Eliminate about 13 mEq of hydrogen ions (H^+) daily, as opposed to only 40 to 80 mEq excreted daily by kidneys
- Act promptly to correct metabolic acid-base disturbance; regulate H^+ concentration (pH) by controlling the level of CO_2 in the ECF as follows:
  - Metabolic alkalosis causes compensatory hypoventilation resulting in CO_2 excretions (increased acidity of the ECF)
  - Metabolic acidosis causes compensatory hyperventilation, resulting in CO_2 excretion (decreased acidity of the ECF)
  - Remove approximately 300 mL of water daily through exhalation (insensible water loss) in the normal adult.

Adrenal glands
- Regulate blood volume and sodium and potassium balance by secreting aldosterone; a mineral corticoid secreted by the adrenal cortex
  - The primary regulator of aldosterone appears to be angiotensin II which is produced by the renin-angiotensin system. A decrease in blood volume triggers this system and increases aldosterone secretion, which causes sodium retention (and thus water retention) and potassium loss
  - Decreased secretion of aldosterone causes sodium and water loss and potassium retention.
- Cortisol, another ACTH, has only a fraction of the potency of aldosterone
- However, secretion of cortisol in large quantities can produce sodium and water retention and potassium deficit.

Pituitary gland
- Stores and releases ADH, which makes the body retain water. Functions of ADH include to maintain osmotic pressure of the cells by controlling renal water retention or excretion
  - When osmotic pressure of the ECF is greater than that of the cells (as in hypernatremia or hyperglycemia). ADH secretions is increased causing renal retention of water
  - When osmotic pressure of the ECF is less than that of the cells, (as in hyponatremia) ADH secretion is decreased, causing renal excretion of water
- Controls blood volume (less influential than aldosterone)
  - When blood volume is decreased, an increased secretion of ADH result in water conservation
  - When blood volume is increased, a decreased secretion ADH results in water loss

Parathyroid glands
- Regulate calcium (Ca_2^+) and phosphate (HPO_4^{2-}) balance by means of PTH; PTH influences bone reabsorption, calcium absorption from the intestines and calcium reabsorption from renal tubules
- Increase secretion of PTH causes the following:
  - Elevated serum calcium concentration
  - Lowered serum phosphate concentration
- Conversely decreased secretion of PTH causes the following:
  - Lowered serum calcium concentration
  - Elevated serum phosphate concentration

hypo-osmolality of the ECF, increased blood volume, exposure to cold, acute alcohol ingestion, carbon dioxide inhalation, administration of some diuretics, lithium and some antipsychotic medications. ADH prevents urine production and promotes water reabsorption from the renal tubules. Stimulation of the thirst mechanism and ADH release usually occur concurrently in response to a body fluid deficit.

Adrenal Gland: Extracellular fluid volume is maintained by a combinations of hormonal influences. ADH affects only water reabsorption. Hormones released by the adrenal cortex helps to regulate both water and electrolytes. Two groups of hormones secreted by the adrenal cortex include glucocorticoids and mineralocorticoids. The glucocorticoids primarily have an anti-inflammatory effect and increase serum glucose, whereas mineralocorticoids (e.g. aldosterone) enhances sodium retention and potassium excretion. When sodium is reabsorbed, water follows as a result of osmotic charges. "Cortisol" is most common hormone which has both gluco and minerlocorticoids properties. Adrenocorticotrophic hormone (ACTH) from the anterior pituitary is necessary for aldosterone secretions.

Hypovelemia is a common clinical condition in which aldosterone is secreted to maintain homeostasis.

Kidneys: The kidneys maintain fluid volume and concentration of urine by filtering the ECF through the glomeruli. Reabsorption and excretion of ECF occur in the renal tubules in response to ADH, aldosterone and ANP (atrial natriuretic peptides). ANP released from the atria in response to atrial distention, vasoconstriction, or direct cardiac failure. These factors increase the excretion of sodium and water and results in vasodilation. Renal prostaglandins and renal renin-kinin system also increases sodium excretion. The major functions of kidneys in maintaining normal fluid balance include the following:
- Regulation of ECF volume and osmolality by selective retention and excretion of body fluids
- Regulation of electrolytes level in the ECF by selective retention of needed substances and excretion of unneeded substances
- Regulation of pH of ECF by retention of hydrogen ions
- Excretion of metabolic wastes and toxic substances.

Parathyroid Gland: The parathyroid glands embedded in the corners of thyroid gland, regulate calcium and phosphate balance by means of parathyroid hormone (PTH). PTH influences bone resorption, calcium absorption from the intestine and renal tubules.

Gastrointestinal Tract: Daily water intake and output are between 2000 mL and 3000 mL. The gastrointestinal tract accounts for the most of the water intake. Water intake includes fluids, water from foods metabolism and water present in solid goods. Lean meal has approximately 70 percent water whereas the water content of many fruits and vegetables approaches 100 percent. Most of the body water is excreted by kidneys. A small amount of water eliminated by GI tract is feces.

Lungs: The lungs are also vital in maintaining homeostasis. Insensible water loss, which is unavoidable vaporization from the lungs and skin assists in regulating body temperature. Normally, about 900 mL of water per day is lost. The amount of water loss is increased by accelerated body metabolism, which occurs with increased body temperature and exercise. Through exhalation, the lungs remove approximately 300 mL of water daily in the normal adult.

Heart and Blood Vessels: The pumping action of the heart circulates blood through the kidneys under sufficient pressure for urine to form, Failure of the pumping action interferes with renal perfusion and thus with water and electrolytic regulation.

Neural Mechanism: In addition, neural mechanisms also contribute to the balance of water and sodium. Mechanoreceptors and baroreceptors are nerve receptors involved in neural mechanism.

Fluid Imbalances

Fluid imbalances occur when the body's compensating mechanisms are unable to maintain homeostatic state. Fluid imbalance may relate to either volume or distribution of water or electrolytes.

Fluid Volume Deficit (FVD)

Fluid volume deficit can be caused by a deficiency in the amount of both water and electrolytes in ECF, but the water and electrolytes proportions remain near normal. The state is commonly known as 'hypovolemia'. Both osmotic and hydrostatic pressure changes force the interstitial fluid into intravascular space. As the interstitial space is depleted, its fluid becomes hypertonic, and cellular fluid is then drawn into the interstitial space, leaving cells without adequate fluid of function properly.

Fluid volume deficit results from the loss of body fluids, especially if fluid intake is simultaneously decreased. The related factors of FVD are as follows:
- (i) Loss of water and electrolytes, as in the cases of:
  - Vomiting
  - Diarrhea
  - Excessive laxative use
  - Fistulas
  - Polyuria
  - Fever
  - Excessive sweating
  - Third space fluid shafts
  - Gastrointestinal suction.
- (ii) Decreased intake, as in the cases of:
  - Anorexia
  - Inability to gain access of fluids
  - Inability to swallow fluids
  - Nausea
  - Depression.

The main characteristics of fluid volume deficits are as follows:
- Weight loss over short period (except in third space losses)
- Decreased skin and tongue turgor
- Dry mucous membranes
- Urine output less than 30 mL per hour in adult
- Postural hypotension (systolic pressure drops by more than 15 mm Hg when client moves from lying to standing or sitting position)
- Weak, rapid pulse
- Slow-filling peripheral veins
- Decreased body temperature, such as 95 to 98°F (38 to 36.7°C) unless infection is present
- CVP less than 4 cm H_2O
- BUN elevated out of proportion to serum creatinine
- Specific gravity (urine) high
- Hematocrit elevated
- Flat neck veins in supine position
- Marked oliguria, late
- Altered sensorium.

Nursing Intervention for FVD

1. Assess for presence or worsening of FVD.
2. Administer oral fluids if indicated.
   - Consider the client's likes and dislikes when offering fluids
   - If the client is reluctant to drink because of oral discomfort select fluids that are non-irritating to the mucosa, and provide frequent mouth care (offer saline gargle and apply lubricant to lips)
   - Offer fluids at frequent intervals
   - Explain the need for fluid replacement to the client
   - Administer p.r.n. medications if nausea is present, to provide relief before fluids are offered.
3. Consider the following interventions for clients with impaired swallowing:
   - Assess gag reflex and ability to swallow water before offering solid foods; have a suction apparatus on hand
   - Position the client in an upright position with head and neck flexed slightly forward during feeding (tilting the head backward during swallowing predisposes to aspiration because this position opens the airway)
   - Provide thick fluids or semisolid foods (such as pudding or gelatine). These are more easily swallowed because of their consistency and weight than are thin liquids.
4. If the client is unable to eat and drink, discuss possibility of tube feeding or TPN with the physician.
5. Monitor response to fluid intake, either orally or parenterally.
6. Monitor clients with tendency for abnormal fluid retention (such as renal or cardiac problems) for signs of overload during aggressive fluid replacement.
7. Turn client frequently, apply moisturizing agents on the skin.

Sometimes dehydration is used as synonym for hypovolemia; technically it is wrong. Dehydration refers only to a decreased volume of water; but water is not decreased without electrolyte charges also. Hydration is the union of a substance with water and is often used to indicate that there is normal water volume in the body.

Fluid Volume Excess (FVE)

Excessive retention of water and sodium in ECF in near-normal proportions results in a condition termed as fluid volume excess. It is also called "hypervolemia". Overhydration refers only to above-normal amounts of water in extracellular spaces. Malfunction of the kidneys causing an inability to excrete, the success and failure of the heart to function as a pump resulting in accumulation of fluid in the lungs and dependant parts of the body, are common causes. When water is retained in excessive amount, so as sodium.

Due to increased extracellular osmotic pressure from the retained sodium, fluid is pulled from the cells to equalize the tonicity. By the time intracellular and extracellular spaces are isotonic to each other, an excess of both water and sodium are in ECF, while the cells are nearly depleted. The excessive ECF may accumulate in tissue spaces, thus is known as edema: Edema can be observed around eyes, fingers ankles and sacral space and also accumulate in or around body organs. It may result in a weight gain in excess of 5 percent. When the excess fluid remains in the intravascular space, the 'concentration of solids in the blood is decreased.

Interstitial to plasma shift is the movement of fluid from the space surrounding the cells to the blood. The shift, also called hypervolemia is a compensatory response to volume or osmotic pressure changes of the intravascular fluid. Although the body attempts to maintain normal balance in all fluid spaces, the intravascular fluid is usually protected at the expense of interstitial fluid and ICF.

The common related factors which lead to fluid volume excess (FVE) are as follows:
- Compromised regulatory mechanisms such as
  - Renal failure
  - Congestive heart failure
  - Cirrhosis of liver
  - Cushing's syndrome.
- Overzealous administration of sodium containing IV fluids
- Excessive ingestion of sodium containing substances in diet or sodium containing medication.

The characteristics of fluid volume excess include the following:
- Weight gain over short period
- Peripheral edema (excess of fluid in interstitial space)
- Distended neck veins
- Distended peripheral veins
- Slow-emptying peripheral veins
- CVP over 11 cm H_2O
- Crackles and wheezers in lungs
- Polyuria (if renal function normal)
- Ascitis, pleural effusion (when FVE is severe, fluid transudates into body cavities)
- Decreased BUN (due to plasma dilution)
- Decreased hematocrit (due to plasma dilution)
- Bounding, full pulse
- Pulmonary edema, if severe.

Nursing Intervention for FVE

- Assess the presence or worsening of FVE
- Encourage adherence to sodium restricted diet, if prescribed
- Teach client requiring sodium restrictions to avoid over-the-counter drugs without first checking with the healthcare adviser/nurse
- When fluid retention persists despite adherence to dietary sodium intake, consider hidden sources of sodium, such as water supply or use of water softener
- When indicated, encourage rest period, lying down favors diuresis of edema fluid
- Monitor the client's response to diuretics
- Discuss significant findings with physician
- Monitor the rate of parenteral fluids and the client response. Discuss significant finding with physician

- Teach self-monitoring of weight and intake and output measurements to clients with chronic fluid retention (such as those of ECF, renal failure, cirrhosis of liver)
- If dyspnea or orthopnea are present, position the client in semi-Fowler's position to facilitate lung expansion
- Turn and position the client frequently, beware that edematous tissue is more prone to skin breakdown than in normal tissue.

Electrolytes

Electrolytes are substances whose molecules dissociate or split into ions when placed in water. These substances are found in ECF and ICF that dissociate into electrically charged particles known as 'ions'. 'Cations' are positively charged ions. For example, sodium (Na^+), potassium (K^+), calcium (Ca^{2+}) and magnesium (Mg^+), hydrogen (H^+) ions. 'Anions' are negative charged ions. For example, bicarbonates (HCO_3^-), chloride (Cl^-) and phosphate (PO_4^3) ions and proteins. The ionic charge is termed 'valence'. Cations and anions combine according to their valency.

The concentration of electrolytes can be expressed in mol per deciliter (mol/dL), millimol per liter (mmol/L) or milliequivalent per liter (mEq/L). See the normal level of electrolytes in appendix. The role of electrolytes in cellular functions include the following:

- Regulation of water distribution, and osmolality.
- Regulation of acid-base balance.
- Transmission of nerve impulses, i.e. neuromuscular activity.
- Contraction of muscles.
- Clotting of blood.
- Enzyme reaction.

Regulation of Electrolytes

Electrolytes regulate water distribution, regulate acid-base balance and maintain a balanced degree of neuromuscular excitability. There are many different kinds of electrolytes in the body. These include sodium (Na^+), potassium (K^+), calcium (Ca^{++}), magnesium (Mg^{2+}), chloride (Cl^-), bicarbonate (HCO_3^-), phosphate (PO_4^-), etc.

Sodium

Sodium is the chief electrolyte of ECF. It moves. easily between intravascular and interstitial spaces and moves across cell membrane by active transport. Many chemical reactions in the body are influenced by sodium, particularly in nervous tissue cells and muscle tissue cells.

The functions of sodium are as follows:
- It controls and regulates the volume of body fluids
- It maintains water balance throughout the body
- It is the primary regulator of ECF volume
- It influences ICF volume
- It participates in the generation and transmission of nerve impulses
- It is an essential electrolyte in the sodium potassium pump

Sources and Losses of Sodium

- An average daily intake is not known, but the average adult intake is eliminated to be between 6 and 15 mg and the RDA for sodium for adults is approximately 500 mg for 0.5 gm
- Sodium is found in many foods, particularly bacon, ham, sausage, catsup, mustard, relish, processed cheese, canned vegetables, bread, cereal, and salted snack food. It is found in table salt ($NaCl$) which has about 46 percent sodium
- Sodium excess are eliminated primarily by the kidneys, small amounts are lost in feces and perspiration.

Regulation of Sodium

- Sodium normally is maintained in the body within a relatively narrow range, and deviations quickly result in a serious health problem
- Salt intake regulates sodium concentrations
- Sodium is conserved through reabsorption in the kidneys, a process of stimulation by aldosterone
- The normal extracellular concentrations of sodium is 135 to 145 mEq/L (mmol/L).

Potassium

Potassium is the major cation of ICF. Potassium and sodium work reciprocally. For example, an excessive intake of sodium results in an excretion of potassium and vice versa. The functions of potassium are as follows:

- It is the chief regulator of cellular enzyme activity and cellular water content
- It plays a vital role in such process as the transmission of electric impulses, particularly in nerve, heart, skeletal, intestinal, and lung tissue; protein and carbohydrate metabolism and cellular building
- It assists in regulation of acid-base balance by cellular exchange with H^+.

Sources and Losses of Potassium

- An average daily requirement of K^+ is not known; but an intake of 50 to 100 mEq daily maintains potassium balance
- A well-balanced diet contains adequate quantities of potassium. Major sources include bananas, peaches, kiwi, figs, dates, apricots, oranges prunes, melons, raising, broccoli, and potatoes. Meat and dairy products also provide adequate amounts of potassium
- Potassium excreted primarily by the kidneys. The kidneys have no effective method of conserving potassium. Therefore, deficits develop readily if excreted in excess amount without being replaced simultaneously
- Gastrointestinal secretions contain potassium in large quantities. Some is also found in perspiration and saliva.

Regulation of K^+

- Cellular potassium is conserved by the sodium pump when sodium is excluded
- The kidneys conserve potassium when cellular K^+ is decreased

- Aldosterone secretions trigger potassium excretion in urine
- The normal range for serum potassium is 3.5 to 5 mEq/L.

Calcium

Calcium is the most abundant electrolyte in the body. Up to 99 percent of the total amount of calcium in the body is found in bones and teeth in ionized form. There is close link between concentration of calcium and phosphorus. The functions of calcium are as follows:

- It is necessary for nerve impulse transmissions and blood clotting
- It is catalyst for muscle contraction. Strength of contractions (especially cardiac muscle contraction) is directly related to the serum concentration of calcium ions
- It is needed for vitamin B_{12} absorption and for its use by body cells
- It acts as a catalyst for many cell chemical activities
- It is necessary for strong bones and teeth
- It establishes thickness and strength of cell membrane.

Sources and Losses of Calcium
- The average daily requirements for calcium is about 1 gm for adults. Higher amounts are required according to body weight; for children, for pregnant and lactating women, and postmenopausal women
- Calcium is found in milk, cheese and dried beans. Some calcium is present in meats and vegetables
- Use of calcium is stimulated by vitamin D. The most active form of vitamin D (calcifriol) promotes calcium absorption and limits calcium excretion when levels are inadequate
- It leaves bones and teeth to maintain normal blood calcium levels, if necessary
- It is excreted in urine, feces, bile, digestive secretion and perspiration.

Regulation of Calcium
- When ECF calcium levels decrease, the parathyroid glands increase the secretions of PTH, which acts on bones to increase the release of calcium into the blood and acts on the kidney, tubules and the intestinal mucosa to increase the absorption of calcium from the kidneys and the intestine
- A high serum phosphate concentration increases serum calcium; a low serum phosphate concentration decreases serum calcium
- Calcitonin, a hormone secreted by the thyroid gland has an opposite effect on calcium than PTH. Increase in calcitonin reduce the serum calcium concentration primarily by opposing osteoclast bone resorption.

Magnesium

Most of the cation magnesium is found within body cells. It is present in heart, bone, nerve, and muscle tissues. Magnesium is the second most important cation of ICF. The functions of magnesium are as follows:

- It is important for the metabolism of carbohydrates and proteins
- It is important for many vital reactions related to the body's enzymes
- It is necessary for protein and DNA synthesis, DNA and RNA transcription, and translation of RNA
- It maintains normal intracellular levels of potassium
- It serves to help or maintain electric activity in nervous membranes and muscle membranes.

Sources and Losses of Magnesium
- The average daily adult requirement for magnesium is about 18 to 30 mEq. Children are required larger amount
- Magnesium is found in most foods but especially in vegetables, nuts, fish, whole grains, peas and beans.

Regulation of Magnesium
- Magnesium is absorbed by the intestines and secreted by the kidneys
- Plasma concentration of magnesium range from 1.3 to 2.1 mEq/L with about one third of that amount bound to plasma proteins.

Chloride

Chloride the chief extracellular anion is found in blood, interstial fluid, and lymph and in minute amounts in intracellular fluid. The functions of chlorides are as follows:

- It acts with sodium to maintain the osmotic pressure of the blood
- It plays a role in the body's acid-base balance
- It is important in buffering action when O_2 and CO_2 exchange in RBCs
- It is essential for the production of HCl in gastric juices
- The average daily requirement of chlorides is unknown. It is found in foods rich in sodium, in dairy products and meat.

Regulation of Chloride
- It is normally paired with sodium and excreted and conserved with sodium by the kidneys
- Chloride deficit leads to potassium deficit and *vice-versa*
- Normal serum chloride levels range from 95 to 105 mEq/L.

Bicarbonate

The bicarbonate molecule is an anion. It is the major chemical base buffer within the body and is found in both ECF and ICF. It is essential for acid-base balance. Bicarbonate and carbonic acid constitute the body's primary buffer systems.

Phosphate

The phosphate ion is the major anion in body cells. It is a buffer anion in both ICF and ECF. The functions of phosphate are as follows:

- It helps maintain acid-base balance

- It is involved in important chemical reactions in the body. For example, it is necessary for many B vitamins to be effective; helps promote nerve and muscle action, and plays role in carbohydrate metabolism
- It is important for cell division and for the transmission of heredity or hereditary traits.

An average daily requirement for phosphorus are similar to those for calcium. It is found in most foods by especially in beef, pork, and dried peas and beans. It is metabolised in the same manner as calcium.

Phosphate is regulated by PTH and by activated vitamin D. Calcium and phosphates are inversely proportional and increase in one results in a decrease in the other. The normal range of phosphate is 2.5 to 4.5 mEq/L (mmol/L).

Electrolyte Imbalances

Human body contains quite large volume of water as ICF and ECF and the fluid contains several inorganic ions such as sodium, potassium, chloride, bicarbonate, sulfate, phosphate, calcium and magnesium. The complex mechanism of human life maintains the concentration and volume of the body fluids at a constant level and in general, it is not influenced by dietary intake and metabolism, while kidneys playa vital role in maintaining the balance. When clients present with deficit or excesses of sodium, potassium, calcium, magnesium or phosphate, special nursing care is required. A brief description of the common electrolyte imbalances are as follows.

Hyponatremia

Hyponatremia refers to a sodium deficit in ECF caused by loss of sodium or a gain of water. It is a condition on lowered level of plasma volume. In this condition, osmotic pressure changes result in ECF, moving into the cells. When this occurs, an examiner's fingerprints tend to remain on the client's skin over the sternum where pressure is applied with the fingers.

The related factors leading to hyponatremia are as follows:
- Loss of sodium as in: loss of GI fluids, use of diuretics; adrenal insufficiency
- Gains of water as in: excessive administration of Ds W, diseases associated with SIADH; pharmacological agents that impair renal water excretion
- Hyponatremia or sodium depletion occurs from loss of body fluids through sweating, vomiting, diarrhea, intestinal fistula, dialysis and from aspiration of gastric contents
- Chronic pyelonephritis, chronic uremia, diuretic phase of acute renal failure, diabetic ketoacidosis, cystic diseases of the kidney, and excessive or prolonged use of diuretics result in excessive loss of sodium through urine
- Endocrine diseases show as myxoedema, Addison's disease, hyperaldosteronism, and uncontrolled diabetes mellitus also lead to sodium depletion
- Excessive loss of sodium can also occur through the skins as in extensive burns, generalized dermatitis and, etc. in children with cystic fibrosis.

Sodium is mainly an extracellular ion, and its depletion causes migration of water in the intracellular compartments, making the extracellular fluid hypotonic. Consequently, plasma becomes hypo-osmolar and plasma volume falls.

Main Characteristics

- Anorexia
- Fingerprint over sternum
- Nausea and vomiting
- Muscular twitching
- Lethargy
- Seizures
- Confusion
- Coma
- Muscle cramps
- Serum sodium below 135 mEq/L.

This condition presents with tiredness, lethargy, muscular weakness, mental confusion, and in severe cases, convulsions and coma. The skin appears cold, pale and inelastic. Tongue is dry. Reduction in plasma volume causes reduction in cardiac output and results tachycardia, fall of blood pressure and raising pulse rate. The eyeballs become soft due to reduced intraocular pressure, urine output is reduced and soon oliguria supervenes and finally leads to uremia. When the plasma serum concentration falls exaggeratedly to 120 mmol/L of blood or less, muscle cramps occur. It can produce acidosis and circulatory failure as complication.

Treatment

Mild cases are treated with frequent drink of water with added sodium chloride or with isotonic (0.9%) saline solution by IV injection. In other cases, 2-4 liters of isotonic saline solution is given IV infusion over 6-12 hours. More severe cases are treated with 2-3 liters of IV isotonic solution in first 2-3 hours, followed by further 2-5 liters within 24-48 hours. If there is associated water intoxication, water intake is restricted to 500-1000 mL in 24 hours. In addition, the client is given treatment for the underlying condition.

Nursing Intervention

- Identify clients at risk for hyponatremia
- Monitor fluid losses and gains. Look for loss of sodium containing fluids, particularly in conjunction with low sodium intake
- Monitor presence of gastrointestinal symptoms, such as anorexia, nausea, vomiting, and abdominal cramping
- Monitor laboratory date for serum sodium levels less than normal
- Check specific gravity of urine
- With clients able to consume a general diet, encourage foods and fluids with high sodium content
- Be familiar with the sodium content of commonly used parenteral fluids. Monitor client with cardiovascular disease receiving sodium-containing fluids closely for sign of circulatory overload, such as moist rales in the lungs

- Use extreme caution when administering hypertonic saline solution (3 to 5% NaCl). Beware that these fluids can be lethal if infused carelessly
- Avoid giving large water supplements to clients receiving isotonic tube feedings, particularly if routes of abnormal sodium loss are present or water is being retained abnormally.

Hypernatremia

Hypernatremia or sodium excess refers to surplus of sodium in ECF that can result from excess water loss or overall excess of sodium. Because of the increased extracellular osmotic pressure, fluids move from the cells, leaving them without sufficient fluid. It is a condition which excess of sodium occurs in the ECF, giving rise to cellular dehydration.

The related factors which lead to hyponatremia are as follows:

- Deprivation of water, most common in those unable to perceive or respond to thirst
- Hypertonic tube feeding with inadequate water supplements
- Increased insensible water loss (as in hyper ventilation)
- Ingestion of salt in unusual amounts
- Excessive parenteral administration of sodium-containing solution:
  - Hypertonic saline (3 or 5% NaCl)
  - 7.5 percent sodium bicarbonate
  - Isotonic saline
- Profuse sweating
- Diabetes insipidus
- Heat stroke
- Drowning in sea water
- Hypernatremia also occurs when water losses of the body exceed sodium loss as that is seen in diabetes insipidus, marked glycosuria, hypercalcemia, hypokalemia, chronic renal failure, and recovery phase of acute renal failure
- Sodium excess may occur along with water excess when due to inadequate clearance of the kidneys both sodium and water accumulate in the extracellular space, leading to edema, for example, nephrotic syndrome, cardiac failure, nutritional or thiamine deficiency, cirrhosis of liver, and in cases of usage of drugs such as corticosteroids, androgens, phenylbutazone, oral contraceptive and carbenoxelone.

It causes retention of sodium, increased volume of ECF and edema in the interstitial compartment.

Main Characteristics

- Thirst
- Elevated body temperature
- Tongue dry and swollen, sticky mucous membranes
- In severe hypernatremia:
  - Disorientation
  - Hallucinations
  - Lethargy when disturbed
  - Irritable and hyperreactive when stimulated
  - Focal or grandmal seizures, coma, low blood pressure, tachycardia

- Serum sodium above 145 mEq/L
- Urinary specific gravity .015 provided water loss from nonrenal route.

It may produce hyponatremia, hyperglycemia and shock as complication.

Treatment

Management of the condition calls for an immediate attention and treatment instituted within 24-48 hours can avoid occurrence of cerebral edema.

Mild cases are given IV infusion 5 percent dextrose solution. Other cases need restriction of water and salt by mouth. Management of the condition depends upon the underlying condition. Diuretics and other measures are taken on the advice of the physician according to condition of patient.

Nursing Intervention

- Identify clients at risk of hypernatremia
- Monitor fluid losses and gains. Look for abnormal losses of water or low water intake, and for large gains of sodium as might occur with ingestion of proprietary drugs with high sodium content. And also consider that prescription drugs may have high sodium content. Of course one should look for excessive intake of high sodium foods
- Monitor changes in behavior–such as restlessness, disorientation and lethargy
- Look for excessive thirst, and elevated body temperature. If present, evaluate in relation to other signs
- Monitor serum sodium level
- Prevent hyponatremia in debilitated clients unable to perceive or respond to thirst by offering them fluids at regular intervals. If fluids intake remains inadequate, consult the physician in order to plan and alternate route for intake, either by tube feedings or by the parenteral route
- If tube feedings are used, give sufficient water to keep the serum sodium and the BUN level within normal limits. Beware that the higher the osmolity of the feeding, the greater the need for water supplements.

Hypokalemia

Hypokalemia refers to a potassium deficit in ECF. When the extracellular potassium level falls, potassium moves from the cell, creating an intracellular potassium deficiency. Sodium and hydrogen ions are then retained by the cells to maintain isotonic fluids. These electrolyte shifts influence normal cellular functioning, the pH of ECF, and function of most of the body systems. Skeletal muscles are generally the first to demonstrate a potassium deficiency. It is a condition associated with depletion of potassium characterized by muscular weakness, leg cramps, apathy, mental confusion and paralysis.

The related factors leading to hypokalemia are as follows:

- It develops from excessive loss of potassium in the urine and stool and from severe water depletion
- Potassium-losing diuretics, i.e. frusemide, thiazide, etc.
- Steroid administration

- Use of carbenicillin, sodium penicillin, amphoterecin B
- Hyperaldosteronism
- Hyperalimentations
- Poor intake as in anorexia nervosa, alcoholism, potassium-free parenteral fluids
- Osmotic diuresis (as occurs in uncontrolled diabetes mellitus or mannitol administration).

Main Characteristics
- Fatigue
- Anorexia, nausea and vomiting
- Muscle weakness
- Decreased bowel motility (intestinal ileus)–paralytic ileus
- Cardiac arrhythmia
- Increased, i.e. sensitivity to digitalis
- Polyuria, nocturia, dilute urine (if hypokalemia prolonged)
- Mild hyperglycemia
- Serum K below 3.5 mEq/L
- Paresthesis or tender muscles
- ECG changes–flatened T waves, ST segment depressions
- Respiratory hyperventilation.

Treatment

Management of the condition requires adequate management of the underlying conditions.

Nursing Intervention
- Beware of clients at risk for hypokalemia and monitor for its occurrence
- Assess digitalized clients at risk for hypokalemia especially closely for symptoms of digitalis toxicity
- Take measures to prevent hypokalemia when possible
    - Prevention may take the form of encouraging extra potassium intake for at-risk patient (when the diet allows)
    - When hypokalemia due to abuse of laxatives or diuretics education of the client may help alleviate the problems
- Administer oral potassium supplement when prescribed
- Beware that clients may not need potassium supplements if they are using salt substitutes because these substances usually contain sizable amounts of potassium
- Be thoroughly familiar with the critical facts related to administering potassium intravenously

Hyperkalemia

Hyperkalemia refers to a condition with excess of potassium in ECG, characterized by conduction defect in the heart and myoneural junction of the muscle.

The related factors which lead to hyperkalemia are as follows:
- Decreased potassium excretions as in:
    - Oliguric renal failure
    - Potassium-conserving diuretic usage
    - Hypoaldosteronism
- High potassium intake, especially in presence of renal insufficiency
- Improper use of oral potassium supplements
- Rapid excessive administration of IV potassium
    - High-dose potassium penicillin
    - Foods high in potassium (such as dried apricots)

- Shift of potassium out of cells due to acidosis, tissue trauma, and malignant cell lysis
- Potassium excess also occur in acute renal failure, severe crush injuries and burns. Severe hemorrhages and adrenal insufficiency
- It is also seen in diabetic ketoacidosis.

Main Characteristics
- Vague muscular weakness is usually first sign
- Cardiac arrhythmias, bradycardia and heart block can occur
- Paresthesias of face, tongue, feet and hands . Flaccid muscle paralysis (spreads from legs to trunk and arms, respiratory muscle may be affected)
- Gastrointestinal symptoms such as nausea, intermittent intestinal colic, or diarrhea may occur
- ECG changes falls, peaked T waves, absent P waves widened QRS complex
- Serum K, above 5.0 mEq/L (mmol/L).

It can produce cardiac arrest, metabolic acidosis and respiratory acidosis as complications.

Treatment

Management of the condition is done by replacement of water loss and correction of electrolyte imbalance, the client is given diet with restricted protein but with as much as fat and carbohydrate and also managing the underlying condition.

Nursing Intervention
- Beware of clients at risk for hyperkalemia and monitor for its occurrence. Hyperkalemia is life-threatening; it is imperative to detect it easily
- Take measures to prevent hyperkalemia when possible by following guidelines for administering potassium safely both intravenously or orally:
    - Follow rules for safe administration of potassium
    - Avoid administration of potassium conserving diuretics, potassium supplements or salt substitutes to client with renal insufficiency
    - Caution client to use salt substitute sparingly if they are taking other supplementary form of potassium or taking potassium-conserving diuretics (e.g. spironolactone, triamaterine, and amiloride)
    - Caution hyperkalemic clients to avoid foods high in potassium content. Some of these are coffee, cocoa, tea, dried fruits, dried beans, whole grain breads.

Hypocalcemia

Hypocalcemia refers to a calcium deficit in ECF. If the condition is prolonged calcium is taken from bones. This results in osteomalacia, which is characterized by soft and pliable bones. Common signs and symptoms for hypocalcemia include numbness and tingling of fingers, muscle cramps and tetany.

The related factors leading to hypocalcemia are as follows:
- Surgical hypoparathyroidism (may follow thyroid surgery or radical neck surgery for cancer)

- Malabsorption
- Vitamin D deficiency
- Acute pancreatitis
- Excessive administration of citrated blood
- Primary hypothyroidism
- Alkalitic states (decreased ionized calcium)
- Hyperphosphatemia
- Medullary carcinoma of thyroid
- Hypoalbuminemia (as in cirrhosis, nephrotic syndrome and starvation)
- Hypomagnesemia
- Increased/Decreased ultraviolet exposure.

Main Characteristics
- Numbness, tingling fingers, circumoral region and toes
- Cramps in the muscle of extremities
- Hyperactive deep tendon reflexes (such as patellar and triceps)
- Trousseau's sign
- Chvostek's sign
- Mental changes such as confusion and alteration in mood and memory
- Convulsions, usually generalized but may be focal
- Spasm of laryngeal muscles
- ECG shows prolonged QT interval
- Spasms of muscles in abdomen (can simulate acute abdo-emergency)
- Total calcium level below 8.5 mg/ dL or ionized level below normal (below 50%)
- Hypocalcemic state occurs when calcium loss occurs causing a fall in serum calcium level. This may eventually cause tetany and teath
- It is usually asymptomatic and the neurological manifestation develop slowly
- It then gives rise to diffuse encephalopathy, depression and psychosis
- In severe cases there may be laryngiospasm and general convulsion
- It may also give rise to papilloedema and cataract.

Treatment

Most cases respond well to adequate or supplement calcium and phosphorus. The patient may be given calcium carbonate, 2.52 to 3.78 gm daily orally or calcium gluconate 0.5–1.5 gm along with calciferol 15.45 mg daily orally. Otherwise, 10 mL of 10 percent calcium gluconate is given by slow IV. Adequate management and control of predisposing causes, can prevent the occurrence of the condition.

Nursing Interventions
- Beware of clients at risk for hypocalcemia and monitor its occurrence
- Be prepared to take seizures precautions
- Monitor condition of airway closely because laryngeal stridor can occur
- Take safety precautions if confusion is present

- Beware of factors related to the safe administration of calcium replacement salts
- Educate people in high-risk groups for osteoporosis (especially postmenopausal women not on estrogen therapy). If adequate amounts are not consumed in the diet (as is often the case), calcium supplements should be considered
- Educate people at risk for osteoporosis about the value of regular physical exercise in decreasing bone loss
- To prevent osteoporosis in later years, educate young women about the need for a normal diet to ensure adequate calcium intake. Also discuss the calcium-losing aspects of alcohol and nicotine use.

Hypercalcemia

Hypercalcemia refers to an excess of calcium in ECF. It presents an emergency situation because this condition often leads to cardiac arrest. It is a condition of excess of calcium and is characterized by polyuria, polydipsia, skeletol muscle weakness and hypertension.

The related factors that lead to hypercalcemia are as follows:
- Hyperparathyroidism
- Malignant neoplastic disease
- Prolonged immobilization
- Large doses of vitamin D
- Overuse of calcium containing antacids or calcium supplements thiazide diuretics
- Milk-alkali syndrome
- Sarcoidosis
- It is also seen in person with Paget's disease, myxoedema, Addison's disease and osteoporosis in aged persons.

Main characteristics
- Muscle weakness
- Tiredness, restlessness, lethargy
- Constipation
- Anorexia, nausea, and vomiting
- Decreased memory span, decreased attention span, and confusion
- Polyuria, and polydipsia
- Renal stones
- Neurobic behavior progressing to frank psychosis may occur (reversible with correction of hypercalcemia)
- Cardiac arrest may occur in hypercalcemic crisis
- ECG shows shortened QT interval
- Serum calcium over 10.5 mg/dL
- It may produce renal failure, shock and death in complication.

Treatment

In mild cases, adequate rehydration is often effective. Management of the condition also includes management of the underlying conditions. In other cases, intravenous infusion of isotonic saline is given to promote calciuria. Calcium is also eliminated or maintained in the lower level by giving sodium phosphate 1-2 gm orally daily, and client is encouraged to take more fluids.

Nursing Intervention
- Beware of clients at risk for hypercalcemia and monitor its occurrence
- Increase client mobilization when feasible
- Encourage the oral intake of sufficient fluids to keep the client well hydrated
- Discourage excessive consumption of milk products and other high calcium foods
- Encourage adequate bulk in the diet to offset the tendency for constipation
- Take safety precautions if confusion or other mental symptoms by hypercalcemia are present
- Beware that cardiac arrest can occur in clients with severe hypercalcemia be prepared to deal with this emergency
- Beware that bones may fracture more easily in clients with chronic hypercalcemia because bone resorption has been excessive, weakening the bony structure. Transfer clients cautiously
- Educate home-bound oncology clients with a predisposition for hypercalcemia and their families, to be alert for symptoms that occur with this condition and to report them to the healthcare providers before they become severe
- Be alert for signs of digitalis toxicity when hypercalcemia occurs in digitalized clients
- Help prevent formation of calcium renal stones in clients with longstanding hyper calcemia or immobilization by:
  - Forcing fluids to maintain a dilute urine, thus avoiding supersaturation of precipitates
  - Encouraging fluids that yield an acid ash (prune or cranberry milk) because a urinary pH less than 6.5 favors calcium deposits
- Preventing urinary stasis by turning the immobilized client, elevating head of the bed and having the client sit up if this can be tolerated.

Hypomagnesemia

Magnesium is an important and plentiful cation, and is essential for many enzymatic system associated with protein, carbohydrate and lipid metabolism.

Hypomagnesemia refers to magnesium deficit. It is condition of low plasma concentration of magnesium, characterized by neuromuscular and CNS hyperirritability.

The related factors which lead to hypomagnesemia are as follows:
- Chronic alcoholism
- Intestinal malabsorption syndrome
- Diarrhea
- Nasogastric suction–prolonged
- Aggressive refeeding after starvation (as in TPN)
- Prolonged administration of magnesium–free IV fluids
- Uncontrolled diabetes mellitus–diabetic ketoacidosis
- Hyperaldosteronism
- Drugs–prolonged use of:
  - Diuretics, aminoglycoside, antibiotics (e.g. gentamycin), cisplatin

- Excessive dose of vitamin-D or calcium supplements
  - Citrate preservative in blood products
  - Pancreatitis, thyrotoxicosis, hyper-parathyroiders
- Severe osteotis fibrosa, PEM.

Main Characteristics
- It presents with multiple metabolic and nutritional deficiency
- It gives rise to anorexia, lethargy, vomiting, weakness, and tetany
- Neuromuscular irritability
  - Increased reflex
  - Course tremors
  - Positive Chvostek's and Trousseau's signs
  - Convulsions
- Cardiac manifestations will include:
  - Tachyarrhythmias
  - Increased susceptibility to digitalis toxicity
- ECG changes in severe cases, PR and QT interval prolongation, widened QRS complex, ST segment depression and T -wave inversion
- Mental changes
  - Disorientation in memory
  - Mood changes
  - Intense confusion
  - Hallucination
- Serum magnesium level below 1.3 mEq/L.

Treatment
Repletion of the cases are done through magnesium sulfate and chloride. It is customary to give double the amount required because half of magnesium given excreted by the kidneys. The repletion is done gradually and is given orally or intravenously; in severe cases, IV only.

Nursing Intervention
- Beware, client at risk for hypomagnesemia, especially closely for symptoms of digitalis toxicity because a deficit of magnesium predisposes to toxicity
- Be prepared to take seizure precautions when hypomagnesemia, especially closely for symptoms of digitalis toxicity, because a deficit of magnesium predisposes to toxicity
- Monitor condition of airway, because laryngeal stridor can occur
- Take safety precautions if confusion presents
- Be familiar with magnesium replacement salts and factors related to these safe administration
- Beware that magnesium-depleted clients may experience difficulty in swallowing
- When magnesium deficit is due to abuse of diuretics in laxatives, educating the client may help alleviate problem
- Beware that most commonly used IV fluids have either no magnesium or relatively small amount. When indicated, discuss the need for magnesium replacement with physicians
- For clients experiencing abnormal losses, but able to consume a general diet, encourage intake of magnesium–rich foods (such as green-leafy vegetables, nuts, legumes and fruits such as bananas, oranges, and grape fruits).

Hypermagnesemia

Hypermagnesemia refers to a magnesium excess. It can occur especially in end stage renal failure. When kidneys fail to excrete magnesium and excessive amounts are administered therapeutically. It is a condition associated with excess of magnesium and is characterized by muscular weakness and ECG changes.

The related factors which lead to hypermagnesemia are as follows:

- Renal failure (particularly when magnesium containing medications are administered)
- Adrenal insufficiency
- Excessive magnesium administration during treatment of eclampsia
- Hemodialysis with excessively hard water or with dialysate inadvertantly high in magnesium content.

Magnesium has a direct action on the myoneural junction. Its excess produces blockage causing impairment of neuro-muscular transmission and that results diminished excitability of the muscle cells.

Main Characteristics
- Early signs (serum level of mg of 3 to 5 mEq/L)
- Flushing and a sense of skin warmth (due to peripheral vasodilation)
- Hypotension (due to blockage of sympathetic ganglia)
- Depressed respiration
- Drowsiness, hypoactive reflexes and muscular weakness
- Cardiac abnormalities–cardiac arrest may develop
- Weak or absent cry in newborn
- ECG shows prolonged PR interval, widened QRS complex and elevated T-wave amplitude
- Elevated serum magnesium level.

Treatment
In severe cases and also in other cases cardiac and respiratory support are given by IV injection of 10-20 mL of 10 percent calcium gluconate. Maintenance of adequate hydration is essential. The client is also given frusemide by IV injection to promote excretion of magnesium. In more severe cases, hemodialysis is done.

Nursing Intervention
- Beware of client at risk for hypermagnesemia and assess for its presence. When it is suspected assess the following parameters:
  - Vital signs–look for low blood pressure and shallow respirations with periods of apnea
  - Level of consciousness–look for drowsiness, lethargy and coma
- Do not give magnesium containing medication to clients with renal failure or compromised renal function
- Be particularly careful in following 'standing order' for bowel preparation for X-ray because some of these include the use of magnesium citrate

- Caution clients with renal disease to check with their healthcare providers before taking over the counter medication
- Beware of factors related to safe parenteral administration of magnesium salts.

Hypophosphatemia

Hypophosphatemia refers to a below normal serum concentration of inorganic phosphorus. It is a clinical manifestation of phosphate depletion, characterized by progressive encephalo-pathy and osteomalacia.

The related factors which lead to hypophosphatemia are as follows:

- Inadequate intake or absorption of phosphorus–malabsorption
- It is associated with vomiting and diarrhea
- Prolonged injection of aluminum hydroxide or bicarbonate
- It is also seen in:
  - Prolonged use of glucose insulin, fructose, administrations
  - Refeeding after starvation
  - Hyperalimentation
  - Alcohol withdrawal
  - Diabetic ketoacidosis
  - Respiratory alkalosis
  - Phosphate-binding antacids use
  - Recovery phase after severe burns
  - Use of anabolic steroids
  - Chronic hemodialysis.

Main Characteristics
- Progressive encephalopathy
- Paresthesias
- Muscle weakness
- Muscle pain and tenderness
- Mental changes, such as apprehension, confusion, delirium coma
- Cardiomyopathy
- Acute respiratory failure
- Seizures
- Decreased tissue oxygenation
- Joint stiffness
- Serum phosphate below 2.5 mg/dL
- Phosphate compounds are present in all normal foods and are essential for metabolism of carbohydrate, protein and fat. They are also responsible for changes, transfer, or depletion occurs from prolonged negative phosphate balance and form chronic malnutrition.

Treatment
Management of the condition includes treatment of the underlying cause, repletion of phosphate, and maintenance of body fluids.

Nursing Intervention
- Identify clients at risk for hypophosphatemia
  - Severely malnourished clients

– Alcoholic clients
– Clients with diabetic ketoacidosis
* Monitor clients at risk for the presence of hypophosphatemia
* Beware that severely hypophosphatemic clients are thought to be greater risk for infection because of changes in WBCs
* Administer IV phosphate products cautiously
* Beware that in adults the usual maintenance dose of phosphorus is 10 to 15 mmol/L of TPN solution
* Beware of the need to introduce hyperalimentation gradually in clients who are malnourished
* Because it is possible to give too much phosphorus when administering phosphate solutions, monitor for signs of hyperphosphatemia and of the salt in which it is administered
* Monitor for diarrhea in clients taking oral phosphorus supplements; consult physician if it persists or is severe
* Powdered oral phosphorus supplements with chilled or ice water to make them more palatable.

Hyperphosphatemia

Hyperphosphatemia refers to above normal serum concentrations of inorganic phosphorus. It is a condition associated with increased level of phosphate and is characterized by hypocalcemia.

The related factors which lead to hyperphosphatemia are as follows:
* Excessive intake of phosphate
* Hypervitaminosis D–large vitamin D intake
* Acute renal failure
* Chronic renal insufficiency
* Chemotherapy, particularly for acute lymphoblastic leukemia and lymphoma
* Large intake of milk
* Use of cow's milk in infants
* Excessive intake of phosphate containing laxatives
* Overzealous administration of phosphorus supplements (oral or IV)
* Excessive use of fleets phospho soda as enema solution particularly in children and people with slow bowel elimination
* Hypoparathyroidism
* Hyperthyroidism.

Main Characteristics
This condition by itself does not give rise to any symptoms but manifested with that of hypocalcemia, which includes:
* Short-term consequences–symptoms of tetany, such as tingling of fingertips and around mouth, numbness and muscle spasms
* Long-term consequences–precipitation of calcium phosphate in nonosseous sites; such as kidney, joints, arteries, skin of cornea
* Serum phosphate above 4.5 mg/dL.

Treatment
Management of the condition requires correction of underlying condition.

Nursing Intervention
* Identify clients at risk for hyperphosphatemia
* Monitor signs of tetanus and other features of hypocalcemia
* Beware that soft-tissue calcification can be long-term complication of a chemically elevated serum phosphate level. Calcification may occur in site such as kidney, arteries, joints, etc.
* Administer prescribed oral or IV phosphate supplements cautiously and monitor serum phosphorus levels periodically during their use
* When appropriate, instruct clients that use of phosphate, containing laxatives may result in acute phosphate poisoning
* Beware that phosphate containing enema can result in hyperphosphatemia if used injudiciously, particularly in children and those with slow bowel emptying, instruct clients accordingly
* When low-phosphorus diet is prescribed, instruct clients to avoid foods high in phosphorus content. Such foods include hard cheese or cream, nuts and nut products; whole grain cereals (e.g. bran and catmeal), dried fruits, dried vegetables; special meats such as kidneys, sardines, and sweet breads and desserts made with milk.

Acid-base Imbalances

Arterial blood gases (ABGs) are most commonly used to assess and treat acid-base imbalances. Results from venous blood are only specific for particular extremity or area where the blood was sampled and do not provide information on how well the lungs oxygenating the blood. The pH of plasma indicates balance or impending acidosis or alkalosis. In addition, however, a study of the blood oxygen and carbon dioxide gases is important. The partial pressure (indicated by 'P') of these gases, or their tensions are determined by the use of a nomogram, which reflects the chemical and physical activities of two gases. The partial pressure of carbon dioxide $PaCO_2$; for oxygen, it is PaO_2. The "a" indicates an arterial specimen. When the PaO_2 is low, hemoglobin carries less than/normal amounts of oxygen, when the PaO_2 is high, the hemoglobin carries more oxygen, oxygen saturation readings (SaO_2) reveal the percentage of O_2 in the blood that combines with hemoglobin. The $PaCO_2$ is influenced almost entirely by respiratory activity. When $PaCO_2$ is low, carbonic acid leaves the body in excessive amounts; when the $PaCO_2$ is high, there are excessive amounts of carbonic acid in the body.

Acid-base imbalance occurs when the carbonic acid or bicarbonate levels become disproportionate. When there is a single primary cause, these disturbances are known as respiratory acidosis or alkalosis and metabolic acidosis or alkalosis. These disturbances (result of an upset in acid-base balance) are as follows:
* Respiratory disturbance alters carbonic acid portion:
  – Respiratory acidosis and alkalosis are the results of respiratory disturbances

- Compensation occurs to resolve balance in the kidneys by either conserving or excreting more bicarbonate
- A metabolic disturbance alters the bicarbonate portion
  - Metabolic acidosis and alkalosis are almost entirely the result of metabolic processes
  - The primary organs for compensation to restore balance are lungs, which either try to conserve or excrete more CO_2 which is available in weakly ionized carbonic acid.

The brief descriptions of management of acidbase imbalances are as follows.

Respiratory Acidosis (Carbonic Acid Excess)

Respiratory acidosis is primary excess of carbonic acid in ECF. Any decrease in alveolar ventilations that result in retention of CO_2 can cause respiratory acidosis. Because the lungs are the source of the problem, they are unable to participate in compensation. As the carbonic acid content increases, the kidney attempts to retain more bicarbonate and increase their hydrogen excretion. It is a clinical state of altered hydrogen ion concentration characterized by hypoventilation.

RA = high $PaCO_2$ because of alveolar hypoventilations.

The related factors for respiratory acidosis (RA) are as follows:

1. Acute respiratory acidosis
   - Acute pulmonary edema
   - Aspiration of a foreign body
   - Atelectasis
   - Pheumothorax, hemothorax
   - Overdose of sedatives or anesthetic
   - Position on operative room table that interferes with respiration
   - Cardiac arrest
   - Severe pneumonia
   - Laryngospasm
   - Mechanical ventilation improperly regulated
   - Chronic respiratory acidosis
   - Emphysema
   - Cysticfibrosis
   - Advanced multiple sclerosis
   - Bronchiectasis
   - Bronchial asthma.
2. Factors favoring hypoventilation
   - Obesity
   - Tight abdominal binders and dressings
   - Postoperative pain (as in high abdominal or chest incisions)
   - Abdominal distention from cirrhosis or bowel obstruction.

Main Characteristics
1. Acute respiratory acidosis
   - Mental cloudiness–Ventricular fibrillation may be the first sign in anesthetized patient (related to hypokalemia)
   - Dizziness

- Palpitations
- Muscular twitching
- Arterial blood gases (ABGs)
- Convulsions
- pH below 7.35
- Warm flushed skin
- $PaCO_2$ over 45 mm Hg (primary)
- Unconsciousness
- HCO_3 normal or only slightly elevated.

2. Chronic respiratory acidosis
   - Weakness
   - Dull headache
   - Symptoms underlying disease process
   - ABGs
   - pH below 7.35 or within lower limits of normal
   - $PaCO_2$ over 4.5 mm Hg (primary)
   - HCO_3^- over 26 mEq/L (compensatory).

Treatment
Administer respiratory stimulants, i.e. nikethamide 2-4 mL of 25 percent solution by IV repeated everyone or two and treating the underlying condition.

Nursing Intervention
- Treatment is directed improving ventilation; exact measures vary with the cause of inadequate ventilation
- Pharmacological agents are used as indicated. For example, bronchodilators help to reduce bronchial spasm; antibiotic for infection
- Pulmonary hygienic measures are used when necessary to rid the respiratory tract of mucous and purulent drainage
- Adequate hydration (2 to 3 L/day) is indicated to keep mucous membranes moist and thereby facilitate removal of secretions. Supplemental oxygen is used as necessary
- A mechanical respirator, used cautiously, may improve the pulmonary ventilation. One must remember that overzealous use of a mechanical respirator may cause rapid excretion of CO_2 the kidneys will be unable to eliminate excess bicarbonate with sufficient rapidly to prevent alkalosis and convulsion. For this reason the elevated $PaCO_2$ must be decreased slowly.

Respiratory Alkalosis (Carbonic Acid Deficit)

Respiratory alkalosis is a primary deficit of carbonic acid in ECF. It is the result of the increased alveolar ventilation and therefore, a decrease in CO_2. An increase in respiratory rate and depth cause the CO_2 loss because the CO_2 is excreted faster than normal. Because of the deficit of the CO_2, which is a respiratory stimulant sensed in the medulla of the brain. Depression in cessation of respiration eventually can occur. Because the lungs are the source of the problem, they are unable *to* participate in compensation. Therefore kidneys attempt *to* alleviate the imbalance by increasing bicarbonate excretion and by retaining more hydrogen.

Respiratory alkalosis = Low $PaCO_2$ because of alveolar hyperventilation.

It is a clinical disorder of altered hydrogen's ion concentration, that is developing from hyperventilation.

The related factors which lead to respiratory alkalosis are:

- Extreme anxiety (most common cause)
- Hypoxemia
- High fever
- Early salicylate intoxication (stimulates respiratory center)
- Gram-negative bacteremia
- CNS lesions involving respiratory center, meningitis, encephalitis
- Pulmonary emboli, pneumonia
- Thyrotoxicosis
- Excessive ventilation by mechanical ventilators
- Pregnancy (high progesterone level sensitizes the respiratory center to CO_2: physiologic).

Main Characteristics

- The condition presents with anxiety
- Light headedness (a low $PaCO_2$ causes cerebral vasoconstrictions and thus decreased cerebral blood flow)
- Respiratory symptoms–frequent, deep, sighing, or rapid and deep breathing
- Hyperventilation syndrome, i.e. tinnitus, palpitations, sweating, dry mouth, tremulousness, precordial pain (tightness), nausea and vomiting, epigastric pain, blurred vision, convulsions and loss of consciousness
- ABGs
  - pH over 7.45
  - $PaCO_2$ below 35 mm Hg (primary)
  - HCO_3^- under 22 mEq/L (compensatory).

Treatment

Treatment is given by correction of underlying causes.

Nursing Intervention

- If the cause of respiratory alkalosis is anxiety, the client should be made aware that the abnormal breathing practice is responsible for the symptoms accompanying this condition
- Instruct the client *to* breathe more slowly (to cause accumulation of CO_2) or to breathe in closed system (such as paper bag)
- Usually sedative is required to relieve ventilation in very anxious patients (if alkalosis severe enough to cause fainting, the increase ventilation ceases and respiration reverts to normal)
- Treatment for other causes of respiratory alkalosis is directed at correcting for the underlying problem.

Metabolic Acidosis (Base Bicarbonate Deficit)

Metabolic acidosis is a proportionate deficit of bicarbonate in ECF. The deficit can occur as the remit of an increase in acid components or an excessive loss of bicarbonate. The lungs attempt *to* increase the CO_2 excretion by increasing the rate and depth of respirations. The kidneys attempt *to* compensate by retaining bicarbonate and by excreting more hydrogen. If the body is unable *to* achieve normal balance, the person may lose consciousness as metabolic acidosis increases and death eventually results. Thus,

Metabolic acidosis = Low bicarbonate, non-volatile acid present used.

HCO_2^- in disproportionate amounts

It is a condition of hydrogen ion concentration characterized by rise of hydrogen ion and reduction in plasma bicarbonate level.

The related factors which lead to metabolic acidosis are as follows:

- Normal anion gap related to
  - Diarrhea
  - Intestinal fistulas
  - Ureter sigmoidostomy
  - Hyperalimentation–vomiting excessively
  - Acidifying drugs (such as ammonium chloride)
  - Renal tubular acidosis (RTA).
- High anion gap related to:
  - Diabetic ketoacidosis
  - Starvational ketoacidosis
  - Lactic acidosis
  - Renal failure
  - Ingestion of toxins (such as salicylates, ehylene glycol, and methanol)
  - Acute alcoholic.

Main Characteristics

- Headache, confusion, drowsiness
- Increased respiratory rate and depth (may not become clinically evident until HCO_3^- is quite low)
- Nausea and vomiting
- Peripheral vasodilation (may be present, causing warm flushed skin)
- Decreased cardiac output when pH below 7 Bradycardia may present
- ABGs
  - HCO_3^- under 22 mEq/L (primary)
  - $PaCO_2$ under 35 mm Hg (compensatory by lungs)
  - Base excess always negative
- Hypokalemia frequently present
- Hyperapnea-Kussmaul's respiration
- It eventually produces circulatory shock in complication.

Treatment

Salt and water repletion, and treating underlying conditions. Treatment is directed toward correcting the metabolic defect. If the cause of the problem is excessive intake of chloride, treatment obviously focuses on eliminating the source, when necessary, bicarbonate is administered.

Control of the condition requires avoidance of and adequate management of the conditions which gives rise to the condition.

Metabolic Alkalosis (Base Bicarbonate Excess)

Metabolic alkalosis is a primary excess of bicarbonate in ECF. This may be the result of excessive acid losses or increased base ingestion or retention. The body attempts to compensate by retaining CO_2. The respirations become slow and shallow, and periods of breathing may occur. The kidneys attempt to excrete potassium and sodium with the excessive bicarbonate, and retain hydrogen in carbonic acid. Thus,

Metabolic alkalosis =

High bicarbonate.

Nonvolatile acid is lost and it is not using up HCO_3^- or HCO_3^- gained is in disproportionate amount

It is a disorder of hydrogen ion concentration disturbance characterized by hypocalcemia and hypokalemia.

The related factors which lead to metabolic alkalosis are as follows:
- Vomiting or gastric suction
- Hypokalemia
- Hyperaldosteronism
- Cushing's syndrome
- Potassium losing diuretics (e.g. thiazide, frusamide, ethacrynic acid)
- Alkali ingestion (bicarbonate containing antacids)
- Parenteral $NaHCO_3$ administration for cardiopulmonary resuscitation
- Abrupt relief of chronic respiratory acidosis.

Main Characteristics
- Irritation and neuromuscular excitation
- Those related to decreased calcium ionization are:
  - Dizziness, tingling of fingers and toes, circumoral paresthesia, carpopedal spasm, hypertonic muscles
- Depressed respiration (compensatory action by lungs)
- ABGs
  - pH above 7.45, bicarbonate over 26 mEq/L
  - $PaCO_2$ over 45 mm Hg (compensatory)
  - Base excess is always possible
- Hypokalemia often present
- Serum CI is relatively lower than Na.

Treatment
Correction of the underlying cause is essential for proper management of condition. Treatment is aimed at reversal of the underlying disorder. Sufficient chloride must be supplied to the kidney to absorb sodium with chloride (allowing the excretion of excessive bicarbonate).

Treatment also includes restoration of normal fluid volume by administration of sodium chloride fluids because continued volume depletion serves to maintain the alkalosis.

Nurses wishing to get role model of selfcare behaviors that promote fluid, electrolyte, and acid-base balance should meet the following goals:
- The nurse daily ingests the quantity and type of fluids (to include six to eight glasses of water) that promote healthy hydration and urinary functioning
- The nurse evaluates use of food diets, diuretics, laxatives, and alcohol, identifying potential risks to health
- The nurse identifies situations of high risk for fluid and electrolyte imbalance and intervene appropriately

Responsibilities of a Nurse in Maintaining Fluid and Electrolyte Balance

Important nursing functions include:
1. Assisting the doctor in evaluating patients fluid and electrolyte status.
2. Helping in prevention of fluid and electrolyte imbalance by replacement therapy and relief of symptoms.
3. Recognition and reporting early symptoms of fluid and electrolyte imbalance.
4. To keep a fluid balance chart.

Fluid Balance Chart									
Sl No.	Time	Intravenous Fluid		Oral		Urine	Aspiration	Vomit	Others
		Type	Amount	Type	Amount				

24 hours
Total

Determination of Fluid and Electrolyte Balance

Every patient who are receiving IV fluids should have a chart of fluid intake and output. This record should be accurate. It is critically studied to determine whether there is the expected ratio between intake and output or there is excess or deficit. Any marked change in ratio should be reported to the doctor.

The intake record should show the type and volume of all fluids the patient has received and the route by which they are administered. The time should be noted. The output record includes urinary output, vomiting, gastric suction and drainage from any body cavity or wound. Blood loss from any part of the body should be measured carefully.

Though diaphoresis is difficult to measure yet careful note of heavy perspiration and its duration should be recorded (accurate recording of body temperature helps the doctor to determine how much fluid the patient needs). Since fluid loss through the skin and lungs increases the temperature rises.

Daily weight record is a good indication of the onset of dehydration or of the accumulation of fluid. The patient must be weighed on the same time and each day with the same clothings.

Prevention of electrolyte and fluid imbalance by:

1. *Oral rehydration therapy:* The best way to restore water and electrolytes to the body is to give them by mouth. Oral rehydration therapy is based on the observation that glucose given orally enhances the intestinal absorption of salt and water

and is capable of correcting the electrolyte and water deficit. The composition of oral fluid as suggested by WHO is as follows:

Sodium Chloride (table salt)	3.5 g.
Potassium Chloride	1.5 g.
Sodium citrate	2.9 g.
Glucose (Dextrose)	20.0 g.
Potable water	1 liter

Oral rehydration mixtures are now freely available. The contents of the packet are dissolved in one litre of drinking water and should be used within 24 hours.

2. *Parenteral:* If oral route is not possible then the commonest method of replacement is by intravenous infusion. In case of infant it may be given into subcutaneous tissue if venous route is not possible. Concentrated solution of glucose should always be given IV in small amounts at time and slowly because they will pull fluid from the body to dilute themselves. Normal saline solution may cause fluid to diffuse from the tissues to equalize the concentration of salt in the fluid compartments. If any of these concentrated solutions flow quickly into the vascular system pulmonary edema can develop rapidly. The initial signs of pulmonary edema are bounding pulse, engorged peripheral veins, hoarseness, dyspnea, chest pain, cough, etc.

Common solutions used parenterally:

(i) Glucose 5% in distilled water is often used to maintain fluid intake or to re-establish blood volume.

(ii) 4.3% Dextrose and 0.18% saline may be used as Dextrose-saline. It is isotonic.

(iii) Isotonic solution of sodium chloride (0.9%) usually is given to re-establish the blood volume.

(iv) One-sixth molar lactate solution may be used when sodium but not chloride needs replacement.

(v) Balance solution containing several electrolytes may be used. Ringer's lactate solution. Hartmann's solution, Darrows solution are examples.

Recognition of Various Common Conditions

1. **Water depletion (dehydration):** Occurs due to diminished intake, severe diarrhoea. vomiting, intestinal obstruction.
Features are: (*a*) Thirst (*b*) Weakness, exhaustion (*c*) Low urine volume (*d*) Dry wrinkled skin and mouth (*e*) Vertigo (*f*) Sunken eyes (*g*) Mental confusion, delirium (*h*) Coma.

2. **Water intoxication (water excess):** Occurs when excessive amount of water is given orally, intravenously or by other routes.
Features: (*a*) Drowsiness, weakness (*b*) Headache (*c*) Giddiness, nausea, vomiting (*d*) Breathlessness (*e*) Abdominal cramps (*f*) Confusion (*g*) Pitting edema (late) (*h*) Pulmonary edema (*i*) Convulsion and coma (*j*) Low serum sodium concentration.

3. **Hyponatremia (Low sodium-ion in plasma):** Common causes are intestinal obstruction, severe diarrhea, dysentery, cholera, ulcerative colitis, bilious, pancreatic or intestinal fistula.
Features: (*a*) Headache (*b*) Nausea and vomiting; (*c*) Muscular cramp, convulsion (*d*) Weakness (*e*) Abdominal cramps (*f*) Less sweating (*g*) Sunken eyes (*h*) Loss of elasticity of skin (*i*) Cold extremities (*j*) Fall of BP.

4. **Hypernairemia (Sodium excess):** When excess of normal saline or hypertonic saline has been given IV.
Features: (*a*) Puffiness of face, weakness (*b*) Accumulation of fluid in the various serous sacs and pitting edema (*c*) In infancy - increased tension in anterior fontanelle, edema and increase in the number of urination.

5. **Hypokalaemia (Postassium depletion):** Observed in ulcerative colitis, intestinal fistula, when intravenous alimentation is continued for more than 72 hours, in diabetic coma treated by insulin, in prolonged saline infusion together with nasogastric aspiration.
Features: (*a*) Lethargy, drowsiness, slurred speech (*b*) Anorexia (*c*) Constipation (*d*) Polyuria due to incontinence (*e*) Muscular weakness (*f*) Mental confusion (*g*) Distension of the abdomen (*h*) Shock (*i*) Weakness of heart muscles causing circulation to slowed down which may lead to cardiac arrest.

6. **Hyperkalaemia (Postassium excess)** viz. in renal failure.
Features: (*a*) Nausea (*b*) Weakness of the muscles (*c*) Colic (*d*) Spasticity of muscles due to overstimulation, skeletal muscle spasm (*e*) Irregular and slow heart beat due to overstimulation of cardiac muscle (*f*) Sudden cardiac arrest.

7. **Metabolic alkalosis** (Bicarbonate excess) accompanies with electrolyte imbalance.
Features: (*a*) Slow and shallow breathing (*b*) Tetany (*c*) Convulsion (*d*) Confusion (*e*) Coma.

8. **Metabolic acidosis** (Bicarbonate deficit) viz., in renal failure, shock.
Features: (*a*) Dyspnea, tiredness, weakness (*b*) Deep and periodic breathing (*c*) Stupor (*d*) Coma.

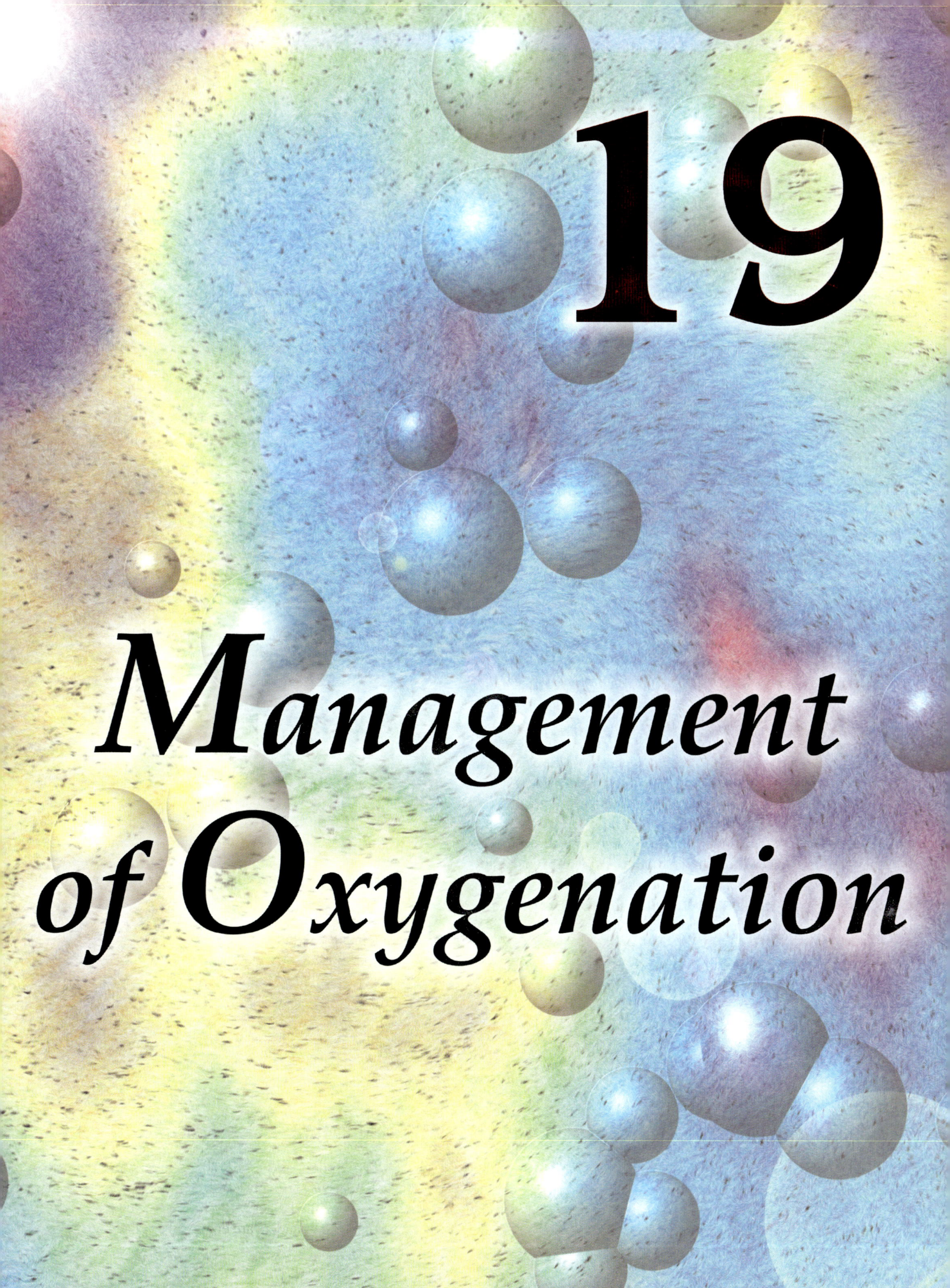

19
Management
of Oxygenation

Introduction

Oxygen is a basic need and is required to sustain life. The nurse often encounters clients who are unable to independently meet oxygen needs; the nurse must understand cardiac and respiratory physiology.

The function of the cardiac system is to deliver oxygen, nutrients, and other substances to the tissues, and remove the waste products of cellular metabolism. The objective is achieved through the cardiac pump, the circulatory vascular system, and the integration of other systems, i.e., respiratory, digestive and renal. Cardiac physiology involves the delivery of oxygenated blood to the tissues and the delivery of deoxygenated blood to the pulmonary system. Once the blood is delivered to the pulmonary circulation, the lungs oxygenate the blood and this oxygenated blood is returned to the left side of the heart and then delivered to the tissues.

Normal functioning of the respiratory system depends essentially on the following factors:

- The integrity of the airway system to transport air to and from the lungs
- A properly functioning of cardiovascular system to carry nutrients and wastes to and from body cells

Respiratory physiology involves oxygenation of the body through the mechanism of ventilation, perfusion, and transport of respiratory gases.

In addition, neural and chemical regulators control fluctuations in respiratory rate and depth to meet tissue oxygen demands. Together, the cardiac and respiratory system function to supply the body's demands of oxygen.

Administration of oxygen must be ordered by the physician or qualified medical practitioner. Some areas will have protocols that govern oxygen therapy and allow the nurse to begin therapy independently. Oxygen is a drug, so medication administration criteria are followed in addition to the steps unique to oxygen therapy. Clients unable to maintain adequate PO_2 and O_2 saturation levels on room air are candidates for oxygen therapy. An adequate airway is essential to effectiveness of the treatment. It is best to treat the hypoxia with the lowest oxygen dose possible. Some clients with a normal oxygen level are also given oxygen if they are at risk for complications related to hypoxia; for example, the myocardial infarction client often receives oxygen therapy to prevent dysrhythmias.

Factors Affecting Oxygenation

Adequate of circulation, ventilation, perfusion and transport respiratory gases to the tissues are influenced by four types of factor.

Physiological Factors: Any condition that affects cardiopulmonary functioning directly affects the body's ability to meet oxygen demand. The general classification of cardiac disorders includes disturbance in condition, impaired valvular function, myocardial hypoxia, cardiomyopathic conditions and peripheral tissue hypoxia, respiratory disorders include hyperventilation, hypoventilation and hypoxia. Other physiologic process which affects oxygenation will include anemia, toxic inhalatent (CO), airway obstruction, high altitude fever and decreased chest wall movement due to musculoskeletal impairments, pregnancy and obesity.

Developmental Factors: The developmental stage of the client and the normal aging process can affect tissue oxygenation, e.g. children are at risk of acute upper respiratory tract infections and exposure to these infections. Affects the tissue oxygenation; young and middle-aged persons are exposed to multiple cardiopulmonary risk factors; a nonhealthy diet, lack of exercise, stress and smoky which affect tissue.

Behavioral Factors: A person's behavior or lifestyle may directly or indirectly affect the body's ability to meet oxygen requirements. Lifestyle factors that influence respiratory functioning include, nutrition (e.g. obesity and malnutrition), exercise (lack of exercise), cigarette smoking, substance abuse (excessive alcohol, drug addiction), and stress (severe anxiety).

Environmental Factors: The environment can also influence oxygenation. The incidence of pulmonary disease is higher in smoggy, urban areas than rural areas. In addition client's workplace may increase the risk for pulmonary disease. Occupational pollutions include asbestos, talcum powder, dust and airborne fibers leads to occupation diseases.

Oxygen Therapy Administration

Administration of oxygen is a major part of nursing procedure. A nurse should be well-acquainted with various aspects of oxygen therapy.

Indications of Oxygen Therapy

- Obstruction in air-passage like foreign body, growth, enlarged thyroid
- Bronchial asthma
- Pneumonia and pulmonary edema
- Cardiac insufficiency
- Peripheral circulatory failure
- Asphyxia of various causes
- Poisoning
- Drowning
- Chest injuries
- During operation

Oxygen Cylinder and Fittings (Fig. 19.1)

- Oxygen cylinders and other gas cylinders and painted in distinctive color for ready identification. Oxygen cylinders are actually painted black with white value end:
- Sometimes the cylinders are engraved or labeled oxygen.

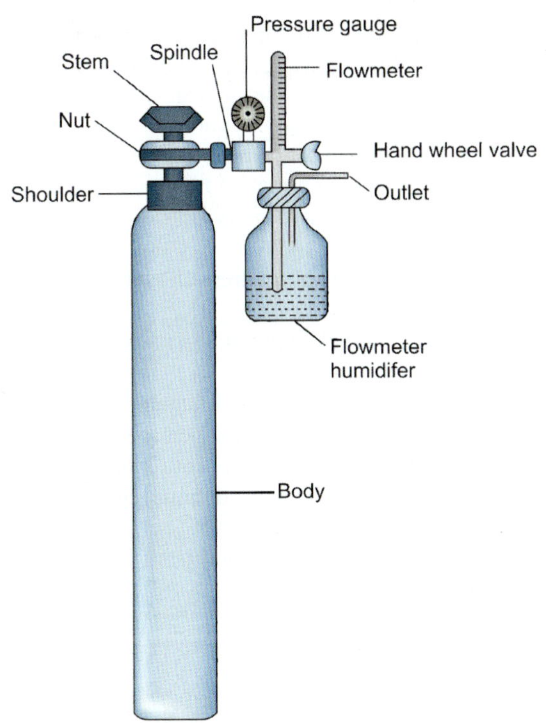

Figure 19.1: Oxygen cylinder

- The gas is compressed in cylinder when the cylinder is filled to accommodate more gas in small space. The small cylinder of 2½ feet × 5″ diameter contains 24 cubic feet or oxygen while big cylinders of 4 feet × 8″ diameter contains about 120 cubic feet of oxygen.
- As the gas is with pressure, a valve is attached to the mouth of cylinder for controlled related of gas. A gauze attached to the valve measure the amount of oxygen in cylinder.
- The cylinder is opened by means of metal key.
- A flowmeter is a piece of apparatus attached to valve for easy adjustment and control of flow of oxygen.
- A rate of 6 to 8 liters per minute is normally given if face mask is used. Higher rate may be given if oxygen tent is used.
- All empty cylinder should be kept labeled "empty" inward.
- The cylinder is usually kept in a wheeled stand for easy transport from patient to patient.

Precautions for Handling Oxygen Cylinder

- No naked light, cigarette, mechanical toy which produces sparks must be allowed anywhere near oxygen tent or specially when it is in use for patient.
- No electrical bells, lights or healing pads should be allowed near oxygen tent.
- Patient should be rubbed with oil or spirit while the tent is being operated.
- Grease must not be used on the valve or flowmeter.
- There is a risk of explosion if grease is used.

- When the tent is used the cylinder should be carefully watched and not allowed to be empty as it may cause dangerous effect on patient as oxygen supply fails.
- The nozzle of cylinder must be cleaned before attaching to the regulator.
- Place 'NO SMOKING' notice on cylinder.
- Store cylinder in a cool place.
- Warn visitors regarding dangers of oxygen.
- Check cylinder of gauze intermittently and also the masks or nasal tubes.

Different Modes of Administration of Oxygen

Oxygen may be given by means of the following:
 (i) A mask
 (ii) Oxygen tent
 (iii) Through nasal tube or catheters

Masks: There are different varieties of masks. The commands used as a given below:

Disposable polythene mask: A polythene mask is light and handy and is cheaper. It is disposed off after use. So no sterilization is required. When the mask is connected to oxygen supply, the flow of oxygen inflates a cuff round the edge of the mask, which then fits closely and comfortably. When the oxygen supply is by any means stopped the cuff will deflate and draws attention of nurse or relatives.

The vent mask: The vent mask is designed to provide accurate control of oxygen concentration so that it does not rise high enough to cause respiratory depression but it is sufficient to relieve anoxia. The range of controlled concentration is 24 to 35 percent. The disposable face piece is edged with foam rubber so that it fits closely and comfortably round the patient's nose.

Tracheostomy mask: When a tracheostomy is done on a patient it is of no use to give oxygen by nasal route as upper respiratory passage is already blocked. A special type of mask is used for oxygen therapy to tracheotomy patient, which fits to the tracheotomy patient, which fits to the tracheotomy opening. This also allows suction to be carried out when the mask is in position. There are perforations on side of mask for carbon dioxide expulsion.

Oxygen tent: Oxygen tent is a thin plastic tents like structure which is suspended over patient and the sides are tucked in firmly under bed clothings of patient. As it is air-proof material the temperature inside tent rises, for cooling the inside temperature either electrically cooling system is done or ice is kept in basin. The inside temperature is not allowed to rise above 70°F. For measuring the temperature, a thermometer is suspended inside the tent, preferably near the patient. The concentration of oxygen is maintained at constant rate. The patients or children who cannot use mask or tubes, oxygen tent is very useful. A special humidifier is also incorporated into tent to maintain humidity of oxygen. The disadvantages of tent are as follows:

 (i) The patient may get cut off contact with others.

 (ii) The patient may get panicky.

(iii) Excess oxygen may be given by this method.

(iv) There may be insufficient carbon dioxide to provide necessary stimulating effect for respiration. The patient should be taken out of tent at regular intervals.

Nasal Tubes: The nasal tubes or nasal catheters, though commonly used in hospitals for oxygen therapy, is not a good method. By this method, there is a great waste of oxygen and there is no control for concentration and rate. When given by nasal tube the oxygen must pass through a humidifier system (A bottle containing water in which oxygen is passed through). Dry, oxygen is irritating to nasal passage.

It is better to insert two small catheters rather than single one. A spectacle frame is a convenient way to use two nasal catheters. The catheters are cleaned and lubricated before introducing into nostril.

Procedures of Material Required for Oxygen Administration

 1. Oxygen cylinder with regulator fitments
 2. Opening key
 3. Humidifier
 4. Nasal tubes
 5. Rubber tubing
 6. Lubricant lotion
 7. Adhesive tape
 8. Cylinder strep
 9. Oxygen mask, if available
10. Cotton swabs to clean nostrils
11. A bowl containing water to check flow of oxygen

The points to be considering oxygen administering are:

- In a conscious patient, explain the procedure and why it is required
- Check the cylinder, open the valve away from patient and observe gauze reading to ensure the amount to oxygen
- Fill humidifier with water
- Attach the tubing of humidifier to oxygen cylinder and outlet of humidifier for patient
- Unscrew regulator and allow release of oxygen from cylinder which can be observed
- Now check nasal catheter by dipping in a bowl of water and see for bubbling. Now you are sure that the flow of oxygen is correct
- Now close the regulator to stop flow of oxygen
- Lubricate the catheter
- Determine the approximate depth to which the catheter is to be inserted by measuring distance from external nostril, to tragus of ear and mark the distance of catheter (about 8 cm). clean the nostrils by swab

- Now release and adjust regulator to provide 4 to 8 liter of oxygen per minute
- Insert the catheter slowly and gently with oxygen flowing through nostril into oropharynx until patient swallows bolus of oxygen and then withdraw about half an inch
- Bring catheter up along bridge of nose and over forehead or bring it across the neck and apply adhesive tape to secure in place
- Pin the tubing to pillow or mattress allowing patient to more freely
- A fresh catheter should be put in other nostril after 12 hours and the old one can be removed
- Check the flow of oxygen, humidification every one hourly
- Watch the gauze for amount of oxygen spent. Timely ask for and make ready a second cylinder for replacement
- Where therapy is ordered to discontinue, close regulator and remove nasal catheters gently
- The humidifier may be cleaned or dried if immediate oxygen therapy is not required
- Record the time of oxygen therapy of administration, time of discontinuing oxygen, etc.

Producers of Administering Oxygen (Table 19.1)

The health care provider orders the oxygen delivery system and flow rate, and the nurse monitors response to the therapy. The dosage of oxygen may be ordered as an FIO_2 (fraction of inspired oxygen), which is expressed as a percentage or as liters per minute (L/min). Respiratory therapists may be available to assist in the administration of oxygen therapy and client assessment. Before administration of oxygen the nurse should

1. Determine client history and acute and chronic health problems. Clients with carbon dioxide retaining chronic obstructive pulmonary disease (COPD) will need lower amounts of oxygen so as not to obliterate their hypoxic respiratory drive. They may already be on oxygen and need long-term continuous therapy.

2. Assess the client's baseline respiratory signs; including airway, respiratory pattern, rate, depth, and rhythm, noting indications of increased work of breathing. Helps determine the client's need for oxygen as well as response to the therapy.

3. Check the extremities and mucous membranes closely for color. Gives some indication of oxygenation, although problems with circulation and tissue perfusion can also alter these factors.

4. Review arterial blood gas (ABG) and pulse oximetry results. These are the most important determinants of the effectiveness of the pulmonary system and determine the need for therapy as well as changes in therapy.

5. Note lung sounds for wheezes/crackles. Secretions will interfere with airway patency and diffusion of oxygen and carbon dioxide across the alveolar-capillary bed.

6. Assess the nares, behind the earlobes, cheek, tracheostomy site, or other places where oxygen tubing or equipment is in constant contact with the skin to look for signs of skin irritation or breakdown.

The objectives of oxygen administration will include:

- Oxygen level will return to normal in blood and tissues as evident by oxygen saturation = 92% skin color normal.
- Respiratory rate, pattern and depth will be within the normal range for client.
- The client will not develop any skin or tissue irritation or breakdown.
- The client will demonstrate methods to clear secretions and maintain optimal oxygenation.
- Breathing efficiency and activity tolerance will be increased.
- The client will understand the rationale for the therapy.

Equipment needed for oxygen administrator are:

- Stethoscope
- Oxygen source – portable or in-line
- Oxygen flow meter
- Oxygen delivery device; nasal cannula, mask, tent or T-tube with adapter for artificial airway
- Oxygen tubing
- Pulse oximeter
- Humidifier and distilled or sterile water (not needed with low flow rates per nasal cannula)

Table 19.1: Oxygen Administration			
	Nursing actions		*Rationales*
	Check clients identification band Explain procedure before beginning		To identity right patient To get cooperation and reduce anxiety
1.	Cleanse hands.	1.	Reduces the transmission of microorganisms.
2.	Verify the health care provider's order.	2.	Ensures correct dosage and route.
3.	Remind clients who smoke of the reasons for not smoking while O_2 is in use.	3.	Increases compliance with procedures. Oxygen supports combustion.
4.	If using humidity, fill humidifier to fill line with distilled water and close container.	4.	Prevents drying of the client's airway and thins any secretions.
5.	Attach humidifier to oxygen flow meter.	5.	Allows the oxygen to pass through the water and become humidified.
6.	Insert humidifier and flow meter into oxygen source in wall or portable unit. Many institutions also have compressed air available from outlets very similar in appearance to oxygen outlets. Green always stands for oxygen. Be sure to plug the flow meter into the green outlet.	6.	Gives access to oxygen. Reduces possibility of inserting into wrong outlet.
7.	Attach the oxygen tubing and nasal cannula to the flow meter and turn it on to the prescribed flow rate (1 to 5 L/min). Use extension tubing for ambulatory clients so they can get up to go to the bathroom.	7.	Rates above 6 L/min are not efficacious and can dry the nasal mucosa.
8.	Check for bubbling in the humidifier.	8.	Ensures proper functioning.
9.	Place the nasal prongs in the client's nostrils (Fig. 19.2). Secure the cannula in place by adjusting the tubing around the client's ears and using the slip ring to stabilize it under the client's chin (Fig. 19.2).	9.	Keeps delivery system in place so client receives the amount of oxygen ordered.
10.	Check for proper flow rate every 4 hours and when the client returns from procedures.	10.	Ensures that client receives proper dose. The nasal cannula is a low-flow system because it administers oxygen while the client also inspires room air. The actual dose of oxygen received by the client will vary depending on the client's respiratory pattern.
11.	Assess client's nostrils every 8 hours. If the client complains of dryness or has signs of irritation, use sterile lubricant to keep mucous membranes moist. Add humidifier if not already in place.	11.	Dry membranes are more prone to breakdown by friction or pressure from nasal cannula.

Contd...

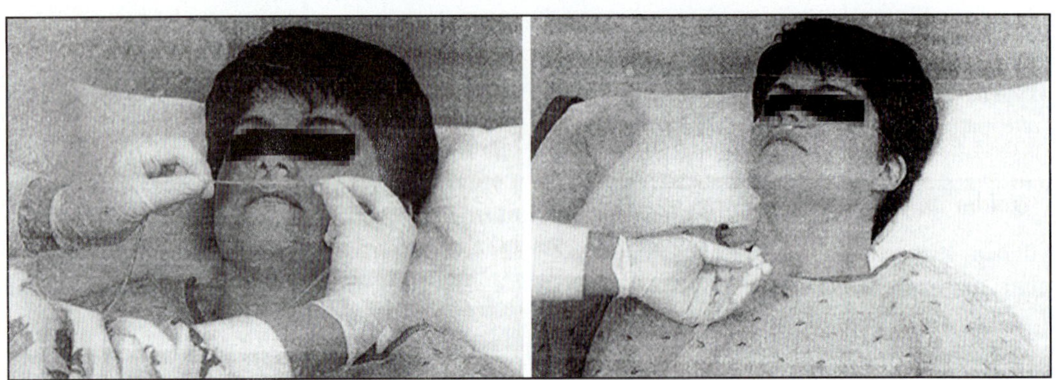

**Figures 19.2 A and B: A. Insert cannula prong into nostrils
(gloves are optional) B. Adjust tubing**

<table>
<tr><td colspan="4" align="center">Table 19.1: Contd...</td></tr>
<tr><td colspan="2">Nursing actions</td><td colspan="2">Rationales</td></tr>
<tr><td>12.</td><td>Monitor vital signs, oxygen saturation, and client condition every 4 to 8 hours (or as indicated or ordered) for signs and symptoms of hypoxia.</td><td>12.</td><td>Detects any untoward effects from therapy.</td></tr>
<tr><td>13.</td><td>Wean client from oxygen as soon as possible using standard protocols.</td><td>13.</td><td>Oxygen is not without side effects and should be used only as long as needed. Problems with reimbursement may develop if criteria for therapy are not met.</td></tr>
<tr><td colspan="4">Mask: Venturi (high-flow device), simple mask (low flow), partial rebreather mask, nonrebreather mask, and face tent</td></tr>
<tr><td>14.</td><td>Repeat Actions 1–6.</td><td>14.</td><td>See Rationales 1–6.</td></tr>
<tr><td>15.</td><td>Attach appropriately sized mask or face tent to oxygen tubing and turn on flow meter to prescribed flow rate. The venturi mask will have color-coded inserts that list the flow rate necessary to obtain the desired percentage of oxygen. Allow the reservoir bag of the nonrebreathing or partial rebreathing mask to fill completely.</td><td>15.</td><td>Ensures proper fit; size needed is based on the client's size. Checks the oxygen source and primes the tubing and mask or tent.</td></tr>
<tr><td>16.</td><td>Check for bubbling in the humidifier.</td><td>16.</td><td>Ensures proper functioning.</td></tr>
<tr><td>17.</td><td>Place the mask or tent on the client's face, fasten the elastic band around the client's ears, and tighten until the mask fits snugly.</td><td>17.</td><td>Prevents loss of oxygen from the sides of the mask.</td></tr>
<tr><td>18.</td><td>Check for proper flow rate every 4 hours.</td><td>18.</td><td>Ensures that client is receiving the proper dose.</td></tr>
<tr><td>19.</td><td>Ensure that the ports of the venturi mask are not under covers or impeded by any other source.</td><td>19.</td><td>Air must be entrained to mix room air and oxygen coming from source to ensure proper oxygen percentage (FIO_2).</td></tr>
<tr><td>20.</td><td>Assess client's face and ears for pressure from the mask and use padding as needed.</td><td>20.</td><td>Provides client comfort and prevents skin breakdown.</td></tr>
<tr><td>21.</td><td>Wean client to nasal cannula and then wean off oxygen per protocol.</td><td>21.</td><td>Oxygen is not without side effects and should be used only as long as needed. The nasal cannula provides a lower FIO_2 thank the mask. Problems with reimbursement may develop if criteria for therapy are not met.</td></tr>
</table>

After O_2 administrator nurse should see than:
- Oxygen level returned to normal in blood and tissues as evident by oxygen saturation = 92%; skin color normal for client.
- Respiratory rate, pattern, and depth are within the normal range.
- The client did not develop any skin or tissue irritation or breakdown.
- Breathing efficiency and activity tolerance are increased.
- The client understands the rationale for the therapy.

And do document the nurses' notes as given below:
- O_2 saturation and respiratory status
- Method of oxygen delivery and rate
- Client's assessment parameters and response to treatment
- Changes in mental status

Performing Nasopharyngeal and Oropharyngeal Suctioning (Table 19.2)

Suctioning secretions is necessary to maintain a patent airway for a client who is unable to effectively clear secretions by coughing. It is considered a sterile procedure, thereby preventing the introduction of microorganisms into the client's airway and lungs.

Suctioning is performed as often as necessary to remove excess secretions, depending on the amount of secretions the client is generating and client's ability to clear the airway. The client's airway and oxygenation are evaluated to determine the need for suctioning.

Wall suction should be set at 100 to 120 mm Hg for adults, 50 to 100 mm Hg for children, and 40 to 60 mm Hg for infants. Portable suction should be set at 8 to 15 mm Hg for adults, 5 to 8 mm Hg for children, and 3 to 5 mm Hg for infants.

Before performance the nurse should:
- Assess respirations for rate, rhythm, depth, and bubbling or gurgling noises to evaluate airway.
- Auscultate lung fields to evaluate airway and determine need for suctioning.
- Monitor arterial blood gases and/or pulse oximetry values to determine oxygen level and adequate air exchange.
- Assess for anxiety and restlessness, which may be signs of airway distress and/or hypoxia.
- Address the client's understanding of the suctioning procedure to decrease the client's anxiety.

The objective of this procedure will be:
1. The client will have no coarse bubbling or gurgling noises with respirations.
2. The client will report breathing comfortably.
3. The client will have no apparent anxiety or restlessness.
4. The client will have arterial blood gases and pulse oximetry values within normal limits.
5. The client will express understanding of the suctioning process.

Equipment needed for the procedures are:
- Suction source (wall or portable with collection bottle)
- Sterile suction kit
- Sterile gloves (if not in kit)

	Table 19.2: Performing Nasopharyngeal and Oropharyngeal Suctioning		
	Nursing actions		*Rationales*
	Check clients identification band Explain procedure before beginning		To identity right patient To get cooperation and reduce anxiety
1.	Choose the most appropriate route (nasopharyngeal or oropharyngeal) for your client. If nasopharyngeal approach is considered, inspect the nares with a penlight to determine patency. Alternately, you may assess patency by occluding each nare in turn with finger pressure while asking the client to breathe through the remaining nare.	1.	The oropharyngeal approach is easier but requires that the client cooperate; it may also produce gagging more readily. The nasopharyngeal route is more effective for reaching the posterior oropharynx but is contraindicated in clients with a deviated nasal septum, nasal polyps, or any tendency toward excessive bleeding (low platelet count, use of anticoagulants, and recent history of epistaxis or nasal trauma).
2.	Advise the client that suctioning may cause coughing or gagging but emphasize the importance of clearing the airway.	2.	Promotes cooperation and reduces anxiety.
3.	Cleanse hands.	3.	Reduces transmission of microorganisms.
4.	Position the client in a high Fowler's or semi-Fowler's position.	4.	Maximizes lung expansion and effective coughing.
5.	If the client is unconscious or otherwise unable to protect his or her airway, place in a side-lying position.	5.	Protects the client from aspiration in the event of vomiting.
6.	Connect extension tubing to suction device if not already in place, and adjust suction control to between 100 and 120 mm Hg for adult.	6.	Excessive negative pressure can cause tissue trauma, whereas insufficient pressure will be ineffective.

Contd...

Table 19.2: *Contd...*

	Nursing actions		Rationales
7.	Put on gown and mask and goggles or face shield.	7.	Protects nurse from splattering of body fluids.
8.	Using sterile technique, open the suction kit. Consider the inside wrapper of the kit to be sterile, and spread the wrapper out carefully to create a small sterile field.	8.	Produces an area in which to place sterile items without contaminating them.
9.	Open a packet of sterile water-soluble lubricant and squeeze out the contents of the packet onto the sterile field.	9.	Lubricant will be used to further lubricate the catheter tip if the nasopharyngeal route is used.
10.	If sterile solution (water or saline) is not included in the kit, pour about 100 mL of solution into the sterile container provided in the kit.	10.	Will be used to lubricate the catheter and to rinse the inside of the catheter to clear secretions.
11.	If gloves are wrapped, carefully lift the wrapped gloves from the kit without touching the inside of the kit or the gloves themselves. Lay the wrapped gloves next to the suction kit, and open the wrapper. Put on the gloves using sterile gloving technique (Procedure 27-2).	11.	Keeps gloves sterile for handling the sterile suction catheter to avoid introducing pathogens into the client's airway.
12.	If a cup of sterile solution is included in the suction kit, open it.	12.	Will be used to lubricate the catheter and to rinse the inside of the catheter to clear secretions.
13.	Designate one hand as *sterile* (able to touch only sterile items) and the other as *clean* (able to touch only unsterile items).	13.	Usually, the dominant hand is the sterile hand, while the nondominant hand is clean. This prevents contamination of sterile supplies while allowing unsterile items to be handled.
14.	*Using your sterile hand,* pick up the suction catheter. Grasp the plastic connector end between your thumb and forefinger and coil the tip around your remaining fingers.	14.	Prevents accidental contamination of the catheter tip.
15.	Pick up the extension tubing *with your clean hand* connect the suction catheter to the extension tubing, taking care not to contaminate the catheter (Fig. 19.3).	15.	The extension tubing is not sterile.
16.	Position your clean hand with the thumb over the catheter's suction port.	16.	Suction is activated by occluding this port with the thumb. Releasing the port deactivates the suction.
17.	Dip the catheter tip into the sterile solution, and activate the suction. Observe as the solution is drawn into the catheter.	17.	Tests the suction device as well as lubricates the interior of the catheter to enhance clearance of secretions.
18.	For oropharyngeal suctioning, ask the client to open his or her mouth. Without activating the suction, use sterile hand to gently insert the catheter and advance it until your reach the pool of secretions or until the client coughs. Do not poke catheter in oropharynx.	18.	To minimize trauma, do not apply suction while the catheter is being advanced.

Contd...

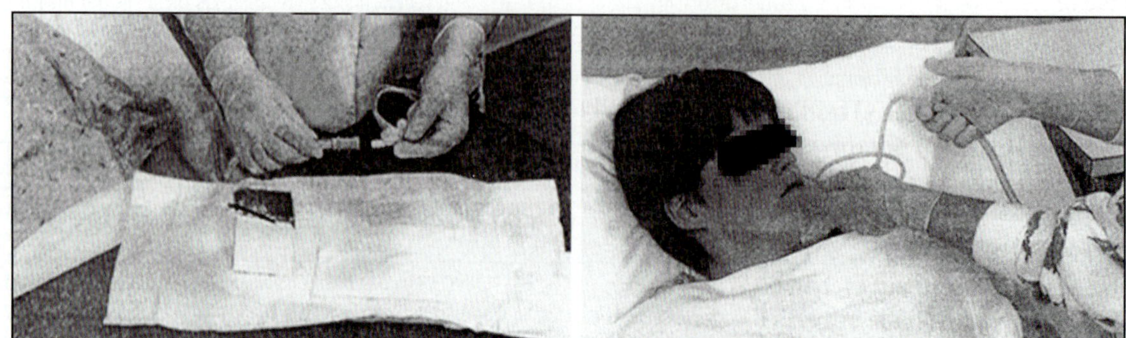

Figures 19.3A and B: A. Attach catheter to tubing. B. Insert catheter into nostril (This nurse is left-handed)

Table 19.2: Contd...			
	Nursing Actions		*Rationales*
19.	For nasopharyngeal suctioning, estimate the distance from the tip of the client's nose to the earlobe and grasp the catheter between your thumb and forefinger at a point equal to this distance from the catheter's tip.	19.	Ensures placement of the catheter tip in the oropharynx and not in the trachea.
20.	Dip the tip of the suction catheter into the water soluble lubricant to coat catheter tip liberally.	20.	Promotes the client's comfort and minimizes trauma to nasal mucosa.
21.	Use *sterile* hand to insert the catheter tip into the nostril with the suction control port uncovered. Advance the catheter gently with a slight downward slant. Slight rotation of the catheter may be used to ease insertion. Advance the catheter to the point marked by your thumb and forefinger.	21.	Guides the catheter toward the posterior oropharynx along the floor of the nasal cavity.
22.	If resistance is met, *do not force the catheter.* Withdraw it and attempt insertion via the opposite nostril.	22.	Forceful insertion may cause tissue damage and bleeding.
23.	With *clean* hand, apply suction by occluding the suction control port with your thumb; at the same time, slowly rotate the catheter by rolling it between your thumb and fingers while slowly withdrawing it. Apply suction for no longer than 15 seconds at a time.	23.	Prolonged suction applied to a single area of tissue can cause tissue damage.
24.	Repeat steps 23 until secretions have been cleared, allowing brief rest periods between suctioning episodes.	24.	Promotes complete clearance of the airways.
25.	Withdraw the catheter by looping it around your fingers as you pull it out.	25.	Allows you to maintain control over the catheter tip as it is withdrawn.
26.	Dip the catheter tip into the sterile solution and apply suction.	26.	Clears the extension tubing of secretions that would promote bacterial growth and could block tubing.
27.	Disconnect the catheter from the extension tubing. Holding the coiled catheter in your gloved hand, remove the glove by pulling it over the catheter. Discard catheter and gloves in an appropriate container.	27.	Contains the catheter and secretions in the glove for disposal.
28.	Discard remaining supplies in the appropriate container and wash your hands.	28.	Prevents transmission of microorganisms.
29.	Provide the client with oral hygiene if indicated or desired.	29.	Suctioning and coughing may produce an unpleasant taste.

- Sterile water-soluble lubricant
- Small bottle of sterile water or normal saline (if not in kit)
- Tubing connected to suction source
- Personal protective equipment: gown, mask, and goggles or face shield

After procedure nurse should:
- Check breath sounds for a patent airway.
- Ask client if breathing is easier.
- Assess client for signs of dyspnea.
- Review arterial blood gases and/or pulse oximetry results.

And do documents on nurses' notes:
- Date and time of suctioning procedure
- Client's tolerance of the procedure
- Amount, consistency, color, and odor or secretions
- Arterial blood gases and/or pulse oximetry results

Performing Tracheostomy Care (Table 19.3)

A tracheotomy is an incision made into the trachea with insertion of a cannula for airway management. Tracheostomy is the creation of an opening into the trachea through the neck. The two terms can be used interchangeably. A tracheostomy is performed for the client with potential or present airway obstruction, for ventilatory assistance, to provide pulmonary hygiene, to decrease the anatomic dead space in the client with chronic obstructive pulmonary disease, to provide pulmonary hygiene, to decrease the anatomic dead space in the client with chronic obstructive pulmonary disease, to avoid prolonged endotracheal intubation, and to provide an airway for clients with severe obstructive sleep apnea syndrome. The tracheostomy is performed below the level of the vocal cords and allows air to enter and exit the tracheostomy rather than through the upper airway. The tracheostomy tube can have a single or double cannula. The determination of the tube design used is based on the needs of the client. The double cannula tube allows for the tube to be cleaned to prevent obstruction caused by dried secretions. During the acute phase after a tracheostomy has been performed, all care must be performed using sterile technique.

Once care of the tracheostomy tube becomes a client procedure, a clean technique is used.

Before performance the nurse should
- Assess respirations for rate, rhythm, depth, to evaluate airway.
- Assess the client's lung sounds to determine the need for suctioning.
- Assess the client's arterial blood gases and/or pulse oximetry values to evaluate air exchange and blood oxygen levels.
- Assess the movement of air through the tracheostomy tube to evaluate the air exchange through the tube and determine whether there is any obstruction.
- Assess the amount and color of tracheal secretions to evaluate for bleeding, infection, and the need for suctioning.

Table 19.3: Performing Tracheastomy Care

	Nursing Actions		*Rationales*
	Check clients identification band Explain procedure before beginning		To identity right patient To get cooperation and reduce anxiety
1.	Cleanse hands and apply clean gloves.	1.	Reduces transmission of microorganisms.
2.	Remove soiled dressing and discard inside gloves as they are removed.	2.	Prevents contamination of other areas.
Conventional/Reusable Inner Cannula			
3.	Open tracheostomy care set.	3.	Provides sterile equipment for use in the procedure.
4.	Apply sterile gloves.	4.	Uses aseptic technique.
5.	Place hydrogen peroxide solution in one basin and sterile water or saline in a second basin.	5.	Prepare solutions prior to applying gloves.
6.	Dip the applicator in the basin of hydrogen peroxide.	6.	Prevents contamination of the applicator.
7.	Remove inner cannula.	7.	Allows for cleaning.
8.	Place inner cannula in basin of hydrogen peroxide.	8.	Loosens secretions.
9.	Clean the area under the neck plate of the tracheostomy tube using a cotton applicator moistened with hydrogen peroxide (Fig. 19.4A).	9.	Decreases microorganisms and removes crusting.
10.	Rinse area under neck plate with cotton applicator moistened with sterile water or saline.	10.	Removes hydrogen peroxide from the skin.

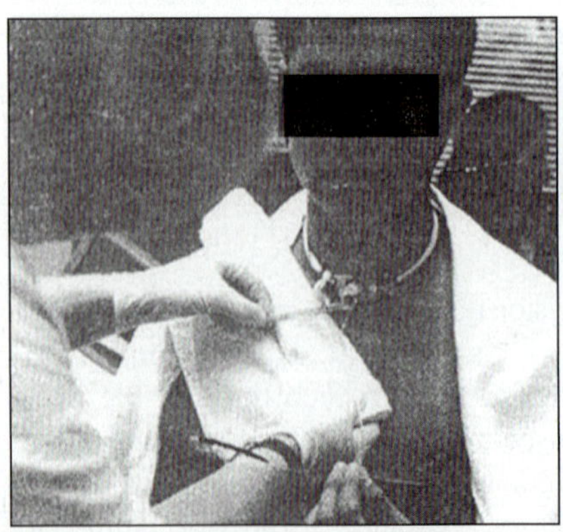

Figure 19.4A: Clean the area under the neck plate with a cotton applicator moistened with hydrogen peroxide

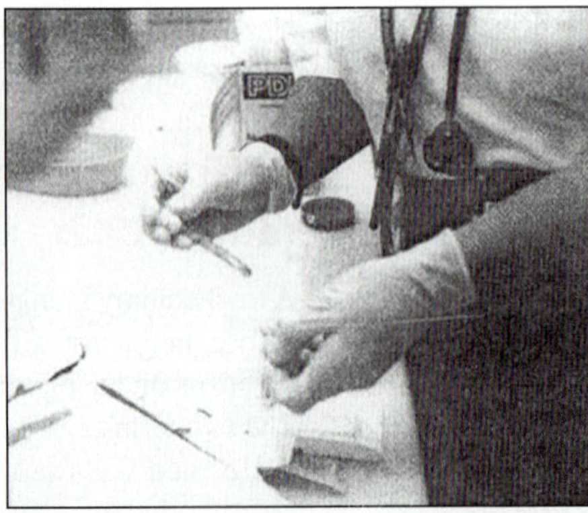

Figure 19.4B: Use a sterile cotton-tipped applicator to clean the inner cannula area and remove crusted secretions

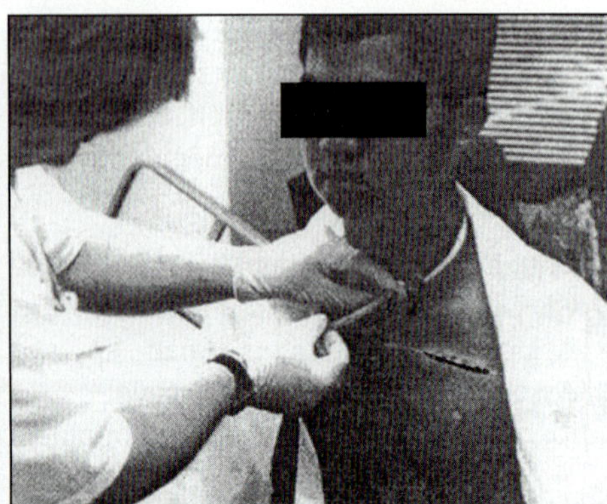

Figure 19.4C: Carefully reinsert inner cannula and lock into place

Table 19.3: Contd...

	Nursing Actions		Rationales
11.	Dry skin under neck plate with cotton-tip applicator.	11.	Prevents skin excoriation from moisture.
12.	Use a tracheostomy brush or sterile cotton-tip applicator to clean inner cannula (Fig. 19.4B)	12.	Removes crusted secretions.
13.	Rinse inner cannula with sterile water or sterile saline.	13.	Removes hydrogen peroxide from inner cannula.
14.	Dry inner cannula.	14.	Prevents introduction of solutions into the trachea.
15.	Reinsert inner cannula and lock it into place (Fig. 19.4C).	15.	Prevents accidental removal of the inner cannula during coughing.
16.	Remove gloves and cleanse hands.	16.	Reduces transmission of microorganisms.
Disposable Inner Cannula			
17.	Cleanse hands. Open disposable cannula container without touching cannula.	17.	Reduces transmission of microorganisms.
18.	Apply sterile gloves.	18.	Uses aseptic technique.
19.	Remove inner cannula and discard.	19.	Disposable inner cannulas are not to be reused.
20.	Replace inner cannula with new disposable cannula.	20.	Provides a clean open cannula.
21.	Remove gloves and cleanse hands.	21.	Prevents transmission of microorganisms.
Two-Person Technique of Changing Tracheostomy Ties			
22.	Cut two pieces of twill tape about 12 to 14 inches in length.	22.	Prepares equipment before beginning procedure.
23.	Make a fold about 1 inch below the end of each piece of twill tape and cut a half-inch slit lengthwise in the center of the fold.	23.	Prepares tape for insertion.
24.	Have a second person gently hold the tracheostomy tube in place with fingers on both sides of the neck plate.	24.	Prevents accidental movement of the tracheostomy tube resulting in coughing and accidental decannulation.
25.	Untie old tracheostomy ties and discard.	25.	Removes tracheostomy ties.
26.	Insert the split end of the tracheostomy tape through the opening on one side of the tracheostomy tube neck plate. Pull the distal end of the tracheostomy tie through the cut end and pull tightly.	26.	Secures tracheostomy tie within neck plate.
27.	Repeat procedure with second piece of twill tape.	27.	Secures tracheostomy tube.
28.	Tie tracheostomy tapes with a double knot at the side of the neck.	28.	Secures tracheostomy tube.
29.	Insert one finger under tracheostomy tapes.	29.	Ensure that tube has been tied securely.
30.	Insert tracheostomy gauze under neck plate of tube.	30.	Prevents irritation of skin from secretions and rubbing of tracheostomy tube.
31.	Discard all used materials and cleanse hands.	31.	Reduces transmission of microorganisms.
One-Person Technique of Changing Tracheostomy Ties			
32.	Follow Actions 22-23 and 26-28.	32.	See Rationales 22-23 and 26-28.
33.	Hold the neck plate firmly with one hand; untie and remove old tracheostomy ties.	33.	Prevents dislodgment while untying and removing old tracheostomy tapes.
34.	Place one finger under tracheostomy ties.	34.	Checks for tightness and security.
35.	Discard all used materials and cleanse hands.	35.	Reduces transmission of microorganisms.

- Assess for anxiety, restlessness, and fear. Anxiety and restlessness may be symptoms of airway distress and hypoxia.
- Assess the client's understanding of the procedure to determine client education and support needed.

The objective of this procedure includes:

1. The client's airway will be free of obstruction.
2. The procedure will be performed with a minimum of client anxiety.
3. The client's skin will remain intact and free of redness and excoriation.
4. The client will remain free of signs and symptoms of infection.
5. The client will have cannulas free of secretions and clean, securities.

Equipment Needed for the procedure for Cleaning the Inner Cannula

- Sterile gloves
- Disposable inner cannula (if available)
- Tracheostomy care kit: 2 basins, tracheostomy brush, tracheostomy ties
- Hydrogen peroxide
- Sterile water or sterile saline

After procedure nurse has to monitor:

- Airway is free of obstruction.
- Client anxiety was minimal during procedure.
- There is no evidence of infection.
- Airway is patent.
- Cannulas free of secretions, and clean, secured ties.
- Client's skin intact and free of redness and excoriation.

And do documents in Nurses' Notes as follows:

- Date, time, procedure performed, and client's tolerance of the procedure
- Size and type of tracheostomy tube in place
- Amount and consistency of any secretions
- Condition of the client's skin
- Client teaching and participation

Performing Tracheostomy Suctioning (Table 19.4)

Suctioning secretions is necessary to maintain the airway of a client who is unable to clear his or her own secretions by coughing. Some clients may be able to cough but not effectively enough to expel the secretions. Suctioning the client's airway is considered a sterile procedure. Using sterile technique prevents the introduction of contagion into the client's airway and lungs.

Suctioning is performed as often as necessary to remove excess secretions. The procedure may be performed as often as

Table 19.4: Performing Tracheostomy Suctioning			
Nursing Actions		*Rationales*	
*Check clients identification band * Explain procedure before beginning		* To identity right patient * To get cooperation and reduce anxiety	
1.	Assess depth and rate of respirations; Auscultate breath sounds.	1.	Determines need for suctioning.
2.	Assemble supplies on bedside table.	2.	Organizes work.
3.	Cleanse hands.	3.	Reduces transmission of microorganisms.
4.	Position the client in a high Fowler's or semi-Fowler's position.	4.	Maximizes lung expansion and effective coughing.
5.	Connect extension tubing to suction device, if not already in place, and adjust suction control to between 100 and 120 mm Hg.	5.	Excessive negative pressure can cause tissue trauma, hypoxemia, and atelectasis, whereas insufficient pressure will be ineffective.
6.	Put on gown and mask and goggles or face shield.	6.	Protects from splattering body fluids.
7.	Using sterile technique. Open tracheostomy care kit. Consider the inside wrapper of the kit to be sterile, and spread the wrapper out carefully to create a small sterile field. Add sterile suction catheter if not in kit.	7.	Produces an area in which to place sterile items without contaminating them.
8.	If gloves are wrapped, carefully lift the wrapped gloves from the kit without touching the inside of the kit or the gloves themselves. Lay the wrapped gloves down and open the wrapper. Put on the gloves using sterile gloving technique.	8.	Reduces introduction of pathogens into the client's airway.
9.	Pour hydrogen peroxide in one basin and sterile water or saline in the other.	9.	Provides solution to clean inner cannula and to lubricate the catheter and rinse the inside of the catheter to clear secretions.

Contd...

Table 19.4: *Contd...*

	Nursing Actions		Rationales
10.	Designate one hand as *sterile* (able to touch only sterile items), usually the dominant hand, and the other as *clean* (able to touch only nonsterile items), the nondominant hand.	10.	Prevents contamination of sterile supplies while allowing you to handle unsterile items.
11.	*Using your sterile hand,* pick up the suction catheter. Grasp the plastic connector end between your thumb and forefinger and coil the tip around your remaining fingers.	11.	Prevents accidental contamination of the catheter tip.
12.	Pick up the extension tubing *with your clean hand.* Connect the suction catheter to the extension tubing, taking care not to contaminate the catheter.	12.	The extension tubing is not sterile.
13.	If client is not receiving oxygen, administer oxygen or use Ambu-bag with *clean* hand before beginning procedure.	13.	Hyperoxygenates clients and prevents hypoxia during suctioning.
14.	Remove inner cannula and place in basin of hydrogen peroxide to loosen secretions, if reusable, or set aside if disposable. Do not dispose of disposable cannula until new inner cannula is securely in place.	14.	Allows easier passage of the suction catheter. Retain old cannula until you are sure the new cannula fits correctly.
15.	Position your clean hand with the thumb over the catheter's suction port, dip the catheter tip into the sterile solution is drawn into the catheter.	15.	Tests the suction device as well as lubricating the interior of the catheter to enhance clearance of secretions.
16.	Remove thumb from suction port.	16.	Deactivates the suction.
17.	Using your *clean* hand, remove the oxygen delivery device from the tracheostomy tube and place it on a clean surface.	17.	Permits access to the tracheostomy tube. Placing the oxygen device on a clean surface reduces contamination (the sterile glove wrapper may be used for this purpose).
18.	Without occluding the suction control port, insert the catheter tip into the tracheostomy tube and advance it until the client coughs or resistance is met (Fig. 19.5) and withdraw slightly.	18.	Minimizes trauma when suction not applied while the catheter is being advanced.
19.	Apply suction by occluding the suction control port with your thumb, while slowly rotating the catheter between your thumb and finger and slowly withdrawing it. Apply suction for no longer than 15 seconds at a time.	19.	Prolonged suction can cause tissue damage, atelectasis, and hypoxemia.
20.	Repeat step 19 until all secretions have been cleared, allowing brief rest periods between suctioning episodes. Encourage client to breathe deeply between suctioning episodes. Provide oxygen between passes of the suction catheter.	20.	Promotes complete clearance of the airway.

Contd...

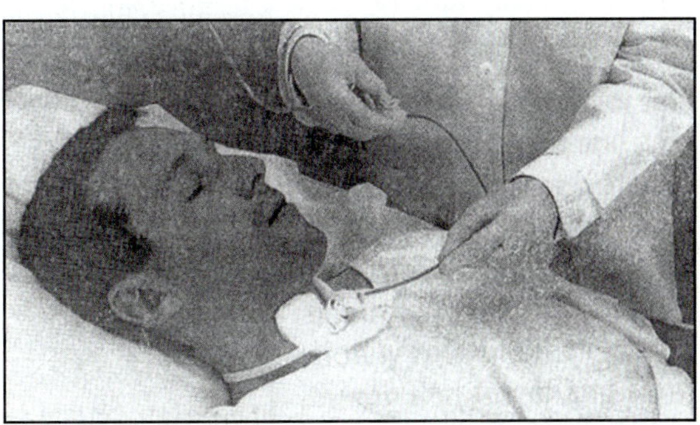

Figure 19.5: Suction tracheostomy

<table>
<tr><td colspan="2" align="center">**Table 19.4:** *Contd...*</td></tr>
<tr><td>*Nursing Actions*</td><td>*Rationales*</td></tr>
<tr><td>21. Withdraw the catheter and dip it into the cup of sterile saline, applying suction.</td><td>21. Cleans suction catheter of secretions.</td></tr>
<tr><td>22. Clean inner cannula using tracheostomy brush and rinse well in sterile water or sterile saline. Dry (or open new disposable inner cannula).</td><td>22. Removes secretions and maintains patent inner cannula.</td></tr>
<tr><td>23. Reinsert inner cannula and lock into place.</td><td>23. Prevents secretions from obstructing outer cannula.</td></tr>
<tr><td>24. Reapply oxygen delivery device.</td><td>24. Reoxygenates the client and restores supplemental oxygen and humidification.</td></tr>
<tr><td>25. Dip the catheter tip into sterile solution and apply suction.</td><td>25. Clears the extension tubing of secretions, which would promote bacterial growth.</td></tr>
<tr><td>26. Disconnect the catheter from the extension tubing. Holding the coiled catheter in your gloved hand, remove the glove by pulling it over the catheter. Discard catheter and gloves in an appropriate container.</td><td>26. Contains the catheter and secretions in the glove for disposal.</td></tr>
<tr><td>27. Discard remaining supplies in the appropriate container.</td><td>27. Follow institutional policy regarding disposal of client care supplies.</td></tr>
<tr><td>28. Cleanse hands.</td><td>28. Prevents transmission of the pathogens.</td></tr>
<tr><td>29. Provide the client with oral hygiene if indicated/desired.</td><td>29. Suctioning and coughing may produce an unpleasant taste.</td></tr>
</table>

every 5 minutes or as infrequently as every few hours, depending on the amount of secretions the client is generating and the client's ability to clear his or her own airway. Evaluate the client's airway and oxygenation to determine the need for suctioning. Wall suction should be set at 100 to 120 mm Hg for adults, 50 to 100 mm Hg for children, and 40 to 60 mm Hg for infants. Portable suction set at 8 to 15 mm Hg for adults, 5 to 8 mm Hg for children, and 3 to 5 mm Hg for infants.

Before procedure the nurse has to:

1. Assess respirations for rate, rhythm, and depth to evaluate airway.
2. Auscultate lung fields to evaluate airway and determine need for suctioning.
3. Monitor arterial blood gases and/or pulse oximetry values to determine oxygen levels and adequate air exchange.
4. Assess passage of air through the tracheostomy tube to determine air exchange and obstruction of the tube.
5. Monitor tracheal secretions for amount, color, consistency, and odor to assess for evidence of bleeding or signs of infection and need for suctioning.
6. Assess for anxiety and restlessness, which may be signs of airway distress and/or hypoxia.
7. Assess the client's understanding of the suctioning procedure to decrease the client's anxiety.

The objective of this procedure includes:

1. The client will have no crackles or wheezes in large airways and the absence of cyanosis.
2. The client will report breathing comfortably and will have no apparent anxiety or restlessness.
3. The client will have minimal amount of thin, normal colored secretions.
4. The client will maintain a patent airway.

Equipment Needed for the procedure are

- Sterile gloves
- Mask, eye protection, and gown if appropriate
- Source of negative pressure (suction machine or wall suction)
- Sterile suction catheter
- Oxygen or Ambu-bag
- Equipment for tracheostomy care or tracheostomy care tray

After procedure nurse has to monitor as given below:

- Ask client whether breathing is easier.
- Auscultate breath sounds for a patent airway.
- Review arterial blood gases and/or pulse oximetry values.
- Assess client for signs of dyspnea.
- Evaluate consistency, color, amount, and odor of secretions.

And do documents in Nurses' Notes as follows:

- Date, time of suctioning procedure.
- Client's tolerance of the suctioning procedure
- Amount, consistency, color, and odor of secretions
- Arterial blood gases and/or pulse oximetry values

In addition, certain simple procedure performed earlier days shown in following,

Procedures for Administering Oxygen by Mask (Table 19.5)

Table 19.5: Procedures for Administering Oxygen by Mask	
Equipment	
• Flowmeter connected to pad elastic • Face mask specified by physician	• Humidifier with sterile oxygen supply band (optional) • Gauze to distilled water
Nursing Actions	*Rationales*
1. Explain procedure to client and review safety precautions necessary when oxygen is in use. Place 'NO SMOKING' sign in appropriate areas.	1. Oxygen supports combustion. Explanation alleviates anxiety.
2. Wash your hands.	2. Handwashing deters the spread of microorganisms
3. Attach the face mask to the oxygen set-up with humidification. Start the flow of oxygen at the specified rate.	3. Oxygen forced through a water reservoir is humidified before it is delivered to the client, thus preventing dehydration of the mucous membranes.
4. Position the face mask over the client's nose and mouth. Adjust it with the elastic strap so that the mask fits snugly but comfortably on the face.	4. A loose or poorly fitting mask will result in oxygen loss and decreased therapeutic value. Masks may cause feeling of suffocation, and client needs frequent attention and reassurance.
5. Use gauze pads to reduce irritation on the client's ears and scalp.	5. Pads reduce irritation and pressure and protect the skin.
6. Wash your hands.	6. Hand washing deters the spread of microorganisms.
7. Remove the mask and dry the skin every 2 to 3 hours if the oxygen is running continuously. Do not powder around the mask.	7. The tight-fitting mask and moisture from condensation can irritate the skin on the face. There is danger of inhaling powder if it is placed on the mask.
8. Assess and chart client's response to therapy.	8. Client respiratory rate and pattern, color, and so forth, indicate effectiveness of oxygen therapy.

Procedures for Oxygen by Tent (Table 19.6)

Table 19.6: Procedures for Administering Oxygen by Tent	
Equipment	
• Oxygen tent with tubing flow, elastic regulator, and oxygen analyzer • Sterile distilled water • Ice	• Oxygen source • Humidifier • Gauze to pad
Nursing actions	*Rationales*
1. Explain procedure to client and family.	1. This reassures client and facilitates cooperation
2. Gather equipment.	2. This provides for organized approach to task.
3. Wash your hands.	3. Hand washing deters the spread of microorganisms.
4. Use bath blanket to cover plastic mattress. Place second bath blanket over bottom sheet.	4. Bath blanket minimizes potential for static electricity from plastic mattress. Additional bath blanket is used to provide warmth and absorb moisture
5. Prepare tent and position over bed. Attach to oxygen source.	5. Tent allows oxygen to be delivered in a confined environment.
6. Fill ice trough or start refrigeration component	6. Ice or refrigeration unit cools the air in the tent.

Contd...

Table 19.6: Contd...

	Nursing actions		Rationales
7.	Fill nebulizer or humidifier to recommended level with sterile distilled water. Turn on flow-meter and adjust oxygen flow to deliver required amount. Use oxygen analyzer now and recheck at least every 4 hours.	7.	Humidification of oxygen prevents excessive drying of the respiratory tract. Oxygen analyzer measures oxygen concentration.
8.	Place client in tent. Observe all safety precautions.	8.	Oxygen supports combustion.
9.	Secure tent between folded top sheet and under mattress.	9.	Oxygen is heavier than air. If tent is not secure, oxygen content may be decreased.
10.	Wash your hands.	10.	Hand washing deters the spread of microorganisms.
11.	Open tent as little as possible by organizing nursing care.	11.	This maintains oxygen content in tent.
12.	Assess client at frequent intervals (vital signs, color, response to therapy). Monitor equipment on a frequent basis.	12.	Oxygen toxicity may develop in response to exposure to a high concentration of oxygen.
13.	Change gown and linens as necessary. Edges of tent may be loosened, and tent may be secured with bath blanket under client's chin when performing hygienic care or other procedures.	13.	This provides warmth and comfort.
14	Record type of therapy and client response.	14.	Keeping records provides accurate documentation of procedure.

Procedures for Using a Pulse Oximeter (Table 19.7)

Table 19.7: Procedures for Using a Pulse Oximeter

Equipment			
• Pulse oximeter • Nailpolish remover (if necessary)		• Alcohol • Dry washcloth or towel	
	Nursing actions		Rationales
1.	Explain procedure to client.	1.	An explanation relieves anxiety and facilitates client cooperation.
2.	Wash your hands.	2.	Handwashing deters the spread of microorganisms.
3. (a) (b) (c) (d)	Select an adequate site for application of the sensor; Use the client's index, middle, or ring finger Check the proximal pulse and capillary refill at the pulse closest to the site If circulation at site is inadequate, the earlobe, forehead, or bridge of nose may be considered Use a toe only if lower extremity circulation is not compromised.	3. (a) (b) (c) (d)	Inadequate circulation can interfere with the SaO_2 reading Brisk capillary refill and a strong pulse indicate that circulation to the site is adequate. — These alternate sites are highly vascular alternatives. Peripheral vascular disease is common in lower extremities.
4. (a) (b) (c)	Use the proper equipment: If one finger is too large for the probe, use a smaller one. A pediatric probe may be used for a small adult. Use probes appropriate for client's age and size. Check if client is allergic to adhesive. A nonadhesive finger.	4. (a) (b) (c)	— Inaccurate readings can result if probe or sensor is not attached correctly. — A reaction may occur if client is allergic to adhesive substance.
5. (a) (b)	Prepare the monitoring site: Cleanse the selected area with an alcohol prep. Allow site to dry. Remove nailpolish and artificial nails after checking manufacturer's instructions.	5.	Skin oils, dirt, or grime, or site; polish; and artificial nails can interfere with the passage of light waves. Never oximeters can read through red and pink nail polish and some artificial nails. Blue, green, gold, black, and brown polish should always be removed.

Contd...

Table 19.7: *Contd...*			
	Nursing actions		*Rationales*
6.	Apply the probe securely to the skin. Make sure that the light-emitting sensor and the light-receiving sensor are aligned opposite to each other (not necessary to check if placed on the forehead or bridge of the nose).	6.	Secure attachments and proper alignment of the marking for the light-emitting and light-receiving sensor promote satisfactory operation of the equipment and accurate recording of the SaO_2.
7.	Connect the sensor probe to the pulse oximeter and check operation of the equipment (presence of audible beep and fluctuation of bar of light or waveform on the face of the oximeter).	7.	Audible beep represents the arterial pulse and fluctuation waveform indicates strength of the pulse. A weak signal will produce an inaccurate recording of the SaO_2.
8.	Set the alarms on the pulse oximeter. Check manufacturer's alarms on the pulse oximeter. Check manufacturer's alarm limits for high and low pulse rate settings.	8.	Alarm provides additional safeguard for client and signals when high or low limits have been surpassed
9.	Check oxygen saturation at regular intervals as ordered by physician and necessitated by alarms. Monitor client's hemoglobin level.	9.	Monitoring SaO_2 provides ongoing assessment of client's condition. A low heimoglobin level may be satisfactorily saturated yet not be adequate to meet a client's oxygen needs.
10.	Remove sensor or a regular basis and check for skin irritation or signs of pressure (every 2 hr for spring tension sensor or every 4 hr for adhesive finger or tow sensor).	10.	Prolonged pressure may lead to tissue necrosis and adhesive sensor may cause skin irritation
11. (a) (b) (c)	Evaluate any malfunctions or problems with equipment For absent or weak signal check the client's vital signs and conditions. If satisfactory, check connections and circulation to site. For inaccurate reading check prescribed medications and history of circulatory disorders. Try device on a healthy person to see if problem is equipment related or client-related. If bright light (sunlight or fluorescent light) is suspected of causing equipment malfunction, cover probe with a dry washcloth.	11. (a) (b)	— Hypotension makes an accurate recording difficult. Equipment (restraint, BP cuff) may compromise circulation to site and cause venous blood to pulsate, giving an inaccurate reading. Drugs that cause vasoconstriction interfere with accurate recording of oxygen saturation.
12.	Document and report SaO_2, appropriately Home care consideration.	12.	Ensure continuity of care and ongoing assessment record. Portable units are available for use in the home or an outpatient setting.

Procedures for Administering Oxygen by Nasal Cannula (Table 19.8)

Table 19.8: Procedures for Administering Oxygen by Nasal Cannula			
Equipment			
• Flowmeter connected to oxygen supply • Dry washcloth or towel		• Humidifier with sterile distilled water (optional with low-flow system) • Gauze to pad tubing over ears (optional)	
	Nursing actions		*Rationales*
1.	Explain procedure to client and review safety precautions necessary when oxygen is in use. Place 'NO SMOKING' sign in appropriate areas.	1.	Oxygen supports combustion.
2.	Wash your hands.	2.	Handwashing deters the spread of microorganisms.
3.	Connect the nasal cannula to the oxygen set up with humidification, if one is in use. Adjust the flow rate as ordered by physician. Check that oxygen is flowing out of prongs.	3.	Oxygen forced through a water reservoir is humidified before it is delivered to the client, thus preventing dehydration of the mucous membranes. Recent research has questioned the necessity of humidification with low-flow oxygen delivery by way of cannula.

Contd...

Table 19.8: *Contd...*

	Nursing actions		Rationales
4. (a) (b)	Place the prongs in the client's nostrils. Adjust according to type of equipment. Over the behind each ear with adjuster comfortably under chin, or Around the client's head.	4.	Correct placement of the prongs and fastener facilitates oxygen administration and comfort for the client
5.	Use gauze pads at ear beneath the tubing as necessary.	5.	Pads reduce irritation and pressure and protect the skin
6.	Encourage client to breathe through his or other nose with mouth closed.	6.	Provides for optimal delivery of oxygen to client
7.	Wash your hands.	7.	Handwashing deters the spread of microorganisms
8.	Assess and chart client's response to therapy.	8.	Client's respirations, color, breathing pattern, and chest movements indicate effectiveness of oxygen therapy
9.	Remove and clean the cannula and assess nurses at least every 8 hours or according to agency recommendations. Check nares for evidence.	9.	The continued presence of the cannula causes irritation and dryness of the mucous membranes. Lubricant counteracts the drying effects of oxygen or irritation

Home care considerations: Clients may require oxygen administration to continue in the home setting. Portable oxygen cylinders are used most frequently and an indicator on the set-up alerts the client or family member to call for a refill. Caregivers require instruction concerning safety precautions with oxygen use and an understanding of the rationale for the specific liter flow of oxygen.

Suctioning the Naso/Oropharyngeal Areas (Table 19.9)

Table 19.9: Procedures for Suctioning the Nasopharyngeal and Oropharyngeal Areas

Equipment		
• Portable or well suction unit with tubing • Sterile suction catheter with Y-port • Towel or waterproof pad	• Sterile water on saline • Sterile disposable container • Sterile gloves	

	Nursing actions		Rationales
1.	Determine the need for suctioning. Administer pain medication before suctioning to postoperative client.	1.	Suctioning should be done only when secretions have accumulated or adventitious breath sounds are audible. This minimizes trauma to airway mucosa. Suctioning stimulates coughing which is painful for clients with surgical incisions.
2.	Explain procedure to client.	2.	This provides reassurance and promotes cooperation.
3.	Assemble equipment.	3.	This provides for organized approach
4.	Wash your hands.	4.	Hand washing deters the spread of microorganisms.
5.	Adjust bed to comfortable working position. Lower side rail closer to you. Place the client in a semi-Flower's position if conscious. An unconscious client should be placed in the lateral position facing you.	5.	Having the client in a sitting position helps him or her to cough and makes breathing easier. Gravity also facilitates the insertion of the catheter. Lateral position prevents the airway from becoming obstructed and promotes drainage of secretions.
6.	Place towel or waterproof and across client's chest	6.	This protects bed linens.

7.	Turn suction to appropriate pressure:
	(a) Wall unit
	    Adult: 100 to 120 mm Hg
	    Child: 95 to 110 mm Hg
	    Infant: 50 to 95 mm Hg
		7.	Negative pressure must be at a safe level of pneumothorax may occur.

Contd...

Table 19.9: Contd...

	Nursing Actions		*Rationales*
	(b) Portable unit Adult: 10 to 15 mm Hg Child: 5 to 10 mm Hg Infant: 2 to 5 mm Hg		
8.	Open sterile suction package. Set up sterile container touching only the outside surface, and pour sterile saline or water into it.	8.	Sterile normal saline or water is used to lubricate the outside of the catheter, thus minimizing irritation of mucosa as it is being introduced.
9.	Don sterile gloves. The dominant hand that will handle the catheter must remain sterile while the nondominant hand is considered clean rather than sterile.	9.	Handling the sterile catheter with a hand wearing a sterile glove helps prevent introducing organisms into the respiratory tract and the clean glove protects the nurse from microorganisms.
10.	With sterile gloved hand, pick up sterile catheter and connect to suction tubing that is held with unsterile hand.	10.	Sterilization can be maintained.
11.	Moisten the catheter by dipping it into the container of sterile saline. Occlude Y-tube to check suction.	11.	Lubricating the inside of the catheter with saline helps move secretions in the catheter.
12.	Estimate the distance from the earlobe to the nostril, and place thumb and forefinger of gloved hand as that point on the catheter.	12.	Ensures that catheter remains in pharynx rather than trachea.
13.	Gently insert the catheter with the suction off by leaving the vent on the Y-connector open. Slip the catheter gently along the floor of an unobstructed nostril toward the trachea to suction the nasopharynx. Or, insert the catheter along the side of the mouth toward the trachea to suction the oropharynx. Never apply suction as the catheter is introduced	13.	Using suction while inserting the catheter can cause trauma to the mucosa and removes oxygen from the respiratory tract. Coughing is induced when the trachea is touched. This helps the client raise secretions.
14	Apply suction by occluding the suctioning port with your thumb and gently rotate the catheter as it is being withdrawn, do not allow the suctioning to continue for more than 10 to 15 seconds at a time.	14.	Turning the catheter as it is withdrawn helps clean all surfaces of the respiratory passageways. Suctioning the client for longer than 10 to 15 seconds robs the respiratory tract of oxygen, which may result in hypoxia.
15.	Flush the catheter with saline and repeat suctioning as needed and according to client's toleration of procedure.	15.	Flushing cleans and clears catheter and lubricates it for next insertion.
16.	Allow at least 20 to 30 seconds' interval if additional suctioning is needed. The nares should be alternated when repeated suctioning is required. Do not force catheter through the nares. Encourage client to cough and deeply breathe between suctioning.	16.	Normal breathing between suctioning helps compensate for any hypoxia induced by the previous suctioning.
17.	When suctioning is completed, remove gloves inside out and dispose of gloves, catheter, and container with solution in proper receptacle. Wash your hands.	17.	Handwashing prevents transmission of microorganisms.
18.	Use auscultation to listen to chest and breathing sounds to assess the effectiveness and suctioning.	18.	Listening to chest and breathing sounds helps determine whether the respiratory passageways are clear of secretions are present.
19.	Record the time of suctioning and the nature and amount of secretions. Also note the character of the client's respirations before and after the suctioning.	19.	Records of nursing measures used help assess, evaluate, and coordinate care.
20.	Offer oral hygiene after suctioning.	20.	Respiratory secretions that are allowed to accumulate in the mouth are irritating to mucous membranes and unpleasant for the client.

Suctioning the Tracheostomy (Tables 19.10 and 19.11)

Table 19.10: Procedures for Suctioning the Tracheostomy	
Equipment	
• Portable or well suction device with connecting tubing • Sterile suction kit containing the following or gather separately • Sterile suction catheter of appropriate size with Y-port • Resuscitation bag connected to 100 percent oxygen 　Infant: 6-8 F 　Child: 8-19 F 　Adult: 12-16 F	• Sterile container • Sterile glove • Sterile normal saline • Clean towel or sterile drape (optional) • Goggles (or glasses) and mask • Gown (optional)
Nursing actions	*Rationales*
1. Explain procedure to client and reassure him or her that you will interrupt procedure if the client indicates respiratory difficulty. Administer pain medication before suctioning to postoperative client.	1. Explanation facilitates cooperation and provides reassurance for client. Any procedure's that compromise respiration is frightening for the client. Suctioning stimulates coughing which is painful with surgical incisions.
2. Gather equipment and provide privacy for client.	2. This provides for organized approach to task.
3. Wash your hands.	3. Hand washing deters the spread of microorganisms.
4. Assist the client to a semi-Fowler's or Fowler's position if conscious. An unconscious client should be placed in the lateral position facing you.	4. Sitting position helps client to cough and breathe easier. This position also used gravity to aid in the insertion of catheter. Lateral position prevents the airway from becoming obstructed and promotes drainage of secretions.
5. Turn suction to appropriate pressure: 　(a) Wall unit 　　　Adult: 100 to 120 mm Hg 　　　Child: 95 to 110 mm Hg 　　　Infant: 50 mm Hg 　(b) Portable unit 　　　Adult: 10 to 15 mm Hg 　　　Child: 5 to 10 mm Hg 　　　Infant: 2 to 5 mm Hg	5. Negative pressure must be at safe level or damage to tracheal mucosa may occur.
6. Place clean towel, if being used, across client's chest. Don goggles, mask, and gown, if necessary	6. Towel protects client and bed linens. Wearing protective equipment prevents contamination of the caregiver's mucous membranes.
7. Open sterile kit or set up equipment, and prepare to suction: (a) Place sterile drape, if available, across client's chest. (b) Open sterile container and place on bedside table or overbed table without contaminating inner surface. Pour sterile saline into it. (c) Hyperoxygenate client using manual resuscitation bag or sigh mechanisms on mechanical ventilator. (d) Don sterile gloves or one sterile glove on dominant hand and clean glove on nondominant hand. (e) Connect sterile suction catheter to suction tubing that is held with unsterile gloved hand.	7. — (a) Drape protects client and bed linens. (b) This maintains sterile set-up. (c) This prevents hypoxemia that can occur during suctioning. (d) Gloves maintain sterility of procedure and protect the nurse from microorganisms. (e) Sterile technique helps prevent introducing organisms into the respiratory tract.
8. Moisten the catheter by dipping it into the container of sterile saline unless it is one of the newer silicone catheters that do not require lubrication.	8. Lubricating the inside of catheter with saline helps move secretions into the catheter. Silicone catheters do not require lubrication.
9. Remove oxygen delivery set-up with unsterile gloved hand if it is still in place.	9. This exposes tracheostomy tube.

Contd...

Table 19.10: *Contd...*

	Nursing actions		Rationales
10.	Using sterile gloved hand, gently and quickly insert catheter into the trachea. Advance about 10 to 12.5 cm (4 to 5 inches) or until client coughs. Do not occlude Y-port when inserting catheter.	10.	Using suction while inserting catheter can cause trauma to the mucosa and removes oxygen from the respiratory tract.
11.	Apply intermittent suction by occluding Y-port with thumb of unsterile gloved hand. Gently rotate the catheter is being withdrawn. Do not allow the suctioning to continue for more than 10 seconds. Encourage client to cough and deeply breathe between suctioning.	11.	Turning the catheter while withdrawing it helps clean surfaces of respiratory tract and prevents injury to tracheal mucosa Suctioning for longer than 10 seconds may result in hypoxia.
12.	Flush the catheter with saline and repeat suctioning as needed and according to client's toleration of procedure. Allow client to rest at least for a minute between suctioning, and replace oxygen delivery set-up, if necessary.	12.	Flushing cleans and clears catheter and lubricates it for next insertion. Allowing time interval and replacing oxygen delivery set-up helps compensate for hypoxia induced by the previous suctioning.
13.	When procedure is completed, turn off suction and disconnect catheter from suction tubing. Remove gloves inside out and dispose of gloves, catheter, and container with solution in proper receptacle. Wash hands.	13.	This prevents transmission of microorganisms.
14.	Adjust client's position. Auscultate chest to evaluate breathe sounds.	14.	Auscultation helps determine if respiratory passage ways are cleared of secretions.
15.	Record the time of suctioning and the nature and amount of secretions. Also note the character of the client's respirations before and after the suctioning.	15.	This provides accurate documentation and provides for comprehensive care.
16.	Offer oral hygiene.	16.	Respiratory secretions that accumulate are irritating to mucous membranes and unpleasant for the client.

Table 19.11: Modified Procedures for Suctioning the Tracheostomy

Equipment

- Disposable gloves
- Sterile gloves
- Goggles or face shield (optional)
- Sterile tracheostomy cleaning it (if available) or
- Sterile basins(2)
- Sterile brush/pipe cleaners
- Scissors

- Sterile cotton-tipped applicators
- Sterile cleaning solutions: Hydrogen peroxide Normal saline solution
- Replacement inner cannula (if available)
- Commercially prepared trache-stomy dressing or sterile non-cotton-filled 4 × 4 gauze pad
- Tracheostomy ties (twill tape or Velcro)
- Plastic disposal bag

	Nursing actions		Rationales
1.	Explain procedure to client.	1.	Explanation facilitates cooperation and provides reassurance for client.
2.	If tracheostomy tube has just been suctioned, remove soiled dressing from around tube and discard with gloves when they are removed.	2.	Suctioning prevents secretions from accumulating in inner cannula and occluding airway.
3.	Wash your hands and open necessary supplies.	3.	Hand washing deters the spread of microorganisms.
Cleaning a nondisposable inner cannula			
4. (a)	Prepare supplies prior to cleaning inner cannula: Open tracheostomy care kit and separate basins touching only the edges. If kit is not available, open two sterile basins.	4. (a) (b)	— Basins are sterile receptacles for cleaning solutions. Hydrogen peroxide facilitates removal of dry, encrusted secretions.

Contd...

Table 19.11: *Contd...*

	Nursing actions		*Rationales*
(b)	Fill one basin ½ in (1.25 cm) deep with hydrogen peroxide.	(c)	Saline rinses and removes hydrogen peroxide and lubricates
(c)	Fill other basin ½ IN (1.25 cm) deep with saline.		the outer surface of the inner cannula for easier reinsertion
(d)	Open sterile brush or pipe cleaners if they are not	(d)	Sterile brush or pipe cleaner provides friction to clean inner
	already available in a cleaning kit.		surface of cannula.
5.	Don disposable gloves.	5.	Gloves protect from exposure to blood and body substances.
6.	Remove the oxygen source if one is present. Rotate the lock on the inner cannula in a counter clockwise motion to release it.	6.	Releasing the lock permits removal of the inner cannula.
7.	Gently remove the inner cannula and carefully drop it in the basin with hydrogen peroxide. Remove gloves and discard.	7.	Soaking in hydrogen peroxide loosens dry, hardened secretions.
8.	Clean the inner cannula:	8.	—
(a)	Don sterile gloves	(a)	Sterile gloves maintain surgical asepsis.
(b)	Remove inner cannula from soaking solution. Moisten brush or pipe cleaners in saline and insert into tube, using back-and-forth motion	(b)	Movement of brush creates friction and aids in removal of accumulated secretions.
(c)	Agitate cannula in saline solution. Remove and tap against inner surface of basin.	(c)	Saline rinses inner cannula. Tapping tube against basin removes excess saline in inner tube.
9.	Replace inner cannula into outer cannula. Turn lock clockwise and check that inner cannula is secure. Reapply oxygen source if needed.	9.	Clockwise motion secures inner cannula is in place.
Replacing a disposable inner cannula			
10.	Release lock. Gently remove inner cannula and place in disposable bag. Replace with appropriately sized new cannula. Engage lock on inner cannula.	10.	Disposable cannulas, although more costly, ensure that airway is clean and patent.
Applying clean dressing and tape			
11.	Dip cotton-tipped applicator in saline and clean stoma under faceplate. Use each applicator only once, moving from softly site outward.	11.	Saline is nonirritating to tissue. Cleansing from stoma outward and using each applicator only once promotes aseptic technique.
12.	Apply hydrogen specify to area around stoma faceplate, and outer carefully if secretions prove difficult to remove. Rinse area with saline.	12.	Hydrogen peroxide may cause tissue damage and needs to be removed from skin and surrounding area.
13.	Pat skin gently with dry 4 × 4 gauze.	13.	Gauze removes excess moisture.
14.	Slide commercially prepared tracheostomy dressing of refolded non-cotton-filled 4 × 4 dressing under faceplate	14.	Lint or fiber from cotton-filled gauze pad can be aspirated into the trachea and cause irritation.
15.	Change the tracheostomy tape:	15.	—
(a)	Leave soiled tape in plate until new one is applied.	(a)	Ensure that tracheostomy will not be expelled if client coughs or moves.
(b)	Cut piece of tape that is twice the neck circumference plus 4 in (10 cm) ends of tape on the diagonal	(b)	Provides for secure attachment with not in front at neckplate. Diagonal cut facilitates insertion of tape into openings on faceplate.
(c)	Insert one end of tape through faceplate opening alongside old tape. Pull through until both ends are even.	(c)	Provides attachment for one side of faceplate.
(d)	Slide both tapes under client's neck and insert one end through remaining opening on other side of faceplate. Pull snugly and tie ends in double square knot.	(d)	A secure tape prevents accidental expulsion of the tracheostomy tube. Neck flexion that is comfortable assures that tape will not compromise circulation to the area.
(e)	Carefully remove old tape. Reapply oxygen source if necessary	(e)	New tape provides for secure attachment.
16.	Remove gloves and discard. Wash hands. Assess the client's respirations. Document assessments and completion of procedure.	16.	Assessment and accurate documentation provide for comprehensive care.

Home care considerations: The client and home caregiver are given instructions on how to perform tracheostomy care. The nurse also observes the return demonstration and provides feedback. Clean rather than sterile technique can be used in the home setting. Sterile saline can be made by mixing one teaspoon of table salt in one quart of water and boiling for 15 minutes. The solution is cooled and stored in a clean dry container. Saline is discarded at the end of each day to prevent growth of bacteria. If the client is performing self-care, the nurse recommends the use of a mirror to view the steps in the procedure.

Wolff's Humidifier Bottle

This is a simple glass bottle with a rubber cork having two glass tubes. One glass tube is short and one is long. Water is filled in bottle by removing cork and then fitting the cork with two glass rods so that long glass rod is inside water. The short one remains above water untouched to the water level. The long one is fitted by rubber tubing to oxygen cylinder and the short one to nasal tube of the patient. Oxygen enters into water bubbles gets into short tube and then to nasal tube of patient.

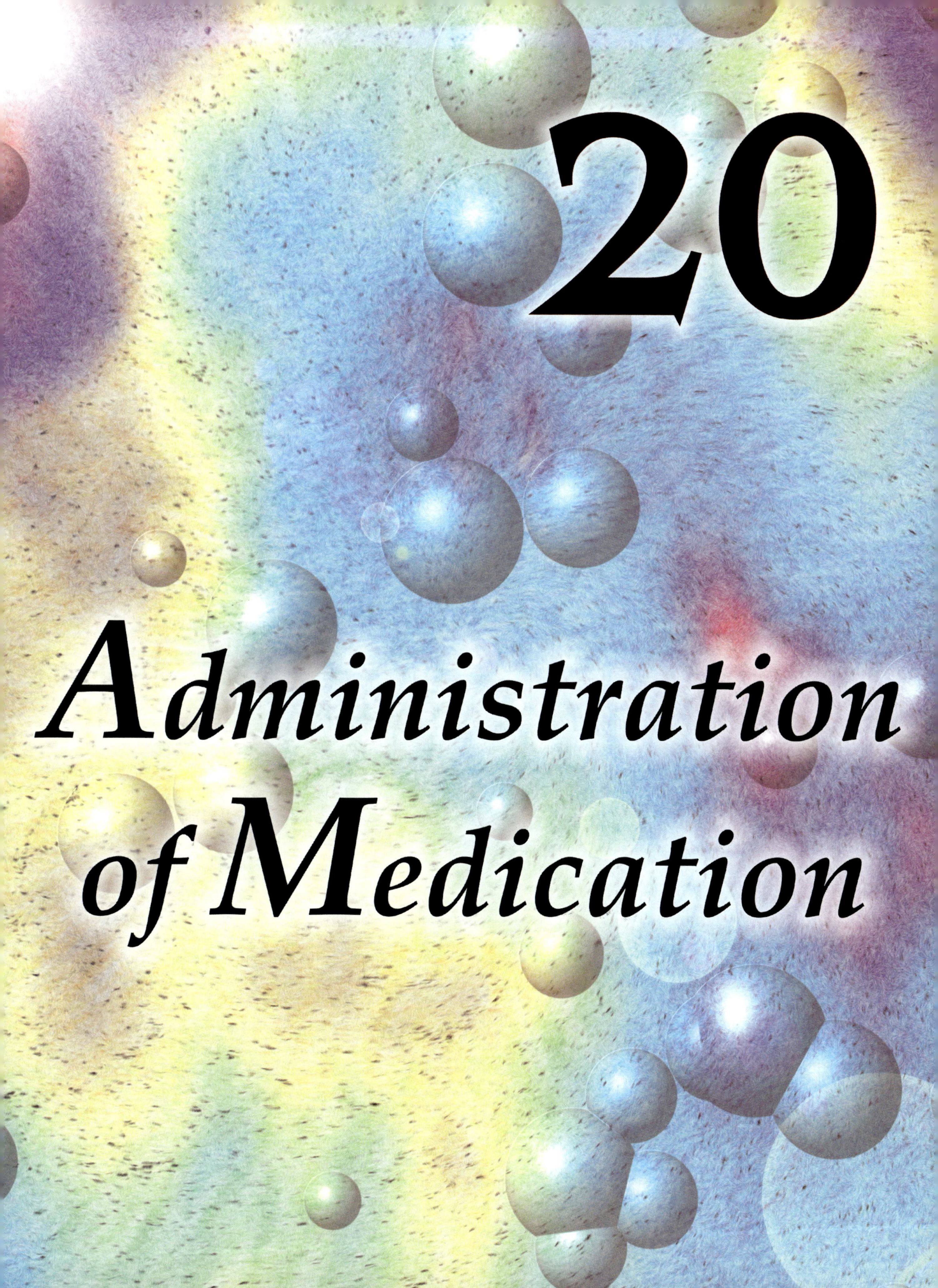

20
Administration
of Medication

Introduction

Medication or a drug is a substance used in the diagnosis, treatment cure, relief or prevention of disease. A drug or medication is any substance that modified body function when taken into the living organisms. The study which deals with chemicals that affect the body function is called pharmacology. The person having license to prepare and design drugs is pharmacist. The physician and dentists are legally responsible for prescribing medication. In some countries legislation granted-to nurses also to prescribe certain drugs. The physician or nurse practitioner conveys the medication plan to other by an order called prescription.

Administration of medication is a basic nursing function that involves skillful technique and consideration of the patient progress and safety. The safe and accurate administration of medication is one of the nurse's most important responsibilities. Drugs are primarily means of therapy for patients with health problems, but any drug has the potential for causing harmful effects when administered improperly. The nurse administering medication is expected to a knowledge basic concerning drugs, including names, preparation, classifications, adverse effect and physiologic factors that affect drugs action.

Drug Names (Nomenclature)

A single drug may have as many as four different names:

1. The chemical name is a precise description of the drugs' chemical composition; it identified the drugs atomic and molecular structure, e.g. acetylsalicylic acid (aspirin).
2. The generic name is the name assigned by the manufacturer that first develops the drug. Often the generic name derived from the chemical name, e.g. aspirin (acetylsalicylic acid).
3. The official name is the name by which the drug is identified in the official publications, e.g. BP (British Pharmacopoeia), USP (United States Pharmacopeia), NF (National Formulary).
4. The trade name also referred to as the brand name or proprietary name is selected by the drug company that sets the drug and is copyrighted.

Drug Preparation/Forms

Drugs are available in many forms or preparations. The forms of the drug determine its route of administration. For example, capsule (oral), ointment (topical). The drugs preparation or forms commonly used by the nurses are as follows.

Tablet: Solid dosage form for oral use; shaped like a capsule and coated for ease of swallowing.

Capsule: Solid dosage form for oral use; medication in power, liquid or oil or gel form of an active drug enclosed in a gelatinous container or shell; capsule colored to aid in product identification.

Elixir: Medication in a clear liquid/fluid containing water and/or alcohol, sweetness and flavors designed for oral use.

Enteric coated tablet: Tablet for oral use coated with materials that do not dissolve in stomach; coatings dissolve in intestine, where medication is absorbed.

Extended release: Preparation of a medication that allows for slow and continuous release over a predetermined period, may now be referred to as CR or CRT (controlled release), SR (sustained or show release), SA (sustained action), LA (long acting) or TR (timed release).

Extract: Concentrated drug form made by removing active portion of the drug from its other components (e.g. fluid extract in the drug made into solution from vegetable sources).

Glycerine: Solution of drug combined with glycerine for external use contains at least 50 percent glycerine.

Liniment: Medication mixed with alcohol, oil or soapy emollient that applied to skin or rubbed on the skin.

Lotion: Drug is liquid suspension or drug particles in a solution for topical use, i.e. applied externally to protect skin.

Lozenge: Small oval, round and oblong preparation containing a drug in a flavored or sweetened base, which dissolves in the mouth and releases medication, also called troche.

Ointment (salve): It is also called unguentum. It is semisolid preparation usually containing one or more drugs, to be applied externally.

Paste: Semisolid preparation; thickest and stiffer than ointment; absorbed through skin more slowly than ointment.

Pill: Mixture of powered drug with a cohesive material. It is a semisolid dosage containing one or more drugs, shaped of lobules (round), ovoids (oval), or oblonged shapes; true pills are rarely used because they have been replaced by tablets.

Powder: Single or mixture of finally ground drugs.

Solution: A drug dissolved in another substance (e.g. in an aqueous solution the drug has been dissolved in water). It is a liquid preparation that may be used orally, parentally or externally, can also instilled into body organ cavity (e.g. bladdery irrigation); contain water with one or more dissolved compounds; must be sterile for parental use.

Suppository: An easily melted medication preparation in a firm base such as gelatin that is inserted into the body. They are solid dosage form mixed with gelatin and shaped in form of pellet for insertion into body cavity (rectum or vagina or urethra); melts when it reaches body temperature, releasing drug for absorption.

Suspension: Finally divided drug particles dispersed in a liquid medium; when suspension is left standing, particles settle to bottom of container, should be shaken before use.

It is commonly oral medication and not given intravenously.

Syrup: Medication dissolved in concentrated sugar solution; may contain flavoring to make drug more palatable.

Tablet: Small, solid -powered dose of medication, form compressed into hard disks or cylinders or molded, may be any color, size or shape. In addition to primary drug contains bindness (adhesive to allow powder to stick together), disintegrator (to promote tablet dissolution), lubricants (for ease of manufacturing), and fillers (for convenient tablet size).

Transdermal disk or patch: Medication contained within semipermeable membrane disk or patch, which allows medication to be absorbed through skin slowly over long period. It is a unit dose of medication applied directly to skin for diffusion through skin and absorption into the blood stream.

Tincture: Alcohol or water alcohol drug solution.

Troche (Lozenge): Flat, round dosage form containing drug, flavoring, sugar and mucilage, dissolves in mouth to release drug.

Drug Classification

Drugs can be classified from different perspectives. For example, drugs may be classified by body system (e.g. drugs that affect the respiratory system, drugs that affect cardiovascular system, etc), by the symptoms relieved by the drug or by the clinical indigestion of the drug (e.g. at analgesics, antibiotic, etc.). Nurses categorize medications with similar characteristics by their class. Drug classification indicates the effect on body system, the symptoms relieved, or the desired effect. Each class contains drugs prescribed for similar types of health problems. The class is not necessary the same. A drug may also belong to more than one class. For example, aspirin is an analgesic, an anti-pyretic and an anti-inflammatory drug.

Nurses should know the general characteristic of drugs in each class. Each class has nursing implications for proper administration and monitoring. For example, nursing implication related to diuretic administration includes monitoring intake and output, weighing the client duly, assessing the development edema in body tissues, and monitoring serum-electro level. Nursing implications of all medications within a class provide guidelines for safe and effective care.

Mechanism of Drug Action

Medications act to produce therapeutically useful effects. Drugs act at the cellular level to achieve their desired effects. The process by which drugs alter cell physiology is called 'pharmacodynamics'. One mechanism of drug action is a drug receptor interaction in which the drug interacts with one or more cellular structures to alter cell function. These specialized structures are called 'receptors sites'. The drug fits the receptor as a key fits a lock. Drug may also combine with enzymes to achieve the desired effect, which is referred to as a drug-enzyme

interaction. Some drugs act on the cell membrane or alter cellular environment. So the drugs produce actions by altering body fluids or cell membrane or interacting with receptors sites (e.g. antacids altering body fluids her, general anesthetic gases interact with cell membrane, and digitals interacting with receptor sites).

'Pharmacokinetics' is the study of the movement of the drug molecules in the body in relation to the drugs absorption, distribution, metabolism and excretion (Fig. 20.1).

Absorption: It is the process by which a drug is transferred from its site of entry into the body to the bloodstream. Absorption of a drug is influenced by several factors which include route of administration (injected drugs absorb quickly their drug solubility; liquid drugs well absorbed in stomach), local condition at the site of administration, and drug dosage.

Distribution: After a drug is absorbed into the blood stream, it is distributed throughout the body. It is distributed within the body tissues and organs and ultimately to its specific site of action. Distribution depends upon the rate of perfusion and capillary permeability to the drug. The rate and extent of distribution depend on physical and chemical properties of the drug and physiological make-up of the person consuming drugs, i.e. body size, circulatory dynamics and protein binding.

Metabolism: After drug reaches its sites of action, it is metabolized into the inactive form that is more easily excreted, i.e. biotransformation occurs, i.e. the breakdown of the drug to an inactive form. The biotransformation occurs under the influence of enzymes, that detoxify, degrade and remove biologically active chemicals. The liver is the primary site for drug metabolism. Physiologic changes associated with aging and the presence of liver disease may complicate the (process. Most biotransformations occur within the liver, although the lungs, kidneys, blood and intensive also metabolize drugs. If any of the organs that participate in drug metabolism are altered, the client is at risk for drug toxicity.

Excretion: After the drug is metabolized, they exist the body through the kidney, liver, bowel, lungs and exocrine glands. Most drugs are excreted by the kidneys. The lungs are primary route for the excretion of gaseous substances, such as inhalation of anesthetics alcohol (deep breathing and coughing help the postoperation patient). Many drugs are excreted through the intestines. The sweat, salivary and mammary glands also are routes of drug excretion.

Pharmacokinetics refers to the absorption, distribution, metabolism, and excretion of a drug (Table 20.1).

Absorption of the Drug

Absorption refers to the movement of the drug from the site of administration into the bloodstream. The rate of absorption determines when a drug becomes available to exert its action; thus, absorption also influences metabolism and excretion. Absorption depends on the route of administration, form of the drug, drug solubility, effects of pH, blood flow to the area, and body surface area.

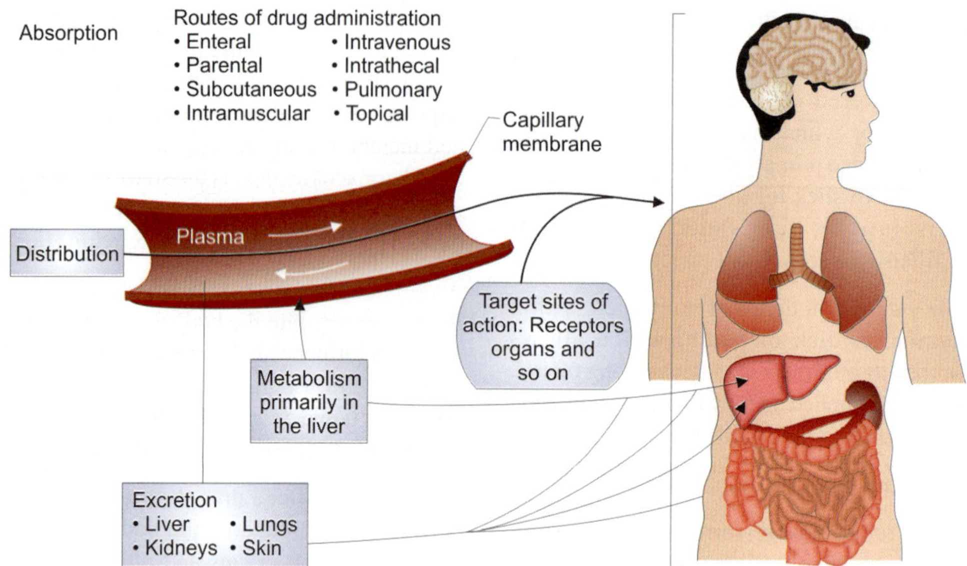

Figure 20.1: Pharmacokinetics

- ***Route of Administration:*** Drugs are given for either local or systemic effect. The local effects of a drug occur at the site of application (e.g. certain topical applications of drugs to the skin), so no absorption occurs. When a medication is given for a systemic effect, the drug must be absorbed into the bloodstream before it can be distributed to a distant location. A drug may enter the circulation either by injection into a vein or by absorption from other areas into which it has been placed (e.g. muscle, mucous membranes, skin).

Drugs are designed for a specific route of administration: oral, sublingual, buccal, topical, enteral, and parenteral. Drugs are absorbed at different rates from each of these routes. The form (preparation) of a drug usually determines its route of administration. Medications are available in a variety of forms.

The choice of route is crucial in determining the suitability of the drug for an individual patient. For example, if patient is vomiting, an oral drug will not be absorbed in the stomach and will likely be expelled during vomiting. If the patient has diarrhea, the rapid motility of the gastrointestinal tract will decrease absorption.

- ***Solubility of the Drug:*** Solubility refers to ability of a medication to be transformed into a liquid form that can be absorbed into the bloodstream. Enteric-coated drugs cannot be decomposed by gastric secretions; the coating thus prevents the medication from being diluted before it reaches the intestines. The coating thereby provides delayed action of the medication. It also decreases irritating effects of the medication on the stomach. Timed-release (sustained-release) medications are formulated to dissolve slowly, releasing small amounts for absorption over several hours.

To be absorbed, oral preparations must be water soluble so that they can dissolve in the *aqueous* (watery) contents of the gastrointestinal (Gl) tract. *Liquids* (e.g. suspensions or solutions) are absorbed faster than tablets or capsules because the medications are already dissolved. To cross the lipid-rich cell membrane, drugs must also be at least somewhat lipid-soluble. Lipid solubility depends partly on the drug's chemical structure and partly on the environment at the site of absorption. Lipid-soluble drugs can penetrate fat-containing cells, whereas water-soluble drugs, such as penicillin, cannot penetrate these areas. That is why a highly fat-soluble drug, such as nitrous oxide, can cross the blood-brain barrier and effect sedation.

- ***Effects*** of ***pH and Ionization:*** The **pH** (relative acidity or alkalinity) of the local environment also affects the absorption of a drug. The acid content of the stomach aids in transporting the medication across the mucous membrane, so *acidic* medications, such as aspirin, are more readily absorbed in the stomach than *basic* (alkaline) medications, such as amphetamines, which are readily absorbed in the more alkaline small intestine.

In solution, some of a drug's molecules are in ionized (electrically charged) form, and others are nonionized (neutral or noncharged). The ionized molecules are lipid insoluble and, thus, cannot pass easily through the phospholipid layer of cell membranes. Drug molecules can be converted easily from one form to the other, depending primarily on the pH of the environment. For example, when aspirin is dissolved in the stomach acid, most of its molecules remain nonionized, so they easily pass through the membranes of the gastric mucosa and enter the bloodstream. If the person ingests an antacid before taking aspirin, however, it will likely reduce the effects of the aspirin.

- ***Blood Flow to the Area:*** Medications are absorbed rapidly in areas where blood flow to the tissue is greatest (e.g. oral mucous membranes). Areas with poor vascular supply (e.g. the skin, scarred areas) experience delayed absorption.

Distribution of Drugs

Distribution involves the transportation of a drug in body fluids (usually the bloodstream) to the various tissues and organs of the body. Because blood goes to all parts of the body, theoretically a drug can produce effects (intended or unintended) anywhere. The rate of distribution depends on the adequacy of local blood flow in the target area (the site where the drug effects occur), the permeability of capillaries to the drug's molecules, and the protein-binding capacity of the drug.

- ***Local Blood Flow:*** The vascularity of the target site affects distribution. For example, it is difficult to deliver a systemic-medication to the skin and toes, where the blood vessels are very small. Circulation in the tissues is affected by a variety of factors. Factors that cause vasodilation in an area (e.g. application of warmth to an injection site, fever, and rest) increase circulation to area tissues. Factors that cause vasoconstriction (e.g. shock and chilling of the body) decrease circulation to the target tissue.
- ***Membrane Permeability:*** Drug molecules must leave the blood and cross capillary membranes to reach their sites of action. Some capillary membranes act as barriers. The capillary networks in some organs consist of tightly packed endothelial cells that prevent some drugs from crossing them. For example, the *blood-brain barrier* allows distribution into the brain and cerebrospinal fluid of only those drugs that are (1) lipid soluble (e.g. anesthetics and barbiturates) and (2) not tightly bound to plasma proteins. Many antibiotics are only water soluble and thus cannot be used to treat infections of the central nervous system. This barrier can be bypassed by injecting medications intrathecally (via the spinal canal) into the cerebrospinal fluid.
- ***Protein-Binding Capacity:*** A drug's tendency to bind to plasma proteins in the blood also affects distribution. For a given amount of a drug some molecules bind to plasma proteins, and the remainder will be "free." For example, nearly all acetaminophen (Tylenol) molecules are free in the bloodstream and are therefore pharmacologically active. By contrast about 99% of the anticoagulant warfarin (Coumadin) bound in the blood; its effects are produced by only the 1% of free warfarin molecules. Only free (unbound) drug molecules can produce pharmacological effects, because only free molecules can be metabolized or excreted drug's tendency to bind to plasma proteins depend mostly on its chemical structure. Some medical conditions also affect protein binding. For example, malnourishment and liver disease reduce the amount of protein (serum albumin) available for binding.

Metabolization of Drugs

Metabolism (or biotransformation) is the chemical inactivation of a drug through its conversion into a water-soluble compound or into metabolites that can be excreted from the body. Once a medication reaches its site of action, it is metabolized (changed into the inactive form) in preparation for excretion.

Metabolism takes place mainly in the liver, but medications also can be detoxified in the kidneys, blood, plasma, intestinal mucosa, and lungs. If there is a disease in liver function (e.g. due to liver disease or aging), the drug will be eliminated more slowly, and toxic levels may accumulate. Disease states also affect drugs metabolism. For example, patients with diabetes do not metabolize sugar well, so they should not be given elixirs, which are high in sugar content.

Oral medications are absorbed from the gastrointestinal (GI) tract and circulate through the liver before they reach the systemic circulation. Many oral medications can be almost completely inactivated in this way. This inactivation is known as the first-pass effect. For this reason, oral medications are formulated a higher concentration of the drug than are parenteral medications. Alternatively, some medications can be given parenterally, allowing the drug to be distributed directly to target sites before it passes through the liver. For example, nitroglycerine undergoes this first-pass effect when taken orally; therefore it is given sublingually or intravenously so that it bypasses the stomach and liver and reaches therapeutic levels in the blood.

Excretion of Drug

A drug continues to act in the body until it is excreted. For excretion to occur, drug molecules must be removed from their sites of action and eliminated from the body. Drugs may be metabolized completely, partially, or not at all when they are excreted. The following are common organs of excretion.

- *Kidneys*: This is the primary site of excretion. Adequate fluid intake facilitates renal excretion. If patient has decreased renal function (e.g. as indicated by an elevated creatinine level), you should monitor for medication toxicity; if signs of toxicity are present, obtain orders for adjusted dosing.
- *Liver and GI tract:* Some drugs broken down by the liver are excreted into the GI tract and eliminated in the feces. Others (e.g. fat-soluble agents) are reabsorbed by the bloodstream, distributed to the target site, and returned to the liver. This is called enterohepatic recirculation. The kidneys later excrete these compounds. Anything that increases peristalsis (e.g. diarrhea, laxatives, or enemas) accelerates drug excretion via feces. Inactivity, poor diet, and decreased peristalsis delay excretion, increasing the effects of a drug.
- *Lungs:* Most drugs removed by the lungs are not metabolized first. Gases and volatile liquids (e.g. general anesthetics) administered by inhalation usually are exhaled through the lungs. Other volatile substances, such as ethyl alcohol and paraldehyde, are highly soluble in blood and are excreted in limited amounts by the lungs. Exercising and deep breathing increase pulmonary blood flow and thereby promote excretion. By contrast, decreased cardiac output (as in shock) prolongs the period of time for drug elimination.
- *Exocrine glands:* Drug excretion through the exocrine (sweat and salivary) glands is limited. The elimination of metabolites in sweat is frequently responsible for such side effects as dermatitis. Drugs excreted in the saliva are usually swallowed and undergo the same fate as other orally administered agents.

In addition to the processes of absorption, distribution, metabolism, and excretion, you need to understand four other concepts related to a drug's effectiveness: (1) onset, peak, and duration of drug action; (2) therapeutic range; (3) bioavailability of the drug; and (4) concentration of the drug at target sites.

The *onset of action* is the time needed for drug concentration to reach a high enough blood level for its effects to appear. This is the minimum effective concentration. When the concentration of medication is highest in the blood, the medication has reached its peak action. The *duration of action* is that period of time in which the medication has a pharmacological effect (before it is metabolized and excreted). If the serum level of a medication falls below the minimum effective concentration, then the drug is not effective during that time. If the drug level exceeds the peak level, toxicity occurs.

When giving an ongoing medication (e.g. an antibiotic), the goal is to achieve a constant, therapeutic blood level. Because a fraction of the drug is constantly being excreted, repeated doses of the medication are given to achieve and maintain a constant therapeutic concentration. Even after absorption stops, distribution, metabolism, and excretion continue.

- **Therapeutic level** is the concentration of a drug in the blood serum that produces the desired effect without toxicity.
- **Therapeutic range** of a drug is a *range* of therapeutic concentrations. At *onset,* serum drug level is minimal.

- **Peak level** occurs when the drug is at its highest concentration (when the rate of absorption is equal to the rate of elimination). After that, metabolism and excretion begin to remove the drug from the tissues and blood.
- **Trough level** occurs when the drug is at its lowest concentration, right before the next dose is due.

A medication's *biological half-life* is the amount of time it takes for half of the drug to be eliminated. For example tramadol, an analgesic, has a half-life of approximately 6 hours. This means if you take a 50 mg dose at 8:00 AM, by 2:00 PM half of that dose (25 mg) will still be left in your body. In 12 hours, one-fourth of the initial dose (12.5 mg) will be left in your body. Because of their effect on metabolism and excretion, the following prolong half-life: liver and kidney disease, aging, absence of food, and slowed metabolic rate. Drug composition and distribution also affect half-life.

The effectiveness of a medication depends ultimately on its *concentration* at the intended site. For example, a medication such as nitrofurantoin may be ordered to treat a urinary tract infection. This drug is used because it is highly soluble in urine and therefore tends to accumulate and concentrate in the bladder and kidneys, where the infection exists.

Table 20.1: Pharmacokinetics Process Across the Life Span		
Pharmacokinetics	*Children*	*Older Adults*
Absorption	• Exaggerated in infants as a result of lack of gastric acidity and shorter intestines. • More complete topical absorption resulting from a larger body surface and thinner epidermis. • Enteral route is unpredictable. • Decreased muscle tone makes absorption of parenteral drugs unpredictable. • Gastric pH is higher, so that medications absorbed in acid environments are absorbed much more slowly.	• Delayed but more complete. • Gastric pH is less acidic because of decreased acid production in the stomach. • Decreased gastric pH delays absorption of medications absorbed in acid environments. • Because of decreased intestinal motility, drugs remain in the system longer, allowing for more absorption.
Distribution	• Protein binding may be a problem. • Greater chance of toxicity because of low albumin levels. • Water content in the child's body is higher than in adults, so water-soluble drugs are less concentrated in the child and fat-soluble drugs are more highly concentrated.	• Low albumin level could create a problem with plasma protein binding. • Increased risk of toxicity due to multiorgan slowdown. • Altered because of less lean mass. • Less body water, greater body fat. • Dehydration, poor nutrition, and electrolyte imbalances decrease absorption.
Metabolism	• Metabolism may be altered because of immature liver. • Best to base dosage on body weight to avoid toxicity.	• Presence of diseases may decrease metabolism of the drug. • Changes due to age, higher blood concentration, and less excretion cause greater chances of toxicity. • Some drugs interfere with the liver's ability to metabolize another drug.
Excretion	• Delayed as result of immature kidneys. • Repeat dosing may cause problems.	• Decreased glomerular filtration rate inhibits excretion from the kidneys. • Diminished renal function inhibits excretion, thereby increasing the risk of toxicity.

Factors when Affect Pharmacokinetics

A drug's pharmacokinetics and, therefore, its effectiveness and safety are affected by the following factors:

- *Age:* Infants and young children need smaller doses because of their smaller body mass and immature body systems. Older adults may have declining liver and kidney function and are therefore at higher risk for drug toxicity. Table 20.1 summarizes life span variations in pharmacokinetics.
- *Body mass (weight):* The average adult dose is based on the drug quantity that will produce a particular effect in 50% of people 18 to 65 years of age and weighing 150 lb. Obviously, a person who is much larger or smaller than this "average" requires an adjusted dose.
- *Sex:* Women are smaller than men and have different proportions of body fat and water, which affect drug absorption.
- *Pregnancy:* Most drugs are contraindicated during pregnancy because of their possible adverse effects on the embryo or fetus. Drugs that are known to cause developmental defects are called teratogenic drugs. Examples are alcohol and the anticonvulsant phenytoin (Dilantin).
- *Environment:* For example, heat and cold affect peripheral circulation. A noisy environment may interfere with a person's response to antianxiety, sedative, or pain medications.
- *Timing of administration:* The presence or absence of food in the GI tract affects an oral drug's pharmacokinetics. Biorhythms and cycles (e.g. drug-metabolizing enzyme rhythms, blood pressure cycles) also influence drug action.
- *Fluids:* Insufficient fluid intake affects the absorption of solid dosage forms.
- *Pathological states:* Intense pain decreases the effect of opioids; diseases causing circulatory, hepatic, or renal dysfunction interfere with pharmacokinetic processes.
- *Genetic factors:* Abnormal susceptibility to certain chemicals is genetically determined. Enzyme deficiencies and altered metabolism change a patient's responses to a drug. For example, African Americans respond better to diuretics for blood pressure control than do other racial groups; and people of Asian descent metabolize some opioids at a slower rate. Use your critical thinking now. What important nursing intervention should you perform after you administer an opiate to an Asian patient?
- *Psychological factors:* Some patients have the same response to a *placebo*–a pharmacologically inactive substance–as they do to the active drug. If a person has faith that a drug will help him, a *placebo effect* similar to the effect of an active drug may occur. Emotional states, such as anxiety, may cause resistance to tranquilizing drugs. Hostility toward or mistrust of medicine or health personnel can also interfere with a drug's effectiveness.

Pharmacodynamics

Pharmacodynamics is the study of *how* medications achieve their effects at various sites in the body–how specific drug molecules interact with target cells and how biological responses occur.

Primary Effects

Primary or therapeutic effects of medications are those effects which are predicted, intended, and desired. The primary effects, in short, are the reason the drug was prescribed. All other consequences are secondary effects (unintended, non therapeutic). Both primary and secondary effects are dose related, so increasing the dose increases the effects. Medications are given for the following effects:

- **Palliative effects** relieve the signs and symptoms of a disease but have no effect on the disease itself. For example, morphine sulfate may be given to a patient with cancer to manage pain, but it does not destroy cancer cells. The goal of palliative therapy is to make the patient as comfortable as possible when treatment options have been exhausted.
- **Supportive effects** support the integrity of body functions until other medications or treatments can become effective. For a patient with a bacterial infection, you may give acetaminophen (Tylenol) to control fever until blood levels of the prescribed antibiotic are effective in combating the infection causing the fewer.
- **Substitutive effects** replace either body fluids or a chemical required by the body for improved functioning. You may, for example, administer insulin to a diabetic patient to replace the insulin no longer produced by the pancreas.
- **Chemotherapeutic effects** destroy disease-producing microorganisms or body cells. Two examples are (1) antibiotics, used to treat infections by killing if or limiting the reproduction of certain bacteria; and (2) antineoplastic drugs, used to treat cancer by limiting cell reproduction and destroying malignant cells.
- **Restorative effects** return the body to or maintain the body at optimal levels of health. For example vitamin and mineral supplements are administered to many patients recovering from surgery.

Secondary Effects

All medications can cause secondary effects (e.g. side effects, adverse reactions, allergic reactions), which can either be harmless or cause injury and which can sometimes be predicted.

- *Side Effects:* Side effects are unintended, often predictable, physiological effects that are usually well tolerated by patients. They occur at the usual prescribed dose and may be immediate (e.g. dizziness) or delayed (e.g. constipation). For hospitalized patients, you will most often see side effects caused by analgesics, antibiotics, antipsychotics, and sedatives. The most common side effects are nausea, vomiting, diarrhea, dizziness, drowsiness, dry mouth, abdominal distention or distress, and constipation.

If side effects are serious enough, the physician may discontinue the medication. For example, lanoxin (Digoxin), which is given to regulate and strengthen the heartbeat, can cause cardiac irregularities, a side effect that can be lethal. Persistent or troublesome side effects may require symptom management with laxatives, antidiarrheals, and antiemetics. For example, levofloxacin (Levaquin), an antibiotic, may cause diarrhea, which is treated with antidiarrheals (e.g. loperamide [Immodium]). Teach your patients what side effects to anticipate with medications and how to manage them.

- **Adverse Reactions:** Adverse reactions are harmful, unintended, usually unpredicted reactions to a drug administered at the normal dosage. They are more severe than side effects and often require discontinuation of the drug.
  - When adverse reactions are *dose related,* the undesired effects result from known pharmacological effects of the medication. For example, a diabetic patient treated with insulin may develop very low blood sugar if too much insulin is administered or he doesn't eat.
  - Adverse reactions also occur because of *patient sensitivity,* meaning that the patient is unusually susceptible to the effects of the drug.

Risk factors for adverse drug reactions includes:
- Receiving treatment from two or more physicians at the same time
- Concurrent illnesses (e.g. diabetes and renal failure)
- A change in the ability to metabolize or excrete the drug
- Taking multiple prescription drugs in addition to over the-counter preparations
- Taking a drug inconsistently
- History of allergies
- History of previous adverse drug reactions
- Long-term use of a drug (may promote accumulation, leading to toxicity)
- Very old or very young age
- Obesity or extreme thinness
- Impaired hepatic and renal function

Severe reactions as those that (1) are life-threatening, (2) require intervention to prevent permanent impairment or death, or (3) lead to congenital anomaly, disability, hospitalization, or death. You must document serious adverse reactions according to agency policy and report them.

- **Toxic Reactions:** Toxic reactions are dangerous, damaging effects to an organ or tissue. They are more severe than adverse reactions, sometimes even causing permanent damage or death. It may help to think of toxicity as poisoning. Antidotes are available for some medications; for example, naloxone (Narcan) is given for opiate toxicity. Toxicity may be caused by any of the following:
  - *Overdosing* (e.g. respiratory depression from excessive morphine or hypoglycemia from too much insulin)
  - *Accumulation* of the drug in the tissues (related to long-term use or incomplete metabolism/excretion)
  - *Abnormal sensitivity* to the drug

    Toxic reactions are usually localized, reversible, and immediate. However:
  - They can be localized to a particular tissue or organ, or they can affect several organ systems.
  - They may be reversible (e.g. tinnitus caused by aspirin) or permanent (e.g. hearing loss caused by aminoglycoside antibiotics).

- They usually occur soon after administration; but, some require months or even years to develop (e.g. drug-induced cancers).

- **Allergic Reactions:** In an allergic reaction, the immune system identifies a medication as a foreign substance that should be neutralized or destroyed. The patient experiences no problems with the first dose of the medication, but it acts as an antigen, activating the formation of antibodies against the drug. When the drug is again administered, the antigen-antibody binding prompts an allergic reaction.

  Allergic reactions range from minor to serious; however, even a small amount of a medication has the potential to cause a severe reaction. Urticaria (hives), pruritus (itching), and rhinitis (inflammation of the nasal mucosa) usually occur within minutes to 2 weeks after exposure and are considered mild. Such reactions often disappear after the medication is discontinued and the blood level of the drug falls. Table 20.2 shows some drugs most frequently in allergic reactions

Table 20.2: Drugs Leads to Allergic Reactions	
Antibiotics	Cephalosporins Erythomycin Neomycin Penicillin Streptomycin Sulfonamides Tetracycline Vancomycin
Biological agents	Antibiotics, antitoxins, corticotropin (ACTH), enzymes, gamma globulin, insulin, vaccines
Diagnostic agents	Iodinated media contrasts, intravenous pyelogram (IVP) dye
Other drugs	Acetaminophen (Tylenol), aspirin, benzocaine, dextran, histamines, iodines, iron, phenothiazides, quinidine, tranquilizers; anesthetic agents, such as tetracaine, phenylbutazone, procaine, lidocaine, cocaine

An *anaphylactic reaction* is a life-threatening allergic reaction. It occurs immediately after administration, with sudden constriction of bronchioles, edema of larynx and pharynx, severe shortness of breath, wheezing, and severe hypotension (low blood pressure). Immediate treatment includes discontinuing the medication, giving epinephrine, IV fluids, steroids, and anti-histamines. Respiratory support ranging from oxygen to intubation and ventilation may also be required. A patient who is allergic to one drug may also be allergic to other medications in the same class. For example, many patients who are allergic to penicillin are also allergic to cephalexin (Keflex), a synthetic penicillin.

Allergic reactions occur with 5 to 10% of all prescriptions, so always explore the patient's allergy history use Allergy Alert bracelets and stickers, and document allergies in the patient's chart and care plan. People with severe allergic reactions should wear a MedicAlert bracelet.

- ***Idiosyncratic Reactions:*** Idiosyncratic reaction is an unexpected, abnormal, or peculiar response to a medication. Idiosyncratic reactions may take the form of extreme sensitivity to a medication, lack of response, or a paradoxical (opposite of expected) response, such as agitation in response to a sedative. In children, for example, diphenhydramine (Benadryl) has been known to cause agitation or excitability instead of the expected drowsiness.
- ***Cumulative Effect:*** Cumulative effect is the increased response to repeated doses of a drug when the rate of administration is greater than the rate of metabolism and excretion. This occurs when (1) the body cannot metabolize a dose of the medication before the next dose is given, (2) excretion is slowed but absorption is normal or rapid, or (3) absorption is slowed. Unless the dose is changed, the medication accumulates in the system until a toxic level is reached. Opiates and barbiturates are known for their cumulative effects.

Interaction of Drugs and/or Nurse

When one drug alters or modifies the action of another, a drug interaction occurs. In an antagonistic drug relationship, one drug interferes with the actions of another and decreases the resultant drug effect–that is, the combined effect is less than one drug given alone. In a synergistic drug relationship, there is an additive effect; that is, the effect of both drugs together is greater than the individual effects. Drug incompatibilities occur when multiple drugs are mixed together, causing a chemical deterioration of one or both the drugs. The result is an incompatible solution that should not be administered. Nurses can usually recognize an incompatibility when the mixed solution takes on a change in appearance. However, nurse should always consult medication resources and compatibility charts *prior* to mixing medications. Then, after mixing, double-check the medication for changes in appearance.

Nurses must be knowledgeable of drug interactions and monitor their patients for them.

The more drugs a patient takes, the higher the risk of a drug interaction. Other variables influence drug interactions: intestinal absorption, competition for protein binding, drug metabolism, renal excretion, and alteration of electrolyte imbalance.

Drugs may also interact with certain foods. For example,
- Fatty foods and foods low in fiber will delay stomach emptying and medication absorption by up to 2 hours.
- Acidic citrus fruits and juices enhance absorption of Iron.
- Carbonated soft drinks can cause medications to dissolve faster, be neutralized, or experience a change in absorption rate in the stomach.
- When dairy products are taken with an antibiotic such as tetracycline, there is decreased absorption of the drug in the stomach.
- When foods containing tyramine (e.g. aged, dried, or fermented products) are ingested with MAO inhibitors, a hypertensive crisis may result.

A drug may produce more than one effect due to its chemical make-up and physiological action, which are classified as follows:

Therapeutic effect: It is an intended or produced physiological response that a drug causes. Each drug has a desired effect.

Side effects: These may be harmless or injurious. They have predictable responses to a drug which causes unintended secondary effects.

Toxic effects: These develop after prolonged intake of high doses of medications or after prolonged use of a drug intended for external application or after a drug accumulates the blood because of impaired metabolism or excretion.

Idiosyncratic reactions: Idiosyncratic effect occurs when a client overacts or underacts to a drug or has a reaction different from normal. It is unpredictable.

Allergic reactions: It is another unpredictable response to a drug, which includes urticaria (hives), eczema (rash), pruritis, and rhinitis. These may lead to anaphylactic shocks (sudden constriction of broncholar muscles, edema of the pharynx and larynx, and severe wheezing or ghortress of breath, hypotension) which need immediate attention.

Drug tolerance: According the unusual low metabolism or response to a drug. An increase in dosage may be needed to cause a therapeutic effect.

Drug interaction: If a drug modifies the action of another, drug interaction occurs. Drug interactions are common in individuals taking many medications. When two drugs are given simultaneously they can have a synergistic or addictive effect. With a synergistic effect, the physiological action of the two drugs in combination is greater than the effects of the drugs when given separately. For example, administration diuretic and vasodilators for moderate hypertension.

The factors that affect drug action are as follows:
- *Developmental consideration:* A child's dose for medication is smaller than adult dose. Infants are responsive to drugs because of the immaturity of the organ. Older people are responsive to drugs according to experience and aging process.
- *Weight:* The drug dose is calculated according to body weight and body surface, particularly in children. The nurse should be aware of the usual dose for particular medication.
- In addition to genetic and cultural factors, psychologic factors, pathology, diet, environment and time of administration also are the factors affecting drug action.

Medication Order

No drug may be given to a client without a medication order from a medically qualified doctor. Safe practice dictates that a nurse follows only a written order. A written order by a physician is least likely to result in an error or misunderstanding. Under certain circumstances such as in an emergency, a verbal order may be followed but should be recorded accordingly in the nurses notes. There are several types of orders:

- A standing order is carried out as specified until it is canceled by another order or upto specified period
- As needed (p.r.n.) order. The client relieves medication when it is requested or needed (pain relief measure for PO cases)
- Single order that carried out only once
- A state order is also single order but one that is carried out at once

The medication order consists of several parts, which includes the followings:

- Client's name
- Date and time, the order is written
- Name of drug to be administered
- Dosage of the drug
- Route by which the drug is to be administered
- Frequency of administration of the drug
- Signature of person writing the order

Common types of medication orders are based on the duration, frequency, and/or urgency of the order.

- **Standard written orders** apply indefinitely until the prescriber writes an order to alter or discontinue the medication or indicates on the original order a specific stop date. For example, "Give Lasix 20 mg IV twice a day for 5 days."
- **Automatic stop dates** are protocols that hospitals use for discontinuing medications after a certain length of time. Most narcotic orders are in effect only for 7 days. If the medication is needed after the automatic stop date, the care provider must write another order.
- **A STAT order** means that a single dose of medication is to be given immediately and only once. The word *stat* or *now* should appear in the order, for example, "Give Lasix 20 mg IV STAT," or "Give Ativan 1 mg IV now."
- **A single order,** or *one-time order*, indicates that the medication is to be given only once at a specified time. Preoperative medications, given prior to surgery or diagnostic procedures or treatments, are single orders. For example:
  - Versed 25 mg intramuscularly on call for OR [i.e., when the OR notifies you]
  - Tetanus toxoid 0.5 mL intramuscularly before discharge
- **Standing orders:** When a unit frequently provides care to a standard population of patients-for example, coronary care patients or knee replacement patients-the physician may develop a set of *standing orders*. These are officially accepted sets of orders to be applied routinely by nurses for the care of patients under certain conditions or under certain circumstances. They establish guidelines for treating a particular disease or set of symptoms. For example:
  - Coronary care or intensive care units (CCUs or ICUs) may have standing orders for the administration of nitroglycerine (NTG) or morphine for chest pain (e.g. "Give NTG 0.4 mg sublingually q3-5 min for chest pain, to a maximum of 3 doses in 15 min").

- Many postoperative patients receive a set number of doses of ketorolac (Toradol), an injectable analgesic medication. So, for all the postoperative patients on a unit, standing orders would include, "Toradol 30 mg IV q12hr × 2 days."
- **PRN orders:** The care provider may order a medication to be given whenever the patient requires (PRN). A PRN order requires the nurse to determine, in collaboration with the patient, when the medication is to be given. The order specifies (1) the condition for which the medication is to be given and (2) the minimum time intervals between doses. The medication cannot be given any more frequently than prescribed, even if symptoms persist. Pain medications, antiemetics (antinausea medications), and laxatives are usually given PRN. For example:
  - Morphine 10 mg intramuscularly q3–4hr P incisional pain.
  - Tylenol 650 mg po q4hr PRN for temp >101° F.

Communicating Medication Orders

Medication orders can be communicated in various ways. The nursing implications are slightly different for each.

- **Written orders** are those written (or preprinted) on a standard medication order form. Some agencies permit the physician to **fax orders** to the nurse and bring the original copy later. Although this step may save time, the risk of errors is greater because faxed copies may be illegible.
- **Verbal orders** are given orally rather than in writing, while the physician is present with the nurse. When nurse receives a verbal order, she/he will write the order and sign it with the physician's name followed by her/his name and credentials. Nurse should then repeat the order to the physician to ensure accuracy. Avoid taking verbal orders and tell them only in urgent situations, because they increase the risk for miscommunication and errors.
- **Telephone orders** are those that the physician gives you via a telephone. Usually this will be response to a call the nurse have placed to report a change in the patient's condition or the results of laboratory or other tests. The physician usually must cosign verbal and telephone orders within 24 hours.

Legal Responsibilities in Medication

Nurses are legally responsible for medications they administer, as a nurse, if you believe an order incorrect, perform the following steps:

- Ask another nurse to check the order.
- Look up the medication in a reliable resource to verify spelling, usage, dosages, and routes.
- Contact the ordering physician for clarifications, concerns, or questions.
- Do not assume you are correctly interpretating the order if you have any question at all.

As a nurse, use your knowledge, common sense, and intuition when administering medications. To avoid errors, you must know and understand the procedures at your facility, be familiar with the medications you give and always check the orders.

Nursing interventions also include activities to address specific nursing diagnoses and, for all patients, the following activities to ensure safe administration of medications.

Preventing Medication Errors

Errors included giving the dose at the wrong time, omitting doses, giving the wrong dose, and giving the dose without authorization. Seven percent of the errors were clinically significant. To help prevent errors, perform "three checks" and "six rights" when giving medications.

(i) Three Checks

Check each medication three times as a nurse:

1. *BEFORE you pour, mix or draw up a medication,* check its label against the entry on the MAR. Be sure that the name, route, dose, and time match the MAR entry. (Medication administration record)
2. *AFTER you prepare the medication,* and before returning the container to the medication cart or discarding anything, check the label against the MAR entry again.
3. *AT THE BEDSIDE, check the medication again* before actually administering it.

Observing the "three checks" rule will help you to practice the "six rights."

(ii) Six Rights

Practicing the "six rights" will help to ensure accurate administration. This means that nurse will give the right medication to the (2) right patient in the (3) right dose using the (4) right route at the (5) right time. Nurse will also carry out (6) right documentation of the medication administration. Nurses regard these safeguards as the minimum requirements for safety and error prevention.

Right drug: Obviously, you must always administer the correct medication. That is one reason for reading each label three times (see the "three checks"). The following are other ways to ensure that you give the correct drug:

- Always check the order (especially after days off, after working a different shift, and after lunch) to see whether there have been changes in the medication dosage, route, and so forth.
- Select the ordered medication from the *patient's* drug drawer (unless it is a stock drug). Do not substitute one medication for another.
- Avoid selecting medications based on size and color, because many medications are the same size, shape, and color as others. Similarly, be alert for similar-looking labels and similarly spelled names.

- Always repeat back verbal orders to be sure you have heard correctly. Spell the medication name, medication names that sound the same can be very confusing and lead to administering the wrong drug.
- Review abbreviations that may be confusing. Clarify dose form, especially with time-released drugs.
- If a label is hard to read or comes off the container, return the container to the pharmacy. Never give a medication from such a container.
- Do not transfer medications from one pharmacy container to another.

Right dose: The right dose is the dose prescribed for the particular patient. Be sure that the dose is within the recommended range for the patient's age and condition. Perform the "three checks" of the container against the MAR If the pharmacist has sent a dose different from the one ordered, you may need to calculate how much of it to give. It is a good idea to have another nurse check your calculations.

How you prepare medications can affect the dose. When you must break a tablet, use a knife or a cutting device. If the tablet does not break evenly, you should discard it. Also, when crushing a tablet to mix with liquid or food, clean the crushing device completely before using it to remove any pieces of a previously crushed drug. Clean it after using it, as well.

Right time: Check the order against the time to give the drug, and document the exact time of administration on the MAR. Medications are administered at specific times to maintain constant therapeutic blood levels.

- Scheduled medications may be given within a "window" of one-half hour before and one-half hour after the scheduled time.
- "Right time" also includes timing of oral medications in relation to meals. Give drugs that are irritating to the stomach (e.g. potassium, aspirin) with food; give drugs that absorb better on an empty stomach (e.g. tetracycline) before meals.
- Determine whether your patient is scheduled for any diagnostic procedures, surgery, or blood tests that require him to remain NPO.

Right route: Recall that drug absorption is highly dependent on the route of administration. Perform the "three checks," and be sure that the drug is in the proper form for the route ordered. Many medications are available in multiple forms; others are made for one specific route. For example, cephalcxin (Keflex), an antibiotic, comes in capsules, suspensions for oral use, and injectable forms for intramuscular and intravenous administration. By contrast, the antibiotic penicillin G procaine (Crystacillin) is prepared for intramuscular injection and is *nut* to be given intravenously.

Right patient: Just before giving the medication, always double-check the patient's identification (ID) bracelet to ensure that you have the correct patient. So, ask the patient to state his name. It is best to say, "Please tell me your name," because patients with hearing problems and confused patients may respond yet incorrectly when asked and use your own sense to identify the person.

Right documentation: Some nurses consider documentation the sixth right. After administering a medication, document it immediately on the patient's MAR. Be sure to document the following information:
- Name of medication given
- Dose of medication given
- Route of administration and injection site for parenteral medications
- Date and time administered
- Your name or initials as administering nurse

Most MARs are preprinted with the patient's name, name of the medication, dosage, and route administered (e.g. intramuscular, oral, or intravenous). If so you need only to write the time you actually gave the medication, initial each medication, and sign the form of one time. As for all charting, write legibly in ink.

If for some reason you do not administer an ordered medication, document that information on the MAR and write a nurse's note explaining the reason it was not given. Reasons may include patient's refusal, NPO for surgery, tests, or procedures being performed. For example:

06/20/06 0800–Pt NPO for surgery this ordered by Dr. Chenna Naik

0800 meds held as ordered by Lalitha R.N.

When giving a PRN medication, in addition recording on the MAR, you should write a nurse's note documenting your assessment and the time the drug was given. Then, after allowing time for the medication to be absorbed and take effect, evaluate and document the patient's responses. For example:

0800–Pt c/o #6 (scale of 1-10) abd pain at incision site. Active bowel sounds auscultated. Resp 16, BP 130/84. Morphine 10 mg given intramuscularly in right vastus lateralis **(Signature of RN)**

0900–States pain relieved; "about 3" (scale of 1–10). Resp 14. BP 126/80. **(Signature of RN)**

Nurses are responsible for documenting the client's responses to all medications, including therapeutic effects, side effects, and unexpected or adverse reactions.

In addition to the "six rights" already discussed, patients also have the following rights:
- **Right reason:** This includes the right to *not* receive unnecessary medications. For example, a tranquilizer or sleeping pill should be given because the patient is very anxious or cannot sleep, not for the convenience of caregivers who are weary of his.
- **Right to know:** This means that you tell the patient the name of the medication, why it is being given, its actions, and potential side effects.
- **Right to refuse:** The patient always has a right to refuse a medication regardless of her reasons and regardless of the consequences.

Routes of Administration of Medication (Table 20.3)

Administering Oral Medications

- Observe the "three checks"; before and after drawing up the medication, and at the bedside.
- Observe the "six rights" of medication of administration.
- *Tablets and capsules*: Pour the correct number into the medication cup.
- *Liquids*: Hold the plastic medication cup at eye level to measure the dose.
- Assist the patient to a high-Fowler's position, if possible.
- For enterically administered medications, check for correct placement of the nasogastric or gastric.
- Correctly administer the medication.
  Powder: Mix with liquid, and give it to the patient to drink.
  Lozenge: Instruct the patient not to chew or swallow it.
  Tablet or capsule: Place the tablet or medication cup in the patient's hand or mouth, and have the patient swallow with sips of liquid.
  Sublingual: Have the patient place the tablet under the tongue and hold it there until it is completely dissolved.
  Buccal: Have the patient place the tablet between the cheek and teeth hold it there until it is completely dissolved.
- Stay with patient until medications have been swallowed or dissolved.

The oral route is the easiest and the most commonly used in which drugs are given by mouth and swallowed. Oral route drugs are usually less expensive and has a slower onset of action and more prolonged effect. The oral route involves sublingual and buccal routes. There are sublingual drugs that are designed to be readily absorbed after being placed under the tongue to dissolve (e.g. nitroglyceria tubes, i.e. called sublingual route). Administration of dreg by the buccal route involves placing the solid medication against the mucus membranes of the cheek until the drug dissolves. Here the clients-should be taught to alternate cheeks with subsequent dose to avoid mucosal irritation and also warned not to chew or swallow the drug or to take liquids. A buccal medication acts locally on the mucosa or systematically as it is swallowed as solids.

These oral, buccal, sublingual routes are convenient and comfortable for the client and are also economical. Medication may produce local and systematic effects. These routes are avoided when client has alteration in gastrointestinal function, i.e. nausea and vomiting reduced mobility (after general anesthesia and surgery of the GI tract). Some drugs are destroyed by gastric secretion, oral administration is contraindicated and clients:
- Who are unable to swallow, e.g. neuromuscular disorder
- Who has gastric suction and before some tests or surgery
- Who are unconscious or confused, unwilling to swallow, etc.

Table 20.3: Forms of Drug and its Advantages and Routes of Administration		
Form of the drug	*Advantages*	*Disadvantages*
1. Oral Route: The drug is swallowed and absorbed from the stomach or small intestines.		
Capsule–A gelatinous container that holds the liquid, powder, or oil form of the swallowed, the gelatin container gastric juices. **Pill–**This term is rarely used now. *Tablet* is the preferred term. **Tablet–**A powdered drug is compressed into a hard, compact form (e. g., round, oval) that is easy to swallow and then breaks up into a fine powder in the stomach. The tablet is the most common oral preparation. *Enteric-coated tablets* have an acid-insoluble coating to keep them from dissolving in the stomach; they disintegrate in the alkaline secretions of the small intestine. **Time-released tablet or capsule–**A tablet *or* capsule formulated so that it does not dissolve all at once, but gradually releases medication over a few hours. **Elixir–**A liquid containing water and about 25% alcohol that is sweetened with volatile oils (e.g., aromatic elixir); not as sticky or as sweet as syrups. **Extract–**A very concentrated form of a drug made from animals or vegetables; may be a syrupy liquid or a powder. **Fluid extract–**An alcohol-based solution of a drug from a vegetable source (e.g., belladonna); the most concentrated of the fluid preparations. **Spirits–**A concentrated alcohol-based solution *of* a volatile (easily evaporated) substance or oil (e.g., ammonia, peppermint oil, orange oil); it contains larger amounts of the substance than can be dissolved in water. **Syrup–**An aqueous solution of sugar, used to disguise unpleasant taste of drugs. **Tincture–**An alcohol or water-and-alcohol (with a high percentage of alcohol) solution made by extracting potent plants; may also be used externally (e.g., tincture of iodine). **Powder–**Finely ground drug(s), usually mixed with a liquid before ingesting; some are used internally, others externally. (Some are mixed with a diluent for parenteral injection.) **Solution–**Drug(s) dissolved in a liquid carrier. *Aqueous solutions* are medications dissolved in water. (May be used orally, externally, and parenterally.) **Suspension–**Drug(s) that are suspended (not completely dissolved) in a liquid. *Aqueous suspensions* are suspended in water. *Never* used *for* IV or intra-arterial routes.	• Convenient • Sterility is not needed for oral use • Economical • Noninvasive, low-risk procedure • Easy to administer, good for self-administration • Capsule can mask unpleasant taste of a drug	• Unpleasant taste may cause noncompliance • May irritate gastric mucosa • Patient must be conscious • Digestive juices may destroy drug • Cannot use if patient has nausea and vomiting or decreased gastric motility • Cannot use if patient has difficulty swallowing • Potential for aspiration • May be harmful to teeth • Onset of action is slow

Contd...

Table 20.3: *Contd...*

Form of the drug	*Advantages*	*Disadvantages*
2. Enteral Route: The drug is given directly into the stomach or intestine (e.g., through a nasogastric or gastrostomy tube).		
Same as for oral medications	• Can be used for patients with Impaired Swallowing as an alternative to parenteral administration	• Not all pills can be crushed; medications can clog the NG tube • NG tube itself presents some risk of aspiration
3. Sublingual Route: (a variation of transmucosal administration) – Drug is held under the tongue and absorbed across the sublingual mucous membrane.		
Lipid-soluble lozenge (troche)–A flat, round preparation that dissolves when held in the mouth. May act locally or be absorbed through mucosa for systemic effect. **Tablet** (see oral route).	• Used for local or systemic effects • Convenient • Sterility not needed • Quick delivery to general circulation • Bypasses stomach and intestines; absorbed directly into bloodstream	• May inadvertently be swallowed in the saliva • Not useful for drugs with unpleasant taste • May irritate oral mucosa • Patient must be conscious • Useful only for highly lipid soluble drugs • Patient must hold the drug in place until it is dissolved, which may take a few minutes • Limited period of effective ness, requiring frequent redosing
4. Buccal Route: Transmucosal administration: medication is held against mucous membrane of cheek until it dissolves.		
Lipid-soluble lozenge or tablet (see oral and sublingual routes).	• Same as sublingual	• Same as sublingual
5. Topical (Skin) Route: Drug acts locally or is absorbed directly through skin (transdermal or percutaneous absorption).		
Aerosol spray or foam–A liquid or foam that is sprayed by air pressure onto the skin. **Cream–**A non-oily, semisolid substance applied to the skin. **Gel or jelly–**A clear or translucent semisolid substance that liquefies when applied to the skin. **Liniment–**An oily liquid to rub into the skin. **Lotion–**An *emollient* (softening or soothing agent) for use on the skin; may be a clear solution, suspension, or emulsion. **Ointment–**A semisolid, fatty (usually petroleum jelly- or lanolin-based) substance for skin or mucous membranes; usually not water soluble. **Paste–**Similar to an ointment, but thicker and stiffer. **Tincture** (see oral route). **Transdermal patch–**Releases constant, controlled amounts of medication, for systemic effect.	• Continuous dosing • Sterility is not needed • For local or systemic effects • Long-acting systemic effect • Useful if patient is unable to take oral medications • Acceptable to most patients	• Effective only for lipid-soluble drugs and must be specially formulated • May cause local irritation, especially if the patient is allergic to latex or tape • Discarded patches may pose danger of poisoning • Leaves residue on skin • Accurate doses can be difficult to obtain when the drug is in a tube or jar
6. Tropical: Instillations Route: The drug is placed into a body cavity (e.g., urinary bladder, rectum, vagina, ears, nose, eye).		
Solutions (for nose ears, eyes; enemas per rectum)–Drug(s) dissolved in a liquid carrier. **Suppositories (for nose ears, eyes; enemas per rectum)–**Drug(s) mixed with a glycerin-gelatin or cocoa butter base and shaped for insertion into the body. It dissolves gradually at body temperature. **Jellies, creams (for vagina and rectum)** see skin route.	• Continuous dosing • Sterility is not needed • Useful if patient is unable to take oral medications • May be used for local or systemic effects	• May be embarrassing for patient • Drugs may be poorly, absorbed from the rectum if stool is present or if patient defecates before suppository melts

Contd...

Table 20.3: *Contd...*

Form of the drug	Advantages	Disadvantages
7. Tropical: Inhalation Route: A device (e.g., nebulizer, face mask) breaks the drug into finely dispersed particles, which are breathed into the respiratory passages. Some drugs are intended for local effects in the respiratory passages; others (e.g., anesthetic gases) are for systemic effects; especially in the brain.		
Aerosols–Aerosols are liquids in very fine particles that can be inhaled into the lungs; they are sprayed under air pressure. **Gases**–Gas is a basic form of matter (i.e., solid, liquid, and gas). A gas must be kept in a closed container; otherwise, the fast-moving molecules escape into the air. Examples are oxygen, nitrogen, carbon dioxide, and anesthetic gases.	• Quick and efficient local and systemic route through the lungs • May be given to unconscious patient • Allows continuous dosing, and dosage can be easily modified	• Requires special equipment • May irritate lung mucosa • Useful only for drugs that are gases at room temperature • May have unexpected systemic effect when only local effect is desired
8. All Parenteral Routes:		
Dependent on Route	• Patient may conscious or unconscious	• Requires sterile procedure • Poses risk for infection because skin is broken • Requires skill • May cause some pain • Produces anxiety • More expensive than oral administration
9. Parenteral: Intravenous Route: The drug is injected directly into the vein, either by bolus or slow infusion.		
Aqueous solutions–Drug(s) dissolved in water.	• Rapid effect because absorption is bypassed; therefore, good for emergency situations • Patient needs only one needle-stick, even for multiple doses	• Poses risk of transient drug concentrations if drug is injected too rapidly • Limited to highly soluble medications • Poses risk for sepsis because pathogens may be introduced directly into blood stream • Patient must have usable veins • Cost of supplies and medications
10. Parenteral: Intrmuscular Route: The drug is injected into muscle mass.		
Primarily aqueous solutions (see intravenous route), although some preparations (e.g., penicillin) suspensions	• Rapid absorption, except for oily preparations or suspensions • Allows uses of drugs pain (than do subcutaneous injections) from irritating drugs because they are deep in muscle • Allows administration of a larger volume than does subQ administration • Allows more rapid absorption than does subQ or oral administration	• May cause irritation and local reactions • Poses risk for tissue and nerve damage if site is improperly located • Cannot be used where tissue is damaged (e.g., bruised) or peripheral circulation is decreased
11. Parenteral: Subcutaneous Route: Drug is injected into the subcutaneous tissue under the skin.		
Primarily solutions–Drugs dissolved in a liquid carrier.	• Allows faster action than does oral administration • Allows better absorption of lipid-soluble drugs than does intramuscular administration	• Only very small amounts can be given • Absorption is relatively slow and often confined to the injected area

Contd...

Table 20.3: *Contd...*		
Form of the drug	*Advantages*	*Disadvantages*
12. Parenteral: Intradermal Route: The drug is injected under the skin, into the dermis. Most commonly used for diagnostic testing or screening or for injecting local anesthetic.		
13. Parenteral Route: • **Intraspinal**–Injection of drug into spinal canal. • **Intrathecal**–Injection of drug into subarachnoid space around the spinal cord. • **Epidural**–Injection of drug between the vertebral spines into the extradural space. Most commonly used for regional anesthesia.		

Administering Medications

Pouring Liquid Medications

Liquid medications are frequently used for children and older adults. They usually come in multiple-dose bottles, so you will need to pour individual doses into a disposable, calibrated cup. When pouring, hold the bottle so the liquid does not run over the label, making it difficult to read.

• Measure the dosage with the calibrated cup at eye level.
• Read the dosage where the lowest part of the concaved surface (meniscus) of the fluid is on the line.
• When you are finished, wipe the rim of the bottle with a clean tissue or paper towel before replacing the cap.

If the patient has difficulty taking liquids from a cup, you can use a syringe without a needle to place the medication in his mouth. Place the patient in a side-lying or upright position to help prevent choking and aspiration. Place the syringe between the gum and cheek, and slowly push the plunger to administer the liquid slowly.

Buccal and Sublingual Medications

Buccal and sublingual medications, although placed in the mouth, are intended for absorption in the saliva rather than in the GI tract. Some medications and enzyme preparations are administered by this route and are rapidly absorbed, some within seconds. Buccal medications are held in the cheek; sublingual medications are held under the tongue.

Enteral (Nasogastric and Gastrostomy) Medications

For patients who cannot swallow or who have feeding tubes, you can give oral medications through nasogastric (NG), gastrostomy, or jejunal tubes. Observe the following precautions when administering enteral medications:

• Do not give hydrophilic medications, such as Metamucil, through feeding tubes because they attract water and will solidify in the tube.
• Some tablets should not be crushed, because crushing changes aspects of their action. Be sure to check that crushing is acceptable. Never crush an enteric-coated medication.

• Give medications separately, and flush with water between each. Some medications are less effective when given in combination with others.
• If the patient is receiving a continuous tube feeding, disconnect it before giving the medications; leave the tube clamped for a few minutes after administering the medication, according to agency protocol.
• If the enteral tube is connected to suction, you will usually discontinue the suction for 20 to 30 minutes after administration and keep the tube clamped, to allow tune for the drug to be absorbed.
• Be sure to document on the intake and output record the amount of liquid medication and the water used for flushing.
• If the patient is on fluid restrictions, use the smallest amount of water possible to dissolve tablets and flush the tube.

Special Situations

Some oral medications can discolor or damage the enamel of the teeth. Mix these drugs with a liquid and have the patient drink it through a straw and drink water afterward. For medications (usually in liquid form) that have an objectionable taste, the following methods help to disguise the taste:

• Unless contraindicated, have the patient drink a liberal amount of flavored liquid (e.g. juice) or water to dilute the medication.
• Have the patient suck on ice chips for several minutes before taking the medication. Ice numbs the taste buds.
• Store the medication in the refrigerator. Especially if it is an oily liquid, its smell and taste will be less objectionable.
• Use a syringe to place the medication on the back of the patient's tongue. There are fewer taste buds there.
• Regardless of method, offer oral hygiene immediately after giving the medication.

Some patients have difficulty swallowing medications; they gag, or the pills become "stuck" in their throat. It may help to crush soluble tablets and place them in liquids or in a small amount of applesauce or pudding. Remember that some forms (e.g. time-released tablets) should not be crushed, so check your drug reference sources to be certain. Remember that you cannot give oral medications to patients who:

• Cannot swallow fluids. The risk for aspiration is too great.

- Have nausea or vomiting. The medication would be lost in the emesis.
- Are NPO.

In these situations you should obtain a medical order for an alternative route or, in the case of NPO, permission to give the medication with small sips of water.

Medicating Children

Young children present unique challenges because they cannot be motivated by logic. They cannot grasp the cause and effect of "Take this; it will make you feel better." If they do not like the taste, they will not swallow it. Another challenge is that before the age of 5 years, children may not be able to swallow tablets and capsules. For these reasons, most oral medications for children are prepared as sweetened liquids. For very young children and infants, you must take care to prevent choking and aspiration. Parents can often suggest the best methods for getting their child to take medicines. For other parents, you may need to teach techniques for administering medications at home.

Teaching Parents about Medicating Children

- If the child is old enough to understand, warn him when a medication has an objectionable taste (e.g. "Raghu, this doesn't taste very good, but you can have a big drink of juice as soon as you swallow it"). You will lose his trust if you surprise him with a bad taste.
- Give the child a frozen fruit bar or frozen flavored ice pop just before the medication. This helps to numb the taste buds to weaken the taste of the medication.
- To mask bad-tasting medicines, you can crush tablets or empty the contents of a capsule and mix with soft foods, such as applesauce, hot cereal, or pudding. This is helpful for patients who might aspirate liquids, as well. *(Caution:* Check with a pharmacist or physician before crushing a tablet or emptying a capsule. Some medications should not be crushed.)
- Do not use essential foods in the child's diet (e.g. milk or orange juice) to mask the taste of medications. The child may later refuse a food that he associates with the medicine.
- Take care to prevent choking or aspiration. When giving liquids to infants and toddlers, hold the child in a sitting or semi-sitting position. Use a medicine dropper or syringe to place the medication between the gum and cheek. Apply gentle pressure; avoid giving too much medication too fast.
- Always praise the child after she swallows the medication.

Medicating Older Adults

As you already know, because of physiological changes associated with aging, older adults usually require smaller dosages of drugs. In addition, their reactions to some medications are unpredictable. Therefore, you will need to observe carefully for both therapeutic and undesired effects. Other problems include the following:

- *Difficulty swallowing medications:* It may help to crush tablets or give drugs in liquid form. Gently massaging the area just below the chin may help to initiate swallowing. Consult a speech therapist for other suggestions.
- *Slow reflexes and reasoning ability:* You may need to allow more time to explain and administer medications to older adults. Some may not understand exactly what you want them to do.
- *Forgetting to take the medications:* Impaired memory is more common with age, so clients need simple plans that they can follow at home. A written schedule may help, especially if you schedule the drugs to be taken at mealtimes and at bedtime. Many people take their medication, only to forget shortly thereafter whether or not they did so. Advise the patient to use a divided pill container or a small glass filled with the medications for each dosage time during the day. If the A.M. container is empty, that means the person has taken the morning drugs.
- *Impaired visual acuity.* For patients who cannot see well, write out the home medication schedule in large letters, or ask family members to help.
- *Difficulty opening containers and administering medications:* Because of pain or stiffness in the hands and fingers, and also because of decreased visual acuity, older adults often find it difficult to open containers or to administer their own insulin injections, inhalers, eye medications, and so on. Help them find solutions or assistance from family and friends.
- *Lack of understanding of the need for the medication:* Some older adults accept unquestioningly everything a physician says, but they may not understand what each drug is for. For example, suppose a patient's tranquilizer is not effective. The physician prescribes a new one, but the patient does not understand that he should stop taking the old one; so for a period of time, he takes both medications. This type of situation can happen, too, when patients are being treated by more than one physician.

However, some patients do not see the need for the medication ("I don't feel any better when I take all this stuff"), so they simply do not take it. In the hospital, they may refuse to take medications, or they may put the tablets in their mouth but spit them out when you leave the room. You should stay with the patient until you see that he has swallowed the medications.

Administering Respiratory Inhalations

Nebulization is the production of a fine spray, fog, powder, or mist from a liquid drug. The patient inhales the medication mixture by breathing deeply through a mouthpiece attached to the nebulizer. The airways and alveoli are highly vascularized and therefore absorb inhaled medications rapidly.

Types of Nebulizers

The following are four types of devices for achieving nebulization:

- *Atomizers* disperse the medication in the form of large droplets.
- *Aerosol sprayers* suspend the droplets of medication in a gas (e.g. oxygen).
- An *ultrasonic (hand-held) nebulizer* mixes a small volume of medication, usually less than 1 mL, with 3 mL of normal saline. The device forces air through the nebulizer and delivers medication and humidity as a fine mist. Because the particles are so small, the mist can be inhaled deep into the lungs.
- A *metered-dose inhaler (MDI)* is a type of nebulizer that delivers measured doses of a nebulized drug. A dry powder inhaler (DPI) is a type of MDI.

No matter which device is used, the smaller the droplets, the farther the medication can be inhaled into the respiratory tract.

Metered-Dose Inhalers

A *metered-dose inhaler (MDI)* is a pressurized container prefilled with several doses of a drug and a gas propellant. The patient inhales while pushing the canister's pump to release a measured dose of medication through a nosepiece or mouthpiece. Sometimes an extender (spacer) is attached to the mouthpiece. The medication is pumped into the extender instead of directly into the patient's mouth. The patient inhales the drug from the chamber. Use of a spacer prevents coughing that may be triggered by the propellant.

A *dry powder inhaler (DPI)* does not have a propellant, but instead is activated by inhalation. Each powdered dose is in a blister pack that is activated according to the manufacturer's instructions. Once the dose is loaded, the patient simply takes a deep breath. Examples are Turbuhaler, and Diskhaler.

Patients frequently self-administer inhalations (most often bronchodilators or steroids) using an MDI. However, you may need to teach your patients how to use the device correctly.

The advantage of MDIs is that high doses of medication can he rapidly instilled in the lungs, producing local effects and avoiding systemic side effects. Disadvantages are the need for manual dexterity, which is often compromised in the older adult; skill in coordinating the inhaling of the medication and the pushing of the canister to administer the dose; and the ability to inhale and exhale deeply enough to allow penetration of the medication in the more distal bronchioles.

Teaching the Use of a Metered-Dose Inhaler (MDI)

Before teaching the steps of the procedure:

- Obtain the appropriate supplies for the procedure, including the inhaler and tissues.
- Explain to the patient when to use the inhaler and what side effects to anticipate.
- Demonstrate how the inhaler fits into the canister.

Then teach the following steps:

- Sit upright, preferably in a straight-backed chair.
- Remove the cap, and hold the canister upright in your dominant hand.
- Shake the canister several times to mix the medication in the canister.
- With a new inhaler, or when using an inhaler that you haven't used for a week or so, discharge the first two puffs into the air. Otherwise, you get a mouthful of the propellant instead of medication.
- Open your mouth, and hold the inhaler according to the care provider's or manufacturer's instructions. Either:
  Hold the mouthpiece 1 to 2 inches in front of your open mouth
  Or
  Place the mouthpiece over your tongue and into your mouth. Close your teeth and lips tightly around the mouthpiece. This is the method to use for all MDIs with a spacer or extender.
- Take a deep breath and breathe out until you can expel no more air from your lungs.
- Press the top of the canister firmly with your fore finger while inhaling deeply.
- Continue to inhale so the medication is drawn deep into your lungs. Then hold that breath as long as possible. Try to count to 10 seconds if possible.
- Exhale slowly through pursed lips to keep the small airways open during exhalation.
- Remove the inhaler from your mouth, and breathe normally.
- Wait at least 1 minute before giving the second puff, or 5 minutes before giving another inhaled medication, so the medication can enter the bloodstream and the canister can recharge.
- If you are using an inhaled steroid, rinse your mouth or gargle with water to prevent the steroid from being absorbed in the mouth.
- Clean the mouthpiece with a tissue, and replace the cap.

When inhaler is empty user should observe:

- Each container is clearly marked with the number of sprays per container (30 to 100, usually); make a mark each time you use it. Or
- Remove the container from the plastic holder and place in a bowl of water. It will sink to the bottom when it is full and float more to the top as it empties. This method is imprecise and works only with MDIs.

Administering Parenteral Medications

Parenteral medications include those that are injected by the intradermal, subcutaneous, intramuscular, or intravenous routes. Parenteral injections are absorbed faster and more completely than drugs given by other routes; the results are more predictable; and the dosage can be measured more accurately. In addition, they can be used for patients who cannot take oral medications. However, injectable medications have some disadvantages:

1. They bypass the skin barrier, making infection more likely if aseptic technique is not used.
2. Tissue damage may result if the pH, osmotic pressure, or solubility of the medication is not appropriate to the tissue where the medication is given. For example, medications intended for injection into muscle may damage subcutaneous tissue.
3. Preparation and administration must be performed accurately, because the onset of action is relatively rapid and the medications, once given, cannot be retrieved.

The term internal means within the intestine. Parenteral means outside the intestines or alimentary canal. Most people use the term parenteral to refer to injection routes only. Medication may be injected to an artery, the peritoneum, heart tissues, the spinal cord and bones.

Preparing Medication for Administration by Injections

Drugs may be dispensed in single dose of glass ampules, single dose rubber capped vials, multidose rubber capped vials, and prefilled cartridges.

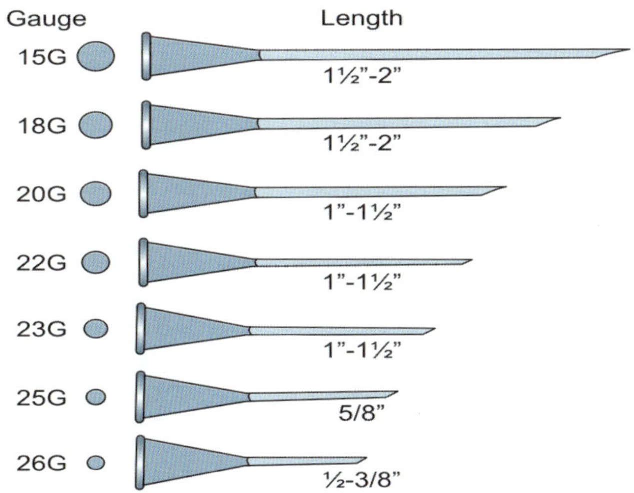

Figure 20.2: Needle length and gauge

Preparing Injectable Medications

Injectable medications are those that are injected or infused into body tissues or into the bloodstream. When administering them, as a nurse you must know about various kinds of needles and syringes. You will need to decide, based on each situation, what size and type of needle and syringe to use.

Needles

Needles are disposable, stainless steel sheaths that attach to a syringe. Needles are made in various lengths and gauges and with different bevel sizes (Fig. 20.2).

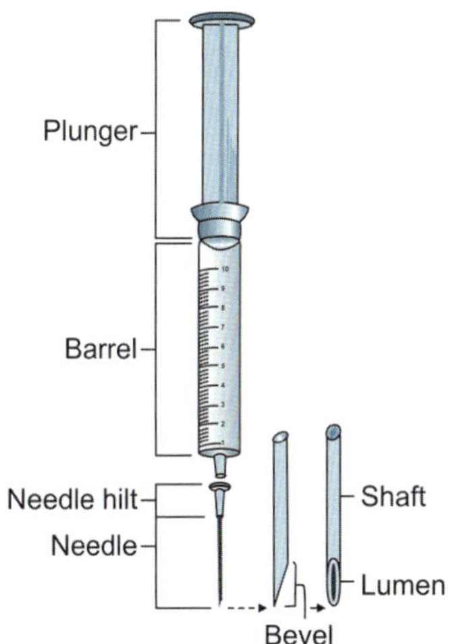

Figure 20.3: Parts of needle and syringe

The gauge refers to the inside diameter of the needle lumen. The smaller the gauge, the larger the diameter (i.e., a 16-gauge needle has a larger diameter than a 20-gauge needle). Needle gauges are numbered 14 through 30. Choose the gauge based on the patient's size and skin condition, the viscosity of medication used, and the speed of administration desired. Smaller needles (26 to 30 gauge) cause less pain and trauma to the tissue, so they are especially useful for patients who must have frequent or long-term injections (e.g. for insulin and heparin). Larger needles (14 to 18 gauge) are used for blood and more viscous medications, such as penicillin, to mix intravenous (IV) medications, or for rapid infusion of IV medications.

The bevel is the slanted tip with a narrow slit. The slant is designed to make an opening that will close quickly to prevent leakage of medication, blood, and serum. A long bevel tip is sharper and narrower and therefore causes less discomfort during injection. Long bevels are usually used for subcutaneous (subQ) and intramuscular injections. Short bevels are used for intradermal or IV injections.

The needle length (commonly 3/8 to 3 inches) is the distance from the tip to the hub (bottom) of the needle. Use a longer needle for subQ and intramuscular injections, and a shorter one for intradermal and IV injections. Vary the length according to the thickness of the patient's muscle and adipose tissue. Although a 1½ inch needle is common for intramuscular injections, you would use a shorter one for a child or a very thin person.

Filter needles and filter straws are used to trap rubber or glass fragments when drawing up a medication from a vial or an ampule. Nurse must replace the filter needle with a regular needle before injecting the medication into the patient or into the IV solution.

Syringes

A syringe consists of a barrel, plunger, and syringe tip. Because injections require strict sterile technique, nurse may touch the outside of the barrel and end of the plunger but not the inside of the barrel, hub, shaft of the plunger or needle (Fig. 20.3).

Syringes are usually made of plastic and are disposable. Some have the needle attached; others do not. The syringe tip, either Luer-Lok (twist on) or non-Luer-Lok (slip on), fits into the needle hub. Syringes are made in various sizes, from 0.5 mL to 60 mL. The larger sizes are used for adding medications to IV solutions and for irrigating wounds. As nurse you will usually use a 2 mL or 3 mL syringe for intramuscular injections. Syringes larger than 5 mL are used for IV administration, instillations, and irrigations.

Five syringes are shown in Figure 20.4. Standard syringes are supplied in 3, 5, and 10 mL sizes. They are commonly supplied without needles or with 18-, 21-, 23-, or 25-gauge needles that are 0.5 to 3 inches long. They are calibrated and marked in 0.1 mL and 1 or 2 mL increments so that drugs can be measured accurately. Tuberculin syringes have a 1 mL capacity and are calibrated in 0.01 mL increments; they come with a small (usually 26- to 28-) gauge, short (0.5 to 0.625 inch) needle. Use tuberculin syringes to administer small, precise doses of medication (e.g. when medicating infants or children, for allergy tests, or when administering potentially dangerous medications, such as heparin). Insulin syringes are calibrated in units and are used to administer insulin. Insulin syringes are calibrated in 100 units per milliliter. They are made in 0.3, 0.5, or 1 mL sizes with very small-gauge needles (26 to 30 gauge).

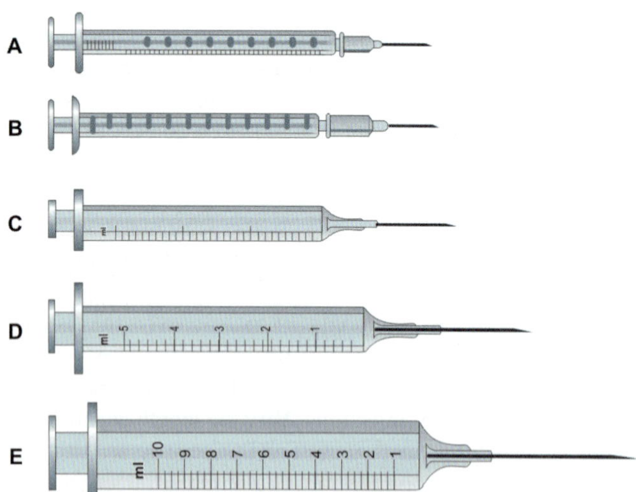

Figures 20.4A to E: A. Insulin syringe marked in units (100), B. 1 mL tuberculin syringe marked in 0.01 (hundredths) and minims, C. 3 mL syringe, D. 5 mL syringe, E. 10 mL syringe

Drawing Up Medications from an Ampule

An ampule is a thin-walled, disposable glass container with a narrow neck that you must snap off to access the medication. To prevent injuries, use an ampule opener to snap the glass. Each ampule holds a single dose of a liquid medication, usually 1 mL to 10 mL, but some hold 50 mL. Because glass fragments may be introduced into the medication, most agencies require you to

use a filter needle or filter straw to draw up the medication. The critical aspects are as given below:
- Maintain sterile technique.
- Recap the needle or injection cannula using a needle recapping device or the one-handed method.
- Change the needle, if indicated.

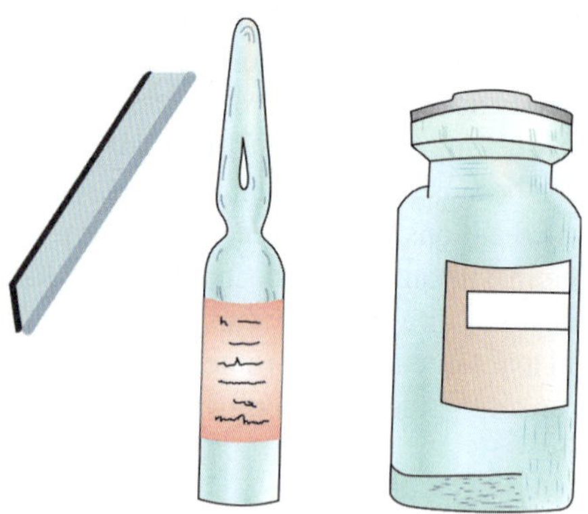

Figure 20.5: Ampule, vial and ampule cutter

Ampule

An ampule is a glass flask that contains a single dose of medication for parenteral administration (Fig. 20.5). Care must be taken not to contaminate the needle by touching the rim of the ampule. Following procedure helps to know how to remove medication from an ampule (Table 20.4):

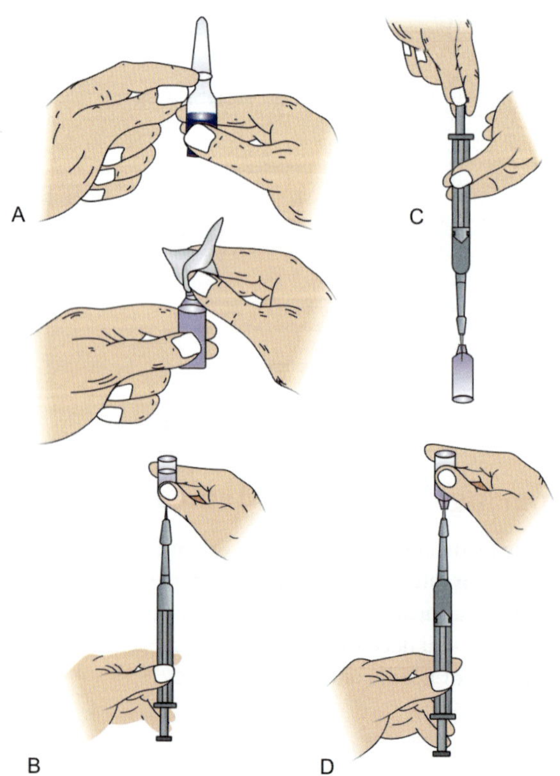

Figure 20.6: Removing medication from ampule

Table 20.4: Procedures for Removing Medication from an Ampule

	Nursing actions		*Rationales*
1.	Gather equipment, check the medication order against the original physician order according to hospital policy.	1.	This comparison helps to identify errors that may have occurred when orders were transcribed.
2.	Wash your hands.	2.	This prevents spread of organism.
3.	Tape the stem of the ampule or twist your wrist quickly while holding the ampule vertically.	3.	This facilitates movement of medication in the stem to the body of the ampule.
4.	Wrap a small gauge pad or dry alcohol swab around the neck of the ampule.	4.	This protects the nurses finger's from the glass as the ampule is broken.
5.	Use a snapping motion to break off the top of the ampule along the prescribed line at its neck. Always break away from your body.	5.	This protects the nurse's face and fingers from any shattered glass fragments.
6.	Remove the cap from the needle by pulling it straight off. Insert the needle into the ampule, being careful not to touch the rim. (Or use filter needles when withdrawing solution from an ampule).	6.	The rim of the ampule is considered contaminated (use of filter needle prevents the accidental withdrawing of small glass particles with the medication).
7.	Withdraw medication in the amount ordered. Do not inject air into solutions. Use either of the following methods (Fig. 20.6): (a) Insert the tip of the needle into the ampule which is upright on a flat surface and withdraw fluid into the syringe. Touch plunger at knob only. (b) Insert the tip of the needle into the ampule, and invert the ampule. Keep the needle centered and not touching the sides of the ampule. Touch plunger at knob only.	7.	(a) The contents of the ampule are not under pressure; therefore, air is unnecessary and will cause the contents to overflow. Handling plunger at knob only with keep shaft to plunger sterile. (b) Surface tension holds the fluid in the ampule when inverted. If the needle touches the side or is removed and then reinserted into the ampule, surface tension is broken and fluid run out. Handling plunger at knob only will keep shaft and plunger sterile.
8.	Do not expel any air bubbles that may form in the solution. Wait until the needle has been withdrawn to tap the syringe and expel the air carefully. Check the amount of medication in the syringe and discard any surplus.	8.	Injecting air into the solution increases pressure in the ampule and can force the medication to spill-out over the ampule.
9.	Discard the ampule in a suitable container after comparing with medication cart or kardex.	9.	If all the medication has been removed the ampule, it must be discarded because there is no way, to maintain sterility of contents in an opened ampule.
10.	Cap the needle on the syringe the nurse against inadvertent needle sticks.	10.	This prevents contamination of the needle and protects.
11.	Wash your hands.	11.	This deters the spread of microorganism.

Equipments needed are as follows:
- Sterile syringe and needle (depending upon size)
- Ampule of medication
- Medication cart or kardex
- Alcohol swab or gauze paid
- Filter needle

Vial

Vial is a glass bottle with self sealing stopped through which medication is removed. For safety and transporting and shorting, the single dose rubber capped vials is usually covered with a soft metal cap that can be easily removed. The rubber stopper that is then exposed in the means of entrance into vial. Some drugs are dispensed in. vials that contain several doses of medication. This means that the nurse can remove several doses from the same container. To facilitate removal of medication, the nurse injects air into the vial. The amount of air is in the same as the desired quantity. The following procedures show how to remove medication from vial (Table 20.5).

Table 20.5: Procedures for Removing Medication from Vial

	Nursing actions		Rationales
1.	Gather equipment, check medication order against original physician's order.	1.	This comparison helps to identify errors that may occur when orders were transcribed.
2.	Wash your hands.	2.	It prevents spread of microorganism.
3.	Remove the metal or plastic cap on the vial that protects the rubber stopper.	3.	The metal cap prevents contamination of the rubber top.
4.	Swab the rubber top with alcohol is not necessary, the first time rubber stopper is entered but subsequent re-entries into the vial requires the use of alcohol cleaning.	4.	Alcohol removes surface bacteria contamination.
5.	Remove the cap from the needle by pulling it straight off (use filter needle).	5.	Before fluid is remove injection of an equal amount of air is required to prevent the formation of partial enough air is injected, the negative pressure makes it difficult to withdraw medication (use of filter needles prevents any solid material being withdrawn).
6.	Pierce the rubber stopped in the center with the needle tip and inject the measured air into the space into the space above the solution (do not inject air into solution). The vial may be positioned upright or flat surface or inverted (Fig. 20.7A).	6.	Air bubbles through the solution could result in withdrawal of an inaccurate amount of medication.
7.	Invert the vial and withdraw the needle tip slightly so that it is below the fluid level.	7.	This prevents air from being aspirated into the syringe.
8.	Draw up the prescribed amount of medication while holding the syringe at eye level and vertically. Be careful to touch the plunger at knob only (Fig. 20.7B).	8.	Holding the syringe at eye level facilitates accurate reading, and the plunger at knob only makes the removal of air bubbles from the syringe easy. Handling plunger at knob only will keep shaft of plunger sterile.
9.	If any air bubble accumulates in the syringe, tap the barrel of the syringe sharply and move the needle past the fluid into the air space to reinject the air bubble into the vial. Return the needle tip to the solution and continue withdrawal of the medication.	9	Removal of the air bubbles is necessary to ensure accurate dose of medication.
10.	Once the correct dose is withdrawn, remove the needle from the vial and cap it.	10.	This prevents contamination of the needle and protects the nurse against accidental needle sticks.
11.	If a multidose vial is being used, store the vial containing the remaining medication according to hospital policy.	11.	Because the vial is sealed the medication inside remains sterile and can be used for future injections.
12.	Wash your hands.	12.	It deters the spread of microorganism.

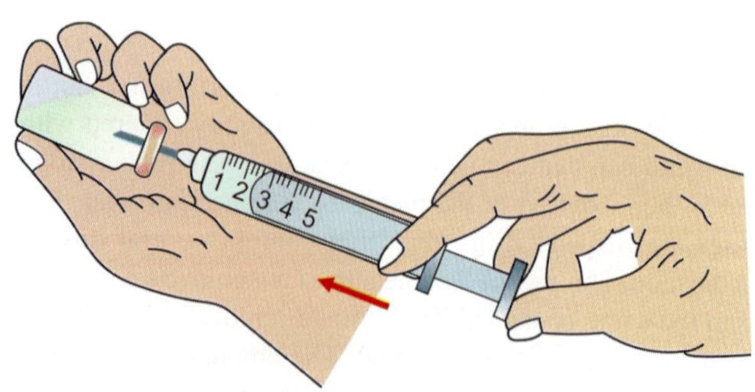

Figure 20.7A: Insertion of air into vial

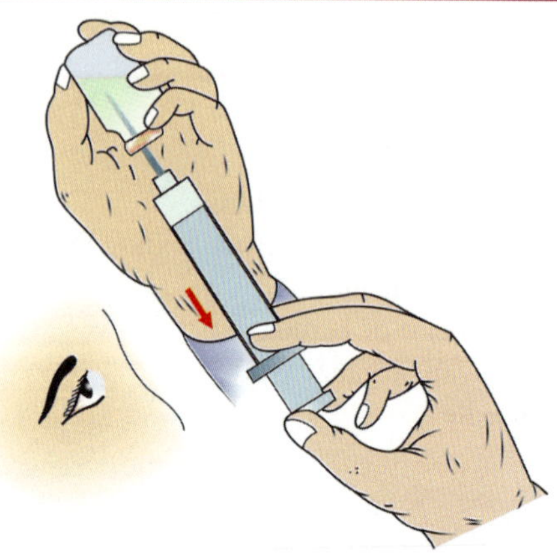

Figure 20.7B: Withdrawing from vial

Equipments needed are as follows:

- Sterile syringe (size depends on drug being administered to client)
- Vial of medication
- Medication cart, kardex
- Alcohol swab
- Filter needle (optional)

A. Ampules (Fig. 20.8A)

- Tap the ampule to remove medication trapped in the top of the ampule.
- Use an ampule opener to break the ampule neck. If one is not available, wrap gauze around the neck of the ampule, and snap the ampule away from you.
- Use a filter needle or filter straw to withdraw the medication.
- Withdraw all of the medication from the ampule by inverting or tipping the ampule (Fig. 20.9).
- Dispose of the top and bottom of ampule and filter needle in a sharps container.

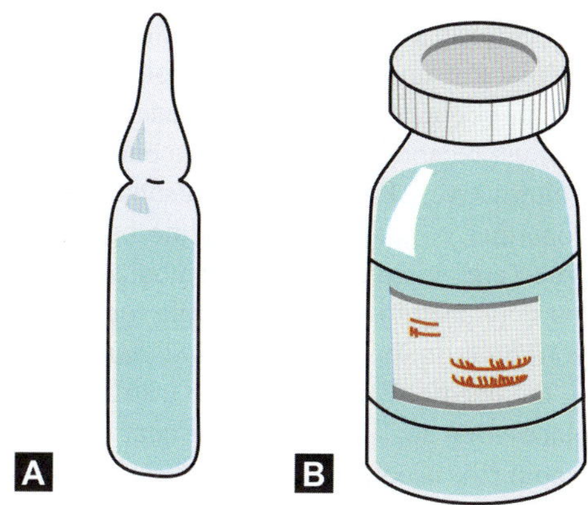

**Figures 20.8A and B: Parenteral medication containers.
A. Ampule; B. Vial**

B. Vials (Fig. 20.8B)

- Thoroughly clean the rubber top of the vial with an alcohol prep pad (for a multiple-dose vial only).
- Draw air into the syringe equal to the amount of medication to be withdrawn.
- When inserting the needle through the rubber top of the vial, avoid coring by inserting the needle at a 45 to 60° angle, bevel up, or by using a filter needle.
- Keeping the needle above the fluid line, inject air into the vial before withdrawing the medication.
- Remove bubbles, hold the vial at eye level, and check that the dose is correct before removing the needle.

Drawing Up Medications from a Vial

A vial is a single-dose or multidose plastic or glass container with a rubber stopper that seals the top. A plastic or metal cap covers the rubber stopper to protect it until it is used. Because the vial is a closed system, you must inject air into it to withdraw the solution. Otherwise, a vacuum is created in the vial that makes withdrawal difficult.

Nurses traditionally wipe the rubber stopper after removing the cap, even on a single-dose vial. However, there is little, if any, scientific justification for this practice. At least one study concluded that it is unnecessary as an infection control measure.

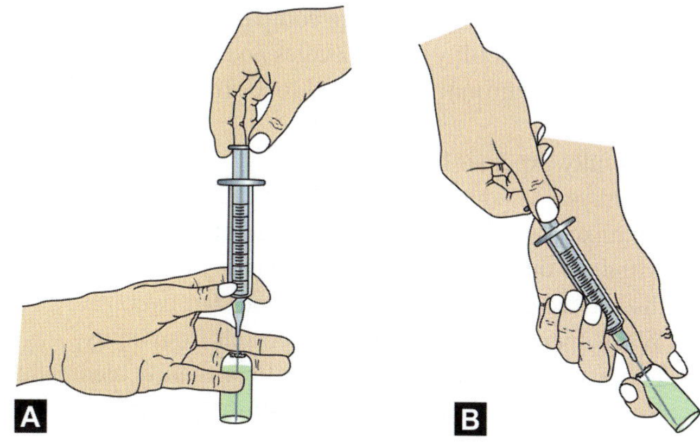

Figure 20.9: Withdrawing medication from ampule

Reconstituting Medications

Medications that are not stable in solution are dispensed as powders in vials. You must add a diluent or solvent to the powder to create a solution for injection. The diluent is usually sterile water or saline; however, each packaged vial includes the manufacturer's instructions for the amount and kind of solvent to add. For safety, use a plastic vial access cannula instead of a needle when possible.

Mixing Medications in the Same Syringe

You can mix two medications in the same syringe (1) if they are compatible, (2) if the total dose is within accepted limits, and, obviously, (3) if they are both to be given by the same route. This technique allows for efficient use of supplies and allows the patient to receive fewer injections.

Medications are *compatible* if they can be mixed without affecting their constituents or actions. Package inserts and medication references usually include compatibility information. Always check the compatibility before mixing medications together. If the contents of the syringe become discolored, there are particles floating in the solution, or there is a change in consistency, do not administer the medications. When mixing medications in one syringe, you must follow these principles:

- Maintain sterile technique.
- Do not contaminate one container with medication from the other container. You must use a separate needle to withdraw from each vial (unless both are single-dose vials).
- Ensure that the dosage of *each* medication is accurate. Calculate each dose before beginning, and draw the second drug up slowly and carefully. If you draw up too much of the second drug, you must discard the syringe and medication and begin again.
- Ensure that the total, final, dosage is correct. Add the volumes calculated in step 3; when you have drawn up both

medications, that total volume should be the amount you have in the syringe. Be sure at each measurement step either to expel or to account for air in the syringe.

The critical aspects of mixing for guidelines are as given below:
- Make sure the medications are compatible.
- Maintain the sterility of the needles and medication.
- Avoid contaminating a multidose vial with a second medication.
- Carefully expel air bubbles.
- When you withdraw the second medication, the medications are mixed as you pull back the plunger; therefore, you must withdraw the exact amount. If there is any excess, you must discard the contents of the syringe and start over.
- When opening ampules, protect yourself from injury.
- Use a filter needle or filter straw to withdraw medication from ampules; change to a needle of the proper length and gauge for administering the medication.
- When drawing up from a single-dose vial and ampule, draw up from the vial first.
- Do not use prefilled cartridges for intramuscular injections unless they have a safety device; transfer the medication to a syringe with a safety device before administering.
- Always recap a sterile needle using a needle capping device or the one-handed scoop method.

Accounting for Needle "Dead Space"

Some nurses believe that a small amount of the patient's medication remains in the needle when an injection is given. Therefore, in the past, some recommended adding 0.2 mL of air to the syringe after measuring a medication for IM injection. Nurses are not in agreement about the need for adding air and unfortunately, there is scant research to settle the question. Theoretically, on injection the air clears the needle of medication, ensuring that the patient receives the entire dose. However, because syringes are calibrated to account for medication left in the needle and because the medication left in the needle after injection is the same amount as before the injection, many believe that air should not be added. We recommend that you add air only in the following situations:

1. *When the medication is irritating to subcutaneous tissues,* add 0.2 mL of air after measuring proper dose. The air drives the medication deep into the muscle tissue; the air injected into the tissue creates an air lock above the medication, preventing it from tracking through subcutaneous tissue.
2. *When you change needles after drawing up the medication.* For example, when you draw up the dose using a filter needle, then replace it with the new needle, the new needle has air in it instead of medication. If you push the plunger until you see a drop of medication at the tip of the needle, you will see that you no longer have a complete dose in the syringe. Adding a 0.2 mL air lock will drive the entire dose into the patient's tissue.

Preventing Needlestick Injuries

Healthcare workers suffer up to 1 million injuries per year from needles and other "sharps," putting them at risk for infectious diseases such as hepatitis B and AIDS. For this reason, special safety devices have been designed to reduce the risk of needlestick injuries. One such device is a special syringe with a guard that covers the needle immediately after it is withdrawn from the skin. Then dispose of both needle and sheath in a "sharp" container. Most systems involve adapters that can be used with regular intravenous tubing and medication vials, permitting access through a valve system without a needle.

Always dispose of needles, glass, and other "sharps" in clearly marked, usually red, puncture-proof containers. Never force a needle into an already full container; you may be injured by sharps protruding from the top. Never put a needle or other sharp in a wastebasket, in your pocket, or at the patient's bedside.

Recapping Contaminated Needles

You should never recap a contaminated needle (e.g. after giving an injection); place it uncapped, needle pointing downward, directly into a sharps container. However, you may occasionally find that you must recap a contaminated needle when there is "no feasible alternative." For example, in some patient rooms the sharps container is not located near the bed. If there are several people (e.g. visitors) between you and the sharps container, you may need to recap the needle for their safety as well as for your own. In this case, use a *one-handed technique* for recapping the needle. For step-by-step instructions,
- Do not place your nondominant hand near the needle cap when recapping the needle or engaging the safety mechanism.
- If you are using a safety needle, engage the safety mechanism to cover the needle.
- If available, place the needle cap in a mechanical recapping device.
- If recapping devices are not available and you must recap the needle for your own and/or the patient's safety, use the one-handed scoop technique.

Recapping Sterile Needles

Authorities do not advise against recapping sterile needles (e.g. after drawing up a medication), except to recommend needleless systems and safety systems. We suggest that you not use the one-handed "scoop" technique to recap a sterile needle, because the risk of contaminating it is high.
- Be sure to keep the needle and cap sterile.
- Do not place your nondominant hand near the needle cap when recapping the needle or engaging the safety mechanism.
- Use one of the following methods:
  - Place the needle cap in a medication cup, and recap the needle.
  - Place the cap on a clean surface so that the end of the needle cap protrudes over the edge of the counter or shelf, and scoop with the needle.

– Use a hard syringe cover: Insert the needle cap into the cover, and then insert the needle.
– Place the needle cap on a sterile surface, such as on open alcohol prep pad, and use the one-handed scoop technique (this is the least desirable method).

Administering Parenteral Injections

Parenteral techniques are invasive. They carry the potential for tissue trauma and provide a portal of entry for pathogens through the skin. Therefore, you must maintain strict aseptic (sterile) technique to minimize the risk of infection. When you choose a site for injection, consider the type of medication to be administered, the viscosity of the medication, the volume of the medication, the anatomical landmarks underlying injection sites, and the patient's situation (e.g. the condition of the tissues at the injection site, the accessibility of certain sites). Your injection technique is critical to patient safety. The following are examples of some errors and their consequences:

- Injecting a large volume of medication into a small muscle causes pain and may damage the tissues.
- Injecting into the wrong tissue (e.g. giving an intra muscular medication too shallowly into the subcutaneous tissue) may

(1) accelerate or delay the rate of absorption and (2) cause tissue injury and pain.
- Incorrectly locating an injection site may result in bone or nerve injury when you insert the needle.
- If you fail to hold the needle and syringe steady while injecting the drug, you may cause pain and tissue trauma.
- If you fail to aspirate before injecting the medication, you risk injecting it into an artery or vein; with some medications, this could be fatal.

Tissue penetration by injections shown in Figure 20.10.

Minimizing Discomfort

The discomfort associated with an injection comes from three sources: the prick of the needle, the pressure of the volume of the drug in the tissues, and chemical irritation caused by some drugs. Fear and anxiety magnify discomfort. Use the following techniques to reduce discomfort:

- Use the smallest needle suited for the site and medication.
- Use two needles when drawing up medications: one to withdraw the medication from the container, and the second one for the injection. If the needle is not free of medication, it may irritate tissues as it is inserted.

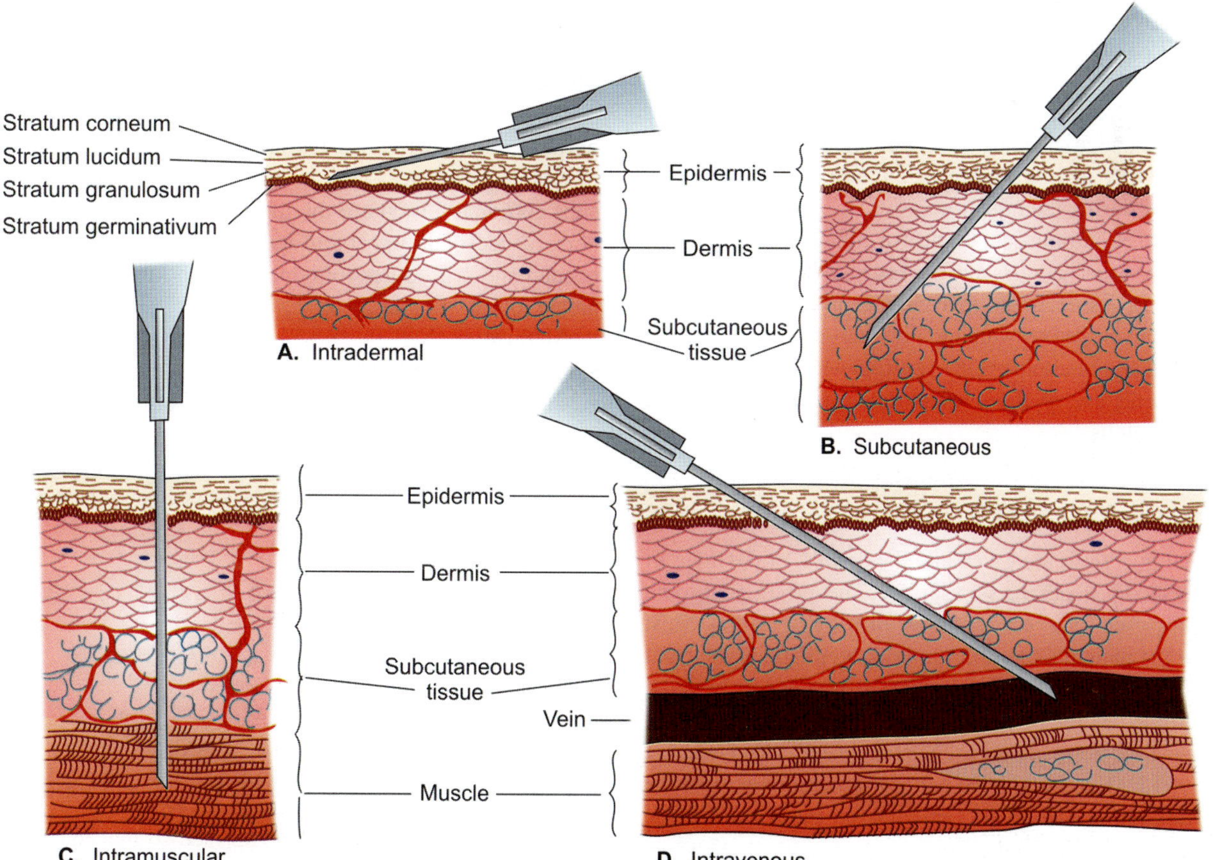

Figure 20.10: Tissue penetration by injection

- Do not administer too much solution into an injection site. If the total volume is more than the recommended amount, give it in two injections and two sites.
- For intramuscular injections, help the client to assume a position that reduces muscle tension.
- For intramuscular injections, use the Z-track technique. This prevents leakage of the medication up through the needle track after the needle is withdrawn.
- Pull the skin taut, and insert the needle quickly to avoid pulling the tissues. Remove the needle quickly and at the same angle you inserted it.
- Steady the syringe with one hand while injecting the medication.
- Inject the medication slowly, about 10 seconds per mL.
- Distract the client from the procedure by talking to her.
- Apply gentle pressure (not massage) after injection unless contraindicated.
- Especially with children, acknowledge that they will feel some pain (e.g. "This may hurt a little bit."). If you deny or minimize the pain, the patient will lose trust in you and be even more anxious about future injections.
- After injecting a child, pat or hug him, speak softly to him, and perhaps play with him, so that he does not associate you only with pain.

Developmental Considerations

Because older adults may experience muscle atrophy or have decreased muscle mass, you may need to use a shorter needle. Infants and children also require shorter (5/8 to 1 inch), thinner (e.g. 22- to 25-gauge) needles. Also, you should ask a parent or another caregiver to immobilize an infant or young child to prevent injury during the injection.

The preferred intramuscular site for infants 7 months and younger is the vastus lateral is muscle, because there are no major nerves or blood vessels in the area and the gluteal muscles have not yet been developed by walking. For children over the age of 7 months, the site of choice is the ventrogluteal muscle. We do not recommend use of the dorsogluteal site even for older children and adults.

Intradermal Injections

Intradermal injections are given into the dermis, or the layer of the skin located beneath the skin surface. The intradermal route is commonly used for allergy or tuberculosis (TB) testing. Most nurses use the patient's left arm for TB screening and the right arm, chest, or upper neck for all other tests. Give only small amounts of medication by this route–about 0.1 mL. Use a 1 mL syringe and a short, small (26- to 28-gauge) needle, and insert at an angle of 15° (Fig. 20.11). Do not apply pressure or massage the injection site, because the capillaries in the dermal tissue will quickly absorb the medication.

The critical aspects for critical elements of intradermal injections are as given below:

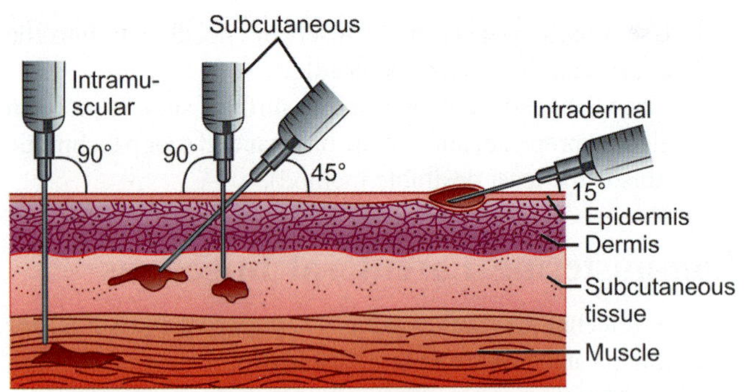

Figure 20.11: Standard angels of insertion for intramuscular, subcutaneous, and intradermal injections

- Maintain sterile technique and standard precautions.
- Use a 1 mL syringe and a 25- to 28-gauge, ¼ to 5/8 inch needle.
- Be aware that an intradermal dose is small, usually about 0.01 to 0.1 mL.
- Administer the injection on the ventral surface of the forearm, upper back, or upper chest.
- Hold the syringe parallel to the skin at a 5 to 15° angle, with the bevel up.
- Stretch the skin taut to insert the needle.
- Do not aspirate.
- Inject slowly, and create a wheal or bleb.
- Do not massage the site.

Administering an Intradermal Injection

The intradermal route has the longest absorption time of all parenteral routes. Intradermal injection is used for diagnostic purpose (e.g. tuberculosis test) to tests to determine sensitivity to various substances (e.g. giving test dose of penicillin). The sites commonly used are the inner surface of the forearm, the dorsal aspect of the upper arm and the upper back. The equipment needed and procedures for administering intradermal injection are as follows (Table 20.6).

- Medication
- Medication card
- Sterile syringe and needle (tuberculosis syringe, calibrated 10th and 100th of m.litre
- Alcohol swab
- Acetone and 2 × 2 sterile gauge square (optional)
- Disposable gloves

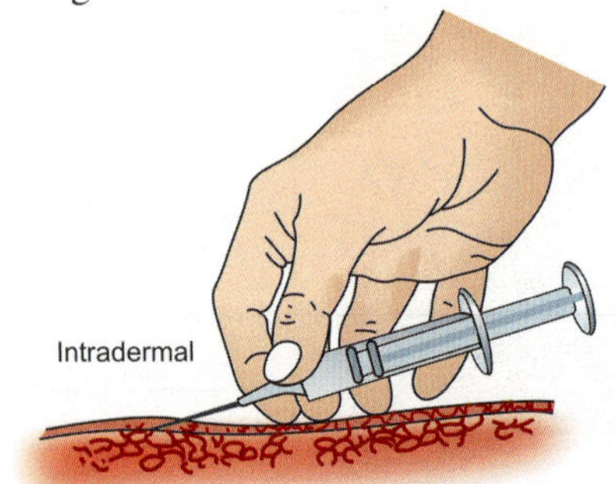

Figure 20.12: Administration of intradermal injection (Step 9)

Table 20.6: Procedures for Administering Intradermal Injection

	Nursing actions		*Rationales*
1.	Assemble equipment and check the physician order.	1.	This ensures that the client is receiving the right medication at the right time by right route. Many intradermal drugs are potent allergies and may cause a significant reaction if given in incorrect dose.
2.	Explain the procedure to the client.	2.	It encourages cooperation and reduces apprehension.
3.	Wash your hands and don disposable gloves.	3.	This prevents spread of microorganism. Gloves act as a barrier and protects the nurse's hands from accidental exposure to blood during injecting procedure.
4.	If necessary, withdraw medication from ampule or vial.		
5.	Select an area on the inner aspect of the forearm, that is not heavily pigmented or covered with hair. The upper chest or upper breath the scapula also are sites for intradermal injection.	5.	The forearm is convenient and easy location for introducing an agent intradermally. Hour or lesions at the injection site may interfere with assessment of skin changes at the site.
6.	Cleanse the area with an alcohol swab while wiping with a firm, circular motion and moving outward from the injection site. Allow the skin to dry. If the skin is only, clean the area with a pledget moistened with acetone.	6.	Pathogens on the skin can be forced into the tissues by the needle. Introducing alcohol into tissue irritates the tissues and is uncomfortable for the patient. Acetone is effective for remaining oily substances from the skin.
7.	Use the nondominant hand to spread the skin taut over the injection site.	7.	Taut skin provides an easy entrance into intradermal tissue.
8.	Remove the needle cap with the nondominant hand by pulling it straight off.	8.	The cap protects the needle from contact with micro-organism. This technique lessens the risk of an accidental needle stick.
9.	Place the needle almost that against the clients skin, bevel side up and insert the needle into the skin so that the paint of the needle can be seen through the skin. Insert the needles only about 1/8 inch (Fig. 20.12).	9.	Intradermal tissue is entered when the needle is held as nearly parallel to the skin as possible and is inserted about 1/8 inch.
10.	Slowly inject the agent while watching for a small wheal or blister to appear. If nothing appears, withdraw the needle slightly.	10.	If a small wheel or blister appears, the agent is in intradermal tissue.
11.	Withdraw the needle quickly at the same angle that it was inserted.	11.	Withdrawing the needle quickly any at the angle at which it entered the skin minimized tissue damage and discomfort for client.
12.	Do not massage the area after removing the needle.	12.	Massaging the area where an intradermal injection is given may interfere with test results by spreading medication to underlying substances tissue.
13.	Do not recap the used needle. Discard this needle and syringe in appropriate receptacle.	13.	Proper disposal of the needle, protects the nurse from accidental injection. Most accidental puncture wound occurs when recapping needles.
14.	Assist the client to a position of comfort.	14.	This provides for the well-being of the client.
15.	Remove gloves and dispose them properly.	15.	This deters the spread of microorganism.
16.	Chart the administration of the medication.	16.	Accurate documentation is necessary to prevent medication error.
17.	Observe the area for signs of a reaction at ordered intervals, usually at 24 to 72 hours period. Inform the client of this inspection. The circle may be drawn on the skin around the injection site.	17.	This easily identifies the site of intradermal injection and allows for careful observation of the exact area.

Subcutaneous Injections

Subcutaneous (subQ) injections are given into the subcutaneous tissue, the layer of fat located below the dermis and above the muscle tissue. Absorption is slower than through the intramuscular route because subQ tissue does not have as rich a blood supply as muscle. However, speed of absorption varies with the subQ site selected. Sites on the abdomen and arms offer fastest absorption; those on the thigh and upper buttocks, the slowest absorption. Medication is absorbed more evenly from the abdomen than from the thighs and buttocks because it is less affected by activity (Fig. 20.13).

Conventional techniques call for the nurse to aspirate before injecting medication; if there is no blood return, the nurse is assured that the medication will not be injected into a blood vessel. Some nurses aspirate before injecting a medication subcutaneously; others do not. It has been stated that there are no clinical studies to confirm the need for aspiration and further, that it "is cumbersome, rarely yields blood, and isn't a reliable indicator of correct needle placement."

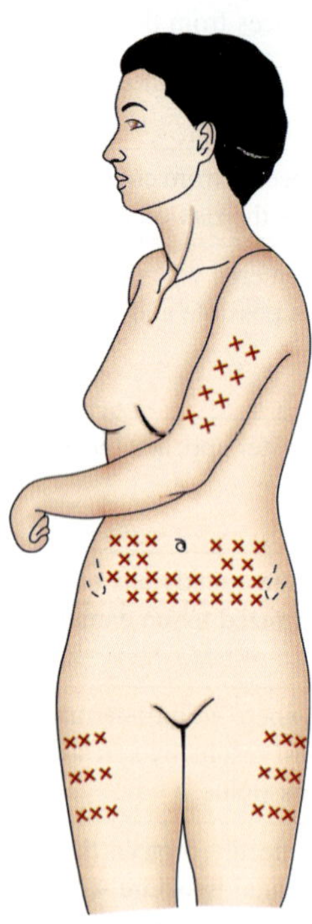

Figure 20.13: Sites used for subcutaneous injections A. Upper outer arm, B. Lower abdomen, C. Upper outer thigh

- Maintain sterile technique and standard precautions.
- Use a 1 mL syringe and a 25- to 27-gauge needle that is less than 1 inch long (usually 3/8 to 5/8 inch).
- A subcutaneous dose must be no more than 1 mL.
- Injection sites: Use the outer aspect of the upper arms, abdomen, anterior aspects of the thighs, or the scapular area on the upper back.
- Pinch the skin to inject as a general rule.
- For an average-weight or thin client, inject at a 45° angle. For an obese client, inject at a 90° angle.

- Aspiration is optional, but do not aspirate when injecting heparin or insulin.
- Do not massage the site.

Choosing a Subcutaneous Site

Avoid sites of abnormal subcutaneous tissue, such as areas lying beneath burns. birthmarks, inflamed tissue, or scars. Do not use sites with lesions or sites over bony prominences, large underlying vessels, or nerves. When using the abdominal site, do not inject any closer than 5 cm (2 inches) from the umbilicus. For repeated injections, rotate sites to minimize tissue damage, aid absorption, and decrease discomfort.

Choosing a Subcutaneous Needle

As a general rule, use a syringe with a short (3/8 to 5/8 inch) and small (25- to 30-gauge) needle; insert a 5/8 inch needle at a 45° angle; insert a 3/8 inch needle at a 90° angle. Vary the needle length and angle of insertion according to how much subcutaneous tissue the client has (e.g. for an obese patient you might use a 1 inch needle). The following are two methods of determining needle length and angle of insertion:

- Pinch up the tissue, and choose a needle length that is half the width of the pinched-up skin.
- Or, if you can grasp 2 inches of tissue, insert the needle at a 90° angle to ensure that it enters subcutaneous tissue; if you can grasp only 1 inch of tissue, insert at a 45° angle.

Administering a Subcutaneous (SC) Injection (Fig. 20.14)

Subcutaneous tissue lies between the epidermis and the muscle. Because there is subcutaneous tissue all over the body, various sites used for 'subcutaneous injection'. These sites are the outer aspect of the arm, anterior aspect of the thigh, lower abdominal

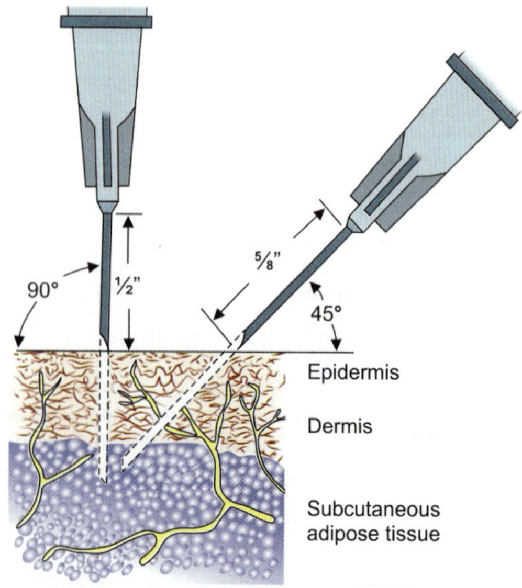

Figure 20.14: Administering subcutaneous injection

<table>
<tr><td colspan="4" align="center">Table 20.7: Procedures for Administering Subcutaneous Injection</td></tr>
<tr><td colspan="2">Nursing actions</td><td colspan="2">Rationales</td></tr>
<tr><td>1.</td><td>Assemble the equipment and check the physician order.</td><td>1.</td><td>This ensures that the client receives the right medication at the right time by right route.</td></tr>
<tr><td>2.</td><td>Explain the procedure to the client.</td><td>2.</td><td>An explanation encourages client cooperation and reduces apprehension.</td></tr>
<tr><td>3.</td><td>Wash your hands.</td><td>3.</td><td>It deters the spread of microorganism.</td></tr>
<tr><td>4.</td><td>If necessary, withdraw medication from an ampule or vial.</td><td></td><td></td></tr>
<tr><td>5.</td><td>Identify the client carefully close curtain to provide privacy on disposable gloves.</td><td>5.</td><td>It is the nurse's responsibility to guard against error. Gloves act as a barrier and protect the nurse's hands from accidental exposure to bleed during procedure.</td></tr>
<tr><td>6.</td><td>Have the client assume a position appropriate for the site selected.
(a) Outer aspect of upper arm-the client's arm should be relaxed and at the side of the body.
(b) Anterior thigh-the client may sit or lie with the leg relaxed.
(c) Abdomen-the client may lie to semirecumbent position.
(d) Scapular-the client may be prone, onside or in a sitting position.</td><td>6.</td><td>Injection into a tense muscle causes discomfort.</td></tr>
<tr><td>7.</td><td>Locate the site of choice, according to directions given. Ensure that the area is not tender and is free of lumps or nodules.</td><td>7.</td><td>Good visualization is necessary to establish the correct location of the site. This avoids damage to the tissues. Nodules or lumps may indicate a previous injection site where absorption was inadequate.</td></tr>
<tr><td>8.</td><td>Clean the area around the injection site with an alcohol swab. Use a firm, circular motion while moving outward from the injection site. Allow the antiseptic to dry. Leave the alcohol swab in a dean area for reuse when withdrawing the needle.</td><td>8.</td><td>Friction helps to clean skin. A clean area is contaminated when a solid object is rubbed over its surface.</td></tr>
<tr><td>9.</td><td>Remove the needle cap with the nondominant hand, pulling it straight off.</td><td>9.</td><td>The cap protects the needle from contact with microorganism. This technique lessens the risk of an accidental needlestick.</td></tr>
<tr><td>10.</td><td>Group and bunch the area surround the injection site or spread the skin at the site.</td><td>10.</td><td>This provides for easy, less painful entry into the subcutaneous tissue. The decision to pinch or spread tissue at time of injection depends on the size of the client. If the client is obese, skin needs to be bunched to allow the needle to penetrate below the fatty layer in the SC tissue.</td></tr>
<tr><td>11.</td><td>Hold the syringe in the dominant hand between the thumb and forefinger. Inject the needle quickly at an angle at 45° to 90°, depending upon the amount and turgor of the tissue and the length of the needle (Fig. 20.14).</td><td>11.</td><td>Subcutaneous tissue is abundant in well-nourished, well-hydrated persons and space is emaciated, dehydrated of very thin persons.</td></tr>
<tr><td>12.</td><td>After the needle is in place, release the tissue and immediately move your non dominant hand to steady the lower end of the syringe. Slide your dominant hand to the tip of the barrel.</td><td>12.</td><td>Injecting the solution into compressed tissue results in pressure against nerve fibers and creates discomfort. The nondominant hand secures the syringe and allows for smooth aspiration.</td></tr>
<tr><td>13.</td><td>Aspirate by pulling back gently on the plunger of the syringe to determine whether the needle is in a blood vessel (optional). If blood appears, the needle should be withdrawn, and the medication syringe, e.g. needles are discarded and new syringe with new medication prepared (heparin should be aspirated).</td><td>13.</td><td>Discomfort and possibly a serious reaction may occur if a drug intended for subcutaneous use is injected into a view. Heparin is an anticoagulant and may cause bruising if aspirated. Aspiration is recommended for children, thin adults, and athletic individuals who may have more superficial blood vessels.</td></tr>
<tr><td>14.</td><td>If no blood appears, inject the solution slowly.</td><td>14.</td><td>Rapid injection of the solution creates pressure in the tissues resulting in discomfort.</td></tr>
</table>

Contd...

Table 20.7: *Contd...*			
	Nursing actions		*Rationales*
15.	Withdraw the needle quickly at the same angle at which it was inserted.	15.	Slow withdrawal of the needles pulls the tissues and causes discomfort. Applying counter-reaction around the injection site helps to prevent pulling on the tissue as the needle is withdrawn. Removing the needle at the same angle at which act was inserted to minimize tissue damage and discomfort to client.
16.	Massage the area gently with the alcohol swab (Do not massage a SC heparin or insulin site).	16.	Massaging helps to distribute the solution and hastens its absorption. Massaging the site of heparin injection causes additional brushing. Massaging, after insulin injection may contribute to unpredictable absorption medication.
17.	Do not recap the used needle. Discard the needle and syringe in the appropriate receptile.	17.	Proper disposal of the needle protects the nurse from accidental agents. Most accidental puncture wounds occur when recapping needles.
18.	Assist the client to position of comfort.	18.	This provides for the well-being of the client.
19.	Remove gloves and dispose them properly and wash hands.	19.	It deters spread of microorganisms.
20.	Chart the administration of medication.	20.	Accurate documentation is necessary to prevent medication error.
21.	Evaluate the response of the client to medication within an appropriate timeframe.	21.	Reaction to medication given by the parental route may occur within 15 to 30 minutes after injection.

wall, and upper back. This route is used for administering insulin, heparin and for certain immunizations. The equipment used for SC injection depends upon medication to be given. For insulin, insulin syringe; for heparin, tuberculin syringe is used. A ½ to 1½, 25 gauge needle is used for this route. The equipment needed and procedures for administering subcutaneous injection are as follows (Table 20.7).

- Medication
- Medication cart
- A sterile syringe needle
- Alcohol swab
- Disposable gloves

Prepacked Medications (Fig. 20.15)

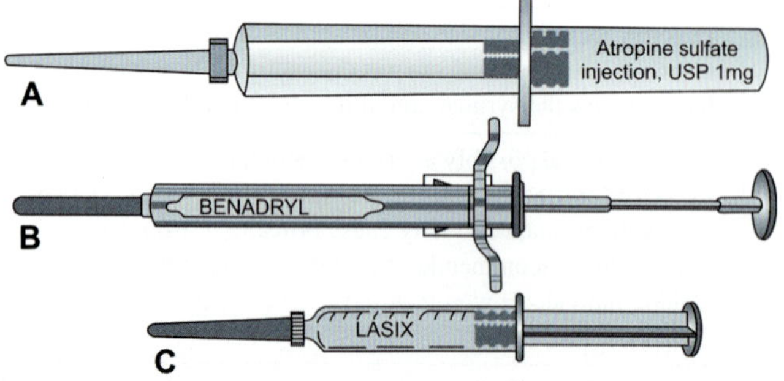

Figures 20.15A to C: Types of prepacked medications. A. Emergency medications are available in prefilled cartridges for use with a plastic barrel and attached needle. B. Reusable metal or plastic syringes are used with prefilled medication cartridges. C. Commonly used medications are available in convenient prefilled syringes

Reusing Needles and Syringes

Many people (e.g. those who have diabetes) must give themselves repeated injections, perhaps several each day. Supplies for home use are expensive. Insurance may or may not cover the cost, or the person may not have insurance. Therefore, although manufacturers recommend that disposable syringes and needles be used only once, some people find it practical to reuse needles and syringes.

- Assess the patient to determine that he is capable of safely recapping a syringe. This requires adequate vision, manual dexterity, and no obvious tremor.
- Assess for contraindications to needle reuse. Patients with poor personal hygiene, an acute illness, open wounds on the hands, or decreased resistance to infection should not reuse a syringe or needle.
- Instruct the patient in a recapping technique: Hold the syringe in one hand, and with the other, replace the cap with a straight motion of the thumb. Advise the patient not to guide both the needle and cap to meet in midair, because this frequently results in needlestick injury.

Teach your patient the following:
- Consult your healthcare provider before beginning this practice.
- Discard needles when they become dull. (Usually they cannot be used more than 10 times)
- Examine the needle carefully before reusing it. The new 30- and 31-gauge needles can easily be bent at the tip to form a hook, which can lacerate tissue or break off within the skin. Never reuse a needle that is deformed in any way.

- Do not reuse a needle if it has come in contact with any thing other than the skin.
- Recap the needle immediately after use if you plan to use it again.
- Do not use alcohol to cleanse the needle. Alcohol may remove the silicon coating that makes for less painful skin puncture.
- The syringe and needle may be stored at room temperature. The potential benefits or risks of refrigerating the syringe are unknown.
- Be aware that reusing needles and syringes increases the risk of infection, although most insulin preparations have bacteriostatic additives that inhibit growth of bacteria commonly found on the skin.
- Inspect injection sites for redness or swelling. If these signs are present, do not reuse a needle; consult your healthcare provider.
- Never share syringes or needles with another person. This poses a risk of acquiring a bloodborne viral infection (e.g. hepatitis).
- Dispose of needles safely. Do not bend or break a needle; doing so increases the chance of injury. Use a coffee can or other puncture-proof container with a lid to dispose of needles.

The medication you are giving influences your choice of syringe. Recall that there are special insulin syringes and that you will use a tuberculin syringe or prefilled cartridge when giving heparin. Inject only small amounts (0.5 to 1 mL) of water-soluble medication subcutaneously to avoid creating sterile abscesses (hardened, painful lumps under the skin).

Administering Insulin

Insulin must be administered subcutaneously or intravenously because it is a protein and would be destroyed in the gastrointestinal tract. Recall that insulin is administered using a special insulin syringe (Fig. 20.16). The physician will prescribe the number of units rather than the number of milliliters or milligrams. Insulin vials contain 100 units/mL. Insulin may be ordered in specific dosages at specific times or by a sliding scale. A sliding scale prescribes the dosage on the basis of the patient's blood glucose level. For example:

Give regular insulin subQ:

4 units for glucose 200 to 240 mg/dL

6 units for glucose 241 to 250 mg/dL

8 units for glucose 251 to 300 mg/dL

For glucose 300 mg/dL or higher, notify physician

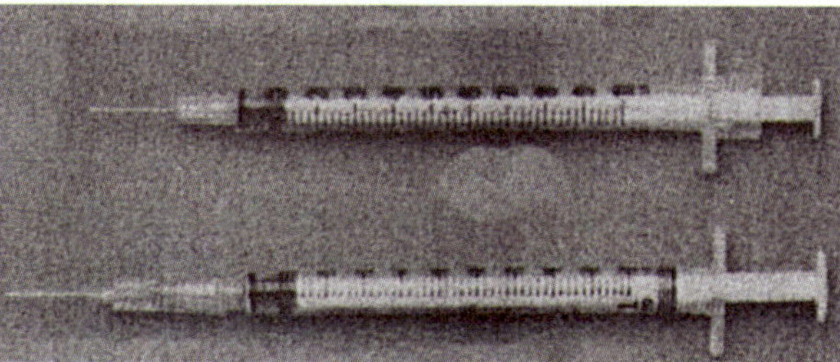

Figure 20.16: Insulin syringe

Regular (unmodified) insulin is rapid acting. It is a clear solution. Other types of insulin (e.g. Lente, semi-Lente, and neutral protamine hagedorn [NPH]) are cloudy because of the addition of proteins, which slow the absorption of the drug, giving the insulin an intermediate to long duration of action. If a vial of regular insulin is cloudy, you should discard it. Insulin is potent for 1 month after the vial is opened.

As a rule, remember "clear before cloudy"; that is, draw up the regular (clear) insulin first, and then draw up the modified (cloudy) insulin. Actually, though, you will rarely need to mix insulins because stable premixed insulins are available (e.g. 70% NPH and 30% regular, or 50% of each).

People with diabetes usually administer their own insulin injections. They should rotate injection sites to promote absorption and minimize tissue damage. Insulin is absorbed at different rates from different parts of the body, so the client should rotate injections within an anatomical area. For example, if the morning dose of insulin is given in the abdomen, the evening insulin should also be given in the abdomen, but at least 2.5 cm (1 inch) away from the morning site. The injection site should not be used again for at least 1 month. For hospitalized patients, you should document site rotation (usually on a diagram of the body) to prevent repeated use of the same site.

Administering Heparin

Heparin is a fast-acting medication that interrupts the blood clotting process. It may be used for clients at risk for clot formation, for example, those who are immobile after major surgery, have undergone vascular surgery, or have problems related to blood clotting, such as cerebrovascular accident (stroke) or myocardial infarction (heart attack). Because heparin is absorbed poorly from the gastrointestinal tract, it is given intravenously or subcutaneously. If mistakenly given intramuscularly, it will cause hematoma and pain. Dosage is based on the patient's weight and results of blood coagulation studies, so always check laboratory values for coagulation studies before giving.

Give the injection deep into the subcutaneous tissue of the abdomen, at least 5 cm (2 inches) away from the umbilicus. Rotate sites, as with insulin administration. Because of the anticoagulant properties of heparin, you will need to modify your injection technique. Primarily, this means:

- Add 0.2 mL air after drawing up the correct dose.
- Do not aspirate before injecting the patient.
- Do not massage the site after the injection.

Intramuscular Injections

Intramuscular injections (injections into muscle tissue) are absorbed faster than subcutaneous medications because of the rich blood supply in the muscles. Muscles can also tolerate more fluid-you can give as much as 3 or 4 mL of liquid in the large vastus lateralis and ventrogluteal muscles. The smaller the muscle, the less fluid it can tolerate. For example, you should usually give no more than 0.5 to 1 mL in the average deltoid muscle.

A disadvantage of this route is that there a risk of inadvertently injecting a medication into a blood vessel; therefore, always aspirate before injecting an IM medication. You should know, however, that there are no research data to document the necessity of aspirating. Nevertheless, most experts recommend it on a theoretical basis to ensure that the needle tip is not in a blood vessel.

Choosing an Intramuscular Site

When selecting an IM site, you should look for a site that is:
- A safe distance from nerves, large blood vessels, and bones
- Free from injury, abscesses, tenderness, necrosis, abrasion, or other pathology
- Large enough to accommodate the volume of medication to be given

Muscles that have commonly been used are ventrogluteal, deltoid, vastus lateralis, rectus femoris, and dorsogluteal. However, the rectus femoris and dorsogluteal are no longer recommended sites, and they should be used only if other sites are not available. Advantages and disadvantages of each site are given in the following sections. The critical aspects are as follows:
- Always palpate the landmarks and the muscle mass to ensure correct placement.
- *Deltoid:* The injection site is an inverted triangle. The base is two to three fingerbreadths below the acromion process, and the tip is even with the top of the axilla.
- *Vastus lateralis:* Midlateral thigh: On adults, one handbreadth below the head of the trochanter and one handbreadth above the knee. The site is the middle third of this area. This is the preferred site for infants under 7 months.
- *Ventrogluteal:* On adults, a triangle formed between your fingers when you place your palm on the head of the trochanter, index finger on the anterior superior iliac spine, and middle finger on the iliac crest. This is the preferred site for adults and children over 7 months.
- *Dorsogluteal:* Locate the site by drawing an imaginary line between the head of the trochanter and the posterior superior iliac spine. At the middle of the line, go up approximately 1 inch. Use this site only if no others are accessible.
- *Rectus femoris:* Middle third of the anterior thigh. Use this site only if no others are accessible.

Choosing an Intramuscular Needle (Fig. 20.17)

Although a 1½ inch needle is considered "standard" for intramuscular injections, you should choose the needle gauge and length based on the size of the muscle, the amount of medication to be given, and the amount of adipose tissue over the muscle. In the deltoid muscle, for example, you might use a 23- or 25-gauge, I-inch needle. But if the solution is viscous,

you would need a larger needle (e.g. 20-gauge). For a very thin person, you could use a 1-inch needle, even when injecting into the larger muscles. For an obese person, you might need a needle as long as 3 inches to penetrate adipose tissue and reach the muscle (unfortunately, long needles may not be available in some settings). As a rule, the angle of insertion for an intramuscular injection is 90º.

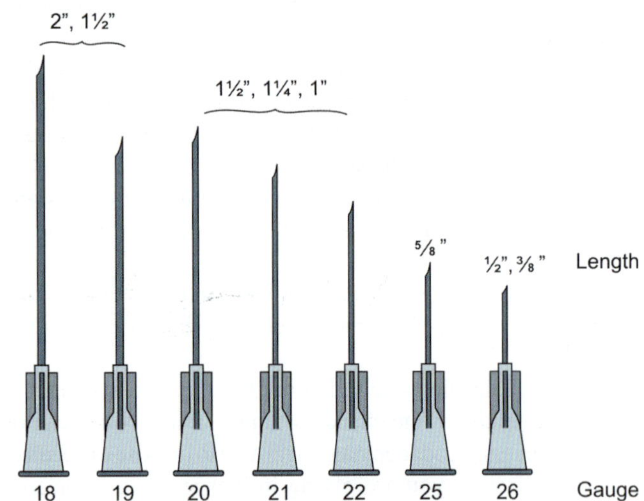

Figure 20.17: Needle gauges and lengths. Each gauge is supplied in a limited number of lengths

Z-Track Technique (Fig. 20.18)

The procedure for using the Z-track technique for intramuscular injections. This technique seals the needle track and prevents medication from leaking out of the muscle up through the needle track and into the subcutaneous tissues. You must use this technique for irritating medications, such as Vistaril and iron. It is recommended for all intramuscular injections, because it is less painful and helps to prevent irritation of subcutaneous tissues. For this technique, it is best to use the larger muscles: the ventrogluteal, vastus lateralis, and dorsogluteal sites. (Use the dorsogluteal site only if other sites are not available.)

Ventrogluteal Muscle–Site of Choice (Figs 20.19A to C)

Whenever possible, use the ventrogluteal site for intramuscular injections; it is the site of choice of adults and infants over 7 to 12 months old (Figs 20.24A and B). The ventrogluteal site, located on the lateral muscles (Fig. 20.19). Because it is located away from major blood vessels and nerves, it is the safest and least painful site for intramuscular injections. This site is also less likely to be contaminated if the patient is incontinent.

When learning to locate this site, many students notice that it feels "hard" to palpation and worry that the needle will hit the bone. In part, the muscle feels hard because there is little subcutaneous tissue over it. To reassure yourself that it is safe, examine a skeleton model with the muscles attached. Notice that the ilium is concave (curves in) and that the muscle lies

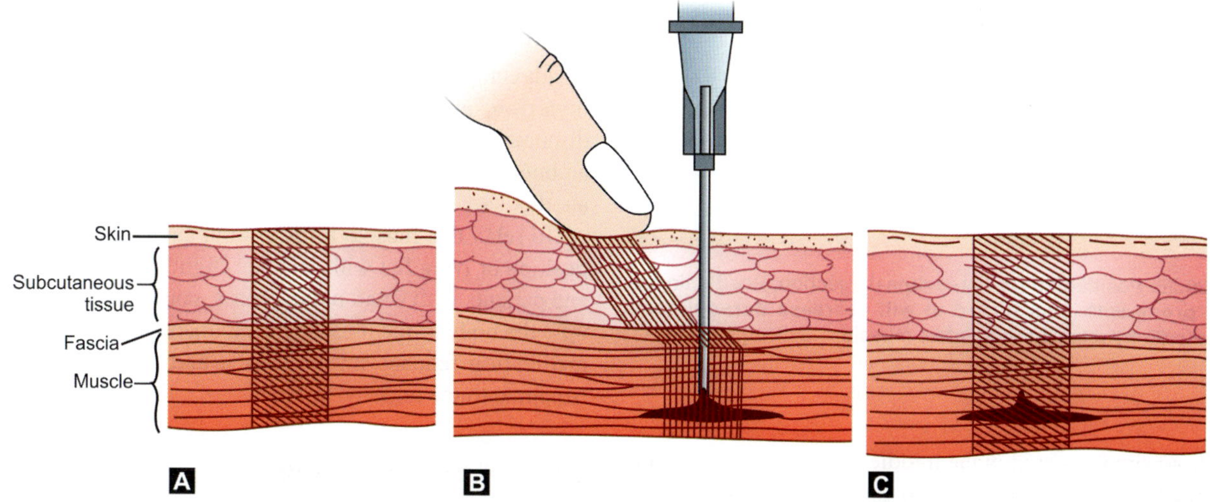

Figures 20.18A to C: Z-track technique. A. Normal tissue relationship prior to injection. B. Altered tissue relationship during injection. Retract tissue, insert needle, administer injection, wait 10 seconds, remove needle, and release tissue. C. Normal relationship following injection. Note: angled "Z" track left by needle

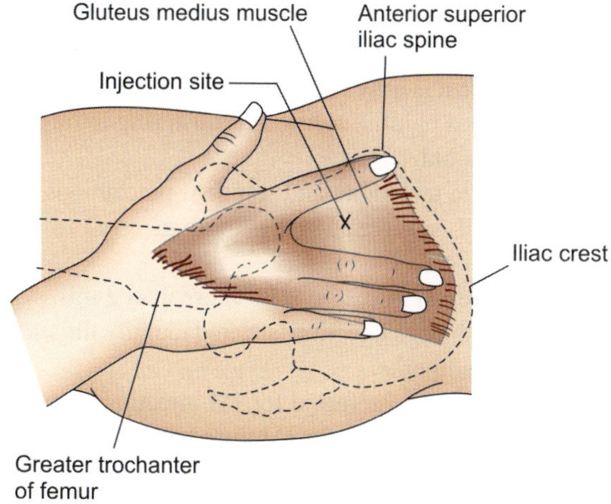

Figure 20.19A: Ventrogluteal injection site in a supine client

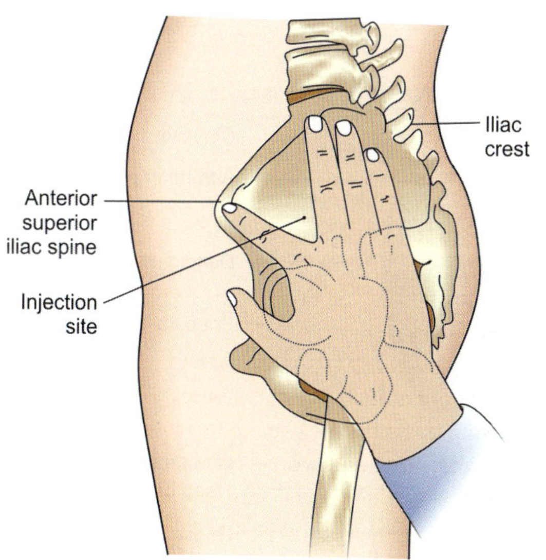

Figure 20.19B: Locating the ventrogluteal site

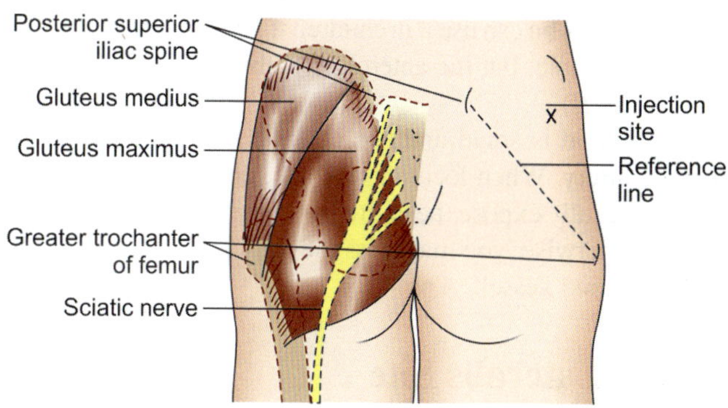

Figure 20.19C: Ventrogluteal injection site

deep down in the "cup" it forms. If you are sure you have located the anterosuperior iliac spine and if you follow the procedure steps, you will not hit a bone. In fact, you are less likely to do so than if you use other sites.

Dorsogluteal Site (Fig. 20.20)

The dorsogluteal site consists of the gluteal muscles of the buttocks (Figs 20.25A and B). Because of its close proximity to the sciatic nerve and superior gluteal artery, we do not recommend this site for use; it is always contraindicated for use in infants or children. Using this site increases the risk of injection into a major blood vessel, as well as damage to the sciatic nerve, which can cause permanent or partial paralysis of the leg involved. Furthermore, the site is difficult to identify accurately in older adults or people with flabby skin. We include this site only because you may rarely encounter a patient in whom all of the other sites are unusable.

You may observe in your practice that some nurses continue to use the dorsogluteal site because they were taught to use it long ago and have not learned how to locate the ventrogluteal site. This gives you the opportunity to improve practice by demonstrating correct technique for locating the preferred site.

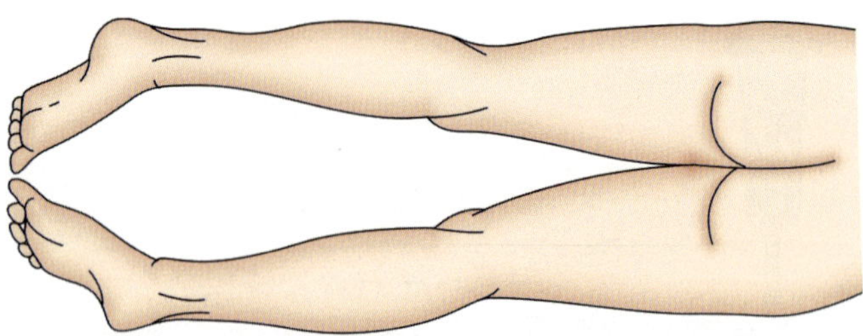

Figure 20.20: Positioning for dorsogluteal injection. Positioning a person prone with toes turned in will decrease dorsogluteal injection pain by relaxing the gluteal muscle

Deltoid Site

The deltoid site is located in the middle third of the upper arm (Fig. 20.21). The area has a small muscle mass with little subcutaneous tissue, so medications are absorbed rapidly. This muscle is easily accessible but is not well developed in many adults; so, you should use it only for small amounts of up to ½ to 1 mL or when other sites are inaccessible. Avoid using the deltoid site in infants; you can use it in children if you are sure the muscle mass is adequate, but the anterolateral thigh is preferred (Figs 20.28A and B).

The deltoid is small and lies close to the radial nerve and brachial artery. When locating this site, do not merely roll up the sleeve; fully expose the entire upper arm and shoulder (Fig. 20.29). Otherwise, you may miss the muscle mass and injure a nerve or blood vessel.

Vastus Lateralis Site

The vastus lateralis muscle, located in the anterolateral thigh (Fig. 20.22), is another site used for adults, and it is the preferred site for infants and children (Figs 20.26A and B) (Saari & Committee on Infectious Diseases, 2003). Its main advantage is that drugs are rapidly absorbed from this area. Moreover, it can

accommodate a larger volume of medication than the deltoid, and it is not near any major blood vessels or nerves. A disadvantage is that the patient can see you administer the injection, and the psychological effect may create some discomfort. Also, because this muscle is used in walking, an ambulatory client may notice more residual soreness than in another site.

To relax this muscle for injection, have the client in sitting position or lying flat with his knee slightly flexed. For children and patients with small muscle mass, you should grasp ("pinch up") the body of the muscle during injection to be sure that the medication reaches muscle tissue and the needle does not penetrate to the underlying bone.

Rectus Femoris Site

The rectus femoris site, located in the anterior thigh, is no longer recommended for infants and children. You may occasionally use it for adults when rapid absorption is needed or other sites are inaccessible (Figs 20.27A and B). This area contains no large blood vessels or nerves, so it is safe for intramuscular injections. It is often used by clients who self-administer their intramuscular injections because it is easy for them to reach. A disadvantage is that it is sometimes painful. While administering intramuscular injections you should

- Maintain sterile technique and standard precautions.
- Use a 1 to 3 mL syringe and a 21- to 25-gauge, 1 to 1½ inch needle.
- The usual dose per injection is no more than 3 mL.
- Select an appropriate injection site, and identify the site using anatomical landmarks:
- Ventrogluteal site is preferred for IM injections.
- Deltoid site is acceptable for IM doses of 1 mL or less.
- Aspirate before injecting. If blood appears, remove the needle, discard it, and start over.
- Inject at a 90° angle.

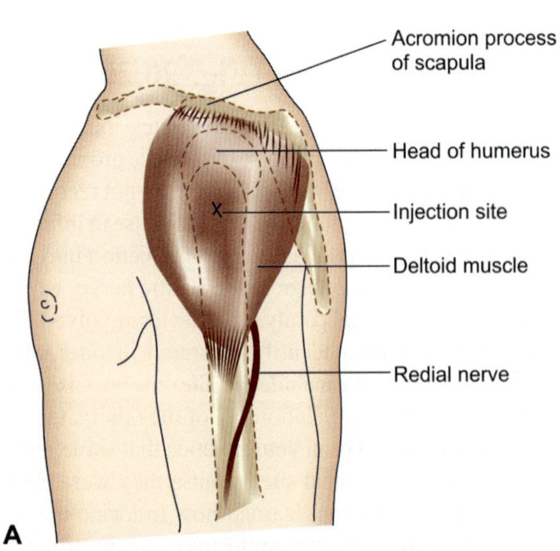

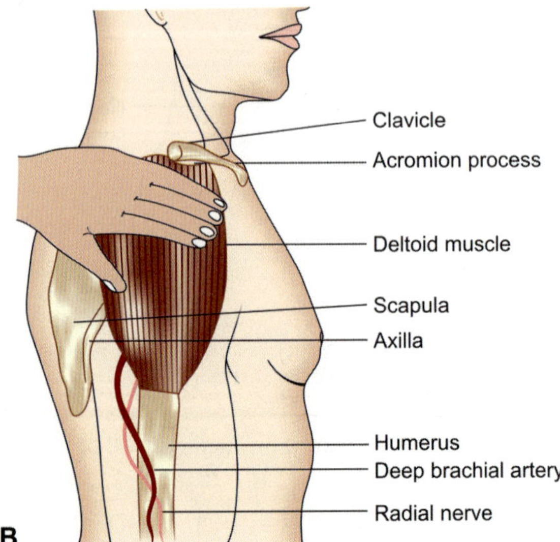

Figure 20.21: Locating the deltoid site

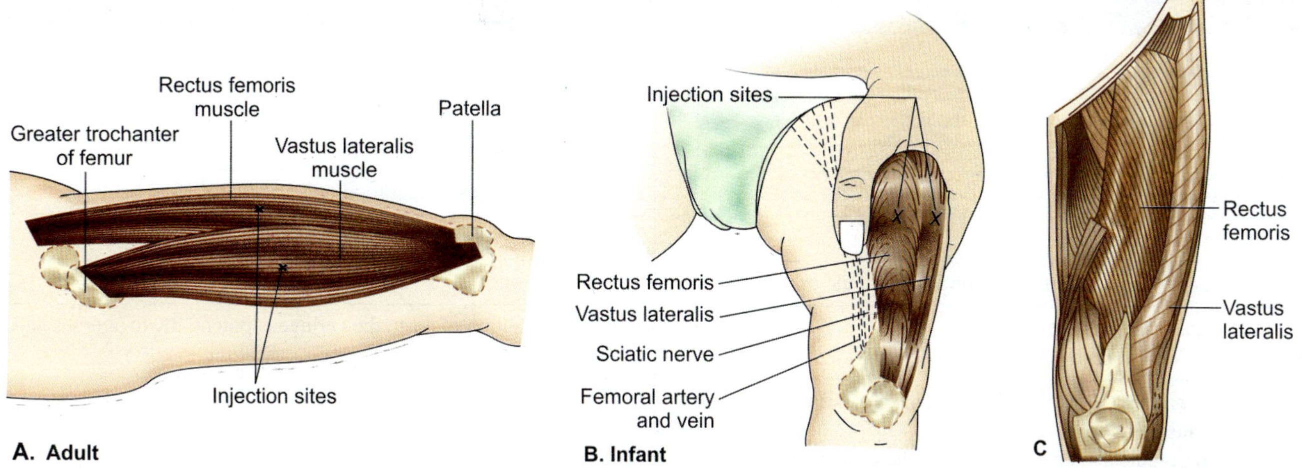

Figure 20.22: Locating the vastus lateralis site

- Z-track technique is recommended. Mnemonic:

Deliver	**D**isplace
All	**A**spirate
Injections	**I**nject (wait 10 seconds)
With	**W**ithdraw
Responsibility	**R**elease

Administering an Intramuscular (IM) Injection

The intramuscular route often is used for drugs that are irritating because there are few nerve endings in deep muscle tissue. Absorption occurs as in subcutaneous administration but more rapidly because of the greater vascularity of muscle tissue. The amount of 4 mL is considered the maximum to be given in one site for an adult with well-developed muscles. An important point to note while administering IM injection is the selection of safe site; one that is away from large nerves, bone and blood vessels. When care is not taken, common complications include abscesses, necroses and skin slough nerve injuries, lingering pain, and periostitis. The site for injecting intramuscular medication should be routed when therapy required repeated injection. The usual sites for IM injection are ventrogluteal, dorsogluteal, vastus lateral is, rectus femoris and deltoid muscle. The procedures and equipment needed for administering an intramuscular injection are as follows (Table 20.8):

- Medication
- Medication chart
- Sterile syringe and needle
- Alcohol swab
- Dry sponge
- Disposable gloves

General guidelines to reduce discomfort in subcutaneous and intramuscular administration of medication are as follows:

- Select a needle of the smallest gauge that is appropriate for the site and solution to be injected and select the correct needle length
- Be sure the needle is free of medication that may irritate superficial tissues as the needle is inserted. Recommended procedure is to use two needles, one to remove the medication from the vial or ampule and a second one to inject the

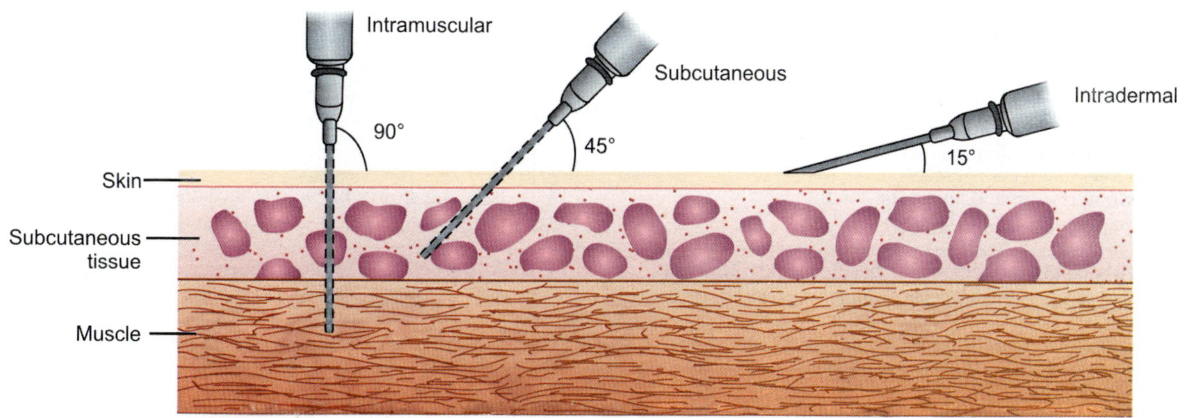

Figure 20.23: Different degrees of angle of administering medication (IM, SC, ID)

Table 20.8: Procedures for Administering Intramuscular Injections

	Nursing actions		*Rationales*
1.	Assemble equipment and check the physician's order.	1.	This ensures that the client receives the right medication at right time by right route.
2.	Explain the procedures to the client.	2.	It encourages cooperation and eliminates apprehension.
3.	Wash your hands.	3.	It deters spread of microorganism.
4.	If necessary, withdraw medication from ampule or vial.		
5.	Do not add air to the syringe.	5.	The addition of air to the syringe is potentially dangerous and may result in an overdose of medication.
6.	Provide privacy. Have the client assume a position appropriate for the site selected: (a) Ventrogluteal–a client may lie on the back or side with the tip hip and knee flexed. (b) Dorsogluteal–a client may be prone with toes tainting inward or on the side with the upper leg flexed and placed in front of the lower leg. (c) Vastus lateralis–the client may lie on the back or may assume a sitting position. (d) Deltoid–the client may sit or lie with arm relaxed.	6.	Injection into a tense muscle causes discomfort.
7.	Locate the site of choice according to direction and ensure that the area is non-tender and free of lumps or nodules. Don disposable gloves (Fig. 20.23).	7.	Good visualization is necessary to establish the correct location of the site and avoid damages to tissues. Nodules or lumps may indicate previous injection side, where absorption was inadequate. Gloves act as a barrier and protects nurse's hands from accidental exposure to blood.
8.	Clean the area thoroughly with an alcohol swab, using friction. Allow alcohol to dry.	8.	Path of germs present on the skin and alcohol can be forced into the tissue by the needle.
9.	Remove the needle cap by pulling it straight off.	9.	The cap protects the needle from contact with microorganism. This technique lessens the risk of accidental needlestick.
10.	Displace the skin in a Z-track manner or spread the skin at the site using your nondominant hand.	10.	This makes the tissue tact the minimized discomfort. Z-track prevents seepage of the medication into the needle track and is less painful.
11.	Hold the syringe in your dominant hand between the thumb and forefinger. Quickly dart the needle into the tissue at a 90° angle.	11.	A quick injection is less painful. Inserting the needle at a 90° angle facilitate entry into muscle tissue.
12.	As soon as the needle is in place, use your nondominant hand to hold the lower end of the syringe. Slide your dominant hand to the tip of the barrel.	12.	This acts to steady the syringe and allows for smooth aspiration.
13.	Aspirate by slowly (for at least 9 seconds) pulling back on the plunger to determine whether the needle is in a blood vessel. If blood is aspirated, discard the needle and syringe and medication. Prepare new medication with new sterile syringe needle and look for another site.	13.	Discomfort and possibly a serious reaction may occur if a drug intended for IM use as injected into a hard or tender areas. Allowing at least 5 seconds for aspiration facilitates back flow of blood even if needle is small, low flow blood vessel.
14.	If no blood is aspirated, inject the solution slowly (10 seconds) per mL of medication.	14.	Injecting slowly helps to reduce discomfort by allowing time for the solution to disperse in the tissues.
15.	Wait 10 seconds and remove the needle quickly. Release displaced tissue if Z-track technique was used.	15.	A 10 seconds delay allows the medication to begin to be diffused through muscle. Removing the needle quickly is less painful.
16.	Apply gentle pressure at the site with a small, dry sponge.	16.	Light pressure causes less fravima and irritation to the tissues.

Contd...

<table>
<tr><td colspan="2" align="center">**Table 20.8:** *Contd...*</td></tr>
<tr><td>*Nursing actions*</td><td>*Rationales*</td></tr>
<tr><td>17. Do not recap the used needle. Discard the needle and syringe in the appropriate receptile.</td><td>17. Proper disposal of the needle protects the nurse from accidental injuries. Most accidental puncture wound occurs when recapping.</td></tr>
<tr><td>18. Assist the client to a position of comfort, encourage client to exercise leg, if possible.</td><td>18. Exercise promotes absorption of the medication.</td></tr>
<tr><td>19. Remove gloves and dispose them properly. Wash hands.</td><td>19. This deters to spread of microorganism.</td></tr>
<tr><td>20. Chart the administration of medication.</td><td>20. Accurate documentation is necessary to prevent medication error.</td></tr>
<tr><td>21. Evaluate the client response to the medication within an appropriate timeframe. Assess site, if possible within 2-4 hours after administration.</td><td>21. Reaction to medication given by the parenteral route is possible. Assessment also allows for visualization of the site for any untoward effects.</td></tr>
</table>

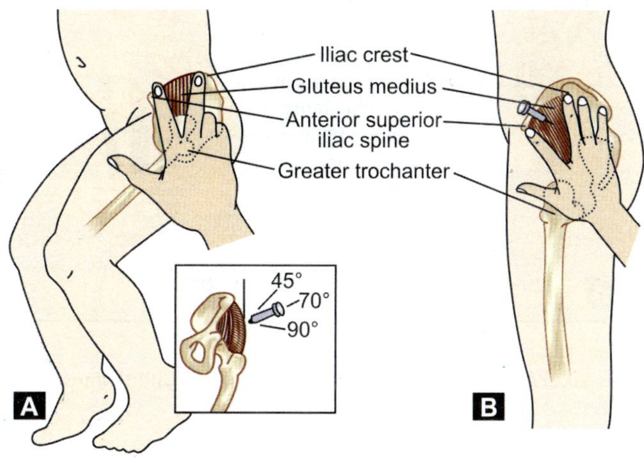

Figures 20.24A and B: Ventrogluteal site: A. Child/infant, B. Adult

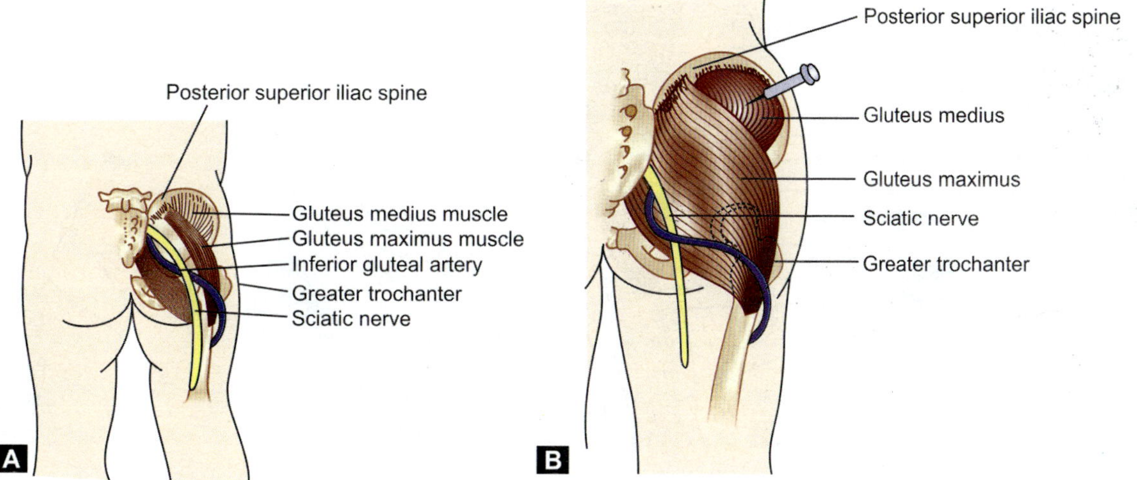

Figures 20.25A and B: Dorsogluteal site: A. Child/infant, B. Adult

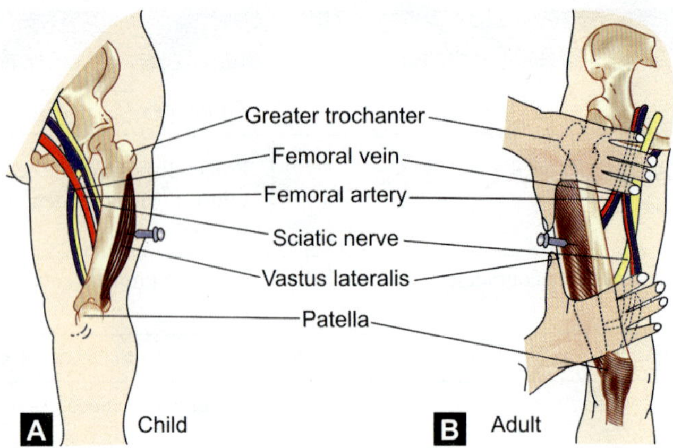

Figures 20.26A and B: Vastus lateralis: A. Child/infant, B. Adult

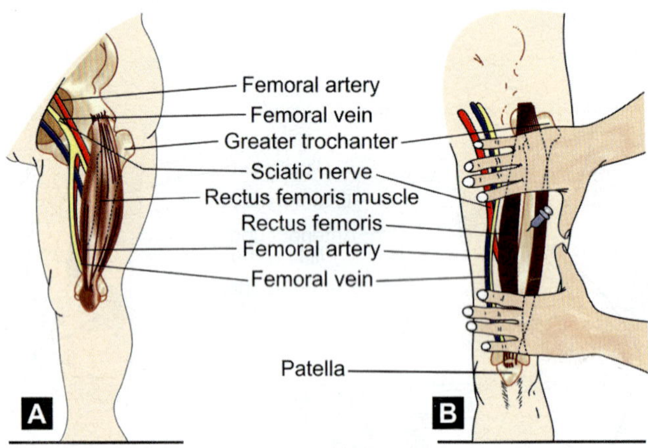

Figures 20.27A and B: Rectus femoris muscle: A. Child/infant, B. Adult

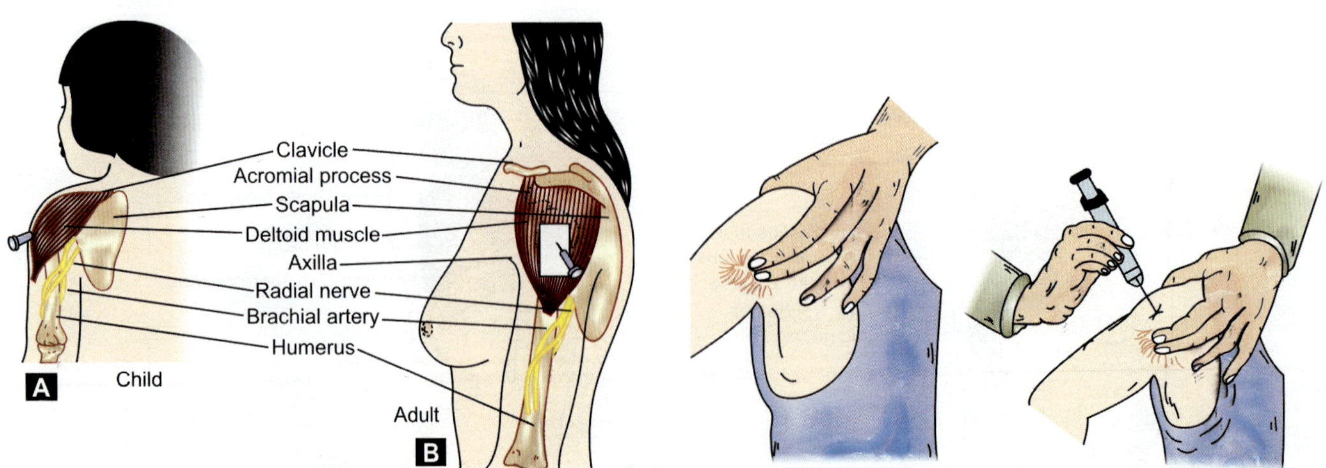

**Figures 20.28A and B: Deltoid muscle site:
A. Child/infant, B. Adult**

Figure 20.29: Technique of intramuscular injection

medication, if medication is in a prefilled syringes with a nonremovable needle and has dripped back on the needle dummy preparation and dry needle with sterile gauge

- Use the Z-track technique for intramuscular injections to prevent leakage of medication into the needle track, thus minimizing the client's discomfort
- Inject the medication into relaxed musculature. There is more pressure and discomfort when the medication if injected into a contracted muscle
- Do not inject areas that feel hard on palpation or tender to the client
- Insert the needle with a darlike motion without hesitation, and remove it quickly at the same ample at which it was inserted. These techniques help to reduce discomfort and tissue irritation
- Do not administer more solution in one injection than is recommended for the site. Injecting more solution creates excess pressure in the area and increases discomfort
- Inject the solution slowly so that it may be dispersed more easily into the surrounding tissue (10 second/1 mL)
- Apply gentle pressure after injection, unless this technique is contraindicated
- Allow the client who is fearful of injections to talk about the fears. Answer the client's questions, truthfully and explain nature and purpose of injection, which reduces fears
- Rotate the sites when the client is to receive repeated injections. Injection On the same sites may cause undue discomfort, irritation and abscesses in tissues.

Teaching Patient about Self-Medication

- Do not take medications prescribed to others, and do not share your medications with others.
- Keep a list of your medications, including doses and times taken. Take this list with you when you visit any physician or an emergency department.
- If you are on a variety of medications, post a list of them in a prominent place for easy access in the event of an emergency.
- Wear a MedicAlert bracelet or necklace if you are a diabetic, take anticoagulants, or have severe allergies.
- When you are prescribed a new medication, ask why you are taking it, what side effects should you expect, whether you should take it with food, and whether there are any special precautions.
- Be sure to read the label carefully on the bottle each time you take the medication so that you take the correct medication. Many pills look alike, and you do not want to take the wrong medication.
- Take only the amount and dose prescribed. If you have questions, call your prescriber.
- To measure liquids, use kitchen measuring spoons rather than tableware, which can vary in volume.
- Take the medication for the prescribed length of time to make certain you receive the full benefit of the drug. For example,

some patients may take only part of an expensive antibiotic, hoping to "save it for later." If you do not take the full course of medication, the infection may recur.

- Notify your prescriber if you have any side effects or adverse reactions.
- Do not store your medication in a different container from the one it came in. The medication may lose its strength, or you may take the wrong medication.
- Store all your medication in a dry place out of the sunlight and away from the heat. If a medication requires a cold storage, be sure you return the medication to the refrigerator immediately after use.
- Check expiration dates, and discard any medications that are outdated.
- Do not take expired medications; they may have lost their strength.
- Do not place expired medications in the trash within the reach of children. Disposing of expired medications in the sink or toilet is not environmentally sound. Some communities sponsor an "old medications discard day" or provide a place to discard them to avoid contamination.
- Use child-proof lids if children have access to your medications.
- Monitor your prescription amounts, and get refills before you run out. If you get medications by mail, be sure you send for them in plenty of time.
- If you become pregnant, notify your physician as soon as possible so your medications can be discontinued or adjusted.

Intravenous Medications

Intravenous medications are given through a catheter or cannula inserted into a vein. The onset of medication action takes place within seconds, so IV administration is especially useful in emergencies. However, because an IV drug begins to act immediately, there is no way for you to stop its action if an adverse reaction occurs.

IV medications may be administered by a variety of programmable electronic pumps and infusers. To prevent complications, when administering IV medications, you should:

- Use scrupulous sterile technique.
- Administer the medication slowly.
- Be aware that in addition to the effects of the medicine, the volume of fluid infused has possible consequences.
- Observe the patient carefully for signs of adverse reactions.
- Have an antidote on hand if the drug has potentially serious side effects.
- Assess the client before, during, and after giving the medication.
- Determine that the drug is compatible with the fluid that is infusing; consult a pharmacist if necessary.
- Determine that the drug is compatible with the plastic IV bag and tubing; you may occasionally, need to use a glass IV bottle and special tubing.
- Observe the insertion site often; ensure that the cannula is in the vein before administering a medication.

Setting Volume to be Infused

When setting the volume to be infused (e.g. 1.000 mL), set It slightly lower (e.g. 950 mL) so the alarm goes off before the fluids are completely gone. This practice provides time to have the next bag of fluids ready when all 1,000 mL has been infused. This is especially helpful when having to warm refrigerated fluids. Report to the next shift that the alarm is set to go off early.

Because venous blood flows upward toward the heart, select a vein for an IV at its most distal end to maintain the integrity of the vein. When a vein is punctured with a needle, fluids can infiltrate (leak from the vein into the tissue at the site of puncture). When IV therapy is discontinued for infiltration, it can only be restarted above the initial puncture site. Generally, it is best to begin with the hand and advance up the arm if new sites are needed. Figure 20.30 illustrates common peripheral sites for initiating IV therapy.

Locating Vein: With the client's arm extended on a firm surface, place a tourniquet on the arm, tight enough to impede venous flow yet loose enough that a radial pulse can still be palpated.

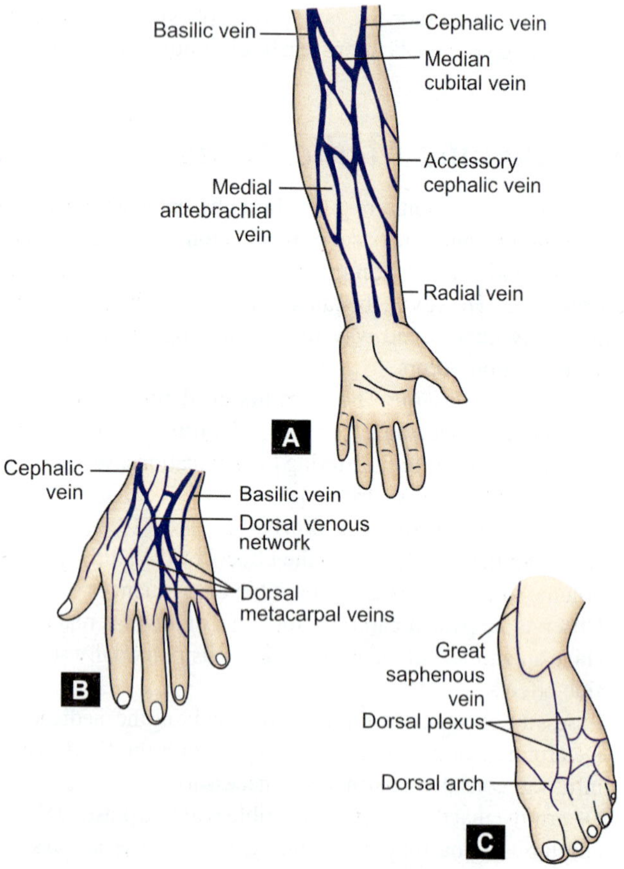

Figure 20.30: Peripheral Veins Used in Intravenous Therapy: A. Forearm; B. Dorsum of the hand; C. Dorsal plexus of the foot

Next, the index and middle fingers of the nondominant hand are used to palpate a vein. It should feel soft and resilient and not have a pulse. If no vein can be seen or felt, a warm, moist compress may be applied for 10 to 20 minutes, the area may be massaged toward the heart, or the client may open and close the fist.

Placing the Needle: After hand hygiene and gloving is completed, prepare the selected site according to agency policy. Without touching the prepared site, stabilize the vein by placing your thumb beside the vein and pulling down. Hold the needle at a 10- to 30-degree angle, bevel up to puncture the skin then lessen the angle to prevent puncturing the back of the vein. Secure the needle in place according to agency policy.

Infection Control: Venipuncture

Administering *IV Therapy:* When the solution has been prepared and the rate calculated, explain the procedure to the client. Administration may be continuous over a 24-hour period, or intermittent, 1,000 mL once in a 24-hour period. Although fluids may be continuous, the type of fluids can change over a 24-hour period. For example, an order might read: Add 40 mEq of KCl to first bag of 1,000 mL of normal saline.

Intravenous medications may be piggybacked, connected to an existing IV to infuse concurrently. Refrigerated solutions and medications should be warmed to room temperature before administration (usually for 30 minutes) for client comfort.

Regulating IV solution Flow Rate: The flow rate for IV solutions can be regulated by calculating the drops per minute and adjusting the drip rate to that number or by the use of volume controllers and pumps.

Volume Controllers and Pumps: Controllers are devices dependent on gravity to maintain a preselected flow but do not add pressure to overcome resistance (e.g. Dial-a-Flo or Buretrol). Resistance may develop from the use of a large catheter in a small vein, high venous pressure, infusing a viscous solution, or a decrease in the height of the container from the IV site.

This chapter will explain how to administer IV medications by (1) adding medication to the large-volume primary or maintenance fluids, (2) IV push or bolus, (3) intermittent infusion (piggyback or tandem setups), and (4) volume-control infusion sets.

Adding Medications to Large-Volume (Primary) Infusions

The safest and easiest way to administer a drug intravenously is to mix it into a bag of fluid that is already infusing. This is often normal saline or lactated Ringer's solution or, sometimes, glucose. Vitamins, potassium chloride, oxytocin (Pitocin), and several blood pressure and cardiovascular drugs are commonly given this way. This method is useful when the drug can be infused continuously over a long period of time or when it must be given continuously to achieve the desired effect. The main disadvantage is the danger of infusing too much fluid, especially for children, older adults, and people with cardiac or renal disease. In some instances, the drug may be premixed with the IV fluid in the pharmacy. Or you may need to add a drug to a bag before you hang it or to one that is already infusing.

A safe method for adding medications to an IV container is to use a *transfer needle* or *cannula*–a blunted plastic needle with a double beveled tip. One end is inserted into the powdered or liquid medication and the other end is inserted into a port of the IV bag. Solution is transferred from the IV bag into the medication vial, which you shake lightly to mix the medication. Then the medication is transferred back into the IV bag for administration.

The critical aspects of adding medications to large-volume infusions is as follows:

- Check the compatibility of the intravenous solution and medication.
- Assess the patency of the intravenous site.
- Maintain the sterility of intravenous fluids and medication admixture.
- Affix the medication label to the bag, with the name and amount of medication, date and time administered, and your name or initials.

IV Push Medications

IV push (bolus) medications are injected undiluted directly into the systemic circulation. Many drugs given by IV push have a package insert that contains specific guidelines for their administration rate (usually between 1 and 10 minutes). It is safer if the physician writes an order specifying the rate (e.g. "IV over 2 minutes") instead of ordering "IV push." Two minutes can seem like a very long time when you are pushing a medication, so don't guess–look at your watch! Take note that "IV push" does not mean the same thing as "give rapidly." If given too rapidly, IV drugs can be quite dangerous.

Because you cannot retrieve the medication once it is injected, there is no margin for error. Observing the six rights will help ensure that you are administering the correct dose and the correct medication.

Because many IV push medications can irritate tissues, you must confirm that the IV cannula is in the vein before injecting the drug. If the medication is accidentally injected into tissues, sloughing, pain, and abscesses may occur. The medications may also be irritating to the lining of the vein, so evaluate the condition of the injection site frequently.

The critical aspects of IV push medications are as follows:
- Determine the type and amount of dilution needed for the medication.
- Determine the amount of time needed to administer the medication.
- Ensure the patency of the line prior to administration.
- Flush the line before and after administering the medication.
- Maintain sterility.

Intermittent Infusion

Many medications, such as antibiotics, are administered intravenously by intermittent infusion. Intermittent infusions may be given through the port of a running IV line or, if the patient does not need the IV fluids, through an intermittent injection port, also called a saline or heparin lock.

Most intermittent infusion medications are supplied in bags containing 50 to 250 mL of 5% dextrose in water (D_5W) or normal saline. The drug is given over a period of time, usually 30 to 60 minutes, and at regular intervals (e.g. every 6 hours). The small bag of diluted medication (the "secondary" bag) is attached to the primary IV infusion line for administration. There are two types of setups for intermittent infusion using a primary IV line:

1. A **tandem setup** is connected to the primary IV line at the lower (secondary) port (Fig. 20.31). The medication can be given intermittently or at the same time as the primary IV infusion-both bags can infuse at the same time.

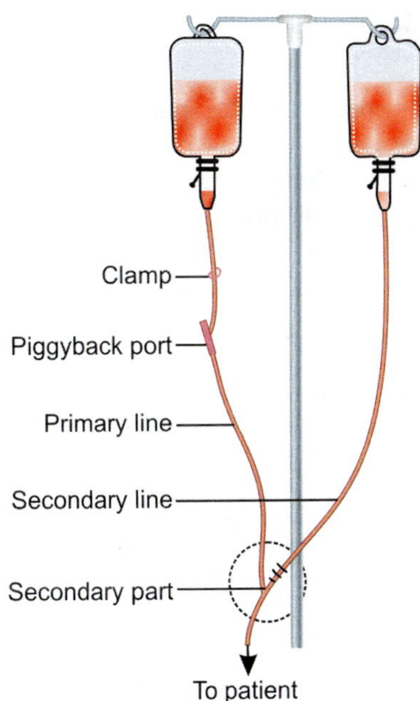

Figure 20.31: A tandem setup is attached to the primary (continuous infusion) IV line at the lower port, allowing for both intermittent and simultaneous infusion

2. With an **IV piggyback setup** the smaller (secondary) container is connected to the primary (continuous) infusion line at the upper (primary) port (Fig. 20.32). This setup allows for intermittent use only.

Traditionally, the secondary tubing was attached to the primary set tubing by inserting a needle into the port and taping it in place most agencies now use needleless systems, which use a threaded or lever-type lock to make the connection. In addition to helping prevent needlestick injuries, a needleless system prevents touch contamination at the IV connection site.

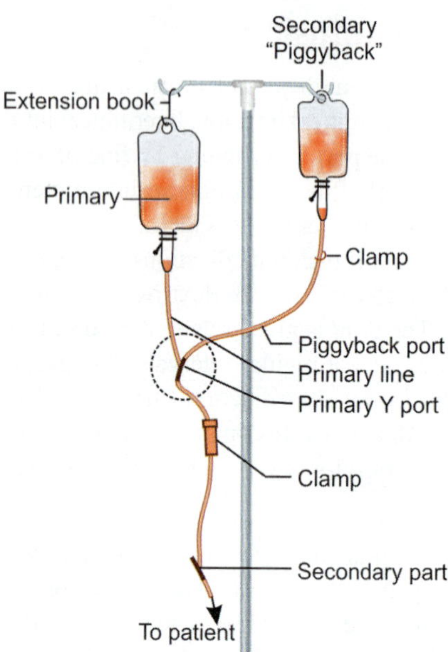

Figure 20.32: A piggyback setup is attached to the primary (continuous infusion) IV line at the upper port, allowing for intermittent infusion only

The critical aspects provides guidelines for administering intermittent infusions as given below:

- Ensure the compatibility of the IV solution and medication, both the solution in the primary IV system and the diluent in the secondary system.
- Assess the IV site and the patency of the line.

- Calculate amount of medication to add to the solution.
- Use the correct amount and type of diluent solution.
- Use the correct rate of administration.
- Determine the correct primary line port in which to infuse the medication.
- Affix the correct label to the secondary bag, with start date and hour, discard date and hour, and your initials.

Volume-Control Infusion Set

To effectively control the infusion of smaller amounts of solutions, particularly with pediatric patients, a volume-control infusion set (e.g. the Buretrol, Soluset, Volutrol, or Pediatol) may be used. These are small fluid containers (100 to 150 mL) that are attached directly below the primary fluid container. The medication and the desired amount of IV fluid are added to the volume-control container and administered through the primary line. This system decreases the risk of overhydration because the amount of fluid that can infuse into the client is limited to the amount that you place in the small container.

Nurse's Responsibilities for Administering Medication

Medications are administered in a variety of ways. Preparing and administering medications require accuracy by the nurse. The nurse must pay full attention in preparing medications and

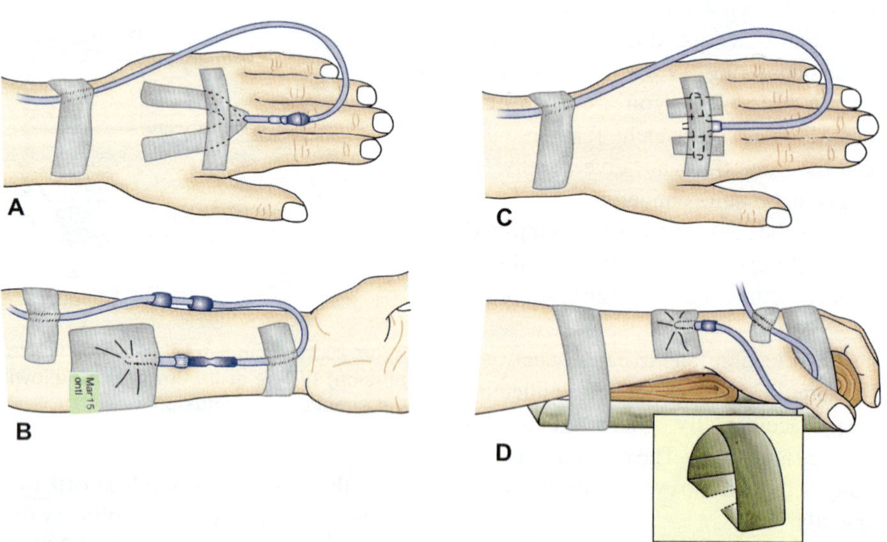

Figures 20.33A to D : Methods of securing intravenous catheters and butterfly needle. (A) Using tape to secure catheter in hand. A ½-inch strip of tape is placed under the hub of the catheter, sticky side up, and then criss-crossed over the top like a chevron stripe. A small bandage is then placed over the top of the tape. The tubing is then taped at one or two places on the arm for additional security. (B) Using transparent dressing to secure the catheter (least recommended). (C) Using tape to secure a butterfly needle. Place one piece of 1-inch tape on each wing in line with the needle and tubing, then place a third piece of tape across the wings, forming an H, or use the chevron method as described in A, placing a piece of tape across the wings. (D) Use an amboard to secure the catheter near a joint. Note the padding to protect the hand and arm. In the inset, note the shorter strip of tape placed in the center of the sticky side of the longer strip to prevent the longer strip of tape from adhering to hair on the arm while the sticky ends of the longer strip remain free to adhere to the armboard

must not attempt to do other tasks simultaneously. The nurse uses the principles or guidelines (which include 'six rights' and 'three label checks' and universal precautions) while administering drug in anyone of the routes. They are as follows:

Six Rights

Six rights refer to give the right medication in the right dose to the right patient at the right time by the right route to ensure safe drug administration.

Right medication: When drugs are first ordered, the nurse must make sure the drug given is correct, by checking the label on its container three times.
- When taking the medication from its storage area.
- When removing the medication from its container.
- When discarding or replacing the medication container.

Right dose: The nurse should check the physical order to verify the dosage of drugs before administering.

Right patient: The nurse should identify the client, to whom the drug is prescribed. Since so many clients admitted in the ward/ unit for which is responsible to check the name, number, bed number, etc.

Right time: The nurse is responsible for placing the drug order on the right time schedule.

Right route: The nurse should see that the drug order which indicates the preferred route of drug administration.

Right Documentation

In brief, the nursing responsibilities while administering drug will include the following:
- Assessment for the client and clear understanding of why the client is receiving particular medication.
- Preparing medication to be administered (i.e., checking labels, preparing infections, observing proper aseptic technique with needles and syringes).
- Accurate dosage calculations.
- Administration of medication (proper injection techniques, aids to help swallowing; topical methods, etc.)
- Documentation of medication given.
- Observing the client reactions and evaluating the client's response.
- Educating the client regarding his or her medications and medication regimens.
- Most medication errors occur when a nurse fails to follow routine procedure. The following precautions to be taken to avoid errors during administration of medication (Table 20.9). When giving medication to the children or adults some special techniques have to be followed:

For Oral Medication
- Liquid forms are safer to swallow to avoid aspiration
- Juice, a soft drink or a frozen juice, is offered after a drug is swallowed
- Allow the child to have such a small piece of ice for a few minutes before taking medication. The ice numbs the taste buds and objectionable taste will be less discernible

Table 20.9: Taking Precautions to Avoid Errors in Drug Administration

	Precautions		Rationales
1.	Read drugs label carefully.	1.	Many products come in similar containers, colors and shapes.
2.	Question administration of multiple tablets or vials for single dose.	2.	Most dosages are one or two tablets or capsules or one single dose vial. Incorrect interpretation of order may result in excessively high dose.
3.	Be aware of drugs with similar names.	3.	Many drugs named sound alike, e.g. digoxin and digitoxin, orinase and orinade.
4.	Check decimal point.	4.	Some drugs come in quantities that are multiples of one another.
5.	Question abrupt and excessive increase in dosage.	5.	Most dosages are made gradually so that physician can monitor therapeutic effect and response.
6.	When new or unfamiliar drug is ordered consult resource.	6.	If physician is also unfamiliar with drug, there is greater risk of inaccurate dosage being ordered.
7.	Do not administer a drug ordered by nickname or unofficial.	7.	Many physicians refer to commonly ordered medications by nicknames or unofficial abbreviations. If nurse is unfamiliar with name, wrong drug may be administered.
8.	Do not attempt to decipher illegible writing.	8.	When is doubt, ask physician, unless nurse question order that is difficult to read, chance of misinterpretation is great.
9.	Know clients with same last names, also have clients state their full names, check name carefully.	9.	It is common to have two or more clients with same and similar last names.
10.	Do not confuse with equivalents, e.g. milligram instead milliliter.	10.	When in hurry, it may be easy to misread equivalents.

- When mixing the drugs with palatable flavorings such as syrup or honey, the nurse uses only a small amount. The child may refuse to take all of the larger mixture. The nurse avoids mixing a drug with food or liquid
- A plastic disposal syringe is the most accurate devise for preparing liquid dosages, especially those less than 10 mL (cups, teaspoons and droppers are inaccurate)
- When administering liquid drugs–a spoon, plastic cup or oral syringe without needle are useful.

For Injection

- The nurse is very careful when selecting IM injection sites, as infants and small children have underdeveloped muscles
- Children can be unpredictable and uncooperative, someone should be available to restrain a child, if needed
- The nurse always should awake a sleeping child before giving injection
- Distracting the child with conversation or any toy may reduce pain perception
- The nurse should give the injection quickly and should not fight with the child.

Older people also require special consideration while administering the drugs to them, because age factor is one which has an effect on the absorption, distribution, metabolism and excretion of drugs.

Administering Oral Medication (External Route)

The term internal means within the intestine. Administering medication in oral route is most commonly used route, because it is more convenient and safest for the client. Drugs given orally are intended for the absorption in the stomach and small intestine. Oral medications are available in solid (tablets, pills, capsules) and are liquid form (elixir, suspensions, spirit and syrup). The equipment needed for oral medication are as follows:

- Medication kardex, cards or computer gene rated MARK
- Medication cart or tray
- Medication cups (disposable)
- Straws
- Water or juice

The steps to be followed in administration of oral medication are given in Table 20.10.

Administering Medications Intravenously

The intravenous route is the most dangerous route, but it leads to an immediate effect of the medication on clients. Because the drug is placed directly into the blood stream. Intravenous routes can be chosen in an emergency situation. When immediate

Table 20.10: Steps for Administering Oral Medication

	Nursing actions		Rationales
1.	Gather equipment, check each medication order against the origined physician order according to policy of the hospital. Clarify any inconsistencies, check the patient for allergy.	1.	This comparison helps to identify error that, may have occurred when orders were transcribed. The physician order is the legal record of medication order.
2.	Know the actions, special considerations, safe dose ranges, purpose of administration, and adverse effect, effect of medication to be administered.	2.	This knowledge helps the nurse evaluating the therapeutic effect of the medication in relation to the client diagnosis.
3.	Wash your hands.	3.	This prevents spread of microorganism.
4.	Move the medication cart to the outside of the clients room or prepare for administration in the medication area.	4.	Organization facilitates error-free administration and saves time.
5.	Unlock the medication cart or drawer (if tray-set tray). supply.	5.	Locking the cart or drawer safeguards each client's medication
6.	Prepare medication for one client at a time.	6.	This prevents errors in medication administration.
7.	Select the proper medication from the drawer or stock or tray and compare with kardex or order. Check expiration date or perform calculation, if necessary. (a) Place nil-dose-packed medication in a disposable cup-do not open wrapper until at bedside. Keep narcotics and medication that require special nursing assessment and a separate container. (b) When removing tablets or capsules from a bottle, pair and necessary number into the bottle cap and then placed the tablet in a medication cup. Break the scored tablet, if necessary to obtain the proper dose.	7.	Comparison of medication to physician order reduces error in medication administration. Verify calculation with another nurse if necessary. This is the first safety check. (a) The label is needed for an additional safety check. Prerequisites in giving certain medication may include monitoring of client visual signs. (b) Pouring medication into the cap allows for easy return of excess medication to bottle. Pouring tablets or capsules into the nurses hand is unsanitary.

Contd...

Table 20.10: *Contd...*		
Nursing actions		*Rationales*
	(c) Hold the liquid medication bottles with the label against the palm. Use the appropriate measuring device when pouring liquids, and read the amount of medication at the bottom of the meniscus at eye level. Wipe the lip of the bottle with paper towel.		(c) Accuracy is possible when the appropriate measuring device is used and then read accurately, liquid that may drop into the label makes the label difficult to read.
8.	Recheck each medication package card or preparation with the order as it is poured.	8.	This is second check to guard against a medication error.
9.	When all medications for one client have been pre-prepared, recheck once again with the medication order before taking them to client.	9.	This is a third check to ensure accuracy and to prevent errors.
10.	Transport medication to the client, bedside carefully, and keep the medications in sight at all times.	10.	Careful handling and close observation prevent accidental or deliberate disarrangement of medications.
11.	See that the client receives medication at the correct time.	11.	Check hospital policies, which may allow for administering within a period of 30 minutes before and 30 minutes after designated time.
12.	Identify the client carefully. There are three correct ways to do this: (a) Check the name on the client's identification band. (b) Ask the of the client name. (c) Verify the client's identification with a staff member who knows the client.	12.	Identifying the client is the nurse's responsibility to guard against error. (a) This is the most reliable method, replaced the identification band if it is missing or inaccurate in anyway. (b) This requires response from the client but illness and strange surroundings often makes client confused. (c) This is another way to doublecheck identity. Do not use the name on the door or over the bed because these may be inaccurate.
13.	Complete the necessary assessment before administering medication. Check allergy bracelet or ask client about allergies. Explain the purpose and action of each medication to the client.	13.	Assessment is a prerequisite of administration of medication.
14.	Assist the client to be an upright or lateral position.	14.	Swallowing is to be made in proper positioning. An upright of sidelying position protects the client from aspiration.
15.	Administer medication: (a) Offer water or other permitted fluids, with pills, capsules, tablets and some liquid medications. (b) Ask the client's preference regarding medication to be taken by hand or in a cup and one at a time or all at once. (c) If the capsule or tablet falls to the floor it must be discarded and a new one should be administered. (d) Record any fluid intake if intake output measurement is ordered.		(a) Liquids facilitate swallowing of solid drugs. Some liquid drugs are intended to adhere to the pharyngeal area in which case liquid is not offered with the medication. (b) This encourages client participation in taking the medication. (c) This prevents contamination. (d) This provides accurate documentation.
16.	Remain with the client until each medication is swallowed. Unless the nurse has seen the client swallow the drug, it cannot be recorded that the drug was administered.	16.	The client's chart is a legal record, only with the physician order can medication be left at the bedside.
17.	Wash your hands.	17.	This prevents spread of microorganism.
18.	Record each medication given on the medication chart using the required formula: (a) If the drug is refused or omitted, record this in the appropriate area on the medicard. (b) Recording of administration of narcotic drugs requires additional documentation on narcotic record and other specific information. (c) Check the client within 30 minutes to verify response to medication.	18.	Prompt recording avoids possibility of accidentally repeating the administration of drug. (a) This verifies reason why medication was omitted. (b) Controlled substance laws necessitate careful recording of narcotic use. (c) This provides opportunity for further documentation and additional assessment.

Table 20.11: Procedures for Administering Medication Infusion Intravenously

	Nursing actions		Rationales
1.	Gather all equipment and bring to the bedside. Check IV solution and medication additives with physician order.	1.	Having equipment available saves time and facilitate accomplishment of tasks. Ensure that client receives the correct IV solution and medication as ordered by the physician.
2.	Explain the procedure to the client.	2.	Explanation allays client's anxiety.
3.	Wash your hands.	3.	It deters spread of microorganism.
4.	Prepare IV solution and tubing. (a) Maintain aseptic technique when opening sterile. Packages and IV solution. (b) Clamp tubing uncap spike, and insert into entry site on bag or bottles as manufacture directs. (c) Squeeze drip chamber and allow it to fill at least half way. (d) Remove cap at end of tubing, release clamp, and allow fluid to move through tubing. Allow fluid to flow until all air bubble, have disappeared. Close clamp and recap end of tubing maintaining sterility of set up. (e) If an electronic device is to be used, follow manufacturer instructions for inserting tubing and setting infusion route. (f) Apply label if medication was added to container (Pharmacy may have added medication and applied label). (g) Place time tape on container.	4.	 (a) This prevents spread of microorganism. (b) This puncture the seal in the IV bag or bottle. (c) Such an effect causes fluid to move into drip chamber. Also prevents air from moving down the tubing. (d) This removes air from tubing that can, in larger amounts, act as an air embolus. (e) This ensures correct flow rate and proper use of equipment. (f) Provide for administration of correct solution with presented medication or additive. (g) Permit immediate evaluation of IV according to schedule.
5.	Have the client in a low Fowler's position in bed. Place protective towel or pad, under clients arm.	5.	The supine position permits either arm to be used and allows for good body alignment. The low Fowler's position is usually most comfortable for the client.
6.	Select an appropriate site and palpate accessible veins.	6.	The selection of an appropriate site decreases discomfort for the client and possible damage to the body tissues.
7.	If the site is hairy and agency policy permits, shave or clip 2-inch area around the intended site of entry.	7.	It is difficult to clean the site of entry in the presence of hair because, hair can harbor microorganism. Adhesive tape will adhere better and may be removed more easily if hair is removed from the site.
8.	Apply tourniquet 5 to 6 inches above the venipuncture site to obstruct venous blood flow and distend the view. Direct the ends of the tourniquet away from the site of entry. Check to be sure that the radial pulse is still present.	8.	Interrupting the blood flow to the heart causes the vein to distend. Interruption of the arterial flow impedes various filling. Distended veins are easy to see, palpate and enter. The end of the tourniquet could contaminate the area of injection if directed toward the site of entry.
9.	Ask the client to open and close his or her fist. Observe and palpate for a suitable vein. Try the following techniques if a vein cannot be felt. (a) Release the tourniquet and have the client lower his or her arm below the level of the heart to fill the veins. Reapply tourniquet and gently tap over the intended vein to help distend it. (b) Remove tourniquet and place warm compresses over the intended vein for 10 to 15 minutes.	9.	Contraction of the muscles of the forearm forces blood into the veins, thereby distending them further. Lowering arm below the level of the heart, tapping the vein, and applying warmth help distend veins by filling them with blood.
10.	Don clean gloves.	10.	Care must be taken when handling any blood or body fluids to prevent transmission of HIV and other blood -borne infections.
11.	Cleanse the entry site with an antiseptic solution (alcohol swab) followed by antimicrobial solution (povidone-10 dine) according to hospital policy. Use circular motion to move from the center outward for several inches.	11.	Cleansing that begins at the site of entry and moves outward in a circular motion carries organisms away from the site of entry. Organisms on the skin can be introduced into the tissues or the bloodstream with the needle.

Contd...

	Table 20.11: *Contd...*		
	Nursing actions		*Rationales*
12.	Use the nondominant hand, placed about 1 inch or 2 inches below entry site, to hold the skin taut against the vein.	12.	Pressure on the view and surrounding tissue helps prevent movement of the vein as the needle or catheter is being inserted.
13.	Enter the skin gently with the catheter held by the hub in the dominant hand, bevel side up, at a 25° to 45° angle. The catheter may be inserted from either directly over the vein or the side of the vein. While following the course of the vein, advance the needle or catheter into the vein. A sensation can be felt when the needle enters the vein (Fig. 20.34).	13.	This allows needle or catheter to enter the vein with minimal trauma and deters passage of the needle through the vein.
14.	When blood returns through the lumen the needle or the flashback chamber of the catheter, advance either device further into vein. A catheter needs to be advanced until the hub is at the venipuncture site but the exact technique depends on the type of device used.	14.	The tourniquet causes increased venous pressure resulting in automatic backflow. Having the catheter placed well into the vein helps to prevent dislodgement.
15.	Quickly remove protective cap from the IV tubing and attach the tubing to the catheter or needle. Stabilize the catheter or needle with nondominant hand and release the tourniquet with your other hand.	15.	Bleeding is minimized and patency of the vein is maintained if the connection is made smoothly between the catheter and tubing.
16.	Start the flow of solution promptly by releasing the clamp on the tubing. Examine the tissue around the entry site for signs of infiltration.	16.	Blood clots readily if intravenous flow is not maintained. If catheter accidentally slips out of the vein, solution will accumulate and infiltrate into the surrounding tissue.
17.	Support the catheter with small piece of gauge under the hub.	17.	This helps maintain the catheter in proper position in the vein.
18.	Secure the catheter with narrow tape (½ inch) placed sticky side-up under the hub and crossed over the top of the hub (Fig. 20.33A).	18.	The smooth structure of the vein does not offer resistance to the movement of the catheter. The weight of the tubing is sufficient to pull it out of the vein if it is not well anchored.
19.	An antiseptic ointment may be applied to the catheter site of entry if a gauze dressing will be applied.	19.	Antiseptic ointment reduces skin contamination and protects against infection.
20.	Place sterile dressing over venipuncture site. Hospital policy may direct nurse to use gauze dressing or transparent dressing. Apply tape to dressing if necessary. Loop the tabing near the site of entry, and anchor to dressing (Fig. 20.33B).	20.	Transparent dressing allows easy visualization of site but may place client at increased risk of infection. Gauze dressing absorbs drainage and may have a decreased infection rate, discussion continuous about effectiveness of type of dressing.
21.	Mark the date and time, venipuncture site and type and size of the catheter used for the infusion on the tape anchoring the tubing.	21.	Personnel working will know what type of device is used, the site and when it was needed. This protects clients and IV site from infections.
22.	Anchor arm to an armboard for support, if necessary (Fig. 20.33D).	22.	An armboard protects against change in the position of the vein and acts as a reminder to the client to minimize movements of his or her arm.
23.	Adjust the rate of solution flow according to the amount prescribed or follow manufacturers directions for adjusting flow rate on infusion pump.	23.	The physician prescribes the rate of flow.
24.	Remove all equipments and dispose in proper manner. Remove gloves and wash hands.	24.	It deters spread of microorganism.
25.	Document the procedure and client's response chart time, site, device and solution, medication (if).	25.	This provides accurate documentation and ensures continuity of care.
26.	Return to check flow rate and observe for infiltration 30 minutes after starting in fusion.	26.	This documents client's response to infusion.

Note:
1 Remove air trapped in during an IV infusion as shown in Figure 20.35.
2 There are three methods of administering IV infusion as shown in Figures 20.36A to C.

absorption is required. It is relatively common form of therapy for handling fluid disturbances in the use of the various solutions infused by vein (IV). Sterile technique is observed when a vein is entered. Disposable infusion tabing and needles are used to help eliminate many possible sources of contamination and to reduce the cost of equipment aftercare. The following procedures and equipment need starting an IV infusion (Table 20.11):

- IV solution
- Cleaning swabs (alcohol, povidone-1)
- IV infusion set
- Towel or disposable pad
- IV tubing
- Gauze or transparent dressing
- IV catheter or butterfly needle
- Antiseptic ointment (optional)
- Tourniquet
- Time tape or label (for IV container)
- Tape
- Electronic infusion device (if ordered)
- Arm board
- Clean gloves
- IV pole or stand.

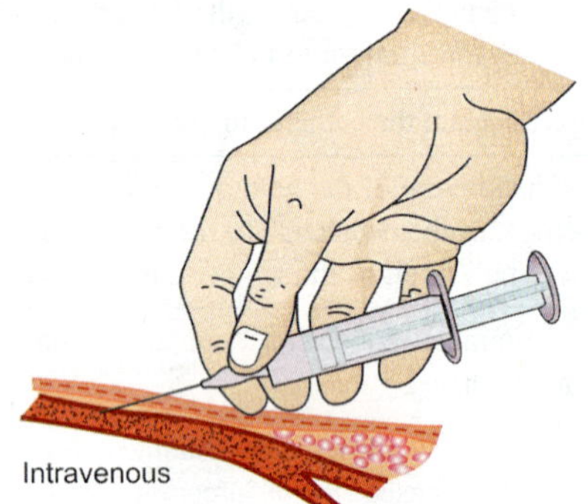

Figure 20.34: Administering intravenous injection (step 13)

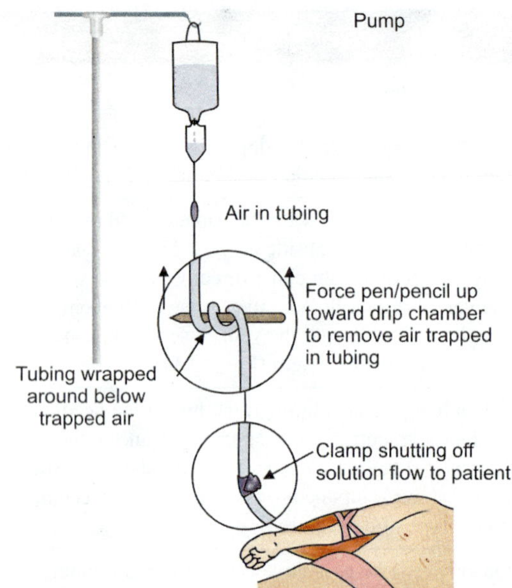

Figure 20.35: Removing air-trapped in tube during an IV infusion. The air is between the patient and the drip chamber with the flow clamp below the trapped air. The clamp is tightened to shut off the flow of solution to the patient and to prevent blood from being drawn up into the tubing as the nurse compresses the tubing with a pencil, forcing out the trapped air

Adding Medication to an IV Solution Container

The following equipment and procedures are needed (Table 20.12):

- Medication prepared in a syringe with 19-21 gauge needle or needless device
- Alcohol swab
- IV fluid container (bag or bottle)
- Label to be attached to the IV container

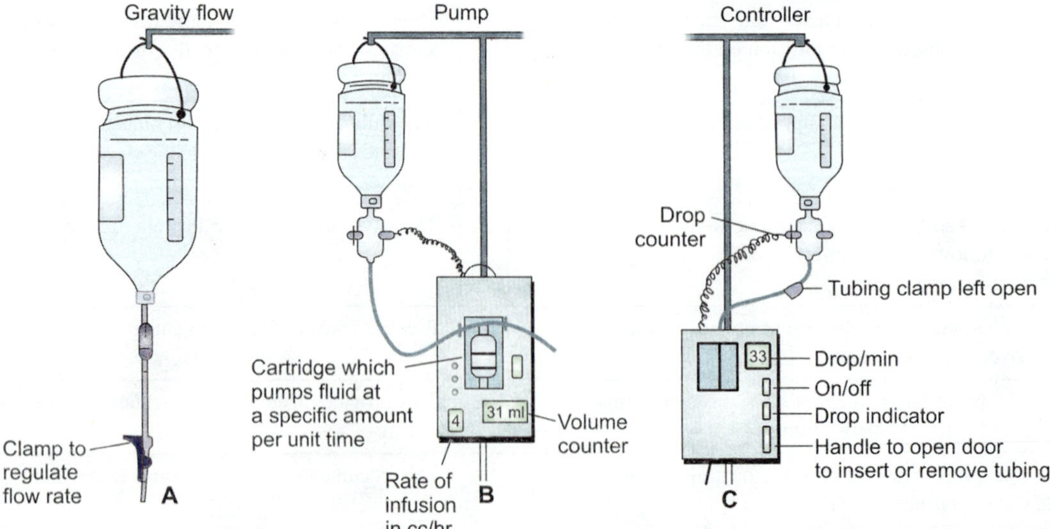

Figures 20.36 A to C: Three methods for administering intravenous fluids: (A) Gravity flow using tube clamp to regulate flow. (B) Infusion pump using a syringe device to measure volume of fluid infused. (C) Controller using a drop counter around the drip chamber to regulate flow in drops per minute

Table 20.12: Procedures for Adding Medication to an IV Solution Container

	Nursing actions		*Rationales*
1.	Gather all equipment and bring to the clients bedside. Check the medication order with the physician order.	1.	Having equipment available saves time and facilitates performing task. Checking the orders ensure that client receives correct medication.
2.	Explain the procedure to the client.	2.	Explanation allays the clients anxiety.
3.	Wash your hands.	3.	It deters spread of microorganism.
4.	Identify the client by checking the band on the clients wrist and asking the client his or her name.	4.	This ensures that medication is given to the right person.
5.	Add the medication to the IV solution that is infusing (a) Check that the volume in the bag or bottle is adequate. (b) Close the IV clamp. (c) Clean the medication part with alcohol swab. (d) Study the container, uncap the needle, and insert the needle into the part, inject the medication. (e) Remove the container from the IV pole and gently rotate the solution. (f) Rehang the container, open the clamp and readjust the flow rate. (g) Attach the label to the container so that the dose of medication that has been added is apparent.	4.	 (a) The volume should be sufficient to dilute the drug. (b) This prevents backflow directly to the client of improperly diluted medication. (c) This deters entry to microorganism when the needle puncture the part. (d) This ensures that the needle enters the container and medication can be dispersed into the solution. (e) This mixes the medication with the solution. (f) This ensures the infusion of the IV with medication as the prescribed rate. (g) This confirms that the prescribed dose of medication has been added to the IV solution.
6.	Add the medication to the IV solution before infusion. (a) Carefully remove any protective cover and locate the injection part. Clean with an alcohol swab. (b) Uncap the needle and insert the spike into the part-inject the medication. (c) Withdraw the needle and insert the spike into the proper entry site on the bag or bottle. (d) With tubing clamped, gently rotate the IV solution in the bag or bottle. Hang the IV. (e) Attach the label to the container so that the dose of medication that has been added is apparent.	6.	This deters entry to microorganism when the needle punctures the part. (a) This ensures that the needle enters the container and that medication can be dispersed into the solution. (b) This punctures the seal in the IV bag or bottle. (c) This mixes medication with the solution. (d) This confirms that the prescribed dose of medication has been added to the IV solution.
7.	Dispose the equipment according to hospital policy.	7.	This prevents inadvertent injury from the equipment.
8.	Wash your hands.	8.	It deters spread of microorganism.
9.	Chart the addition of medication to the IV solution.	9.	Accurate documentation is necessary to prevent medication errors.
10.	Evaluate the client's response to medication within the appropriate timeframe.	10.	Clients require careful observation because of medication given by the IV route may have a rapid effect.

Adding a Bolus IV Medication to an Existing IV

The following procedures and equipment are needed for this medication (Table 20.13):
- Medication is prepared in a syringe with 23 to 25 gauge, 1 inch needle (or needleless device)
- Alcohol swab
- Watch with second hand
- Disposable gloves

Introducing Drugs through a Heparin or Intravenous Lock using the Saline Flush

The procedures and equipment needed are as follows (Table 20.14):
- Medication
- Alcohol swabs
- Medication card digital reaction
- Watch with secondhand or
- Saline vial

Table 20.13: Procedures for Adding a Bolus IV Medication to an Existing IV

	Nursing actions		Rationales
1.	Gather all equipment and bring to the clients bedside. Check the medication order with the physician order.	1.	Having equipment available saves time and facilitates performing task. Checking the orders ensure that client receives correct medication.
2.	Explain the procedure to the client.	2.	Explanation allays the client's anxiety.
3.	Wash your hands.	3.	It deters spread of microorganism.
4.	Identify the client by checking the band on the clients wrist and asking the client his or her name.	4.	This ensures that medication is given to the right person.
5.	Assess the IV site for the presence of the inflammation or infiltration.	5.	Intravenous medication must be given directly into a view for safe administration.
6.	Select the injection part on the tubing that is closest to the venipuncture site, clean the port with an alcohol swab.	6.	Using the part closest to the needle insertion site minimizes dilution of the medication. Cleaning with alcohol deters entry to microorganism when the needle puncture the part.
7.	Uncap the syringe, steady the port with your nondominant hand while inserting the needle into the center of the port.	7.	This supports the injection part and lessens the risk of accidentally distorting the IV or entering the part incorrectly.
8.	Move your nondominant hand to the section of IV tubing just beyond the injection part. Fold the tubing between your fingers to temporarily stop the flow of the IV solution.	8.	This minimizes the dilution of the IV medication with an IV solution.
9.	Pull back slightly on the plunger just until blood appears in the tubing.	9.	This ensures injection of medication into a vein.
10.	Inject the medication at the prescribed rate.	10.	This delivers the correct amount of medication at the proper interval.
11.	Remove the needle. Do not cap it. Release the tubing and allow the IV flow at proper rate.	11.	This prevents accidental needledstick.
12.	Dispose the needle and syringe in the proper receptacle.	12.	Proper disposal of the needle prevents accidental injury and spread of microorganism.
13.	Remove gloves and wash hands.	13.	It deters spread of microorganism.
14.	Chart the administration of the medication.	14.	Accurate documentation is necessary to prevent medication error.
15.	Evaluate the client's response to the medication within the appropriate timeframe.	15.	The client requires careful observation because medication given by an IV bolus injection may have rapid effect.

- Disposable glove
- Sterile syringe
- 25 gauge needle or needleless device
- *For bolus injection:* Sterile syringe with medications and 25 gauge needle or needleless *device*
- *For intermittent IV devices*: IV set up 25 gauge needle or needleless device alternate tubing
- Additional sterile 25 gauge needle or needleless device
- Adhesive tape
- IV pump or infusion controller (optional)

Monitoring an IV Site and Infusion

See Table 20.15.

Changing an IV Dressing

See Table 20.16.

Converting a Primary Intravenous Access to a Heparin or Saline Lock

See Table 20.17.

Table 20.14: Procedures for Iintroducing Drug Through a Heparin or IV Lock Using Saline Flush

	Nursing actions		*Rationales*
1.	Assemble equipment and check-up physician prescription at the right time and right level.	1.	This ensures that client receives the right medication.
2.	Explain the procedure to the client.	2.	This alleviates the client apprehension.
3.	Wash your hands.	3.	It deters spread of microorganism.
4.	Withdraw 1 to 2 mL of sterile saline from the vial into the syringe.	4.	Using saline eliminates concern about drug incompatibilities and effect on systemic circulation that exists with heparin flush.
5.	Don the cleaned gloves.	5.	Gloves protect the nurse's hands from contact with the client blood.
6.	Administer the medication.		

For bolus IV inject

(a)	Check the drug package for the correct injection rate for the IV push route.	(a)	Using the correct injection rate prevents occurrence of speeds hock.
(b)	Clean the port of the lock with alcohol swab.	(b)	Remove surface bacteria at the heparin lock entry site.
(c)	Gently inject the medication, using a watch to verify correct injection rate. Do not force if resistance is felt. If the lock is jogged, it has to be changed. Remove the medication syringe and needle when administer is completed.	(c)	Easy instillation of the medication usually indicates that the lock is still patent and in the vein.

For administration of a drug by way of an intermittent delivery system

(a)	Use a drug resource book to check for the correct flow rate of medication (the usual rates 30 to 60 minutes).	(a)	Using the correct injection rate prevents occurrence of speed.
(b)	Connect the infusion tubing to the medication set-up, accordingly. Hang the IV set-up on a pole. Open clamp and allow solution to clear IV tubing of air reclamp tubing.	(b)	This removes air from the tubing and preserves the sterility of the set-up.
(c)	Attach sterile 25 gauge needle to the end of the infusion tubing.	(c)	A small gauge needle prevents damage to the lock.
(d)	Clean the port of the lock with an alcohol swab. Stabilize the port with your nondominant hand and insert the needle on the tubing into the port secure with tape.	(d)	Cleaning removes surface batches at the lock entry site. Tape secures the needle in the lock part.
(e)	Open the clamp and regulate the flow rate or attach to IV pump or controller according to manufacture direction close clamp when infusion is complete.	(e)	This ensures that the client receives the medication at the correct rate.
(f)	Remove the needle from lock. Carefully replace the uncapped used needle on the tubing with a sterile covered needle. Allow the medication set-up to hand on the pole for future use accordingly.	(f)	This prevents possible needle stitch with contaminated needle.
(g)	Dispose of uncapped used needle appropriately.	(g)	This prevents possible needless injury.
7.	Insert the needle of the syringe contain saline and flush the reservoir with 1 to 2 mL of sterile saline. Remove the syringe and needle and discard in the appropriate recepticle. Remove gloves and discard appropriately.	7.	Saline clears the line of medication with less of the systematic effects of the heparin flush.
8.	Wash your hands.	8.	It deters the spread of microorganism.
9.	The injection site and IV lock should be checked at least every 8 hours and a small amount of saline is administered if medication is not given at least that time.	9.	This ensures the patency of the system for continuing injections.
10.	The heparin lock should be changed at least every 48 hours or according to hospital policy. A clogged lock should be changed immediately.	10.	Changing a heparin lock regularly and having it free of clotted blood reduces dangers of infection and emboli in the circulating blood.
11.	Chart the administration of medication or saline flush.	11.	Accurate documentation is necessary to prevent medication error.

Table 20.15: Procedures for Monitoring an IV Site and Infusion

	Nursing actions		*Rationales*
1.	Monitor IV infusion at least once every hour. More frequent checks may be necessary if medication is being infused. (a) Check physician's order for IV solution. (b) Check drip chamber and time drops if IV is not regulated by an infusion control device. (c) Check tubing for anything that might interfere with flow. Be sure that clamp is in the open position. Observe dressing for leakage of IV solution. (d) Observe settings, alarm, and indicator lights on infusion control device if one is being used.	1.	Promotes safe administration of IV fluids and medication. Two rapid administration of medications can result in the development of speed shock. (a) This ensures that correct solution is being given at the correct rate and in the proper sequence with the correct medications. (b) This ensures that flow rate is correct. (c) Any kind of pressure on tubing may interfere with flow. Leakage may occur at connection of tubing with hub of needle or catheter and allow for loss of IV solution. (d) Observation ensures that infusion control device is functioning and that alarm is in ON position.
2.	Inspect site for swelling, pain, coolness, or pallor at site of insertion, which may indicate infiltration of IV. This necessitates removing IV and restarting at another site.	2.	Needle may become dislodged from vein, and IV solution may flow into subcutaneous tissue.
3.	Inspect site for redness, swelling, heat, and pain at the IV site, which may indicate phlebitis is present. IV will need to be discontinued and restarted at another site. Notify physician if you suspect that phlebitis may have occurred.	3.	Chemical irritation or mechanical trauma cause injury to the vein and can lead to the development of phlebitis.
4.	Check for local or systemic manifestations that indicate an infection present at the site. IV will be discontinued and physician notified. Never disconnect IV tubing when putting on client's hospital.	4.	Poor aseptic technique may allow bacteria to enter the needle or catheter insertion site or tubing connection.
5.	Be alert for additional complications of IV therapy (a) Circulatory overload can result in signs of cardiac failure and pulmonary edema. Monitor intake and output during IV therapy. (b) Bleeding at the site is most likely to occur when the IV is discontinued.	5.	 (a) Infusing too much IV solution results in an increased volume of circulating fluid. (b) Bleeding may be caused by anticoagulant medication.
6.	If possible, instruct client to call for assistance if any discomfort is noted at site, solution container is nearly empty, or flow has changed in any way.	6.	This facilitates cooperation of client and safe administration of IV solution.
7.	Document IV infusion, any complications of therapy, and client's reaction to therapy.	7.	This provides accurate documentation as ensures continuity of care.

(*Note:* Changing the tubing during the IV infusion, if necessary, is to be done as shown in Figure 20.37).

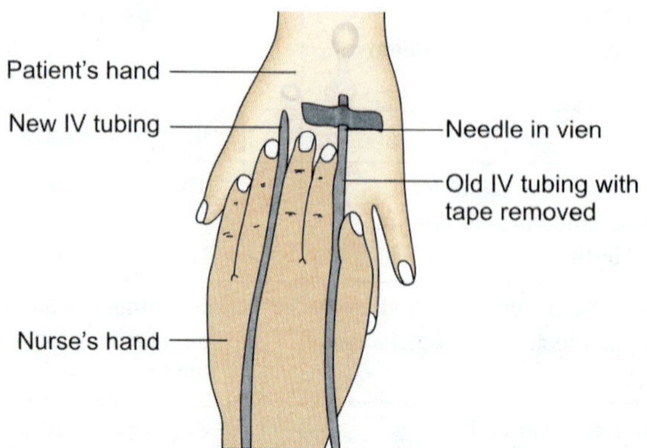

Figure 20.37: Changing tubing during an IV infusion. Care must be taken not to contaminate new tubing while removing old tubing from needle hub

Table 20.16: Procedures for Changing an IV Dressing

Equipment

- Sterile gauze (2 × 2 or 4 × 4) or transparent polyurethane dressing
- Povidone-iodine (betadine) solution or swabs
- Alcohol swabs
- Clean gloves
- Adhesive remover Povidone-iodine ointment (or other antiseptic ointment) recommended by agency)
- Tape
- Towel or disposable pad

	Nursing actions		*Rationales*
1.	Assess client's need for dressing change.	1.	Agency policy determines interval for dressing change (every 24 to 72 hours). The presence of moisture or a nonadhering dressing increases risk of bacterial contamination at the site.
2.	Gather equipment and bring to bedside. Place towel or disposable pad under extremity.	2.	Having equipment available saves time and facilitates the performance of the task.
3.	Explain procedure to client.	3.	Explanation allays client's anxiety.
4.	Wash your hands. Don clean gloves.	4.	Handwashing deters the spread of microorganism. Gloves prevent transmission of HIV and other blood-borne infections.
5.	Carefully remove old dressing but leave tap that anchors IV needle or catheter in place. Discard in proper manner.	5.	This prevents dislodging of IV needle or catheter.
6.	Assess IV site for presence of inflammation or infiltration. Discontinue and relocate the IV, if noted.	6.	Inflammation or infiltration causes trauma to tissues and necessitates removal of the IV needle or catheter.
7.	Loosen tape and gently remove, being careful to steady catheter or needle hub with one hand.	7.	Tape stabilizes needle and prevents inadvertently dislodging it.
8.	Use adhesive remover to initiate cleansing procedure at site.	8.	Process removes adhesive residue and facilitates attachment of new dressing.
9.	Cleanse the entry site with povidone-iodine solution. Use a circular motion to move from the center outward. Follow with alcohol cleansing according to agency policy.	9.	Cleansing in a circular motion while moving outward carries organisms away from the entry site. Use of antiseptic solutions reduces the number of microorganisms on the skin surface.
10.	Reapply tape strip to needle or catheter at entry site.	10.	Tape anchors needle or catheter to prevent dislodgement.
11.	Apply povidone-iodine ointment to the entry site, if agency policy recommends this.	11.	Antiseptic ointment reduces skin contamination and protects against infection.
12.	Apply sterile gauze or transparent polyurethance dressing over entry site. Remove gloves and dispose of properly.	12.	Dressing protects site and deters contamination with microorganisms.
13.	Secure IV tubing with additional tape is necessary. Label dressing with date, time of change, and initials. Check that IV flow is accurate and system is patent.	13.	Label documents IV dressing change.
14.	Discard equipment properly and wash.	14.	Handwashing protects against spread.
15.	Record client's response to dressing change and observation of site.	15.	This provides accurate documentation and ensures continuity of care.

Table 20.17: Procedures for Converting a Primary IV Access to a Heparin or Saline Lock

Equipment	
• Lock device (also caned male adaptor or Luer-Lok) • Clean gloves • 4 × 4 gauze pad • Tape	• Saline (non preservative saline) or heparin flush (1 mL) prepared in a syringe with a 25-gauge needle or according to agency policy • Alcohol wipe • Plastic clamp or hemostat

	Nursing actions		*Rationales*
1.	Gather equipment and verify physician's order.	1.	Having equipment available saves time and facilitates the task; ensures that the procedure has been ordered by the physician.
2.	Explain the procedure to the client.	2.	Explanation allays the client's anxiety.
3.	Wash your hands.	3.	Handwashing deters the spread of microorganism.
4.	Assess the IV site.	4.	Complications such as infiltration or phlebitis necessitate discontinuation of the IV infusion at that site.
5.	Use a plastic clamp or hemostat to close off primary line.	5.	This protects client and nurse from inadvertent blood loss when IV and tubing are disconnected.
6.	Don clean gloves.	6.	Gloves protect the nurse from contact with the client's blood.
7.	Place gauze 4 × 4 sponge underneath IV connection hub between IV catheter and tubing.	7.	Gauze absorbs any blood leakage when IV and tubing are disconnected.
8.	Stabilize hub of IV catheter with nondominant hand. Use dominant hand to quickly twist and disconnect IV tubing from the catheter, discard it, and attach heparin device to hub without contaminating the tips of the catheter and the lock.	8.	This maintains sterility of IV set-up.
9.	Cleanse lock entry with an alcohol wipe.	9.	Cleansing removes surface bacteria at the heparin lock entry site.
10.	Insert the syringe needle into the heparin lock part and gently flush catheter with saline, nonpreservative saline, or heparin flush as per agency policy. Remove syringe carefully.	10.	This maintains patency of the IV access line. Clinical evidence had demonstrated that a saline flush is as effective as heparin for peripheral IVs and avoids the adverse effects of heparin, in less expensive, and prevents drug incompatibilities.
11.	Tape heparin lock securely in place.	11.	Tape secures the heparin lock and IV in place.
12.	Chart on IV administration record or medication kardex per institutional policy.	12.	Accurate documentation is necessary to prevent errors.

Blood Transfusion

Definition

Blood transfusion is a process by which transplantation of blood (tissue) can be done into the human circulation. The person giving blood is called the 'Donor' and the person receiving is called the 'Recipient'.

Indications

1. Hemorrhage
A. Traumatic
  (i) Operative - (a) In patients below 9 gm%-Hb pre or post operatively; (b) Where much blood loss is expected, e.g. Partial gastrectomy, Hemicolectomy, Nephrectomy.
  (ii) Nonoperative - In accidental loss.
B. Erosion and rupture of blood vessels: (a) Peptic ulcer (b) Hemorrhoids.
C. Hemorrhagic conditions
  (i) Disturbance of coagulating mechanism - (a) Hemophilia, (b) Thrombocytopenic purpura, (c) Prothrombinopenia, (d) Obstructive Jaundice, (e) After excessive administration of anticoagulants.
  (ii) Local vascular disorder, e.g. Scurvy.
2. Peripheral circulatory failure
  (a) Secondary shock viz. dehydration
  (b) Burns.
3. Blood dyscrasia
  (a) Leukemia
  (b) Purpura
  (c) Hemolytic anemia

4. In severe infection: e.g., septicemia, gas gangrene, *E. coli*, shock, in strangulated gut.
5. Miscellaneous: (i) Corrosive poisoning viz. Carbon monoxide poisoning. (ii) Erythroblastosis fetalis.

Contraindications

1. Congestive cardiac failure
2. Pulmonary edema
3. Gross renal damage
4. Increased intracranial tension

Blood grouping: Many different antigens have been recognised in human RBC. For practical purposes according to the presence or absence of A and B antigen human blood group is classified because there are only two antigens to which antibodies occur naturally. There are thus four major human blood groups.

Group 'O': RBC does not contain either A or B antigen. Serum contains Anti 'A' and Anti 'B' antibodies.

Group 'A': RBC contains A but not B antigen. Serum contains Anti 'B' but not Anti 'A' antibody.

Group 'B': RBC contains B but not A antigen serum contains Anti 'A' but not Anti 'B' antibody.

Group 'AB': RBC contains both A and B antigen. Serum contains neither Anti 'A' nor Anti 'B' antibody.

Rh system: The Rh(D) factor is an antigen other than A and B when injected into patients without them produce antibodies. When the red cells contain the Rh(D) the patient is Rh-positive and when they do not the patient is Rh-negative.

Investigations and Precautions during Blood Transfusion

1. Examination of recipient
2. Examination of donor
3. Examination of blood before transfusion
4. Precaution during the method of transfusion.

1. Recipient
(a) Prior clinical examination and investigation to exclude contra indication.
(b) Should not have any allergic manifestation.
(c) Grouping and cross matching must be done.
(d) Should be in empty stomach to avoid nausea and vomiting.

2. Donor
(a) History—Donor should not have history of infective hepatitis, syphilis, recent impetigo, malaria, brucellosis and cytomegalo-virus inclusion disease.
(b) Must not take protein food before 24 hrs (to prevent allergic reaction).
(c) Examination of blood for VDRL and WB Test (ELISA).
(d) Blood grouping and cross matching.

3. Examinations of blood before transfusion
(a) Name, age, sex, bed no, group, date of expiry, (Rh confirmation factor).
(b) Blood bottle should be checked twice before transfusion.
(c) Any evidence of haemolysis to be checked.
   (i) Normally there is a clear line between cell and serum.
   (ii) Haziness in fluid is abnormal.
(d) Clot formation - Blood containing clots should not be used.

Precaution during the Method of Transfusion

1. Proper aseptic technique.
2. Slow rate of transfusion unless specially indicated.
3. If any reaction the blood transfusion must be stopped immediately.
4. During transfusion half hourly pulse and hourly temperature are to be recorded.
5. Refrigerated blood must not be transfused till the temperature of stored blood is almost in room temperature.

Common Sites for Blood Transfusion

1. Vein—Cephalic vein, Basilic vein, Saphenous vein.
2. Bone marrow—rarely.

Method of Administration of Blood

1. Indirect: This method being simpler is commonly used. It may be of two types:
   (a) Closed type
   (b) Open type
2. Direct: In emergency direct method may be used by the doctor.

Procedure for Blood Transfusion

1. Articles for blood transfusion should be ready at bed side and the patient is to be screened.
2. The procedure is to be explained to the patient if possible.
3. A bedpan may be offered as it is going to be a long procedure.
4. An antihistamine is preferred.
5. The patient should be in comfortable position.
6. The bed has to be protected with a mackinosh and towel.

Responsibilities of Nurse

A. Before transfusion
1. The blood transfusion form must be checked carefully regarding name, age, sex, bed number, blood group and date of expiry.
2. Strict aseptic technique has to be followed throughout the procedure.

3. No substantial food should be taken within 2 hours before transfusion.
4. The blood should be transfused at room temperature. Too cold blood must not be given.

B. During transfusion
1. The flow, the desired rate, any extravasation or dislodgement of needle must be watched.
2. A close vigilance should be kept to the patient regarding any untoward features.
3. If there is any untoward symptom it should be reported immediately.
4. Intake and output chart must be maintained.
5. Vital signs.

C. After transfusion
1. The amount of blood transfused should be noted.
2. Starting time and time of discontinuation of transfusion is to be recorded.
3. If there is any complication after the transfusion is over it must be recorded.
4. No substantial food should be taken within 2 hours after the transfusion.
5. Pulse, respiration and temperature has to be recorded.
6. First sample of urine after transfusion has to be checked macroscopically for evidence of hematuria or any other abnormality.
7. A close vigilance to the patient.
8. The patient should be comfortable after the transfusion.

Complications

Complications may be grouped as follows:
  (a) Associated with donor: (i) Transfusion of disease - hepatitis, malaria, syphilis etc. as mentioned. (ii) Allergic reaction.
  (b) Associated with blood: (i) Febrile reaction; (ii) Incompatibility.
  (c) Associated with storage: (i) Hemorrhagic tendency (ii) Infection (iii) Citrate intoxication (iv) Subnormal temperature.
  (d) Associated with administrations: (i) Thrombophlebitis (ii) Overloading (iii) Embolism.
  (e) Other common complications: (i) Anaphylactic shock (ii) Sepsis of the area.

Prevention and Management of Complications

A. Associated with donor
1. Transmission of disease, e.g., (a) Viral hepatitis, (b) Malaria etc.
   Preventions: By careful screening of the donor.
2. Allergic reaction: commonly follows repeated transfusion from same donor.
   Antihistaminic group of drugs has to be given.

B. Associated with blood itself
1. Febrile reaction-factors are pyrogens, infected blood, dirty apparatus and rapid rate of transfusion.

Prevention: By adopting disposable sets and plastic apparatus. Pyrogen free solution and slow rate of transfusion.

Treatment: As it is difficult to distinguish between febrile reaction and incompatibility it is better to regard febrile reaction as evidence of incompatibility. Blood transfusion must be stopped and arrangements for further grouping and cross matching of blood is made. Analgesics, antipyretics and antibiotics are given.

Incompatibility: If antibodies present in the recipients serum are incompatible with donor's cells a transfusion reaction will set up. This is due to agglutination and haemolysis of donor's cells. This may lead to acute renal tubular necrosis and renal failure.

Feature: There is rigor, temperature, pain in the loins. There may be hematuria, chest pain, dyspnea and the patient becomes extremely alarmed.

Treatment:
  (i) Transfusion must be stopped immediately.
  (ii) Furesemide—80-120 mg IV to provoke diuresis and may be repeated if there is anuria.
  (iii) Steroid.
  (iv) Sodium bicarbonate 40 meq. with administration of 1000 ml of Ringer's lactate solution.
  (v) Fresh specimen of venous blood for further blood transfusion.
  (vi) Urine from patient together with the residue of used blood should be sent for examination.
  (vii) Patients pulse, BP and urinary output should be under close watch.

C. Associated with storage
1. Hemorrhagic tendency: Particularly with massive blood transfusion.
2. Hypothermia: Due to massive transfusion of a cold blood this can be prevented by warming up blood to body temperature by running it through several extension coils of plastic transfusion tubing immersed in a heated water bath. Excessive warming causes hemolysis. So warming above 98°F is not desirable.
3. Infection: Inspite of best care bacteria may enter the container and some organisms can multiply at 4°C-6°C: Transfusion of such blood will cause septicaemia or toxaemia.
4. Citrate intoxication: Large volume of transfusion of blood (stored with acid citrate dextrose) contain citrate in high concentration which bind free calcium in blood diminishing ionised calcium which may lead to cardiac arrest.
   Treatment: 13 ml of 10% calcium gluconate or chloride IV to every 2 pint of blood.

D Associated with administration

1. Thrombophlebitis: Factors are (a) long continued transfusion (site should be changed) (b) Irritating substance 10% glucose (c) Infection.
   Treatment: Avoidance of factors.
2. Overloading of circulation:
   Diagnosis: (i) Sensation of tightness of chest (ii) Cough (iii) Dyspnoea, cyanosis (iv) Engorgement of neck veins (v) Tachycardia (vi) Pulmonary edema.
   Prevention:
   1. Limiting blood transfusion in anaemia to 300 ml. or packed cell transfusion.
   2. Observation during transfusion.

Treatment:

1. Stopping of transfusion
2. Digitalization
3. Oxygen
4. Aminophyllin
5. Propped up position
6. Furesemide 40 ml IV stat or at the onset of transfusion as a preventive measure.

Administering a Blood Transfusion

See Table 20.18.

Table 20.18: Procedures for Administering a Blood Transfusion

Equipment

- Blood product
- Blood administration set (tubing with IV) line filter and Y for saline administration)
- Disposable gloves
- 0.9 percent normal saline
- IV pole
- Intravenous line with a 18 or 19 gauge needle or catheter
- Tape

	Nursing actions		*Rationales*
1.	Determine if client knows reason for transfusion. Ask if the client has had a transfusion or transfusion reaction in the past.	1.	This directs teaching before beginning transfusion.
2.	Explain procedure to client. Check for signed consent for transfusion if required by agency. Advise client to report any chills, itching, rash, or unusual symptoms.	2.	Explanation provides reassurance and facilitates cooperation for the client; prompt reporting of any reaction to transfusion necessitates stopping immediately.
3.	Wash your hands and put on clean gloves.	3.	Handwashing deters the spread of microorganisms. Gloves protect against accidental exposure to the client's blood.
4.	Hang container of 0.9 percent normal saline with blood administration set to initiate IV infusion and follow administration or blood.	4.	Dextrose may lead to clumping of red blood cells and hemolysis. Filter in blood administration removes particulate material formed during storage of blood.
5.	Start intravenous in fusion with 18- or 19-gauze catheter if not already present. Keep IV in fusion open by starting flow of normal saline.	5.	Large bore needle or catheter is necessary for infusion of blood products. The lumen must be large enough not to cause damage to red blood cells.
6.	Obtain blood product from blood bank according to agency policy.	6.	Blood must be stored in refrigerated unit at carefully controlled temperature (4°C).
7.	Complete identification and checks as required by agency: (a) Identification number. (b) Blood group and type. (c) Expiration date. (d) Client's name. (e) Inspect blood for clots.	7.	Some agencies require two registered nurses to verify information: (a) That unit numbers match. (b) That ABO group and Rh type are the same. (c) Safe storage of blood is limited to 35 days before red blood cells begin to deteriorate. (d) Never administer blood to a client without a name band. (e) If clots are present, blood should be returned to blood bank.
8.	Take baseline set of vital signs prior to beginning transfusion.	8.	Any change in vital signs during the transfusion may indicate a reaction.
9.	Start infusion of the blood product: (a) Prime in-line filter with blood.	9.	 (a) Priming is necessary if blood is to flow properly.

Contd...

<table>
<tr><td colspan="4" align="center">**Table 20.18:** *Contd...*</td></tr>
<tr><td colspan="2">*Nursing actions*</td><td colspan="2">*Rationales*</td></tr>
<tr>
<td></td>
<td>(b) Start administration slowly (no more than 10-25 mL for the first 15 minutes). Stay with the client for the first 15 minutes of transfusion.</td>
<td></td>
<td>(b) Transfusion reactions typically occur during this period, and a slow rate will minimize the volume of red blood cells infused. If there have been no adverse effects during this time, the infusion rate is increased.</td>
</tr>
<tr>
<td></td>
<td>(c) Check vital signs at least every 15 minutes for the first half hour after the start of the transfusion and then every half hour or a hour after the transfusion depending on agency policy.
(d) Observe client for flushing, dyspnea, itching, hives, or rash.</td>
<td></td>
<td>(c) If complications occur, they can be observed, and the blood can be stopped immediately.

(d) These symptoms may be early indication of a transfusion reaction.</td>
</tr>
<tr>
<td></td>
<td>(e) Use a blood warming device, if indicated, especially with rapid transfusions through a CVP catheter.</td>
<td></td>
<td>(e) Rapid administration of cold blood can result in cardiac arrhythmias.</td>
</tr>
<tr>
<td>10.</td>
<td>Maintain the prescribed flow rate as ordered and assess frequently for transfusion reaction. Stop blood transfusion and allow saline to flow if you suspect a reaction. Notify physician and blood bank.</td>
<td>10.</td>
<td>Rate must be carefully controlled, and client's reaction must be monitored on a frequent basis.</td>
</tr>
<tr>
<td>11.</td>
<td>When transfusion is complete, infuse 0.9 percent normal saline.</td>
<td>11.</td>
<td>Saline prevents hemolysis of red blood cells and clears remainder of blood in IV line.</td>
</tr>
<tr>
<td>12.</td>
<td>Record administration of blood and client's reaction as ordered by agency. Return blood transfusion bag to blood bank according to agency policy.</td>
<td>12.</td>
<td>This provides for accurate documentation of client's response to blood transfusion.</td>
</tr>
</table>

Special considerations Electronic infusion devices may be used to maintain prescribed rate but must be specifically designed for use with blood transfusions.

Home care considerations Home care agencies evaluate clients who are candidates for a blood transfusion at home. Home transfusion if not appropriate for clients who are actively bleeding, require more than 4 hours for the transfusion, or recently had a reaction to a blood transfusion. Written consent must be obtained from the client and the physician. The nurse transports the blood product to the client's home in a special cooler.

The nurse and client's caregiver check serial number and other identification information together.

Administering Topical Medications

When a drug is applied directly to the body site, it is called a topical application. Other terms used include the dermal and mucosal route. Topical applications are usually intended for direct action on a particular site, although some systematic effect may also occur. The action depends on the type of tissue and the nature of agent of the site of application is readily accessible, such as the skin, as agent can easily be placed on it. If it is a cavity, such as the nose, or is enclosed, such as the eye, it is necessary to use a mechanical applicator for introducing the drug.

Skin Applications

The skin is a mechanical and chemical barrier that protects the underlying tissues. It is a sense organ, having receptors that respond to touch, pain, pressure and temperature. The "kin helps in excretion and regulating body temperature, and in storing essentials to the body such as water, salt and glucose. When a drug is incorporated in an agent, such as ointment, and rubbed onto the skin for absorption, the procedure is referred to as 'Inunction'. The following are the topical preparation applied to skin areas, their primary purposes, and specific nursing action:

- Powders are used to promote drying of the skin and prevent friction on the skin, use caution when applying to prevent inhalation of the medicated powder.
- Ointments provide prolonged contact of a medication on the skin and soften the skin. They are usually thoroughly massaged into intact skin.
- Creams and boils lubricate and soften the skin and prevent drying of the skin. The preparation should be warmed in the hands or fingers if a large part of the body is to be covered, to prevent chilling.
- Lotions protect and soothe the skin. Shake lotions thoroughly before using and apply with cotton balls or gauze.

Eye Applications

The eye is a delicate organ, highly susceptible to infection and injury. Although the eye is never free of microorganism, the secretions of the conjunctiva have a protective action against many pathogens. A common medication used by client is eyedrops and ointment including over-the-counter preparation such as artificial tears and vasoconstrictor. For maximum safety of the client, equipment, solutions and ointment introduced into the conjunctival sac should be sterile. If this is not possible, the most careful measures of medical asepsis should be followed. When administering medication following principles should be followed by the nurses:

- The cornea of the eye is richly supplied with pain fibers and thus is very sensitive to any thing applied to it. For this reason the nurse avoids instilling any form of eye medication directly into the cornea.
- The risk of transmitting infection from one eye to other is high. The nurse avoids touching eyelids or other eye structures with eyedroppers or ointment tube.
- The nurse uses eye medication only for the affected eye.
- The nurse never allows a person to use another's eye medication.

Topical medications are applied directly to a body site or placed m body cavities by irrigation or instillation. They are usually used for their local effects (e.g. zinc oxide ointment to protect the skin against chafing and chapping associated with bowel and bladder incontinence), but some are absorbed through the skin and mucous membranes for their systemic effects (e.g. estrogen patches), depending on the drug preparation. Most require application to the skin two to three times per day for maximum effect.

Skin Applications: Lotions, Creams, and Ointments

To enhance absorption, cleanse the skin with soap water and pat dry before applying lotions, creams, and ointments. If you warm the medication in your gloved hands, it will be more comfortable for the patient and make the preparation easier to apply. Use a sterile cotton swab, tongue blade, or gloved finger to apply corticosteroid creams and other topical medications so that your skin does not absorb them.

Transdermal Medications

Designed to be absorbed through the skin, transdermal medications are prepared as patches that are made of a special membrane. Patches allow constant controlled amounts of medications to be released over 24 hours or more, giving a prolonged systemic effect. Nitroglycerine (used to control angina or chest pain), scopolamine (used to treat motion sickness), nicotine (used to control smoking urges), and Fentanyl (used treat chronic pain) are examples of drugs administered by patch. Most patches are made with the correct dose already applied; however, you must apply nitroglycerine (NTG) paste to NTG paper, wearing gloves to protect yourself from the medication.

Also wear gloves when applying other transdermal patches. Avoid placing the patch on areas where there are skin lesions.

When removing and discarding patches, be aware that they may still contain medication. Wear gloves, fold the medicated side to the inside, and dispose of the patches where they are not accessible to children or pets.

Performing Irrigations Instillations

Washing out a body cavity with a steady stream of fluid or water is called irrigation. Sterile water, saline, or antiseptic solutions are flushed into the eye, ear, throat, vagina, rectum, or urinary tract to wash out the cavity. Instillation is the insertion of medication into a body cavity (e.g. eye drops) so that the medication can be retained or absorbed through that body cavity. Some medications should remain in the body cavity for a period of time for maximum absorption and effect.

Irrigations and instillations are performed to remove discharge or foreign bodies (e.g. from the eye or ear), to apply heat and cold to an area, to apply medications such as antiseptics, and to prepare an area for surgery (e.g. an enema for cleansing the bowels). You will usually not use sterile technique unless there are breaks in the skin. Several types of syringes are used for irrigating and instilling medications and fluids. Each is calibrated to allow you to control the amount and speed of solution delivered into the cavity (Fig. 20.38).

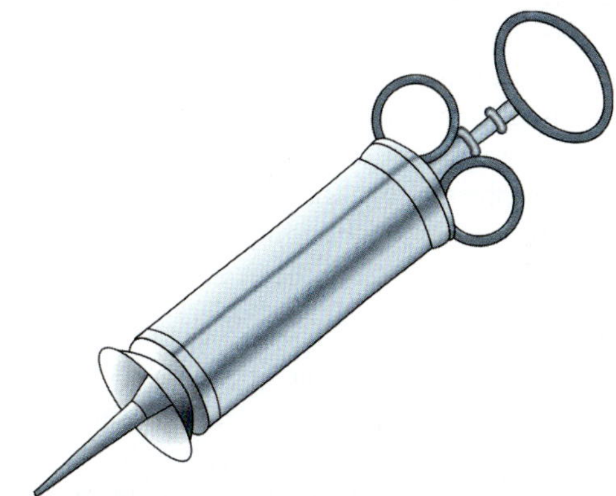

Figure 20.38: Syringe for administering enteral medications and performing irrigations and instillations

Ophthalmic Medications

Ophthalmic ointments or solutions are used for their local effects, for example, to treat eye irritations, infections, and glaucoma or to lubricate the eye. During an eye examination, eye medications may also be used to anesthetize the eye, dilate the pupil, or stain the cornea to identify abraded areas. Eye irrigation may be performed to remove foreign bodies, secretions, or harmful chemicals.

All ophthalmic medications are packaged in small bottles or tubes, which state, *"For ophthalmic use only."* Do not place any medication in the eye unless this statement appears on the container. The cornea the transparent part of the sclera in front of the iris and pupil) is easily injured, so you should not place medications directly onto the eyeball. Take care to not touch the tip of the dropper or tube to the eye or conjunctiva; doing so may lead to bacterial growth on the container.

The critical aspects of administering ophthalmic medications are as follows:

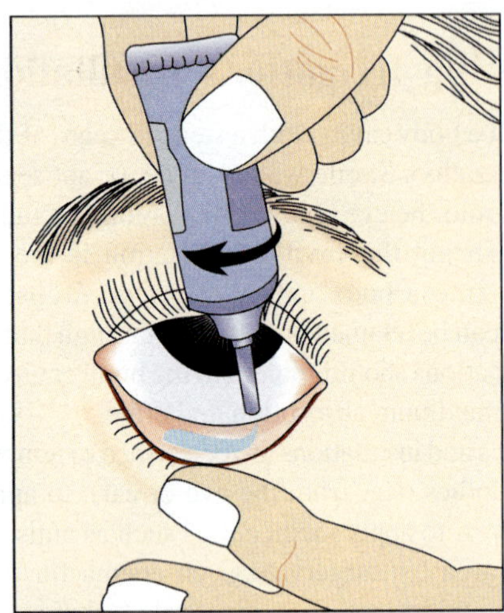

Figure 20.39: Administering eye ointment

For Instillations (Fig. 20.39)
- Assist the patient to high-Fowler's position, with head slightly tilted back.
- If necessary, clean the edges of the eyelid from the inner to outer canthus.
- Apply the medication into the conjunctival sac.
- Do not apply the medication to the cornea.
- Do not let the dropper or tube touch the eye.
- For eye drops, press gently against the same side of the nose for 1 to 2 minutes to close the lacrimal ducts. For eye ointment, ask the patient to gently close the eyes for 2 to 3 minutes.

For Irrigations
- Assist the patient to low-Fowler's position.
- Check the pH in the conjunctival sac, if indicated.
- Use a Morgan lens or IV tubing to irrigate the eyes.
- For direct-flow irrigation, irrigate from the inner canthus to the outer canthus.
- Irrigate for 20 minutes or until desired pH is reached.

Otic Medications
Medications or solutions may be dropped into the ear to treat internal and external ear infections, to apply heat to the area, and to soften and remove earwax. Using sterile technique when administering otic medications will help prevent infection if the eardrum has been ruptured. Use solutions at room temperature, because a solution that is too hot or too cold may cause vertigo, nausea, and pain.

The critical aspects of administering otic medications are as given below:
- Warm the solution to be instilled.
- Assist the patient to a side-lying position, with the appropriate ear facing up.
- Straighten the ear canal. For an adult client, pull the pinna up and back; for a child 3 years or younger, down and back.
- Instill the ordered number of drops into the ear canal.
- Do not force the solution into the ear or occlude the ear canal with the dropper.
- Instruct the patient to remain on his side for 5 to 10 minutes.

Nasal Medications
Clients usually self-administer "nose drops" and sprays. The most frequently used nasal medications are used to shrink swollen mucous membranes and to loosen secretions and drainage for treatment of nasal cavity or sinus infections. Because many nasal medications are available without prescription, caution the patient regarding overuse. Long-term use of decongestants may cause a rebound effect; that is, they will be effective immediately after administration, but the nasal congestion will recur and even increase when the effects of the drug wear off. Frequent use of or swallowing excess decongestant can also cause systemic side effects, such as increased heart rate and increased blood pressure. These effects can be serious in children; saline drops are safer for them.

The critical aspects of administering nasal medications are as given below:
- Determine head position: Consider the indication for the medication and the patient's ability to assume the position.
- Explain to the patient that the medication may cause some burning, tingling, or unusual taste.
- Position the patient with the head down and for ward or supine with the head back.
- Have the patient blow his nose, occlude one nostril, and exhale.
- Administer the spray or drops while the patient is inhaling.
- Repeat for other nostril.
- If nose drops are used, ask the patient to stay in the same position for approximately 5 minutes.

Vaginal Medications
Vaginal medications come in various forms: foams, jellies, liquids (douches) creams, tablets, and suppositories. They may be used for contraception, to destroy bacteria in the vaginal area before gynecological surgery, to treat vaginal itching or infection, or to induce labor. Store suppositories in the refrigerator to keep them firm enough to insert. Insert them with a lubricated, gloved finger. After insertion, the body temperature causes the suppository to melt. Foams and jellies are inserted using an applicator or inserter. Apply a clean perineal pad if there is heavy drainage or if the woman is ambulatory (the medication may melt and drain from the vagina by gravity).

A douche is a vaginal irrigation using low pressure. Vaginal irrigations are used to administer antimicrobial solutions to prevent infection (e.g. before surgery), to remove irritating discharge, and to apply heat or cold (e.g. to reduce inflammation). In the acute care setting, you will usually use sterile supplies. However, this is not usually necessary when the irrigation is self-administered at home because people usually have some resistance to the microorganisms in their daily environment. Teach women that douching is not necessary for ordinary female hygiene and that it may even be harmful because it disturbs the normal balance of microorganisms in the vagina.

The critical aspects provides guidelines for administering vaginal medications as given below:

For Instillation
- Position the patient in a dorsal recumbent or Sims' position.
- Inspect and cleanse the vaginal area before administering the medication.
- Insert the suppository or applicator along the posterior vaginal wall about 8 cm (3 inches).
- Instruct the client to maintain the position for 5 to 15 minutes after the medication is inserted.

For Irrigation (Douche)
- Warm the irrigation solution to approximately 105°F (40.6°C).
- Hang the irrigation solution approximately 30 to 60 cm (1 to 2 ft) above the level of the patient's vagina.
- Position the patient in a dorsal recumbent position on a waterproof pad and bedpan.
- Insert the nozzle approximately 7 to 8 cm (3 inches) into the vagina, and start the flow of irrigation solution.

Rectal Medications

Rectal suppositories and liquid instillations (enemas) are used to encourage bowel movements or to treat systemic complaints. For example, antiemetic suppositories are often used to treat nausea. Absorption is slow and erratic because of rectal contents, local drug irritation, and uncertainty of drug retention in the rectum. Other disadvantages include embarrassment to the patient and possible rectal pain if the patient has hemorrhoids. However, the rectal route may provide for higher blood levels of the medication than does the oral route because the venous blood from the rectum does not pass through the liver before entering the general circulation (review the discussion of the , first-pass effect, as needed). Also, rectal administration may be preferred when a drug has an unacceptable taste or odor or when it is not safe to use the oral route, as with a patient who is vomiting or unconscious. As a rule, rectal medications are contraindicated when there is active rectal bleeding.

The critical aspects provides guidelines for administering a rectal suppository as given below:
- Before inserting the suppository, assess for contraindications, such as rectal surgery, rectal bleeding, or cardiac disease.
- Position the client in Sims' position (left lateral with the upper leg flexed).
- Lubricate the suppository.
- Never force the suppository during insertion.
- Insert the suppository past the internal sphincter about 10 cm (4 inches).

Have the client stay on his side for 5 to 10 minutes and retain (not expel) the suppository for about 30 minutes.

Administering Eye Drops and Ointment

See Table 20.19.

Table 20.19: Procedures for Application of Eye Drops Ointment

Equipment
• Medication bottle with sterile eye dropper or ointment tube • Medication cart • Cotton ball or tissue • Wash basin filled with warm water and wash cloth • Eye pad and tape optional • Disposable glove

	Nursing actions		*Rationales*
1.	Assemble equipment.	1.	This provides for an organized approach to task.
2.	Wash hands.	2.	Reduces transmission of microorganism.
3.	Review the medication order.	3.	Ensures correct administration of medication.
4.	Check client's identification.	4.	Ensure that client receives correct medication.
5.	If eye pad is present, remove it.		
6.	Assess the condition of external eye structure.	6.	Provides baseline to later determine whether local to response medication occurs indicate need to clean eye.
7.	Explain the procedure.	7.	Reduces anxiety of the client.
8.	Arrange supplies at bedside and apply gloves.	8.	Ensures smooth, orderly procedure glove reduces to exposure infectious drainage.
9.	Ask client to be supine or sit back in chair with head slightly hyperextended.	9.	Provides easy access to eye for instillation and minimizes drainage for medication through tear duct.

Contd...

Table 20.19: *Contd...*

	Nursing actions		Rationales
10.	If crusts or drainage present along eyelid margins, or inner canthus, gently wash away. Soak crusts that are dried and difficult to remove by applying damp wash cloth or cotton ball over eye for few minutes. Always wipe clean from inner to outer canthus.	10.	Crusts and drainage harbor organism. Soaking allows, easy removal, thus being applied directly over eye. Cleaning for inner to outer canthus avoids entrance of micro-organisms into lacrimal duct.
11.	Hold cotton balls or clean tissue in nondominant hand on clients. Check bone just below lower lid.	11.	Cotton or tissue absorbs medication that escapes eye.
12.	With tissue or cotton resting below lower lid, gently press downward with thumb or forefinger against bony orbit.	12.	Technique exposes lower conjunctival sac. Retraction against body orbit prevents pressure and trauma to eyeball and fingers from touching eye.
13.	Ask client to look at ceiling.	13.	Action retracts sensitive cornea up and away from conjunctival sac and reduces stimulation of blink reflex.
14.	Instill eyedrops: (a) With dominant hand resting on clients forehead, hold filled medication eyedropper 1 to 2 cm above conjunctival sac (Fig. 20.41). (b) Drop prescribed number of drops into conjunctival sac. (c) If client blinks or closes eye or if drops land on outer lid margin repeat procedure. (d) When administering drugs that cause systemic effects, protect your finger with clean tissue and apply gentle pressure of client's nasal lacrimal duct for 30 to 60 seconds. (e) After instilling drops, ask client to close eye gently.	14.	(a) Helps prevent accidental contact of eyedropper with eye structures, thus reducing risk of injury to eye and transfer of infection to dropper. (b) Conjunctival sac normally hold 1 to 2 drops. Applying drops to sac provides even distribution across eye. (c) Therapeutic effect is obstructed only when drops enters conjunctival sac. (d) Prevents overflow of medications into nasal and pharyngeal passages, prevent absorption into systemic circulation. (e) Helps distribute medication, squinting or squeezing of eyelids forces medication from conjunctival sac.
15.	Instill eye ointment: (a) Holding ointment applicator above lid margin, apply thin stream of ointment evenly along inside edge or lower lid on conjunctiva (Fig. 20.40A). (b) Ask client to look down. (c) Apply thin stream of ointment along upperlid margin on inner conjunctiva (Fig. 20.40B). (d) Have client close eye and rub lid lightly in circular motion with cotton ball.	15.	(a) Distributing medication as evenly accord eye and lid margin. (b) Reduces blinking reflex during ointment application. (c) Distributes medication evenly according to eye and lid margin. (d) Further distribute medication without treatment.
16.	If excess medication is on eyelid, gently wipe it from inner to outer canthus.	16.	Promotes comfort and prevents trauma to eye.
17.	If client has eyepatch, apply clean one by replacing it over affected eye so that entire eye is covered. Tape securely without applying pressure to eye.	17.	Reduces chances of infection.
18.	Dispose of solid supplied in proper receptile. Remove and dispose gloves, wash hands.	18.	Maintains clean environment at bedside and reduces transmission of microorganism.
19.	Observe responses to medication noting signs and systemic effects and conditions of eye.	19.	Evaluates reaction to medication.
20.	Record drug, concentration, number of drops, time of administration and eyes (left or right or both) that receive medication.	20.	Timely documentation preventing medication errors.

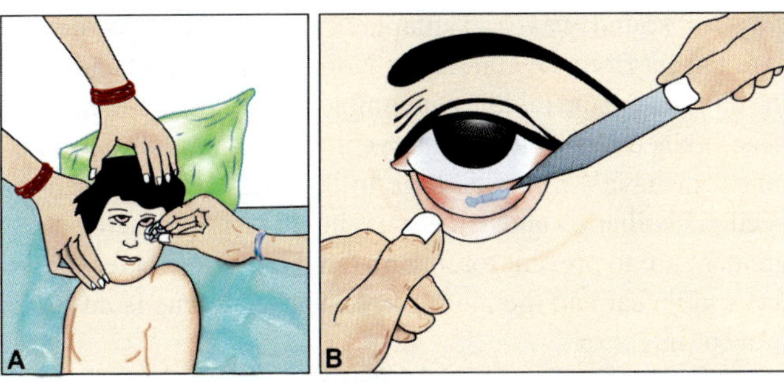

Figures 20.40A and B: Instillation of eye ointment

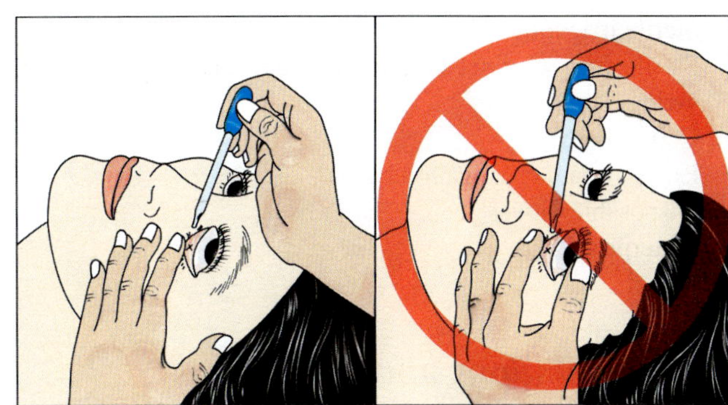

Figure 20.41: Administering eye drops

Administration of an Eye Irrigation

An eye irrigation is performed to remove secretions from the eye. In an emergency, eye irrigation can be used to remove chemicals that may bum to eye. Copious amounts to tap water should be used to remove chemical such as acid. The irrigation should continue for at least 15 minutes. The technique for administering a conjunctival irrigation as follows. The equipment needed and procedures for eye irrigation are as follows (Table 20.20)

	Table 20.20: Procedures or Techniques for Eye Irrigation		
	Nursing actions		*Rationales*
1.	Explain procedures to client.	1.	It facilitates cooperation and reassures client.
2.	Assemble equipment.	2.	This provides for an organized approach to task.
3.	Wash your hands.	3.	It deters spread of microorganism.
4.	Have the client sit or lie with the head tilted towards the side of the affected eye. Protect the client and the bed with a waterproof pad.	4.	Gravity helps the flow of solution away from the unaffected eye and from the inner canthus, if the affected eye toward the outer canthus.
5.	Don disposable gloves. Clean the lids and the lashes with a cotton ball moistened with normal saline or the solution ordered for the irrigation. Wipe from inner canthus to outer canthus. Discard the cotton ball after each wipe.	5.	Materials lodged on the lid of or in the lashes may be washed into the eye. This cleaning motion protects the nasolacrimal duct and the other eye.
6.	Place the cured basin at the cheek on the side of the affected eye to receive the irrigating solution. If the client is sitting up, ask him or her to support the basin.	6.	Cavity aids the flow of solution.
7.	Expose the lower conjunctival sac and hold the upper lid open with your non dominant hand.	7.	The solution is directed on to the lower conjunctival sac because the cornea is sensitive and easily injured. This also prevents reflex blinking.
8.	Hold the irrigator about 2.5 cm (1") from the eye. Direct the flow of the solution from the inner to the outer canthus along the conjunctival sac.	8.	This minimized the risk of injury to the cornea. Solution directed toward the outer canthus helps prevent lacrimal sac, the lacrimal duct and the nose.
9.	Irrigate until the solution is clear or all of the solution has been used. Use only sufficient force gently to remove secretions from the conjunctiva. A void touching any part of the eye with the irrigating tip.	9.	Directing solution with forced injury to the tissues of the eye as well as to the conjunctiva.
10.	Have the client close the eye periodically during the procedure.	10.	Movement of the eye when the lids are closed helps to move secretions from the upper to the lower conjunctival sac.
11.	Dry the area after the irrigating with cotton balls or gauze sponge after a towel to the client if the face and neck are wet.	11.	Leaving the skin most after an irrigation is uncomfortable for the client.
12.	Remove gloves, wash hands.	12.	It deters spread of microorganism.
13.	Chart the irrigating, appearance of the eye, drainage and the client's response.	13.	This provides accurate documentation.

- Sterile irrigating solution (warmed to 37°C or 98.6°F)
- Sterile irrigation set (sterile container and irrigating bulb syringe)
- Cotton balls
- Emesis basin or irrigation basin
- Disposable gloves
- Waterproof pad
- Towel

Ear Instillations and Irrigations

Medication or irrigation are instilled into auditory canal of ear. Medications in solution are placed in auditory canal for their local effects. They are used to soften wax, relieve pain, apply local anesthesia, destroy organism or destroy insect lodged in the ear, which can cause almost intolerable discomfort.

The ear contains the receptions for hearing and for equilibrium. It consists of the external ear, the middle ear and the inner ear. The external ear consists of auricle or pinna in the exterior auditory canal. The auditory canal serves as a passage way for sound waves. Tymapanic membrane separates the external ear from the middle ear. Normally it is intact and closes the entrance to the middle ear completely. If it is ruptured or has been opened by sufficient intervention, the middle ear and the inner ear have a direct passage to the external ear. When this occurs, instillation and irrigations should be performed with the greater care to prevent forcing materials from the outer ear into the middle ear and the inner ear. Sterile technique is needed to prevent infection.

Instillation of Eardrops

The equipments needed for instillation of ear drops are as follows:
- Medication bottle and dropper
- Medication cart
- Cotton tipped applicator (used to remove cerumen or drainage)
- Tissue
- Cotton ball (optional)
- Disposable gloves

	Table 20.21: Procedures for Instilling Eardrop		
	Nursing actions		*Rationales*
1.	Review medication order.	1.	Ensures safe and correct administration
2.	Wash hands.	2.	Reduces transmission of microorganism.
3.	Assemble equipment.		
4.	Identify the client.	4.	Ensures correct client receives medication.
5.	Apply gloves if client has ear discharge.	5.	Reduces exposure to microorganism.
6.	Assess condition of external ear structure and canal.	6.	Provides baseline to determine when the local response to medication.
7.	Explain procedures to the client.	7.	Reduces anxiety.
8.	Arrange supplied at bedside.	8.	Ensures smooth procedure.
9.	Have client assume side lying position with ear to be treated facing up.	9.	Provides easy access to ear instillation of medication. Ear canal is in position to receive medication.
10.	If cerumen or drainage occludes outer most portion of ear canal, wipe out gently with cotton tipped applicator. Do not force wax inward to block ear canal.	10.	Cerumen and drainage harbor microorganism and can block distribute of medication to canal. Occlusion of canal interferes with normal sound conduction.
11.	Straighten ear can by pulling auricles down and back (children) (Fig. 20.42) or upward and outward (adults) (Figs 20.43A and B).	11.	Straightening of ear canal provides direct access to deeper external ear structure.
12.	Instill prescribed drops holding dropper 1 cm (½ inch) above ear canal (Figs 20.44A and B).	12.	Forcing drops into occluded canal can cause injury to eardrum.
13.	Ask client to remain in sidelying position 2 to 3 minutes. Apply gentle massage or pressure to tragus of ear with finger.	13.	Allows complete distribution of medication. Pressure and message move medication inward.
14.	At times, physicians order, placement of cotton ball into outermost part of canal. Do not press cotton into innermost part of canal.	14.	Inserting cotton into outercanal prevents escape of medication. When client site or stands. Cotton should not block canal to impair hearing.

Contd...

<table>
<tr><td colspan="2" align="center">Table 20.21: Contd...</td></tr>
<tr><td>Nursing actions</td><td>Rationales</td></tr>
<tr><td>15. Remove cotton in 15 minutes.</td><td>15. Promotes drug distribution and absorption.</td></tr>
<tr><td>16. Dispose soiled supplies and gloves and wash hands.</td><td>16. Keeps bedside clean. Reduces transmission of microorganism.</td></tr>
<tr><td>17. Assist client to comfortable position after drops are absorbed.</td><td>17. Restores comfort.</td></tr>
<tr><td>18. Evaluation condition of external ear between drug instillation.</td><td>18. Determines response to medication.</td></tr>
<tr><td>19. Record drug, concentration, number of drops, time administered and ear into which drops were instilled on medication form.</td><td>19. Timely documentation prevents drug errors, i.e. repeated dose.</td></tr>
<tr><td>20. Record condition of ear canal in nurse notes.</td><td>20. Documents client status and response to therapy.</td></tr>
</table>

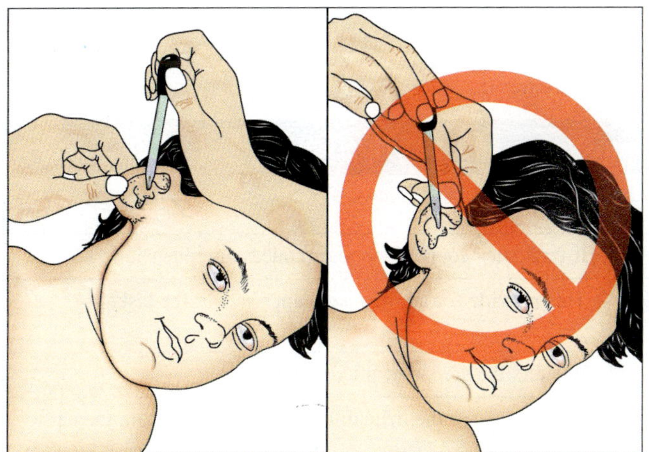

Figure 20.42: Administering eardrops to infant or toddler

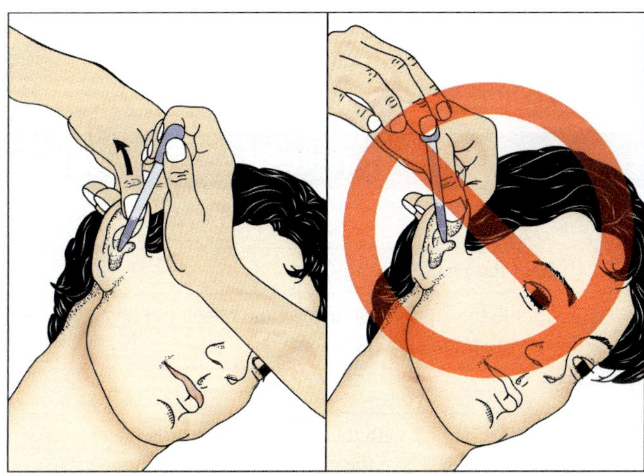

Figure 20.43: Administering eardrops to an adult

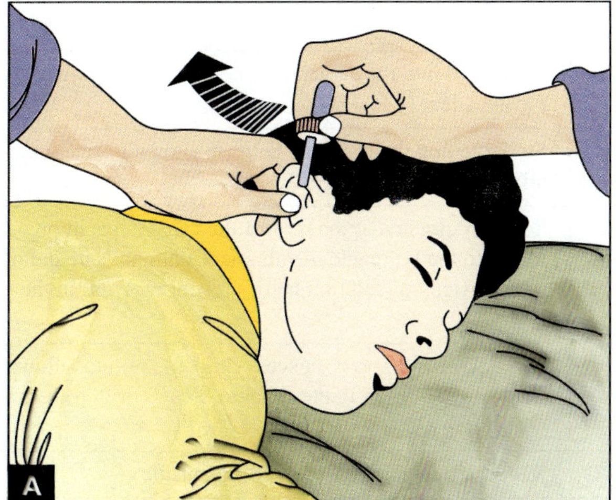

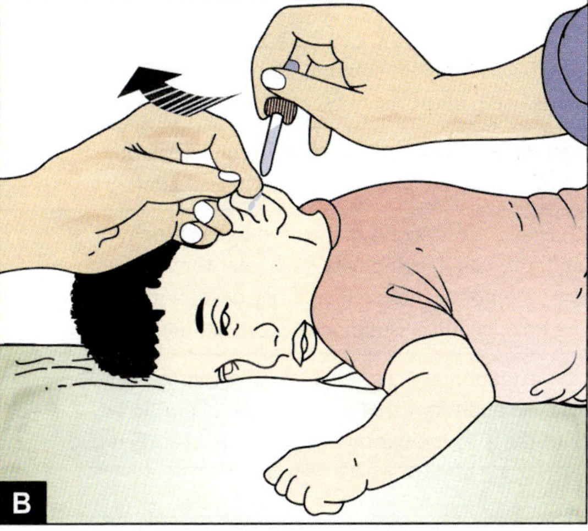

Figures 20.44A and B: Instillation of eardrops

Administering an Ear Irrigation

Irrigation of the external auditory canal is ordinarily for cleaning purposes or for applying heat to the area. Typically normal saline solution is used, although an antiseptic solution may be indicated for local action. The technique of administering of an ear drops are enlisted in Table 20.22.

Equipment: The equipment and techniques of administration of ear irrigation are as follows:
- Presented irrigating solution (warmed to 37°C)
- Irrigation set (container and irrigating or bulb syringe)
- Emesis basin
- Cotton tipped applications
- Disposable gloves (optional)
- Cotton balls
- Water proof pad

Nasal Instillations

Nasal instillation is used to treat sinus infections and nasal congestions. Medications that have a systematic effect such as vasopresin, may also be prepared as nasal instillation. The nose usually is not sterile cavity, but because of its connection with the sinus, medical asepsis should be carefully observed when using nasal instillation. The techniques of administration of nasal drops are enlisted in Table 20.23.

Equipments: These are as follows:
- Prepared medication with clean dropper
- Medication card/form
- Facial tissue
- Small pillow (optional)
- Wash cloth (optional)

Table 20.22: Procedures for Administering an Ear Irrigation

	Nursing actions		*Rationales*
1.	Explain the procedures to client.	1.	It facilitates cooperation and reduces apprehension.
2.	Assemble the equipment, protect the client and bed linen, with a moisture proof pad.	2.	This provide for an organized approach to the task.
3.	Wash your hands.	3.	It deters the spread of microorganism.
4.	Have the client lie with the head tilted towards the side of the affected ear. Have the client support a basin under the ear to receive the irrigating solution.	4.	Gravity causes the irrigating solution to flow from the ear to the basin.
5.	Clean the pinna and the meatus at the auditory canal as necessary with the applicators dipped in normal saline or the irrigating solution.	5.	Materials lodged on the pinna and meatus may be washed into the ear.
6.	Fill the bulb syringe with solution, if an irrigating container is used, allow air to escape from the tubing.	6.	Air forced into the ear canal is noisy and therefore unpleasant for the client.
7.	Straighten the auditory canal by pulling the pinna down and back for an infant and up and back for an adult.	7.	Straightening the ear canal helps in allowing solution to reach all areas of the canal easily.
8.	Direct a steady, slow steam of solution against the roof of the auditory canal, using only sufficient force to remove secretions. Do not occlude the auditory canal with the irrigating nozzle. Allow solution to flow out unimpeded.	8.	Solution directed at the roof of the canal helps in preventing injury to the tympanic membrane. Continuous in and outflow of the irrigating solution helps prevent pressure in the canal.
9.	When the irrigation is completed, place a cotton ball loosely in the auditory canal and have the client lie on the side of the affected ear on a towel or an absorbed pad.	9.	The cotton ball absorbs excess fluid and gravity allows the remaining solution in the canal to escape from the ear.
10.	Wash hands.	10.	Reduces transmission of microorganism.
11.	Chart the irrigation, the appearance of the drainage, and the client's response.	11.	This provides accurate documentation.
12.	Return in 10 to 15 minutes and remove the cotton ball and assess drainage.	12.	Drainage or pain may indicate to the tympanic membrane.

Table 20.23: Techniques of Instilling Nasal Drops

	Nursing actions		Rationales
1.	Review physician's order.	1.	Ensures safe and correct administration.
2.	Refer to medical card to determine which sinus is affected.	2.	Will affect posting that client for instillation.
3.	Wash hands.	3.	Reduces transmission of microorganism.
4.	Assemble equipment.		
5.	Check client identification.	5.	Ensures that the client receives correct medication.
6.	Inspect the condition of nose and sinuses, palpate sinuses for tenderness.	6.	Finding provides baseline for effect of medication. Discharges will interfere with drug absorption.
7.	Explain the procedure regarding positioning and sensations to expect, such as burning or straining of mucosa or choking sensation as medication trickes into throat.	7.	Helps reduce anxiety.
8.	Arrange supplies and medications at bedside.	8.	Ensure smooth, orderly procedure.
9.	Instruct the client to blow nose unless contraindicate (e.g. intracranial pressure or epistaxis).	9.	Removes mucus and secretion that can block distribution of medication.
10.	Administer nasal drops (Fig. 20.45): (a) Assist client to have supine position. (b) Position head properly. • Posterior pharynx–tilt client's head backward • Ethmoid or spheroid–tilt the head back over edge of bed or place pillow under shoulder and tilt head back • Frontal and maxillary sinus tilt head back over-edge of bed or pillow with head turned toward side treated • Support client's head with nondominant hand (c) Instruct client to breath through mouth. (d) Hold dropper 1 cm above nose and instill prescribed number of drops toward midline of the ethmoid bone. (e) Have client remain in supine position for 5 minutes. (f) Offer facial tissues to bolt running nose, but caution against blowing nose.		(a) Position provides access to nasal passages. (b) Position allows medication to drain into affected sinus. • Prevents staining neck muscle. (c) Reduces chance of aspirating nasal drop into trachea and lungs. (d) Avoid contamination of drops and proper distribution of drops. (e) Prevents loss of drops. (f) Allows maximum amount of absorption.
11.	Assist client to be comfortable position after drug absorption.	11.	Restores comfort.
12.	Dispose soiled supplies properly and wash hands.	12.	Prevents spread of microorganism.
13.	Record medication, administration, name numbers of drops, nostril used.	13.	Timely documentation prevents medication error.
14.	Observe client for side effects 15 to 30 minutes after administration.	14.	Drug absorbed through mucosa can cause systemic reaction.

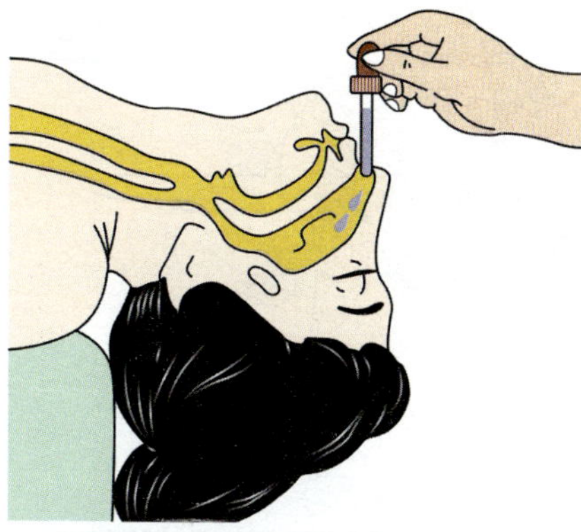

Figure 20.45: Instilling nasal drop

Vaginal Applications

A healthy vagina contains few pathogens but also many nonpathogenic organism. The nonpathogenic organisms are important because they protect the vagina from the invasion of pathogens. The normal secretions of the vagina are acidic which further serve to protect the vagina from microbial invasion. Therefore, the normal mucus membrane is its own best protection.

Vaginal medications are available as suppositories, foam, jellies or creams. Creams can be applied intravaginally, using a narrow, tubular applicator with an attached plunger. Suppositories come individually packaged in foil wrappers.

Suppositories that melt when exposed to body heat are also prepared for vaginal insertion. Suppositories should be refrigerated for storage.

Inserting Vaginal Suppository or Creams

A suppository is given with a gloved hand, clients often prefer administering their own vaginal medication and should be given privacy. The client should be asked to void before inserting the medication. The client is positioned lying on her back with knees flexed. Privacy should be maintained with draping. Adequate light should be available to visualize the vaginal opening. After instillation client may wish to wear perineal pads to collect excess drainage. Because vaginal medications are given to treat infection, any discharge may have foul smelling.

Good aseptic technique should be followed, and clients should be offered frequent opportunities to maintain perineal hygiene. The techniques for inserting vaginal suppository or cream are as follows (Fig. 20.46).

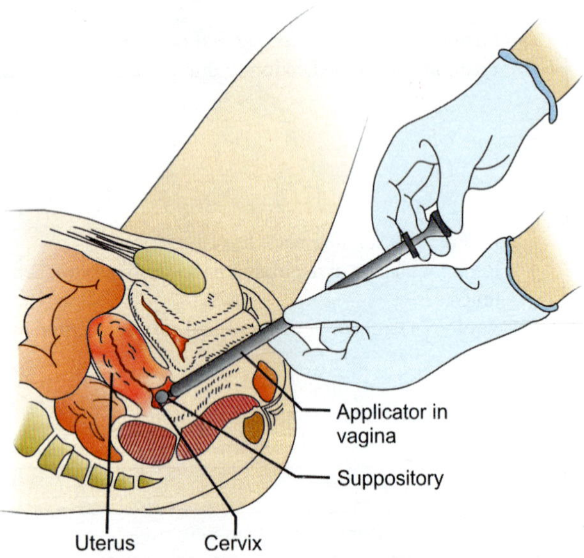

Figure 20.46: Insertion of vaginal suppository

- Fill a vaginal applicator with the prescribed amount of cream or have a suppository ready.
- Lubricate the applicator with water, as necessary. A suppository may be lubricated with a water soluble gel. Ordinarily lubrication is necessary but may be used to reduce friction while inserting the applicatory or suppository.
  - Wear disposable gloves
  - Use clean aseptic technique to administer the medication.
- Spread the labia well with fingers, and clean the area at the vaginal orifice with cotton balls and warm water to remove discharge, as necessary. With each cotton ball, use a single stroke moving from above the orifice downward sacrum. These techniques prevent contamination of the vaginal orifice with debris surrounding the anus.

- Introduce the applicator gently in a rolling manner. While directing it downward and backward to follow the normal contour of the vagina for its full length. Push the plunger to its full length, and then gently remove the applicator with the plunger depressed. After the applicator is properly positioned the labia may be allowed to fall in place to free the nurse's hand for manipulating the plunge. Insert a suppository with a gloved fingers well into the vagina.
- Ask the client to remain in the supine position for 5 to 10 minutes for insertion.
- After the client a perineal pad to collect excess drainage.
- Teach proper techniques to the client who wants to administer vaginal suppositories and creams herself.

Rectal Applications

Rectal suppositories are used primarily for that local action such as laxative and fecal softener (Fig. 20.47). Rectal suppositories differ in shape from vaginal ones. They are thinner and bullet shaped. They are rounded and prevent trauma during insertion. Rectal suppositories contain medications that exert local effects, such as promoting defecation, or systemic effects such as reducing nausea. Acetaminophen suppositories are used for an antipyretic effect and many anti emetics are available in suppository form to relieve nausea and vomiting. Rectal suppositories are stored in the refrigerator until they are administered.

When inserting rectal suppository, be sure to use a clean disposable glove to protect your hand and prevent contamination with face and microorganism. Following guidelines to be followed during inserting rectal suppositories:

- Use the glove for protection while inserting suppository.
- Have the client lie on either side, and pie fold top linens over him or her.
- Lubricate the suppository and fingertips to reduce irritation an intestinal mucosa, while inserting the suppository.
- Separate the buttocks and then have the client relax by breathing through the mouth while the suppository is inserted.

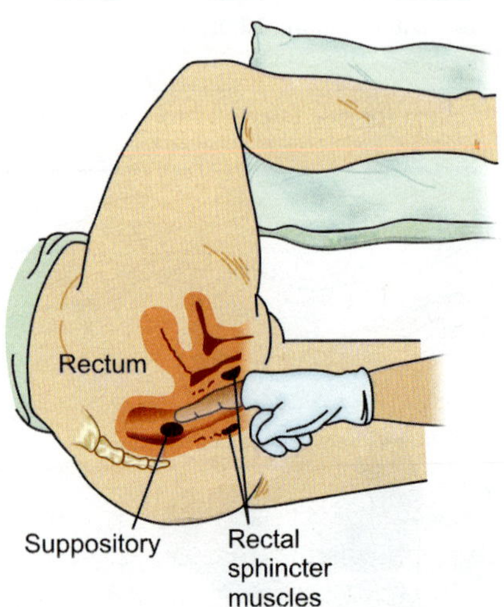

Figure 20.47: Insertion of rectal suppository

- Introduce the suppository well beyond the internal sphincter (4 inches for adults and 2 inches for children and infants) so that the suppository reaches the rectum, where its effect is desired.
- Avoid embedding the suppository in the fecal mass, correct placement when there is stool in the rectum between the stool and the rectal mucosa.
- Be sure the client understands that he or she is to retain the suppository, usually for 30 to 45 minutes after insertion.
- Encourage the client to walk about if ambulatory that often helps promote perisvalisis.

During administration of rectal suppositories, the nurse must place the suppository part the internal anal sphincter and against the rectal mucosa. Otherwise the suppository may be expelled before it can dissolve and be absorbed into the mucosa. With practice a nurse learns to recognize the sensation of the sphincter relaxing around the fingers. The suppository should not be forced into a mass of fecal matter. It may be necessary to clear the rectum with a small cleaning enema before a suppository can be inserted.

Medications Errors

All medications are ordered, prepared, and administered with the best intentions. However, errors occur with surprising frequency. One observational study found that 19% of drug doses administered by nurses were erroneous. Of these, 43% were given at the wrong time; 30% were simply omitted or missed doses; 17% were the wrong dose, and 4% were an unauthorized drug.

The following are a number of reasons why nurses make medication errors:
- Written order is not clear, is illegible, or is transcribed incorrectly.
- Telephone order is taken incorrectly.
- Wrong equipment is used to administer the drug.
- Equipment malfunctions or is not used properly.
- Medication is improperly handled or stored.
- Medication is given to a patient with contraindicating condition.
- Protocol is not understood or is violated.
- A drug is ordered for the wrong patient (written on the wrong patient's chart).
- The wrong dosage is ordered.
- The correct drug or dosage is ordered, but because of poor penmanship the wrong drug or dosage is administered.
- An error in calculating the dosage is made so the patient receives the wrong dose.
- A drug is given by the wrong route.
- The patient's identity is not checked, and the wrong patient receives the medication.
- The first person that administers the medication fails to record it immediately afterward. A second person checking the patient's chart thinks the drug has not been given so administers a dose. The patient receives a double dose.

Techniques to Avoid Errors

To prevent making a medication error, you should develop a set routine for administering medications. Practice this routine scrupulously when you are administering medications. Finally, learn from your mistakes and the mistakes of others. To administer medications safely, incorporate the following actions into your practice:
- Always practice the "three checks" and "six rights" of medication administration.
- Ask another nurse to check your calculations when you must calculate a dosage.
- Look at all medications closely for similar containers, colors, and shapes.
- Question orders of multiple tablets or vials as a single dose; most doses are one or two tablets or one single-dose vial.
- Beware of drugs with similar names (e.g. Keflex and Keflin).
- Check the decimal point! For example, Coumadin comes in both 1 mg and 10 mg sizes.
- Always write a zero before a decimal point (e.g. write "Lanoxin 0.125 mg," *not* "Lanoxin .125 mg"), and carefully read orders without a zero. It is easy to mistake .15 for 115 if the decimal point is written large or the 1 is written small.
- Question abrupt and excessive increases in dosage; most dosages increase gradually.
- When new or unfamiliar drugs are ordered, consult your resources for current information about the medication.
- Do not administer a drug ordered by a nickname or an unofficial abbreviation. Many providers refer to certain drugs by nickname (e.g. "MOM" for "mille of magnesia"); if you aren't familiar with the nickname used, then clarify the order so you select the correct medication.
- Do not attempt to decipher illegible handwriting. The chance of misinterpretation is great, so when in doubt, ask the prescriber to clarify.
- Be alert for patients with the same last names, and check arm bands carefully. It is common to have two patients with same or similar last names (e.g. Wilkinson, Wilson, Wilkerson). Special alerts on charts and MARs are helpful to prevent giving the medication to the wrong patient.
- Do not confuse measurements. It is easy to misread "mg" instead of "mL." There is a significant difference between 1 mg and 1 mL of intravenous morphine, for example.
- Double-check all orders transcribed to the MAR.
- Frequently review orders to make sure there have been no changes.

Steps during Commitment a Medication Error

Here are some steps to follow if you make a medication error:
- First check the patient. Take his vital signs, and perform assessments related to the medication that was given.
- If you are unfamiliar with the side effects of the medication, consult a drug reference source.

- Verify that you have made a medication error, and identify the type of error.
- Notify the nurse in charge for guidance if this is your first error.
- Notify the physician and follow her orders for intervention.
- Document on the chart that the medication was given, but do not indicate that the medication was given in error. This alerts anyone reviewing the chart that an error was made.
- Complete an incident report according to the facility's policies. Ask for assistance the first few times you complete this form so that the information you provide concerning the error is factual and accurate. Do not document in the patient's chart that an incident report was filed. This, again alerts anyone reviewing the chart and makes the incident report available for legal review in the event of a lawsuit.
- Finally, when you have time to think carefully, critically review the error. Identify the influences that led to your making the error. Were you rushed? Did you check the order? Did you follow the six rights? Whatever the reason, use this situation as a learning experience to improve your practice.

21

Infection Control Measures in Nursing

A client entering a healthcare setting is at risk for acquiring infections because of lowered resistance to infection, microorganisms and invasive procedures. The nurse comes in contact with a variety of microorganisms and thus health care workers must practice 'infection control' techniques to avoid spreading them to clients. The nurse is responsible for teaching clients about infection, mode of transmission, reasons for susceptibility, and infection control.

Nurses are responsible for providing quality care that incorporates infection-control principles. These principles are a major component of a safe environment. Here we are discusses the infection-control principles including naturally occurring microorganisms, pathogens, infection and colonization, chain of infection, body defenses, stages of the infectious process, and nosocomial infections. And of the nurse's role in controlling infections is emphasized.

Types of Microorganisms

Flora are microorganisms that occur or have adapted to live in a specific environment, such as intestinal, skin, vaginal, or oral flora. There are two types of flora: resident and transient. **Resident (normal) flora** are microorganisms that are always present, usually without altering the client's health; an example would be *proprionibacterium* on the skin. Resident flora prevent the overgrowth of harmful microorganisms; only when the balance is upset does disease result. **Transient flora** are microorganisms that are episodic (of limited duration); an example would be *staphylococcus aureus*. They attach to the skin for a brief period of time but do not continually live on the skin. Transient flora are usually acquired from direct contact with the microorganisms on environmental surfaces. Although most microorganisms found in the environment do not cause disease and infection, some do. Disease-producing microorganisms are called **pathogens; pathogenicity** refers to the ability of a microorganism to produce disease. **Virulence** refers to the frequency with which a pathogen causes disease. The factors affecting virulence are the strength of the pathogen to adhere to healthy cells; the ability of a pathogen to damage cells or interfere with the body's normal regulating systems; and the ability of a pathogen to evade the attack of white blood cells (WBCs).

Five types of microorganisms can be pathogenic: bacteria, viruses, fungi, protozoa, and Rickettsia.

Bacteria: Bacteria are small, one-celled microorganisms that lack a true nucleus or mechanism to provide metabolism. Therefore, bacteria need an environment that will provide food for survival. Bacteria can be spherical, rod-like, spiral, or curving in shape, usually appearing as single cells, pairs, chains, or groups. Although most bacteria multiply by simple cell division, some forms of bacteria produce **spores,** a resistant stage that withstands unfavorable environments. When proper environmental conditions return, spores germinate and form new cells. Spores are difficult to kill because of their resistance to heat, drying, and disinfectants. The growth rate of bacteria is affected by environmental factors such as changes in temperature and nutrition. The optimal temperature for pathogenic bacteria is 98.6°F. Bacteria can be found in all environments, yet not all bacteria are harmful or cause disease. Only a small percentage of bacteria are actually pathogenic. Common bacterial infections include diarrhea, pneumonia, sinusitis, urinary tract infections, cellulites, meningitis, gonorrhea, otitis media, and impetigo.

Viruses: Viruses are organisms that can live only inside cells. They cannot get nourishment or reproduce outside cells. Viruses contain a core of deoxyribonucleic acid (DNA) or ribonucleic acid (RNA) surrounded by a protein coating. Some viruses have the ability to create an additional coating called an envelope, which helps protect the cell from attack by the immune system. Viruses damage the cells they inhabit by blocking the normal protein synthesis of the cells and by using the cell's mechanism for metabolism to reproduce.

The same viral infection may cause different symptoms in different individuals, based on the individual's immune response to the invading virus. Some viruses will immediately trigger a disease response, whereas others may remain latent for many years. Common viral infections include influenza, measles, common cold, chickenpox, hepatitis B, genital herpes, and HIV.

Fungi: Fungi grow in single cells, as in yeast, or in colonies, as in molds. Fungi obtain food from dead organic matter or from living organisms. Most fungi are not pathogenic and make up many of the body's normal flora. Disease from fungi is found mainly in individuals who are immunologically impaired. Fungi can cause infections or the hair, skin, nails, and mucous membranes.

Protozoa: Protozoa are single-celled parasitic organisms with the ability to move (Fig. 21.1). Most protozoa obtain their nourishment from dead or decaying organic matter. Infection is spread through ingestion of contaminated food or water or through insect bites. Common infections include and vaginal infections.

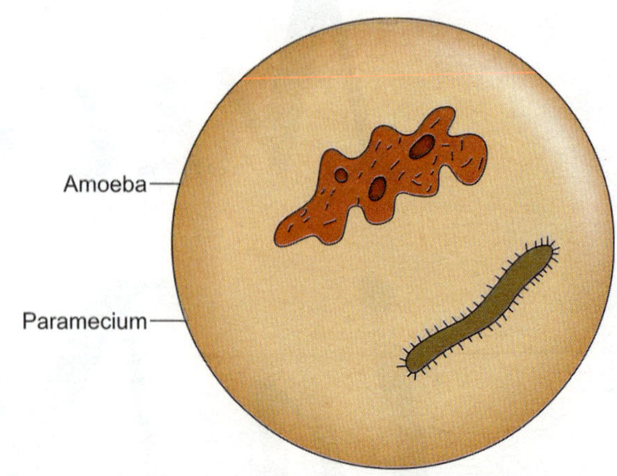

Figure 21.1: Protozoa

Rickettsia: Rickettsia are intracellular parasites that need to be in living cells to reproduce. Infection from *rickettsia* is spread through fleas, ticks, mites, and lice. Common *rickettsia* infections include typhus, Rocky Mountain spotted fever, and Lyme disease.

Infection Process

Colonization is the multiplication of microorganisms on or within a host that does not result in cellular injury; an example of colonization is the normal flora (microorganisms) in the intestines. However, if host susceptibility increases or the microorganism's virulence creases, colonized microorganisms on a host may be a potential source of infection.

Infection is the invasion and multiplication of pathogenic microorganisms in body tissue that results in cellular injury; an example is strep throat. These microorganisms are called **infectious agents.** Infectious agents capable of being transmitted to a client by direct or indirect contact, through a vehicle (or vector) or airborne route are called **communicable agents.** Diseases produced by these agents are referred to as **communicable diseases.**

An infection is an invasion of the body by pathogens, or microorganism capable of producing disease. The development of an infection occurs in a cyclical process that depends on the following six elements (Fig. 21.2).

An infection will develop if this cyclical chain remains intact. To prevent the spread of microorganism, the cycle must be interrupted. Nurses use respective practices to break the chain, so that infection will not occur.

Neither a susceptible host nor the presence of a pathogen means that an infectious process will occur. The **chain of infection** describes the development of an infectious process. An interactive process involving an agent, host, and environment is required. This interactive process involves several essential elements, or "links in the chain," for transmission of microorganisms to occur. Figure 21.2 identifies the six essential links (elements) in the chain of infection. An infectious process cannot occur without the transmission of microorganisms.

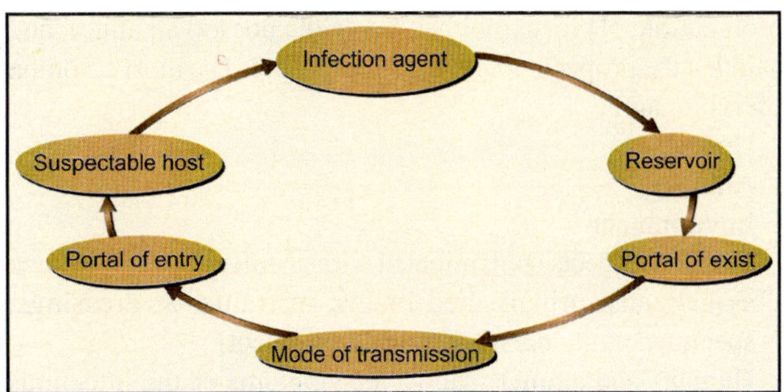

Figure 21.2: Elements of infection process

Therefore, knowledge about the chain of infection facilitates control or elimination of microorganism transmission by breaking the links in the chain. Breaking the chain of infection is achieved by altering the interactive process of the agent, host, and environment. Each of the six links in the chain of infection is discussed above.

Agent

An agent is an entity that is capable of causing disease. Agents that cause disease may be as follows:

- **Biological agents:** Living organisms that invade the host, causing disease, such as bacteria, viruses, fungi, protozoa, and *rickettsia* (Table 21.1).
- **Chemical agents:** Substances that can interact with the body, causing disease, such as food additives, medications, pesticides, and industrial chemicals.
- **Physical agents:** Factors in the environment that are capable of causing disease, such as heat, light, noise, and radiation.

In the chain of infection, the main concern is biological agents and their effect on the host.

Reservoir: The reservoir is a place where the agent can survive. Colonization and reproduction take place while the agent is in the reservoir. A reservoir that promotes growth of pathogens must contain the proper nutrients (such as oxygen and organic matter), maintain proper temperature, contain moisture, maintain

	Table 21.1: Common Pathogens and Infections Organisms Affected Organs			
	Agents	*Organisms*	*Affected organs*	*Infections*
1.	Bacteria	Escherichia coli Staphylococcus aureus Mycobacterium tuberculosis Neisseria gonorrhoeae	Colon Skin Lungs Genito-urinary tract Eye	Enteritis Wound infection Tuberculosis Gonorrhea Conjunctivitis
2.	Viruses	Hepatitis A virus Hepatitis B virus HIV	Feces, blood, urine Body fluids and excretion Blood, semen	Infection hepatitis Serum hepatitis AIDS
3.	Fungi	Aspergillus organism Candida albicans	Mouth, skin, GI tracts Soil, dust	Aspergillosis Thrush, dermatitis
4.	Protozoa	Pl. falciparum	Mosquito	Malaria

a compatible pH level (neither too acidic nor too alkaline), and maintain the proper amount of light exposure. The most common reservoirs are:

- Humans
- Animals
- Environment
- Fomites (objects contaminated with an infectious agent. such as bedpans. urinals. bed linens, instruments. dressings. specimen containers. and other equipment).

Humans and animals can have symptoms of the infectious agents or can be strictly carriers of the agent. **Carriers** have the infectious agent but are symptom free. The agent can be spread to others in both instances.

Portal of Exit: The portal of exit is the route by which an infectious agent leaves the reservoir to be transferred to a susceptible host. The agent leaves the reservoir through body secretions including:

- Sputum, from the respiratory tract
- Semen, vaginal secretions, or urine, from the genitourinary tract
- Saliva and feces, from the gastrointestinal tract
- Blood
- Draining wounds
- Tears.

Modes of Transmission

The mode of transmission is the process of the infectious agent moving from the reservoir or source through the portal of exit *to* the portal of entry of the susceptible "new" host. Most infectious agents have a usual or primary mode of transmission; but some microorganisms may be transmitted *by* more than one mode (Table 21.2). Depending on the agent, almost anything in the environment can become a potential mode of transmission.

Contact Transmission: The most important and frequent mode of transmission is contact transmission. This involves the transfer of an agent from an infected person to a host by direct contact with the infected person, indirect contact with the infected person through a fomite, or close contact with contaminated secretions. Sexually transmitted diseases are spread by direct contact, common viral infections (cold, measles, flu) are spread by close contact with contaminated secretions.

Airborne Transmission: Airborne transmission occurs when a susceptible host contacts droplet nuclei or dust particles that are suspended in the air. Particle size influences the length of time that the organism can remain airborne. The longer the particle is suspended, the greater the chance it will find an available port of entry to the human host. A disease that relies on airborne transmission is measles. Contaminated droplets containing the measles virus are found in the spray from sneezing. The droplet can find a portal entry through the mucous membranes or conjunctiva. Droplets that do not remain airborne or settle out are excluded from this category.

Table 21.2: Modes of Transmission

Mode	Examples
Contact	Direct contact' of health care provider with client: • Touching • Bathing • Rubbing • Toileting (urine and feces) • Secretions from client Indirect contact with fomites: • Clothing • Bed linens • Dressings • Health care equipment • Instruments used in treatments • Specimen containers used for laboratory analysis • Personal belongings • Personal care equipment • Diagnostic equipment
Airborne	Inhaling microorganisms carried by moisture or dust particles in air: • Coughing • Talking • Sneezing
Vehicle	Contact with contaminated inanimate objects: • Water • Blood • Drugs • Food • Urine
Vector borne	Contact with contaminated animate hosts: • Animals • Insects

Vehicle Transmission: Vehicle transmission occurs when an agent is transferred to a susceptible host by contaminated inanimate objects such as water, food, milk, drugs, and blood. Cholera is transmitted through contaminated drinking water, and salmonellosis is transmitted through contaminated meat.

Vectorborne Transmission: Vectorborne transmission occurs when an agent is transferred to a susceptible host by animate means such as mosquitoes, fleas, ticks, lice, and other animals. Lyme disease, malaria, and West Nile are examples of diseases spread by vectors.

An organism may be transmitted from its reservoir by various means of routes. Some organisms can be transmitted by more than one route.

1. *Contact*
   - Direct contact, e.g. *Staphylococcus, T. palladium,* herpes simplex
   - Indirect contact, e.g. Measles virus, HBV, *Enterococcus* and pseudomonal organisms.
   - Droplet contact, e.g. influenza virus, *M. tuberculosis.*

2. *Air*
   - Droplet nuclei, e.g. influenza virus, *Pneumococcus*, V-Z virus
   - Dust, e.g. *Aspergillus-organisms.*
3. *Vehicles*
   - Contaminated items, e.g. M. *tuberculosis*
   - Liquids:
     - water, e.g. *Vibrio cholerae*
     - drugs solution, e.g. *Pseudomonas* organism
     - blood, e.g. hepatitis B virus
     - food, e.g. *Salmonella, Staphylococcus, Enterobacter,* etc. and *Klebsiella* organism.
4. *Vectors*
   - Insects, e.g. mosquitoes–e.g. falciparum
   - Fleas, ticks, e.g. *Rickettsia typhi and* R. *prowazekii*
   - Cows, Dogs, e.g. *Brucella* organisms

A portal of entry A portal of entry is the route by which an infectious agent enters the host. Portals of entry include the following:
- *Integumentary system,* through a break in the integrity of the skin or mucous membranes (e.g. infections of surgical wounds)
- *Respiratory tract,* by inhaling contaminated droplets (such as cold, influenza, measles)
- *Genitourinary tract,* through contact with infected vaginal secretions or semen (as in sexually transmitted diseases)
- *Gastrointestinal tract,* by ingesting contaminated food or water (e.g. typhoid, hepatitis A)
- *Circulatory system,* through the bite of insects (such as mosquito bites resulting in malaria)
- *Transplacental,* through transfer of microorganisms from mother to fetus via the placenta and umbilical cord (including HI V, hepatitis B)

Host

A host is an organism that can be affected by an agent. A human being is usually considered a host. A **susceptible host** is a person who has no resistance to an agent and thus is vulnerable to disease. For example, an individual who has not received the measles vaccine is more likely to contract the infection because of the lack of immunity to the infectious agent. A **compromised host** is a person whose normal body defenses are impaired and is therefore susceptible to infection. For example, a person with a common cold or superficial burns is at greater risk for infection because of the impaired state of the body system mechanisms.

Characteristics of the host influence the susceptibility to and severity of infections. These include:
- *Age:* As a person ages, immunity declines, thus increasing susceptibility to infection.
- *Concurrent diseases:* The existence of comorbid diseases indicates an environment susceptible to infection.
- *Stress:* An individual experiencing a compromised emotional state may have altered or decreased immune system response.
- *Immunization/vaccination status:* Individuals who are not fully immunized are at greater risk for infection.
- *Lifestyle:* Lifestyle practices such as having multiple sex partners or sharing intravenous drug needles increase an individual's potential for illness.
- *Occupation:* Forms of employment that involve an increased exposure to pathogens might include dealing with chemical agents (such as asbestos) or handling sharp instruments (such as scalpels).
- *Nutritional status:* Individuals who maintain targeted weight for height and body frame are less prone to illness.
- *Heredity:* Some individuals are naturally more susceptible to infection than others.

Interaction between agent and host occurs in the environment, which is everything other than the agent and host. Many of the conditions promoting transmission of microorganisms reflect changes in the relationship between humans and their environments.

For microorganism to continue to exists, they must find a source that is acceptable (a host) and overcome any resistance mounted by the host defenses. Susceptibility is the degree of resistance and individual has to pathogens. An organism or parasite potential to produce disease depends on a variety of factors which includes following:
- Number of organisms or parasites
- Virulence of organism or its ability to cause disease
- Competence of a person's immune system
- Ability to enter and survive in the host
- Length and intimacy of the contact between a person and the microorganisms
- Susceptibility of the host.

Sources of Infection

Some infections cause harm in a limited region of the body, such as the upper respiratory tract, the urethra, or a single bone or joint. Such infections are said to be local. In contrast, systemic infections occur when pathogens invade the blood or lymph and spread throughout the body. Bacteremia is the clinical presence of bacteria in the blood, whereas septicemia is symptomatic systemic infection spread via the blood.

In addition, it is helpful for health care providers to distinguish between primary and secondary infections. A primary infection is the first infection that occurs in a patient. Following a primary infection, especially in immunocompromised patients, may be one or more secondary infections. For example, a frail client infected with pneumonia develops herpes zoster (a viral infection related to past infection with varicella) related to the stress of illness.

Healthcare providers also need to determine the source of pathogens in a patient infected while he is in the facility. In exogenous nosocomial infections, the pathogen is acquired from the healthcare environment. In endogenous nosocomial infections, the pathogen arises from the patient's normal flora, and some form of treatment (e.g. chemotherapy or antibiotics) causes the normally harmless microbe to multiply and cause infection. For example, candidal vaginitis (yeast infection) may develop in a client receiving antibiotics after abdominal surgery.

Infections that have a rapid onset but last only a short time, such as a head cold, are said to be *acute.* In contrast, *chronic* infections develop slowly and last for weeks, months, or even years. Some chronic infections, such as relapsing fever, recur after periods of remission. *Latent* infections cause no symptoms for long periods of time, even decades. Human immunodeficiency virus (HIV) is an example. It typically causes an initial, brief illness that is then followed by about 6 years of latency before the patient begins to experience symptoms of AIDS.

A nosocomial infection is an infection acquired in a hospital or other health care facility that was not present or incubating at the time of the client's admission. They also include those infections that become symptomatic after the client is discharged and infections passed among medical personnel. Nosocomial infections are also called *hospital-acquired infections.* These types of infections typically fall into four categories: urinary tract, surgical wounds, pneumonia, and septicemia. Most nosocomial infections are transmitted by health care personnel who fail to practice proper hand hygiene or who fail to change gloves between client contacts. The hospital environment provides exposure to a variety of organisms to which the client has not typically been exposed in the past. Therefore, the client has no resistance to these organisms. Illness impairs the body's defenses.

The term 'nosocomial' is taken from the Greek word *nosocomium* meaning healthcare facility. A nosocomial infection is one that is acquired in a hospital or other health agency. This is a far reaching and serious problem. A hospital is one of the most likely places for acquiring an infection because it harbors a high population of virulent stains of microorganisms that are usually resistant to antibiotics. Nosocomial infections not only extend hospital care for the patient but also increase cost for both patient and hospital.

Iatrogenic infection is a type of nosocomial infection resulting from the diagnostic or therapeutic procedure, e.g. insertion of catheter in urinary tract may develop infection. Nosocomial infection may be exogenous or endogenous. An exogenous infection caused by microorganism from another person, may exist as normal flora (e.g. *S typhi, Cl tetani*). An endogenous is an infection caused by the patients own normal microorganism becoming altered and overgrowing or being transferred from and body site to another. Nosocomial infections are most commonly transmitted by direct contact between health personnel and patient or from patient to patient.

The nurse is responsible for providing the patient with a clean and safe environment. The conscientiousness and accuracy of the nurse in performing clean and aseptic procedures increases the effectiveness of infection control.

Stages of Infections

Infection is the result of tissue invasion and damage by an infectious agent. There are two types of infections:

1. **Localized infections** are limited to a defined area or single organ with symptoms that resemble inflammation (redness, tenderness, and swelling), such as a cold sore.
2. **Systemic infections** affect the entire body and in organs, such as AIDS.

An understanding of the course of infection by stages in the development of an infection is necessary if the nurse is to intervene and disrupt the infection cycle. All infections progress through four stages: incubation, prodromal, illness, and convalescence.

Incubation Stage: The incubation period is the time between entry of an infectious agent in the host and the onset of symptoms. During this time, the infectious agent invades the tissue and multiplies to produce an infection. The client is typically infectious to others during the latter part of this stage. For example, the incubation period for varicella (chickenpox) is 2 to 3 weeks; the infected person is contagious from 5 days before any skin eruptions to no more than 6 days after the skin eruptions appear. Incubation period is the interval between the invasion of the body by the pathogen or entrance of pathogen into the body and the appearance the first symptoms of infection, e.g. chickenpox 2-3 weeks, common cold 1-2 days, tetanus 2 to 21 days. Always verify the incubation period of a suspected infection. Remember that a client may be able to transmit the infection to another person before the onset of symptoms.

Prodromal Stage: The prodromal stage is the time from the onset of nonspecific symptoms until specific symptoms begin to manifest. The infectious agent continues to invade and multiply in the host. A client may also be infectious to other persons during this time period. In the client with chickenpox, a slight elevation in temperature will occur during this stage, followed within 24 hours by eruptions on the skin. A person is most infectious during this stage. It is an internal from onset of nonspecific signs and symptoms (malaise, low grade fever, fatigue) to more specific symptoms. During this time, microorganisms grow and multiply and client is more capable of spreading disease to others.

Illness Stage: The illness stage is the time when the client has specific signs and symptoms of an infectious process. The client with chickenpox will experience a further rise in temperature and continued outbreaks of skin eruptions for at least 2 to 3 more days. Full stage of illness is an interval when client manifests signs and symptoms specific type of infection. The presence of specific signs and symptoms indicates the full stage of illness. The types of infection determine the length of illness and the severity of manifestations. Symptoms that are limited or restricted to a discrete area are referred to as localized symptoms, whereas systematic symptoms are manifested throughout the entire body.

Convalescent Stage: The convalescent stage is from the beginning of the disappearance of acute symptoms until the client returns to the previous state of health. The client with chickenpox will see the skin eruptions and irritation begin to resolve during this stage. Convalescent period represents recovery from the infection. It is an interval when acute symptoms of infection disappear and the person returns to healthy state–length of recovery depends on severity of infection and clients general state of health; recovery may take several days to months.

Defenses Against Infection

The human body has three "lines of defense" against infectious disease. First, certain anatomical features limit the entry of pathogens. Second, protective biochemical processes fight pathogens that do enter. Third, the presence of pathogens activates immune responses against specific, recognized invaders.

The first two lines of defense are nonspecific; that is, they have no means of adapting their response to each specific invader. Instead, they act in precisely the same way against any and all intruders, from a simple cold virus to deadly fungal spores.

Primary Defenses

The "soldiers" in the first line of defense are the structural barriers of the human body. These primary defenses prevent organisms from entering the body.

- *Skin:* The surface of intact, healthy skin is tough and resilient and prevents entry of many pathogens.
- *The respiratory tree:* The nares, trachea, and bronchi are covered with mucous membranes that trap pathogens, which are then expelled. The nose contains hairs that filter the upper airway, and the nasal passages, sinuses, trachea, and larger bronchi are lined with cilia, tiny hair like cells that sweep microorganisms upward from the lower airways. Coughing and sneezing forcefully expel organisms from the respiratory tract.
- *Eyes:* The lacrimal glands produce tears that contain lysozyme, an antimicrobial enzyme. Thus, tears help the body wash infective organisms from the eyes.
- *The mouth:* The mouth normally has a large number of pathogenic microorganisms, but saliva, like tears, contains lysozyme and helps continually wash microbes from the teeth and gums. The rich blood supply of the mouth swiftly transports defensive blood cells that keep the microorganisms in check. In addition, normal flora of the mouth compete for nutrition with invading organisms, thereby limiting the number of pathogens.
- *The gastrointestinal tract:* Many pathogens that reach the stomach are destroyed in its acidic environment. Those that successfully enter the small intestine face the antimicrobial action of bile. Simple peristalsis, as well as diarrhea and vomiting, are other first-line defense mechanisms for pathogens that invade the gastrointestinal tract.
- *The genitourinary tract:* Like the respiratory tree, the genitourinary tract is protected with mucous membranes. The epithelial cells lining the urethra and anus secrete mucus, which adheres to pathogens to promote their excretion through urine and stool. Urine itself is highly acidic and contains lysozyme. Mucous membranes lining the vagina also inhibit establishment of pathogens. In addition, the high acidity and normal flora of the vagina hold pathogens in check.

Secondary Defenses

Pathogens that dodge the primary defenses and gain entry into the body begin to release wastes and secretions and to cause the breakdown of cells and tissues. The presence of such chemicals activates a set of secondary defenses.

- *Phagocytosis*—the process by which white blood cells (WBCs) called *plagocytes* engulf and destroy pathogens directly. Phagocytic white blood cells include neutrophils, monocytes, and eosinophils. Monocytes also have the ability to differentiate into macrophages that specialize in cleaning up sites of injury or infection by phagocytizing pathogens, used WBCs, and cellular debris. Eosinophils are occasionally phagocytic; however, they are responsible mainly for binding to helminths and releasing harmful toxins onto their surface.
- *The complement cascade*—a process by which a set of blood proteins called complement triggers the release of chemicals that attack the cell membranes of pathogens, causing them to rupture. Complement also signals white blood cells called basophils to release a chemical called histamine, which prompts inflammation.
- *Inflammation*—a process that begins when histamine and other chemicals are released either directly from damaged cells, or from basophils in response to the activation of complement. Histamine and other inflammatory chemicals cause dilation and increased permeability of blood vessels, increasing the flow of phagocytes, antimicrobial chemicals, oxygen, and nutrients to the damaged area.
- *Fever*—a rise in core body temperature that increases metabolism, inhibits multiplication of pathogens, and triggers specific immune responses (discussed shortly). Believing that low-grade fevers are a necessary natural defense mechanism, many clinicians do not treat a fever lower than 102°F (38.9°C).

The classic signs and symptoms of inflammation are localized heat and erythema (redness), which develop as blood flow is increased. In addition, fluid leaking from the more permeable blood vessels accumulates in the surrounding tissue, causing edema, which in turn prompts pain as pressure is exerted on nerve endings.

Table 21.3 summarizes the types of white blood cells and their roles in defending against infection.

Tertiary Defenses

Why is it that people who recover from an infectious disease like measles or chickenpox never get the disease again, even if they are repeatedly exposed to the virus? The answer lies in specific immunity: the process by which the body's immune cells "learn" to recognize and destroy pathogens that they have encountered before.

Table 21.3: Types and Functions of White Blood Cells

Type	Function
Granular	
Basophils: 0.5–1% of total WBCs	Release histamine and heparin granules as part of the inflammatory response
Eosinophils: 1–3% of total WBCs	Destroy helminths; mediate allergic reactions; have limited role in phagocytosis
Neutrophils: 55–70% of total WBCs	Phagocytize pathogens
Agranular	
Lymphocytes: 20–35% of total WBCs	T cells–responsible for cell-mediated immunity; recognize, attack, and destroy antigens B cells–responsible for humoral immunity; produce immunoglobulins to attack and destroy antigens
Monocytes: 3-8% of total WBCs	Able to phagocytize directly as well as to differentiate into macrophages, which help clean up damaged or injured tissue

The cells involved in specific immunity are white blood cells called lymphocytes, which are produced from stem cells in the red bone marrow. Lymphocytes that grow to maturity in the bone marrow are designated *B lymphocytes,* or *B cells,* whereas those that mature in the thymus are designated *T lymphocytes,* or *T cells.* After they have matured, most B cells and T cells travel to the lymph nodes, spleen, and other sites of lymphatic tissue. Some circulate in blood and lymph. From all of these locations, lymphocytes seek out foreign cells and other matter to target for destruction. Lymphocytes recognize foreign substances by the molecules that they present on their surfaces. These molecules that trigger a specific immune response are called antigens.

B cells are involved in the humoral immune response. T cells are responsible for cell-mediated immunity. These two types of specific immunity are discussed next.

Humoral Immunity

The humoral immune response acts directly against antigens. In response to the presence of antigens, macrophages and a class of T cells called *helper T cells* stimulate B cells to become plasma cells and produce **antibodies,** also called **immunoglobulins** (Ig). Antibodies are proteins with a base region and two arms (somewhat like the letter Y). They bind to target antigens and destroy them by any of the following methods.

- *Phagocytosis:* Antibodies do not phagocytize directly, but instead signal leukocytes (macrophages and neutrophils) to phagocytize the pathogens to which the antibodies are bound.
- *Neutralization:* By binding to a pathogen's attachment sites, antibodies disable the pathogens' machinery for adhering to and invading body cells; thus, although they are not destroyed, the pathogens are effectively neutralized.
- *Agglutination:* Antibodies have two attachment sites, and therefore each antibody can attach to two pathogenic cells in a population. This quality causes the cells to dump together (agglutinate), reducing the cells' activity and increasing the likelihood that the group will be detected by leukocytes and phagocytized.

- *Activation of complement and inflammation:* Antibodies trigger the complement cascade and stimulate the release of inflammatory chemicals to destroy the antigen.

Immunoglobulins are antibodies secreted by B lymphocytes. Five classes of immunoglobulins (Ig) are formed.
- *IgM:* IgM is produced when an antigen is encountered for the first time. This is a large molecule and cannot pass through the placenta to protect a fetus.
- *IgG:.* IgG is the most common immunoglobulin in the body. Once the body recognizes the antigen and produces IgG, special B memory cells are formed that remember the antigen and rapidly produce IgG in response to subsequent infection. However, it takes at least 10 days for IgG to be produced in response to an initial infection. Eventually the IgG response fades. The length of time the body remembers how to produce IgG for a specific pathogen depends on the characteristics of the pathogen, the strength of the initial response, and the health of the person.

  IgG is small enough to pass through the placenta. If the mother has developed IgG through previous exposure, IgG will pass through the placenta and provide protection from the pathogen. Infants are born with **passive immunity** from their mother's IgG. Additional IgG is passed to the child through breast feeding. Passive immunity can also be given to individuals by administering immune globulins (an injectable medication). Passive immunity is maintained only as long as the IgG molecule exists.
- *IgE:* IgE is the immunoglobulin primarily responsible for the allergic response. The body identifies an allergen as a potential pathogen and begins efforts to destroy or excrete the allergen. Subsequent exposure to the allergen results in a more severe response. Individuals vary in their response to allergens, but a typical allergic response includes some or all of the following symptoms: increased production of mucus, itching (this is actually a defense designed to stimulate the person to rub off the allergen), hives, rashes, eczema, sneezing (to clear the upper airway), wheezing (caused by constriction of the

airways in an effort to prevent further penetration of the allergen into the lungs), and in the most severe responses, a life-threatening anaphylactic shock.
- *IgA:* The mucous membranes secrete IgA around the body openings. They provide additional protection for these vulnerable portals of entry.
- *IgD:* These antibodies form on the surface of B cells and trap the potential pathogen to prevent it from replicating and causing disease.

Cell-Mediated Immunity

Whereas the humoral immune response acts directly against antigenic cells, the cell-mediated immune response acts to destroy body cells that have become infected, in most cases by viruses. T cells are responsible for the cell-mediated immune response. Four types of T cells playa role:
- *Cytotoxic (killer) T cells* directly attack and kill body cells infected with pathogens.
- *Helper T cells* help regulate the action of B cells in humoral immune responses, and of cytotoxic T cells in cell-mediated responses.
- *Memory T cells:* The first time an antigen invades the body, T cells form that respond to that specific antigen. With subsequent infections, the memory T cells are able to increase the speed and amount of the T cell response.
- *Suppressor T cells* are thought to stop the immune response when the infection has been contained.

Support of the Host Defenses

Efforts to promote wellness help break the chain of infection by strengthening an individual's defenses against invading pathogens. Lifestyle factors essential for promoting host defenses are healthful nutrition, adequate hygiene, rest and exercise, stress reduction, and immunizations.

Nutrition: Adequate nutrition, including protein, vitamins, minerals, and water, is essential for combating infection. An acute infection depletes the body's nutritional stores. Nutrients are required to replace these lost stores, to maintain production of white blood cells, and to repair damaged tissues. Fever and increased mucus secretions, which are common defenses against infection, increase water losses. Additional water is needed to supplement this lost fluid and to support the increased metabolic rate.

Hygiene: Hygiene is a crucial aspect of maintaining skin integrity. Intact skin is one of the best defenses against infection. Frequent hand washing, as well as regular showering or bathing, decreases the bacterial count on the skin. However, overzealous cleanliness diminishes the skin's natural oils and may lead to cracking of the skin.

Rest and Exercise: Both rest and exercise are necessary to rejuvenate the body. Adequate rest and sleep renew the body

and mind and conserve strength. Sleep needs vary among individuals. There is really no "correct" amount or pattern of sleep. However, sleep of 7 to 8 hours per night is considered fully restorative. Research demonstrates that exercise is just as important. Too little activity causes circulation to slow and the lungs to supply less oxygen. Excessive exercise leads to fatigue.

Stress Reduction: Stress, whether physical or mental, decreases the body's immune defenses. Numerous studies demonstrate a correlation between increased stress and increased disease. Laughing, in contrast, increases oxygenation, promotes body movement, and increases immune responses.

Immunizations: Immunization via vaccination can protect against several infectious diseases, Immunizations expose the body to weakened or killed pathogens, stimulating an immune response, At a later date, if the body encounters the pathogen, immune cells are available to ward off an infection. Unfortunately, some pathogens, like the virus that causes the common cold, mutate too rapidly for an immunization to be developed.

Factors Increase the Risk for Infection

Anything that weakens the defenses makes a person more susceptible to infection. In addition, any factors that increase the person's exposure to pathogens, such as working at a day care center or being a nurse, increase the risk for infection. Some of the most common factors are discussed below.
- *Developmental stage:* Young children are vulnerable because their immune systems are immature and have had limited exposure to pathogens. Children frequently have an increased number of infections when they start interacting with people outside their family (e.g. when they begin child care or start school). This is a natural process known as acquiring **active immunity.** Also, older adults are more susceptible hosts because their immune response declines with aging. Skin, a primary defense, becomes less elastic and more prone to breakdown with aging. Elders also tend to be less active, and their nutrition may be inadequate.
- *Break in the first line of defense:* A break in the skin, whether caused by a surgical procedure, skin break-down, or insertion of an intravenous device, creates a portal of entry for infectious microorganisms.
- *Illness or injury:* Recuperation from infection or injury limits the physical resources available to combat a new pathogen.
- *Smoking:* Smoking is a major risk factor for pulmonary infections. Smoking interferes with normal respiratory functioning, including the ability to move the chest, cough, sneeze, or have full air exchange. Chemicals in tobacco paralyze cilia; thus, secretions pool in the lower airways, creating a hospitable environment for bacterial growth. Although smokers are most profoundly affected by these changes, people exposed chronically to secondhand smoke,

(e.g. bartenders, children of smokers) are also affected by these changes and are at increased risk for infection.

- *Substance abuse:* Alcohol curbs hunger because it contains many calories. As a result, many chronic alcohol users do not consume an adequate diet. Alcohol is also directly toxic to the liver and to the cells lining the intestinal mucosa. Smoked substances, such as marijuana and cocaine, affect respiratory cilia in a manner similar to tobacco. Any substances that affect orientation and energy level will negatively alter food intake, activity, rest, and hygiene–factors that support host defenses. Injecting substances leads to breaks in skin integrity, increasing the risk of infection.
- *Multiple sexual partners:* The number of sexual partners is directly related to the risk of sexually transmitted infections and cervical cancer.
- *Environmental factors:* Increased exposure to pathogens in one's work situation (e.g. kindergarten teacher, healthcare worker), living situation (e.g. nursing home, parents with young children who are in preschool), and other environmental factors increase one's risk for infection.
- *Chronic disease:* Many chronic diseases diminish the body's ability to fend off infection. Diseases that impair peripheral circulation, such as uncontrolled hypertension (high blood pressure) and diabetes mellitus, make the patient prone to infection in the extremities. Poor circulation prevents antibodies and T cells from reaching the pathogens and damages tissue, making it easier for pathogens to enter. Leukemia, a form of cancer, increases the production of abnormal white blood cells, but these cells are ineffective in fighting infection. Because HIV infects T cells, a patient with AIDS has a reduced ability to fight off secondary infections.
- *Medications:* Some medications are given for the purpose of reducing the immune response, for example, to patients receiving organ or tissue transplants. For most patients, however, decreased immunity is a side effect of treatment. Even common medications, such as nonsteroidal anti-inflammatory agents (e.g. ibuprofen, aspirin) decrease the immune response. As a side effect, *some* medications, such as chemotherapeutic agents, decrease the production of white blood cells or cause the cells produced to he abnormal. Even antibiotics can increase the risk for infection. For example, an antibiotic given for a respiratory infection may cause a vaginal yeast infection because it destroys colonies of normal flora, allowing the harmful microbes to thrive. Such infections are called **superinfections** (opportunistic growth of harmful transient pathogens that are normally kept in check), and some can be extremely challenging to treat.
- *Nursing and medical procedures:* Several procedures are associated with an increased risk of infection. For example, urinary catheterization may damage the fragile urethral mucosa, provide a direct pathway for pathogens into the bladder, and prevent the normal flushing of the urethra. Also an IV line inserted to infuse an antibiotic may serve as a portal of entry for pathogens to enter a patient's body.

Concepts of Asepsis

The nurses efforts to minimize the onset and spread of infection are based on the principles of aseptic technique.

Asepsis is the absence of germs or pathogens. Aseptic technique is the efforts to keep a client as free from hospital microorganisms as possible. The two types of aseptic techniques, the nurses usually practice, are medical and surgical asepsis.

Medical asepsis: Medical asepsis or clean technique includes procedures used to reduce the number of microorganisms and prevent their spread. Changing a clients bed linen daily, hand washing and using clean medicated cups are example of medical asepsis. The practicing basic principles of medical asepsis in client care are as follows:

- Wash hands frequently but especially before handling foods, before eating, after using a handkerchief, after going to the toilet, before and after each client contact, and after removing gloves
- Keep solid items and equipment from touching the clothing, carry soiled linen or other used articles so that they do not touch the uniform
- Do not place solid bed linen or any other items on the floor, which is grossly contaminated, it increases contamination of both surfaces
- Avoid having clients, cough, sneezing, or breath directly on others. Provide them with disposable tissues, and instruct them as indicated to cover their mouth and nose to prevent spread by airborne droplet
- Move equipment away from you when brushing, dusting or scrubbing articles. This helps prevent contaminated particles from settling on the hairs, face and uniform
- Avoid raising dust use a specially treated cloth or a dampened cloth. Do not shake linens. Dust and thin particles constitute a vehicle, by which organisms may be transported from one area to another
- Clean the least soiled areas first and then the more soiled ones. This helps prevent having the cleaner areas soiled by the dirtier areas
- Dispose of soiled or used items directly into appropriate containers. Wrap items that are moist from body discharge or drainage in water proof containers such as plastic bags, before discarding into the refuse holder so that handler will not come in contact with them
- Pour liquids that are to be discarded, such as bath water, mouth rinse and the like directly into the drain so as to avoid splattering in the sink and on to you
- Sterilize items that are suspected of containing pathogen. After sterilization, they can be managed by clean technique
- Use practices of personal grooming that help prevent spready microorganism, i.e. shampooing, nail cutting, avoid wearing rings, etc.
- Follow guidelines conscientiously for isolation in barrier technique as prescribed by agency.

Surgical asepsis: Surgical asepsis or sterile technique, includes procedures used to eliminated microorganisms from an area. Sterilization destroys all microorganisms, and their spores sterile techniques is practiced by nurses in the operating room and treatment areas, where sterile instruments and supplies are used, i.e. care of surgical wounds, urinary catheter insertion, invasive procedures and surgery.

The practicing basic principles of surgical asepsis are as follows:
- Only a sterile object can touch another sterile object, unsterile touching sterile means contamination has occurred
- Open the sterile packages so that the first edge of the wrapper is directed away from the worker to avoid the possibility of a sterile surface touching unsterile clothing. The outside of the sterile package is considered contaminated
- Avoid spilling any solution on a cloth or paper used as a field for a sterile set up. The moisture penetrates through the sterile cloth or paper and carries organism by capillary action so contaminate the field. The wet field is considered contaminated if the surface immediately below it is not sterile
- Hold sterile objects above the level of the waist. This will help ensure keeping the object within sight and prevent accidental contamination
- Avoid talking, coughing, sneezing or reaching over a sterile field or object. This helps prevent contamination by droplets, from the nose and the mouth or by particles dropping from the worker's arms
- Never walk away from or turn your back on a sterile field. This prevents possible contamination while the field as out of the worker's view
- All items brought into contact with broken skin, or used to penetrate the skin in order to inject substances into the body, or to enter normally sterile body cavities, should be sterile. These items include dressing used to cover wounds and incisions, needles for injections and tubes, catheter used to drain urine from the bladder, etc.
- Use dry, sterile, forceps when necessary, forceps soaked in disinfectant are not considered sterile
- Consider the edge (outer one inch) of a sterile field to be contaminated
- Consider an object contaminated if you have any doubt as to its sterility.

Role of the Nurse in Infection Control

The roles and responsibilities of the nurses in infection control are as follows:
- Providing staff education on infection control
- Reviewing infection control policies and procedures
- Reviewing client medical records and laboratory reports to recommend appropriate isolation procedures
- Screening client record for community acquired infection
- Consulting with employer health departments concerning recommendation to prevent and control the spread of infections among personnel such as tuberculosis testing
- Gathering statistics regarding the epidemiology of nosocomial infections
- Notifying public health department of incidences of communicable diseases
- Conferring with all hospital departments to investigate unusual events or clusters of infection
- Educating clients and families
- Identifying infection control problems with equipment
- Checking microorganism sensitivity to antibiotics in use and reminding medical staff of resistance.

Teaching about Infection Control

Clients should be taught to use basic principles of asepsis at home and in public facilities. Teaching about medical aspects and infection control is a challenging nursing responsibility.

The following are examples of medical aseptic practices used in home:
- Wash hands before preparing food and before eating
- Prepare food at temperature sufficiently high to ensure that they are safe to eat
- Use care with cutting boards and utensils and wash hands, before and after handling raw meat
- Keep food refrigerated, especially those containing mayonnaise
- Wash raw fruits and vegetables before serving them
- Use pasteurized milk
- Wash hands after using the bathroom
- Use individual personal care items, such as wash cloths, towels, tooth brushes

Observe infection prevention in public facilities by following these guidelines:
- Wash hands after using any public bathroom
- Use paper towels or hot air dryers in restroom
- Use individually wrapped drinking straws
- Use tongs to lift food from common service trays in caterings food stores, and salad bars

The community reinforces medical aseptic practices in several ways which includes the following:
- Use of sterilized combs and brushes in barber and beauty shops
- Examination of food handlers for evidence of disease
- Enforcement of frequent hand washing by food handlers.

Breaking the Chain of Infection

Nurses focus on breaking the chain of infection by applying proper infection-control practices to interrupt the transmission of microorganisms. Hand hygiene is the first line of defense against infection and is the single most important practice in preventing the spread of infection. Specific strategies can be directed at breaking or blocking the transmission of infection from one link in the chain to the next. A discussion regarding each of the six links follows (Fig. 21.3.).

1. Link between Agent and Reservoir

The first link in the chain of infection is between the agent and the reservoir. The keys to eliminating infection at this point in the chain are cleansing, disinfection, and sterilization. These practices prevent the formation of a reservoir where infectious agents can live and multiply.

(a) Cleansing is the removal of soil or organic material from instruments and equipment used in providing client care. Nurses often cleanse instruments after assisting or performing invasive procedures. To reduce the amount of contamination and loosen the material on reusable objects, the objects are cleansed before sterilization or disinfection. Cleansing involves the use of water, mechanical action, and, sometimes, a detergent. Contaminated objects are cleansed using a soft-bristled brush to scrub the surface. The steps for proper cleansing are:

- Wet the object with *cold* water; warm water coagulates the proteins in organic material and makes them stick.
- Apply detergent and scrub the object under running water using a soft-bristled brush.
- Rinse the object under warm running water.
- Dry the object before sterilization or disinfection.

Cleansing is a potential hazard to the nurse from the splashing of contaminated material onto the body. Nurses should wear gloves, masks, and goggles during cleansing,

(b) Disinfection is the elimination of pathogens, except spores, from inanimate objects. Disinfectants are chemical solutions used to clean inanimate objects. Bedpans, thermometers, and some types of endoscopes are disinfected. Common disinfectants are alcohol, sodium hypochlorite, quaternary ammonium, phenolic solutions, and glutaraldehyde.

A germicide is a chemical that can be applied to both animate (living) and inanimate objects to eliminate pathogens. Antiseptic preparations such as alcohol and silver sulfadiazine are germicides.

(c) Sterilization: Sterilization is destroying all microorganisms including spores. Equipment that enters normally sterile tissue or blood vessels must be sterilized. Methods of achieving sterilization are moist heat (steam), dry heat, and ethylene oxide gas. The method of sterilization depends on the object to be sterilized and the kind and amount of contamination.

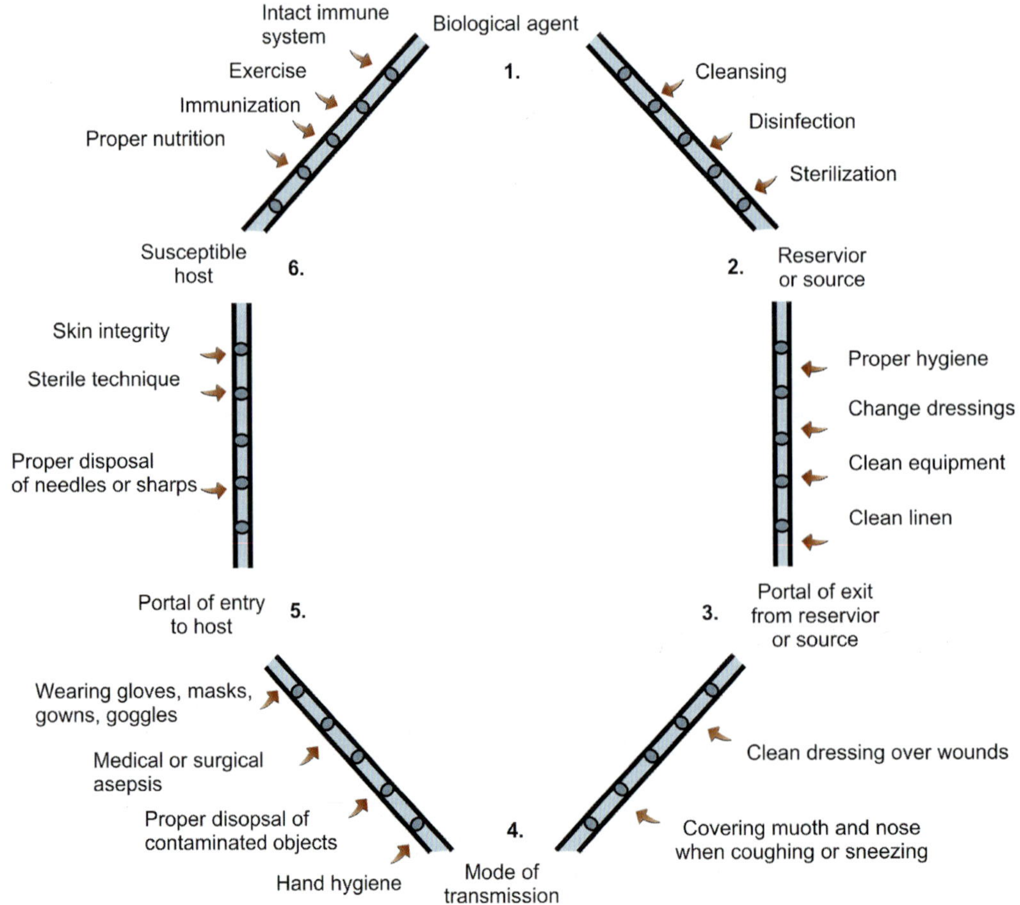

Figure 21.3: The chain of infection: Preventive measures follow each link of the chain

Autoclaving sterilization, which uses moist heat or steam, is the most common sterilization technique used in the hospital setting. Boiling water is not an effective sterilization measure, because some viruses and spores can survive boiling water. Objects that have been boiled in water for 15 to 20 minutes at 121°C (249.8°F) are considered clean but not sterile.

Sterilization is killing of all sorts of microorganisms including bacteria, viruses, spirochaete, fungi, parasites and spores.

Disinfection: It is killing of all organisms except spores.

Disinfectant: It is a chemical substance of germicidal nature used to kill pathogenic microorganisms of inanimate objects.

Antiseptic: It is also a chemical agent but differs from disinfectant in a sense that these inhibit growth of microorganisms so long they are in contact with them.

Methods of Destruction of Bacteria

All pathogenic organisms can be destroyed by any of the following methods as given below:

Natural Method

Sunlight: The heat of sunlight have a drying or dehydrating effect on the organisms which enables it to destroy the germs. This method is not effective unless the contaminated articles are exposed for 2-3 days continuously and hence is not usually applicable.

Physical Methods

1. *Dry heat*
   (a) *Electric (hot air oven)* – By special electric ovens in the form of hot air at 121°C for 6 hours (commercial).
   Materials – Glasswares, vaselin, fats, talc, oil, carbon steel materials.
   Linen, rubber or plastic articles are not sterilized in this method.
   (b) *Flaming* – Contaminated noninflammable articles are sometimes disinfected by smearing with methylated spirit and then flaming. This method destroys only surface bacteria and can be used in case of grave emergency or when no other way of disinfection is possible, e.g. tray, blunt instruments.
   (c) *Burning or incineration* – Contaminated articles of highly infectious diseased patients are burnt to kill the microorganisms and prevent spread of infection e.g.; mattress, pillow, bed linens used by tetanus or gas gangrene patient.

2. *Moist heat*
   (a) *Boiling* – This is one of the commonest method of destruction of micro-organisms. In this, bacteria are killed within 5 to 30 minutes, e.g. syringe. Almost all instruments except sharp, rubber goods, silk, nylon, etc.
   (b) *Chemical method* – Chemical substances, called disinfectants are also used to kill pathogenic organisms. The stronger the chemical the lesser is the time required for disinfection. Common disinfectants are Iysol, carbolic acid, formalin.

The choice and action of disinfectants depend on:
(i) The type of article to be disinfected *e.g.,* metal, rubber or linen.
(ii) The nature and strength of agent used and its effect on the qualities, e.g. effect of lysol 1:20 and carbolic 1: 40 and its stability in the presence of organic matter.
(iii) Time required for disinfection by the chemical to act effectively.
(iv) Nature of solvent used and its temperature.
(v) Nature of contamination, the number and virulence of organisms.
(vi) The cost of the chemical to be used.

For practical purposes- Two common methods are there for sterilization – chemical and heating. A combination of pressure and heat is undertaken for a special advantage that pressure increases heat and power of penetration is more. The different methods are briefly tabulized.

Autoclaving – For materials that will stand up to heat and moisture. In this method with Increased pressure, temperature of water can be raised. This is the most reliable method because of the power of penetration, microbiologic efficiency, easy control, and economy. 15 Ib pressure per sq. inch for 15-45 minutes at 121°C destroys all forms of organisms.

Materials sterilized – Almost all materials except glass wares, vaseline, fats, talc, oils, etc.

There are two types:
1. Those with gravity displacement of air.
2. Those with high vacuum sterilizer.

Steam with – Formaldehyde at subatmospheric pressure sterilization is done at a temperature below 90°C at 10 Ibs pressure for 10 mts. All spores are killed when formaldehyde vapour is used. It is a modified autoclave system.

Pasteurisation – Is the method where materials are sterilized in a thermostatically controlled water bath at 75-80°C for 10 minutes, e.g. Endoscope.

Irradiation – Gamma ray is used for sterilization in industry - Irradiation is from a cobalt 60 source or electron bombardment from a linear accelerator.

Materials sterilized – viz. disposable hospital supplies, plastic, syringes, sutures-catgut, etc.
Ethylene oxide gas – for heat labile article – This is also commercial.
Materials – delicate surgical instruments with optical lenses, plastic parts of heart lung machine, etc.
Chemicals – common solutions used are iodine, Iysol, carbolic acid, hibitane, cetrimide 1%, 2% glutaraldehyde.
Materials
(i) For sterilization of living tissues catguts, etc.
(ii) Sharp Instruments in pure lysol for half an hour, etc.

Methods

Heat sterilization
1. Autoclaving (steam under pressure)
2. Dry heat by oxidation
3. Steam with formaldehyde at subatmospheric pressure

Heat disinfection
1. Steam at subatmospheric pressure
2. Pasteurization
3. Boiling most bacteria are killed within 5 minutes except some spore formings

Cold sterilization
1. Irradiation
2. Ethylene oxide gas
3. Ultraviolet light radiation
4. Chemical—2% glutaraldehyde

Cold disinfection
1. Various chemicals

2. Link between Reservoir and Portal of Exit

Promoting proper hygiene, changing dressings and liens, and ensuring that clean equipment is used in client care are ways to break the chain of infection between the reservoir and the portal of exit. The goal is to eliminate the reservoir for the micro-organism before a pathogen can escape to a susceptible host.

Proper Hygiene: Educate clients on the importance of maintaining the cleanliness and integrity of the skin and the mucous membranes. Clean skin, hair, and nails maintain the body's normal flora and eliminate transient flora from the client's system. Bathing and hand hygiene are important ways to eliminate the potential for infection. Clients should be encouraged to practice daily bathing and teeth brushing. Clients who are unable to perform these activities independently should be assisted.

Change Dressings: Any open injury or other break in skin integrity represents a potential reservoir for infectious agents and portal of exit for a pathogen to be transferred to another individual. Dressings on open or oozing wounds must be changed regularly. To protect both yourself and the client from infection, follow proper aseptic technique when changing dressings. This technique is discussed in detail later in this chapter.

Clean Linens: Bed linens, gowns, and towels are catch-alls for bodily secretions. Infectious agents can be easily transferred from one individual to the next through contact with a client's linens. Linens must be changed regularly, and soiled linens must be properly disposed. When changing linens, take care to keep the soiled articles from contact with your uniform. This will prevent being infected from the soiled linens or passing the infection on to other clients.

Clean Equipment: All equipment used in the care of a client must be cleansed and disinfected after each use. Although many items such as disposable gowns can be discarded after use, items such as beds must be thoroughly cleansed after each use. Clients should be instructed never to share care items. Any nondisposable equipment used in an invasive procedure (such as equipment used in the operating room [OR]) must be sterilized before being used again. Wear gloves and masks when cleansing equipment to avoid being splashed with contaminated waste products or secretions.

3. Link between Portal of Exit and Mode of Transmission

The goal in breaking the chain of infection between the portal of exit and the mode of transmission is to prevent the exit of the infectious agents. Clean dressings must be maintained on all wounds. Clients should be encouraged to cover their mouths and noses when sneezing or coughing, and the nurse must do so as well. Gloves must be worn when caring for a client who may have infectious secretions, and care must be taken to properly dispose of any contaminated article.

4. Link between Mode of Transmission and Portal of Entry

To break the chain of infection between the mode of transmission and the portal of entry, asepsis must be ensured and barrier protection worn when the care of clients involves contact with body secretions. Gloves, masks, gowns, and goggles are barrier protection that can be used. Proper hand hygiene and proper disposal of contaminated equipment and linens are ways to prevent transmission of microorganisms to other clients and health care workers. A thorough discussion of asepsis and disposal of contaminated items is included later in this chapter.

5. Link between Portal of Entry and Host

Maintaining skin integrity and using sterile technique for client contacts are methods of breaking the chain of infection between portal of entry and host. Avoiding needle sticks by properly disposing of sharps also reduces the potential for infection by denying a portal of entry. The goal at this point in the chain is to prevent the transmission of infection to a client or health care worker who is not infected.

6. Link between Host and Agent

Breaking the chain of infection between host and agent means eliminating infection before it begins. There are many ways to reduce the risk of acquiring infection: Proper nutrition, exercise, and immunizations allow an individual to maintain an intact immune system, thus preventing infection.

(a) **Proper nutrition:** Proper nutrition assists the body's immune system to function properly. Clients need adequate amounts of protein in their diets to maintain and repair tissue as well as to produce the antibodies needed to fight infection. A balanced diet also allows the body to maintain appropriate acid-base balance.

(b) **Exercise:** Exercise maintains the body's metabolic rate and, therefore, allows the body to maintain the antibodies and energy necessary to ward off infection.

(c) **Immunization:** Immunization is the process of creating immunity, or resistance to infection, in an individual. Many immunizations are given in early childhood (e.g. measles, mumps, and rubella). Immunization for the flu must be given every year, and for tetanus every 10 years.

(d) A host's immune system is a defense against infectious agents. The immune system is able to recognize "self" and "nonself"; that is, the immune system recognizes what is not consistent with the genetic composition of the host (self). These agents are called antigens (non-self). An immune response against an antigen protects the body from infection. Immune defenses are identified as nonspecific and specific and work together to defend the host from pathogens.

Body Defences

(i) Nonspecific Immune Defense:

The nonspecific immune defense protects the host' from all microorganisms; it does not depend on prior exposure to an antigen. Nonspecific immune defenses are skin and normal flora; mucous membranes; coughing, sneezing, and tearing reflexes; elimination and acidic environment; and inflammation.

- **Skin and Normal Flora:** The skin, the first line of defense against infection, serves as a physical barrier to infectious agents. Skin cells, shed daily, remove potentially harmful microorganisms. Sebum, a substance produced by the skin, contains fatty acids that kill some bacteria. The normal flora residing on the skin and in the body compete with pathogenic flora for food and inhibit pathogen multiplication. The balance of normal flora may become disrupted, allowing pathogenic organisms to proliferate, causing infection or superinfection.
- **Mucous Membranes:** Mucous membranes also are a physical barrier to infectious agents. Mucus produced by these membranes entraps infectious agents and inhibits bacterial growth. For example, the cilia of the respiratory tract trap and "propel mucus and microorganisms away from the lungs, thereby reducing the potential for infection.
- **Coughing, Sneezing, and Tearing Reflexes:** The cough and sneeze reflexes forcibly expel mucus and microorganisms from the respiratory tract. Tears protect the eyes by continually flushing away microorganisms. Tears also contain bactericides, which are bacteria-killing chemicals.
- **Elimination and Acidic Environment:** Elimination and an acidic environment usually prevent growth of pathogenic organisms. Resident flora of the large intestines prevent the growth of pathogens. The mechanical process of defecation removes microorganisms with the feces. Urine acidity prevents microbial growth. Urination flushes and cleans the bladder neck and urethra of microorganisms and prevents microorganisms from ascending into the urinary tract.

  Normal vaginal flora prevent growth of several pathogens. At puberty, lactobacilli ferment and produce sugars in the vagina that lower the pH *to* an acidic range. The acidic environment of the vagina prevents pathogenic growth.
- **Inflammation:** Inflammation is a nonspecific cellular response to tissue injury. Tissue injury caused by bacteria, trauma, chemicals, heat, or any other occurrence releases substances, producing dramatic secondary changes in the injured tissue. This entire complex of tissue changes in response *to* injury is called the *inflammatory process* (Table 21.4). The body's response *to* injury produces characteristic local and systemic signs of inflammation.

Inflammation, while not necessarily the result of invading microorganisms, does have signs and symptoms similar *to* those of an infection. The primary signs of inflammation and infection arc as follows:

- Redness (erythema), results from increased blood flow to the area
- Heat results from increased blood flow and metabolism in the area
- Pain results from increased pressure on pain sensors in the area
- Swelling (edema, a detectable accumulation of increased interstitial fluid) results from fluid and leukocytes entering the tissues from the circulatory system
- Loss of function results from both pain and swelling, is the body's way of resting the injured part

Table 21.4: Stages of the Inflammatory Process	
Description	*Response/Outcome*
Initial injury causes release of chemicals: histamine, bradykinin, serotonin, prostaglandins, and Iymphokines.	Initiates the inflammation process.
Blood flow increases to the injured area.	Produces characteristic redness and warmth.
Increased capillary permeability leaks large amounts of plasma into the damaged tissue; tissue spaces and lymphatics are blocked by fibrinogen clots.	"Walls off" infection; results in nonpitting edema.
Leukocytes infiltrate damaged tissue and engulf the bacteria and necrotic tissue. After several days, these leukocytes die and form a cavity of necrotic tissue and dead leukocytes.	Produces purulent exudate (pus).
Destroyed tissue cells are replaced by identical or similar structural and functioning cells and/or fibrous tissue.	Promotes tissue healing or the formation of fibrous (scar) tissue, which may reduce the functional capacity of the tissue.

- Pus (purulent exudate), resulting from infection, a secretion made up of white blood cells, dead cells, bacteria, and other debris.

The inflammatory process intensity is usually in proportion to the degree of tissue injury.

(ii) Specific Immune Defense

The specific immune defense is a response specific to the invading antigen. It is activated when phagocytes fail to completely destroy the antigen. This causes production of T lymphocytes (T cells), which regulate the immune response by activating other cells. The T cells move to the injured area and release chemical substances called lymphokines. Lymphokines attract other phagocytes and lymphocytes to the injured area and assist in antigen destruction.

The T cells also stimulate the production of B cells, which become plasma cells, producing antibodies specific to the antigen. Antibodies are protein substances that destroy the antigen. The stimulation of B cells and the production of antibodies are collectively known as humoral immunity. Memory B cells are formed to remember the antigen and prepare the host for future antigen invasion. When the antigen enters the body again, the immune response occurs faster by rapidly producing antibodies. The formation of these antibodies is referred to as **acquired immunity,** which protects the individual against future invasions of already experienced antigens such as lethal bacteria, viruses, toxins, and even foreign tissues.

The process of **vaccination** (inoculation with a vaccine to produce immunity against specific diseases) provides acquired immunity. There are three types of vaccines:

- Dead organisms that are no longer capable of causing disease but still have their chemical antigen such as typhoid, whooping cough, and diphtheria
- Toxins that have been chemically treated so their toxic nature is destroyed but their antigens are still intact, such as for tetanus and botulism
- Live organisms that have been attenuated (rendered incapable of causing the disease yet still have the specific antigen, such as for poliomyelitis, yellow fever, measles, smallpox, and many other viral diseases.

Standard Precautions for Infection Control

1. Wash Hands (Plain Soap)
- Wash after touching blood, body fluids, secretions, excretions, and contaminated items.
- Wash immediately after gloves are removed and between patient contacts. Avoid transfer of microorganisms to other patients or environments.

2. Wear Gloves
- Wear when touching blood, body fluids, secretions, excretions, and contaminated items. Put on clean gloves just before touching mucous membranes and nonintact skin. Change gloves between tasks and procedures on the same patient after contact with material that may contain high concentrations of microorganisms. Remove gloves promptly after use, before touching noncontaminated items and environmental surfaces, and before going to another patient, and wash hands immediately to avoid transfer of microorganisms to other patients or environments.

3. Wear Mask and Eye Protection or Face Shield
Protect mucous membranes of the eyes, nose and mouth during procedures and patient-care activities that are likely to generate splashes or sprays of blood, body fluids, secretions, or excretions.

4. Wear Gown
Protect skin and prevent soiling of clothing during procedures that are likely to generate splashes or sprays of blood, body fluids, secretions, or excretions. Remove a soiled gown as promptly as possible and wash hands to avoid transfer of microorganisms to other patients or environments.

5. Patient Care Equipment
Handle used patient-care equipment soiled with blood, body-fluids, secretions, or excretions in a manner that prevents skin and mucous membrane exposures, contamination of clothing, and transfer of microorganisms to other patients and environments. Ensure that reusable equipment is not used for the care of another patient until it has been appropriately cleaned and reprocessed and single use items are properly discarded.

6. Environmental Control
Follow hospital procedures for routine care, cleaning, and disinfection of environmental surfaces, beds, bedrails, bedside equipment and other frequently touched surfaces.

7. Linen
Handle, transport, and process used linen soiled with blood, body fluids, secretions, or excretions in a manner that prevents exposures and contamination of clothing, and avoids transfer of microorganisms to other patients and environments.

8. Occupational Health and Bloodborne Pathogens
- Prevent injuries when using needles, scalpels, and other sharp instruments or devices; when handling sharp instruments after procedures; when cleaning used instruments; and when disposing of used needles.
- Never recap used needles using both hands or any other technique that involves directing the point of the needle towards any part of the body; rather, use either a one-handed "scoop" technique or a mechanical device designed for holding the needle sheath.
- Do not remove used needles from disposable syringes by hand, and do not bend, break, or otherwise manipulate used needles by hand. Place used disposable syringes and needles, scalpels blades, and other sharp items in puncture-resistant sharps containers located as close as practical to

the area in which the items were used, and place reusable syringes and needles in a puncture-resistant container for transport to the reprocessing area.

- Use resuscitation devices as an alternative to mouth-to-mouth resuscitation.

9. Patient Placement

Use a private room for a patient who contaminates the environment (or who does not or cannot be expected to) assist in maintaining appropriate hygiene or environmental control. Consult Infection Control if a private room is not available. In addition some precautions to be taken as given below.

Transmission-Based Precautions

Recall from the discussion on the chain of infection that pathogens may be transmitted by contact, droplet, or air. Each mode of transmission requires a different approach to prevent infection. For a summary of precautions to take for each mode of transmission,

1. Contact Precautions

Contact precautions are used when direct contact with the organism can lead to spread of the pathogen. This is the most common form of transmission. Draining wounds, dressings, patient supplies, and secretions are sources of infection. Indirect contact, or contact with fomites, can also transmit pathogens that spread by this method.

Contact precautions include the following:
- Follow all standard precautions.
- Place the patient in a private room or in a room with a patient with an active infection caused by the same organism and no other infections.
- Wear a clean gown and gloves when you anticipate any contact with the patient or with any contaminated items in the room.
- Either dispose of all items entering the room within the room, or disinfect them per institution policy prior to removing them from the room.
- Double bag all linen and trash, and clearly mark them contaminated.
- Follow any additional precautions specific to the microorganism.

2. Droplet Precautions

Droplet precautions are used when the pathogen can be spread via moist droplets (e.g. sneezing, coughing, talking). Droplets can spread infection by direct contact with mucous membranes or through indirect contact, for example, touching a bedside table that was contaminated with moist droplets and then rubbing your eyes.

Droplet precautions include the following:
- Follow all standard precautions.
- Follow all contact precautions.
- Wear a mask and eye protection when working within 3 feet of the patient.

3. Airborne Precautions

Airborne precautions are used to control the spread of infections that are transmitted on air currents. Airborne infections include tuberculosis, varicella (chickenpox), severe acute respiratory syndrome (SARS), and rubeola (measles). Pathogens that are spread by this method are very small and can be easily transmitted through ventilating systems as well as by any activities that stir the air, such as fanning sheets, shaking out towels, or sweeping the floor.

Airborne precautions include the following:
- Follow all standard precautions.
- Follow all contact precautions.
- Place the patient in a private room or in a room with a patient with an active infection caused by the same organism and no other infections. Make sure that the room has negative air pressure and that the air is discharged through a filtration system.
- Wear a clean gown and gloves when you anticipate any contact with the patient or with any items in the room.
- Wear a special mask (N95 respirator) if the patient is suspected of having pulmonary tuberculosis.
- If the patient is known to have or is suspected of having measles (rubeola) or varicella (chickenpox), only immune caregivers should provide care. Immune caregivers do not need to wear masks.

Protective Isolation

Patients at high risk for infection are placed in a special form of isolation called **protective** (or reverse) **isolation.** The goal of protective isolation is to protect an unusually vulnerable patient from organisms brought in by healthcare workers and visitors. This type of isolation may be used for clients with low Wile counts, clients undergoing chemotherapy, or clients with large open wounds or weak immune systems. Some units, such as neonatal intensive care units, burn units, and labor and delivery suites, may follow some aspects of protective isolation all the time. Protective isolation includes the following:
- Follow all standard precautions.
- Healthcare workers caring for patients in protective isolation should not also be providing care for other patients with active infections.
- When patients in protective isolation need to leave the room, they should wear a mask and have minimal contact with others.
- All persons entering the patient's room should wear a mask and wash their hands thoroughly with soap and water.
- After hand washing, caregivers and visitors should put on a clean or sterile gown over clothing and take care to keep the outside of the gown from any contact with surfaces outside the room.
- Once the gown is placed, don gloves.
- If the mask or gown becomes wet while you provide care, change it.
- On exiting the room, remove the mask, gloves, and gown. Do not use them again.

Nursing Process and Infection Control

Quality nursing care requires the reduction of microorganism transmission in the health care environment. Infection-control practices are directed at controlling or eliminating sources of infection in the health care agency or home. Nurses are responsible for protecting clients and themselves by using infection-control practices.

Assessment

Assessment data guides the prioritization of the client's problem and identification of appropriate nursing diagnoses. Clients at risk for infection require frequent reassessment followed by appropriate changes in the plan of care, goals, and nursing interventions. The health history and physical examination data correlated with the laboratory results identify those clients at risk for infection. Appropriate risk appraisals may be incorporated into the nursing health history interview.

Subjective Data: Relevant data regarding the client at risk for infection are obtained in the health history. A comprehensive assessment also involves appraising the client's environment to detect potential hazards and the client's self-care abilities. Reviewing such factors as work environment, immunization status, and other health-related issues may help identify actual or possible infection risks.

Objective Data: Objective data are gathered through the physical examination and the diagnostic and laboratory findings.

- A complete *health assessment* includes a systematic physical examination, generally conducted from head to toe, to obtain objective data relative to the client's health status and presenting problems. When assessing the client to determine the level of risk for infection, *focus* the physical examination on:
  Range of motion and mobility (A client with limited mobility is at risk for developing joint contractures, skin breakdown. and muscle atrophy.)
  Localized redness, warmth, swelling, pain, and loss of use in a specific body part.
  Fever with an increase in pulse and respirations; weakness; anorexia, nausea, vomiting, and/or diarrhea: enlarged and/or tender lymph nodes
  Secretions or exudate of the skin or mucous membranes; hydration status
  Auscultation of the lungs for crackles or wheezes
- The *laboratory indicators* for an infection are:
  An elevated leukocyte (white blood cell [WBC]) and WBC differential:

Neutrophils: Increased in acute, severe inflammation

Lymphocytes: Increased in chronic bacterial and viral infections

Monocytes: Increased in some protozoan and rickettsial infections and TB

Eosinophils and basophils: Unaltered in an infectious process
- An elevated erythrocyte sedimentation rate (ESR): increased in the presence of inflammation
- An elevated pH of involved body fluids (gastric, urine, or vaginal secretions): indicative of microorganism presence
- Positive cultures of involved body fluids (blood, sputum, urine, or other drainage): indicative of microorganism growth

Nursing Diagnosis

After data collection and analysis, identify a nursing diagnosis. The North American Nursing Diagnosis Association (NANDA) identifies one nursing diagnosis related to infection: *Risk for Infection.*

Risk for infection is an increased risk for being invaded by pathogenic organisms. The risk factors that increase a client's susceptibility to infections are as follows:
- Inadequate primary defenses (broken skin. traumatized tissue. decrease in ciliary action, stasis of body fluids. change in pH of secretions. and altered peristalsis)
- Inadequate secondary defenses (decreased hemoglobin, leukopenia. suppressed inflammatory response)
- Inadequate acquired immunity
- Immunosuppression
- Tissue destruction and increased environmental exposure
- Chronic disease
- Malnutrition
- Invasive procedures
- Pharmaceutical agents
- Trauma
- Rupture of amniotic membranes
- Insufficient knowledge to avoid exposure to pathogens.
  Clients who are at risk for infection may have other associated physiologic and psychological concerns. The common nursing diagnoses that often accompany *risk for infection* include:
- Imbalanced nutrition: Less than body requirements or more than body requirements
- Ineffective protection
- Impaired tissue integrity
- Impaired oral mucous membrane
- Impaired skin integrity
- Deficient knowledge (specify).
  This list indicates several related problems that must be considered when planning care for the client at risk for infection.

Planning

The nurse collaborates with the client and other health care providers to determine goals, outcomes, and interventions to reduce the risk of infection. Outcomes provide direction for nursing care to reduce the risk of infection. Client and caregiver education about identifying potential hazards and health-promotion practices is another critical element of the care plan.

Implementation

Nurses are responsible for providing the client with a safe environment, including prevention of nosocomial infections. Nursing interventions to reduce the risk of infection center around ensuring asepsis and properly disposing of infectious materials to reduce or eliminate infectious agents. Asepsis refers to the absence of microorganisms. Aseptic technique is the infection-control practice used to prevent the transmission of pathogens. The use of aseptic technique decreases the risk and spread of nosocomial infections. There are two types of asepsis: medical and surgical.

(i) Medical Asepsis: The term medical asepsis refers to those practices used to reduce the number, growth, and spread of micro-organisms. It is also called clean technique. In medical asepsis, objects are generally referred to as "clean" or "dirty." Clean objects are considered to have the presence of some micro-organisms that are usually not pathogenic. Dirty (soiled) objects are considered to have a high number of microorganisms, some being potentially pathogenic. Common medical aseptic measures used for clean or dirty objects are hand hygiene, daily changing of linens, and daily cleansing of floors and hospital furniture.

Hand Hygiene: Hand hygiene is a general term that includes *handwashing* (using plain soap and water), *antiseptic handwash* (using antimicrobial substances and water), *antiseptic hand rub* (using alcohol-based hand rub), and *surgical hand antisepsis* (using antiseptic handwash or antiseptic hand rub preoperatively by surgical personnel to eliminate transient and reduce resident hand flora). Perform hand hygiene after arriving at work, before leaving work, before and after each client contact, after removing gloves, when hands are visibly soiled, before eating, after excretion of body waste (urination and defecation), after contact with body fluids, and after handling contaminated equipment. When hands are visibly dirty, wash hands with soap (plain or antimicrobial) and water. If hands are not visibly soiled, and alcohol-based hand rub may be used.

Handwashing is the rubbing together of all surfaces and crevices of the hands using plain soap and water, followed by rinsing in a flowing stream of water. Friction physically removes soil and transient flora, and a flowing stream of water rinses it all away. To remove transient flora from the hands, a washing time of 15 seconds is recommended. High-risk areas such as nurseries usually require a handwash of approximately 2 minutes duration. Soiled hands usually require more time. Handwashing is the most basic and effective infection-control measure to prevent and control the transmission of infectious agents. It is the single most important procedure for preventing nosocomial infections.

Antiseptic hand rub uses an alcohol-containing preparation designed to reduce the number of viable microorganisms on the hands. In the United States, these preparations usually contain 60 to 95% ethanol or isopropanol. Apply product to palm of one hand and rub hands together, covering all surfaces of hands and fingers, until hands are dry. Follow the manufacturer's recommendation for the amount of product to use.

(ii) Surgical Asepsis: Surgical asepsis or sterile technique, consists of those practices that eliminate all microorganisms and spores from an object or area. Surgical asepsis related to surgical handwashing, establishing and maintaining sterile fields, donning surgical attire (caps, masks, and eyewear), and sterile gloves, gowning, with closed gloving.

Surgical asepsis is practiced in the OR, in labor and delivery, and for many therapeutic and diagnostic interventions at the client's bedside. Common nursing procedures requiring sterile technique are:

- All invasive procedures, either entry into a bodily orifice (tracheobronchial suctioning, insertion of a urinary catheter) or intentional perforation of the skin (injections, insertion of intravenous needles catheters)
- Nursing interventions when there is a disruption of skin surfaces (changing a surgical wound or intra-venous site dressing) or destruction of skin layers (trauma and burns)

(iii) Surgical Hand Antisepsis: Surgical hand antisepsis scrub removes soil and microorganisms from the skin. Workers in the OR do surgical hand antisepsis to minimize the client's risk for infection. The skin on the hands and arms should be intact (free of lesions). Agency policy determines the method and timing for the scrub.

(iv) Sterile Field and Equipment: Establish and maintain a sterile field when performing procedures that require sterile technique, such as inserting a urinary catheter or changing wound dressings. Before preparing the sterile field, review the agency's policy and gather all the necessary supplies.

(v) Donning Surgical Attire: Surgical nurses are required to wear a surgical mask and a clean cap covering all of the hair. Protective eyewear (glasses or goggles) is worn during all procedures posing a threat of body fluids splashing into the eyes. Masks, caps, eye-wear, gowns, and gloves are considered barrier precautions because they are a physical impediment to the spread of microorganisms.

(vi) Donning Sterile Gloves: There are two methods of applying sterile gloves: open and closed. The open method is used when performing procedures requiring sterile technique, such as dressing changes. The closed method is used when the nurse wears a sterile gown, as in the OR.

(vii) Gowning with Closed Gloving: When donning a sterile gown, nurses in the OR and special procedure areas such as cardiac cath labs use the closed gloved method. After the surgical scrub, don the sterile gown and gloves using the closed method. The sterile gown serves as a barrier to decrease the risk of wound contamination and also allows the nurse to move freely in the environment of sterile fields.

(viii) Disposal of Infectious Materials: All health care facilities must have guidelines for the disposal of infectious-waste materials as required. The types of materials included are:

- Laboratory wastes
- All body fluids including blood, blood products

- Client care items (soiled bed linen and protection pads, urinals, and bedpans)
- Disposable instruments
- Medication and soiled treatment items
- Surgical wastes.

All health care workers must be diligent in observing the biological hazard symbol and handling all infectious materials as hazardous.

When disposing of infectious waste, all personnel must be sure to:

- Wear gloves.
- Use the proper containers (red or one labeled with the biological hazard symbol as required by the facility), sharps containers for needles, scalpels, and other sharp instruments or devices; and leak proof plastic bags for waste from client areas (soiled dressings, gloves, linen).
- Ensure that all infectious waste is properly labeled.
- Carefully handle plastic bags to avoid punctures and tearing.
- Disinfect carts used to carry infectious waste.
- Dispose of waste only in designated areas.
- Wash hands after disposing of hazardous materials.

Containers for contaminated sharps should be readily accessible to personnel and maintained in an upright position.

Evaluation

Evaluation of the effectiveness of nursing care is based on the achievement of goals and expected outcomes. Keeping the client free from infection requires frequent reassessment followed by timely adjustments made in the plan of care in order for nursing interventions to be effective. It is important for the client to remain free of infection during hospitalization as well as develop a true awareness of the factors that increase the risk for infection.

Maintaining Hand Hygiene

Hand hygiene is a general term that includes handwashing (using plain soap and water), *antiseptic handwash* (using antimicrobial substances and water), antiseptic hand rub (using alcohol-based hand rub), surgical hand antisepsis (using antiseptic handwash or antiseptic hand rub preoperatively by surgical personnel to eliminate transient and reduce resident hand flora). Procedure for maintaining hand hygiene is enlisted in Table 21.5. When hands are visibly dirty, wash hands with soap (plain or antimicrobial) and water. If hands are not visibly soiled, an alcohol-based hand rub may be used.

Handwashing is the rubbing together of all surfaces and crevices of the hands using a soap or chemical and water. Handwashing is a component of all types of isolation precautions and is the most basic and effective infection-control measure to prevent and control the transmission of infectious agents.

The three essential elements of handwashing are soap or chemical, water, and friction. Soaps that contain antimicrobial agents are frequently used in high-risk areas such as emergency departments and nurseries. Friction is the most important element of the trio because it physically removes soil and transient flora.

Handwashing should be performed after arriving at work, before leaving work, between client contacts, after removing gloves, when hands are visibly soiled, before eating, after excretion of body waste (urination and defecation), after contact with body fluids, before and after performing invasive procedures, and after handling contaminated equipment. The exact duration of time required for handwashing depends on the circumstances. A washing time of 10 to 15 seconds is recommended to remove transient flora from the hands. High-risk areas, such as nurseries, usually require about a minimum 2-minute handwash. Soiled hands usually require more time.

Equipment Needed

- Soap
- Paper or cloth towels
- Sink
- Running water.

The hand hygiene was adequate to control topical flora and infectious agents on the hands. The hands were not recontaminated during or shortly after the hand hygiene.

Use of Protecting (Gowns, Masks, Gloves, Cap)

Infection control is an essential area of concern for the nurse in any setting. Effective implementation prevents or reduces the incidence of nosocomial infections. The hospitalized client is at increased risk for infection because of added exposure to pathogens, compromised immunologic state, and potential invasive procedures, Development of infection can delay healing, prolong hospital slay, or cause permanent disability, or even loss of life. The hand hygiene was adequate to control topical flora and infectious agents on the hands. The hands were not recontaminated during or shortly after the hand hygiene.

Medical asepsis is the process *of* reducing microorganisms and preventing their spread, Hand hygiene is the single most important technique for infection control. Surgical asepsis takes this further with procedures implemented to eliminate any microorganisms. This is practiced in the surgical arena to reduce the risk of infection for the client. Use of protective equipments for infection control is enlisted in Table 21.6.

Standard Precautions consider all clients and their bodily fluids (except sweat) to be potentially infectious, thereby replacing the term Universal Precautions, which applied only to blood and visibly bloody fluids (CDC, 2002).

- Gloves are required when hand contact with any body fluids is anticipated. This includes touching mucous membranes and nonintact skin. Latex- and powder-free gloves are recommended. Hands should be cleansed after the gloves are removed.
- Impervious gowns must be worn by health care workers to prevent soiling of clothing by splashes of blood or body fluids, and masks, along with eye protection, are mandated if splashes toward the face are anticipated.
- Masks are worn when caring for clients on airborne and/or droplet precautions and immunocompromised clients.

- Hair should be covered by a cap when in the semirestricted and restricted areas of the surgical suite and in areas of the hospital where special procedures are done (i.e., bone marrow transplant).
- Eye protection (goggles) or face shields should be worn during care activities that may be associated with splashes or sprays of blood or body fluids.
- Soiled protective items should be removed promptly after use and disposed of as appropriate. Handle and process soiled gowns to the laundry according to facility protocol.

Before the use of protective equipment, the nurse should:

Assess if standard precautions are being followed or if specific isolation precautions are needed for the client's condition. The type of microorganism and mode of transmission determine the degree of precautions.

Assess what nursing measures are required before entering the room to have all the necessary equipment ready.

Assess the client's knowledge for the need to wear a cap, gown, and mask during care to direct client teaching.

Assess whether the isolation is airborne, droplet, or contact and which isolation attire is necessary.

Equipment Needed

- Gloves, clean–sterile if necessary
- Gown, sterile or clean
- Cap
- Mask
- Goggles
- Face mask

Table 21.5: Procedure for Hand Hygiene			
Nursing action			*Rationale*
Handwashing			
1.	Remove jewelry. Wristwatch may be pushed up above the wrist (midforearm). Push sleeves of uniform or shirt up above the wrist at mid forearm level.	1.	Provides access to skin surfaces for cleaning. Facilitates cleaning of fingers, hands, and forearms.
2.	Assess hands for hangnails, cuts, or breaks in the skin, and areas that are heavily soiled.	2.	Intact skin acts as a barrier to microorganisms. Breaks in skin integrity facilitate development of infection and should receive extra attention during cleaning.
3.	Turn on the water. Adjust the flow and temperature. Temperature of the water should be warm.	3.	Running water removes microorganisms. Warm water removes less of the natural skin oils.
4.	Wet hands and lower forearms thoroughly by holding under running water. Keep hands and forearms in the down position with elbows straight. Avoid splashing water and touching the sides of the sink.	4.	Water should flow from the least contaminated to the most contaminated areas of the skin. Hands are considered more contaminated than arms. Splashing of water facilitates transfer of microorganisms. Touching of any surface during cleaning contaminates the skin.
5.	Apply about 5 ml (1 teaspoon) of liquid soap. Lather thoroughly.	5.	Lather facilitates removal of microorganisms. Liquid soap harbors less bacteria than bar soap.
6.	Thoroughly rub hands together for about 10 to 15 seconds. Interlace lingers and thumbs and move back and forth to wash between digits. Rub palms and back of hands with circular motion. Special attention should be provided to areas such as the knuckles and fingernails, which are known to harbor organisms.	6.	Friction mechanically removes microorganisms from the skin surface. Friction loosens dirt from soiled areas.
7.	Rinse with hands in the down position, elbows straight, Rinse in the direction of forearm to wrist to fingers.	7.	Flow of water rinses away dirt and microorganisms.
8.	Blot hands and forearms to dry thoroughly, Dry in the direction of fingers to wrist and forearms. Discard the paper towels in the proper receptacle.	8.	Blotting reduces chapping of skin. Drying from cleanest (hand) to least clean area (forearms) prevents transfer of microorganisms to cleanest area.
9.	Turn off the water faucet with a clean, dry paper towel.	9.	Prevents contamination of clean hands by a less clean faucet.
10.	Apply the recommended amount of product to one hand (Alcohol based hand rub)	10.	Amount of rub required varies by product.
11.	Rub hands together, covering hands and fingers on all sides.	11.	Spreads rub to cover all aspects of hands and fingers.
12.	Continue rubbing until hands are dry.	12.	Allows the rub to work.

<table>
<tr><td colspan="4" align="center">Table 21.6: Use of Protective Equipments</td></tr>
<tr><td colspan="2">Nursing action</td><td colspan="2">Rationale</td></tr>
<tr>
<td>1.</td>
<td>Cleanse hands.</td>
<td>1.</td>
<td>Reduces the transmission of microorganisms.</td>
</tr>
<tr>
<td>2.</td>
<td>The first item of apparel donned should be the cap or surgical hat/hood. Hair should be tucked in a manner so that all hair is covered.</td>
<td>2.</td>
<td>Because hair acts as a filter when left uncovered, it collects bacteria in proportion to its length, curliness, and oiliness. Loose hair may fall in the surgical area. Shedding hair may lead to surgical wound infection.</td>
</tr>
<tr>
<td>3.</td>
<td>Apply mask around mouth and nose and secure in a manner that prevents venting. For masks with strings:
(a) Hold mask by top and pinch center (metal strip) over bridge of nose.
(b) Pull top two strings over ears and secure at top, bock of head.
(c) Tie two lower ties around back or nape of neck so bottom of mask fits snugly under chin.</td>
<td>3.</td>
<td>Masks are worn to contain and filter droplets of microorganisms that are expelled when talking, sneezing, or coughing. Masks prevent the transmission of oral and nasopharyngeal organisms between the nurse and client.</td>
</tr>
<tr>
<td>4.</td>
<td>Open gown, slip arms into sleeves, and secure at neck and side.</td>
<td>4.</td>
<td>Gowns act as a protective barrier and should be worn to reduce exposure to blood, body fluid, or other potentially infectious liquids.</td>
</tr>
<tr>
<td>5.</td>
<td>Protective eyewear should be worn whenever health care provider or client are at risk for splash and contamination. These are applied as goggles/glasses or face shields, which have elastic ties for around the ears.</td>
<td>5.</td>
<td>Protective eyewear reduces the incidence of contamination to the eyes. If eyewear or face shields become contaminated, they should be discarded immediately and replaced with a clean barrier.</td>
</tr>
<tr>
<td>6.</td>
<td>Don clean gloves. If sterile gloves are required for a procedure, use open or closed method.</td>
<td>6.</td>
<td>Gloves are worn to prevent gross contamination of the hands. They should be changed between clients and hands cleansed. The open method is used when performing procedures that require sterile technique but do not require donning a sterile gown or when both gloves need to be changed without assistance during a surgical procedure. The closed method is used by scrubbed personnel in the operating room.</td>
</tr>
<tr>
<td>7.</td>
<td>The open glove technique:
(a) Slide the hands into the gown all the way through the cuffs on the gown.
(b) Pick up the cuff of the left glove using the thumb and index finger of the right hand.
(c) Pull the glove onto the left hand, leaving the cuff of the glove turned down.
(d) Take the gloved left hand and slide the fingers under the cuff of the right glove, keeping the gloved fingers under the folded cuff.
(e) Pull the glove onto the right hand.
(f) Rotate the arm as tile cuff of tire glove is pulled over the gown.</td>
<td>7.</td>
<td>The open glove method is commonly used for sterile procedures or when both gloves need to be changed without assistance during a surgical procedure.</td>
</tr>
<tr>
<td>8.</td>
<td>The closed glove technique:
(a) Slide the hands in to the gown all the way through the cuffs on, the gown.
(b) Use right hand to pick up left glove.
(c) Place the glove on the upward-turned left hand–palm side down thumb to thumb with the fingers extending along the forearm pointing toward the elbow.
(d) Hold the glove cuff and sleeve cuff together with the thumb of the left hand.
(e) The right hand stretches the cuff of the left glove over the opened end of the sleeve.
(f) Work the fingers into the glove as the cuff is pulled onto the wrist.
(g) The right glove is done in the same manner.</td>
<td>8.</td>
<td>The closed glove technique is used by the scrubbed personnel in the operating room. This is preferred because the possibility of the glove touching the skin is eliminated.</td>
</tr>
</table>

Contd...

<table>
<tr><td colspan="4" align="center">Table 21.6: Contd...</td></tr>
<tr><td colspan="2">Nursing action</td><td colspan="2">Rationale</td></tr>
<tr><td>9.</td><td>Enter the client's room and explain the rationale for wearing the attire.</td><td>9.</td><td>Minimizes anxiety and feelings of isolation.</td></tr>
<tr><td>10.</td><td>After performing necessary tasks, remove gown, gloves, mask, and cap before leaving the room.</td><td>10.</td><td>Reduces transmission of organisms.</td></tr>
<tr><td>11.</td><td>Removal of gown: Untie gown and remove from shoulders. Fold and roll gown down in front into a ball, so contaminated area is rolled onto center of gown. Dispose in approved receptacle.</td><td>11.</td><td>Reduces transmission of organisms.</td></tr>
<tr><td>12.</td><td>Removal of gloves:
(a) Grasp outside cuff of one glove and pull off, turning, inside out. Hold it with the remaining gloved hand.
(b) Pull the second glove off without touching the outside of the second glove. Turn the second glove as it is removed. Dispose into receptacle with first glove.</td><td>12.</td><td>(a) Reduces risk of contamination.
(b) Reduces risk of contamination.</td></tr>
<tr><td>13.</td><td>Removal of mask: Untie bottom strings of mask first, then top strings, and lift off face. Hold mask by strings and discard.</td><td>13.</td><td>Prevents contaminated surface of mask from contacting uniform.</td></tr>
<tr><td>14.</td><td>Removal of cap: Grasp top surface of cap and lift from head.</td><td>14.</td><td>Minimizes contact of hands to hair.</td></tr>
<tr><td>15.</td><td>Cleanse hands.</td><td>15.</td><td>Reduces transmission of microorganisms.</td></tr>
</table>

Donning and removing gloves, caps, and masks is a skill that is required of all personnel, including ancillary personnel. Proper technique should be monitored by the nursing staff.

Gowning for Isolation

The use of gowns in isolation is important primarily to protect clothing from getting soiled while administering patient care. The gown also prevents contact with infections microorganisms that could have exited from the patient. Donning, and isolation gown, is indicated when caring for patients with diseases characterized by heavy drainage, infectious and acute diarrheal and other gastrointestinal disorders, respiratory disorder, skin wounds or bums and urinary disorders.

The supply needed for gowning for isolation is as 'isolation gown'. Isolation gowns open at the back with ties at the neck and the waist. This keeps the gown securely closed, protecting the back of the uniforms, as well as the fronts. The gown should be long enough to cover the uniform and have a long sleeves with cuffs for added protection.

The nurse gowns for isolation for the following reasons:

To prevent the nurse from contracting an infection from patients.

To prevent medical personnel from contaminating the patient who has a disease affecting the immune system.

The steps for gowning for isolation are discussed in Table 21.7.

<table>
<tr><td colspan="4" align="center">Table 21.7: Steps for Gowning for Isolation</td></tr>
<tr><td colspan="2">Nursing actions</td><td colspan="2">Rationales</td></tr>
<tr><td>1.</td><td>Remove watch and push up long sleeves.</td><td>1.</td><td>Ensures that uniform sleeve is under gown sleeve for protection.</td></tr>
<tr><td>2.</td><td>Place watch on a paper towel before taking vital sign.</td><td>2.</td><td>Prevents cross contamination of watch.</td></tr>
<tr><td>3.</td><td>Wash hands.</td><td>3.</td><td>Inhibits spread of microorganism.</td></tr>
<tr><td>4.</td><td>Don gown by securely typing gown at neck and waist.</td><td>4.</td><td>Provides protective covering of the entire uniform.</td></tr>
<tr><td>5.</td><td>Remove gown.</td><td>5.</td><td>Protects nurse.</td></tr>
<tr><td>6.</td><td>Wash hands.</td><td>6.</td><td>Prevents spread of microorganisms.</td></tr>
</table>

Donning Gloves

Nurses or healthcare personnel wear/don gloves if there is any possibility of contact with infectious material. Nurses wear gloves for all types of patient care for the following reasons:
- To protect the nurse and the nurses family from disease
- To protect the patient from the nurse, who may be considered a contaminator to the patient
- To protect the personnel from contact with the infectious microorganism.

The supply needed for donning gloves is a 'pair of gloves'. The steps of the donning gloves are discussed in Table 21.8.

Donning a Mask

A mask should be worn for the following purposes:
- To prevent the wearer from inhaling microorganism that travel on airborne droplets for short distances or that remain suspended in the air for longer periods
- To prevent inhaling pathogens if resistance is reduced or if being transported to another area (patient use)
- To discourage that wearer from touching the mouth, nose, or eye and from transmitting infection material.

The steps of donning 'isolation mask' are enlisted in Table 21.9.

Double Bagging

A single bag is adequate if the contaminated articles can be placed in the bag without contamination of the outside of the bag. Double bagging is recommended when it is impossible to keep the outer surface of the single bag, free from contamination. The second bag should be labeled for color coded to alert nursing personnels and to prevent contamination of housekeeping personnels when handling contaminated material. Double bag can be used for safe removal of any article from room.

Double bagging has purposes, i.e. to prevent spread of microorganism to the surrounding area and to prevent potential accidental exposure of personnel to contaminated article. The supplies and equipment needed for double bagging are as follows:
- Single isolation bag
- Special color coded bag
- Holder for isolation bag
- Isolation gown, mask and clean gloves
- Holder for laundry bags

<table>
<tr><td colspan="4">Table 21.8: Steps for Donning Gloves for Isolation</td></tr>
<tr><td colspan="2">Nursing actions</td><td colspan="2">Rationales</td></tr>
<tr><td>1.</td><td>Remove gloves from dispenser.</td><td>1.</td><td>Keeps gloves readily available for use.</td></tr>
<tr><td>2.</td><td>Don gloves when ready to begin patient care.</td><td>2.</td><td>Provides protection for the patient and nurse.</td></tr>
<tr><td>3.</td><td>Inspect gloves for possibility of perforation.</td><td>3.</td><td>Perforated gloves can allow entry of pathogenic microorganism.</td></tr>
<tr><td>4.</td><td>Change gloves after direct handling of infection drainage.</td><td>4.</td><td>Prevents contamination of patient.</td></tr>
<tr><td>5.</td><td>Remove gloves by grasping at cuff/edge and turning gloves inside out and drop into waste container.</td><td>5.</td><td>Prevents nurse from touching outside area of gloves, which is considered contaminated.</td></tr>
<tr><td>6.</td><td>Wash hands thoroughly.</td><td>6.</td><td>Removes microorganism that could be on nurses hands.</td></tr>
</table>

<table>
<tr><td colspan="4">Table 21.9: Steps for Donning Mask for Isolation</td></tr>
<tr><td colspan="2">Nursing actions</td><td colspan="2">Rationales</td></tr>
<tr><td>1.</td><td>Remove mask from container.</td><td>1.</td><td>Keeps mask readily available for use.</td></tr>
<tr><td>2.</td><td>Don mask when ready to begin patient.</td><td>2.</td><td>Provides protection from microorganism care by covering nose and mouth with the mask secure mask in place with elastic band or by tying the stringes behind the head.</td></tr>
<tr><td>3.</td><td>Wear mask until it becomes moist out no longer than 20 to 30 minutes.</td><td>3.</td><td>Moisture renders mask ineffective.</td></tr>
<tr><td>4.</td><td>Remove masks by untying the stringes or moving the elastic. Make certain not to touch contaminated area.</td><td>4.</td><td>Protects nurse from coming into contact with contaminated mask.</td></tr>
<tr><td>5.</td><td>Dispose of soiled mask.</td><td>5.</td><td>Protects other healthcare workers.</td></tr>
<tr><td>6.</td><td>Wash hands thoroughly.</td><td>6.</td><td>Removes microorganism.</td></tr>
</table>

Table 21.10: Steps for Double Bagging			
	Nursing actions		*Rationales*
1.	Don gown, mask and glove before entering patient room.	1.	Prevents contact with contaminated article.
2.	Collect all contaminated disposable article in isolation bag.	2.	Prepare for double bagging.
3.	Summon second healthcare worker to remain outside patient area.	3.	Prevents risk of contamination of personnel.
4.	Second person holds double bag with top edge of bag covering hands.	4.	Prevents risk of contamination of personnel.
5.	First person drops contaminated bag in double bag, without touching edges of bag.	5.	Outside of double bags remain clean.
6.	Bags are sealed or tied and labeled.	6.	Prevents spread of microorganism.
7.	First person places new bags in holders.	7.	Keeps articles ready for use.
8.	Remove gloves, gown and mask without contamination.	8.	Prevent spread of pathogens.
9.	Wash hands thoroughly.	9.	Prevents contamination of nurse and others.

The steps to be followed for double bagging are given in Table 21.10

Isolation Technique

The type of isolation technique followed will depend on transmissibility of the pathogen. The use of environmental barriers will keep pathogens in a confined care, i.e. private room, isolation room, closed door, protective gown, masks and gloves and shoe covers.

The nurse follows isolation technique to prevent the transmission of infection from microorganisms by preventing pathogens from leaving the room of the infected patient or from entering the room of a highly susceptible patient.

The supplies and equipment needed for isolation technique are as follows:
- Isolation/gown, masks, gloves
- Clean linen
- Single and double isolation bags
- Paper towels
- Running water
- Soap with dispenser
- Holder for isolation bag and laundry bag.

The steps to be followed in an isolation technique are enlisted in Table 21.11.

Preparing for Disinfection and Sterilization

There are two methods of sterilization and disinfection, i.e. physical method and chemical method:
- Physical method will include steam under pressure (autoclave), boiling water, radiation, dry heat
- Chemical method will include gas (ethylene oxide) and chemical solutions.

The nurse follows basic clean or aseptic technique to interrupt the infection process in order to prevent and control the spread of infections. The supplies and equipment needed for preparing for disinfection are gloves, running water, scrub brush and for sterilized clean cloth wrapper.

The step to be followed in preparing for disinfection and sterilization are enlisted in Table 21.12.

Medical Handwashing

Handwashing is a vigorous, brief rubbing together of all surfaces of hands lathered in soap, followed by rinsing under a steam of water. The purpose is to remove soil and transient organisms from the hands and to reduce total microbial counts over time. It is the most important preventive technique for interrupting the infection process.

Handwashing is the single most important means for preventing the spread of infections. It is frequently, however, incorrectly or inadequately done in an attempt to save time. Unfortunately, this may cause increased infections and longer patient hospitalization at increased cost. Contaminated hands are a prime cause of cross infection.

The need for handwashing depends on the type, intensity, duration and sequence of activity. Handwashing of nurses recommended the following situations:
- Upon arising at the clinical unit prior to beginning a period of duty. This will serve to decrease the microorganism transported to the hospital from external environment. Nurses also wash their hands prior to leaving the area for rest and meal break in order to decrease the special of microorganism to other areas of the hospital and to themselves.
- Before contact with clients who are susceptible to infections, e.g. newborn infants, clients with leukemia, organ transplant recipients and HIV +ve cases, in order to prevent the spread of microorganisms.

Table 21.11: Steps for Isolation Technique

	Nursing actions		Rationales
1.	Determine causative organism or effectiveness of patients immune system.	1.	Helps nurse know virulence of causative pathogen.
2.	Recognize the mode of transmission and show microorganism exist in the body.	2.	Determine categories or types of isolation to use.
3.	Follow hospital policy for specific type of isolation used.	3.	Increases awareness of isolation categories available in hospital.
4.	Provide environment with adequate equipment and supplies. (i) Private room for isolation with anteroom. (ii) Sign stating isolation category. (iii) Adequate handwashing facility. (iv) Special containers for trash, soiled linen and sharp instruments, such as needles.	4.	 (i) reduces possibility of transmission of microorganism. (ii) Alert personnel, patient family and visitors about special precaution to be followed. (iii) Handwashing can easily be performed on entering and leaving the area. (iv) Ensures safe disposal of contaminated articles.
5.	Plan time to explain isolation technique to patient family and visitors.	5.	Relieve apprehension and promotes cooperation of those involved.
6.	Postcard on door of patients room or wall outside room stating the protective measure in use for patient care.	6.	Informs those entering room of precautions to be followed and encourages cooperation.
7.	Supply the room with designated lined containers for soiled linens and for trash.	7.	Prevents transmission of pathogens from see page through container

Table 21.12: Steps Preparing for Disinfection and Sterilization

	Nursing actions		Rationales
1.	Prepare equipment and supplies: (a) Disinfectant to use for cleaning. (b) Material of sterilization. (c) Gloves. (d) Running water. (e) Scrub brush. (f) Cloth wrapper.	1.	Ensures organization taste: (a) Helps in appropriate care of equipment and reusable supplies. (b) Ensures that appropriate method is used. (c) Protect nurse from contamination. (d) Helps in cleansing and rinsing. (e) Articles in cleansing grooves. (f) Provides means for wrapping articles requiring sterilization.
2.	Don gloves.	2.	Protects nurse from contamination.
3.	Rinse articles under cool running water.	3.	Emulsifies or softens dirt for easy removal.
4.	Wash articles with detergent.	4.	Emulsifies and softens dirt for easy removal.
5.	Use scrub brush to remove material in grooves.	5.	Friction loosens material in corners and grooves.
6.	Dry articles thoroughly.	6.	Prevents growth of microorganism.
7.	Prepare articles for sterilization by wrapping it in cloth wrappers.	7.	Ensures appropriate sterilization of the article.

- After caring for an infected clients.
- Prior to performing any clean duties such as preparing medications, handling food trays, assembling equipment or selecting clean linen.
- After touching organic material, i.e. after performing any duties involving contaminated articles such as bedpans, surgical dressings, soiled tissues or dirty linen.
- Before performing invasive procedures such as administration of injections, catheterization and suctioning.
- Before and after handling dressing or touching open wounds.
- Between contact with different clients in high risk units.

- After removing disposable gloves or handling contaminated equipment.

The supplies needed for handwashing are as follows:
- Soap as provided by the hospital; this may be liquid in a foot controlled dispenser, bar soap or a paper sheet with soap in it
- Stick or brush for cleaning fingernails
- Warm running water, preferably with foot or knee control
- Disposable towels or warm air dryer.

The steps to be followed while medical hand washing are enlisted in Table 21.13.

Table 21.13: Steps for Medical Handwashing

	Nursing actions		Rationales
1.	Use easy to reach sink with warm running water soap or disinfectant, paper towels.	1.	Running water facilitates removal of organism, paper towels are easy to disposed.
2.	Push wristwatch and long uniform sleeves about wrist. Avoid wearing rings and jewellery, if worn remove during washing.	2.	Provides complete access to fingers, hands increases of microorganisms in hands, jewellery harbors microorganisms and is difficult to clean.
3.	Keep finger nails short and filed.	3.	Most microbes on hands come from beneath fingernails.
4.	Inspect hands, observing for visible soiling, breaks or cuts in the skin and cuticles, i.e. determine contamination of hands.	4.	Poor personal hygiene and open cuts or wounds can harbor high concentration of microorganisms and may serve as portal exist.
5.	Stand in front of sink, keeping hands and uniform away from sink surface.	5.	Inside of sink is contaminated area. Reaching over sink increases risk of touching edge which is contaminated.
6.	Turn on water. Press pedals with foot to regulate flow and temperature. Push knee pedals laterally to control flow and temperature. Turn on hand operated faucets by covering faucets with paper towel.	6.	Water is too hot which can chap skin, and too much how will cause splashing and spread of microorganisms to other areas. When hands contact faucet they are contaminated. Organisms spread easily from hands to faucets and heat opens pores and also removes protective oils on the nurses hands.
7.	Avoid splashing water against uniform.	7.	Microorganism travel and grow in moisture.
8.	Wet the hands thoroughly by holding hands below the level of the elbows.	8.	In this manner, the water will flow from the least contaminated areas (arms) to the most contaminated areas (finger tips) because hands are the most contaminated par of the arms, water should flow from the wrist, over the hands and then down the drain.
9.	Apply soap, if bar soap is used, the bar is rinsed prior to returning it to the soap dish or lather hands with liquid soap (about 1 tea spoon).	9.	Soap emulsifies fat and acids in cleansing. Most hospital soap kills some microorganisms, i.e. it is bacteriostatic. Soap is rinsed to prevent the spread of microorganisms since microbes grow on the wet surface of the soap.
10.	Wash hands using plenty of lather and friction for atleast 10 to 14 sec. Interlace fingers and rub palms and back of hands with circular motions atleast 5 times each.	10.	Soap cleanses by emulsifying fat and oil and lowering surface tension. Friction and rubbing mechanically loosen and remove dirt and transient bacteria. Interlacin fingers and thumbs ensures that all surfaces are cleansed.
11.	Wash each hand, finger and nail separately paying special attention to the webbed areas between fingers, wash for one full minute.	11.	These area frequently missed till washing times vary. A full minute is required for the first washing of the duty period and for heavily soiled hands.
12.	Rinse wrists and hands completely, keeping hands lower than elbows, i.e., keeping hands down and elbows up. Rinse so that water flows down from the wrist area off the finger tips.	12.	Water should run from cleaner area (the wrists) over the hands, and then down the drain, rinsing the dirt and microorganism away. Water flows from the least contaminated area (wrist) to the most contaminated area (finger tips).
13.	Clean fingernails under running water using finger nails of other hands or blunt end of an orange stick.	13.	Reduces chances of microorganisms remaining under nails.
14.	Dry hands thoroughly from finger to wrist and forearms.	14.	Drying from cleanest (fingertips) to least clean forearm area avoids contamination. Drying hands prevents chapping and roughened skin.
15.	Turn off water with foot and knee pedals or turn off hand faucet, use clean dry paper towel.	15.	Clean hands prevent touching contaminated handles. Wet towel and hands allow transfer of pathogens by capillary actions.
16.	Use hand lotion if desired.	16.	Keeps skin soft and lubricated so skin will not crack easily.
17.	Inspect hands and nails for cleanliness.	17.	Ensures cleanliness of hands and nails.

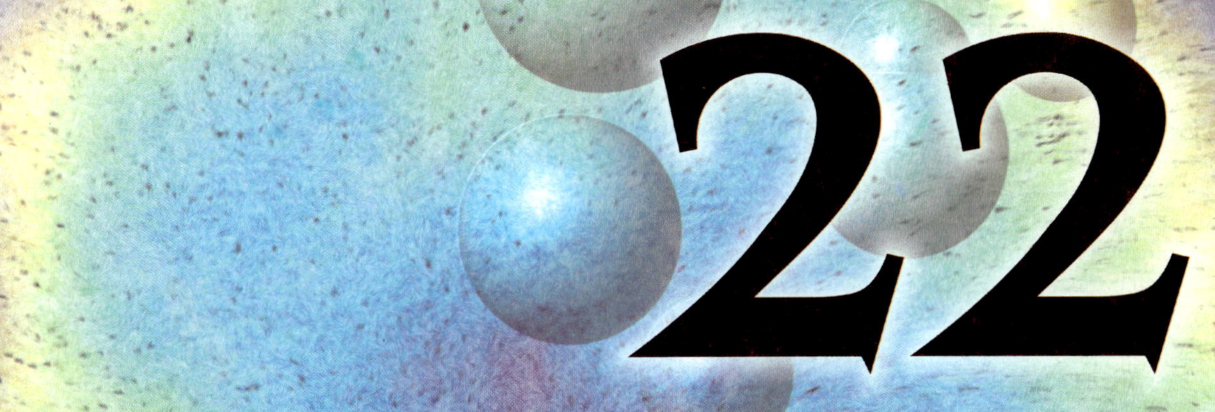

22

Biomedical Waste Management

The management of Biomedical waste or Hospital waste has assumed great importance the world over because of the serious hazards it poses to the environment in general and the public in particular. Although hospital waste management has become serious concern throughout the world, in India, only ten states and districts have given adequate thought to manage properly the collection and disposal of waste from hospitals. Authorities are still not familiar with proper waste classification: segregation, handling and disposal of the waste generated in the hospitals.

A hospital is an institution which produces many types of waste material. Housekeeping activity generates considerable amount of trash, the visitors and others bring with them food, fruits and other materials which must in some way be disposed off. In addition to waste that is produced in all residential buildings, hospitals generate pathological waste (blood soaked dressings, carcasses and similar waste). These waste materials must be suitably disposed of immediately *lest* they putrefy, emit foul smells, act as a source of infection, disease and become a public health hazard. Hospital waste still finds its way to roadside heaps of rubbish, where it mixes with municipal or corporation solid waste, rendering it hazardous for the environment and the public. All these years, the management of hospital waste was relegated to the hands of nurses, wardboys, ward ayahs, sweepers and sanitary workers. Now the 'hospital waste' also termed as 'Biomedical waste' and the management of biomedical waste shall be the duty of every person who has control over an institution or its premises of an institution generating biomedical waste, which includes a hospital, nursing home, clinic, dispensary, veterinary institution, animal house, pathological laboratory, blood bank by whatever name called to take all steps to ensure that such waste is handled without any adverse effect to human health and the environment.

Nurses are responsible and accountable for professional behavior that involves application of the nursing process and cooperation with appropriate others within current legislation affecting the practice of nursing according to professions code of ethics and practice with the context of the policies and practices of the employing agency, and within the customs and values of the society in which the nursing care is being provided. This has direct application to hospital nursing practice, which includes biomedical waste management.

Concepts of Waste

As we know that "waste" constitutes an important part of the environment to which man is continuously exposed, which includes refuse or solid wastes, excreta or night soil and sullage. The term 'refuse' is applied to all solid waste from human habitations that is not covered by the sewers, i.e. all wastes other than sullage (waste water or slop water and comprises all liquid wastes including industrial waste but excluding night soil) and night soil. It includes public refuse (originating from homes, hotels, institutions, street, stables and markets) and industrial refuse. The solid waste originating from homes or domestic refuse consists or garbage, rubbish and ash.

- *Garbage* is the waste from food during its handling at various stages including preparation, cooking and serving.
- *Rubbish* comprise of dirt, dust and bits of paper, wood, clothing, glass, rubber, plastic, metal, etc.
- *Ash* is the residue after burning of fuel.

Different types of wastes impinge upon physical, mental and social health in various ways. For example, solid waste if allowed to accumulate is a health hazard, because,

- It decomposes and favours fly breeding (Flies may help to spread certain diseases like diarrheal disease).
- It attracts rodents (for example, rats may help to spread dengue fever or plague, etc.) and also attracts vermin (for, e.g. mosquito, help to transmit malaria or filaria).
- The pathogens which may be present in the solid waste, may be conveyed back to man's food through flies and dust; dust may harbour tubercle bacilli and other microorganisms which cause diseases accordingly).
- There is a possibility of water and soil pollution may lead to many infections and infestations. (ex. soil polluted with night soil may be rich in tetanus spores).
- Heaps of refuse present an unsightly appearance and nuisance from bad odors.

Type of Waste

Wastes are divided into following types which include:

Type '0' waste refers to a waste which is a mixture of highly combustible as paper, cardboard, cartons, wooden boxes and combustible, floor sweeping from commercial, industrial and housekeeping activities. The mixture contains upto 10 percent weight of plastic bags, coated paper, laminated paper, treated corrugated paper, oily rags and plastic and rubber scraps. This type of waste contains 10 percent of moisture, 5 percent incombustible solids and has heating value of 8.500 BTU/lb fired.

Type 1 waste is a rubbish consisting of combustible waste such as paper cartons, rags, wood scrap, saw-dust, foliage, and floor sweeping from domestic, commercial and industrial activities. This type of waste contains 25 percent moisture, upto 10 percent incombustible solids, and has heating value of 6.500 BTU/lb as fired.

Type 2 waste is a refuse consisting of approximately even mixture of rubbish and garbage by weight. This type of waste is common to residential blocks, and contains upto 50 percent of moisture, 7 percent incombustible solids and has a heating value of 4.300 BTU/lb as fired.

Type 3 waste is a garbage consisting of animal and vegetable wastes from restaurants, cafeterias, hotels, hospitals, markets and similar establishments. This type of waste contains upto 70 percent of moisture, upto 5 percent incombustible solids and has a heating value of 2,500 BTU/lb as fired.

Type 4 waste is pathological waste, i.e. human and animal remains consisting of carcasses, organs, and solid organic wastes from hospitals, laboratories, abattoirs, animal pounds and similar source containing upto 85 percent moisture, 5 percent incombustible solids and having a heating value of 1000 BTU/lb as fired.

Type 5 and 6 waste are byproduct waste, gaseous, liquid, semiliquid, and solid from industrial operations. Calorific value must be determined for the individual material to be destroyed.

Classification of Hospital Waste

Hospital waste can be defined as any discarded, unwanted residual matter arising from the hospital or activities related to the hospital 'Disposal' covers the total process of collecting, handling, packing, storage, transportation and final treatment of wastes. Hospital waste can be classified into two major groups-solid wastes and liquid wastes.

The *solid wastes* of a hospital includes the following:
- Dry garbage: Ordinary floor refuse, papers, flowers, fresh.
- Wet garbage: Waste from kitchen (fruit peels, left over food, etc).
- Wet tissues and bones: From operation theatre, labor rooms, mortuary laboratory.
- Plaster casts from plaster room.
- Packing materials: Cardboard, Cartons, paper packets, etc.
- Surgical waste: Dressing, Cotton pads.
- Metal waste: Tins, cans, bottle caps, needles.
- Glass: Broken bottles, syringes.
- Disposal plastic items: From all areas in hospital.

The *liquid wastes* cover sullage and sewage which emanate from bathrooms, lavatories, toilets, kitchen, pantries, operation theatre, dressing room, laboratory and laundry, and waste from radiology department comprising of chemical developer and fixer solutions. The quantity of total liquid waste is estimated at 300 to 400 litres per bed per day.

The Radioactive waste from Radiotherapy and Nuclear Medicine Department.

Biomedical Waste (BMW)

In daily usage "Waste" refers to pieces of paper, pieces of cloth, left over food, portion of commodity, ashes, animals droppings, animals' dead bodies including unused articles swept from roads, markets, hospitals, etc. 'Hazardous wastes' refers to waste or parts of waste, according to their physical, chemical components and their infection that could cause sickness, death or possibility of being harmful to health of animate things and environment if its collection, transportation and disposal are inappropriately managed.

Now the term 'hospital waste' replaced by the term 'BIOMEDICAL WASTE'. According to World Health Organization, "Medical Waste" refers to that portion of a health care or research facilities total waste stream that contains potentially infectious agents, hazardous chemicals or radioactive materials" which includes:

- *Solid medical waste*: Wastes such as needles, infusion sets, bandages, anatomical wastes, isolation wastes and all other materials contaminated or potentially contaminated with blood and/or body fluids from medical diagnoses, treatment or research.
- *Liquid medical waste*: Wastes such as blood, body fluids, dialysis solutions, chemical reagents, solvents, acids, heavy metal solutions, film developers, cytotoxic and other pharmaceuticals resulting from medical treatment or research.
- *Isolation waste*: All disposable materials associated with a medical patient isolated from other patients to prevent transmission of a very infectious disease.
- *Household waste (domestic)*: Solid wastes that do not contain solid biomedical waste, household waste originating from medical treatment or research centers includes uncontaminated wastes such as office paper and packaging material.

According to the Gazette of India "Biomedical Waste" means any waste, which is generated during diagnosis, treatment or immunization of human beings, or animals or in research activities pertaining there to or in the production or testing of biologicals and including categories mentioned in Schedule 1 (Union Ministry of Environment and Forest, Gazette Notification dated 20 July, 1998) which includes the following:

Category No. 1

Human anatomical waste: Human tissues, organs, body parts.

Category No. 2

Animal waste: Animal tissues, organs, body parts, carcasses bleeding parts, fluids, blood and experimental animals use in research, waste generated by veterinary hospitals, colleges, discharges from hospitals, animal house.

Category No. 3

Microbiology and biotechnology waste: Waste from laboratory cultures, stocks or specimen of microorganisms live or attenuated, vaccines, human and animal cells culture used, infections agents from research and industrial laboratories, waste from production of biologicals, toxins, dishes, devices used for transfer of cultures.

Category No. 4

Waste sharps: Needles, syringes, scalpels, blades, glass, etc. that may cause puncture and cuts. This includes both used and unused sharps.

Category No. 5

Discarded medicine and cytotoxic drugs: Wastes comprising outdated, contaminated and discarded medicines.

Category No. 6

Solid waste: Items contaminated with blood and fluids including cotton, dressings, soiled plaster casts, linen beddings, other material contaminated with blood.

Category No. 7

Solid waste: Wastes generated from disposable items other than the waste sharp such as tubings, catheters, intravenous sets, etc.

Category No. 8

Liquid waste: Waste generated from laboratory washing, cleaning, housekeeping, and disinfecting activities.

Category No. 9

Incineration ash: Ash for incineration of any biomedical waste.

Category No. 10

Chemical: Use in production of biologicals, chemicals, used in disinfection as insecticides, etc.

(For further details please read the Biomedical Waste Managements and Handling Rules 1998 at the end of the chapter).

Thus, Biomedical Waste refers to any waste that consists wholly or partly human tissue or animal tissue, blood and other body fluids, excretions, drugs or other pharmaceutical products including antineoplastic drugs, swabs, dressings, syringes, needles or other sharp instruments being waste which unless rendered safe, may prove hazardous to any person coming in contact with it and any other waste arising from medical, nursing, dental, pharmaceutical or similar practice, investigation including radioactive waste, treatment, care, teaching or research or collection of blood and blood product from transfusion, being waste which may cause infection to any person coming in contact with it.

Ill Effects of Biomedical Waste

Waste generated from different health care facilities will have different character in the composition of biomedical waste. Although medical waste stream represents only a small fraction of the total municipal waste however, it is most visible and critical in public opinion.

- Foul odor is emitted at the disposable site due to continuous decomposition of organic matter and emission of methane, hydrogen sulphide, ammonia, etc. The problem is intensified if proper mitigation measures are not adopted/taken.
- Odor is also emitted at the collection points if quick removal of wastes is not practised. Spreading of the waste in the area adjacent to the local collection point due to the activity of the rag pickers cause degradation of aesthetic quality. Uncontrolled disposal and open burning of wastes at the local dumping site create unpleasant visions.

- Domestic rats, birds and other scavenging animals besides being aesthetically unpleasant also act as reservoirs for many organ is transmissible to people, including plague, forms of typhus, leptospirosis, trichinosis, psittacosis, and Salmonella infection.
- Chemical control of both house flies and rodents is not very effective, because of widespread resistance to insecticides. The essential basis of control remains denial of access to food and harborage by covered storage bags and efficient removal of waste.
- Aedes mosquitoes, vectors of dengue fever and yellow fever, breed prolifically in discarded containers that trap rain water. Culex mosquitoes, vectors of filariasis, breed in polluted stagnant water. Such breeding sites often occur where hospital drains are blocked by solid waste.
- Hospital acquired infection (nosocomial infections) have shown increase in incidence due to mismanagement of hospital wastes, e.g. hospital gangrene, hepatitis B and C, HIV and AIDS, tuberculosis, cholera, diphtheria, etc. and transfusion associated virus.
- Psychological and emotional distress related to the recognizable body parts like amputed limbs, abortus and dead feature thrown with the waste. Waste handlers working at the municipal dumping site refuse to handle waste which has body parts. Injury to the waste handlers leads to infections.
- It is reported that 60 percent of all hospital staff sustain injuries from sharps, knowingly or unknowingly during various procedures undertaken in the health care facilities. Hospital personnel working in operation theatre, are specially prone to needle injuries while suturing. Injury to the professionals like physician, surgeons, nurses may lead to infection such as hepatitis B and HIV infections because, they handle the waste during performing surgical or diagnostic procedures.

The effects associated with poor hospital waste management include the following:

Health Hazards

- Injuries from sharp to all categories of hospital personnel and waste handlers.
- Nosocomial infections due to poor infection control and poor waste management.
- Risks of infections outside the hospital for waste handlers, scavengers and eventually the general public.
- Risks associated with hazardous chemicals, drugs being handled by persons handling wastes at all levels.
- 'Disposable' being repacked and sold without being even washed.
- Drugs disposed being repacked and sold to unsuspecting buyers.

Environmental Hazards

- Toxic emissions like dioxins, furan gases carbon, sulphur particles from defective and inefficient incineration

- Indiscriminate disposal of incinerator ash and residues.
- Leachate from improper waste residues, leading to contamination of ground water.
- Dangers of Blood Borne Pathogens in Hospital Waste and Laboratory.

At present, most health care workers, managers and administrators are familiar with the risk of disease transmission of blood borne pathogens. The following areas need attention:

- Availability and use of handwashing facilities.
- Identification labelling and disposal of contaminated equipment like used syringes, needles, etc.
- Provision, use, accessibility and condition of PPE (personal protective equipment) as and when required.
- Correct housekeeping practices.
- Establishment and implementation of hepatitis B, C and tetanus vaccination and postexposure evaluation and follow-up.
- Compliance with hazard communication requirements.
  - Proper labels and signs.
  - Information and training.
- Record keeping including.
  - Medical records for employees with occupational exposure.
  - Training records.
  - Hepatitis B, C and tetanus vaccination declaration forms.

Biomedical waste contains (or is likely to contain) blood borne pathogens. All workers who handle it are, therefore, at risk of exposure and are subject to the requirements including training, vaccination, protective equipment and clothing.

Air Contamination

Most biomedical waste treatment and transport systems under normal operating conditions contaminate air, combustion systems and chemical treatment systems all carry the potential to release toxic gases, vapours and particulates into the work area. In addition, systems that pre-shred biomedical waste (e.g., chemical, microwave, autoclave and irradiation systems) also carry the potential to release microbial aerosols into the work area. For working with the incinerator system, a respirator should be worn during manual ash clean out or charging of the incinerator.

Heat and Fire Hazards

All higher temperature thermal systems like boiler, incinerator and autoclave are potential sources of heat and fire at the workplace. Radiant and convective heat can greatly increase temperatures in the work area and may cause worker discomfort, heat stress or serious injury.

During unusually warm weather, operators should be encouraged to take frequent short breaks and drink plenty of fluids. Any behavioral or physical symptoms of fatigue should be immediately brought to the attention of the authorities. Although people usually get used to moderate condition of hot and cold over the course of about two to three weeks, this alone

is rarely sufficient protection. Therefore, the amount of radiant and convective heat escaping to the surrounding work area must be reduced.

Eye Injury Hazards

Fully enclosed safety eye-cover should be routinely worn by all workers handling biomedical waste, specially those working with incinerators. High temperature systems carry the additional hazard of infrared radiation which can cause corneal cataracts and blindness.

Noise

Many biomedical waste treatment systems can be noisy. Noise poses a serious health problem and can cause irreversible hearing loss due to long-term exposure.

Need for Biomedical Waste Management

Now, the number of health care facilities both in the Government and private sectors, have grown considerably. All these health care facilities generate waste as a result of health care activities. No reliable figures about the quantum of waste generated per person per day are available. However, studies have estimated that the quantum of waste generated from hospitals ranges from 1.5 to 2.5 kg per day per patient. It may be more in specialized health care facilities like dialysis centers. In the west, the quantity of water generated is 4 to 5 kg per day per patient.

In a study of pattern of wastes in Indian cities, the quantity of refuse varied from 0.48 to 0.06 kg per capita per day with total compostable matter varying from 30 to 40 percent (Bhide AD 1975). The quantum of domestic waste in advanced countries is six to ten times more. So far as hospitals in advanced countries are concerned, the average refuse in hospitals in Denmark and West Germany is 3 kg per bed per day and in USA upto 14 kg per bed per day (Hansen L and Hansen A 1977). The quantum and type of waste reflects the lifestyle of the society and this fact must be borne in mind in the planning or waste management in hospitals. On an average, the volume of total solid waste in hospitals in India is estimated to range between 1 kg and 3 kg per day on a per bed basis. In a teaching hospital of 700 beds, solid waste averaged 1.5 kg per bed per day (Ray DB, Bhaskaran R *et al* 1978). It is estimated that about 0.75 kg out of this consists of food wastes.

In India many of our hospitals neither have a satisfactory waste disposal system nor a waste management and disposable policy. The disposal of waste is exclusively extrusted to the junior-most staff from the housekeeping department. Without any supervision and even pathological wastes are observed to be disposed off in the available open ground around hospitals with scant regard to aesthetic and hygienic consideration (Sharma *et al* 1993).

Waste management in generally not given the importance it deserves because the intrinsic value of the waste materials as an object further utility has not been fully recognized. The net result is that a hospital tries to cut on the expenditure involved in waste disposal by meagre allotment of resources.

The data available in India regarding the incidence of diseases directly related to poor biomedical waste management is virtually nonexisting. Even so, injuries by sharps are the most common. There have been sporasic reports pointing to a rise in hepatitis B positivity among health care personnel. Disease causing organisms are likely to be transmitted through contaminated waste under climatic, environmental and socioeconomic conditions that exist in the country.

The awareness regarding biomedical waste rules is very low even among qualified medical personnel including Medical Superintendents of hospitals and hospital administrator. The nurse plays an important role in management of respective patient and wards/units and should be well equipped with knowledge and practices of biomedical waste management to maintain safe environment. For the patient as expected and practiced by Florence Nightingale. A clean hospital and good housekeeping have a direct effect on the health, comfort and morale of patients visitors and hospital personal alike. Cleanliness radiates cheer and a well-kept hospital would give the public a feeling of confidence.

Objectives of Biomedical Waste Management

The objectives of the biomedical waste management are grouped as general and specific as given below.

General Objectives

- Reduction of the impact of this waste on the community.
- Reduction of the chances of infection and accidental injury to the workers.
- Reduction of cost of total treatment of waste.

Specific Objectives

- Motivation and sensitization of health care personnel.
- Training of health care personnel.
- Segregation of waste so that each type is treated in a suitable manner and thus minimising harm.
- Using proper disinfection technology, depending on the type of waste.

- Fixing of responsibility in institutions for biomedical waste disposal and treatment.

Elements of Biomedical Waste Management

Biomedical waste management (both infectious and non-infectious) should be managed through a pathway composed of six elements, each must be addressed in terms of personnel and material costs and occupational and safety risks. The six elements are:

- Separation (segregation)
- Identification (different colors-coded bags)
- Handling (collection, measurement, storage, transport)
- Treatment (off-site and on-site)
- Waste reduction (by shredding)
- Disposal

Separation/Segregation

Good segregation practices will lead to decrease in total biomedical waste. There is a significant impact on cost saving by the implementation of street waste segregation practices. Each category of waste (according to Schedule 1, of the rules) has to be kept segregated in proper container or bag as the case may be. Such container must be sturdy enough to contain the designed maximum volume and weight of the waste without damage. It should be without any puncture or leakage. The container should have a cover, preferably operated by foot, if plastic bags are to be used, they have to be securely fitted within a container in such a manner that they stay in place during opening and closing of the lid and can also be removed without difficulty. The sharps must be mutilated by a needle cutter, placed in the department/ward itself before putting them in puncture proof sharp containers. Attempts should be made to designate fixed places for each containers that it becomes a part of regular scenario and practice for the concerned medical as well as nursing staff.

Identification

The color coding and type of container for disposal of biomedical wastes will be made according to Schedule II. (Biomedical Waste Management and Handling Rules 1998) as given in table below.

Color	Type of bag	Waste type	Treatment option	Coding	Container	Category as per schedule I
Yellow	Plastic bag	Category 1,2,3-6	Incinerating			Deep burial
Red	Disinfected container	Category 3,6,7	Autoclaving/ Microwaving/ Chemical treatment			
Blue	Plastic bag/	Category 4 & 7	Autoclaving/ Microwaving/Chemical treatment and destruction/ shedding	White	Puncture proof	
Black	Plastic bag	Category 5,9 and 10 (solid)	Disposal insecured land fill			

When a bag or container is sealed, a tag indicating the name of the department, type of waste, its content/composition, the person responsible and his/her designation, date, shift, time, etc. has to be attached. A water proof marker pen should be used for writing.

Handling

The collection containers for biomedical waste have to be sturdy, leakproof, of adequate size and wheeled; two wheeled bins may be used. The 4 wheeled containers have two fixed wheels and two castors and they are fitted with wheel locking devices to prevent unwanted rollings. There should be not sharp edges or corners, especially metallic bins. Collection timings and duty chart should be pasted in a prominent place with copies given to he concerned waste collectors and supervisors. For general waste from the office, kitchens, garden, etc. normal wheel barrows may be used.

Separate service corridors for taking waste matter from the storage area to the collection room must be provided. These corridors should not cross the paths used by patients and visitors. The waste has to be taken to the common storage area first, from where it is to be taken to the treatment/disposal facility either within or outside premises, as the case may be. The wheel barrows containing general waste may be sent to a dumper container or further segregated as described under the rules of transportation of biomedical waste. It is important that the following points be observed when transporting the waste within the hospital:

- Containers and bags should always be closed during transport.
- The earth used for this purpose will have smooth surface and be easy to clean, e.g. carts made with fibre glass bodies have smooth surface.
- The carts should be used exclusively for transporting waste.
- The carts should be washed daily with water, detergents and disinfectants.
- The waste bags or containers should never be dragged on the floor.
- The waste should never be transferred from one receptacle to another.
- In particular, the thumb rules while handling BMW are as follows:
  - Direct contact with the wastes must be avoided.
  - Bags should not be overfilled so that they may be closed easily.
  - Bags should not be emptied into other bags.

Smaller units such as nursing homes, pathological laboratories, etc. do not have many department/units. In this case, intermediate storage is not required. They should install a needle cutter and a small device for cutting, plastic tubing, gloves, etc. and separate steam autoclave/microwave exclusively established for this purpose. Adequate precaution should be taken for occupation and environmental hazards.

Staff, who handle clinical waste bags and containers should be trained to be aware of the following to avoid injuries and accidents:

- When waste bags/ containers are three fourth full, they should be sealed.
- All bags and containers must conform to the different color coding system. Labelling can be done by writing the information on the bags an outer container.
- Separation of biomedical wastes to be done at source (in different color coding bags).
- Check that waste bags are effectively sealed.
- Origin of the waste is marked on the waste bag or container.
- Bag should be picked up by the neck and placed so that they can be picked up by the neck again for further handling.
- Manual handling of waste bags should be minimized to reduce the black of needle prick injuries.
- Bags should not be clasped against the body and too many bags should not be carried at a time.
- Avoid the bag hitting the body when being carried.
- Yellow bags and blue/white translucent bags should not be thrown or dragged.
- Sharp containers should be picked up and carried by the handle provided. The other hand should not be used to support the bottom of the container.
- Clinical waste should be kept only in a specified storage area.
- Staff should know the appropriate cleaning and disinfection procedures in case of accidental spillage and how to report an incident.
- Simple color coding system for plastic bags.
- Secure plastic color coded bags before waste handling.
- Poster should wear protective clothing like gloves, overall, etc.
- If the bag is soiled, it should be placed in another clean bag of the same color.
- Under no circumstances should any one insert their hands into any waste container.

Treatment

There are five broad categories of medical waste treatment technologies, which include:

- Mechanical process
- Thermal process
- Chemical process
- Irradiation process
- Biological process.

1. *Mechanical process* are used to change the physical form or characteristics of the waste, either to facilitate waste handling or to process the waste in conjunction with other treatment steps. The two primary mechanical processes are compaction and shredding.

Compaction involves compressing the waste into containers to reduce its volume. *Shredding* which also includes granulations, grinding, pulping and the like, is used to break the waste into smaller places. This process is not safe but still can be used accordingly.

2. *Thermal process* use heat to decontaminate or destroy medical waste. Most microorganisms are rapidly destroyed at temperature ranging from 120°F to 195°F and most living organisms are killed at 212°F. The basic thermal treatment processes are—Autoclave, Hydroclave, Incineration.

3. *Chemical process* is a chemical treatment, synonymous with chemical disinfection or simply disinfection. Most chemical waste treatment systems use a disinfectant solution in combination with shredding to provide decontamination and disfigurement. However, several systems feature strong chemical reactions which destroy or disintegrate the waste and a few use chemical polymers to encapsulate the waste. This treatment is recommended for waste sharps, solid and liquid waste, as well as chemical wastes. Chemical treatment involves use of atleast 1 percent hypochlorite solution with a minimum contact period of 30 minutes or other equivalent chemical reagents such as phenolic compound, iodine, hexachlorophene, iodine alcohol, or formaldehyde-alcohol, etc. Pre-shredding of the waste is desirable for better contact with the waste material.

4. *Irradiation process*: Irradiation is synonymous with electromagnetic or ionizing radiation. Currently, one vendor is developing a process utilizing *Cobalt 60* and another bendor is developing a system utilizing an electron beam accelerator unit or electron beam gun for irradiating and sterilizing the medical waste.

5. *Biological process*: In the conveyor transports waste to a shredder. The shredder residue is mixed with water and pumped as a slurry to a tank containing enzymes where biological reaction takes place. Treated residue is pumped from the tank through a screw press to separate solids. Solid residues are compacted and collected in a bin for disposal.

In addition to the above treatment, techniques required for sanitary and secured landfilling and nonhazardous and nontoxic may be taken care by composting and control recycling of packaging material.

Disposal

Biomedical waste can be disposed off in several ways as briefed in treatment. After the disposal treatment, the resultant residual waste may be deposited safely in a landfill designated for this purpose. The establishment requires provision for segregated for this purpose. The establishment requires provision for segregated storage (according to rules which can be packed in sealed containers/sturdy bags and handed over to the agency carrying them to the common treatment/disposal facility.

For more details on Biomedical waste management please refer Authors Text on "Community Health Nursing" revised second edition Jaypee Brother Medical Publication.

Nurses' Role and Responsibility in BMW

- Disinfect the waste so that it is no longer the source of pathogenic organisms.
- Reduce the bulk in order to reduce requirements for storage and transportation.
- Make waste unrecognizable for aesthetic reason.
- Make recyclable items unusable, e.g. cutting up syringes and damaging the needles.
- Recycling of infectious plastic wastes can be considered only after adequate disinfection/sterilization, e.g. glass, paper, corrugated cardboard, aluminium, X-ray film, reclaimed silver from X-ray film, plastics (non-infectious components).
- Disposable items like gloves, syringes, etc. should be mutilated after use to prevent illegal packing and reuse.
- Wastes minimization can be done by:
  Purchase of reusable items made of glass, rubber, metal, etc.
  Select non-PVC plastic.
  Strengthen sterilization procedure.
  Adopt proper procedure and policies of BMW.
  Establish effective sound recycling policy.
- There should be three types of container should be available at each point namely for general waste, infected non-sharp waste and infected sharp waste.
- Color coding of bags be done as per rules.
- Needles, syringes other sharp instruments and objects, should be placed in a puncture-resistant plastic/metal container at the work station.
- Needle syringes and such other should be boiled, hydroclaved/autoclave or chemically disinfected and then disposed.
- Alternatively, transport sharps to a central site for treatment, reused containers if at all only after cleaning and disinfecting.
- 40 percent needle prick injuries are due to resheathing, so do not recap.
- Reusable glass syringes and needles.
  - Aspirate hypochloric solution.
  - Immerse in flat tray for 20 minutes.
  - Rinse with water several times.
- Chemical disinfection prior to disposal is required for sharps, disposable infectious plastics/rubber, infectious glassware, blood and body fluids, by:
  - Using 1 percent hypochlorite or equivalent disinfectant. Proper concentration is essential.
  - Ensuring all surfaces come in contact with chemical (including luman).
  - Contacting time atleast 30 minutes.
  - Changing chemical solutions frequently atleast once a day.
  - Always handling with gloves and masks. Apron and boots to be used if splashing is expected.
  - Use sharp decontaminating unit made up of outer, solid plastic puncture proof and inner perforated container with handles and filled 1/3 with hypochlorite.
- Do not chemically treat incinerable waste.
- Use available chemical disinfectants as per rules.
- Clean air, clean bedding and hygienic method of dust removal by wet mopping of vacuum cleaning must be recognized as basic requirement of housekeeping.
- Mistakes in segregation are to be corrected by housekeeping or nursing staff.

Methods of Protection from BMW Hazard

Hand Protection: Waste treatment systems and waste handling can subject the hands to mechanical, chemical and biological hazards. For protection from minor abrasions and punctures, heavy-duty gloves made from leather or a suitable synthetic fabric are sufficient. For high temperature applications, aluminised reflective gloves and sleeves should be worn to reduce radiant heat transfer. Special care must be taken when removing gloves, since it is possible to contaminate skin and other body parts with the soiled exterior of the gloves.

Protective Clothing: Protective clothing like gloves and aprons, are designed as a barrier to reduce the likelihood of injury and infection. Most health care personnel do not wear aprons and work in ordinary clothes, thereby spreading infection to others and to themselves.

Foot Protection: Foot and toe protection is very essential for all activities that involve heavy objects and sharps. The hospital waste worker must wear gumboots to protect himself from needle prick and sharp injuries, which may lead to AIDS, hepatitis B and C, tetanus and other infections. The worker most affected is innocent and ignorant of the professional health hazards and possible accident.

Physical Exertion: Excessive exertion to muscles and joints must be avoided at all cost. Those workers not in good physical condition can suffer from fatigue and permanent injury. Excessive loading of the wheel barrow from the wards to the dumpsters must be discouraged. Proper lifting techniques must be used, i.e. keeping the object as close to the body as possible, lifting from knees and use of a mechanical aid when objects are routinely heavier 25 to 30 kg. Routine physical examination must be performed with special attention given to the back. In case of over exertion, medical advice must be sought after recovery, specially pertaining to rehabilitation.

The Biomedical Waste (BMW) rules that were first published in Gazette Notification on 27 July, 1998, have regrettably ignored the aspect of safety and training for the workers who handle biomedical waste. During the inspection of some large hospitals in the Capital following PIL by Mr Wadhera vs Government of India, it was found that the poor innocent waste handlers were charging the incinerator with bare feet and bare hands. There was no protective clothing or equipment being worn. The workers raw wounds on the feet, were fatigued and unaware of the hazards they were exposed to. On interrogation, the workers pointed to gumboots given to be and said that he felt uncomfortable wearing them. This is reason for shock and dismay and also points to the growing lacunae of occupational safety and health which has been totally disregarded, not just in the BMW rules but also in the administration of hospitals. The rules have been framed in a manner that speaks of total disregard to the safety of the biomedical waste handler. Clearly, the issue needs to be addressed more seriously and emphasis laid on training and awareness of safety among health care personnel.

Safety and Health Issues in a Nutshell

Personal protective clothing (PPC) and personal protective equipments (PPE) must be available to the staff and its usage ensured for safety as given below.

PPC

1. Gloves
    (a) Disposable vinyl gloves in all patient care areas.
    (b) Latex surgical gloves for operative procedures.
    (c) Heavy duty thick rubber gloves for waste handlers.
2. Masks: Simple, reusable plastic masks to protect health care workers from splashes.
3. Aprons: Full sleeved, knee length cotton aprons must be worn at all times.

PPE

1. Footwear: Gumboots for waste handlers. The trousers must remain outside the gumboots.
2. Eye shield.
3. Apron: A reusable heavy duty, autoclavable rubber apron may be worn where heavy contamination/excessive splashing is expected, e.g. in laborroom, operation theatre, etc.

General

1. Hand washing facility: Soap and water should be available at all time.
2. Drinking water: Safe drinking water must be available for waste handlers, working near boilers to prevent dehydration.
3. Immunization: Tetanus, hepatitis B.
4. Maintenance of health records.

Biomedical Waste (Management and Handling) Rules 1998

Ministry of Environment and Forests Notification
New Delhi, 20th July, 1998

S.O. 630 (E)-Whereas a notification in exercise of the powers conferred by Sections 6, 8 and 25 of the Environment (Protection) Act, 1986 (29 of 1986) was published in the Gazette vide S.O. 746 (E) dated 16 October, 1997 inviting objections from the public within 60 day's from the date of the publication of the said notification on the Biomedical Waste (Management and Handling) Rules, 1998 and whereas all objections received were duly considered.

Now, therefore, in exercise of the powers conferred by section 6,8 and 25 of the Environment (Protection) Act, 1986 the Central Government hereby notifies the rules for the management and handling of biomedical waste.

1. Short Title and Commencement
   - These rules may be called the Biomedical Waste (Management and Handling) Rules, 1998.
   - They shall come into force on the data of their publication in the official Gazette.
2. Application: These rules apply to all persons who generate, collect, receive, store, transport, treat, dispose, or handle biomedical waste in any form.
3. *Definitions*: In these rules unless the context otherwise requires:
   - "Act" means the Environment (Protection) Act, 1986 (29 of 1986);
   - "Animal House" means a place where animals are reared/kept for experiments or testing purposes;
   - "Authorization" means permission granted by the prescribed authority for the generation, collection, reception, storage, transportation, treatment, disposal and/or any other form of handling of bio-medical waste in accordance with these rules and any guidelines issued by the Central Government;
   - "Authorized person" means an occupier or operator authorised by the prescribed authority to generate, collect, receive, store, transport, treat, dispose and/or handle biomedical waste in accordance with these rules and any guidelines issued by the Central Government;
   - "Biomedical waste" means any waste, which is generated during the diagnosis, treatment or immunization of human beings or animals or in research activities pertaining thereto or in the production or testing of biologicals and including categories mentioned in Schedule 1;
   - "Biologicals" means any preparation made from organisms or microorganisms or product of metabolism and biochemical reactions intended for use in the diagnosis, immunization or the treatment of human beings or animals or in research activities pertaining thereto;
   - "Biomedical waste treatment facility" means any facility wherein treatment, disposal of biomedical waste or processes incidental to such treatment or disposal is carried out;
   - "Occupier" in relation to any institution generating biomedical waste , which includes a hospital, nursing home, clinic dispensary, veterinary institution, animal house, pathological laboratory, blood bank by whatever name called, means a person who has control over an institution and/or its premises;
   - "Operator of a biomedical waste facility" means a person who owns or controls or operates a facility for the collection, reception, storage, transport, treatment, disposal or any other form of handling of biomedical waste;
   - "Schedule" means schedules appended to these rules.

4. Duty of Occupier
   It shall be the duty of every occupier of an institution generating biomedical waste which includes a hospital, nursing home, clinic, dispensary, veterinary institution, animal house, pathological laboratory, blood bank by whatever name called to take all steps to ensure that such waste is handled without any adverse effect to human health and the environment.
5. Treatment and Disposal
   - Biomedical waste shall be treated and disposed of in accordance with Schedule 1, and in compliance with the standards prescribed in Schedule V.
   - Every occupier, where required, shall set up in accordance with the time-Schedule VI, requisite biomedical waste treatment facilities like incinerator, autoclave, microwave system for the treatment of waste or ensure requisite treatment of waste at common waste treatment facility or any other waste treatment facility.
6. Segregation, Packaging, Transportation and Storage
   - Biomedical waste shall not be mixed with other wastes.
   - Biomedical waste shall be segregated into containers/bags at the point of generation in accordance with Schedule II prior to its storage, transportation, treatment and disposal. The containers shall be labeled according to Schedule III.
   - If a container is transported from the premises where biomedical waste is generated to any waste treatment facility outside the premises, the container shall, apart from the label prescribed in Schedule III, also carry information prescribed in Schedule IV.
   - Notwithstanding anything contained in the Motor Vehicles Act, 1988, or rules hereunder, untreated biomedical waste shall be transported only in such vehicle as may be authorized for the purpose by the competent authority as specified by the Government.
   - No untreated biomedical waste shall be kept stored beyond a period of 48 hours.

     Provided that if for any reason it becomes necessary to store the waste beyond such period, the authorised person must take permission of the prescribed authority and take measures to ensure that the waste does not adversely affect human health and the environment.

7. Prescribed Authority
   - The Government of every State and Union Territory shall establish a prescribed authority with such members as may be specified for granting authorisation and implementing these rules. If the prescribed authority comprises of more than one member, a chairperson for the authority shall be designated.
   - The prescribed authority for the State or Union Territory shall be appointed within one month of the coming into force of these rules
   - The prescribed authority shall function under the supervision and control of the respective Government of the State or Union Territory.

- The prescribed authority shall, on receipt of Form 1, make such enquiry as it seems fit and if it is satisfied that the applicant possesses the necessary capacity to handle biomedical waste in accordance with these rules, grant or renew an authorisation as the case may be.
- An authorisation shall be granted for a period of three years, including an initial trial period of one year from the date of issue. Thereafter, an application shall be made by the occupier/operator for renewal. All such subsequent authorisation shall be for a period of three years. A provisional authorisation will be granted for the trial period, to enable the occupier/operator to demonstrate the capacity of the facility.
- The prescribed authority may after giving reasonable opportunity of being heard to the applicant and for reasons thereof to be recorded in writing, refuse to grant or renew authorisation.
- Every application for authorisation shall be deposed of by the prescribed authority within ninety days from the date of receipt of the application.
- The prescribed authority may cancel or suspend an authorisation, if for reasons, to be recorded in within, the occupier/operator has failed to comply with any provision of the Act or these rules.

  Provided that no authorisation shall be cancelled or suspended without giving a reasonable opportunity to the occupier/operator of being heard.

8. Authorisation
   - Every occupier of an institution generating, collecting, receiving, storing, transporting, treating, disposing and handling biomedical waste in any other manner, except such occupier of clinics, dispensaries, pathological laboratories, blood banks providing treatment/service to less than 1000 (one thousand) patients per month, shall make an application in Form 1 to the prescribed authority for grant authorization.
   - Every operator of a biomedical waste facility shall make an application in Form 1 to the prescribed authority for grant of authorization.
   - Every application in Form 1 for grant of authorization shall be accompanied by a fee as may be prescribed by the Government of the State or Union Territory.

9. Advisory Committee
   The Government of every State/Union Territory shall constitute an advisory committee. The committee will include experts in the field of medical and health, animal husbandry and veterinary science, environmental management, municipal administration and any other related department or organisation including nongovernmental organisations. The State Pollution Control Board/Pollution Control Committee shall be represented. As and when required, the committee shall advise the Government of the State/Union Territory and the prescribed authority about matters related to the implementation of these rules.

10. Annual Report
    Every occupier/operator shall submit an annual report to the prescribed authority in Form II by 31 January every year, to include information about the categories and quantities of biomedical wastes handled during the preceding year. The prescribed authority shall send this information in a compiled form to the Central Pollution Control Board by 31 March every year.

11. Maintenance of Records
    - Every authorised person shall maintain records related to the generation, collection, reception, storage, transportation, treatment, disposal and/or any form of handling of biomedical waste in accordance with these rules and any guidelines issued.
    - All records shall be subject to inspection and verification by the authority at any time.

12. Accident Reporting
    When any accident occurs at any institution or facility or any other site where biomedical waste is handled or during transportation of such waste, the authorised person shall report the accident in Form III to the prescribed authority forthwith.

13. Appeal
    Any person aggrieved by an order made the prescribed authority under these rules may, within days from the date on which the order is communicated to him, prefer an appeal to such authority as the Government of State/Union Territory may think fit to constitute:

    Provided that the authority may entertain the appeal after the expiry of the said period of thirty days, if it is satisfied that the appellant was prevented by sufficient cause from filing the appeal in time.

Standards for Waste Autoclaving

The autoclave should be dedicated for the purpose of disinfecting and treating biomedical waste,

1. When operating a gravity flow autoclave, medical waste shall be subjected:
   (i) A temperature of not less than 121°C and pressure of 15 pounds per square inch (psi) for an autoclave residence time of not less than 60 minutes; or
   (ii) A temperature of not less than 135°C and a pressure of 31 psi for an autoclave residence time of not less than 45 minutes; or
   (iii) A temperature of not less than 149°C and a pressure of 52 psi for an autoclave residence time of not less than 30 minutes; or

2. When operating a vacuum autoclave, medical waste shall be subjected to minimum of one prevacuum pulse to purge the autoclave of all air. The waste shall be subjected to the following:
   (i) A temperature of not less than 121°C and pressure of 15 psi per an autoclave residence time of not less than 45 minutes; or

SCHEDULE I
(See Rule 5)
CATEGORIES OF BIOMEDICAL WASTE

Option	Waste Category	Treatment and Disposal
Category No. 1	Human anatomical waste (human tissues, organs, body parts)	Incineration[2]/deep burial*
Category No. 2	Animal waste (animal tissues, organs, body parts, carcasses, bleeding parts, fluids, blood and experimental animals used in research, waste generated by veterinary hospitals, colleges, discharge from hospital, animal house)	Incineration[2]/deep burial
Category No. 3	Microbiology and biotechnology waste (waste from laboratory cultures, stocks or specimens of microorganisms live or attenuated, vaccines, human and animal cell culture used in research and infectious agents from research and industrial laboratories, waste from production of biologicals, toxins, dishes and devices used for transfer of cultures)	Local autoclaving/microwaving/ incineration[2]
Category No. 4	Waste sharps (needles, syringes, scalpels, blades, glass, etc. that may course puncture and cuts. This includes both used and unused sharps	Disinfection (chemical treatment @/ autoclaving/microwaving and mutilation/shredding)
Category No. 5	Discarded medicines and cytotoxic drugs (wastes comprising of outdated, contaminated and discarded medicines)	Incineration @ destruction and drugs disposal in secured landfills
Category No. 6	Solid waste (items contaminated with blood, and fluids including cotton, dressings, soiled plaster casts, liner, beddings, other material contaminated with blood)	Incineration @ autoclaving/ microwaving
Category No. 7	Solid waste (wastes generated from disposable items other than the waste sharps such as tubings, catheters, intravenous sets, etc.)	Disinfection by chemical treatment @@ autoclaving/microwaving and mutilation/shredding##
Category No. 8	Liquid waste (waste generated from laboratory and washing, cleaning, housekeeping and disinfecting activities)	Disinfection by chemical treatment @@ and discharge into drains
Category No. 9	Incineration ash (ash for incineration of any biomedical waste)	Disposal in municipal landfill
Category No. 10	Chemical used in production of biologicals, chemicals used in disinfection as insecticides, etc.	Chemical treatment @@ and discharge into drains for liquids and secured landfill for solids

@@ Chemicals treatment using atleast 1% hypochlorite solution or any other equipment chemical reagent. It must be ensured that chemical treatment ensures disinfection.

\#\# Mutilation/shredding must be such so as to prevent unauthorized reuse.

@ There will be no chemical pretreatment before incineration. Chlorinated plastics shall not be incinerated.

[2] Deep burial shall be an option available only in towns with population less than five lakhs and in rural areas.

SCHEDULE II
(See Rule 6)
COLOR CODING AND TYPE OF CONTAINER FOR DISPOSAL OF BIOMEDICAL WASTES

Color Coding	Type of Container	Waste Category	Treatment Options asper Schedule I
Yellow	Plastic bag	Cat.1, Cat.2, and Cat.3, Cat.6	Incineration/deep burial
Red	Disinfected container/ plastic bag	Cat.3, Cat.6, Cat.7	Autoclaving/microwaving/chemical treatment
Blue/white translucent	Plastic bag/puncture proof container	Cat.4, Cat.7	Autoclaving/microwaving/chemical Treatment and destruction /shredding
Black	Plastic bag	Cat.5 and Cat.9 and Cat.10 (solid)	Disposal in secured landfill

Notes:

1. Color coding of waste categories with multiple treatment options as defined in Schedule I, shall be selected depending on treatment option chosen, which shall be as specified in Schedule I

2. Waste collection bags for waste types needing incineration shall not be made of chlorinated plastics.

3. Categories 8 and 10 (liquid) do not require containers/bags.

4. Category 3 if disinfected locally need not be put in containers/bags.

SCHEDULE III
(See Rule 6)
LABEL FOR BIOMEDICAL WASTE CONTAINERS/BAGS

Biohazard Symbol   Cytotoxic Hazard Symbol

Biohazard   Cytotoxic

HANDLE WITH CARE

Note: Label shall be nonwashable and prominently visible.

SCHEDULE IV
(See Rule 6)
LABEL FOR TRANSPORT BIOMEDICAL WASTE CONTAINERS/BAGS

                                                              Day............. Month....................

                              Year..................

Waste category No......   Date of generation...............
Waste class
Waste description
Sender's Name & Address   Receiver's Name & Address
Phone No......   Phone No.....
Telex No.....   Telex No.....
Fax No.......   Fax No.......
Contact Person.......   Contact Person..............
In case of emergency please contact:
Name & Address:
Phone No.
Note: Label shall be nonwashable and prominently visible.

SCHEDULE V
(See Rule 5 and Schedule I)
STANDARDS FOR TREATMENT AND DISPOSAL OF BIOMEDICAL WASTES

Standards for Incinerators:

All incinerators shall meet the following operating and emission standards:

A. Operating Standards

1. Combustion efficiency (CE) shall be atleast 99.00%
2. The combustion efficiency is computed as follows:

$$CE = \frac{\%CO_2}{\%CO_2 + \%CO} \times 100$$

3. The temperature of the primary chamber shall be 800 + 50°C.
4. The secondary chamber gas residence time shall be atleast 1 (one) second at 1050 + 50°C, with minimum 3% oxygen in the stack gas

B. Emission Standards

Parameters	Concentration mg/Nm 3 at (12% CO_2 correction)
1. Particulate matter	150
2. Nitrogen oxides	450
3. HCl	50

4. Minimum stack height shall be 30 metres above ground
5. Volatile organic compounds in ash shall not be more than 0.01%

Note:

- Suitably designed pollution control devices should be installed/retrofitted with the incinerator to achieve the above emission limits, if necessary.
- Wastes to be incinerated shall not be chemically treated with any chlorinated disinfectants.
- Chlorinated plastics shall not be incinerated.
- Toxic metals in incineration ash shall be limited within the regulatory quantities as defined under the Hazardous Waste (Management and Handling Rules) 1989.
- Only low sulphur fuel like LDO/LSHS/Diesel shall be used as fuel in the incinerator.

(ii) A temperature of not less than 135°C and a pressure of 31 psi for an autoclave residence time of not less than 30 minutes;

3. Medical waste shall not be considered properly treated unless the time, temperature and pressure indicators indicate that the required time, temperature and pressure were reached during the autoclave process. If for any reasons, time, temperature or pressure indicator indicates that the required temperature, pressure or residence time was not reached, the entire load of medical waste must be autoclaved again until the proper temperature, pressure and residence time were achieved.
4. Recording of operational parameters:

   Each autoclave shall have graphic or computer recording devices which will automatically and continuously monitor and record dates, time of day, load identification number and operating parameters throughout the entire length of the autoclave cycle.
5. Validation test

   Spore testing

   The autoclave should completely and consistently kill the approved biological indicator at the maximum design capacity of each autoclave unit. Biological indicator for autoclave shall be *Bacillus stearothermophilus* spores using vials or spore strips, with atleast 1×10^4 spores per millilitre. Under no circumstances will an autoclave have minimum operating parameters less than a residence time of 30 minutes, regardless of temperature and pressure, a temperature less than 121°C or a pressure less than 15 psi.

6. Routine test

   A chemical indicator strip/tape that changes color when a certain temperature is reached can be used to verify that specific temperature has been achieved. It may be necessary to use more than one strip over the waste package at different location to ensure that the inner content of the package has been adequately autoclaved.

Standards for Liquid Waste

The effluent generated from the hospital should conform to the following limits:

Parameters	Permissible limits
pH	6.5-9.0
Suspended solids	100 mg/l
Oil and grease	10 mg/l
BOD	30 mg/l
COD	250 mg/l
Bioassay test	90% survival of fish after 96 hours in 100% effluent

These limits are applicable to those hospitals which are either connected with sewers without terminal sewage treatment plant or not connected to public sewers. For discharge into public sewers with terminal facilities, the general standards as notified under the Environment (Protection) Act, 1986, shall be applicable.

Standards of Microwaving

1. Microwave treatment shall not be used for cytotoxic, hazardous or radioactive wastes, contaminated animal carcasses, body parts and large metal items.
2. The microwave system shall comply with the efficacy test/routine tests and a performance guarantee may be provided by the supplier before operation of the unit.
3. The microwave should completely and consistently kill the bacteria and other pathogenic organisms that is ensured by approved biological indicator at the maximum design capacity or each microwave unit. Biological indicators for microwave shall be *Bacillus subtilis* spores using vials or spore strips with atleast 1×10^4 spores per milliliter.

Standards for Deep Burial

1. A pit or trench should be dug about 2 meters deep. It should be half filled with waste, than covered with lime within 50 cm of the surface, before filling the rest of the pit with soil.
2. It must be ensured that animals do not have any access to burial sites. Covers of galvanised iron/wire meshes may be used.
3. On each occasion, when wastes are added to the pit, a layer of 10 cm of soil shall be added to cover the wastes.
4. Burial must be performed under close and dedicated supervision.
5. The deep burial site should be relatively impermeable and no shallow well should be close to the site.
6. The pits should be distant from habitation, and sited so as to ensure that no contamination occurs of any surface water or groundwater. The area should not be prone to flooding or erosion.
7. The location of the deep burial site will be authorized by the prescribed authority.
8. The institution shall maintain a record of all pits for deep burial.

SCHEDULE VI
(See Rule 5)
STANDARDS FOR WASTE TREATMENT FACILITIES
LIKE INCINERATOR/AUTOCLAVE/MICROWAVE SYSTEM

A. Hospitals and nursing homes in towns with   by 31st December, 1999 or earlier
    population of 30 lakhs and above
B. Hospitals and nursing homes in towns
    with population of below 30 lakhs
    a. with 500 beds and above   by 31st December, 1999 or earlier
    b. with 200 beds and above but less than 500 beds   by 31st December, 2000 or earlier
    c. with 50 beds and above but less   by 31st December, 2001 or earlier
      than 200 beds
    d. with less than 50 beds   by 31st December, 2002 or earlier
C. All other institutions generating biomedical   by 31st December, 2002 or earlier
    waste not included in A and B above

FORM I
(See Rule 8)
APPLICATION FOR AUTHORISATION
(To be submitted in duplicate)

To
    The Prescribed Authority
    (Name of the State Govt/UT Administration)
    Address
1. Particulars of applicant:
    i.   Name of the applicant
       (In block letters and in full)
    ii. Name of the institution:
       Address:
       Tele. no., Fax no. Telex no.
2. Activity for which authorization is sought:
        i. Generation
       ii. Collection
       iii. Reception
       iv. Storage
        v. Transportation
       vi. Treatment
       vii. Disposal
       viii. Any other form of handling
3. Please state whether applying for fresh authorization or for renewal:
    (In case of renewal, previous authorisation number and date)
4. i. Address of the institution handling biomedical wastes:
    ii. Address of the place of the treatment facility:
    iii. Address of the place of the disposal of the waste:
5. i. Mode of transportation (in any) of biomedical waste:
    ii. Mode(s) of treatment:
6. Brief description of method of treatment and disposal (attach details):
7. i. Category (see Schedule 1) of waste to be handled:
    ii. Quantity of waste (category-wise) to be handled per month:
8. Declaration:

    I do hereby declare that the statements made and informations given above are true to the best of my knowledge and belief and that I have not concealed any information.

    I do also hereby undertake to provide any further information sought by the prescribed authority in relation to these rules and to fulfill any conditions stipulated by the prescribed authority.

Date: Signature of the applicant

Place: Designation of the applicant

FORM II

(See Rule 10)

ANNUAL REPORT

(To be submitted to the prescribed authority by 31 January every year)

1. Particulars of the applicant:
   - i. Name of the authorized person (occupier/operator):
   - ii. Name of the institution:
     - Address
     - Tel. No.
     - Telex No.
     - Fax No.
2. Categories of waste generated and quantity on a monthly average basis:
3. Brief details of the treatment facility:
   In case of off-site facility
   - i. Name of the operator:
   - ii. Name and address of the facility:
   - iii. Name and address of the facility:
     - Tel. No., Telex No., Fax No.
4. Category-wise quantity of waste treated:
5. Mode of treatment with details:
6. Any other information:
7. Certified that the above report is for the period from

Date:..................................   Signature.........................

Place:.................................   Designation.....................

FORM III

(See Rule 12)

ACCIDENT REPORTING

1. Date and time of accident:
2. Sequence of events leading to accident:
3. The waste involved in accident:
4. Assessment of the effects of the accident on human health and the environment:
5. Emergency measures taken:
6. Steps taken to alleviate the effects of the accident:
7. Steps taken to prevent the recurrence of such an accident:

Date:..................................   Signature.........................

23

Role of Nurses in Diagnostic Examination

Introduction

Diagnostic tests are either noninvasive or invasive. **Noninvasive** means that the body is not entered with any type of instrument; the skin and other body tissues, organs, and cavities remain intact. **Invasive** means that the body's tissues, organs, or cavities are accessed through some type of instrument.

Information from a thorough history and physical examination determines the need for diagnostic testing. Results of diagnostic procedures are used to formulate a medical diagnosis and plan a course of treatment. The challenge of cost-effective health care encourages practitioners to rely on basic assessment and to be selective about expensive diagnostic tests. The emphasis on cost containment has changed the nurse's role from doing for the client to teaching clients to do for themselves. The nurse teachers the client, family, and significant others about the diagnostic testing, how to prepare for the specific test(s), and the care required after the test. Although the primary focus is on teaching, the nurse may assist in performing various diagnostic tests. To deliver appropriate care to the client, nurses must known the implications of diagnostic tests and must know anatomy and physiology to understand the nature of diagnostic tests. Nurses can then relate diagnostic tests to specific disease processes and understand the test results.

Diagnostic testing is a critical element of assessment. In collaboration with the client, assessment data are used to formulate nursing diagnoses, outcome measures, and a plan of care. Evaluation of the client's expected outcomes requires the incorporation of diagnostic findings.

Preparing the Client for Diagnostic Testing

The nurse plays a key role in scheduling and preparing the client for diagnostic testing. Tests not scheduled correctly inconvenience the client and delay interventions, which may place the client's health at risk. The institution is also at risk to lose money. Ensure that the client is wearing an identification band and understands those things to be done. Also see that needed consent forms have been signed.

Nursing measures to ensure client safety are establish baseline vital signs, identify known allergies, and assess teaching effectiveness. In ambulatory and outpatient centers, there might be only one opportunity to assess and record vital signs. It is important to confirm that the vital signs are normal values *for the client.* Compare the vital signs taken during and after the procedure to those obtained before as baseline data to accurately assess the client's response to anesthetic agents and the procedure performed. Advise the client of those things to expect during the procedure. Such teaching can both increase the level of cooperation and decrease the degree of anxiety. The client's family should also be informed of what will happen during the procedure and approximately how long the procedure should last. Know the facility's specific protocols and procedures, because these are not standardized.

The purpose of preparing the client for diagnosing testing is to increase the reliability of the test by providing client teaching on the reason the test is being performed, those things the client can expect during the test, and the outcomes and side effects of the test to decrease the client's anxiety about the test and the associated risks Increase the client's knowledge, thereby promoting cooperation and enhancing the quality of the testing decrease the time required to perform the tests, thereby increasing cost effectiveness Prevent delays by ensuring proper physical preparation

During preparation nurse has to assess the client as follows:

- Ensure that the client is wearing an identification band
- Review the medical record for allergies and previous adverse reactions to dyes and other contrast media; a signed consent form; and the recorded findings of diagnostic tests relative to the procedure
- Assess for the presence location, and characteristics of physical and communicative limitations or pre-existing conditions
- Monitor the client's knowledge of the reasons for the test and things to expect during and after testing
- Monitor vital signs, including pain, of the client scheduled for invasive testing, to establish baseline data
- Assess client outcome measures relative to the practitioner's preferences for preprocedure preparations
- Monitor level of hydration and weakness for clients who are designated nothing by mouth (NPO)

After an assessment nurses has to:

- Notify physician of allergy, previous adverse reaction, or suspected adverse reaction following the administration of drugs
- Notify physician of any client or family concerns not alleviated by discussions with nurse and take following interventions and evaluative measures is given below:
- Clarify with practitioner whether regularly scheduled medications are to be administered
- Implement NPO status, as determined by the type of test
- Administer cathartics or laxatives as noted on the test's protocol; instruct clients who are weak to call for assistance to the bathroom
- Teach relaxation techniques, such as deep breathing and imagery
- Establish intravenous (IV) access if necessary for the procedure

And then

- Evaluate the client's knowledge of those things to expect
- Evaluate the client's anxiety level
- Evaluate the client's level of safety and comfort

Further, nurses has the responsibilities of client teaching, including: discuss the following with the client and family, as appropriate to the specific test:

- The reason for the test and those things to expect
- An estimate of how long the test will take

- Specifics of NPO status, including amount of water to drink if oral medication is to be taken
- Cathartics or laxative: amount, frequency
- Sputum: cough deeply, do not clear throat
- Urine: voided, clean-catch specimen; timing of collection
- Removal of objects (e.g.,) jewellery or hair clips) that will obscure X-ray film
- Contrast medium:
  - Barium: taste, consistency, after-effects (lightly colored stools for 24 to 72 hours; possibly, obstruction/impaction)
  - Iodine: metallic taste, delayed allergic reaction (itching, rashes, hives, wheezing and breathing difficulties)
- Positioning during the test
- Positioning posttest (e.g., immobilize limb after angiography)
- Posttest (encourage fluid intake if not contraindicated)

And perform documentation by record in the clients medical record:

- Practitioner notification of allergies or suspected adverse reaction to contrast media
- Presence, location, and characteristics of symptoms
- Teaching and the client's response to teaching
- Responses to interventions (client outcomes)

Care of the Client during Diagnostic Testing

Client care must be individualized according to the specific procedure, general guidelines for client care during a procedure are outlined in Table 23.2. Protocols are used to assist with client care.

Standard Precautions are used when possible exposure to body fluids may occur. Protective barriers, such as gown, gloves, and goggles, should be used during invasive procedures. Label all specimens with the client's name and room number (for hospitalized clients) and the date, time, and specimen source. Some specimens may need to be taken immediately to the laboratory or placed on ice (e.g., arterial blood gases [ABGs]).

Ongoing assessment of the client is required during any procedure. The patency of the client's airway should be continuously assessed, because it may be compromised by the client's position, by anesthesia, or by the procedure itself. During an invasive procedure, monitor for signs and symptoms of accidental perforation of an organ (e.g., sudden changes in vital signs).

The nurse has the following additional responsibilities:

- Prepare the procedure room (e.g., ensure adequate lighting).
- Gather and charge for supplies to be used during the procedure.
- Test the equipment to ensure it is functional and safe.
- Secure proper containers for specimen collection.

Physicians usually have preference cards within the diagnostic testing area that specify the type of equipment to be used, the position in which to place the client, and the type of sedative or anesthestic agent to be used. Some diagnostic tests are performed with the RN administering IV sedation, also called procedural

sedation. **Procedural sedation** is a minimally depressed level of consciousness during which the client retains the ability to maintain a continuously patent airway and respond appropriately to physical stimulation or verbal commands. The nurse managing procedural sedation functions in an expanded role that requires additional education and demonstrated ability beyond the basic education.

The purpose of care during testing into: to increase cooperation and participation by allaying the client's anxiety and to provide the maximum level of safety and comfort during a procedure

This care which helps to:

- Encourage relaxation of the muscles and thus facilitate instrumentation by increasing the client's participation and comfort
- Ensure efficient use of time during the test and reliable results from the test with proper client preparation

During diagnostic testing nurse has to assess the following:

- Check the client's identification band to ensure the correct client
- Review the medical record for allergies
- Assess the client's reaction to the preprocedure sedatives administered prior to the induction of anesthesia during the procedure
- Assess airway maintenance and gag reflex, if a local anesthetic is sprayed into the client's throat
- Assess vital signs, including pain, throughout the procedure and compare to baseline data
- Assess the client's ability to maintain and tolerate the prescribed position
- Assess the client's comfort level (pain) to ensure the effectiveness of the anesthetic agent
- Assess for related symptoms indicating complications specific to the procedure (e.g., accidental perforation of an organ)

Assessment report should be informed to the physician or practitioner

- Notify the physician of any client concerns or questions not answered in discussions with the nurse
- Notify the practitioner of any family members present and their location during the procedure
- Notify the practitioner when the client is positioned properly and the anesthetic agent has been administered to the client

And take following interventions and evaluation measure

- Institute Standard Precautions or appropriate aseptic technique for the specific test
- Report to all personnel involved in the test any known client allergies
- Place the client in the correct position, drape, and monitor to ensure that breathing is not compromised
- Remain with the client during induction and maintenance of anesthesia
- If the procedure requires the administration of a dye, ensure that the client is not allergic to the dye; if the client has not received the dye before, perform the skin allergy test according to the manufacturer's instructions that accompany the medication

- Monitor the client's airway and keep resuscitative equipment available
- Assist the client to relax during insertion of the instrument by telling the client to breathe through the mouth and to concentrate on relaxing the involved muscles
- Explain what the practitioner is doing so that the client knows what to expect
- Label and handle the specimen according to the type of materials obtained and the testing to be done
- Report to the practitioner any symptoms of complications
- Secure client transport from the diagnostic area
  Posttest in the diagnostic area:
- Assist the client to a comfortable, safe position
- Provide oral hygiene and water to clients who were designated NPO for the test, if they are alert and able to swallow
- Remain with the client awaiting transport to another area
  And
- Evaluate the client's ventilatory status and tolerance to the procedure
- Evaluate the client's need for assistance
- Evaluate the clients understanding of what was performed during the procedure
- Evaluate the client's understanding of findings identified during the procedure
- Evaluate the client's knowledge of what to expect after the procedure
  Further, do the following clinical teaching

Discuss the following with the client and family, as appropriate to the specific test:

- Those things that occurred during the procedure
- Questions and concerns of the client or family member
- Those things to expect during the immediate recovery phase
- Those things to report to the nurse during the immediate recovery phase

And document the details of test by recording the client's medical record as the information as given below:

- Person who performed the procedure
- Reason for the procedure
- Type of anesthestic, dye, or other medications administered
- Type of specimen obtained and where it was sent
- Vital signs and other assessment data such as client's tolerance of the procedure or pain/discomfort level
- Any symptoms of complications
- Person who transported the client to another area (designate the names of persons who provided transport and the destination)

Care of the Client after Diagnostic Testing

Postprocedure nursing care is directed toward restoring the client's prediagnostic level of functioning. Nursing assessment and interventions are based mainly on the nature of the test and whether the client received anesthesia. The client is closely monitored for signs of respiratory distress and bleeding. Some diagnostic tests require vital signs measurement every 15 minutes for the first hour, and then at gradually longer intervals until the client is **stable** (alert and with vital signs within the client's normal range).

Some diagnostic tests use medications that are excreted through the kidneys. The client's intake and output (I&O) is monitored for 24 hours. The client is taught to monitor I&O and to report **hematuria** (presence of blood in the urine). Clients should receive written instructions when discharged after diagnostic testing. Most agencies have discharge forms on which teaching regarding medications, dietary and activity restrictions, and signs and symptoms to be reported immediately to the practitioner are documented.

The purpose of care after diagnosis testing is to restore the client's prediagnostic level of functioning by providing care and teaching relative to both those things the client can expect after a test and the outcomes o side effects of the test.

It helps to decrease client anxiety by increasing the client's participation and knowledge of expected outcome measures after a diagnostic test. Through proper postprocedure care and client teaching, alert the client to those signs and symptoms that must be reported to the practitioner

After diagnostic testing nurse has to assess the following

- Check the identification band and call the client by name
- Assess the client closely for signs of airway distress, adverse reactions to anesthestic or other medications, and other signs that may indicate accidental perforation of an organ
- Assess for bleeding in those areas where a biopsy was performed
- Assess the client's vital signs, including pain
- Assess vascular access lines or other invasive monitoring devices
- Assess the client's ability to expel air, if air was instilled during a gastrointestinal test
- Assess the client's knowledge of those things to expect during the recovery phase
- And notify the physician of any signs of respiratory distress, bleeding, or changes in vital signs; adverse reactions to anesthestic, sedative, or dye; and other signs of complications
- Notify the physician of client or family concerns or questions not answered in discussions with the nurse
- Notify the physician when any results are obtained from the diagnostic test
- Notify the physician when the client is fully alert and recovered (for an order to discharge)
  And take following interventions and evaluation measure
- Implement the physician orders regarding the postprocedure care of the client
- Institute standard precautions or surgical asepsis as appropriate to the client's care needs
- Position the client for comfort and accessibility so as to facilitate performance of nursing measures
- Monitor vital signs according to the frequency required for the specific test
- Observe the insertion site for hematoma or blood loss; replace pressure dressing, as needed

- Monitor the client's urinary output and drainage from other devices
- Enforce activity restrictions appropriate to the test
- Schedule client appointments as directed by the physician and
- Evaluate the client's respiratory status, especially if an anesthetic agent was used
- Evaluate the client's tolerance of oral liquids
- Evaluate the client's understanding of the procedural findings of when the physician expects to receive written results
- Evaluate the client's knowledge of those things to expect after discharge

Further based on client assessment and evaluation of knowledge, teach the client or family about the following:

- Dietary or activity restrictions
- Signs and symptoms that should be reported immediately to the practitioner
- Medications

And document the event as follows including

Record in the client's medical record on the appropriate forms: Assessment data, nursing interventions, and achievement of expected outcomes, Client or family teaching and demonstrated level of understanding. Written instructions given to the client or family members.

Specimen Collection

The nurse is directly responsible for ensuring that specimens are accurately obtained, properly labeled in appropriate container and transported to the laboratory on time for diagnostic purposes. Institutions provide special containers for particular specimen. Some tests require specimens to be placed in chemical preservatives.

While collecting any specimen for diagnostic purposes, nurses have to take certain precautions to protect themselves and others, because certain pathogenic microorganisms can be found in the blood and other body fluids of infected individuals. These pathogens can be transmitted to uninfected individuals from infected ones. All blood and potentially infected materials are to be considered infectious irrespective of perceived status of the source of client. The following precautions should be taken particularly when collecting blood, body fluids and tissues, which include tissues, semen, vaginal secretions, cerebrospinal fluid, synovial fluid, pleural fluid, pericardial fluid, and amniotic fluid.

Precautions in Collection of Specimen

- Wash hands before and after contact with any client whether gloves are worn or not
- Wash hands before and after a procedure performed whether gloves are worn or not
- Always wear gloves when obtaining, handling or testing specimen (body fluids, excretions, secretions) or touching any item or article exposed to substances with contaminated potential

- Change gloves between clients or when soiled or torn
- Wash hands or any skin or mucous membrane area immediately following contact with blood, body fluids, or any potentially infective material; flush with water or wash with soap and water as soon as feasible following the contact
- Gloves are not to be washed or decontaminated for reuse
- Anticipate the kind of client and use appropriate personal protective device
- Anticipate splashing of blood or body fluids, and attempt to eliminate or minimize spills or splashes
- Wear disposable gown, apron or lab coat when in contact or potentially in contact with blood or other infectious materials
- Wear mask, eye protection (goggles with solid side shield), or chin-length face shield, as indicated, to protect skin, eyes and mouth from contact with splashes, sprays, splattering, or droplets of potentially infected body fluids
- All garments contaminated by blood should be removed and disposed properly prior to leaving work
- Wearing apparel that is contaminated with blood and body fluids should be placed in a waterproof labeled bag in a designated area
- Know the limitation of the personal protective equipment being used, when it can protect and when it cannot
- Contaminated needles and other sharps should not be bent, recapped removed, sheared or purposely broken
- Discard used disposable needles, syringes and other sharps in puncture and leak proof containers marked with a biohazard label; the articles should be discarded as soon as feasible following use
- Discard reusable sharps in a color-coded, labeled container for decontamination
- Replace containers when they are three-quarters full, close the full container and place in a designated area/proper place
- Always use disposable supplies to collect specimen when possible
- Avoid accidental sticks form needles when obtaining blood samples
- Mouth pipetting of blood and other potentially reflective materials is prohibited
- Specimens of blood and other potentially infected materials should be placed in a container and then in a biohazard bag that prevents leakage during, the collection, handling, processing storage and transport of the specimens
- Container should be labeled or color-coded. If the outside container is contaminated, it should be placed in a secondary container that is puncture-resistant.
- Specimens that are to be transport outside, the facilities are to be labeled with a biohazard sticker on container
- All microbiologic wastes such as culture and stocks of etiologic agents must be steam-sterilized in the laboratory prior to transport
- All anatomic pathology wastes are placed in a color-coded bag or lined box prior to transport by housekeeping
- All blood product containers are placed in a bag within a biohazard-labeled container

- Cleanse any spills of body fluids during collection or handling by wiping with paper toweling first, then washing with soap and water and washing with a disinfectant solution.

Please note that above precautions will not be applicable to all specimens related to feces, nasal secretions, breast milk, sputum, sweat, tears, urine and vomitus unless they contain visible blood and also do not apply to saliva except in dentistry.

The special points to remember while collecting specimens in general are as follows:

- Always remember five rights, i.e., right patient to be selected to collect right specimen through right method at right time and placed in right container, tested at right time or sent to right laboratory or place at right time
- The patient should be intimated well in advance regarding the procedure and sample of specimen
- Prepare the client according to the specimen required
- Make sure that appropriate specimens containers, clean or sterile are used
- Label the containers clearly indicating patient's name, unit number, name of the specimen, date and ward unit, bed number
- Prevent contamination of specimens. Use aseptic technique to obtain a sterile specimen
- Avoid tilting of test tubes, to prevent wetting the cotton plug.

Procedures for Assisting Diagnostic Examinations

In recent years, many laboratory and diagnostic tests are performed and the nurse must be aware of all aspects of the effect on the patients even though other personnel may be doing the procedure. The nurse must know how to prepare the patient for each test, the appropriate requisition form to complete and where it must be sent, the side effects to each test, nursing measures to perform, how to interpret each test, in order to notify the doctor, what the patient will endure during test, the follow-up care and how to document the tests. For certain tests, informed consent must be obtained from the patient by the nurses. The nurse prepares the patient for test for following purposes (Table 23.1).

- To ensure the patient is ready for the test to be performed
- To avoid prolonging hospital stay because of inadequate test program.

First, the nurses should understand their roles in preparation of patients for diagnostic examinations. The nurses' roles in this respect are enlisted in Table 23.2.

Urine Analysis

Urine Analysis: Urinalysis assists in the diagnosis of various conditions. Substances not normally found in the urine include RBCs, white blood cells (WBCs), protein, glucose, ketones, and casts. Test often performed on a urine specimen are found in Table 23.17.

Urine pH: The hydrogen ion concentration in the urine determines the pH. Diabetes mellitus, diarrhea, dehydration, emphysema, and starvation make the urine acidic. Urinary tract infections, chronic renal failure, renal tubular acidosis, and salicylate poisoning make the urine alkaline.

Specific Gravity: Specific gravity measures the number of solutes in a solution. Urea and uric acid, by-products of nitrogen metabolism, are the greatest influence on urine specific gravity. Specific gravity increases with excess fluid loss from the body. Renal disease decreases specific gravity.

Urine Glucose: Glucose spills into the urine when the blood level of glucose exceeds the renal threshold (180 mg/dL). Measuring urine glucose is not as accurate as measuring the blood glucose level.

Urine Ketones: Products of incomplete fat metabolism, are completely metabolized by the liver under normal conditions.

Table 23.1: Procedure of Preparing Patient for Diagnostic Examination

	Nursing actions		*Rationales*
1.	Read physician's order.	1.	Provides basis for care.
2.	Collect supplies.	2.	Organizes procedure.
3.	Introduce self.	3.	Decreases anxiety level.
4.	Identify the patient by identification band.	4.	Identifies right patient for procedure.
5.	Explain procedure to the patient.	5.	Seeks cooperation and decreases anxiety.
6.	Wash hands, and don clean gloves.	6.	Helps prevent cross-contamination.
7.	Assist physician with procedure.	7.	Provides help to physician while providing support to patients.
8.	Answer questions from patient.	8.	Provides security and emotional support to patient.
9.	Ensure delivery of specimens to lab, when applicable.	9.	Ensures accuracy of appropriate specimen.
10.	Document.	10.	Document procedure and patient response for documentation.

Table 23.2: Nurses' Responsibilities in Preparation of Patient for Diagnostic Examinations

Examination	Before examination	After examination
Urinalysis	Prepare requisition form Explain purpose and specific method of urine collection Wash perineal area, if soiled If patient is menstruating, note this on requisition form	Report results
CBC	Prepare requisition form Explain procedure	Observe site for bleeding Report result
Blood chemistries	Prepare requisition form NPO or hold meal Explain procedure Smoking may be prohibited	Observe site for bleeding Be certain patient's meal is served after test is completed Report results
Glucose tolerance	Prepare requisition slip Explain procedure NPO—encourage H_2O intake so patient can provide urine samples Obtain urine samples at designated times Blood and urine specimen will be collected at the same time The procedure will be as follows: 1. Make certain the patient empties his bladder and 30 minutes later obtain a fasting UA 2. Laboratory will administer 75 grams of dextrose orally 3. The nurse will collect urine specimen ½ hour, 1 hour, 1 ½ hours, 2 ½ hours, 3 ½ hours, up to 5 hours after dextrose, depending on the physician's order	Observe venipuncture site for bleeding Make certain patient received meal when test is completed Report results: An elevated blood glucose level at the 2-hour point usually indicates some disorder of carbohydrate metabolism; depending on the elevation of the blood glucose, there may be glucose present in the urine
Lumbar puncture	Explain before procedure and after procedure routine Obtain written consent Bladder and bowel should be empty if possible Provide necessary equipment Assist patient to assume appropriate position The nurse may be asked to hold manometer straight Label and number specimens	Keep patient flat after procedure Observe patient for mobility of extremities, pain, drainage, and ability to void Notify physician if any unusual occurrences Report results
Chest X-ray	Prepare requisition form Explain procedure Be certain there are no snaps or pins on gown	Report results
Bone scan	Prepare requisition form Explain procedure Instruct patient to remove jewellery or any metal objects Encourage patient to drink several glasses of water Patient should void before examination	Observe injection site for erythema or edema; if hematoma forms, apply warm soaks to the area to relieve pain
Ultrasound/sonogram	Most of these procedures require little preparation Prepare requisition form Explain procedure If a pelvic sonogram is ordered, the patient needs a full bladder If a gallbladder sonogram is ordered, the patient needs to be NPO Signed consent form may be required	Because this procedure is noninvasive no specific follow-up care is needed Usual diet may be resumed after examination

Contd...

Table 23.2: *Contd...*

Examination	Before Examination	After Examination
Bronchoscopy	Prepare requisition form Explain procedure Obtain in informed consent before patient is premedicated Patient is NPO after midnight Administer preoperative mediation is ordered Remove and safely store contact lenses, dentures, glasses Reassure patient	Do not allow patient to eat or drink after procedure until the effect of anesthesia no longer exists and gag reflex has returned-usually about 2 hours Observe any sputum for blood Monitor vital signs frequently, fever is normal within the first 24 hours after bronchoscopy Observe for impaired respirations Observe closely until effects of anesthesia no longer exist If patient complains of sore throat, warm saline gargles and lozenges may be ordered
Myelogram	NPO for 4 hours before examination Explain procedure Obtain written consent	Proper positioning will be prescribed by the physician Observe the patient for fever, stiff neck, occipital headache, or photo phobia Monitor vital signs Monitor ability to void Encourage fluids so patient does not get dehydrated; this will result in a severe headache
Mammography	Prepare requisition form Explain procedure If patient is embarrassed by the procedure, ask patient to verbalize her feelings Provide emotional support. Instruct patient not to wear deodorant, powder, or lotion	Explain how test results can be obtained
Brain scan	Explain procedure Keep patient NPO for 4 hours before examination Instruct patient not to wear wig, hairpins, or clips Observe patient for iodine allergies If ordered, give sedation	No special care required after procedure Encourage fluid intake
Body scan	Prepare requisition form Explain procedure No specific preparation	No specific follow-up care
Abdominal scan	Prepare requisition form Explain procedure Patient is NPO for 4 hours before examination	No specific follow-up care
Lung scan	Prepare requisition form Explain procedure Patient is NPO for 4 hours before examination Observe the patient for allergies to iodine	No specific follow-up care Encourage fluid intake
Endoscopy and gastorscopy	Prepare requisition form Administer pre-examination medication if ordered Explain procedure Obtain written consent	Perform oral hygiene measures Do not allow food or drink until the gag reflex returns (2-4 hours) Explain that drinking cool fluids and gargling will help relieve some soreness
Eye piece	Keep patient NPO after midnight Provide emotional support Remove patient's dentures and eye glasses Perform oral hygiene measures	Observe the patient for bleeding, fever, abdominal pain, dysphagia, and dyspnea Monitor vital signs Observe safety precautions until the effects of the sedatives no longer exist

Contd...

Table 23.2: *Contd...*		
Examination	*Before Examination*	*After Examination*
Colonoscopy	Prepare requisition form Explain procedure Obtain written consent Assist with the bowel preparation Record the results from the cathartics and enemas	Observe the patient for abdominal pain, tenderness, and bleeding Examine stools for gross blood Encourage fluids Offer normal diet A warm bath may be soothing Allow time for rest Take safety precautions until the effects of the medication no longer exist
Proctoscopy and sigmoidoscopy	Prepare requisition form Explain procedure Provide emotional support Obtain written consent Patient is allowed a light breakfast on day of examination Administer enemas as ordered, and record results	Observe the patient for fever, bleeding, abdominal distention, and unusual complaints of pain
Cystoscopy	Explain procedure Obtain written consent Administer enemas as ordered, and record results If patient will be under local anesthesia, a liquid breakfast may be allowed If patient will be under general anesthesia, keep patient NPO Administer preprocedure medications as ordered	Assess patient's ability to void for at least 24 hours after procedure Record urine color-if bright red, report to physician Warm sitz baths may be soothing Encourage fluid intake Observe vital signs Observe for hemorrhage and for sepsis Administer antibiotic as ordered Observe for anaphylaxis (respiratory distress, shock, and drop in blood pressure)
Intravenous pyelogram	Prepare requisition form Be certain IVP is done before barium X-rays are performed Explain procedure Check for allergies to iodine, since the intravenous dye usually contains iodine Administer cathartics or laxatives as ordered (children and infants are not given cathartics or laxatives) Keep patient NPO after midnight (if an intravenous solution is infusing, ask physician if he wishes to decrease IV to a keep-open-rate to prevent hydration: in an IVP the patient needs to have fluid restricted for the dye to be taken up by the kidney)	Allow patient to have normal diet Encourage fluid intake to help eliminate any dye left in body Assess for weakness Encourage to ambulate with assistance unless contraindicated
Electrocardiogram	Prepare requisition form Explain procedure	Remove gel from patient's skin with a tissue
Arteriogram	Explain procedure	Keep patient at bed rest for 8 hours
Femoral angiogram	Provide emotional support Observe patient for allergies to iodine dye Obtain written consent Keep patient NPO after midnight	Observe catheter insertion site for inflammation, hemorrhage, hematoma at the site, or absence of peripheral pulses Observe the involved extremity for numbness, tingling, pain, or loss of function Monitor vital signs Cold compresses to the puncture site may reduce discomfort and edema If patient complains of continuous, severe pain, notify physician

Contd...

Table 23.2: *Contd...*

Examination	Before Examination	After Examination
Endocardiogram	Prepare requisition form Explain procedure Answer questions	Remove the gel from the patient's chest with a tissue
Electroencephalogram	Prepare requisition form Explain procedure Hair should be clean; administer shampoo as necessary Confer with physician if any medications should be discontinued before examination Administer sedatives or hypnotics as ordered Encourage food intake but eliminate coffee, tea, and colas	Assist the patient to remove the electrode paste Shampoo hair Ensure safety precautions until effects of the sedatives no longer exist
Renal angiography	Explain procedure Answer questions Obtain written consent Assess patient for allergy to iodine dye Keep patient NPO after midnight Administer cathartics as ordered Administer preprocedure medications	Observe arterial puncture site frequently Monitor the extremity for adequate circulation Monitor pedal pulses and vital signs frequently Keep patient on bed rest for 12-24 hours Cold compresses to puncture site will help to reduce discomfort and edema Encourage fluids
Amniocentesis	Explain procedure Encourage verbalization Obtain written consent Monitor fetal heart tones	Monitor fetal heart tones If patient complains of vertigo, allow her to rest on her left side for several minutes before leaving examination room If patient has any fluid loss or temperature elevation, instruct her to notify her physician Inform patient to contact her physician to obtain results
Thoracentesis	Explain procedure Obtain written consent Obtain equipment Assist patient to assume the appropriate position (usually sitting) Offer emotional support	Monitor patient for coughing or for hemoptysis Monitor patient for complications notify physician if any unusual signs and symptoms occur Monitor patient's lung sounds If no complaints of dyspnea, normal activity can be resumed in an hour
Paracentesis	Explain procedure Obtain written consent Provide emotional support Obtain equipment Assist physician	Send specimen to laboratory for examination if requested Observe puncture site Observe for syncope Monitor vital signs Encourage a period of rest after examination Send specimen to laboratory for examination if requested
Upper gastrointestinal series	Prepare requisition form Explain procedure Answer questions Offer emotional support Keep patient NPO after midnight	Patient may eat as soon as series is completed unless contraindicated Encourage fluids Monitor stools Administer milk of magnesia, 2 oz, as per hospital protocol
Barium Enema	Prepare requisition form Explain procedure Provide needed emotional support Assist with required preparation – monitor Effecting cathartics and/or enemas Patient in NPO after midnight Some physicians allow liquids for breakfast	Patient may resume regular diet as soon as examination is completed Monitor stools—barium may cause constipation A local anesthetic ointment may be ordered after examination to relieve anal discomfort A warm bath may be soothing Administer milk of magnesia, 2 oz, after

Contd...

	Table 23.2: *Contd...*	
Examination	*Before Examination*	*After Examination*
		examination as per hospital protocol Allow time for rest
Gallbladder series	Prepare requisition form	Monitor patient for side effects to the tablets
Cholecystogram	Explain procedure A fat-free meal is allowed the evening before examination Assess patient for allergy to iodine Administer the iopanoic acid tablets (Telepaque) as ordered the day before the examination – usually early evening A number of tablets are ordered; the tablets should not be crushed and should be taken one at a time, waiting 15 minutes between each tablet	Usual diet may be resumed as soon as series is completed
Bone marrow aspiration	Prepare requisition form Explain procedure Obtain written consent Assist in obtaining specimens Provide needed emotional support	Observe the puncture site for bleeding Monitor patient for signs and symptoms of shock Patient may assume normal activity 30-60 minutes after examination Mild analgesics may be needed for complains of tenderness at the puncture site Explain procedure. No specific follow-up care
Hematest of stools	Assist patient in obtaining specimens Document specimens as sent to laboratory	Read results
Liver biopsy	Explain procedure Obtain written consent NPO before examination Assist physician Send specimens to laboratory promptly Have specimen placed in proper fixative; usually 10% formalin is used but the nurse must consult with the laboratory or pathologist. If the liver specimen is for detection of lymphoma saline solution is used	Keep patient at bed rest for 24 hours Observe for hemorrhage Monitor vital signs Observe biopsy site
Cardiac catheterization	Explain procedure Obtain written consent Provide needed emotional support NPO for 6-8 hours Determine if any dye allergies Administer pre-examination medications as ordered	Monitor vital signs Observe catheter site for bleeding Monitor pedal pulses for adequate circulation Encourage rest Encourage fluids
Lactose tolerance test	Explain procedure Patient will be NPO until after the test except for water Hold medications Instruct patient not to smoke Instruct patient to wear suitable clothing	Diet as usual Resume medication regime Patient to rest several hours after examination and is not to shower immediately after examination

The most common cause of ketonuria (excessive ketones in the urine) is diabetes.

Urine Cells and Casts: The urine is normally free of blood cells and casts. In cases of nephritis, renal damage or failure, and urinary stones or infections, the following can occur:

- Bleeding, resulting in RBCs in the urine
- Accumulation of epithelial cells accompanied by cast formation
- WBCs in the urine, indicating infection

Urine Collection

Urine Collection: Urine can be collected for various studies. The type of testing determines the method of collection. The different methods of urine collection are as follows:

- Random collection (routine analysis)
- Timed collection (24-hours urine)
- Collection from a closed urinary drainage system
- Sterile specimen (catheterized)
- Clean-voided specimen

The client's age and the method of collection determine client teaching. The collection method should be written on the laboratory requisition.

- **Random Collection:** The practitioner writes the order for a UA (routine urine analysis), also called a random collection. The specimen can be collected at any time using a clean, not sterile, cup. The specimen should be taken immediately to the laboratory to prevent bacterial growth and changes in the urine's analytes.
- **Timed Collection:** Timed collection is done over a 24-hours period. The urine is collected in a plastic gallon container that contains preservative(s), some of which are caustic.

For a timed collection, the client is told to **void** (eliminate urine) and discard the specimen at the beginning of the collection. Timing for a 24-hours urine collection begins after the first voiding has been discarded. For example, if the client voids at 1000 hours (24-hours [military] time), that urine should be discarded, but all urine is saved until 1000 hours the following day, when the last urine is saved. The client can void into a clean container and pour the urine into the collection bottle. Toilet issue should not be dropped into the container used to catch the urine. The collection container should be refrigerated or kept on ice the entire 24-hours to stabilize the analytes and retard bacterial growth.

- **Collection from a Closed-Drainage System:** A sterile specimen can be collected from a client with an indwelling Foley catheter and closed-drainage system. A sterile specimen is used for urine culture. The urine specimen should *not* be obtained from the drainage bag because the analytes in the urine drainage bag change, leading to inaccurate results, and bacteria grows quickly in the drainage bag. The closed-drainage tubing has an aspiration port for sterile specimen collection.
- **Sterile Specimen:** When a sterile urine specimen is required and the client does not have an indwelling catheter and closed-drainage system, the client is catheterized. A small amount of urine is allowed to run out of the catheter into a basin, then the urine is allowed to flow into a sterile specimen bottle.
- **Clean-Voided Specimen:** Clean-voided (clean-catch, or midstream) specimen collection is done to have a specimen uncontaminated by skin flora. The collection technique is different for women and men. The female client is instructed to cleanse from the front to the back and then void into the specimen bottle; the male client is instructed to cleanse from the tip of the penis downward and then void into the specimen bottle.

The most common urinary diagnostic study is the urine analysis [The normal and abnormal constituents of the urine]. A urine analysis may be done in relation to conditions of other body system, because of the role of the kidneys in maintaining homeostasis. The nurse may be responsible for collecting urine sample. Depending on the test ordered, the specimen container may contain special chemicals as preservative and/or the urine may need to be kept cold. The nurse should follow the institutional procedure manual. The nurse must know how the specimens are collected and how to instruct the clients on specimen collection.

- *Collection of random specimen:* Random specimen are urine samples that are collected at any time of the day in clean containers. Usually 15 to 60 mL of urine are sufficient for tests performed on random samples. Random samples are used for routine screening tests to detect obvious abnormalities. The client instructed to void directly into the urine container or to void some other type of clean container or to void some other type of clean container, after which the sample is transferred to another type of container. If the sample is collected by the client at home, it must be transported to the laboratory within 2 hours.
- *First morning specimen:* The specimen is collected upon arising in the morning, when urine is most concentrated. Such samples are ideal for screening purposes, as substances may be detectable in them that are not found in more dilute samples. In addition to routine screening test, first morning samples are desirable for pregnancy tests and tests for orthostatic protienuria.

The articles required for routine first morning specimens are as follows (Table 23.3):
- Clean kidney dish
- Sterile cotton pad for female infants, and two artery forceps, clean kidney dish for female infants
- Sterile test tubes for (male infants) and adhesive tape
- Clean and label specimen container
- Screen (for adult bed patients)
- Requisition forms
- *Double-voided specimens:* These specimens are used when testing urine for sugar and acetone. The purpose of this approach is to ensure that the urine tested is fresh, so that it serves as a valid indicator of current blood glucose and ketone level. The client is instructed to empty the bladder and, if possible, to drink a glass of water. Approximately 30 minutes later, the client voids again. The second sample is then tested.
- *Clean-catch midstream specimen:* These specimens are used to avoid contamination of the sample with urethral cells, microorganisms and mucus. The procedure for collecting a midstream urine specimen is discussed in Table 23.4.
- *Collecting a sterile urine specimen (Catheter specimen):* A sterile urine specimen can be obtained either by inserting a straight catheter into urinary bladder and removing urine or obtaining specimen from the port of an indwelling catheter using sterile technique. Procedure for collecting this specimen are as follow.

Follow steps 1 to 6 of previous procedure by collecting supplies required for port collection and straight catheter collections as given below (Table 23.5). The equipment need for Port collection includes:
- Sterile specimen cup
- 20 mL syringe
- 22 or 21 inch needle
- Tube clamp
- Alcohol prep
- Requisition slip.

Table 23.3: Procedures of Collecting First Morning Urine Specimen

	Nursing Actions		*Rationales*
1.	Explain the importance.	1.	Seek cooperation and reduce anxiety.
2.	Screen the bed.	2.	Provide privacy.
3.	Wash hands, don gloves.	3.	Prevent cross-infection.
4.	Clean genitalia before voiding.	4.	Provides cleaner specimens.
5.	For females if menstruating, place clean pad to void into the clean receiver/urinal.	5.	Seeks cooperation and decreases anxiety.
6.	Pour 100 mL of urine into a specimen container without soiling the outerside.	6.	Helps prevent cross-contamination.
7.	In case of male infant, fix the mouth of test tube over the penis and remove as soon as he voids.	7.	Provides help to physician while providing support to patient.
8.	In case of female infant, apply sterile pad over the genital area.	8.	Provides security and emotional support to patient.
9.	Squeeze the urine-soaked pad with artery forceps into the container.	9.	Ensures accuracy of appropriate specimen.
10.	Check the label once again and send to laboratory in time along with requisition forms.	10.	Document procedure and patient response.

Table 23.4: Procedures of Collecting a Midstream Urine Specimen

	Nursing Actions		*Rationales*
1.	Read physician's guidelines.	1.	Provide basis of care.
2.	Collect supplies; sterile cotton balls, antiseptic and sterile specimen container, gloves, kidney dish, bed pan, laboratory requisition form.	2.	Organizes procedure.
3.	Introduce self.	3.	Decreases anxiety level.
4.	Identify patient by Id band.	4.	Identifies correct patient for procedure.
5.	Explain the procedure to patients. Make certain, that patient understands how to perform procedure.	5.	Seeks cooperation, decreases anxiety and ensures accuracy in collecting specimen.
6.	Wash hands and don gloves.	6.	Helps prevent cross-contamination.
7. (a)	If the patient is able, allow patient to cleanse perineum with antiseptic solution. Separate the labia well on a female patient or retract foreskin of an uncircumcised male. Use each cotton ball that is saturated with antiseptic solution one time only. If the patient is unable to cleanse the area, the nurse will don gloves and assist with procedure (please note that is women menstruating she should insert a vaginal tampon before beginning the cleaning process).	7.	Provide a cleaner specimen. Prevents organisms at or near the meatus being washed into the specimen.
8. (a) (b) (c)	Request that patient: Begins to void into container about 30 mL; then place the sterile specimen container to the sides of the labia of the female, do not touch. Without stopping flow, void a small amount into specimen cup. Without stopping flow, finish voiding into toilet seat collector (bedpan).	8.	Collects midstream urine specimen appropriately. The first 30 mL is discarded, so that the organisms at meatus will be washed away.
9.	Secure lid on container.	9.	Prevents spillate.
10.	Cleanse and return toilet.	10.	Readies for next use.
11.	Laboratory specimen appropriately.	11.	Provides accuracy.
12.	Ensure that specimen is taken to laboratory with requisition.	12.	Ensures fresh specimen for testing.
13.	Document-signature, mentioning date and time.	13.	Document procedure and patient's response for communication.
14.	Allow patient to wash hands after procedure.	14.	Prevents cross-contamination.

Table 23.5: Procedures of Catheter Port Collecting

	Nursing Actions		*Rationales*
1.	Clamp just below catheter port for about 30 minutes.	1.	Allows urine to collect for removal.
2.	Return in 30 minutes and cleanse port with alcohol prep.	2.	Cleanse port for needle puncture.
3.	Insert needle into port at 30 degree angle, and with draw 5 to 10 mL: of urine for a specimen.	3.	Provides urine for testing.
4.	Place urine in sterile specimen cup.	4.	Keeps specimen sterile.
5.	Unclamp catheter.	5.	Allows continuous urine flow.
6.	Label specimen, and send to the laboratory with requisition.	6.	Provides accuracy of specimen.
7.	Documents.	7.	Document procedure.

Table 23.6: Procedures of Catheter Port Collecting

	Nursing Actions		*Rationales*
1.	Read physician's order.	1.	Verifies procedure.
2.	Wash hands.	2.	Promotes medical asepsis.
3.	Identify patient.	3.	Ensures accuracy.
4.	Explain procedure.	4.	Ensures patient's cooperation.
5.	Instruct patient about the importance of collecting all urine for a period of 24-hours.	5.	Ensures a valid test can be obtained of 24-hours kidney function.
6.	Instruct patient not to place toilet tissue or fecal material in urine.	6.	Prevents contamination of specimen and alteration in tests.
7.	Have a patient void when the 24-hours specimen collection begins (usually 6 AM to 6 AM) discard this voiding.	7.	This voiding is formed in urinary system before the study began.
8.	Place labeled container (add preservative, i.e. ice if institutional policy permits).	8.	Keeping the specimen cool decreases decomposition and odor.
9.	Save all urines for 24-hours period. Place each voided specimen into the large container with preservative.	9.	All urines must be saved or results will be altered.
10.	Instruct patient to void a few minutes before end of 24 hours, this urine is part of 24-hours specimen.	10.	Empties bladder before the end of testing.
11.	Send the specimen to laboratory promptly with requisition.	11.	Ensures proper identification of specimen.

For straight catheter collection follow procedure and collect sterile specimen.

Suprapubic aspiration: It can be used to collect urine specimen. This involves inserting a needle directly into the bladder to obtain sterile urine sample. In this procedure the skin over the suprapubic areas is cleansed with antiseptic and draped with sterile drapes. A local anesthetic may be injected. The needle is inserted and the sample is removed, after which a sterile dressing is applied and the site is observed for any inflammation.

- *Collecting 24-hours urine specimen* (Table 23.6): Twenty-four-hour (timed) specimens allow for quantification of substances in urine. Methods of preserving the accumulating samples vary among laboratories and therefore, the laboratory should be consulted for advice regarding the use of preservative or the need for refrigeration or both. It is critical that all urine excreted during the 24-hours period is collected. The articles required for 24-hours collection of urine specimen are: Urinals/bed pan/big specimen container with added preservative of agency's choice. A pint jug, clean kidney tray.

As stated earlier, the nurse is frequently responsible for collecting urine specimens for laboratory test. The nurse inspects the client's urine for color, clarity, and odor. The nurse also is responsible for performing certain simple tests of urine, including specific gravity, urine culture, and glucose and ketone tests.

The normal characteristics and values of normal urine are as follows:

(i) *Color:* Normal urine ranges from a pale straw color to amber, depending on its concentration. Dark red urine seen in bleeding and kidney and ureters, bright red urine in bleeding from bladder or urethra.

(ii) *Clarity:* Normal urine appears transparent at voiding. Urine that stands several minutes in container will be cloudy. Thick or cloudy urine seen in bacterial infection and renal disease.

(iii) *Odor:* Urine has a characteristic odor. The more concentrated, the urine, the stronger the odor. A sweaty or fruity odor occurs from acetone or acetoacitonic acid, by-products of incomplete fat metabolism seen in diabetes mellitus or starvation.

(iv) *Normal values:*
- pH value 4.6 to 8.0
- Protein level—up to 10 mg/100 mL
- Glucose level—not normally present
- Ketone level—not normally present
- Blood level—up to two RBCs
- Specific gravity—1.01 to 1.03.

Urinalysis is the physical or macroscopic, chemical and microscopic examination of urine. It is performed to detect any abnormality in urine and to help in diagnosis and treatment of disease. When performing urinalysis, the nurse has to keep following points in her mind.

- Always take a fresh specimen of urine with patient's name and unit number, clearly written on container
- Use clean articles to test urine, especially test tube and dropper
- Ensure that chemical agents are fresh and pure
- Pay special attention to the method and techniques of urine analysis
- Always record the results of the test accurately and report if necessary
- Teach the diabetic patients and close associates the technique of urine testing

Urine Collection in Closed Drainage System

Indwelling catheters are used frequently in acute care settings for episodic or continuous drainage of urine. Specimens may be required to evaluate urine content, such as electrolytes, dilution, hormones, glucose, or abnormal factors, or renal function. Bacteria can be identified in urine specimens to determine if the catheter needs to be removed or if antibiotic therapy is indicated. Catheter tubing is generally designed to allow for access to obtain specimens without disconnecting the catheter from the tubing. Careful technique should prevent contamination of the system and, hence, risk for infection. Urine collection in closed drainage system is enlisted in Table 23.7.

	Table 23.7: Urine Collection in Closed Drainage System		
	Nursing actions		*Rationales*
	Check clients identification band Explain procedure before beginning		To identity right patient To get cooperation and reduce anxiety
1.	Cleanse hands.	1.	Reduces transmission of microorganisms.
2.	Check health care provider's order.	2.	Determines test and container needed for the specimen.
3.	Provide privacy.	3.	Maintains client dignity.
4.	Check for urine in the tubing.	4.	Determines if there is sufficient urine in the collecting tubing for a specimen. *Urine from the collection bag should not be used for sterile specimens.*
5.	If more urine is needed, clamp the tubing using a non-serrated clamp or a rubber band for 10 to 15 minutes	5.	Collects 10 ml of urine, which is needed for most urinalyses.
6.	Put on clean gloves.	6.	Practices Standard Precautions.
7.	Clean sample port with a procidone-iodine swab.	7.	Prevents entrance of microorganisms into the system.
8.	Insert sterile needle of syringe into the sample port of catheter at a 45-degree angle and withdraw 10 ml of urine	8.	Obtains specimen with sufficient volume for most urine tests.
9.	Put urine into sterile container and close tightly, taking care not to contaminate the lid of the container.	9.	Prevents contamination of specimen and spill of urine.
10.	Place needle and syringe into sharps container; *never recap a contaminated needle.*	10.	Prevents accidental needlesticks.
11.	Remove clamp and rearrange tubing avoiding dependent loops.	11.	Reestablishes urine flow and drainage into the system.
12.	Label specimen container, put it in a plastic bag, and transport to the laboratory.	12.	Ensures right test and controls transfer of pathogens.
13.	Cleanse hands.	13.	Reduces transmission of microorganisms.

Prior to Procedure the nurse should
- Identify the purpose of the urine test to determine the amount of urine needed and the proper container to collect it in.
- Assess the client's understanding of the test to determine the amount of instruction needed.
- Identify the type of collecting tubing attached to the indwelling catheter to determine if you need to disconnect the catheter from the system or can obtain the specimen from a closed system.

Equipment needed for this procedure
- Nonserrated clamp or rubber band
- Nonsterile gloves
- 10-cc syringe with needle (1-inch)
- Specimen container, plastic bag, and labels
- Povidone-iodine swabs

After the Procedure nurse should see than:
- Client understands the reason for the specimen
- Specimen was obtained in the proper container in a timely manner
- Specimen remained uncontaminated

And Document in the Nurses' Notes
- Date and time the specimen was sent to the laboratory
- Date, time, client name and room number, and test(s) ordered
- Amount of urine collected for the specimen

Clean Catch Urine Collection – Female/Male

A clean urine specimen to be used for culture and sensitivity can be collected without using an invasive method such as catheterization. This procedure is referred to as a clean-voided, clean-catch, or midstream urine specimen in that it is not a sterile procedure such as catheterization but, rather, a method of obtaining a clean specimen. This procedure is best accomplished with the client on the toilet because the use of a urinal or bedpan increases the risk of contamination. The client is asked to clean him or herself and initiate urination. After the client starts voiding, a sterile collection cup is placed under the stream of urine and a specimen collected. Hence it is called midstream collection. The initial urine is not collected because this portion of the stream flushes the urethral opening and meatus of any bacteria. The end urine is not collected because as the urine stream slows, and increased dripping and contact with the meatus occurs, the chance of contamination increases. The clean-catch specimen is sent to a laboratory for analysis.

Prior to Procedure the nurse should
- Evaluate the client's ability to obtain a clean-catch specimen to determine if the client is able to clean him or herself appropriately and understands the need to obtain a midstream specimen.
- Assess the presence of signs and symptoms of urinary tract infections or other abnormalities because burning or the inability to control urination may hamper the client's ability to obtain a clean specimen.

The Equipment Needed
- Sterile collection container with lid and label
- Sterile midstream kit, antiseptic towelettes, or cotton balls with antiseptic solution
- Toilet paper
- Nonsterile latex-free gloves
- Sterile gauze (optional)

After the Procedure the Nurse should see than
- Clean midstream specimen obtained.
- Client understood procedure.
- Client had no complaints associated with urination, such as burning, pain, or inability to initiate urination.

And Document in the Nurses' Notes
- Procedure.
- Characteristics of urine.
- Clients signs and symptoms associated with urination. Procedure, please refer Table 23.8.

Methods for Urine Analysis
For urine analysis, collect the following articles in a tray:
- Spirit lamp
- Match box
- Set of test tubes in a stand
- Test tubes holder
- Kidney tray
- Two droppers in bowl or jar of water (For urine and reagents)
- Urinometer in a case
- Conical flask
- Reagents
- Benedict's solution
- — acetic acid
- — sodium nitroprusside crystals
- — ammonium sulphate
- — fresh concentrated ammonia sol
- Red and blue litmus paper
- pH paper fresh urine

(i) *Macroscopic examination:* After collecting fresh urine, observe urine is clear and transparent container. Inspect urine for its amount, color, odor, consistency, deposits and presence of blood and record and report if necessary.

(ii) *Test for reaction*
- Take fresh sample of urine in a clean container
- Dip one end of blue litmus paper into the urine, if blue litmus paper turns red, the urine is acid
- If does not turn red, then dip red litmus paper into the urine, if this turns blue, urine is alkaline
- Dip one end of pH paper into the urine and allow it to dry
- Compare color with the standard
- Record the result

(iii) *Test for specific gravity*
- Fill ¾ of conical glass with urine. Ensure that there is no froth
- Place bulb of urinometer in urine. Allow urinometer to float and stand clear of the sides of the glass
- Read the level of urine on urinometer at eye level. Normal specific gravity is 1.010 to 1.020.

Table 23.8: Clean Catch Urine Collection

	Nursing actions		*Rationales*
	Check clients identification band Explain procedure before beginning		To identity right patient To get cooperation and reduce anxiety
1.	Check orders and assess need for the procedure.	1.	Provides understanding of the purpose of the procedure.
2.	Gather equipment.	2.	Provides for organization.
3.	Assess the client's ability to complete the procedure, including understanding, mobility, and balance.	3.	Improves compliance and likelihood of obtaining clean specimen.
4.	If the nurse is to perform the procedure; Cleanse hands and apply gloves. If the client is to perform the procedure, instruct the client to cleanse hands before and after the procedure. If the client wishes, provide a pair of gloves.	4.	Decreases transmission of microorganisms.
5.	Provide privacy.	5.	Decrease embarrassment.
6.	Using sterile procedure, open kit or towelettes. Open sterile container, placing the lid with sterile side up on a firm surface.	6.	Prevents contamination of the specimen.
7.	**Female client:** Sit with legs separated on the toilet. Use the thumb and forefinger to separate the labia, or have the client separate the labia with finger. With the labia separated, use a downward stroke (from the top of the labia down toward the rectal area), and cleanse one side of the labia with the towelette. Discard the towelette and repeat the procedure on the other side with another towelette, keeping the labia separated at all times. With a third towelette, keeping the labia separated at all times. With a third towelette, use a downward stroke from the top of the urethral opening to the bottom. Discard the towelette.	7.	Provides access for cleaning the labia. Cleanses area and prevents contamination of clean area. Prevents contamination by feces. Keeping labia separated avoids contamination and decreases microorganisms in specimen.
8.	**Male client:** Stand in front of toilet. Pull back the foreskin (if present in uncircumcised male) and clean with a single stroke around meatus and glans. Use a circular motion, starting with the head of the penis at the urethral opening, moving down the glans shaft. Discard the towelette and repeat the procedure with another towelette and repeat the procedure with another towelette, keeping the foreskin retracted. Cleanse the head of the penis three times using a circular motion. Use a new towelette each time.	8.	Prevents contamination of microorganisms from foreskin. Single strokes and moving away from opening prevents contamination of the urethral opening.
9.	Ask the client to begin to urinate into the toilet. After the stream starts with good flow, place the collection cup under the stream of urine. Avoid touching the skin with the container. Fill the container before urination ceases. Wipe with toilet paper.	9.	The specimen is collected midstream to avoid contamination of urine that touches the labia. The initial urine flushes bacteria from the orifice and the end urine may have contact with the meatus or labia and, hence, be contaminated.
10.	Place the sterile lid back onto the container and close tightly. Clean and dry the outside of the container with a towelette. Cleanse hands. Label and enclose in a plastic biohazard bag, and follow facility policy for transporting specimen to the laboratory.	10.	Prevents contamination of clean specimen, prevents spillage, and ensures accuracy.
11.	Remove and dispose of gloves and cleanse hands.	11.	Decreases transmission of microorganisms.

(iv) *Test for albumin*
(a) *Hot method*
  • Take a clean test tube and fill 3/4th with urine
  • Fix test tube holder on lower 1/3 of test tube
  • Hold the test tube with test tube holder at an angle to spirit lamp
  • Flame only at the top portion or upper layer by keeping test tube away from you and others
  • Observe the top heated column of urine for any cloudy appearance
  • If cloudy, add five drops of 2% acetic acid; if it becomes clean, it is due to phosphates
  • If the cloudiness persists then it indicates presence of albumin
  • The result may be recorded and reported according to the amount to precipitate one plus (+) to form ++++ (plus)
    — No cloudiness   = No albumin –
    — Slight cloudiness   = Trace of albumin +
    — Heavy cloudiness   = Significant amount of albumin.

(b) *Cold method*
  • Fix a clean and dry test tube on holder
  • Fill ½ inch of test tube with nitric acid
  • Pour equal quantity to urine with dropper gradually from the side of the test tube without shaking it
  • Formation of a white ring at the junction of urine and nitric acid and presence of albumin

(v) Test for acetone (Rothera's test)
  In a confirmed diabetic patient, acetone or ketone bodies may be found. Tests for detection of acetone are as follows:
  • Put 1 mL of ammonium sulphate crystals into a dry test tube
  • Pour 5 mL of urine into it and shake well till it is saturated or until crystals dissolve
  • Add one or two crystals of sodium nitroprusside and shake again
  • Pour 2 mL of concentrated liquor ammonia gently from the side of test tube without shaking it
  • Formation of a purple ring at the junction of the two solutions indicates the presence of acetone
  • If there is no ring, let it stand for 10 minutes and observe again
  • Record and report the result, according to thickness of ring, which may be one plus to four plus.

(vi) *Test for sugar*
  • Take about 5 mL of Benedict's solution in a clean test tube
  • Hold with a test tube holder
  • Heat it over a spirit lamp flame, keeping the open end of test tube away from you, continuously rotating it to avoid breakage.
  • Add 8 drops of urine with dropper into the boiling solution
  • Heat it again for two minutes and let it cool
  • Be careful not to let the urine boil over and spill out of test tube
  • Observe for any change in color; if nor change, it indicates sugar absence
  • If sugar is present, color will be green, yellow, orange or brick red and compare the percentage with scale given as standard.
  • Record the result as:
    — Green color   : Traces of sugar
    — Green turbidity   : Less than 0.5 gm%
    — Yellow turbidity   : 0.51 gm% ++
    — Orange turbidity   : 1-2 gm% ++
    — Brick red   : 2 gm% or more ++++
  In recent days, the uristix method, i.e. dextrose strips and clinitest tablets, may be used to determine sugar in urine and acetone by dipping stick or adding urine to acetone tablets are used in determine acetone and observing the color changes and comparing the color with standard color charts provided by manufacturers are very easy methods.

(vii) *Testing for bile salts (sulphur test)*
  • Take 10 mL of urine in test tube
  • Gently sprinkle few pinches of sulphur powder at the top of urine in test tube
  • If bile salts are present, the amount of sulphur will remain at the top of urine.

(viii) *Testing for bile pigments*
(a) *Iodine test*
  • Take about 5 mL of urine in a clean test tube
  • Add few mL of 10% alcoholic solution of iodine over the urine
  • A green ring indicates presence of bilirubins.
(b) *Paper strip method*
  • By dipping the strip in the urine and matching the color with color chart provided by the manufacturers. After the particular tests of urine is completed, the nurse has to follow the following:
  - Ensure that all reagent/chemical containers are properly closed and replaced
  - Put off the spirit lamp or sources of heat properly
  - Discard the urine samples from containers and test tubes. Thoroughly rinse with soap and brush till they are clear
  - Clean and wash the conical glass, urinometer and kidney tray
  - Keep test tubes inverted in the stand
  - Replace tray for the next time.
  Some more tests performed in urine, please see Table 23.17.

Stool Tests/ Examination

Stool specimens are examined for normal substances (such as urobilinogen) and blood, bacteria, and parasites.
  • **Urobilinogen,** a colorless derivative of bilirubin, is formed by the normal action of intestinal flora on bilirubin. It increases in situations of severe hemolysis and decreases with most biliary obstructions.

- **Occult blood** is invisible blood in the stool that can be detected only be chemical means or with a microscope. The digestive process in the GI tract acts on blood, making it occult. Random sampling for occult blood is done to diagnose gastrointestinal bleeding, ulcers, and malignant tumors.

  To decrease the possibility of a false-positive result when occult blood is to be used to confirm suspicions of a gastrointestinal disorder, the client is placed on a 3-day diet free of meat, poultry, and fish. Drugs causing a false-positive test for occult blood are salicylate, steroids, and indomethacin.

- **Parasites** The gastrointestinal tract can harbor parasites and their eggs (ova). Whereas some of these parasites are harmless, others cause clinical symptoms. Most common parasites except pinworms (which can enter the body through both the oral and anal routes) enter the body through the mouth when contaminated water or food is ingested.

  The reason for collecting a stool specimen should be explained to the client. The client is then instructed to defecate into a clean bedpan or container, and discard used tissue in the toilet. Stools can be collected one time or over 24, 48, or 72 hours. Stools to be collected over a prolonged period must be placed into a container and refrigerated. Once all stools have been collected, the container should be labeled with the client's name, the date and time, and the test to be performed. All stool specimens are placed in a biohazard bag before being transported to the laboratory.

Collecting a Stool Specimen

The nurse is directly responsible for ensuring that specimens are accurately obtained, properly labeled in appropriate containers, and transported to the laboratory on time. Institutions provide special containers for fecal specimens. Some tests require specimens to be placed in chemical preservatives. Medical aseptic technique should be used during collection of stool specimen. Because about 25% of the solid potion of stool are bacterially infected from the colon, so the nurse should wear disposable gloves when handling specimen.

Stool specimens are collected and examined for a variety of reasons including to determine the presence of infection, bleeding, to observe the amount, color, consistency and presence of fats, and to identify parasites, ova, and bacteria. The nurse collects stool specimens to test for abnormal elements in stool and determine malabsorption problems. Procedures for collecting stool specimens are given in Tables 23.9 and 23.11.

Stool specimens are not collected as frequently as urine or blood specimens, but they are extremely valuable in evaluating and diagnosing a variety of gastrointestinal diseases. The most common tests on a stool specimen are occult blood, culture, fecal fat, fecal leukocyte, and OVA and parasite (parasite screen). A stool specimen can help identify GI bleeding; screen for carcinomas, polyps, diverticulitis, and colitis; diagnose and monitor various pathogenic microorganisms; diagnose inflammatory bowel disorders, pancreatitis, and malabsorption syndrome; and identify parasitic infestations. A single specimen is often not diagnostic, and at least three stool cultures are required for a pathogenic diagnosis.

1. Assess the client's or family member's understanding of the need for the test so the nurse can provide needed teaching.
2. Assess the client's ability to cooperate with the procedure to collect the specimen to maintain privacy while a sample is obtained.
3. Assess the client's medical history for bleeding or GI disorders. The nurse can initiate screening tests.
4. Assess any medications the client receives that can cause GI bleeding, such as anticoagulants, steroids, or acetylsalicylic acid, to help determine the need for testing and/or the possible source of bleeding.

Test performed on stool, please see Table 23.18.

Equipment Needed

- Paper towel
- Disposable gloves
- Wooden applicator
- Specimen container
- Gloves
- Clean, dry bedpan, bedside commode, or toilet "hat"

After the Procedure the nurse should
- Note presence or absence of color change in the guaiac paper.
- Note color, character, and consistency of stool.
- Ask the client to explain the rationale and procedure for the stool test.

And document in the Nurses' Notes
- Date and time the collection was obtained
- Color, character, and consistency of the stool
- When the results of the test were reported to the health care provider

Collecting of Sputum Specimens (Table 23.10)

Sputum is mucus from the lung. A sputum specimen must come from deep in the bronchial tree. Many tests can be performed on sputum such as the following.

Culture and sensitivity: Here sputum specimen used to identify specific microorganisms and its drugs resistance and sensitivities.

Cytological examination: Here specimen used to identify abnormal cells and lung cancer by cell type.

Acid-fast-bacilli (AFB) specimen used to identify the presence of tubercle bacilli-M. tuberculis. The AFB specimen obtained 3 consecutive days in early morning.

Early morning is the best time for collecting sputum specimen because the patient has not yet cleared the respiratory passage. When sputum specimens are obtained, the nurse must ensure that specimens consist of mucus deep from the bronchus and not saliva. For which nurse instructs the patient the night before the test to drink extra-fluids, since this assists loosening secretions to more easily expectorate for the specimen.

Table 23.9: Collecting Stool Specimen

	Nursing actions		Rationales
	Check clients identification band Explain procedure before beginning		To identity right patient To get cooperation and reduce anxiety
1.	Cleanse hands and apply gloves.	1.	Reduces transmission of microorganisms from fecal specimen to nurse.
2.	Depending on agency policy, assist client as needed to bedside commode or toilet. Have client void before moving bowels. Then, prepare for specimen collection. If client is not ambulatory, use a bedpan. For the toilet, use "hat"	2.	Allows client privacy and the ability to move bowels in a more normal physiological position.
3.	Instruct the client not to contaminate the specimen with urine, vaginal discharge or toilet paper.	3.	Minimizes risk of skewed laboratory results.
4.	Ask the client to notify you as soon as the specimen is available.	4.	Reduces the risk of contamination of specimen, and reduces embarrassment to client.
5.	Assist the client with hygiene, help the client back to bed (as required), and ensure client comfort before turning attention to specimen.	5.	Promotes client cleanliness and dignity.
6.	Apply gloves and wear gown if client is on isolation or at risk for infectious stool, such as vancomycin-resistant enterococcus (VRE).	6.	Reduces the risk of transmission of microorganisms.
7.	Assess the stool for color, consistency, and odor, and presence or absence of visible blood or mucus.	7.	Facilitates comprehensive client assessment.
8.	Using one or two tongue blades (depending on how much specimen is needed and for which test), transfer a representative sample of stool to the specimen card or container, taking care not to contaminate the outside of the container (or the inside of a sterile specimen cup). If using a culture swab, swab in a representative area of stool, particularly if any purulent material is visible. Check with laboratory regarding the volume of stool needed for a particular test.	8.	Provides a high-quality sample for optimal results.
9.	Close the card, place the lid on the container, or place the swab in the culture tube (according to agency policy) as soon as specimen is collected.	9.	Reduces the risk of spread of microorganisms and reduces odor.
10.	Place the specimen container in a biohazard bag for transport to the lab after proper labeling is done according to agency policy. Be careful not to contaminate the outside of bag. Provide requisition for test according to agency policy.	10.	Properly identifies specimen to client; makes transport of specimen to lab more aesthetic for personnel. Provides client privacy. Reduces spread of microorganisms.
11.	Dispose of rest of stool according to agency policy.	11.	Reduces spread of microorganisms.
12.	Remove gloves and cleanse hands.	12.	Reduces spread of microorganisms.
13.	Send specimen to laboratory immediately.	13.	Maximizes quality of specimen for testing.

Table 23.10: Procedures of Collecting Sputum Specimen

	Nursing actions		*Rationales*
1.	Read the physician's guidelines.	1.	Provides basis of care.
2.	Collect supplies. • Sterile sputum collection • Tissues • Label for specimen • Laboratory requisites • Gloves	2.	Organizes procedure.
3.	Introduce self.	3.	Decreases anxiety.
4.	Identify patient.	4.	Identifies correct patient for procedure.
5.	Explain the procedure to patient.	5.	Seeks cooperation and decreases anxiety.
6.	Wash hands and don gloves.	6.	Helps prevent cross-contamination.
7.	Position patient in Fowler's position.	7.	Assist coughing.
8.	Instruct the patient to take three breaths and force cough into sterile container.	8.	Help patient expectorate mucus.
9.	Close container immediately label specimen container.	9.	Ensures appropriate specimen reaches lab.
10.	Send it to the laboratory with requisition on time.	10.	Ensures specimen to the laboratory.
11.	Remove gloves and wash hands.	11.	Helps prevent cross-contamination.
12.	Record the color, consistency, amount, and odor of the sputum and document.	12.	Identify any abnormalities and communicate to others.

Table 23.11: Procedures of Collecting a Stool Specimen

	Nursing actions		*Rationales*
1.	Read physician's guidelines.	1.	Provides basis of care.
2.	Collect supplies, i.e. • Stool specimen cup • Spatula • Bed pan, urinal, specimen • Culture tube with device or commode, kidney tray sterile swab stick • Gloves • Label • Laboratory requisition	2.	Organizes procedure.
3.	Introduce self.	3.	Decreases anxiety level.
4.	Identify patient.	4.	Identifies correct patient.
5.	Explain procedure to patient.	5.	Seeks cooperation and decreases anxiety.
6.	Wash hands and don gloves.	6.	Helps prevent cross-contamination.
7.	Assist to bathroom when necessary.	7.	Provides patient safety.
8. (a) (b)	Request patient to defecate into commode, specimen device or bed pan and to prevent urine from entering specimen. For female patient, provide bed pan and kidney tray to get urine in kidney tray and stool in the bedpan. Nurse assists for helpless patient. For male patient, provide bed pan and urinal.	8.	Prevents contamination of specimens.
9.	Transfer stool to specimen cup with use of a spatula and close lid.	9.	Protects specimen.
10.	Discard used spatula in the waste bin.	10.	
11.	For culture, specimens can be obtained with the help of sterile swab stick and put into culture tube.	11.	
12.	Remove gloves and wash hands.	12.	Protects nurse from contamination.
13.	Attach label, send specimens to laboratory in time with requisition form.	13.	Identifies specimen for laboratory.
14.	Assist patient to bed.	14.	Provides comfort and safety.
15.	Record procedure response.	15.	Communicating others.

Blood Tests/Examination

Many tests can be performed on the blood. Test specific to the hematologic system are described in Table 23.16.

Type and Crossmatch

A **type and crossmatch** identifies the client's blood type and determines compatibility of blood between a potential donor and recipient (client). There are four basic blood types: A, B, AB, and O. the blood types are determined by the presence or absence of A or B antigens. **Antigens** are substances, usually proteins, that cause the formation of and react specifically with antibodies. **Antibodies** are immunoglobulins produces by the body in response to bacteria, viruses, or other antigenic substances. Type A and type B are antigens that are classified as **agglutinogens,** or substances that cause **agglutination** (clumping of RBCs). **Agglutinis** are specific kinds of antibodies whose interaction with antigens manifests as agglutination.

Blood types are also identified as positive or negative, depending on the presence or absence of the Rh factor. The Rh factor is an antigen that may be found on the RBC. The designation *Rh positive* means the antigen is present; *Rh negative* means the antigen is absent. An individual's blood type and Rh are determined genetically.

Crossmatch identifies the compatibility of the donor's blood with that of the recipient. A sample of the recipient's blood is mixed with the blood of a possible donor in the laboratory. If the mixed sample does not agglutinate, it is compatible.

Blood Chemistry

Blood chemistry tests are often grouped together, requiring one requisition and one venous specimen. Tests performed include glucose, electrolytes, enzymes, lipids, creatinine, and protein values. Other tests that may be performed on a blood specimen are listed in Table 23.16.

Blood Glucose: Blood for measuring glucose is obtained by either skin puncture or venipuncture and is either fasting (FBS) or nonfasting (usually 2 hours postprandial) blood sugar. If the results of this screening test for diabetes mellitus are abnormal, the practitioner may order a glucose tolerance test, the most accurate test for diagnosing hypoglycemia and hyperglycemia (diabetes mellitus).

Serum Electrolytes: An **electrolyte** is a substance that, when in solution, separates into ions and conducts electricity. Some electrolytes act on the cell membrane to allow the transmission of electrochemical impulses in nerve and muscle fibers, whereas others determine the activity of cellular metabolism.

Cations are ions that have a positive charge, such as sodium (Na^+), potassium (K^+), calcium (Ca^{++}), and Magnesium (Mg^{++}). Anions are ions that have a negative charge, including chloride (Cl^-), bicarbonate (HCO_3^-), and phosphate (HPO_4^-),

Blood Enzymes: Enzymes are globular proteins produces in the body that catalyze chemical reactions within the cells. Enzyme tests are key to diagnosing tissue damage, mainly to the myocardium and, to a lesser degree, to the brain.

Plasma levels of intracellular enzymes elevate in the presence of myocardial **necrosis** (tissue death as the result of disease or injury). Enzymes in the blood are directly proportional to the degree of cellular damage. The enzymes are not used alone in determining a diagnosis but, rather, are reviewed with other diagnostic studies.

Blood Lipids: An elevated serum lipid level is one of the controllable contributing risk factors to congestive heart disease (CHD). **Lipoproteins** (blood lipids bound to protein) are measured along with cholesterol.

Laboratory Tests

Common laboratory studies are usually simple measurements to determine the amount or number of **analytes** (i.e., measured substances) present in a specimen. Laboratory tests are ordered by the practitioner to:
- Detect and quantify future disease risk.
- Establish or exclude diagnoses.
- Assess the disease process severity and formulate a prognosis.
- Guide intervention selection.
- Monitor the progress of the disorder.
- Monitor treatment effectiveness.

Blood Specimen Collection

The scheduling and sequencing of laboratory tests are important. All tests requiring **venipuncture** (the use of a needle to puncture a vein to aspirate blood) should be grouped together so the client has only one venipuncture (Table 23.13). Fasting laboratory and radiological studies should be scheduled on the same day so that the client is only required to fact for 1 day. The client's comfort level and satisfaction increases with appropriate scheduling.

Accuracy in laboratory testing requires that:
- The correct requisition form is used.
- All requested information is written on the form (e.g., the client's full name and medical number).
- Pertinent data that could influence the test's results, such as medications taken, is included.
- Specimen collection from the correct client is confirmed by checking the identification band.
- Laboratory results are placed in the correct medical record.

Venipuncture: Various members of the health care team can perform venipuncture. Although laboratories employ **phlebotomists** (individuals who perform venipuncture) to collect blood specimens, nurses must known hoe to perform venipuncture, because they routinely perform venipuncture in hospital critical care units, the home, and long-term care settings.

Venipuncture can be performed by using either a sterile needle and syringe or a vacuum tube holder with a sterile two-ended needle. Test tubes with different colored stoppers are used to collect blood specimens. The stoppers indicate the type of additive in the test tube. The tubes are universally color coded as follows:

- Red: no additive
- Lavender: ethylene diaminote traacetic acid (EDTA)
- Green: sodium heparin
- Gray: potassium oxalate
- Black: sodium oxalate

Arterial Puncture: Arterial blood gases reveal the lung's ability to exchange gases by measuring the partial pressures of oxygen (PaO_2) and carbon dioxide ($PaCo_2$) and evaluates the potential of hydrogen (pH) of arterial blood. Blood gases are ordered to evaluate:

- Oxygenation
- Ventilation and the effectiveness of respiratory therapy
- Acid—base balance in the blood

Arterial blood is drawn from a peripheral artery (e.g., radial or femoral) or from an arterial line. The blood is collected in a 5-3L heparinized syringe. The syringe is then rotated to mix the blood with the heparin to prevent clotting and then placed on ice.

In some agencies, it is within the scope of nursing practice to perform radial artery puncture, but femoral artery puncture is usually performed only by an advanced practitioner because of the associated increased risk of hemorrhage. It is not common practice for student nurses to draw ABG samples, but students often assist with the procedure and care for the client afterward.

The nurse is responsible for assessing the client for symptoms of postpuncture bleeding or occlusion. Apply direct pressure to the puncture site until all bleeding has stopped (a minimum of 5 minutes). Symptoms of impaired circulation include:

- Numbness and tingling
- Bluish color (cyanosis)
- Absence of a peripheral pulse

Capillary Puncture: When small quantities of capillary blood are needed for analysis or when the client has poor veins, a capillary puncture is performed. They are also used for blood glucose analysis. Procedures of obtaining blood by skin puncture is enlisted in Table 23.12.

Central Lines: A blood sample can also be collected from a **central line** (a venous catheter inserted into the superior vena cava through the subclavian or internal or external jugular vein). Central lines are used to treat fluid or electrolyte imbalances, such as severe dehydration caused by vomiting. Central lines are inserted when a peripheral route cannot be obtained, can be used for treatment, and to withdraw blood for analysis.

The first blood sample drawn from a central line cannot be used for diagnostic testing. It must be discarded, with the volume of discard being the same as the dead space (catheter size). Agency protocol should specify the volume to discard relative to the type and size of catheter.

Central line care requires strict sterile technique. The practitioner must write an order for a blood sample to be obtained from a central line.

Implanted Port: Some clients have a **port-a-cath** (a port that has been implanted under the skin) over the third or fourth rib. The port's catheter is inserted into the superior vena cava or right atrium through the subclavian or internal jugular vein. This implanted port is used for the same purpose as a central line. Using strict sterile technique, blood can be withdrawn for analysis by accessing the port. This should be performed only by a nurse who has the education to properly do so. Students are not usually taught how to access an implanted port.

Venous site or heparin lock. If the extremity must be used, obtain the sample from a site distal to the IV or heparin lock.

- The skin is prepared by cleansing with an antiseptic such as betadine (povidone-iodine) or 70% alcohol and allowed to air-dry and dried with sterile gauze.

Culture and Sensitivity Tests

Culture is the growing of microorganisms to identify the pathogen. Culture and **sensitivity** (C&S) tests are performed to identify both the pathogen and its susceptibility to commonly used antibiotics. Sensitivity allows the selection of appropriate antibiotic therapy. All C&S specimens should be immediately taken to the laboratory.

Blood Culture: **Bacteremia** is bacteria in the blood. A blood culture should be procured while the client is having chills and fever. A series of three collections are performed using strict sterile technique. The needle should be changed after the specimen is collected and before injecting the blood sample into the test tube.

Throat (Swab) Culture: The throat normally hosts many organisms. Throat cultures identify such pathogens as beta-hemolytic streptococci. *Staphylococcus aureus,* meningococci, gonococci, *Bordetella pertusis,* and *Corynebacterium diphtheria.* A throat swab is commonly done to identify streptococcal infections, which can cause rheumatic fever or glomerulonephritis if left untreated.

To obtain a throat swab, use a wooden blade to depress the tongue and swab the white patches, exudates, or ulcerations of the throat with a sterile applicator. The applicator should not touch any other parts of the mouth. The applicator is then placed in a sterile container.

Sputum Culture: Sputum tests include culture, smear, and cytology. Sputum, created by the mucous glands and goblet cells of the tracheobronchial tree, is sterile until it reaches the throat and mouth, where it comes in contact with normal flora. For a more accurate identification of pulmonary organisms, sputum can be obtained by tracheo-bronchial suctioning and trabstracheal aspiration.

In addition to the organism(s) found in a culture, a sputum smear identifies eosinophils, epithelial cells, and other substances. Smears helps diagnose asthma (eosinophils) and fungal infections. The specimen must be refrigerated if it cannot be taken immediately to the laboratory.

Table 23.12: Procedures of Obtaining Blood by Skin Puncture

	Nursing actions		*Rationales*
1.	Read the physician's guidelines.	1.	Provides basis for care.
2.	Collect supplies, i.e., • Disposable lancet • Pipette or tubing • Slides • Alcohol sponge • Dry sterile gauze pads • Disposable gloves	2.	Organizes procedure.
3.	Introduce self.	3.	Decreases anxiety.
4.	Identify patient.	4.	Perform procedure with right patient.
5.	Explain the procedure to the patient.	5.	Seek cooperation and decrease anxiety.
6.	Wash hands and put on gloves.	6.	Protects nurse from possible exposure to blood.
7.	Cleanse site with alcohol (spirit swab) and dry with sterile gauze square.	7.	If any alcohol remains, it will alter RBC morphology.
8.	Create stasis by pressing on the distal joint of the finger to produce redness at the end of the finger.	8.	
9.	Use a sterile disposable lancet or an automated lancet.	9.	The avoids the possibility of the transfer of blood-borne viral disease.
10.	Prick the skin sharply and quickly with the lancet.	10.	Pricking quickly and sharply reduces pain and produces free flowing sample.
11.	Release pressure on the finger Wipe off first drop of blood.	11.	Epithelial and endothelial cells may be found in first drop leads to inaccurate counts.
12.	Allow the blood to flow freely with an adequate puncture.	12.	Pressing out the blood dilutes it with tissue fluid.
13.	Obtain the blood sample: a. Fill the pipette or microhematocrit tube. b. Make blood slides according to study required.	13.	Gently touch the drop of blood to glass slides or cover slip.
14.	Apply pressure over the wound with dry gauze sponge until bleeding stops.	14.	
15.	Remove gloves, wash hands. Dispose equipment and supplies in approved container.	15.	Protects nurse and other from exposure to blood.

Table 23.13: Procedures of Obtaining Blood through Venipuncture

	Nursing actions		*Rationales*
1.	Read the physician's guidelines.	1.	Provides basis of care.
2.	Collect supplies. • Seventy percent alcohol or spirit swabs • Iodine • Dry sterile sponges • 5 and 10 mL syringe • tourniquet • disposable gloves • blood sample tube or oxalated bottle	2.	Organizes procedure.
3.	Identify patient and introduce self.	3.	Decreases anxiety.

Contd...

	Table 23.13: *Contd...*		
	Nursing actions		*Rationales*
4.	Reassure the patient and explain that relative little blood will be taken.	4.	The patient is reassured when the nurse displays self assurance and competence in relating to people and when performing technical skill.
5.	Wash hands and don gloves.	5.	Protects nurse from possible exposure to blood.
6.	Instruct the patient to extend his arm, the arm should be held straight at elbow.	6.	—
7.	Apply tourniquet directly above the elbow with just sufficient pressure to prevent venous return.	7.	A tourniquet increases venous pressure and makes the vein more prominent and easier to enter.
8.	Inspect the area to visualize the veins, including anti-cubital area, wrist, dorsum (back) of the hand and top of the foot.	8.	Select the vein that is visible palpable and well fixed to surrounding tissue, so that it does not roll away. Palpate the vein.
9.	Cleanse the skin with iodine and alcohol and dry.	9.	Cleansing the skin reduces pathogens.
10.	Fix chosen vein with the thumb and draw the skin taut immediately below the site before inserting needle to stabilize the vein.	10.	The vein may roll beneath the skin when needle approaches its outer space.
11.	Hold the syringe between the thumb and last 3 fingers with the bevel up and directly in line with the course of vein.	11.	Inserting the needle quickly and smoothly minimizes pain.
12.	Obtain blood sample by gently pulling back on the plunger.	12.	Use of minimal suction prevents hemolysis of blood and collapse of the vein.
13.	Release the tourniquet as soon as specimen is obtained.	13.	
14.	Withdraw the needle away.	14.	Slow withdrawal of needle if less painful.
15.	Apply a sterile dry gauze to puncture site and request patient to apply gentle and firm pressure to site foe 2-4 minutes.	15.	Firm pressure over punctured site prevents leakage of blood into surrounding tissue with subsequent hematoma.
16.	Make the blood smear from the needle as desired. Remove the needle from the syringe. As soon as possible after drawing the blood, gently eject the blood sample into test tube or bottle containing an anticoagulant.	16.	Slowly transfer the blood into the test tube without forming bubbles.
17.	Invert the tube or bottle gently several times to mix blood with anticoagulants.	17.	For some tests, the blood is allowed to coagulate in the test tube or bottle.
18.	Label specimen correctly and send to laboratory immediately with requisition.	18.	Specimen should go to the laboratory with a minimum of delay of optimum reliability.
19.	Dispose needle and syringe in appropriate container. Clean all spills with 10% bleach solution.	19.	The avoid possible spread of blood borne viral disease.
20.	Remove gloves and wash hands.	20.	Protects nurse and others from exposure to blood.

Sputum **cytology** (the study of cells) is performed to diagnose cancer of the lungs. The specimen should be collected early in the morning and after a deep cough.

Urine Culture: Urinary C&S tests are performed whenever a urinary tract infection is suspected.

Stool Culture: Stool C&S is performed to identify bacterial infections. If the client has diarrhea, a rectal swab can be taken and used as a specimen, but fecal material must be visible on the swab for the laboratory to perform the test.

Wound culture: Table 23.14.

Papanicolaou Test

The **Papanicolaou test** (a smear method of examining stained exfoliative cells), commonly called a Pap smear, evaluates the

Table 23.14: Procedures for Collecting a Wound Culture

Equipment	
• Sterile culturette tube with enclosed swab for culture tube with individual swabs • Plastic bag for soiled dressing	• Sterile gloves, clean disposable gloves • Label for culturette tube, laboratory requisition with rubber band or plastic bag

	Nursing actions		*Rationales*
1.	Explain procedure.	1.	An explanation encourages client cooperation and reduces to client apprehension.
2.	Gather equipment.	2.	This provides for organized approach to task.
3.	Wash your hands.	3.	Handwashing deters the spread of microorganisms.
4.	Don clean disposable gloves. Remove dressing and assess wound and drainage.	4.	This protects nurse from handling contaminated dressings.
5.	Using aseptic technique, don sterile gloves And clean wound. Remove sterile gloves.	5.	Previous drainage and skin flora are removed.
6.	Twist cap to loosen swab in culturette, or open separate swab and remove cap from culture tube, keeping inside uncontaminated.	6.	Supplies are within easy reach, and sterility is maintained.
7.	Don clean glove or new sterile glove, if necessary.	7.	Use of culturette tube does not require immediate contact with skin or wound. If contact with wound is necessary to collect specimen, wear sterile glove on that hand.
8.	Carefully insert swab into drainage and roll gently. Use another swab if collecting specimen from another site.	8.	Cotton tip absorbs wound drainage. This prevents cross-contamination of wound.
9.	Place swab in culturette tube, being careful not to touch outside of container. Twist cap to secure.	9.	Outside of container is protected from contamination with microorganisms.
10.	If using culturette tube, crush ampule of medium at bottom of tube.	10.	Swab with drainage can be surrounded by culture medium.
11.	Remove gloves from inside out, and discard them in plastic waste bag.	11.	This prevents spread of microorganisms.
12.	Wash your hands.	12.	Handwashing deters the spread of microorganisms.
13.	Apply clean dressing to wound.	13.	Drainage from wound in absorbed.
14.	Wash your hands. Remove all equipment, and make client comfortable.	14.	Handwashing deters the spread of microorganism.
15.	Label specimen container appropriately (client's name, date, time, nature of specimen). Attach laboratory requisition to tube with rubber band or place tube in plastic bag with requisition attached. Send to laboratory within 20 minutes.	15.	This ensures proper identification of specimen. Over growth of other organisms can interfere with test results if specimen remains at room temperature for extended period.
16.	Record collection of specimen, appearance of wound, and description of drainage in chart.	16.	This provides for accurate documentation of procedure.

metabolic activity, cellular maturity, and morphological variations of cervical tissue. Papanicolaou testing can also be done on specimens from other organs, such as gastric secretions and bronchial aspirations.

Collecting Nose, Throat, and Sputum Specimens

A nose, throat, or sputum specimen is a simple diagnostic tool for clients with signs or symptoms of upper respiratory or sinus infections. Nose and throat specimens are collected from the client using a sterile swab. Sputum specimens are collected in a sterile cup. Sputum specimens can also be obtained via a specimen trap connected to suction. Specimens are sent to the laboratory and placed in a culture medium to allow pathogenic organisms to grow. The type of organism can be identified, thereby enabling diagnosis and appropriate antimicrobial therapy.

Prior to procedure the nurse should
1. Assess the client's understanding of the purpose of the procedure so the client will be able to cooperate.
2. Assess the type of nasal or sinus drainage to determine what kind of collection equipment will be needed.
3. Review the health care provider's orders for the cultures requested so repeat cultures are not done.
4. Assess the client for postnasal drip, sinus headache or tenderness, nasal congestion, or sore throat to know why the procedure is being done.
5. Identify whether the client has received recent antimicrobials and obtain a specimen before treatment, if possible.

For procedure, please refer Table 23.15.

Equipment Needed

- Two sterile swabs in sterile culture tubes or a flexible wire sterile swab with cotton tip for nose or throat cultures
- Tongue blades
- Penlight
- Facial tissues
- Clean, disposable latex-free gloves
- Nasal speculum (optional)
- Emesis basin or clean container
- Sterile specimen cup, or sputum specimen collector

After Procedure the Nurse should see that:
- An adequate specimen was obtained.
- The procedure was performed with a minimum of trauma to the client.

And document the same in Nurses' Notes
- Date, time, and site from which the specimen was obtained.
- Bleeding or obvious trauma as a result of the procedure.
- Description and time the specimen was collected and if the specimen is the first morning specimen, not pooled secretions.

Table 23.15: Nose, Throat, Sputum Specimen for Culture

	Nursing actions		*Rationales*
	Check clients identification band Explain procedure before beginning		To identity right patient To get cooperation and reduce anxiety
1.	Cleanse hands and put on clean gloves.	1.	Reduces transmission of microorganisms.
2.	Ask the client to sit erect in the bed or on a chair facing the nurse.	2.	Provides easy access to the nose or throat.
3.	Prepare a sterile swab for use by loosening the top of the container.	3.	Prevents contamination of the swab.
Collecting Throat Culture			
4.	Ask the client to tilt the head backward, open the mouth, and say "ah."	4.	Promotes visualization of the pharynx, relaxes the throat muscles, and minimizes the gag reflex.
5.	Depress the anterior one-third of the tongue with a tongue blade for better visualization.	5.	Promotes visualization of the pharynx, but may induce the gag reflex.
6.	Insert the swab without touching the cheek, lips, teeth, or tongue.	6.	Prevents contamination of the specimen with oral flora.
7.	Swab the tonsillar area from side to side in a quick, gentle motion.	7.	Ensures collection of microorganisms. Retains microorganisms in the culture tube and ensures the life of bacteria for testing.
8.	Withdraw the swab without touching adjacent structures and place in the culture tube. Crush ampule at bottom of tube and push swab into liquid medium.	8.	Prevents contamination from outside microorganisms and erroneous culture results.
9.	Secure the top to the culture tube and label with the client's name.	9.	Prevents identification mistakes.
10.	Discard the tongue depressor. Remove gloves and discard. Cleanse hands.	10.	Reduces transmission of microorganisms.
Collecting Nose Culture			
11.	Instruct the client to blow nose and check nostrils for patency with penlight.	11.	Clears nasal passages of mucus containing resident bacteria.
12.	Ask the client to occlude one nostril, then the other, and exhale.	12.	Determines the optimal nasal passage from which to obtain the specimen.
13.	Ask the client to tilt the head back.	13.	Promotes visualization of the sinuses.

Contd...

Table 23.15: *Contd...*

	Nursing actions		Rationales
14.	Insert the swab into the nostril until it reaches the inflamed mucosa and rotate the swab.	14.	Ensures the swab will be covered with the appropriate exudates.
15.	Withdraw the swab without touching adjacent structures and place in culture tube. Crush ampule at bottom of tube and push swab into liquid medium.	15.	Prevents contamination from normal nasal flora and erroneous culture results.
16.	Secure the top to the culture tube and label with the client's name.	16.	Prevents identification mistakes.
17.	Remove gloves and discard. Cleanse hands.	17.	Reduces transmission of microorganisms.

Collecting of Nasopharyngeal Culture

18.	Follow Actions 11 to 17, except use a swab on a flexible wire that can reach the nasopharynx via the nose.	18.	Allows for access to the nasopharyngeal area.

Collecting a Sputum Culture

19.	Explain to the client that the specimen must be sputum, coughed up from the lungs.	19.	Promotes client cooperation.
20.	Have a sterile specimen cup ready for the sample and some tissues at hand.	20.	The specimen must be collected in a sterile cup to prevent contamination.
21.	Have the client take several deep breaths and then cough deeply.	21.	Helps loosen secretions so the client will be able to provide a specimen.
22.	Have the client expectorate the sputum into the sterile cup without touching the inside of the cup.	22.	Prevents contamination of the specimen.
23.	Place the lid on the specimen container without touching the inside of the lid or the container.	23.	Prevents contamination of the specimen.
24.	Provide the client with tissues and make him or her comfortable.	24.	Promotes client comfort.

Alternative Sputum Collection Method
Generally used if the client is unable to expectorate an adequate sample

25.	Obtain a sterile suction catheter and an in-line sputum collection container.	25.	Prevents contamination of the specimen.
26.	Provide the client with warm humidified air for about 20 minutes if it is not contraindicated by the client's condition.	26.	Helps loosen secretions in the lungs.
27.	Hook up the sputum collector to the suction tubing and a suction device. Hook up the suction catheter to the sputum collector.	27.	Prepare the equipment before having the client cough.
28.	If the client is able to cooperate, have him or her take several deep breaths and cough.	28.	Loosens the secretions and brings them up to the back of the throat.
29.	As the client is coughing up sputum, carefully insert the catheter either orally or nasopharyngeally into the back of the throat and suction the sputum into the specimen container.	29.	Obtains a sterile specimen that is not contaminated with saliva.
30.	Safely dispose of the suction catheter.	30.	Prevents spread of microorganisms.
31.	Close the specimen container.	31.	Prevents contamination of the specimen.
32.	Provide tissues or other measures for client comfort.	32.	Promotes client comfort.
33.	Cleanse hands.	33.	Reduces transmission of microorganisms.
34.	Label each specimen with the client's name and send to the laboratory.	34.	Promotes the correct diagnosis for the client.

Radiological Studies

Radiography (the study of film exposed to X-rays or gamma rays through the action of ionizing radiation) is used by the practitioner to study internal organ structure. When used in conjunction with a **contrast medium** (a radiopaque substance that facilitates roentgen imaging of the body's internal structures), **fluoroscopy** (immediate, serial images of the body's structure and function) reveals the motion of organs. X-rays are valuable in formulating a diagnosis and helping to determine if other studies (e.g., a lung lesion requiring biopsy to differentiate between a benign or malignant tumor) are necessary.

Some radiological tests require a contrast medium such as barium and iodine that often interferes with other diagnostic studies. Draw a blood sample for thyroid function before beginning an intravenous pyelogram (IVP), where radioactive iodine dye is administered. If a client needs both an IVP and a barium enema, perform the IVP first because the barium is likely to decrease kidney visualization. Commonly performed radiological studies are described in Table 23.19.

Chest X-ray: The chest X-ray is the most common radiological study. Chest X-rays are taken from various views, because multiple views of the chest are needed to assess the entire lung field. To prepare for a chest X-ray, the client should remove all clothing from the waist up and don a gown. The client should also remove all metal objects (jewellery) because metal will appear on the X-ray film, thereby obscuring visualization of parts of the chest. Pregnant women are advised against X-rays; however, if X-ray is absolutely necessary, the woman should be draped with a lead apron to protect the fetus.

Computed Tomography: Computed Tomography (CT) is the radiological scanning of the body. X-ray beams and radiation detectors transmit data to a computer that transcribes the data into quantitative measurement and multidimensional images of the internal structures. Illustrates the sagittal, transverse, and coronal planes used in CT scanning.

The procedure requires the client's informed consent. The client's cooperation is essential during CT scanning because the client will be positioned and asked to remain motionless. Prepare the client by providing an explanation and pictures of what to expect.

Barium Studies: Barium (a chalky white contrast medium) is a preparation that permits roentgenographic visualization of the internal structures of the digestive tract. Barium studies can reveal congenital abnormalities, reflux, spasm, stricture, obstruction, inflammation, ulceration, lesions, varices, and fistula.

Angiography: Angiography allows visualization of vascular structures by using fluoroscopy and a contrast medium.

Arteriography: Arteriography is the radiographic study of the vascular system after radiopaque dye is injected through a catheter. Using fluoroscopy, the catheter is threaded through a peripheral artery into the area to be studied, such as the aorta or the cerebral, coronary, pulmonary, renal, iliac, femoral, or popliteal artery. With the client on a cardiac monitor, dye is injected through the vascular catheter, and a rapid sequence of films is taken.

Dye Injection Studies: Iodine, a common dye used in radiographis studies, might cause the client to experience the following temporary symptoms: shortness of breath, nausea, and a warm to hot flushed sensation. Most dye injection studies are invasive and thus require written informed consent.

Ultrasonography

An ultrasound, also called an echogram or sonogram, is a noninvasive procedure using high-frequency sound waves to visualize deep body structures. To ensure accuracy, this procedure should be scheduled before studies using a contrast medium or air, because the contrast medium would reflect the sound waves differently than body structures do. The client must lie still during the procedure.

Ultrasound is used to evaluate the brain, thyroid, gland, heart, abdominal aorta, vascular structures, liver, gallbladder, pancreas, spleen, and pelvis. During pregnancy, an ultrasound is commonly done to evaluate the size of the fetus and placenta. A full bladder is needed to ensure visualization.

To increase the contact between the skin and the **transducer** (instrument that converts electrical energy to sound waves), a coupling agent (lubricant) is placed on the surface of the body area to be studied. The transducer sends sound waves through the body tissue, which are reflected back and recorded. The varying density of body tissues deflects the waves into a differentiated pattern to an oscilloscope. Photographs are taken of the sound wave pattern on the oscilloscope. Table ___ describes some ultrasound test.

Magnetic Resonance Imaging

Magnetic Resonance Imaging (MRI) uses radiowaves and a strong magnetic filed to make continuous cross-sectional images of the body. During the study, a noniodine IV paramagnetic contrast agent may be used. The study reveals lesions and changes in the body's organs, tissues, and vascular and skeletal structures (Table 23.20).

Nuclear Scans

Radionuclide imaging (nuclear scanning) uses radionuclides (or radiopharmaceuticals) to show morphological and functional changes in the body's structure. A scintigraphic scanner, placed over the area of study, detects emitted radiation and produces a visual image. The results reveal congenital abnormalities, skeletal changes, infections, lesions, and glandular and organ enlargement (Table 23.21). For all nuclear scans, written informed consent is required. The client must remove all jewellery and metal objects.

Electrodiagnostic Studies

Electrodiagnostic tests measure electrical activity of the brain, heart, and skeletal muscles. Electrical sensors (electrodes) are placed at certain points to measure the velocity tone and direction of the impulses. The impulses are then transmitted to an oscilloscope or printed on graphic paper. Table 23.22 describes the various electrodiagnostic studies.

Electroencephalography

An electroencephalography (EEG) is the graphic recording of the brain's electrical activity. During the procedure, electrodes are placed on the client's scalp. The electrodes transmit impulses from the brain to an EEG machine. The machine amplifies the brain's impulses and records the waves on strips of paper. An EEG can reveal not only the presence of a seizure disorder or intracranial lesion but also the type. The absence of the brain's electrical activity is used to confirm death.

Electrocardiography

An electrocardiogram (EKG or ECG) is a graphic, noninvasive recording of the heart's electrical activity.

Lubricated electrodes are applied to the chest wall and extremities. The client is asked to lie still during the test. The pain-free test can reveal abnormal transmission of impulses and electrical position of the heart's axis.

A portable cardiac monitor (Holter monitor) records the heart's electrical activity, producing a continuous recording over a specified time (e.g., 24 hours). It allows the client to ambulate and perform regular activities. Clients keep a log of activities resulting in the heart beating faster or irregularly. The EKG tracing is reviewed in relation to the client's log to determine if certain activities, such as walking, are associated with abnormal transmission of impulses.

Stress Test

A **stress test** measures the client's cardiovascular fitness. It shows the myocardium's ability to respond to increased oxygen requirements (the result of exercise) by increasing the blood flow to the coronary arteries.

The client walks on a treadmill while connected to an EKG machine. Continuous EKG recordings are made during frequent changes in the treadmill's slope and speed. If the client experiences any symptoms of decreased cardiac output (chest pan, dyspnea, fatigue, or ischemic changes revealed by the EKG monitor), the test is stopped immediately.

Thallium Test

Thallium[201] is a radioactive isotope that emits gamma rays and closely resembles potassium. Although a radioactive study, the thallium test is discussed here because it is often performed in conjunction with an EKG. Thallium is rapidly absorbed by normal myocardial tissue but is slowly absorbed by areas with poor blood flow and damaged cells. During the test, thallium is administered intravenously and the scanner detects the radiation and makes a visual image. The light areas on the image represent heavy isotope uptake (normal myocardial tissue), whereas the dark areas represent poor isotope uptake (poor blood flow and damaged cells).

There are two types of thallium test: resting imaging and stress imaging. Resting imaging can detect a myocardial infarction within its first few hours. Stress imaging (thallium stress test) is performed while the client is on a treadmill and being monitored with an EKG. At peak stress, the IV thallium is injected. Scanning is performed in 3 to 5 minutes and again in 2 to 3 hours. The test is stopped immediately if the client becomes symptomatic for ischemia.

Endoscopy

Endoscopy is the visualization of a body organ or cavity through a scope. An endoscope (a metal or fiberoptic tube) is inserted directly into the body structure to be studies. A light and, in some studies, a camera at the end of the scope allow the practitioner to assess, via direct visualization or television picture, for lesions and structural problems. The endoscope has an opening at the distant tip that allows the practitioner to administer an anesthetic agent and to lavage, suction, and biopsy tissue. Common endoscopic procedures are listed in Table 23.16.

Figures 23.1 to 23.4 for some instruments used in endoscopy.

After the procedure, monitor vital signs, observe for bleeding, and assess for procedural risks (e.g., return of the gag and swallowing reflexes following a bronchoscopy performed under local anesthesia).

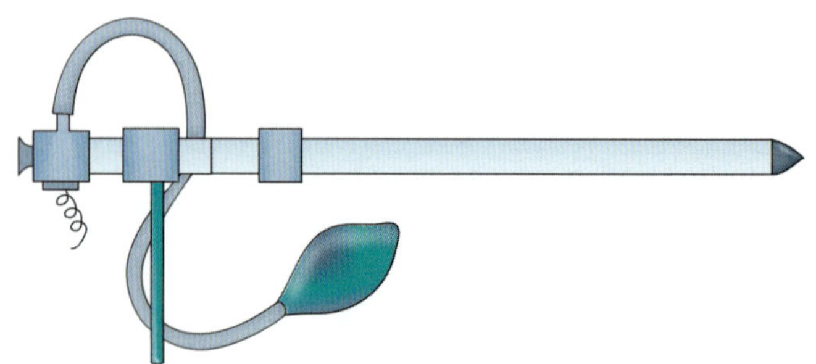

Figure 23.1: Sigmoidoscope

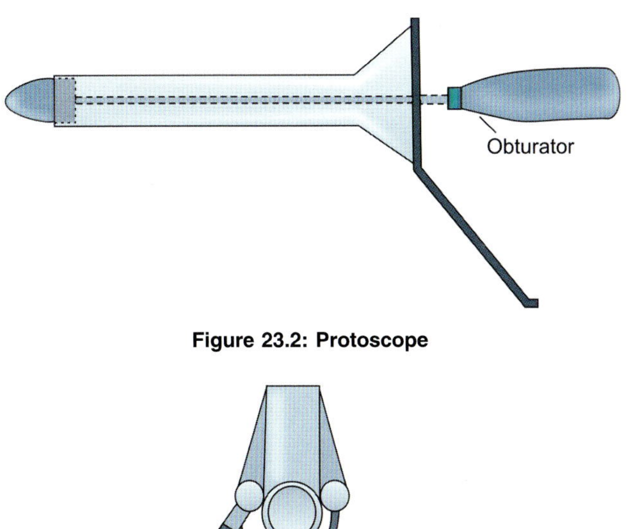

Figure 23.2: Protoscope

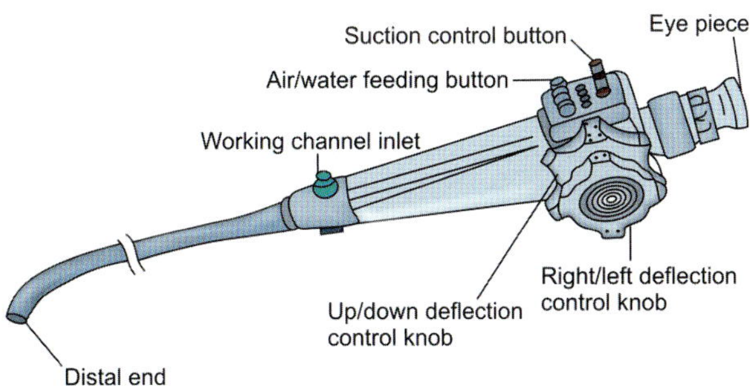

Figure 23.3: Rigid oesophagoscope

Figure 23.4: Gastroscope

A hollow-bore needle with stylet is used to pierce the skin. The stylet is withdrawn once the needle is in place, leaving only the outer needle to aspirate the fluid. A **biopsy** (excision of a small amount of tissue) can be obtained during aspiration or in conjunction with other diagnostic tests (e.g., bronchoscopy). Table 23.16 outlines various aspiration/biopsy procedures.

Bone Marrow Aspiration/Biopsy

The iliac crest and sternum are common sites for bone marrow puncture. A fluid specimen (aspiration) or a core of marrow cells (biopsy) can be obtained. Both tests are often done to obtain the best possible marrow specimen. The test identifies anemia; cancers such as multiple myeloma, leukemia, or Hodgkin's disease; or the client's response to chemotherapy.

Client positioning is determined by the site used: supine for the sternum and side lying for the iliac crest. The site is prepped to decrease the skin's normal flora. Explain to the client that pressure may be experienced as the specimen is withdrawn. The client should hold still because a sudden movement may dislodge the needle.

After the procedure, the client should be kept on bed rest for 1 hour. Monitor vital signs to assess for bleeding (rapid pulse rate, low blood pressure). Instruct the client to report to the practitioner any bleeding or signs of inflammation.

Paracentesis

Paracentesis is the aspiration of fluid from the abdominal cavity. It can be diagnostic, therapeutic, or both. With end-stage liver or renal disease, for instance, **ascites** (an accumulation of fluid in the abdomen) occurs. Pressure from ascities can interfere with breathing and gastrointestinal functioning. In this instance, aspiration is therapeutic. If a specimen for culture is taken, it is also diagnostic.

The client should void and be weighed before the procedure. The client should be placed in a high-Fowler's position in a chair or sitting on the side of the bed. The skin is prepped,

Aspiration/Biopsy

Aspiration is performed to withdraw fluid that has abnormally collected or to obtain a specimen. To minimize client discomfort when the skin is pierced by the needle (Tru-cut biopsy needle, Fig. 23.5), a local anesthetic is administered in the area to be studied.

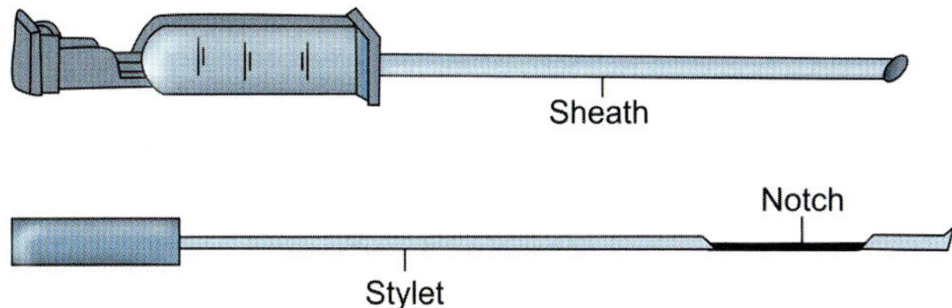

Figure 23.5: Tru-cut biopsy needle

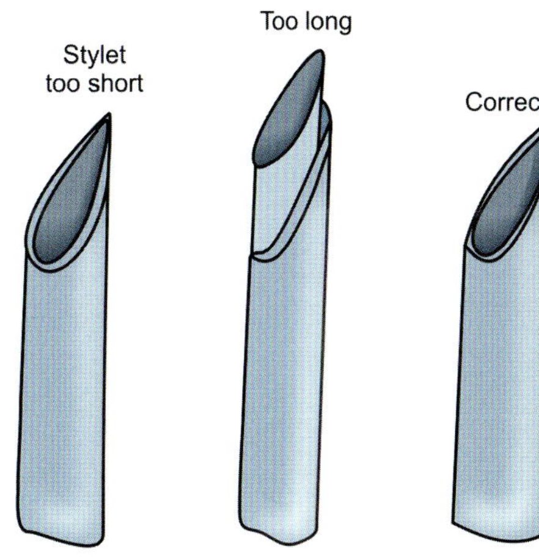

Figure 23.6: Position of the stylet in a needle

anesthetized, and punctured with a **trocar** (a sharply pointed surgical instrument contained in a cannula). (Please see Figures 23.6 and 23.7 for position of the needle and site for puncture during paracentesis). The trocar is held perpendicular to the abdominal wall and advanced into the peritoneal cavity. The trocar is removed when fluid appears, leaving the inner catheter in place to drain the fluid. The client is observed for changes resulting from the rapid removal of fluid.

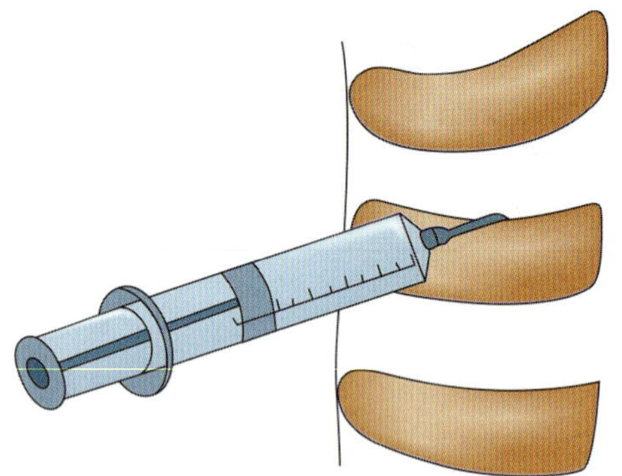
Figure 23.8B: Pleural fluid aspiration–site of needle

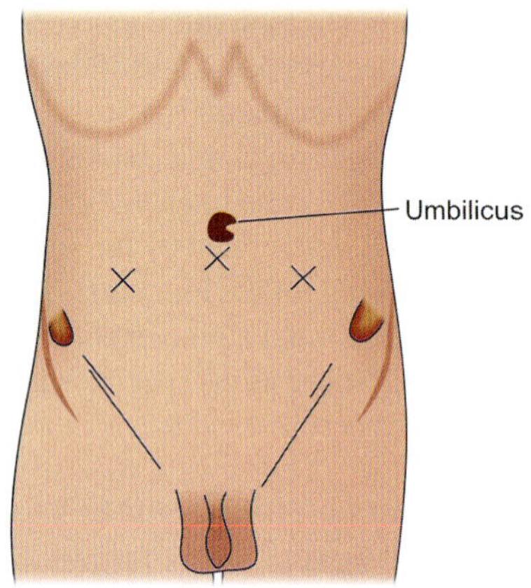

Figure 23.7: Site of puncture

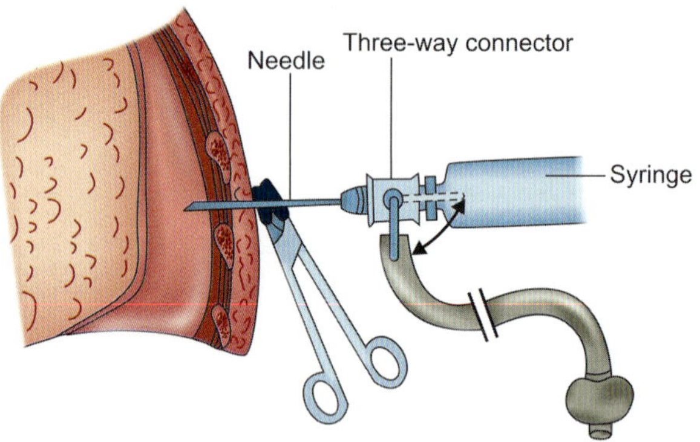

Figure 23.8C: Thoracocentesis

After the procedure, a sterile dressing is applied to the puncture site, and the client is monitored for changes in vital signs and electrolytes. Instruct the client to record the color, amount, and consistency of drainage on the dressing after discharge.

Thoracocentesis

Thoracocentesis is the aspiration of fluids from the pleural cavity (Fig. 23.8C). The pleural cavity normally has a small amount of fluid to lubricate the lining between the lungs and pleura. Inflammation, infection, and trauma may cause increased fluid production, which can impair ventilation.

To facilitate access to the rib cage, position the client with the arms crossed and resting on a bedside table (Fig. 23.8A). The client should not cough during insertion of the trocar. The practitioner selects, preps, and anesthetizes the puncture site. The trocar is usually inserted into the intercostals space at the place of maximum dullness to percussion. This should be above the seventh rib laterally and above the ninth rib posteriorly (Fig. 23.8B).

During the procedure, the client must be carefully monitored for symptoms of a **pneumothorax** (collection of air or gas in the pleural space, causing the lungs to collapse), such as dyspnea, pallor, tachycardia, vertigo, and chest pain. After the procedure, assess for signs of cardiopulmonary changes and a mediastinum shift, as indicated by bloody sputum and changes in vital signs.

Cerebrospinal Fluid Aspiration

Lumbar puncture (LP, "spinal tap") is the aspiration of cerebrospinal fluid (CSF) from the subarachnoid space (Figs 23.9A to C). The specimen is examined for organisms, blood, and tumor cells. A spinal tap is also performed:

- To obtain a pressure measurement when blockage is suspected
- During a myelogram
- To instill medications (anesthetics, antibiotics, or chemotherapeutic agents)

The client assumes a lateral recumbent position, with the craniospinal axis parallel to the floor, the flat of the back perpendicular to the procedure table. The client should assume

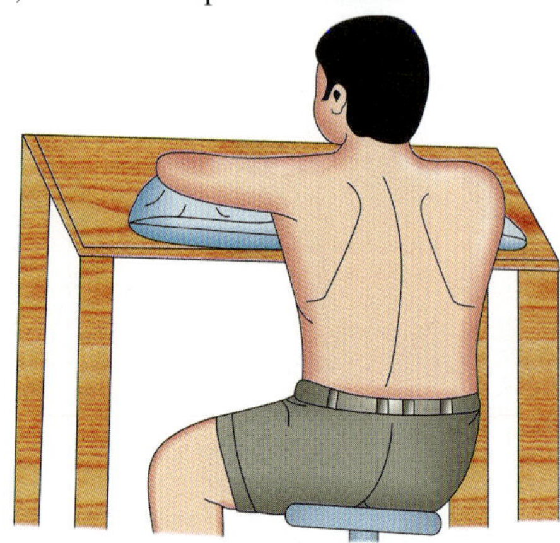

Figure 23.8A: Pleural fluid aspiration–position

a flexed knee-chest position to bow the back, thereby separating the vertebrae (Fig. 23.9B). Most clients require assistance in maintaining this position throughout the procedure. Face the client and place one hand across the client's shoulder blades and the other hand over the client's buttocks.

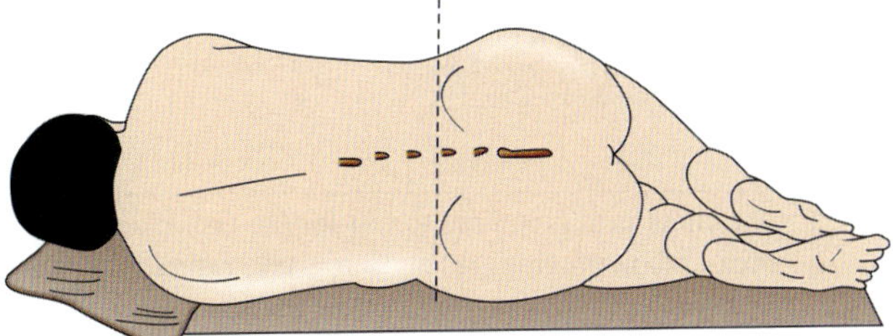

Figure 23.9A: Lumbar puncture, lateral position

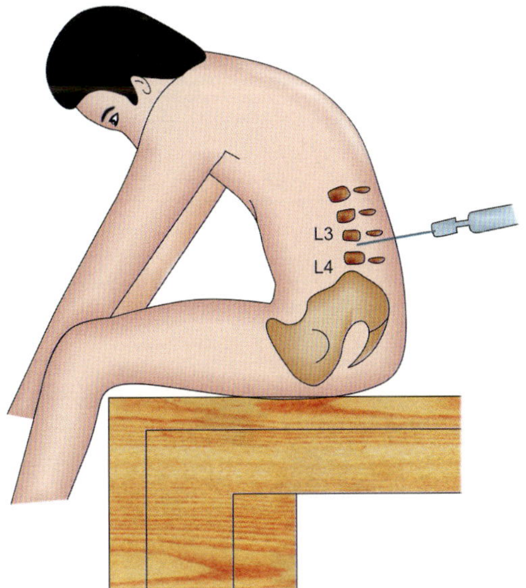

Figure 23.9B: Lumbar puncture, sitting position

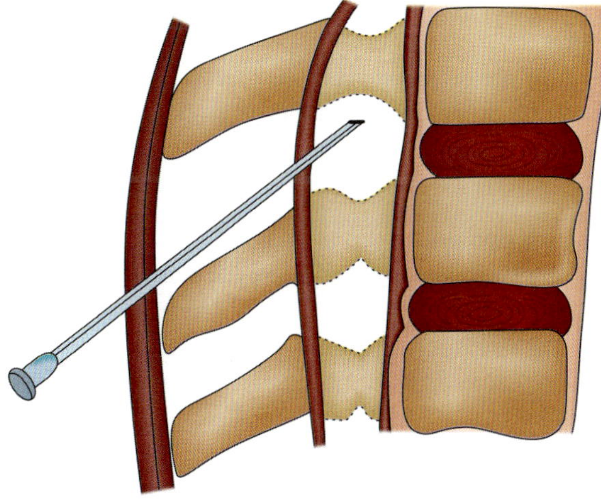

Figure 23.9C: Lumbar puncture

The practitioner selects, preps, and anesthetizes the puncture site (usually interspace L3-L4, L4-L5, OR L5-S1). The needle and stylet are inserted into the midsagittal space and advanced through the longitudinal subarachnoid space.

When positioned, the stylet is removed, leaving the needle in place. An initial CSF pressure reading is taken. If the pressure reading is greater than 200 mm H_2O, an adequate specimen is withdrawn slowly.

After the pressure reading is taken, the stopcock is turned so the CSF slowly flows into a sterile test tube. A sterile cap is placed on the test tube, and the sample is taken to the laboratory. Rapid withdrawal of CSF can cause a transient postural headache. The client's cardiorespiratory status is monitored throughout the procedure.

The list of tests performed on blood specimen, tests performed on urine, tests performed on stool, radiological studies, MRI, Nuclear scans, Electro diagnostic studies, endoscopic procedures, Aspiration/biopsy procedure along with their description and Nurse responsibilities are shown in following tables.
- Test performed to Blood Specimen – Table 23.16
- Tests performed on urine –Table 23.17
- Test performed on stool –Table 23.18
- Radiological studies –Table 23.19
- Magnetic resonance Imaging –Table 23.20
- Nuclear scan –Table 23.21
- Electro diagnostic studies –Table 23.22
- Endoscopic procedures –Table 23.23
- Aspiration/Biopsy procedure –Table 23.24
- Other tests –Table 23.25

The important points to be kept in mind during diagnostic examination of client include the following:
- Most invasive procedures require that the client give written informed consent
- Prepare clients for diagnostic testing by ensuring client under–standing and compliance with preprocedural requirements.
- Clients, families, and significant others must be involved in the testing process; advise them of the estimated procedure time
- To help offset the discomfort and anxiety experienced during procedures, teach the client how to perform relaxation techniques such as imagery
- After a diagnostic test, provide care and teach the client those things to expect, including the outcomes or side effects of the test
- The nurse facilitates the scheduling of diagnostic tests, performs client teaching, performs or assists with procedures and assess clients for adverse responses
- Schedule diagnostic procedures to promote client comfort and cost containment
- Standard precautions are used when obtaining a specimen or assisting with an invasive procedure
- Before a procedure, obtain baseline vital signs and assess the clients preparation for testing
- After a procedure, assess the client for secondary procedural complications and perform any necessary nursing interventions.

	Table 23.16: Tests Performed on Blood Specimen	
Test	*Description*	*Nursing responsibilities*
Red blood cells (RBCs)	Number of RBCs per mm^3 of blood. May be low in clients with rheumatoid arthritis. Clients living in high attitudes may have an elevated RBC level. Normal: Male: 4.6-6.2 million/mm^3 Female: 4.2-5.5 million/mm^3	The client is not required to fast for the test.
White blood cells (WBCs)	Number of WBCs per mm^3 of blood. Elevation is associated with infectious processes. Normal: 4100-10,800 mm^3	The client is not required to fast for the test. Exercise, stress, labor, previous splenectomy, and eating may increase level and alter differential values. Note medications taken that may affect test; aspirin, heparin, and steroids may increase WBC level, whereas antibiotics and diuretics may decrease WBC level.
Differential count	Percentage of types of WBCs in 1 mm of blood.	The client is not required to fast for the test.
Neutrophils	Increase in bacterial infections and trauma. Normal:	
Segs (mature neutrophils)	Segs: 50%-65%	
Bands (immature neutrophils)	Bands: 0%-5%	
Eosinophils	Increased in allergic reactions or parasitic infestation. Normal: 1%-3%	Corticosteroid therapy causes a decreased level.
Basophils	Increased in allergic reactions and during healing periods. Normal: 0.4%-1.0%	Steroids cause a decreased level.
Lymphocytes	Increased in viral infections and other diseases, such as pertussis and tuberculosis (TB). Decreased in acquired immunodeficiency syndrome (AIDS). Normal: 25%-35%	Steroids cause a decreased level.
Monocytes	Increased in chronic diseases, such as malaria, TB, Rocky Mountain spotted fever. May be low in clients with rheumatoid arthritis. Normal: 4% - 6 %	
Hemoglobin (Hgb)	Measures the oxygen-carrying compound in RBCs. Normal: Male: 14-18 g/Dl Female: 12-16 g/dL Critical value: <5 g/dL	The client is not required to fast for the test. Sample may be drawn from a finger of a child or the heel of an infant.
Hemoglobin electrophoresis	Detects abnormal forms of hemoglobin. Performed after positive sickle cell test. If the hemoglobin electrophoresis is negative, the client has the sickle cell trait. If the hemoglobin electrophoresis is positive, the client has sickle cell anemia. Normal: Hgb S: 0% Hgb F: <2% Hgb Ca: 0%	If the client has had a blood transfusion within the last 12 weeks, the results of the test may be altered.

Contd...

<table>
<tr><td colspan="3" align="center">Table 23.16: Contd...</td></tr>
<tr><td align="center">Test</td><td align="center">Description</td><td align="center">Nursing responsibilities</td></tr>
<tr><td>Hematocrit (Hct)</td><td>Measures the percentage of blood cells in a volume of blood. Clients living in high altitudes may have an increased level.
Normal:
    Male: 40%-54%
    Female: 38%-47%
    Critical value: <15% or >60%</td><td>The client is not required to fast for the test.</td></tr>
<tr><td>Platelet count</td><td>Measures the number of platelet per cubic milliliter of blood.
Normal: 150,000-450,000/mm^3</td><td>Instruct the client that strenuous exercise and oral contraceptives increase platelet level.
Instruct the client that aspirin, acetaminophen, and sulfonamides decrease platelet level.</td></tr>
<tr><td></td><td>Critical level: <50,000 and >1 million/mm^3</td><td>If the client has a low platelet count, maintain digital pressure to the puncture site.</td></tr>
<tr><td>Bleeding time</td><td>Measures the length of the time for a platelet plug to occlude a small puncture wound.
Normal: 1-9 minutes (Ivy method)
Critical value: >15 minutes</td><td>Notify the laboratory if the client is taking aspirin, anticoagulants, or other medications that may affect the clotting process.</td></tr>
<tr><td>Prothrombin time (PT, protime)</td><td>Measures the effectiveness of several bloodclotting factors.</td><td>Ensure that the blood specimen is drawn before the daily dose of warfarin (Coumadin) is administered.</td></tr>
<tr><td></td><td>Normal: 10-13.4 seconds</td><td></td></tr>
<tr><td></td><td>INR: 2.0-3.0</td><td>Instruct the client that alcohol intake.</td></tr>
<tr><td></td><td>In the presence of anticoagulant therapy, the values should be 11/2-2 times the normal value.</td><td>May increase PT and that a diet high in fat may decrease PT.</td></tr>
<tr><td></td><td>Critical value: >20 seconds</td><td></td></tr>
<tr><td></td><td>In the presence of anticoagulant therapy, the critical value should be >3 times the normal critical value.</td><td>Note those medications taken that may affect results; salicylates, sulfonamides, and methyldopa (Aldomet), as these may increase PT, whereas digitalis and oral contraceptives decrease the level.</td></tr>
<tr><td></td><td></td><td>Instruct the client not to take any medication without notifying the physician, as medications may affect the PT level.</td></tr>
<tr><td>International normalized ratio (INR)</td><td>Normal: 2-3 (2.5-3.5 for the client with a mechanical prosthetic heart valve).
The INR is more accurate than PT in monitoring warfarin (Coumadin) therapy.</td><td>The daily warfarin (Coumadin) dose should be given after blood has been drawn for the INR.</td></tr>
<tr><td>Partial thromboplastin time (PTT), also called activated partial thromboplastin time (APTT)</td><td>Normal:
  PTT: 60-70 sec
  APTT: 21-35 sec
In the presence of anticoagulant therapy, the normal value is 1.5-2.5 times the control value.</td><td>If the client is receiving intermittent heparin doses, schedule the APTT to be drawn 30-60 minutes before the next heparin dose.
If heparin is given continuously, the blood specimen can be drawn at any time.</td></tr>
<tr><td></td><td>Critical value:</td><td>If PTT is greater than 100 seconds, the client is at risk for bleeding, and the physician is notified.</td></tr>
<tr><td></td><td>APTT: >70 seconds</td><td>The antidote for heparin is protamine sulfate.</td></tr>
</table>

Contd...

Table 23.16: *Contd...*

Test	Description	Nursing responsibilities
	PTT:> 100 seconds	Note whether the client is taking antihistamines, vitamin C, or salicylates, as these prolong PTT time.
D dimmer test (fragment D dimmer, fibrin	Measures a fibrin split product that is released when a clot breaks.	Note whether the client is on thrombolytic therapy, as the results of this test would be increased from negative to positive.
Degradation fragment	Confirms the diagnosis of disseminated intravascular coagulation (DIC). Normal: <10 mg/mL	
Acid phosphatase	Acid phosphatase is an enzyme found in the prostate gland, seminal fluid, and RBCs. An elevated level is seen in clients with prostatic cancer and hemolytic anemias. If tumors are treated successfully, the level will decrease. A rising level may indicate a poor prognosis. Normal: 0-0.80 U/L	Tell the client that no food or drink restrictions are associated with this test. Apply pressure to the venipuncture site. Observe the site for bleeding. Used in rape investigations.
Adrenocorticotropic hormone (ACTH), corticotropin	Determines the function of the anterior pituitary. Because of diurnal variation, specimens should be drawn in both morning and evening. Normal: 4-22 pmol/L	Emotional or physical stress or recent radioisotope scans can interfere with test results. Drugs that may increase ACTH level include corticosteroids, estrogens, ethanol, and spironolactone. Explain the procedure to the client. This is especially important to decrease the client's stress level. Evaluate the client for increased stress level. Initiate NPO status 12 hours before test. The blood specimen must be drawn with a heparinized syringe, chilled by placing the specimen on ice, and immediately transported to the lab.
ACTH stimulation test, cortisol stimulation test, cosyntropin test	Monitors plasma cortisol level to indicate adrenal gland response to ACTH. Normal: 1 hour: ? 20 µg/dL at least above baseline	Note those medications taken that may affect results: cortisone, estrogens, hydrocortisone, and spironolactone may increase plasma cortisol level. Explain the procedure to the client. Initiate NPO status after midnight. For all tests, obtain baseline serum cortisol level. Administer injection of cosyntropin IM or IV. Draw blood specimen 30 to 60 minutes after injection.
Alanine aminotrasferase (ALT, formerly serum glutamic pyruvic transaminase [SGPT]	ALT is an enzyme released in response to liver injury. Normal: varies with testing methods	Note those medications taken that affect results: many medications may increase level, including antibiotics, narcotics, oral contraceptives, and many others.
Alkaline phosphatase (ALP)	Alkaline phosphatase is an enzyme found primarily in the liver, biliary tract, and bone. Detection is important for determining possible liver and bone disease. Normal: varies widely depending on method	Fasting may be required. Apply pressure to the venipuncture site. Observe the site for bleeding.
Alpha-fetoprotein (AFP)	Test for tumor marker; elevated in nonseminomatous testicular cancer. Performed between 16 and 18 weeks of pregnancy. A high level is suggestive of neural tube defects. Normal: 0.9ng/mL 16-18 weeks gestation: 30-43 µg/mL	Apply pressure to site and watch for bleeding or hematoma. Sample must be drawn between 15-20 weeks of gestation.

Contd...

Table 23.16: *Contd...*

Test	Description	Nursing responsibilities
Amylase (AMS)	Amylase is an enzyme secreted by the pancreas. Elevation indicates pancreatitis. Normal: 25-125 IU/L	Note those medications taken that affect test results; steroids, aspirin, alcohol, some narcotics, some diuretics, and other drugs may increase level, whereas citrate, glucose, and oxalates may decrease level.
Antidiuretic hormone (ADH), vasopressin	Determines the production of ADH by the posterior pituitary. Normal: <1.5 pg/L	Explain the procedure to the client. Note those medications taken that may interfere with test results. Drugs that elevate ADH level include acetaminophen, barbiturates, cholinergic agents, estrogen, nicotine, oral hypoglycemic agents, some diuretics such as thiazides, and tricyclic antidepressants. Drugs that decrease ADH level include alcohol, betaadrenergic agents, morphine antagonists, and phenytoin (Dilantin). Client should fast for 12 hours before the test. Evaluate the client for high level of physical or emotional stress.
Antinuclear antibodies (ANAs)	ANAs attack cell nuclei. The result is positive in 95% of clients with systemic lupus erythematosus. Levels are low in clients with mononucleosis, rheumatic fever, and liver diseases. Normal: negative at 1:20 dilution	Fasting is not required. Hydralazine (Apresoline) and procainamide (pronestyl) may increase level. A radioactive scan in the past week may alter results; inform the lab, if applicable.
Antistreptolysin O (ASO)	High titer indicates presence of *beta-hemolytic streptococcus,* which may cause rheumatic fever or acute glomerulonephritis. Upper limit of normal varies with age, season, and geographic area. Normal: Adult: <1:100 12-19 years: <1:200 2-5 years: <1:100	There are no food or fluid restrictions. Antibiotics decrease ASO level. Check urine output if ASO is elevated. Urine output of less than 600 mL/24 h is associated with acute glomerulonephritis.
Antithyroid microsomal antibody, antimicrosomal antibody, microsomal antibody, thyroid autoantibody, thyroid antimicrosomal antibody	Used to detect thyroid microsomal antibodies found in clients with Hashimoto's thyroiditis. Normal: titer <1 : 100	Explain the procedure to the client.
Aspartate aminotransferase (AST, formerly serum glutamic oxaloacetic transaminase [SGOT])	AST is an enzyme that indicates inflammation of heart, liver, skeletal muscle, pancreas, or kidneys. Normal: Male: 8-46 U/L Female: 7-31 U/L	Avoid intramuscular (IM) injections; record date and time of any injections. Avoid hemolysis. Withhold medications that affect results, for 12 hours if possible; several medications, such as antihypertensives, cholinergic agents, anticoagulants, digitalis, and others, may increase level, as may exercise.
Arterial blood gases (ABGs)	Direct measurement of the pH, PaO_2, and $PaCO_2$, and calculated measurement of HCO_3^- and SaO_2 from samples of arterial blood. pH = expresses the acidity or alkalinity of the blood.	Explain that an arterial sample of blood is required. Arterial punctures cause more discomfort than venous. Instruct the client not to move. Assess the adequacy of collateral circulation.
	PaO_2 = partial pressure of oxygen in the blood.	The blood sample is drawn in a syringe containing heparin.

Contd...

<table>
<tr><td colspan="3" align="center">**Table 23.16:** *Contd...*</td></tr>
<tr><td align="center">*Test*</td><td align="center">*Description*</td><td align="center">*Nursing responsibilities*</td></tr>
<tr><td></td><td>$PaCO_2$ = partial pressure of carbon dioxide in the blood.</td><td>After the specimen has been obtained, rotate the syringe to mix the blood and heparin.</td></tr>
<tr><td></td><td>SaO_2 = arterial oxygen saturation.</td><td>The blood sample is placed on ice and taken immediately to the lab.</td></tr>
<tr><td></td><td>HCO_3 = bicarbonate ion concentration in the blood.</td><td>Apply pressure to the arterial site for 3 to 5 minutes or 15 minutes if client is on an anticoagulant. Assess site for bleeding.</td></tr>
<tr><td></td><td>The oxygen content of the blood expressed as a percentage of the oxygen carrying capacity of the blood.
Normal: Critical Level:
pH : 7.35-7.45 <7.2 or >7.6
PaO_2: 75-100 mm Hg <40 mm Hg
$PaCO_2$: 35-45 mm Hg <20 or >70
HCO_3: 22-26 mEq <10 or >40
SaO_2: >95% (at sea level) <60%</td><td></td></tr>
<tr><td>Bilirubin</td><td>Measures bilirubin in the blood. Indicates how well the liver is functioning.
Normal:
Total: 0.1-1.3 mg/dL
Direct: 0.0-0.3 mg/dL
Indirect: 0.1-1.0 mg/dL</td><td>Note those medications taken that affect results; steroids, antibiotics, oral hypoglycemics, narcotics, as well as others may cause increased level, whereas barbiturates, caffeine, penicillins, and salicylates may cause decreased level.
Fasting may be required.
Do not shake the tube; protect the tube from light.</td></tr>
<tr><td>Blood glucose, fasting blood sugar (FBS)</td><td>Measures blood level of glucose (serum values). Results depend on method used by laboratory.
Normal: 70-110 mg/dL
Diabetic: = 126 mg/dL
Critical values:
>400 mg/dL
<50 mg/dL</td><td>Client must fast (except for water) for 12 hours before test. Withhold insulin or oral antidiabetic medications until blood is drawn.
Be certain client receives medications and meal after fasting specimen drawn.
Cortisone, thiazide, and loop diuretics cause increase.</td></tr>
<tr><td>2 hour post prandial glucose (2h PPG) or 2 hour post prandial blood sugar (2h PPBS)</td><td>Measures blood glucose 2 hours after a meal.
Normal: 70-140 mg/dL
Diabetic: >140 mg/dL</td><td>Instruct the client to eat entire meal and then to not eat anything else until blood is drawn.
Notify the laboratory of the time meal was completed.</td></tr>
<tr><td>Blood urea nitrogen (BUN)</td><td>Measures urea, end product of protein metabolism.
Normal: 5-20 mg/dL</td><td>Initiate NPO status 8 hours prior to test, if possible. Note the client's hydration status.
Note those medications taken that may affect results, including phenothiazines, nephrotoxic drugs, diuretics (hydrochlorothiazide [Hydro Diuril], ethacrynic acid [Edecrin], furosemide [Lasiz]); antibiotics (bacitracin, gentamicin, kanamycin, methicillin, neomyclin); antihypertensives (methyldopa [Aldomet], guanethidine [Ismelin]), sulfonamides, propranolol, morphine, lithium, salicylates.</td></tr>
<tr><td>CA – 15-3</td><td>CA – 15-3 (cancer antigen) is a tumor marker for monitoring breast cancer.
Because benign breast or ovarian disease can also cause elevations, it has limited use in diagnosis.
Normal: <22 U/mL</td><td>Fasting is not required.
Apply pressure to the venipuncture site.
Observe the site for bleeding.</td></tr>
</table>

Contd...

Table 23.16: *Contd...*

Test	Description	Nursing responsibilities
CA – 19-9	CA – 19-9 (cancer antigen) is a tumor marker used primarily in the diagnosis of pancreatic carcinoma. Normal: <37 U/mL	Fasting is not required. Apply pressure to the venipuncture site. Observe the site for bleeding.
CA – 125	CA – 125 (cancer antigen) is a tumor marker especially helpful in making the diagnosis of ovarian cancer. Normal: 0-35 U/mL	Fasting is not required. Apply pressure to the venipuncture site. Observe the site for bleeding.
Calcitonin, HCT, thyrocalcitonin	Determines thyroid and parathyroid activity. Also used as a tumor marker to detect thyroid cancer and several other cancer.	Note those medications taken that may increase calcitonin level, including calcium, cholecystokinin, epinephrine, glucagons, pentagastrin, and oral contraceptives. Explain the procedure to the client. The client should fast 8 hours but may have water.
Carcinoembryonic antigen (CEA)	CEA is found in clients with cancer, especially colorectal cancer. It is especially useful in monitoring treatment response and is occasionally the first sign of tumor recurrence. Normal: <5 ng/mL Smoker <2.5 ng/mL Nonsmoker	Fasting is not required. Apply pressure to the venipuncture site. Observe the site for bleeding. Note whether the client smokes or has a disease that will alter results, such as hepatitis, cirrhosis, or colitis.

Cardiac enzymes Serum AST	Indicates possible tissue damage if elevated.
	Normal:
	    Male: 7-21 U/L
	    Female: 6-18 U/L
		Neither fasting nor NPO status is necessary.
		Pattern of elevated levels of AST, CPK, and LDH is indicative of myocardial infarction (MI)

Creatine kinase CPK (CK)	Normal:
	    Male: 55-170 U/L
	    Female: 30-135 U/L
		CPK is the first enzyme elevated after MI, and peaks within the first 24 hours.

CK isoenzymes	Present in skeletal muscle, brain, lungs, and heart muscle. Normal:	Elevation of an isoenzyme indicates damage to tissue in a specific organ; CK-MB is specific for myocardial cells. Level increases 3-6 hours following myocardial infarction, peaks in 12-24 hours and returns to normal in 18-24 hours.
CK-MM (muscle)	100%	
CK-BB (brain)	0%	
CK-MB (heart)	0%	
Lactic dehydrogenase (LDH)	Normal: 45-90 U/L Critical Level: 300-800 U/L following myocardial infarction	LDH_1 value greater than LDH_2 value is indicative of an acute MI. LDH_5 is elevated with congestive heart failure (CHF).
LDH isoenzymes	LDH_1 (heart and erythrocytes)	17.5%-28.3%
	LDH_2 (reticuloendothelial system)	30.4%-36.4%
	LDH_3 (lungs and other tissues)	18.8%-26.0%
	LDH_4 (kidney, placenta, pancreas)	9.2%-16.5%
	LDH_5 (liver and striated muscles)	5.3%-13.4%

Contd...

<table>
<tr><td colspan="3" align="center">Table 23.16: Contd...</td></tr>
<tr><td align="center">Test</td><td align="center">Description</td><td align="center">Nursing responsibilities</td></tr>
<tr>
<td>Cardiac troponin I and T</td>
<td>Proteins found in cardiac muscle. Protein is released when the muscle is injured or dead.
Troponin I elevated level in 4-6 hours
Normal: <1.5 ng/mL
Troponin T elevated level in 1-3 hours
Normal: <0.6 ng/mL</td>
<td>Explain to client that blood sample is needed.
Test very expensive.
Often used in the ED.</td>
</tr>
<tr>
<td>CD4 T- cell count</td>
<td>Predictor of HIV progression; baseline taken after positive HIV test.
Normal: 500-1000/mm^3
Critical value: <200/mm^3</td>
<td>Explain the meaning of the test.
Provide follow-up explanation of test results.</td>
</tr>
<tr>
<td>Cholesterol (lipid profile)</td>
<td>Lipid necessary for steroid, bile, and cell membrane production.
Normal: <200 mg/dL (total)</td>
<td>Have client fast 12-14 hours prior to test.
No alcohol 24 hours prior to test. Diet intake 2 weeks prior to test will affect results. Note those medications taken that may affect results; steroids, phenytoin, diuretics, and others may elevate level, whereas MAO inhibitors, some antibiotics, lovastatin, and others may decrease level.
If elevated, increased risk of coronary artery disease (CAD), hypertension, and MI.</td>
</tr>
<tr>
<td>High density lipoprotein (HDL)</td>
<td>Normal: 30-70 mg/dL</td>
<td></td>
</tr>
<tr>
<td>Low density lipoprotein (LDL)</td>
<td>Normal: 60-160 mg/dL</td>
<td></td>
</tr>
<tr>
<td>Very low density lipoprotein (VLDL)</td>
<td>Normal: 25%-50%</td>
<td></td>
</tr>
<tr>
<td>Triglycerides</td>
<td>Normal: 40-150 mg/dL</td>
<td>Elevated level in CAD; level increases when LDL level increases.</td>
</tr>
<tr>
<td>Complement assay (total complement, C3 and C4)</td>
<td>Decreased levels in autoimmune diseases due to depletion of complement by antibody-antigen complexes.
Normal:
C3: Male: 80-180 mg/dL
Female: 76-120 mg/dL
C4: 15-45 mg/dL</td>
<td>Fasting is not required.</td>
</tr>
<tr>
<td>Coombs' test (direct antiglobulin test)</td>
<td>Detects whether immunoglobulins are attached to RBCs.
Normal: negative</td>
<td>Note whether the client is taking ampicillin (Unasyn), captopril (Capoten), indomethacin (Indocin), or insulin, as these cause false-positive results.</td>
</tr>
<tr>
<td>Cortisol, hydrocortisone</td>
<td>Determines adrenal cortex function. There is normally a diurnal variation, with higher level around 6 to 8 A.M. and lowest levels around midnight.
Normal:
8 A.M.: 6-28 µg/dL, or 170-625 nmol/L
4 P.M.: 2-12 µg/dL, or 80-413 nmol/L</td>
<td>Note whether the client has been under physical or emotional stress as either can artificially elevate plasma cortisol level. Likewise, recent use of radioisotopes can interfere with test results.
Note those medications taken that may affect results. Drugs that may increase plasma cortisol level include estrogen, oral contraceptives, and spironolactone (Aldactone). Drugs that may decrease plasma cortisol level include androgens and phenytoin (Dilantin)
Explain the procedure to the client.</td>
</tr>
</table>

Contd...

<table>
<tr><td colspan="3" align="center">Table 23.16: Contd...</td></tr>
<tr><td>Test</td><td>Description</td><td>Nursing responsibilities</td></tr>
<tr><td></td><td></td><td>Two specimens are drawn – one at 8 A.M. and another at 4 P.M. assess the client for physical or emotional stress and report to the physician.
Indicate times of collection on laboratory requisitions.</td></tr>
<tr><td>C-reactive protein test (CRP)</td><td>An abnormal protein appears in the blood of clients with an acute inflammatory process. Used to monitor the progress of clients with autoimmune disorders such as rheumatoid arthritis. More sensitive than erythrocyte sedimentation rate (ESR).
Normal: less than 6 mg/L</td><td>Fast, except for water, for 8 hours.
Note those medications that may affect results: non-steroidal anti-inflammatory drugs (NSAIDs), steroids, and salicylates may decrease level; oral contraceptives and intrauterine devices (IUDs) may increase level. Inform laboratory, if applicable.</td></tr>
<tr><td>Culture</td><td>Identifies pathogens in blood.
Normal: None</td><td>There are no food or fluid restrictions.</td></tr>
<tr><td>Dexamethasone suppression test (DST), prolonged/ rapid DST, cortisol suppression test (ACTH suppression test)</td><td>Monitors plasma cortisol level to measure adrenal gland function.
Normal: <5 mg/dL</td><td>Stress can interfere with test results.
Note those medications taken that may affect results, including barbiturates, estrogens, oral contraceptives, phenytoin (Dilantin) spironolactone, steroids, and tetracyclines.
Explain the procedure to the client.
Weigh the client for baseline weight.
Rapid test: Adminiter dexamethasone 1 mg orally at 11 P.M. with milk or antacid. Administer sedative, if ordered. At 8 A.M., before client rises, draw plasma cortisol level. Overnight 8-mg dexamethasone suppression test: if no cortisol suppression occurs, repeat test using 8 mg dexamethasone. If there is still no cortisol suppression, a prolonged test over 6 days involving six 24-hours urine collections should be done.</td></tr>
<tr><td>Electrolytes</td><td>Determines blood electrolyte levels.
First four are the most commonly measured.</td><td>Sodium and potassium are necessary for cardiac electrical conduction.</td></tr>
<tr><td>Sodium (Na$^+$)</td><td>Measures level of serum sodium.
Function in the body:
Majore electrolyte in extracellular fluid, regulates fluid balance, stimulates conduction of nerve impulses, helps maintain neuromuscular activity.
Normal: 135-145 mEq/L</td><td>There are no food or fluid restrictions.</td></tr>
<tr><td>Potassium (K$^+$)</td><td>Measures level of serum potassium.
Function in the body:
Major electrolyte in intracellular fluid, maintains normal nerve and muscle activity, assists in cellular metabolism of carbohydrates and proteins.
Normal: 3.5-5.5 mEq/L</td><td>There are no food or fluid restrictions.
If the client has hypokalemia or hyperkalemia, evaluate the client for cardiac dysrhythmias</td></tr>
<tr><td>Chloride (Cl$^-$)</td><td>Measures level of serum chloride
Function in the body:
Major electrolyte in extracellur fluid, functions in combination with sodium to maintain osmotic pressure, assists in maintaining acid-base balance
Normal: 100-110 mEq/L</td><td>There are no food or fluid restrictions.</td></tr>
</table>

Contd...

<table>
<tr><td colspan="3" align="center">Table 23.16: Contd...</td></tr>
<tr><td>Test</td><td>Description</td><td>Nursing responsibilities</td></tr>
<tr>
<td>Calcium, total/ionized Ca^{++}</td>
<td>Indicates parathyroid gland function and calcium metabolism. Because ionized calcium is unaffected by serum albumin, it can give more accurate results; however, most laboratories do not have the equipment to perform the test.
Normal:
Total: 8.5-10.5 mg/dL, or 2.25-2.75 nmol/L
Ionized: 4.5-5.6 ng/dL, or 1.05-1.30 nmol/L</td>
<td>Note those medications taken that may affect results. Drugs that may increase serum calcium salts, hydralazine, lithium, thiazide diuretics, parathyroid hormone (PTH), thyroid hormone, and vitamin D.
Drugs that may decrease serum calcium level include acetazolamide, anticonvulsants, asparaginase, aspirin, calcitonin, cisplatin, corticosteroids, heparin, laxatives, loop diuretics, magnesium salts, and oral contraceptives. Vitamin D and excessive milk ingestion can also interfere with test results.
Explain the procedure to the client.
Fasting is not required for serum calcium, but might be required if other blood chemistry tests are to be drawn.</td>
</tr>
<tr>
<td>Magnesium (Mg^{++})</td>
<td>Measures level of serum magnesium
Function in the body:
Combines with calcium and phosphorous in intracellular bone tissue, essential for neuromuscular contraction, synthesis of protein, and body temperature regulation
Normal: 1.6-2.6 mEq/L</td>
<td>There are no food or fluid restrictions.</td>
</tr>
<tr>
<td>Phosphate (PO_4^-)</td>
<td>Measures level of serum phosphate
Function in the body:
An essential intracellular electrolyte, exists in an inverse relationship with calcium
Normal: 3-4.5 mg/dL</td>
<td>Initiate NPO status after midnight.
Intravenous fluids containing glucose are sometimes discontinued several hours before the test.</td>
</tr>
<tr>
<td>Bicarbonate (HCO_3^-) (total carbon dioxide content or carbon dioxide capacity)</td>
<td>Always in a 20:1 ratio with carbonic acid.
Normal: venous 22-29 mEq/L
Arterial 21-28 mEq/L</td>
<td>There are no food or fluid restrictions.
Loss of gastric contents is the most common reason for increased level.</td>
</tr>
<tr>
<td>ELISA</td>
<td>Screening test used to indicate the presence of HIV
Normal : negative</td>
<td>Inform the client that if the first ELISA test is positive, a second ELISA will be drawn before confirmation is done with Western blot.
Provide pretest counseling. Obtain informed consent.
Provide or arrange for post-test counseling.</td>
</tr>
<tr>
<td>Erythrocyte sedimentation rate (ESR or sed rate test)</td>
<td>Measures, in mm, RBC descent in a normal saline solution after 1 hour. Level is increased in inflammatory, infectious, necrotic, or cancerous conditions, due to increased protein content in plasma. Used to monitor the course of therapy for clients with autoimmune diseases, such as rheumatoid arthritis.
Normal:
Male: 0-13 mm/hr
Female: 0-20 mm/hr</td>
<td>The test should be performed within 3 hours after the blood is drawn.
Menstruation or pregnancy may increase level.
Ethanbutal, quinine, aspirin, cortisone, and prednisone may alter results.</td>
</tr>
<tr>
<td>Folic acid (Folate level)</td>
<td>Measures folic acid level in the blood,
Normal: 5-20 ug/mL, or 14-34 mmol/L</td>
<td>Fasting is not required.
Instruct the client not to drink any alcoholic beverages before the test.
The test is drawn before folic acid medications are administered.
Note whether the client is taking phenytoin (Dilantin), primidone (Mysoline), methotrexate, antimalarial agents, or oral contraceptives as these cause decreased level.</td>
</tr>
</table>

Contd...

Table 23.16: *Contd...*

Test	Description	Nursing responsibilities
Follicle-stimulating hormone (FSH)	Determines anterior pituitary function. Usually measured with luteinizing hormone level. Normal: varies with phase of menstrual cycle Follicular: 5-20 mU/mL Midcycle peak: 15-30 mU/mL Luteal: 5-15 mU/mL Postmenopause: 50-100 mU/mL Male: 5-20 3U/mL	Note whether client is taking estrogen or progesterone, as these may decrease FSH level. Recent use of radioisotopes can also interfere with test results. Explain the procedure to the client. Indicate on the laboratory requisition the date of the last menstrual period (LMP) or that the client is postmenopausal. Indicate use of estrogen or progesterone on laboratory requisition. The client should be relaxed and recumbent for 30 minutes before the test.
Gamma-glutamyl transpeptidase (GGT or GGTP)	Enzyme that detects liver cell dysfunction. Normal: 5-38 IU/L	The client must fast for 8 hours prior to test. Note alcohol, dilantin, and Phenobarbital may elevate results, whereas oral contraceptives and clofibrate may decrease results.
Globulin	Key for antibody production. Indicates how well the liver is functioning. Normal: 2.3-3.5 g/dL	Note those medications taken that affect results (see albumin).
Glucose tolerance test (GTT)	Evaluates blood and urine glucose 30 minutes before, and 1, 2, and 3 hours after a standard glucose load. Normal: fasting 70-110 mg/dL 1 hr 160 mg/dL 1 hr 115 mg/dL 1 hr 70-110 mg/dL	The client must fast (except for water) for 6-8 hours prior to the test. Withhold drugs that interfere with results. After administration of glucose load, withhold all food. The client should drink water, however. Collect urine specimens at hourly periods. Administer meal and medications after test is completed.
Glycosylated hemoglobin (GHB)	Measures glycohemoglobin, evaluating average blood glucose level over 120 days. Normal: nondiabetic 3.5%-6% Good control: 7.5% or less Fair control: 7.6% - 8.9% Poor control: >9% or more	Fasting is not required. Blood can be drawn at any time.
Hepatitis B surface antigen (HB$_S$AG)	A positive result indicates presence of hepatitis or that the person is a carrier. Normal: negative	
Human chorionic gonadotropin (hCG)	Test for tumor market; elevated in germ cell testicular cancer. Normal: negative Female, pregnant: positive, peaks at 8-12 weeks then falls Female, abnormal pregnancy or choriocarcinoma: remains high or increases	Apply pressure to the site and observe for bleeding or hematoma.
Human leukocyte antigen DW4 (HLA-DW4)	Positive (present in 50% of clients with rheumatoid arthritis). Normal: negative	Fasting is not required.
Lupus erythematosus test (LE prep)	Positive in 70%-80% of clients with systemic lupus erythematosus. May be positive in clients with rheumatoid arthritis. Used to diagnose and monitor the course of treatment for clients with systemic lupus erhthematosus. Normal: negative	Fasting is not required. May be ordered daily for 3 days. Note whether the client is taking Apresoline, Pronestyl, oral contraceptives, quinidine, penicillin, Aldomet, tetracycline, isoniazid, or reserpine, as these may cause false-positive results.

Contd...

Table 23.16: *Contd...*

Test	Description	Nursing responsibilities
Luteinizing hormone (LH) assay	Determines anterior pituitary function. It can be used to determine whether ovulation has occurred. Can also determine whether gonadal insufficiency is primary or secondary. Normal: Males: 7-24 mU/mL Females: 6-30 mU/mL	Note whether the client is taking estrogen or progesterone, as these may decrease LH level. Recent use of radioisotopes can also interfere with test results. Explain the procedure to the client. Indicate on the laboratory requisition the date of the LMP or that the client is postmenopausal.
Parathyroid hormone (PTH), parathormone	Measures the quantity of PTH to determine hyperparathyroidism or whether hypercalcemia is caused by parathyroid glands. Normal: 10-60 pg/mL	Recent use of radioisotope can interfere with test results. Explain the procedure to the client. Initiate NPO status after midnight, except for water. Obtain morning blood specimen and indicate time of collection.
Phosphrous	Determines the level of phosphorus in the blood. Normal: 3.0-4.5 mg/dL, or 0.97-1.45 nmol/L	Laxatives or enemas containing sodium phosphate can increase serum phosphorus level. Note those medications taken that may affect results. Drugs that may increase serum phosphorus level include methicillin and excessive vitamin D. Recent carbohydrate ingestion including IV administration causes decreased serum phosphorus level, as do antacids and mannitol. Explain the procedure to the client. Initiate NPO status 12-14 hours before test. Discontinue IV fluids containing glucose for several hours before test, if possible.
Polymerase chain reaction (PCR)	Detects HIV-specific DNA (virus). Normal: negative	Explain the meaning of the test. Provide follow-up explanation of test results.
Progesterone assay	Determines ovulation and function of corpus luteum. Adrenal tumors can elevate level. Normal: Male: <100 ng/dL Female: midcycle: 300-2,400 ng/dL Pregnancy 7-13 weeks, 1,500-5,000 ng/dL 14+weeks 6,500-20,000 ng/dL	Recent use of radioisotopes or hemolysis resulting from rough handling of blood specimen can interfere with test results. Note those medications taken that may interfere with results, including estrogen and progesterone. Explain the procedure to the client. Indicate the date of LMP on the laboratory requisition.
Prolactin level (PRL)	Determines anterior pituitary secretion. Among the problems indicated by an elevated level are pituitary tumors or primary hypothyroidism. Normal: Female, or male: 0-20 ng/mL Pregnant: 20-400 ng/mL	Note those medications taken that may affect results. Drugs that may increase prolactin level include phenothiazines, oral contraceptives, reserpine, opiates, verapamil, histamine antagonists, monoamine oxidase (MAO) inhibitors, and antihistamines. Drugs that may decrease prolactin level include ergot alkaloid derivatives, clonidine, levodopa, and dopamine. Explain the procedure to the client. The blood specimen should be obtained in the morning and placed on ice if not taken immediately to the laboratory.
Prostate-specific antigen (PSA)	PSA is an antigen detected in all males; level increases with prostatic cancer. It is more sensitive and specific than the acid phosphatase. Normal: <4 ng/mL	Fasting is not required. Apply pressure to the venipuncture site. Observe the site for bleeding.

Contd...

Table 23.16: *Contd...*

Test	Description	Nursing responsibilities
Protein	Measures total protein in the blood. Normal: 6-8 g/dL	Note those medications taken that may affect results; steroids and hormones such as insulin, and growth hormones may increase level, whereas oral contraceptives and liver toxic drugs may decrease level.
Rennin assay, plasma rennin activity (PRA)	Measures the amount of rennin and is used as a screening procedure to detect essential or renal hypertension. When combined with plasma aldosterone level, determines adrenal cortex activity. Normal: Upright position, sodium depleted or restricted diet: 20-39 years: 2.9-24 ng/mL/h >40 years: 2.9-10.8 ng/mL/h Upright position, sodium repleted or normal diet: 20-39 years: 0.1-4.3 ng/mL/h >40 years: 0.1-3.0 ng/mL/h	Pregnancy, salt intake, or licorice ingestion can interfere with test results. Time of day (early in the day), a low-salt diet, or an upright position increases rennin value. Note those medications taken that may interfere with test, results, including antihypertensives, diuretics, estrogens, oral contraceptives, and vasodilators. Explain the procedure to the client. The client should maintain a normal diet with sodium restricted to 3 grams per day for 3 days before the test. Drugs and licorice should be discontinued for 2 to 4 weeks before the test. The client should stand or sit upright for 2 hours before blood is drawn. Client position, dietary status, time of day, and drugs should be recorded on the laboratory requisition. Blood specimen should be placed in ice and taken immediately to the laboratory. After blood specimen is obtained, the client may resume a normal diet and restart medications.
Rheumatoid factor (RF)	Abnormal protein in serum of approximately 80% of clients with rheumatoid arthritis. Formed as a result of the reaction of IgM to an abnormal IgG. Also elevated in clients with other autoimmune diseases such as systemic lupus erythematosus. Normal: negative	Fasting is preferred.
Serum acid phosphatase (prostatic) (ACP)	Serum measurement of prostatic acid phosphatase, elevated in malignancy; because it detects cancer in the later stages, no longer commonly used. Normal: 0.0-0.8 U/L	Apply pressure to the site. Observe the site for bleeding or hematoma.
Serum alkaline phosphatase (ALP)	Serum measurement of alkaline phosphates, elevated in malignancy. Normal: 30-120 U/L	Apply pressure to the site. Observe the site for bleeding or hematoma.
Serum creatinine	Specific indicator of renal disease. Normal: 0.4-1.5 mg/dL	Note those medications taken that may affect results, including amphotericin B, cephalosporins (cepfazolin [Ancef], cephalothin [Keflin]), methicillin, ascorbic acid, barbiturates, lithium carbonate, methyldopa (Aldomet), triamterene (Dyrenium).
Sickledex (sickle-cell test)	Screening test to determine the presence of Hgb S. Normal: no Hgb S If results are positive, a hemoglobin electrophoresis test is done.	There are no food or fluid restrictions. Note on the laboratory requisition whether the client had a blood transfusion in the past 3 to 4 months.
Thyroid-stimulating hormone (TSH), thyrotropin	Determines thyroid function as well as monitors exogenous thyroid replacement. Normal: 2-10 µU/mL, or 2-10 mU/L	Recent use of radioisotopes may affect test results. Severe illness may decrease TSH level. Drugs that may increase TSH level include antithyroid drugs, lithium, potassium iodide, and TSH injection.

Contd...

Table 23.16: *Contd...*

Test	Description	Nursing responsibilities
		Drugs that may decrease TSH level include aspirin, dopamine, heparin, steroids, and T_3. Explain the procedure to the client. The client should be relaxed and recumbent for 30 minutes before the test.
TSH stimulation test	Differentiates between primary and secondary hypothyroidism. Normal: none given	Explain the procedure to the client. Obtain baseline level of radioactive iodine intake or serum T4. Administer 5-10 units of TSH intramuscularly for 3 days. Repeat radioactive iodine intake or T4 as indicated for comparison studies.
Thyrotropin-releasing hormone (TRH) test, thyrotropin-releasing factor (TRF) test	Assesses the responsiveness of the anterior pituitary by its secretion of TSH in response to an IV injection of TRH. Also tests the function of the thyroid gland. Normal: undertectable to 15 µU/mL	Pregnancy may increase TSH response to TRH. Note those medications taken that may modify TSH response, including antithyroid drugs, aspirin, corticosteroids, estrogens, levodopa, and T_4. Explain the procedure to the client. Any thyroid preparations should be discontinued for 3-4 weeks before the test.
Thyroxine (T_4) Screen	Directly measures the amount of T_4 present. Normal: radioimmunoassay: 5-12 µg/dL, or 65-155 nmol/L	X-ray iodinated contrast studies may increase T_4 levels. Pregnancy will increase T_4 level. Note those medications taken that may affect results. Drugs that may increase T_4 level include clofibrate, estrogens, heroin, methadone, and oral contraceptives. Drugs that may decrease T_4 level include anabolic steroids, androgens, antithyroid drugs, lithium, phenytoin (Dilantin), and propranolol (Inderal). Explain the procedure to the client. Evaluate the clients drug history. If needed, instruct the client to stop exogenous T_4 medications for 1 month prior to test.
Thyroxine free, FTI, FT_4	Measures the amount of free T_4 that actually enters the cells and is active in metabolism. A true indicator of thyroid activity. Can be used to diagnose thyroid status in pregnant females or clients on drugs that can interfere with results of other tests. Normal: 280-480 pg/dL	Recent radionuclear scans can interfere with test results. Explain the procedure to the client. Blood specimens for T_4 and T_3 uptake must be obtained to calculate T_4.
Total iron-binding capacity (TIBC)	Determines the ability of iron to bind to a protein called transferring. Normal: 300-360 mg/dL	NPO 12 hours prior to the test. A recent blood transfusion or a diet high in iron may affect test results. Note whether the client is taking oral contraceptives, as these increase TIBC level.
Triglycerides	Form of fat produced in the liver. Normal: 30-150 mg/dL	Client to fast 12-14 hours prior to the test, and have no alcohol for 24 hours before. Diet of prior 2 weeks affects results.
Triiodothyronine (T_3) radioimmunoassay (T_3 by RIA)	Determines thyroid gland function Normal: 110-230 mg/dL, or 1.2-1.5 nmol/L	Radioisotope administration may interfere with test results. Pregnancy increases T_3 results. Note those medications taken that may affect results. Drugs that may increase T_3 level include: estrogen,

Contd...

Table 23.16: *Contd...*

Test	Description	Nursing responsibilities
		methadone, and oral contraceptives. Drugs that may decrease T_4 level include anabolic steroids, androgens, phenytoin (Dilantin), propranolol (Inderal), reserpine, and salicylates (high dose). Explain the procedure to the client. Determine whether exogenous T_3 is being taken. With physician's approval, withhold those drugs that would interfere with test results.
Triiodothyronine (T_3) serum free	Measures the amount of free T_3 that actually enters the cells and is active in metabolism. A true indicator of thyroid activity. Can be used to diagnose thyroid status in pregnant females or clients on drugs that can interfere with results of other tests. Normal: 0.2-0.6 ng/Dl	Explain the procedure to the client. Blood specimens for T_3 and T_4 uptake must be obtained to calculate T_3.
Uric acid	Elevated in gout. Normal: Male: 2.1-8.5 mg/dL Female: 2.0-8.0 mg/dL	There are no food or drink restrictions. Note those medications and other substances taken that may affect results, including ascorbic acid, diuretics, levadopa, allopurinol, and Coumadin.
ADRL (Venereal Disease Research Laboratory), RPR (rapid plasma regain), FTSABS (fluorescent treponemal antibody-absorption test), Reiter test, fluorescent antibody Treponema pallidum immobilization (TPI) test (performed only at Centers for Disease Control [CDC] in Atlanta)	Blood tests for presence of syphilis. Normal: negative or nonreactive	Explain the test to the client, including amount of blood to be drawn.
Western blot	Confirmatory test for the presence of antibodies to HIV. Normal: negative	Provide pretest counseling. Obtain informed consent. Provide or arrange post-test counseling.

<table>
<tr><th colspan="3" style="text-align:center">Table 23.17: Tests Performed on Urine</th></tr>
<tr><td>Test</td><td>Description</td><td>Nursing responsibilities</td></tr>
<tr><td>Urinalysis</td><td></td><td>Explain the procedure and purpose</td></tr>
<tr><td>Color</td><td>Clear amber</td><td>to the client and assist with specimen collection, if needed.</td></tr>
<tr><td>Odor</td><td>Pleasantly aromatic until left standing; offensive and unpleasant in kidney infection.</td><td>Ensure that specimen is taken to the laboratory in a timely manner.</td></tr>
<tr><td>pH</td><td>4.6-8.0</td><td></td></tr>
<tr><td>Specific gravity</td><td>1.015-1.030</td><td></td></tr>
<tr><td>Glucose</td><td>Negative</td><td></td></tr>
<tr><td>Acetone (ketone)</td><td>Negative</td><td></td></tr>
<tr><td>Casts</td><td>Rare</td><td></td></tr>
<tr><td>Albumin (protein)</td><td>Negative</td><td></td></tr>
<tr><td>RBCs</td><td>2-3/HPF</td><td></td></tr>
<tr><td>WBCs</td><td>4-5/HPF</td><td></td></tr>
<tr><td>Bilirubin</td><td>Negative</td><td></td></tr>
<tr><td>Bacteria</td><td>Negative</td><td></td></tr>
<tr><td>Aldosterone Assay</td><td>A blood test or 24-hours urine collection to evaluate the adrenal cortex, especially for tumors. The 24-hours urine is more reliable, but the blood specimen is more convenient.
Normal, blood:
Male: 6-22 ng/dL, or 0.17-0.61 nmol/L
Female: 5-30 ng/dL, or 0.14-0.80 nmol/L
Normal, urine: 2-80 µg/24 h, or 5.5-72.0 nmol/24 h</td><td>Strenuous exercise and stress can increase aldosterone level.
Excessive licorice ingestion can decrease aldosterone level.
Client should be upright (sitting or standing) for 4 hours before test.
Explain the procedure to the client.
The client should follow a normal diet with 3 grams of sodium/day and no licorice for at least 2 weeks before the test. Medications should be stopped for at least 2 weeks before the test, if possible.
Initiate 24-hours urine collection. Send collection to laboratory immediately upon conclusion.</td></tr>
<tr><td>Bence Jones Protein</td><td>Bence Jones proteins are immunoglobuins typically found in the urine of clients with multiple myeloma. They may also be associated with tumor metastases to the bone and chronic lymphocytic leukemia.
Normal: negative</td><td>Instruct the client for a clean catch or 24-hours urine specimen.
Instruct the client not to contaminate specimen with toilet paper or stool.</td></tr>
<tr><td>Creatinine clearance</td><td>Normal:
Male: 95-135 mL/min
Female: 85-125 mL/min
Minimum: 10 mL/min to maintain Life</td><td>Instruct the client about the 24-hours urine test.
Encourage hourly water intake. Keep urine on ice or in special refrigerator. Cephalosporins and vigorous exercise affect results.</td></tr>
<tr><td>17-hydroxycorticosteroids (17-OHCS)</td><td>24-hours urine test that measures adrenal cortex function.
Normal:
Male: 3-10 mg/24 h
Female: 2-6 mg/24 h</td><td>Emotional or physical stress or licorice ingestion may increase adrenal activity.
Note those medications taken that may affect results.
Drugs that may increase 17-OHCS level include acetazolamide, chloral hydrate, ascorbic acid, and erythromycin. Drugs that may decrease 17-OHCS level include estrogens, oral contraceptives, phenothiazines, and reserpine.
Explain the procedure to the client.
Initiate 24-hours urine collection.</td></tr>
</table>

Contd...

Table 23.17: *Contd...*		
Test	*Description*	*Nursing responsibilities*
		Send collection to laboratory immediately upon conclusion.
17-ketosteroids (17-KS)	24-hours urine test that measures adrenal cortex function. Normal: Male: 5-23 mg/24 h, or 24-88 μmol/24 h Female: 2-15 mg/24 h, or 14-52 μmol/24 h	Stress may increase adrenal activity. Note medications taken that may affect results. Drugs that increase 17-KS level include antibiotics and dexamethasone. Drugs that may decrease 17-KS level include estrogen and oral contraceptives. Explain the procedure to the client. With physician's approval, withhold all drugs for several days before test. Monitor client for stress and report to physician. Initiate 24-hours urine collection. Send collection to laboratory immediately upon conclusion.
Schilling test	Determines vitamin B_{12} absorption by the intestine. Differentiates between pernicious anemia and gastrointestinal malabsorption problems. Normal: 8%-40% of the radioactive vitamin B_{12} is excreted in the urine within 24 hours.	Collect the urine for a 24- to 48-hour period. Laxatives are not given during the test, as they decrease the absorption of vitamin B_{12}.
Urine cortisol, hydrocortisone	24-hours urine test that measures adrenal cortex function. Normal: 22-69 μmol/24 h, or 8-25 mg/ 24 h	Pregnancy or stress increases cortisol level. Recent radioisotope scans can interfere with test result. Note medications taken that may interfere with test result, including oral contraceptives and spironolactone. Explain the procedure to the client. Assess for stress and report to physician. Initiate 24-hours urine collection. Send collection to laboratory immediately upon conclusion.
Vanillylmandelic acid (VMA) and catecholamines (epinephrine, norepinephrine, metanephrine, normetanephrine, dopamine)	24-hours urine test that diagnoses pheochromocytoma and other adrenal tumors. Normal: VMA: 2-7 mg/24 h, or 10-34 μmol/24 h Epinephrine: 0.5-20.0 μg/24 h, or <275 nmol/24 h Norepinephrine: 15-80 μg/24 h Metanephrine: 24-96 μg/24 h Normetanephrine: 75-375 μg/24 h Dopamine: 65-400 μg/24 h	Certain foods (e.g., tea, coffee, cocoa, vanilla, chocolate), vigorous exercise, stress, or starvation may increase VMA level. Uremia, alkaline urine, or iodinated contrast dyes may falsely decrease VMA level. Note those medications taken that may affect results. Drugs that may increase VMA level include caffeine, epinephrine, levodopa, lithium, and nitroglycerine. Drugs that may decrease VMA level include clonidine, disulfiram (Antabuse), guanethidine, imipramine, MAO inhibitors, phenothiazines, and reserpine. Drugs that may increase catecholamine level include ethyl alcohol, aminophylline, caffeine, chloral hydrate, clonidine (chronic therapy), contrast media (iodine containing), disulfiram (Antabuse), epinephrine, erythromycin, insulin, methenamine, methyldopa, nicotinic acid (large doses), nitroglycerin, quinidine, riboflavin, and tetracyclines. Drugs that may decrease catecholamine level include guanethidine, reserpine, and salicylates. Explain the procedure to the client. The client should be on a VMA-restricted diet for 2-3 days before the test. Items restricted include coffee, tea, bananas, chocolate, cocoa, licorice, citrus fruit, anything with vanilla, and aspirin. Client should not take antihypertensive drugs before the test. Initiate 24-hours urine collection.

Table 23.18: Tests Performed on Stool

Test	Description	Nursing responsibilities
Stool occult blood (guaiac) Fecal occult test (FOBT) Hemoccult	Fecal occult blood screening studies may be utilized as possible indicators of colorectal cancer. Normal: negative for blood	Place a smear of stool on a card. Medications such as anticoagulants, aspirin, iron preparations, NSAIDs, and steroids may cause a false-positive result, whereas vitamin C may cause a false negative. Red meat should not be ingested for 3 days prior to the test. For premenopausal women, wait at least 4 days after menstrual period. Wear gloves when obtaining and handling the specimen.
Stool O & P (ova & parasite)	A positive result indicates infection. Normal: negative	Place the stool specimen in a container and take warm to the laboratory. Usually done 3 times.

Table 23.19: Radiologic Studies

Test	Description	Nursing responsibilities
Radiograph (X-ray)	Most common diagnostic study. Identifies traumatic disorders, i.e., fractures, dislocations, tumors, bone disorders, joint deformities, bone density, and changes in bone relationships. Performed by a technician.	Explain the procedure to the client. Prepare the client as ordered. No specific post procedure care is required. Administer an analgesic, especially for the arthritic client.
Abdominal X-rays	Determines diaphragm position and gas and fluid distribution in the abdomen.	No preparation is required.
Adrenal angiography, Adrenal arteriogram	Study of adrenal glands and arterial system after injection of radiopaque dye to detect benign or malignant tumors or hyperplasia of the adrenal glands. Normal: no growth or enlargement	Assess for allergy to shellfish or iodine; arteriosclerosis; pregnancy; or blood disorders, as they preclude the test. Explain the procedure to the client. Assess for allergies. Informed and written consent must be obtained before the procedure. Note whether client has been taking anticoagulants. Initiate NPO status after midnight. Mark peripheral pulses with a pen before the procedure. Inform the client that a warm flush may be felt when the dye is injected. Observe the puncture site. Monitor vital signs. Monitor peripheral pulses, color, and temperature of extremities. Institute bed rest for 12-24 hours. Apply cold compresses to puncture site, if needed. Force fluids to prevent possible dehydration from the dye.
Adrenal venography	Involves insertion of a catheter through the femoral vein and into the adrenal vein to withdraw a blood specimen to detect the function of each adrenal gland. A contrast dye is injected to visualize size and position of the adrenal glands. Normal: no growth or enlargement	Explain the procedure to the client. Assess for allergies. Obtain informed and written consent. Inform the client that a burning sensation may be experienced when the dye is injected. Although this study involves the venous system, monitor vital signs and injection site as well as pulses, temperature, and color of extremities.

Contd...

Table 23.19: *Contd....*

Test	Description	Nursing responsibilities
Arthrogram (-graphy)	Visualization of a joint. Radiopaque dye or air is injected into the joint cavity to outline soft tissue, usually on knee/shoulder joints. Local anesthetic and sterile technique are used. Performed by a physician; takes approximately 30 minutes. Normal: absence of lesions, fractures, or tears	Explain the procedure to the client. Obtain informed consent. Client wears an elastic bandage for several days; check for edema. Administer a mild analgesic for pain. Monitor for increased pain. Neither fasting nor sedation is required.
Barium enema	An enema of barium is given while X-rays are taken of the large intestine.	Intitiate NPO status the night before. Administer the ordered medication to clean the bowel. Observe the results of the laxatives, and inform the X-ray department if there have been no results. After the test, force oral fluids and administer a cleansing enema, as ordered. Document status of abdomen and stools.
Barium swallow	The client drinks a glass of barium while X-rays are taken of the esophagus and cardiac sphincter.	Initiate NPO status the evening before. Explain the procedure and the time frame for results. Encourage the client to drink fluids and eat fiber after the test. A laxative is sometimes given after the test. The client should be instructed that bowel movements will be white for 1-2 days. During the test, the client will be tilted on the X-ray table in various positions. There may be repeated pictures taken at ½-hour intervals as the barium moves through the bowel. Document the client's tolerance of the procedure and passage of the barium. Because the procedure can be lengthy, encourage the client to take reading material.
Cardiac catheterization (cardiac angiogram, coronary arteriogram)	A catheter is passed into the right and/or left side of the heart to determine oxygen level, cardiac output, and pressure within the heart chambers.	Assess the client for allergy to iodine or shellfish. The client is to fast for 6 hours prior to the test, but medications can be taken with sips of water. Inform the client of the possibility of feeling warm or flushed during the test. After the procedure, assess the peripheral pulses every 15 minutes for 2-4 hours, or according to physician's orders. Assess color, temperature, and pulse in the extremity below the catheter insertion site. Instruct the client to keep the involved extremity straight for 6-8 hours.
Chest X-ray	Provides a two-dimensional image of the lungs without using contrast media. Used to detect the presence of fluid within the interstitial lung tissue or the alveoli; tumors or foreign bodies; and the presence and size of a pneumothorax. The size of the heart can also be determined by chest X-ray.	Explain the test to the client. If appropriate, inquire whether the client may be pregnant, to prevent exposure of the fetus to X-ray. The client is generally required to stand for various views; if the client is unable to stand, views may be obtained with the client in a sitting position, or a portable X-ray may be obtained. Instruct the client to inspire deeply and hold the breath. Instruct the client to remove all metal objects from the chest and neck area and to don a hospital gown that does not have snap closures.

Contd...

Table 23.19: Contd....

Test	Description	Nursing responsibilities
Conduitogram	Radiopaque dye is injected through a catheter into either the conduit or a piece of ileum to assess by means of X-ray the length and emptying ability of the conduit as well as the presence of stricture or obstruction.	A conduit is a connection between the bladder or pouch and the outside of the body. Explain the procedure to the client. Assess the client for allergies to iodine-based dye.
Fistula gram	Radiopaque dye is injected through a catheter into either the conduit or a piece of ileum to assess by means of X-ray the length and emptying ability of the conduit as well as the presence of stricture or obstruction.	Initiate NPO status as ordered. Explain the procedure and the time frame for the results and identify the person who will give the client the results.
Fluoresce in angiography	Radiopaque dye or barium is given to drink, and X-rays are taken as the dye or barium passes through the gastrointestinal tract. The dye shows the location of the fistula and how it is connected to the gastrointestinal tract.	Instill eye drops to dilate the pupils. Start an IV so the sodium fluorescein can be injected. Remove the IV following completion of the test. Inform the client that skin and urine may be yellow for 24-48 hours.
Gallbladder series	X-ray visualization of the gallbladder.	Administer dye tablets the evening before the test. Provide a low-fat or fat-free meal the evening before. Initiate NPO status except for water after taking the dye.
Hysterosalpingogram	Radiopaque dye is instilled through the cervix. Used to diagnose uterine cavity and tubal abnormalities. Performed as a part of an infertility workup.	Explain the procedure and prepare the client in the lithotomy position. The test is done in the radiology department. Inquire about allergies to iodine or other dyes. Assist the physician.
Intravenous pyelogram (IVP)	Infusion of radiopaque dye into a vein, allowing visualization of the urinary system. The renal pelvis, ureters, and bladder can be seen. If BUN is over 40 mg/dL, the test may not be performed.	Explain the procedure to the client. Explain that client will experience a warm feeling during dye injection. Ask the client about allergy to iodine or shellfish. Serve a light supper, then initiate NPO status overnight. Administer a laxative or enema. Schedule test before barium studies. Post-test, observe for untoward reaction to dye. Encourage fluids for 24 hours to eliminate dye.
Kidney-ureter-bladder X-ray (KUB)	Shows abnormalities such as calculi, tumors, or changes in anatomic position.	Explain the procedure to the client. No preparation is required.
Long bone X-rays	Serial X-rays of the long bones to determine bone growth.	Explain the procedure to the client. Instruct the client to keep extremities still while the X-ray is being taken. Shield ovaries, testes, or pregnant uterus. Remove all metallic objects from area being X-rayed.
Lymphangiogram	A contrast dye is injected into the lymph vessels in the hands or feet to examine the lymph vessels and nodes. Used to stage lymphomas and evaluate the effectiveness of chemotherapy and radiation therapy. Normal: Normal-sized lymph nodes with no malignant cells	The dye remains in the lymph nodes for 6 months to 1 year, so disease progress can be evaluated with an X-ray. Obtain informed consent. Inform the client that if a blue-colored dye is used, the skin and urine may have a bluish discoloration. Assess the client's breath sounds after the procedure, as lipoid pneumonia is a possible complication if the dye gets into the thoracic duct.

Contd...

Table 23.19: *Contd....*

Test	Description	Nursing responsibilities
Mammography	Used to diagnose benign and malignant disorders of the breast.	Explain the procedure to the client. The breast will be compressed, possibly causing discomfort for several seconds. Explain that it is important to have a baseline mammogram done between the ages of 35 and 40 and a breast examination done by a physician or nurse practitioner every 3-4 years. For women ages 40-49, a mammogram should be performed every 1-2 years; for those over 50, an annual mammogram is recommended along with an annual breast examination by physician or nurse practitioner.
Myelogram	X-ray of spinal subarachnoid space following injection of an opaque medium.	Follow Nursing responsibilities for lumbar puncture in Table 25-14. Inform the client that the table may be tilted during the procedure. Obtain informed consent according to facility guidelines. Withhold the meal prior to procedure. Administer a light sedative, if ordered. Post-procedure care is determined by the type of medium used; follow physician's orders for activity and fluids.
Pouchogram	Installation of radiopaque dye into the Kock or Indiana pouch. Done with the continent ostomies to determine the state of healing and size of the pouch created.	Assess the client for allergy to iodine. Explain the procedure to the client.
Pulmonary angiography	Assesses the arterial circulation of the lungs. Most often used to detect pulmonary emboli.	Explain the procedure to the client. Assess for allergy to iodine or shellfish. Inform the client that an arterial puncture is required, usually of the femoral artery, and that injection of the dye may cause a flushing or warm sensation due to vasodilation. After the study, assess the arterial puncture site frequently for evidence of bleeding. Assess vital signs and respiratory status. The client may be required to lie flat for up to 6 hours if the femoral artery is used for access. Obtain informed consent per facility policy.
Renal angiography	A catheter is inserted into the femoral artery and threaded into the renal artery. Dye is injected to show blood vessels in the kidney.	Initiate NPO status; administer enema. Assess client for allergy to iodine or shellfish. Check vital signs and peripheral pulses. Institute post-test bed-rest, with leg straight. Monitor vital signs, peripheral pulses, urine output, and puncture site.
Voiding cystourethrography	The bladder is filled with dye, and X-rays are taken to observe bladder filling and emptying. Detects structural abnormalities of the bladder and urethra and reflux into the ureters.	Administer enema. Insert a Foley catheter and inject dye into bladder while X-rays are taken. Remove catheter and ask the client to void while more X-rays are taken. Allow the client to express feelings, as this test may be embarrassing.
Computed tomography (CT) scan	Provides a three-dimensional cross-sectional view of tissues. Computer-constructed picture interprets densities of various tissues. Most useful for viewing tumors in the chest, abdominal cavity, and brain.	Explain the procedure to the client. Obtain informed consent. Remove wigs and hairpins and clips for head CT. Initiate NPO status 8 hours prior to scan.

Contd...

Table 23.19: *Contd....*

Test	Description	Nursing responsibilities
Cardiac positron emission tomography (PET) scan	Radioactive tracers are injected intravenously prior to the test. Nuclear imaging is used to confirm tissue that has adequate blood supply and tissue that has become impaired due to a lack of blood.	Instruct the client not to have caffeine, alcohol, or smoke for 24 hours prior to the test. Initiate NPO status from 10 P.M. the evening before the test, except for medications and water. Obtain informed written consent. Encourage the client to drink fluids after the procedure to facilitate faster excretion of the radioactive material.
Orbital CT scan	Allows visualization of abnormalities not readily seen on standard X-rays, delineating size, position, and relationship to adjoining structures. The orbital CT is a series of images reconstructed by a computer and displayed as anatomic slices on an oscilloscope. It identifies space-occupying lesions earlier and more accurately than do other X-ray techniques. It also provides three-dimensional images of orbital structures, especially the ocular muscles and optic nerve. The enhancement with a contrast agent may help define ocular tissue and circulation abnormalities.	Explain the test and the procedure to the client: that the client is positioned on an X-ray table; that the head of the table is moved into the scanner; that the scanner rotates during the test and may make loud, crackling sounds; that if an IV contrast agent is required, the client may feel flushed and warm or experience a transient headache; and that salty taste, nausea, and vomiting may occur following injection of the IV contrast dye. Reassure the client that the reaction is common and she may signal the technician if she is unable to tolerate the test.
Ultrasound	High-frequency ultrasound waves are sent into the body, and echoes are recorded as they strike tissues of different densities, producing an image or photograph. Useful in distinguishing between cystic and solid masses. Most often used to assess the pelvis, heart, and abdomen. Diagnostic for cysts, tumors, pregnancy, fetal gestational age, and multiple gestation.	Explain the procedure to the client. Most ultrasound tests require no special preparation: Pelvic sonogram: Instruct the client to have a full bladder. Abdominal sonogram: Initiate NPO status at bedtime; prepare bowel as directed. Gallbladder sonogram: Initiate NPO status for 12 hours and institute a fat-free diet the evening before the test. Vaginal sonogram: Client does not need to have a full bladder.
Doppler ultrasound	Determines patency of veins and arteries in conditions such as arterial occlusive disease, arteriodclerotic disease, or Raynaud's disease. Normal: audible "swishing" sound of the Doppler when placed over vessel A Doppler unit with blood pressure cuffs can measure the pulse volume of arteries and veins. An AB index is obtained by dividing the blood pressure reading in the ankle by the blood pressure reading in the arm (brachial artery). This is known as the ankle-to-brachial arterial blood pressure. There should be a less than 20 mm Hg difference between the pressure in the lower extremity as compared to the pressure in the upper extremity. Normal, AB index: 0.85 or greater	Inform the client that the procedure is painless. Remove clothing from the extremity being evaluated. Instruct the client not to smoke for 30 minutes prior to the test, because nicotine causes vasoconstriction of the vessels Remove conductive or acoustic gel from the skin after the test is completed.
Echocardiogram	An ultrasound of the heart to determine hypertrophies, cardiomyopathies, or congenital defects. Very helpful in diagnosing valve abnormalities and pericardial effusion.	Explain the procedure to the client and assure the client that there is no discomfort during the procedure, although some pressure may be felt on the chest wall from the transducer.

Contd...

Table 23.19: *Contd....*

Test	Description	Nursing responsibilities
Thyroid ultrasound	Detects the size, shape, and position of the thyroid gland.	Explain the procedure to the client: that the client will lie supine, with the neck hyperextended; that breathing or swallowing will not be affected by the sound ttransducer; that a liberal amount of lubricating gel will be placed on the neck for the transducer; and that a series of photos will be taken over a 15-minute period. Assist the client in removing the lubricant.
Transrectal bladder ultrasound	Produces an image of the prostate or bladder and surrounding tissue.	Explain the procedure to the client.

Table 23.20: Magnetic Resonance Imaging

Test	Description	Nursing responsibilities
Magnetic Resonance Imaging (MRI)	Uses magnetic field and radio waves to detect edema, hemorrhage, blood flow, infarcts, tumors, infections, aneurysms, demyelinating disease, muscular disease, skeletal abnormalities, intervertebral disk problems, and causes of spinal cord compression. Provides greater tissue discrimination than do chest X-ray or CT scans. Performed by qualified technologist. Takes approximately 1 hour.	Assess the client for the presence of metal objects within the body (i.e., shrapnel, cochlear implants, pacemakers). Explain the procedure to the client: the client will be required to lie still for up to 20 minutes at a time; the client will be placed within a scanning tunnel; sedation may be required if the client has claustrophobic tendencies; the magnet will make a loud thumping noise as images are obtained (provide earplugs as necessary). As the test may require up to 2 hours to perform, have the client void prior to entering the scanning tunnel. Obtain informed written consent, per facility policy.

Table 23.21: Nuclear Scans

Test	Description	Nursing responsibilities
Scan (radioisotope test)	A radioactive substance or isotope is taken up by the part of the body being examined. Organ sites most frequently studied are the liver, spleen, lungs, heart, urinary tract, thyroid, and brain. The radioactive substance is given orally or intravenously by nuclear medicine personnel.	Explain the procedure to the client: that the client must lie still for 30-60 minutes and that the machine makes clicking noise at times. For liver, spleen, lung, thyroid, and brain scans, no special preparation is required. For a heart scan, initiate NPO status the evening before. For a kidney scan, hydrate as ordered.
Radioactive iodine uptake (RAIU), iodine uptake test, [131]] uptake	Uses oral radioactive iodine to determine thyroid function by the thyroid's ability to trap and retain iodine. Normal: 2 hours: 4% -12% absorbed 6 hours: 6% -15% absorbed 24 hours: 8% -30% absorbed	The client who is allergic to iodine or shellfish or is pregnant should not have the test. Client should fast overnight. Drugs that decrease RAIU level include ACTH, antihistamines, saturated solution of potassium iodine, thyroid drugs, antithyroid drugs, and tolbutamide.
Radionuclide angiography (multiplegated radioisotope scan, multigated acquisition scanning, MUGA)	A radioisotope is injected to evaluate the function of the left ventricle. The ejection fraction (a comparison of the volume of blood pumped by the left ventricle to the total volume of blood left in the ventricle) is measured.	
Technetium pyrophosphate scanning	Important in diagnosing acute MIs, with the best accuracy obtained at 48 hours after the client experiences symptoms suggestive of an infarct. A tracer or radioisotope, which is injected intravenously, accumulates in the damaged or infracted tissue areas, called "hot spots."	Instruct the client not to smoke or consume caffeine or alcohol for 3 hours before the test. Inform the client that the test will take 45-60 minutes.
Ventilation-perfusion scan (lung scan)	Assesses ventilation and perfusion of the lungs. Most often used to detect the presence of pulmonary emboli.	Assess for allergy to iodine and shellfish. Explain the procedure to the client: that a radioactive contrast media will be introduced via an IV access and inhalation of radioactive gas and that the client will be required to hold the breath for short periods as images are obtained.

Table 23.22: Electrodiagnostic Studies

Test	Description	Nursing responsibilities
Electrocardiogram (EKG or ECG)	Exectrodes are placed on the skin to record wave patterns of the electrical conduction of the heart. Detects myocardial damage, rhythmic disturbances, and hyperkalemia.	Explain the procedure to the client. Inform the client that the test is painless.
Electroencephalogram (EEG)	Record of electrical activity generated in the brain and obtained through electrodes applied to the scalp or microelectrodes placed in brain tissue during surgery.	Withhold caffeine due to stimulant effect. Serve meal so that blood sugar will not be altered. Shampoo hair night before test. Explain the procedure to the client: that the test takes approximately 45 minutes to 2 hours; the procedure is painless; the client may be asked to open and close the eyes during the test and that there may be flashing lights or small electrical stimulations.
Electromyography (EMG)	Detects primary muscular disorders. A needle electrode is inserted into the muscle being examined. Measures electrical activity of skeletal muscle at rest and during voluntary muscle contraction.	Explain the procedure to the client. Obtain informed written consent. Instruct the client to refrain from consuming caffeine and smoking for 3 hours before the test. Assure client that the needle will not cause electrocution. Inform the client that there will be temporary discomfort when the needle electrode is inserted. Observe the site for hematoma or inflammation after the test. The procedure takes approximately 1 hour.
Electroretinogram (ERG)	A record of the changes in the retina's electric potential following stimulation by light. Clinically useful in some clients with retinal disease. Performed by placing a contact lens electrode on the anesthetized cornea. The electrical potential recorded on the cornea is identical to the response that would be obtained if the electrodes were placed directly on the surface of the retina.	Explain the test and procedure to the client.
Esophageal motility studies (manometry)	Evaluates muscle contractions and coordination by using a tube with transducers. Used as a diagnostic tool for disorders of the esophagus and lower esophageal sphincter (LES).	Initiate NPO status 6—8 hours prior to the test.
Holter monitor	A portable EKG monitors and records the electrical conduction of the heart for a period of 24 hours. The heart rhythm is compared to client activities.	Instruct the client to engage in normal daily activities and to keep a journal of symptoms experienced in performing these activities.
Stress test	An EKG taken as the client exercises. Evaluates the effects of exercise on the heart. Often, the client is asked to walk on a treadmill, the incline of which is elevated at various times throughout the test. Used frequently on clients who have CAD.	Explain the procedure to the client. Encourage the client to wear good walking shoes during the test.
Thallium test (myocardial perfusion scan)	A radioactive tracer (Thallium 201) is injected and accumulates in myocardial tissue that is well perfused. Accumulation is lessened in areas of myocardial tissue that are not well perfused, areas called "cold spots." The client may be asked to perform exercise, such as riding a bike, during the test to evaluate the perfusion of myocardial tissue during exercise.	Instruct the client to refrain from eating and drinking for 3 hours prior to the test.

Table 23.23: Endoscopic Procedures

Test	Description	Nursing responsibilities
Endoscopy	Permits visual examination of internal structures of the body using specially designed instruments. The observation may be done through a natural body opening or through a small incision. A biopsy of suspicious areas may then be done for further study.	Explain the procedure to the client. Initiate NPO status 8-10 hours before test, except for sigmoidoscopy, before which a liquid diet should be followed for several days prior to the examination. Administer a laxative and then a cleansing enema.
Arthroscopy	Endoscopic procedure for direct visualization of a joint. Done in an operating room under sterile conditions and local or general anesthesia.	Perform frequent neurovascular checks. Elevate the client's leg. Apply compression dressing. Administer analgesic for discomfort.
Bronchoscopy	Direct visual examination of the bronchi through a fiber optic scope. Used to remove foreign bodies, for aggressive pulmonary cleansing, and to obtain sputum and tissue specimens.	Obtain written informed consent per facility policy. Explain the procedure to the client: that the client must be NPO for at least 6 hours prior to the test; that, if ordered, preprocedure sedation is administered; that an IV access will be obtained and sedation given during the procedure via this route. Following the procedure, frequently assess vital signs and respiratory status. Assess the client for unusual amounts of bleeding. Inform the client that sputum may be blood tinged initially following the procedure. Maintain the client in a side-lying position until the gag reflex returns. Withhold all food and fluids until the client is fully awake and has a gag reflex.
Colonoscopy	Examination of the rectum, colon, cecum, and ileocecal valve.	Initiate sedation. Cleanse the bowel. Offer only clear liquids after cleansing. Initiate NPO status for 6-8 hours prior to the test. Inform the client that flatulence and cramping will be experienced after the test.
Cystoscopy	A cystoscope is passed through the urethra and into the bladder to examine the interior of the bladder for inflammation, stones, tumors, or congenital abnormalities. A biopsy may be performed, and small stones may be removed. Ureteral catheters may be inserted to obtain urine from each kidney. May require topical, spinal or general anesthesia.	Explain the procedure to the client. Obtain informed written consent. Check vital signs. Instruct in deep breathing, if general anesthesia is to be used. Allow a full liquid diet if topical anesthetic is to be used. Monitor I&O.
Endoscopic retrograde cholangiopancretogram (ERCP)	Examination of the common bile duct (CBD) and biliary and pancreatic systems following injection of dye. Sphincterotomy, stone crushing, and stone removal can be done.	Initiate sedation. X-ray is used in conjunction. Initiate NPO status 6-8 hours prior to examination. Inform the client that the test can last up to 2 hours.
Esophagogastro Duodenoscopy (EGD)	Examination of the esophagus, stomach, and duodenum. Biopsies can be taken, and dilations done.	Initiate sedation. Initiate NPO status 6-8 hours prior to the examination. Remove dentures and eye wear.
Flexible sigmoidoscopy	Examination of the sigmoid colon and rectum.	Sedation is optional. Administer enemas prior to examination. Inform the client to expect some flatulence and cramping after the examination.
Laparoscopy	Examination of the internal pelvic structures by direct visualization with a laparoscope. Usually performed under general anesthesia. Diagnostic for pelvic disorders and infertility problems.	Explain the procedure to the client. Prepare the client, conduct pre- and postoperative assessment, and institute interventions. Provide discharge instructions on activity and follow-up.

Table 23.24: Aspiration/Biopsy Procedures

Test	Description	Nursing responsibilities
Aspiration Procedures		
Arthrocentesis	Procedure to obtain fluid from a joint using strict sterile technique. The knee is anesthetized, the sterile needle is inserted into joint space, and synovial fluid is aspirated. Used to diagnose infections, crystal-induced arthritis, and synovitis, and to inject anti-inflammatory medications. Normal: RBCs, O;WBCs, 0-150/mm^3, neutrophils >25%	Explain the procedure to the client. Obtain written informed consent. Assess site for edema, pain. The client should fast if possible. Apply pressure dressing and ice.
Bone marrow aspiration	Evaluates how well the bone marrow is producing RBCs, WBCs, and platelets. Normal: adequate numbers of RBCs, WBCs, and platelets.	Obtain written informed consent. Inform the client that pressure will be felt when the physician aspirates the bone marrow. Assess the site for bleeding after the procedure is completed. Bed rest for 30 minutes.
Gastric acid stimulation	Determines the amount of hyfrochloric (HCI) acid in the stomach. If no HCI acid is present, that indicates parietal cells are malfunctioning. Parietal cells secrete the intrinsic factor that is essential for vitamin B$_{12}$ absorption. Used to diagnose pernicious anemia. Normal tube test: Basal acid output: 2-6 mEq/h Maximal acid output: 16-26 mEq/h Normal, tubeless test: presence of dye in urine (usually blue or blue-green in color)	If the client is having the tube test, initiate NPO status after midnight and instruct the client, not to smoke prior to the test. Inform the client that a nasogastric tube is inserted prior to the test so that gastric contents can be aspirated after the administration of pentagastrin. If the client is having the tubeless test, inform the client of the possibility of a blue or bluegreen discoloration of urine. Note any medications taken that affect results; antacids, anticholinergics, and cimetidine (Tagamet) decrease HCI level, whereas adrenergic-blocking agents, cholinergics, sterioids, and alcohol elevate HCI level.
Lumbar puncture (LP) (spinal tap)	A needle is inserted into the subarachnoid space to measure CSF pressure and/or to obtain a specimen. Normal pressure: 60-180 mm water pressure Normal specific gravity: 1.007 Normal glucose: 45-100 mg/100mL Normal complete blood count (CBC): 0 Normal WBC: 0-5 cells/mm^3	Obtain informed written consent. Have the client empty the bowel and bladder prior to procedure. Assist in setting up a sterile field and pouring solutions, if not included in the tray. Assist the client to maintain the position. Postprocedure, deliver the specimen to the lab for testing, keep the client flat in bed for 3-24 hours or as ordered by physician; encourage fluid intake to replace fluids lost; and monitor vital and neurological signs.
Paracentesis	Fluid is removed from the pericardial sac for analysis or to relieve pressure.	Obtain written informed consent. Position the client in the semi-Fowler's position during the procedure and attach to an EKG monitor. Postprocedure, take vital signs every 15 minutes and monitor EKG rhythm.
Thoracentesis	Removal of fluid for diagnostic purposes. May also obtain biopsy, instill medications, and remove fluid for client comfort and safety.	Explain the procedure to the client. Obtain written informed consent. Position the client in an upright sitting position, leaning forward.

Contd...

Table 23.24: *Contd....*

Test	Description	Nursing responsibilities
		Have client rest the arms on an overbed table to facilitate this position. Explain to the client that the area will be anesthetized prior to the procedure. Instruct the client to hold as still as possible during the insertion of the thoracentesis needle. Assist the physician during the procedure. Deliver the specimen to the laboratory as soon as possible. Observe the thoracentesis site for bleeding following the procedure. Assess breath sounds before and after the procedure. Report absent breath sounds immediately.
Biopsy procedures	Removal of sample tissue for microscopic study. Tissue may be quickly frozen or placed in formalin before it is chemically stained and thinly sliced for analysis. Frozen section analysis takes only a few minutes and is often completed while a client is still in surgery. The full biopsy analysis takes 24-48 hours to complete but is the most accurate means of establishing a cancer diagnosis. Tissue biopsy is essential to confirming the type of cancer, the amount of lymph node involvement, and whether the cancer was successfully removed.	Explain the procedure to the client. Follow the physician's orders and/or agency protocol for client preparation. Obtain informed written consent.
Breast biopsy	Performed with or without local or general anesthesia and by aspiration, needle biopsy, excision, or incision. Tissue or fluid is obtained and sent to pathology for examination and identification of abnormal cells. New method of obtaining breast biopsies may be done with the stereotactic mammography studies.	Explain the procedure to the client. Have the client undress down to the waist. Cleanse the biopsy region and shave the area, if needed. Drape the breast and adjacent skin. Provide emotional support prior to during, and following the procedure. Monitor vital signs. Apply a sterile dressing or bandage. Instruct the client in postbiopsy wound care.
Cardiac biopsy	Done during a cardiac catheterization. The tissue sample is taken from the apex or septum to determine toxicity related to drugs; inflammation; or rejection of a transplanted heart.	Preparation is the same as for Cardiac Catheterization (see Table 25-8). After the procedure, observe the client for symptoms of a perforation, such as chest pain, decreased blood pressure, or dyspnea.
Endometrial biopsy	Obtained with special biopsy instruments and used to diagnose endometrial tissue abnormalities.	Explain the procedure to the client. Prepare the tissue preservation agent and label and send the sample to pathology. Assist the client in relaxing during the procedure, to offset the discomfort/cramping she may experience.
Liver biopsy	Obtained by inserting a needle into the liver. May be done with ultrasound or CT scan to guide needle placement. Evaluates cirrhosis, cancer, and hepatitis.	Schedule H&H, PT, PTT, and platelet tests prior to the procedure. Instruct the client to refrain from using NSAIDs including aspirin for 1 week prior to the procedure. Prepare the site by scrubbing it with a surgical prep solution and draping with a sterile towel. Monitor for signs of hemorrhage post procedure by frequently monitoring vital signs and pain. Have the client lie on the right side. Support the biopsy site with a towel or bath blanket for 2 hours. Monitor the site for ecchymosis.

Contd...

	Table 23.24: *Contd....*	
Test	*Description*	*Nursing responsibilities*
Prostatic biopsy	Removal of a small piece of tissue for microscopic examination.	Monitor for and educate the client about signs and symptoms of hemorrhage, infection, and postprocedure pain.
Testicular biopsy	Determines presence of sperm and rules out vas deferens obstruction.	Monitor for and educate the client about signs and symptoms of infection or hemorrhage.
Thyroid biopsy	Excision of thyroid tissue for histological examination after noninvasive tests prove abnormal or inconclusive. Can be obtained through needle biopsy or open surgical biopsy under general anesthesia.	Explain the procedure to the client. Obtain informed written consent. Assess for allergies. Have coagulation blood studies done. Assess for bleeding and respiratory and swallowing difficulties after the test. To prevent undue strain on the biopsy site, instruct the client to put both hands behind the neck when sitting up. Warn the client that a sore throat is possible after the biopsy.

	Table 23.25: Other Tests	
Test	*Description*	*Nursing responsibilities*
Arterial plethysmography (pulse volume recorder)	Determinesarteriosclerotic disease in the upper extremities and occlusive disease in the lower extremities. Done by applying three blood pressure cuffs to an extremity. The cuffs are connected to a pulse volume recorder, which records the amplitude of each pulse wave. If there is a decrease in the amplitude of the pulse wave, an occlusion is in the artery proximal to the cuff. A decrease of 20 mm Hg of pressure indicates arterial occlusion. The test is not as reliable as arteriography but also does not have the risks associated with an arteriogram. Normal: normal arterial pulse waves	Explain to the client that the test is painless. Instruct the client to lie still during the test. Instruct the client not to smoke for 30 minutes prior to the test. Instruct the client to remove clothing from the extremity on which the test is to be done.
Audiometric testing	Evaluates both bone and air conduction and determines the degree of hearing loss. The client wears headphones, through which a series of tones is delivered at different frequencies. The client signals to the audiologist when the tones are audible. The results are recorded on an audiogram. The client is kept in a soundproof booth during the test.	Explain the procedure and its purpose to the client. Ensure that the client is not claustrophobic.
Brainstem auditoryevoked response (ErA abd BAER)	Detects hearing dysfunctions of the central nervous system and cochlear nerve (cranial nerve VII). Valuable for testing comatose clients, clients with neurological damage, and children. An altered appearance of the brainstem waveforms or a delay or loss of a waveform indicates an abnormality including a possible cochlear lesion or acoustic neuroma.	Explain the procedure and its purpose to the client particularly that the client will be in a darkened room and will have both electrodes attached to the head and earphones in place.
Caloric test	Assesses alteration in vestibular function. The client is placed in a supine or Fowler's position and each ear is irrigated with cold and then warm water.	Explain the procedure and its purpose to the client. Tell the client that nystagmus, vertigo, nausea, vomiting, and an unsteady gait represent a normal response. Stay with the client and have an emesis basin and tissues available.

Contd...

Table 23.25: *Contd....*

Test	Description	Nursing responsibilities
Color vision tests	Most common color vision tests use pseudo-isochromatic (seemingly the same color) plates comprising patterns of dots of the primary colors superimposed on backgrounds of randomly mixed colors. A client with normal vision can identify the patterns; and client with a color deficiency cannot distinguish between pattern and background.	Explain the test and procedure to the client.
Colposcopy	Direct visualization of the vagina and cervix through a high-powered microscope. Acetic acid is applied to the tissue to dehydrate the cells for improved visualization. Used to diagnose cervical dysplasia or carcinoma in situ of the cervix. Biopsies may be obtained as needed.	Explain the procedure and prepare the client in the dorsal lithotomy position. Assist with the procedure. Prepare biopsy specimens for pathological examination.
Culture and sensitivity (C&S)	Determines presence of microorganism and identifies the antibiotic that will kill or inhibit growth of microorganism. Drainage from infected lesions is obtained with a sterile swab and is incubated in order to identify the causative organism and to determine antibiotic sensitivity. Normal: negative for microorganism growth.	Ensure that the specimen has been obtained before initiating antibiotic therapy. Specimens should be taken to the laboratory within 30 minutes of being obtained.
Cytology	The study of cells and fluids obtained from various organs by scrapings, brushings, or needle aspiration. Cytologic smears, such as the Pap smear, are routinely done to study cells from the female genital tract. A cytological smear showing evidence of malignancy is followed by a biopsy to facilitate a more comprehensive diagnosis.	Explain the procedure to be used for obtaining cells and fluids for study. Follow agency protocol for client preparation.
Dark field examination of wart scrapings	Microscopic examination to differentiate genital warts from syphilis condylomata.	Take a careful client history. Examine the genital area carefully and provide scalpel and slide, if specimen is to be obtained. Explain the procedure thoroughly to the client.
Dilatation and curettage (D&C)	Surgical scraping of the endometrial lining, performed under general, epidural, or paracervical anesthesia and on an outpatient basis. Diagnostic or therapeutic for uterine bleeding disorders.	Explain the procedure to the client. Perform pre- and postoperative assessment and provide care. Provide discharge instructions related to activities and follow-up appointments.
Dynamic infusion cavernosometry and cavernosography (DICC)	Groups of diagnostic tests that measure neurovascular events of penile erection.	Perform baseline assessment, monitor during the procedure, and assess for postoperative complications; advise the client of possible discomfort related to the injection. Explain the procedure to the client. Assess for allergies. If preferred by the laboratory, initiate NPO status after midnight. Restrict iodine and thyroid preparations a week before test. Inform the client that radioactive iodine may be given orally or intravenously. Withhold food for 45-60 minutes after the iodine is given. Provide the client with a list of times to report to radiology. Tell the client that he will lie supine for test, which takes about 30 minutes, and that neither isolation nor specific urine precautions are necessary.

Contd...

Table 23.25: Contd....

Test	Description	Nursing responsibilities
Huhner test (postcoital test)	Performed in the office. The couple has intercourse 2 hours before the appointment. A sample of secretions is removed from the vagina and placed on a microscopic slide. The sperm are observed for number and motility in the cervical mucous. Normal: a minimum of 20 sperm per field that demonstrate good motility	Explain the procedure to the client and schedule it near client's normal ovulation. Prepare the client in the lithotomy position. Assist the physician or nurse practitioner with the procedure. Perform microscopic observations as directed.
Nocturnal tumescence penile monitoring	Various devices are attached to the penis at night to monitor swelling (turnescence).	Explain to the client that the test will require application of a device to the penis and that the device is to be worn while sleeping. Show the client the device and explain how to apply it.
Papnicolaou (Pap) smear	Cells are obtained from the external and internal cervical canal. Screening tool for premalignant and malignant cervical changes.	Explain the procedure. Have client empty bladder and undress. Position client in dorsal lithotomy position. Help client relax during procedure. Prepare microscopic slides for pathology. Instruct the client on the importance of having an annual Pap smear.
Past-point testing	Measures the ability or inability to accurately place a finger on some part of the body, usually the client's or examiner's face and fingers. For example, the examiner will instruct the client to close her eyes and touch her nose, then, with eyes open, touch the examiner's nose or the examiner's index finger.	Explain the procedure and its purpose to the client. Explain that it is painless and represents a helpful measure of vestibular function (coordination).
Patch testing	Allergens within occlusive patches are applied to normal skin (usually the upper back) for 48 hours. If the client is allergic to a specific allergen, an erythematous skin reaction will occur.	Clean and dry the skin where the patches are to be applied. Tell the client that the patches must be left in place for the full 48 hours.
Pelvic examination (recommended annually for women over 18 through menopause)	Performed by a physician or nurse practitioner. The external and internal pelvic structures are visualized, the pelvic organs are palpated via bi-manual examination, and the cervix is examined via a speculum. A Pap smear and rectovaginal exam are also performed, and cultures and wet smears may be obtained.	Explain the procedures to the client; prepare the client by having her void and undress; position the client on the examination table in a dorsal lithotomy position; help the client to relax during the examination, prepare slides and culture medium; obtain other supplies; and assist with the procedure.
Prostatic smears	Microscopic examination of prostatic secretions obtained via rectal massage performed by a physician.	Explain to the client that to obtain the specimen, the prostate must be massaged via the rectum and that this will cause some discomfort.
Pulmonary function tests (PFTs)	A group of studies used to evaluate ventilatory function. Measurements are obtained directly via spirometer or calculated from the results of spirometer measurements. Bronchodilators may be used during the study. Measurements included are: Tidal volume: the amount of air inhaled and exhaled in one breath: 500 mL at rest. Inspiratory reserve volume: the amount of air inspired at the end of a normal inspiration. Expiratory reserve volume: the amount of air expired following a normal expiration. Residual volume: the amount of air left in lungs after maximal expiration.	Explain the procedure to the client, PFTs should not be done within 1-2 hours after a meal. After the test, monitor respiratory status. Advise the client to avoid activity and to rest following the test, as fatigue may result.

Contd...

Table 23.25: *Contd....*

Test	Description	Nursing responsibilities
	Vital capacity: the total volume of air that can be expired after maximal inspiration. Total lung capacity: the total volume of air in the lungs when maximally inflated. Inspiratory capacity: the maximum amount of air that can be inspired after normal expiration. Forced vital capacity: the capacity of air exhaled forcefully and rapidly following maximal inspiration. Minute volume: the amount of air breathed per minute.	
Pulse oximetry	A noninvasive procedure. A transdermal clip is placed on a finger or earlobe to detect the arterial oxygen saturation (SaO_2). Normal:>95% (at sea level)	Explain the procedure to the client. Assess peripheral circulation, as this may alter results. Place the sensor on the earlobe, fingertip, or pinna of the ear. Keep the sensor intact until a consistent reading is obtained. Observe and record readings. Report to the physician measurements below 95%.
Rinne test (tuning fork)	Detects loss of hearing in one or both ears. Tuning fork is struck and placed against the mastoid bone to measure the sound conduction through the bone. The tuning fork is then placed beside and parallel to the ear to test conduction through the air. If the sound is louder when the tines are placed beside the ear, hearing is normal or the hearing loss is sensorineural. If the sound is louder when conducted through the bone, the hearing loss is conductive.	Explain the procedure and its purpose to the client.
Romberg test	Assesses vestibular (balance) function. The client stands with the eyes closed, arms extended in front, and feet together. Normal: slight swaying.	Explain the procedure and its purpose to the client. Stand close and reassure the client that someone will catch him if he begins to fall.
Schiller test	Performed during colposcopy. An iodine solution is applied to the cells of the cervix. Abnormal cells turn white or yellow. Aids in visualization of abnormal tissue and indicates areas for biopsy. Normal: cells turn brown	Explain the reason for the application of the solution. Assist with the biopsy procedure as necessary. Label tissue specimens and send to histology.
Segmented bacteriologic localization cultures	The first 5-10 mL of urine is collected, the next 200 mL is discarded, then 5-10 mL is collected midstream. The prostate is then massaged until prostatic secretions can be collected. Finally, 5-10 mL urine is collected before the bladder is emptied. Four samples are needed in sterile culture tubes.	Ensure that the client is well hydrated and has a full bladder.
Semen analysis	Determines the presence, number, and motility of sperm.	Teach the client about proper collection of sperm.
Skin scrapings	A lesion is scraped with an oiled scalpel blade. The cells are then examined under a microscope. Used to diagnose fungal lesions.	Explain the procedure and its purpose to the client.
Speech audiometry (Spondee threshold)	Evaluates ability to hear and understand the spoken word. A series of two-syllable words commonly recognized by their vowel sounds (like *toothbrush* and *baseball*) are delivered through earphones. When the client correctly repeats the words, the sound intensity is recorded in decibels. The test is normally conducted in a soundproof booth.	Explain the procedure and its purpose to the client. Ensure that the client is not claustrophobic.

Contd...

Table 23.25: *Contd....*

Test	Description	Nursing responsibilities
Sputum analysis	Sputum samples are examined for the presence of bacteria, fungi, molds, yeasts, and malignant cells. Appropriate antibiotic therapy is determined via C&S studies.	Explain the procedure and its purpose to the client. Obtain specimens early in the morning to prevent contamination via ingested food or fluids. Instruct the client to breathe deeply and cough, so as to facilitate collection of a specimen originating from the lower respiratory tract. If necessary, pulmonary suctioning may be used to induce such a specimen. Instruct the client to expectorate sputum into the appropriate container. Deliver specimens to the laboratory as soon as possible.
Tonometry	Used to measure intraocular pressure and to aid in the diagnosis and follow-up evaluation of glaucoma. Two types of tonometric devices are used for assessment; applanation and indentation. An applanation tonometer is the most accurate and commonly used device and measures the force (delineated by the reading on the tension dial on the tonomoter) required to flatten a small, standard area of the cornea. An indentation tonometer measures the deformation of the globe in response to a standard weight placed on the cornea. Before use of wither apparatus, the eyes are anesthetized with a local ophthalmic solution, such as benoxinate with fluorescein or tetracaine, so that the pressure from the tonometer will not be felt. Normal: 20 mm Hg or lower	Explain the procedure and its purpose to the client. Explain to the client that this test measures the pressure within the eyes and that although the test requires the clients eyes to be anesthetized, the anesthesia will wear off shortly after the examination is complete. Reassure the client that the procedure is painless.
Typanometry	Measures the movement of the eardrum in response to air pressure in the ear canal. Evaluates the pressure of fluid in the middle ear and is commonly used to evaluate otitis media in children or adults.	Explain the procedure and its purpose to the client. Inform the client a small burst of air is introduced through the otoscope, which may produce an uncomfortable sensation.
Tzanck smear	Fluid from the base of a vesicle is applied to a glass slide, stained and examined under a microscope. Used to diagnose herpes zoster, herpes simplex, varicella, or pemphigus. Normal: negative	Describe to the client how the laboratory technician will obtain the specimen and that although the procedure will likely not be painful, the client must remain still to prevent injury. Provide scalpel blade, glass slide, and stain for collection.
Urethra pressure profile (UPP)	Assess functional urethral length and general competency of the urethra and sphincter, either at rest or during coughing, straining, or voiding. Functional profile length is the length from bladder outlet to the point in the urethra where urethral pressure equals intravesical pressure. Used to diagnose stress or overflow incontinence or urethral obstruction. Normal: Male: bladder outlet through membranous urethra Female: bladder outlet through Midurethra	Explain the procedure and its purpose to the client: that is often performed when the bladder is empty and the client is at rest; that it may be performed simultaneously with CMG; and that the client may be asked to cough or void. Provide privacy, as the test can be embarrassing.
Uroflowmetry	Noninvasive assessment of urination. An electronic device connected to a funneled commode calculates the rate of urine flow, volume voided, and time taken to void.	Explain the procedure and its produce to the client. Instruct the client to void as usual, leaving client alone to do so, if possible.

Contd...

	Table 23.25: *Contd....*	
Test	*Description*	*Nursing responsibilities*
Weber test (tuning fork)	Detects loss of hearing in one or both ears. Tuning fork is struck and the handle is placed in the middle of the forehead. Clients with normal hearing or bilateral deafness will hear or not hear the sound equally in both ears. Clients with unilateral hearing loss will hear the sound only in the unaffected ear.	Explain the procedure and its purpose to the client
Wood's light examination	Skin and hair are examined under ultraviolet light (black light) in a darkened room. Used a diagnose fungal infections (tinea) of hair and skin.	Explain the procedure and its purpose to the client. Reassure the client that the rays are not harmful.

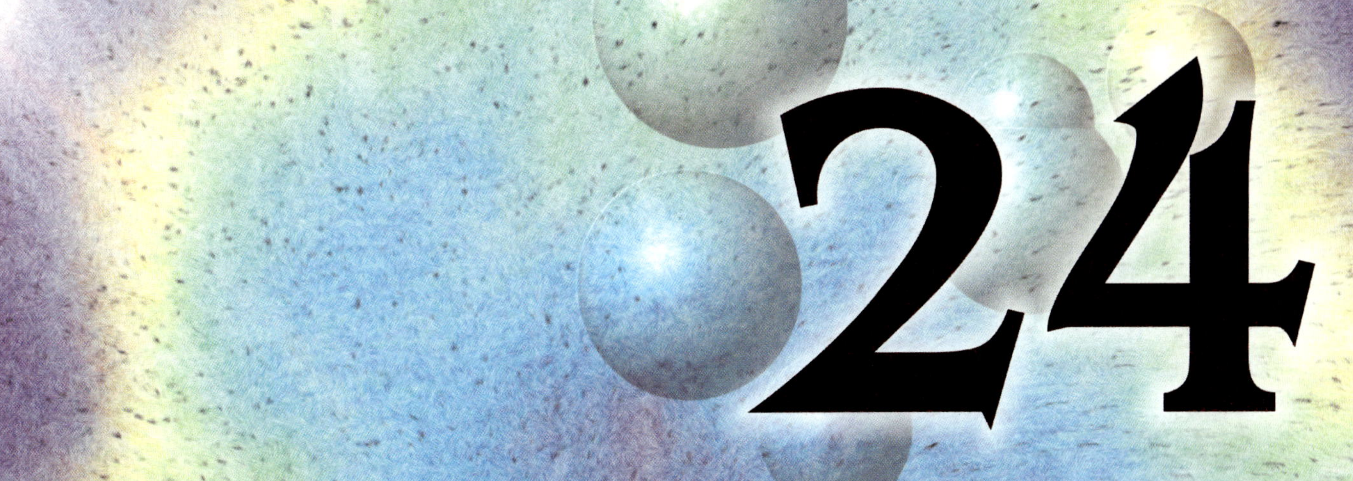

24

Management of Stress

Introduction

Stress is a state produced by a change in the environment that is perceived as challenging, threatening or damaging to the person's dynamic balance or equilibrium. There is an actual or perceived imbalance in the person's ability to meet the demands of the new situation. The change or stimulus that evokes this state is the 'stressor'. The nature of the stressor is variable, i.e. an event or change that will produce stress in one person will be neutral for another, and even that may produce at one time and place for one person may not do so for the same person at another time and place. A person appraises and copes with changing situations. The desired goal is 'adaptation or adjustment' to the energy and ability to meet new demands. This is stress-coping process, a compensatory process with physiologic and psychologic components.

Adaptation is a constant, ongoing process that requires a change in structure, function, or behavior so that the person is better suited to the environment. The process involves an interaction between the person and the environment. The outcome depends upon the degree of fit between the skills and capacities of the person and his or her sources of social support, on the one hand and the types of challenges or stressors being confronted on the other. As such adaptation is an individual process with each individual having different levels of ability to cope and/ or respond. As new challenges are met, this ability to cope and adapt can change, thereby providing the individual with a wide range of adaptation ability from which to draw. Adaptation goes on throughout the life-span and during that process many developmental and situational challenges will be encountered, especially in situations of health and illness. The goal of these encounters is to promote adaptation. In situations of health, and illness, this goal is realized by optional wellness.

Theories/Approaches to Stress

There were three different theoretical approaches which have been used to define stress in nursing.

(i) The first theory conceptualizes **stress as a response** to an environmental stressor. This theory was first proposed by Hano Selye (1956, 1976) who identified/ defined "stress as a nonspecific response of the body to any demand made upon it, regardless of its nature." Selye referred to these stress-inducing demands as 'stressor'. Stressors can be physical (e.g. noise, amphetamines, bums, running a marathon, infectious disease, pain, etc.) or emotional (e.g. diagnosis of cancer, promotion at work, watching a loved one die, failing an examination, financial loss, winning a beauty contest), and pleasant or unpleasant, as long as they require the individual to adapt. In response to either physical or psychologic stressors, a series of physiologic changes occur. Selye called/labeled this pattern of responses as general adaptation syndrome (GAS) (The detailed discussion included in this chapter).

(ii) The second stress theory, views **stress as a stimulus** that causes a response. This theory originated with Holmes TH, (1967), Rahe RH and Masuda (1967, 1975) who developed a tool to assess the effects of life changes on health. Life changes are defined as conditions ranging from minor violation of law to death of a loved one. They define stress as a stimulus, or the cause of the response. In this context, stress is viewed as external to the individual. In this psychosomal model, life events are measured as predictors of illness. Stress is considered as a predisposing or precipitating factor increasing the individual vulnerability to illness. The life events that makes people more vulnerable to illness and their mean values are enlisted in Table 24.1.

The factors that affect individual response to life events indicating the importance of using a holistic approach when assessing the patient/ client.

(iii) The third stress theory focuses on person-environment-transactions and is referred to as the **"transaction or interaction"** theory. In this, stress is defined as "transaction". In the transactive model, there is an exchange or transaction between the persons and the environment, which provides feedback to the person-environment-relationship. The proponent of this theory is Richard Lazarus, who emphasized the role of cognitive appraisal in assessing stressful situations and selecting coping options. Lazarus and Folkman (1984) defined psychologic stress as a particular relationship between the person and the environment that is appraised by the person as taxing his or her resources and endangering his or her well-being.

Lazarus theory focuses on the person-environment-transactions and cognitive appraisal of demands and coping options. Appraisal is a judgment process that includes recognizing the degree of demands or stressors, placed on the individual. The appraisal process also involves the recognition of available resources or options that help when dealing with potential or actual demands.

During primary appraisal, demands are according to the possible impact on the individual well-being. Demands can be judged as irrelevant, benign-positive, or stressful. If demands are appraised stressful, they can be classified as representing harm or loss, threat or challenge. Harm or loss demands involve actual damage and threat demands involve anticipated harm or loss, challenge demand differs from threat and harm or loss because they are viewed as a potential for personal gain or growth.

Secondary appraisal refers to the process of recognizing the coping resources and options that are available. Primary and secondary appraisal often occur simultaneously and interact with each other in determining stress. Cognitive reappraisal is the process of continually relabeling cognitive appraisals. Certain factors influence the labeling of appraisals. Situational factors include the intensity of the external demands, the immediacy of the expected impact, and ambiguity. Person-related factors include motivational characteristics, belief systems and intellectual resources and skills.

Table 24.1: Life Event Stressors and their Mean Values

Sl No	Life event stressors	Mean values
1.	Death of spouse	100
2.	Divorce	73
3.	Marital separation from male	65
4.	Detention	–
5.	Death of a close family member	63
6.	Major personal injury or illness	53
7.	Marriage	50
8.	Being fired at work	45
9.	Marital reconciliation with mate	45
10.	Retirement from work	45
11.	Major changes in health of a family member	44
12.	Pregnancy	40
13.	Sexual difficulties	39
14.	Gaining a new family member (through birth, adoption, etc.)	39
15.	Major business readjustment (merger, reorganization, bankruptcy)	39
16.	Major changes in financial state (worse or better than usual)	38
17.	Death of a close friend	37
18.	Changing to different line of work	36
19.	Major change in number of arguments with spouse	35
20.	Taking out a mortgage or loan for a major purchase	31
21.	Foreclosure on a mortgage or loan	30
22.	Major changes in responsibilities at work (promotions demotions, transfers)	29
23.	Son or a daughter leaving from home	29
24.	Trouble with in-laws	29
25.	Outstanding personal achievement	28
26.	Spouse beginning or ceasing work outside home	26
27.	Beginning or ceasing normal schooling	26
28.	Major change in living conditions (building new house, deterioration of house or neighborhood)	25
29.	Revision of personal habits (dress, manners, association)	24
30.	Trouble with boss	23
31.	Major change in working hours or conditions	20
32.	Change in residence or changing to a new school	20
33.	Major change in usual type and amount of recreation	19
34.	Major change in social activities	17
35.	Taking out a mortgage or loan for a lesser purchase	17
36.	Major changes in sleeping habits	16
37.	Major changes in number of family get together an eating habits	15
38.	Vacation	13
39.	Christmas or any major festival	12
40.	Minor violation of law (traffic tickets, disturbing peace, etc.)	11

Appraisal and coping are affected by the internal characteristics of the person. These include health and energy, as well as the person's belief system including existential belief (faith, religious beliefs) commitments or life goals (motivational properties), and the persons own sense of self including self-esteem, control and mastery. They also include knowledge, problem-solving skills and social skills which include ability to communicate and interact with others.

Some theorists conceptualize stress as a complex, dynamic, and reciprocal transaction between person and environment. Other theorists view stress solely as a stimulus that causes psychological or physiological responses that in turn increase vulnerability to disease. Selye found that physical, emotional, psychological, and spiritual stressors, or the anticipation of a stressor (as in anxiety), can initiate nonspecific physiological *responses*. Selye defined these responses as stress.

Everyone experiences stress as a part of daily life, but we each perceive and respond to stress in our own unique way, Our responses are holistic–that is, physical, psychological, spiritual, and social. As a nurse, you need to understand stress to help your clients cope effectively and adapt to the stressors of illness and caregiving. In addition, you will encounter many stressful situations in your career, so you must develop healthful ways of responding.

Meaning of Stress

Stress is any disturbance in a person's normal balanced state. A stressor is a stimulus that the person perceives as a challenge or threat; it disturbs the person's equilibrium by initiating a physical *or* emotional response. When stress occurs, it produces voluntary and involuntary coping responses aimed at restoring equilibrium (balance, *or* homeostasis), The changes that take place as a result of stress and coping are called adaptation. We can also define adaptation as an ongoing effort to maintain external and internal equilibrium.

Stress is not necessarily bad. It can keep you alert and motivate you to function at a higher performance level. For example, when you are preparing for an examination, your desire to succeed can create just enough anxiety to motivate you to study. On the other hand, if you become too anxious, you may be unable to focus on the task.

Stress and anxiety are universal experiences that can be either a catalyst for positive change or a source of discomfort and pain. Nurses help clients cope with the stress of illness, disability, injury, or treatment approaches. Caring for clients experiencing a high level of anxiety can also be stressful for the nurse. Successful stress management is necessary for everyone's well-being. This chapter discusses the major concepts related to stress and anxiety, including strategies for coping with stress,

According to Hans Selye (1974), stress is a nonspecific response to any demand made on the body, Selye termed such demands stressors. Any situation, event, or agent that produces stress is a stressor. A stressor is a stimulus that evokes the need to adapt. Stressors can be internal or external. For example, pain is an internal stressor, whereas loss of a job is an external stressor.

Even pleasant events can be stressful when they evoke the need to adapt. Stressors themselves are neutral, neither good nor bad. It is the individual's *perception* of the stressor that determines whether the effect is positive or negative. Any event can be stressful, depending on how the person views the event.

Types of Stressors

The sources of stress are infinite; however, stressors are commonly categorized in the following ways:

- *Distress/eustress.* Distress threatens health, and eustress (literally "good stress") is protective. A passionate kiss can produce as strong a stress response as a slap in the face. On the Holmes-Rahe stress scale, for example, marriage and divorce receive similarly high scores.
- *External/internal.* Stressors may be external to the person, for example, death of a family member, a hurricane, or even something as simple as excessive heat in a room. Stressors may also be internal, for example, diseases, anxiety, nervous anticipation of an event, or negative self-talk.
- *Developmental/situational.* Developmental stressors are those that can be predicted to occur at various stages of a person's life. For example, most young adults face the stress of leaving home and beginning a career, and many middle-aged adults must adjust to aging parents and accepting their own physical changes. In a sense, developmental stressors may be easier to cope with because they are expected and the person has some time to prepare for them. Situational stressors are unpredictable. For example, you cannot predict that you will experience an automobile accident, a natural disaster, or an illness. Situational stressors can occur at any life stage and can affect infants, children, and adults equally.
- *Physiological/psychosocial.* Physiological stressors are those that affect body structure or function. They may be chemical (e.g. poison, medications), physical or mechanical (e.g. trauma, cold), nutritional (e.g. vitamin deficiency), biological (e.g. viruses, bacteria) or genetic (e.g. inborn errors of metabolism). Psychosocial stressors are external stressors that arise from our work, family dynamics, living situation, social relationships, and other aspects of our daily lives.

Stressors throughout the Life Span

The following are common developmental stressors. Not everyone will experience these stressors, however.

Childhood
- Stressors occur primarily in the home
- Absence of parental figures
- Failure of parents to meet needs for safety, security, love and belonging
- Failure of parents to meet basic physiological needs for oxygen, food, elimination, rest, and cleanliness

- School-age children may experience stressors at school or among peers.

Adolescence
- Exposure to an expanded environment and a wider circle of friends
- Rapid changes in body appearance
- Need for academic achievement
- Peer pressure
- Maintaining self-esteem while searching for identity
- Decisions about the future in the areas of school, work, and relationships
- Conflicts between standards for behavior and the sex drive
- Decisions about and involvement with drugs.

Young Adult
- Separation from family, starting college
- Making the transition from youth to adult responsibilities
- Preparing for careers: graduation from college, learning a trade
- Establishing career goals and planning progress to move
- Financial stressors around partnerships and providing a home for family
- Parenting children
- Conflicts between responsibilities for work and family or other relationships.

Middle Age
- Career challenges continue
- Child rearing continues; marriage of the children; grandparenting
- Dealing with too many responsibilities: e.g. children, work, elderly parents, community activities
- Empty-nest syndrome when the children leave home
- Being "sandwiched" between caring for aging parents as well as children or grandchildren
- "Mid-life crisis" (wanting to escape from one's present life); the person regresses and tries to recapture youth (e.g. by buying a new sports car, making geographic move, taking an exotic vacation, engaging in an affair, daydreaming about the ideal life in retirement).

Older Adults
- Losses of family and friends, resulting in loneliness and isolation
- Changes in physical appearance and functional abilities
- Major life changes (e.g. retirement, loss of life partner)
- Health problems (e.g. chronic diseases) with accompanying discomfort or pain
- The cost of health care
- Learning to live on a fixed, perhaps inadequate, income
- Adjusting to loss of independence.

Coping and Adaptation to Stress

Coping strategies are those thinking processes and behaviors a person uses to manage stressors. Some examples are problem solving, daydreaming, making changes in lifestyle (e.g. exercising more, eating less), sleeping, and consulting others for support or advice. Coping strategies can be adaptive or maladaptive.

Adaptive (effective) coping consists of making healthy choices that reduce the negative effects of stress (e.g. exercising to relieve tension). Sometimes the difference between effective and ineffective coping is in the degree to which a technique is used.

Maladaptive (ineffective) coping does not promote adaptation. Unhealthful coping choices include overeating, working too much, and substance abuse. Although a maladaptive behavior may temporarily relieve anxiety, it may have other harmful effects. For example, a person who smokes to relieve the tensions of a stressful work situation may experience an immediate decrease in anxiety. However, the person is doing nothing to change or adapt to the stressful situation and, over time, is increasing her risk of respiratory disease.

Approaches to Coping

People use three approaches to cope with stress, at different times and in various combinations:

1. *Altering the stressor:* In some situations, a person takes actions to remove or change the stressor. For example, Ms Gowri a daughter of sick parents might remove one of her stressors by resigning her position as a manager in co.
2. *Adapting to the stressor:* It is not always possible to remove or change a stressor. Adapting involves changing one's thoughts or behaviors related to the stressor. Gowri cannot change the fact that her father needs care and that her mother needs surgery, but as she gains experience as a caregiver, she may find easier and more efficient ways to care for her parents. This would give her a little more time to relax or attend to other responsibilities.
3. *Avoiding the stressor:* Sometimes, it is healthful to avoid a stressor. For example, you may find that being with a certain person is stressful for you, even though you have tried many times to change the dynamics of the relationship. In that case, it may be best to sever your relationship with the person. In other situations, avoidance may be maladaptive. For example, a woman who discovers a lump in her breast becomes anxious that she may have cancer. She copes with her anxiety by putting it out of her mind and avoids seeing her physician. If the lump is cancerous, it will not be treated at an early stage.

The Outcome of Stress

Stress results in either adaptation or disease. Successful adaptation allows for normal growth and development and effective responses to changes and challenges in daily life. The outcome depends on the balance between the strength of the stressors and the effectiveness of the person's coping methods. In the following equation, E is the event (stressor), R is the person's response (which is determined in part by past experiences, perception of the stressor, and coping methods used), and **O** is the outcome.

E	+	R	=	O
stressful event		response (experience perception, coping methods)		outcome (adaptation or disease)

Some events produce more stress than others. However, a person with good coping skills can usually adapt to a single stressful event, even a very demanding one. But suppose several stressors occur in a short period of time. For example, Ms. Lalitha has many stressors, so her coping abilities may be taxed to the limit. When there are many stressors or when stressors continue for a long period of time, adaptation is more likely to fail.

Personal Factors Influence Adaptation

Fortunately, successful adaptation does not depend entirely on being able to alter or avoid stressors. Various personal factors also influence the outcome:

- *Perception of the stressor:* A person's perception may be realistic or exaggerated. Suppose two women with similar coping skills and support systems both must have a mastectomy. Mrs. Indira thinks, ''Yes, I am losing a part of my body, but I am more than just a breast. This will be a difficult adjustment, but I am so grateful to be alive.'' Mrs. Asha thinks, "I will be so ugly. My husband won't want to touch me. I won't be a woman now. This is the worst thing that could ever happen." Which woman do you think is most likely to adapt successfully to this change in her body?
- *Overall health status:* On the one hand, stressors may actually cause a healthy person to engage in constructive adaptive behaviors that improve health. A person who has just discovered that he has hypertension may react by modifying his diet and exercising to lower his blood pressure and prevent complications. On the other hand, a person with severe, chronic arthritis who has been coping for years with pain and immobility may be too overwhelmed and exhausted to take any actions to lower his blood pressure.
- *Support system:* A support system may include friends, family, counseling groups, religious groups, or other like-minded people who share common interests. A good support system can help a person adapt to stress, provide emotional support, encourage expression of feelings, and help the person solve problems. They may also provide financial and other concrete types of support, such as a place to live, meal preparation, household help, child care, and transportation.
- *Other personal factors:* Age, developmental level, and life experiences (e.g. observing how others handle stress) all affect a person's response to stress. For example, infants and the very old may lack the physiological reserve to adapt to physical stressors such as temperature extremes, dehydration, or illness.

Even with a positive attitude and good coping skills, excessive amounts of stress can lead to maladaptation and disease. Some people succumb to illness after only a few stressors, whereas others seem to adapt to multiple, intensely difficult stressors. Each person has a different ability to tolerate stress, but everyone has a breaking point at which stress becomes overwhelming.

Physiological Responses to Stressor

Although Selye's (1974, 1976) response-based model acknowledges physical, emotional, psychological, and spiritual *stressors,* his ideas about responses *(stress)* are primarily physiological. The body has various homeostatic mechanisms for regulating its internal environment to maintain homeostasis. In Selye's theory, physiological responses to stress are described by the general adaptation syndrome (GAS) and the local adaptation syndrome (LAS).

The **general adaptation syndrome (GAS)** is Selye's name for the group of nonspecific responses that all people share in the face of stressors. Regardless of the specific stressor, the responses involve the whole body, especially the autonomic nervous system and the endocrine system. For example, a near-miss automobile accident and kicking the winning field goal at a football game would both produce the same general body responses. The GAS has three stages: (1) the initial alarm stage, (2) resistance (adaptation), and (3) the final stage of either recovery or exhaustion.

Adaptive energy is the term Selye coined to describe the inner force an individual uses to respond or adapt to stress. All persons have adaptive energy, but the amount of adaptive energy varies. When an individual has used all of his adaptive energy, illness, disease, or even death may result, as he is no longer able to adapt. Reactions to stress are typically categorized as either general (affecting the entire body) or local (affecting only the involved body part).

Stressors cause structural and chemical changes in the body as the body attempts to maintain **homeostasis,** which is the balance or equilibrium among the physiologic, psychological, sociocultural, intellectual, and spiritual needs of the body. Selye called these responses to stressors the **general adaptation syndrome** (GAS).

Selye divided the GAS into three stages, as illustrated in Figure 24.1. In the first stage, crisis or alarm, the body readies itself to handle the stressors. The physiologic changes may result in symptoms such as cool, pale skin; shivering; and sweating of the palms and soles of the feet. Severe stress may cause dilated pupils, dry mouth, pounding heart, nausea, and diarrhea.

During the second stage, adaptation or resistance, the body attempts to defend against the stressor through the **fight-or-flight response.** The body becomes physiologically ready to defend itself by either fighting or fleeing from the stressor.

The third stage, exhaustion, occurs if adaptive energy is inadequate to deal with prolonged or overwhelming stress.

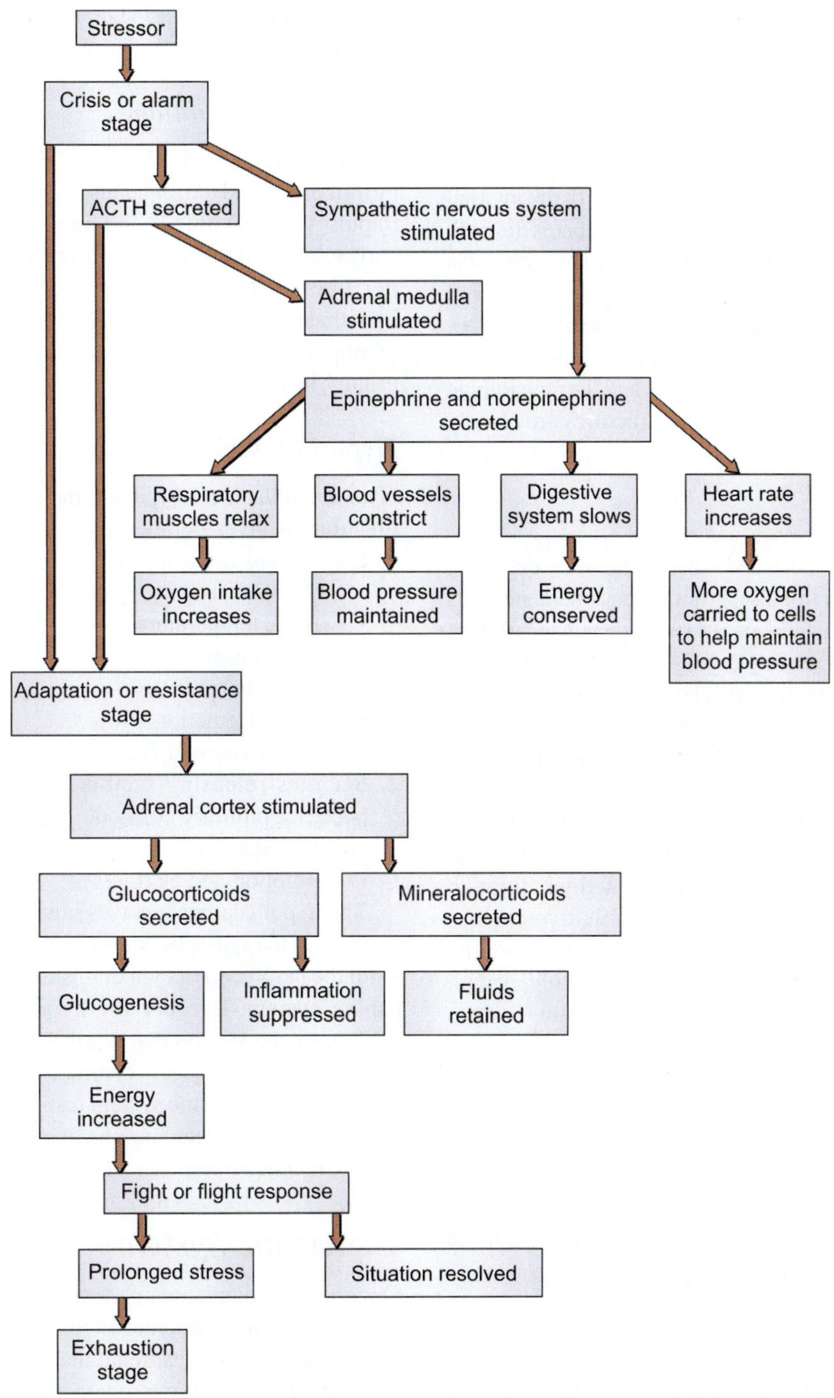

Figure 24.1: Physiological responses of the general adaptation syndrome (GAS)

The physiologic reactions of the body are essentially the same no matter what the source of the stress. For example, an imagined stressor will have the same physiologic response (GAS) as if the stressor had actually been experienced. According to Selye (1976), all stress reactions exhibit similar physiologic reactions.

An understanding of the physiological changes associated with stress provides the foundation for the assessment of the client experiencing stress and the implications for health outcomes. The physiologic response to a stressor is a protective and adaptive mechanism to maintain the homeostatic balance of the body. Stressors or demands may be physical, psychologic or social. The body will respond physiologically to both actual or symbolic stressors. The complex processes by which an event is perceived as a stressor and by which the body responds is not fully understood. However, there are three interrelated systems, viz. nervous system, endocrine system, immune system.

Nervous System

Neural and hormonal actions to maintain homeostatic balance are integrated by the hypothalamus. Hypothalamus is located in the center of the brain, surrounded by the limbic system and the cerebral hemispheres. It integrates autonomic nervous system mechanism, that maintains the chemical constancy of the internal environment of the body. Hypothalamus participates in both emotional and physiologic response to stressors. This control is significant because most stressors precipitate an emotional reaction. In addition to the hypothalamus, other parts of the CNS including cerebral cortex, limbic system and reticular formations are involved in the neural control of emotions and the physiologic responses to stress. The function of these structures are closely interrelated.

Cerebral Cortex

After an external event has occurred, afferent input is sent to the cerebral cortex via sensory impulses from the peripheral nervous system including the eyes and ears. In stress response, afferent impulses are carried from sensory organs (eyes, ear, nose, skin) and internal sensors (baroreceptors, chemoreceptors) to nerve centers to the brain. Afferent impulses that travel to the cortex from the periphery via the spinal cord (spinophthalmic pathway) also activate the reticular formation in the area of the brainstem. The reticular formation then relays input to the thalamus and from the thalamus to the cerebral cortex. The cerebral hemispheres are concerned with cognitive functions, through processes, learning and memory (The limbic system has connection with the both cerebral hemispheres and the brainstem). The network of neurons which is involved with arousal and consciousness is called reticular activating system (RAS). The RAS functions to maintain wakefulness and alertness. The somatic, auditory and visual associative areas and the cerebral cortex receive input from the peripheral sensory fibers and then interpret it. The prefrontal area serves to reduce the speed of the associative functions so that the person has time to evaluate the information in light of the past experiences and future consequences and to plan a course of action. All these functions are involved in the perception of a stressor.

Limbic System

The limbic system, which lies in the inner mid-portion of the brain, near the base includes the septum, cingulate gyrus, amygdala, hippocampus, and anterior muscle of the thalamus. The function of the limbic system is thought to be involved with emotions and behaviors. When these structures are stimulated, emotions, feelings, and behaviors can occur that ensure survival and self-preservation such as feeding, sociability and sexuality (drinking, eating, temperature control, reproduction defense and aggression).

The cerebral cortex and limbic system instruct to serve the experiential and executive functions of emotions. Endorphins are found in this system and around, reduce the perception of painful stimuli.

Reticular Formation

Reticular formation is also located in between the lower end of the brainstem and the thalamus. It contains the RAS, which sends impulses contributing to the limbic system and to the cerebral cortex and thalamus. In addition to receiving input from the periphery, the RAS also receives impulses from the hypothalamus, when the RAS stimulates it increases its output of impulses leading to wakefulness. Both physiologic stress, usually increase the degree of wakefulness.

Hypothalamus

Hypothalamus lies just above the pituitary gland. It has many functions as given below.

1. Coordinates impulse
   - Autonomic nervous system
   - Body temperature regulation
   - Food intake
   - Water balance
   - Urine formation
   - Cardiovascular function
2. Secretes releasing factors – regulation of anterior and posterior pituitary hormone.
3. Affects behavior
   - Emotion and alertness

The hypothalamus receives information regarding traumatic stimuli via the spinophthalmic pathway, pressure-sensitive input from the baroreceptors via brainstem, and emotional stimuli via limbic system. Because the hypothalamus secretes peptide hormones and factors that regulate the release of hormones by the anterior pituitary, it is central to the connection between the nervous and endocrine system responding to stress. In addition, the hypothalamus regulates the function of both sympathetic and parasympathetic branches of the autonomic nervous system.

Endocrine System

Once the hypothalamus is activated in response to stress, the endocrine system becomes involved. The sympathetic nervous system stimulates the adrenal medulla to release the hormones. Epinephrines and the sympathetic nervous system including adrenal-medulla, is referred to as sympathoadrenal response. These hormones prepare the body for the "fight or flight" response. This response is activated by physical stressors such as hypovolemia and hypoxia, and emotional status, particularly anger, excitement and fear.

The hypothalamus released corticotrophin-releasing hormones (CRH) which stimulates the anterior pituitary to release propiomelanocortin (POMC). Both adrenocorticotrophic hormones (ACTH) and endorphins are derived from POMC. ACTH, in turn, stimulates adrenal cortex to synthesize and secretes glucocorticoids, and to a lesser degree aldosterone and androgen. Glucocorticoids in particular, cortisol, are essential for the stress response. Cortisol produces a number of physiologic effects that include increasing the glucose level, potentiatory action of catecholamines on blood vessels and inhibiting inflammatory response. Aldosterone acts to increase sodium reabsorption in the kidney tubules, and as a result increases ECF. During stress, neural stimulation of the posterior pituitary results in the secretion of ADH which also promotes water reabsorption by the distal and collecting tubules of the kidney.

Stimulation of both the adrenal medulla and cortex results in an increased blood glucose level. This elevation provides the additional fuel for the increased metabolism needed for fighting or fleeing. The increased cardiac output, due to increased (HR and ECF) increased blood glucose level, and increased metabolic rate make the physical response possible. In addition, dilatation of the skeletal muscle blood vessels and the brain provide quick movement and increased alertness.

Immune System

Negative stressors lead to alterations in immune functions in humans through processes involving the hypothalamic-pituitary-adrenal axis and the autonomic nervous system that affects immune function. In turn, immune system also affects endocrine and CNS responses. Both corticosteroids and catecholamines are known to suppress immune function. Interleukin-1 (which is released by activated macrophages), on type of cytokine, may directly stimulate the release of ACTH and thus initiate the stress response. Glucocorticoids depress the immune system; when these are present in high concentrations, there is a reduction in the inflammatory response to injury or infection. The steps of inflammation process are inhibited, lymphocytes are destroyed in lymphoid tissues and antibody production is decreased. As a result, the ability of the persons to resist infections is reduced.

Selye's Stages of Stress

In 1936, Selye, experimenting with animals, first described a syndrome consisting of the enlargement of the adrenal cortex, shrinkages, and thymus, spleen, lymph nodes and other lymphatic structures and the appearance of deep bleeding, ulcers in the stomach and duodenum. He identified this as a nonspecific response to diverse, noxious stimuli. From this, he developed a theory of adaptation to biologic stress, which he titled "The general adaptation syndrome" (GAS) (Fig. 24.2).

General Adaptation Syndrome (GAS)

The general adaptation syndrome (GAS) has three phases–alarm, resistance and exhaustion. Once the stressor or stimulus is integrated, into CNS, multiple responses occur because of activation of the hypothalamic-pituitary-adrenal-axis and autonomic nervous system. The nature of these responses, in which the stimulus and its effects successively cause changes in nervous, endocrine and immune systems is fundamental to understanding the physiologic and behavioral changes that occur in an individual experiencing stress.

The Alarm Stage

Imagine this situation: That is dark. You are alone, walking to neighbor house, when you hear footsteps behind you. You stop and look around and see no one. As you begin walking again, the footsteps return. You walk faster; the footsteps are faster. Stop reading, shut your eyes, and use your imagination. How do you feel? Pay attention to your physical and emotional reactions. If you are not feeling a response to this imaginary situation, think back to a time when something similar happened to you-when something frightened you.

- Is your heart pounding?
- Are you breathing fast?
- Is there a flutter in your stomach?

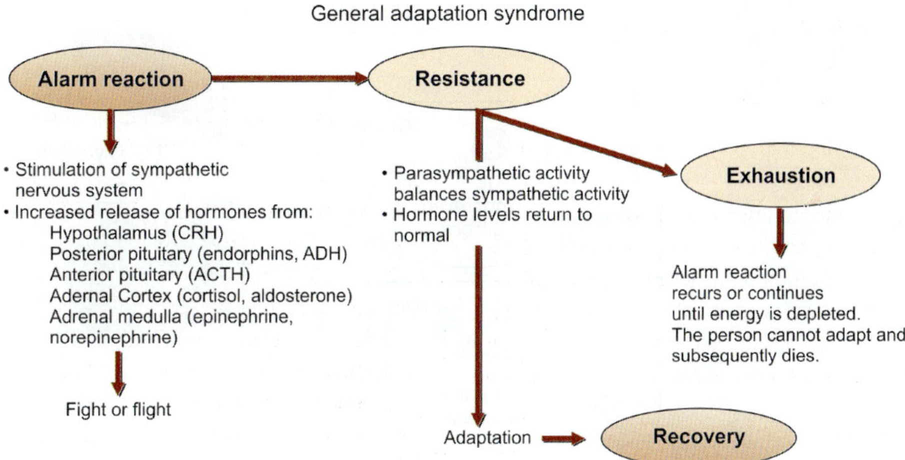

Figure 24.2: The stages of Selye's general adaptation syndrome (GAS)

- What is the physical sensation in your muscles?
- Do you feel frightened?
- What are your emotions?
- Are you straining to hear the footsteps?
- Do you want to run away, or are you "frozen"?
- If someone were to walk into the room where you are studying right now, would it startle you?

This scenario should help you to imagine the experience of the alarm stage, during which the body prepares for *"fight or flight."* The alarm stage has two phases, shock and countershock. The shock phase begins when the cerebral cortex first perceives a stressor and sends out messages to activate the endocrine and sympathetic nervous systems. Large amounts of epinephrine and various other hormones prepare the body for fight or flight. The shock phase does not last long-usually less than 24 hours, and sometimes only a minute or two. In the countershock phase, all the changes produced in the shock phase are reversed, and the person becomes less able to deal with the immediate threat.

Endocrine System Responses

In response to alarm, the following endocrine responses occur:

1. The *hypothalamus* releases corticotropin-releasing hormone (CRH).

2. *CRR,* together with messages from the cerebral cortex, directs the pituitary to release adrenocorticotropic hormone (ACTH) and antidiuretic hormone (ADH).

3. *ACTH* stimulates the adrenal cortex to produce and secrete glucocorticoids (especially cortisol) and mineralocorticoids (especially aldosterone).
   - *Cortisol,* in general, has a glucose-sparing effect. It increases the use of fats and proteins for energy and conserves glucose for use by the brain. Cortisol also has an anti-inflammatory effect. See Figure 24.3 for the effects of cortisol during the alarm reaction of the GAS.
   - *Aldosterone* promotes fluid retention by causing the kidneys to reabsorb more sodium. Thus, it helps to increase fluid volume and maintain or increase blood pressure.

4. *ADH* also promotes fluid retention by increasing the reabsorption of water by kidney tubules. See Figure 24.4 for the effects of aldosterone and ADH.

5. *Endorphins,* secreted by the hypothalamus and posterior pituitary, act like opiates to produce a sense of well-being and reduce pain.

6. *Thyroid-stimulating hormone (TSR)* is secreted by the pituitary gland to increase efficiency of cellular metabolism and fat conversion to energy for cell and muscle needs.

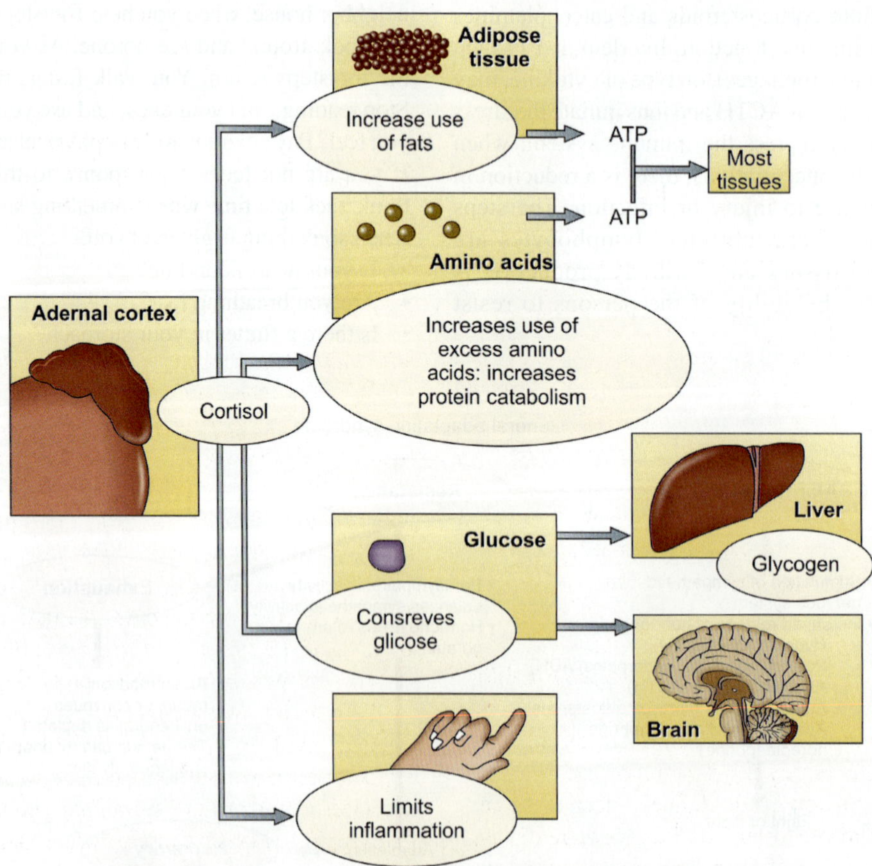

Figure 24.3: Functions of cortisol during the alarm stage of the GAS

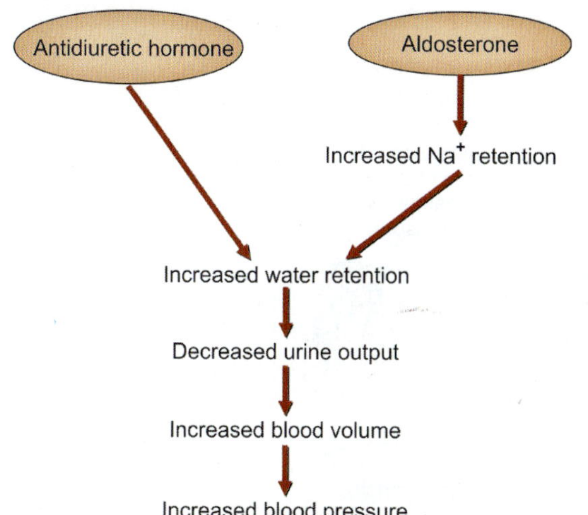

Figure 24.4: The release of ADH (from the posterior pituitary) and aldosterone (from the adrenal cortex) leads to sodium and water retention, increases blood volume, and increases blood pressure

Sympathetic Nervous System Responses

The cerebral cortex also sends messages via the hypothalamus to stimulate the sympathetic nervous system. The sympathetic nervous system stimulates the adrenal glands to secrete adrenaline (epinephrine) and norepinephrine, which increase mental alertness. This allows the person to assess the situation and aids in a decision to stand and fight or run away in flight. Adrenaline also increases the ability of the muscles to contract and causes the pupils to dilate, producing greater visual fields. See Figure 24.5 for the effects of adrenaline during the alarm reaction of the GAS.

(i) Other Body System Responses in the Alarm Stage

The following are some body system responses that occur in the alarm stage as a result of endocrine and sympathetic nervous system activity. Refer to Figures 24.1 through 24.5 to see how these changes are produced.

- *Cardiovascular system:* The heart rate and contraction force increase. Peripheral and visceral vasoconstriction increases blood flow to vital organs (e.g. brain, lungs) and to muscles preparing for flight. Blood volume and blood pressure also increase, and the blood clots more readily.
- *Respiratory system:* The bronchioles dilate, thereby increasing depth of respiration and tidal volume. This makes oxygen available for diffusion to muscle, brain, and cardiac cells.
- *Metabolism:* The rate of metabolism increases. The liver converts more glycogen to glucose *(glycogenolysis),* making it available for energy. Except in the brain, the body uses less glucose for energy. The use of amino acids and the mobilization of fats for energy *(lipolysis)* increase.
- *Urinary system:* Blood flow to the kidneys decreases, and they retain more sodium and water. The kidneys secrete renin, which produces *angiotensin.* In turn, angiotensin constricts the arterioles and tends to increase blood pressure.

- *Gastrointestinal system.* Peristalsis and secretions of digestive enzymes decrease. Blood glucose level increases to fuel the energy needed for fight or flight.
- *Musculoskeletal system.* Blood vessels dilate, increasing flow of blood (and thus oxygen and energy) to skeletal muscles.

(ii) The Resistance Stage

During the second stage of the GAS, **resistance** (or *adaptation),* the body tries to cope, protect itself against the stressor, and maintain homeostasis. Stabilization involves the use of physiological and psychological coping mechanisms. Psychological defense mechanisms for coping will be discussed shortly. Physical adaptations help the heart rate, blood pressure, cardiac output, respiratory function, and hormone levels return to normal. If the person adapts successfully or if the stress can be confined to a small area (as in the inflammatory response, also discussed shortly), the body regains homeostasis. If the stress is too great (as in serious illness or severe blood loss), defense mechanisms fail, and the person enters the third phase of the GAS.

(iii) The Exhaustion or Recovery Stage

If stress continues and adaptive mechanisms become ineffective or are used up, a person enters the final stage, exhaustion. Physiological responses in this stage include vasodilation, decreased blood pressure, and increased pulse and respirations. Physical adaptive resources and energy are depleted. The body is unable to defend itself and cannot maintain resistance against the continuing stressors. Exhaustion usually ends in disease or death.

In contrast, if adaptation is successful, the final stage is recovery. For example, following a miscarriage, a couple participates in a support group and begins to focus more deeply on their relationship with each other. They are able gradually to resolve their grief.

Local Adaptation Syndrome

Seyle also described the *local adaptation syndrome* (LAS), which is the physiologic response to a stressor (e.g. trauma, illness) on a specific part of the body. For example, if a person cuts a hand, the LAS is initiated, inducing localized inflammation. The classic symptoms of inflammation (redness, swelling. and warmth) occur at the injured site. The LAS is usually a temporary process that resolves when the traumatized area is restored to its preinjury state; however, if the inflammation docs not resolve with the LAS, the individual then experiences the GAS as the entire body becomes affected.

Whereas the GAS is a whole-body response to a stressor, the local adaptation syndrome (LAS) is a localized body response; that is, it involves only a specific body part, tissue, or organ. It. is a short-term attempt to restore homeostasis. As a nurse, the two most common LAS responses you will deal with are the reflex pain response and the inflammatory response (others include blood clotting and pupil constriction in response to light).

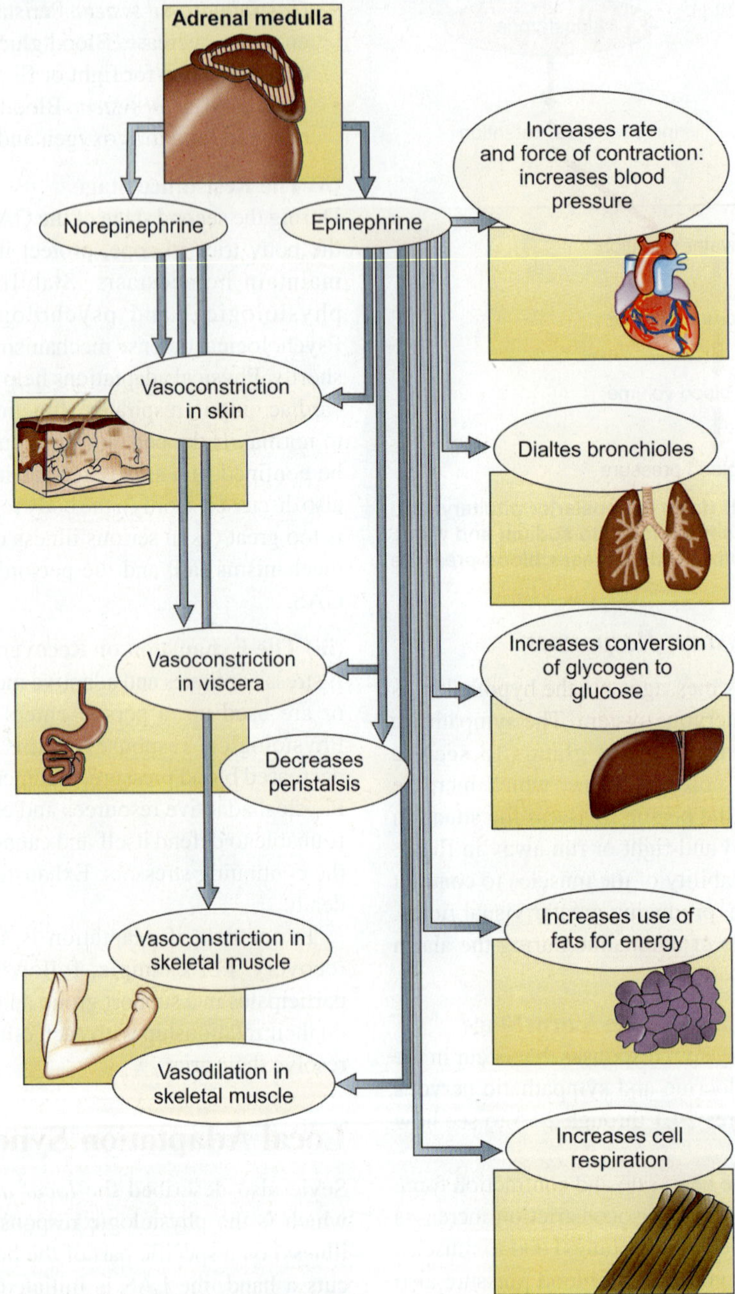

Figure 24.5: Functions of epinephrine and norepinephrine during the alarm stage of the GAS

Reflex Pain Response

When you perceive a painful stimulus, especially in one of your limbs, you immediately and unconsciously withdraw from the source of pain. If you've ever accidentally touched a hot stove, you certainly didn't stop to ponder, "Hmmm, I think I will withdraw my hand." You pulled your hand away before you could even think about it. This is a protective *reflex* (an involuntary, predictable response). Pain receptors send sensory impulses to the spinal cord, where they synapse with the spinal motor neurons. The motor impulses travel back to the site of stimulation, causing the flexor muscles in the limb to contract. This is a local, rather than a whole-body, response.

Inflammatory Response

The inflammatory response is a local reaction to cell injury, either by pathogens or by physical, chemical, or other agents.

The following agents stimulate the inflammatory response by causing cell injury:

- Autoimmune disorders
- Antigen-antibody responses
- Body substances (e.g. digestive enzymes leaking into the abdomen; accumulation of uric acid crystals in joints)
- Chemical injury (e.g. acid or alkali burns)
- Ischemia
- Neoplastic growth (i.e. cancer)

- Pathogens (e.g. bacteria, viruses)
- Physical agents:
  - Heat or cold
  - Radiation
  - Electrothermal injury
  - Mechanical trauma (e.g. abrasion, contusion, laceration, puncture, incision, fractures, sprains).

Its mechanisms are the same, regardless of the injuring agent, and produce the classic symptoms of inflammation: pain, heat, swelling, redness, and loss of function. The inflammatory process includes a vascular response, a cellular response, formation of exudate, and healing.

- *Vascular response:* Immediately after injury, blood vessels at the site constrict (narrow) to control bleeding. After the injured cells release histamine, the vessels dilate, increasing blood now to the area (*hyperemia*). Under the influence of kinins released by the dying cells, the capillaries become more permeable, allowing movement of fluid from capillaries into tissue spaces. The tissue becomes edematous. After leukocytes move into the area, localized blood flow again decreases, to keep them in the area to fight infection.
- *Cellular response:* White blood cells migrate to the site of injury. They phagocytize (engulf) bacteria, other foreign material, and damaged cells and destroy them. Sometimes they form a "wall" around an invading pathogen. The accumulation of dead white cells, digested bacteria, and other cell debris in the presence of infection is called *pus*.
- *Exudate formation:* The fluid and white cells that move from the circulation to the site of injury are called *exudate*. The nature and quantity of exudate depends on the severity of injury and the tissues involved. For example, a surgical incision may ooze serosanguineous (clear or pinkish) exudate for a day or two.
- *Healing:* Healing is the replacement of tissue by regeneration or repair. *Regeneration* is replacement of the damaged cells with identical or similar cells. However, not all cells can regenerate (e.g. some central nervous system neurons and cardiac muscle cells cannot regenerate). Most injuries heal by *repair*, wherein scar tissue replaces the original tissue.

The inflammatory response is adaptive in that it protects the body from infection and promotes healing. However, chronic inflammation, as in arthritis, is itself a stressor.

Do not confuse inflammation with infection. Inflammation is a mechanism for eliminating invading pathogens; therefore, you always see inflammation when there is infection. However, inflammation is stimulated by trauma as well as by pathogens (as in the example of a sprained ankle); thus, it can also occur in the absence of infection.

Psychological Responses to Stress

Recall that stress responses are holistic. That means we respond and adapt to stress psychologically as well as physiologically. Psychological responses are both emotional and cognitive, and they include feelings, thoughts, and behaviors. They may be fleeting, as in a flash of anger that is gone in seconds; or long-term, as in the avoidance of relationships by an adult whose needs for love and security were not met as a child. Examples of psychological responses are as follows:

Cognitive Responses

- Difficulty concentrating
- Poor judgment
- Decrease in accuracy (e.g. in counting money)
- Forgetfulness
- Decreased problem-solving ability
- Decreased attention to detail
- Difficulty learning
- Narrowing of focus
- Preoccupation, daydreaming.

Emotional Responses

- Anger
- Anxiety
- Depression
- Fear
- Feelings of inadequacy
- Low self-esteem
- Irritability
- Lack of motivation
- Lethargy

Behavioral Responses

- Crying, emotional outbursts
- Dependence
- Poor job performance
- Substance use and abuse
- Sleeplessness (or sleeping too much)
- Change in eating habits (e.g. loss of appetite, overeating)
- Decrease in quality of job performance
- Preoccupation (i.e. daydreaming)
- Illnesses
- Increased absenteeism from work or school
- Increased number of accidents
- Avoiding social situations or relationships
- Rebellion, acting out.

As with physical responses, psychological responses can be adaptive or harmful. For example, Mr. Raju and Mr. Kiran have both had heart attacks and are both anxious about the future. To relieve his anxiety, Mr. Raju takes a problem-solving approach, learning about diet, exercise, and lifestyle changes that he must make. Mr. Kiran uses denial; he cannot even accept that he has "really" had a heart attack. He says, "I'm not an invalid. I feel fine. I could follow all those rules and still get hit by a truck and die tomorrow." Both of these responses may relieve the person's anxiety. Which one do you think is more adaptive in the long term?

Anxiety and Fear

As discussed earlier, anxiety is diffuse and not easily defined. NANDA defines it as a "vague, uneasy feeling of discomfort or dread accompanied by an autonomic response (the source often nonspecific or unknown to the individual); a feeling of apprehension caused by anticipation of danger." Notice that the response is not to a danger but to the *anticipation* of danger. An anxious person worries; feels nervous, uneasy, and fearful; may be tearful; and often has physical symptoms, such as nausea, trembling, and sweating.

Fear is an emotion or feeling of apprehension from an identified danger, threat, or pain. The danger may be real or imagined. Anxiety and fear produce similar responses; however, some experts differentiate them as follows:

- Fear is a cognitive response, whereas anxiety is an emotional response.
- Fear is related to a present event, whereas anxiety is related to a future (or anticipated) event.
- The source of fear is easily identifiable, whereas the source of anxiety may not be identifiable.
- Fear can result from either a physical or a psychological event; anxiety results from psychological conflict rather than physical threat.

Mild to moderate anxiety may be adaptive because it motivates and mobilizes the person to action. However, severe anxiety consumes energy and interferes with the person's ability to focus on and respond to what is really happening.

Anxiety and fear initiate release of epinephrine, which stimulates the sympathetic nervous system and prepares the person for fight or flight. Therefore, living with anxiety can be physically, emotionally, and spiritually exhausting.

Ego Defense Mechanisms

Just as the body responds physiologically to stressors, it has psychological responses that protect the person from anxiety and assist with adaptation. *Ego defense mechanisms* are unconscious mental mechanisms that make a stressful situation more tolerable by decreasing the inner tension associated with the stressors. Table 24.2 identifies some common psychological defense mechanisms.

When used in small doses, and for mild to moderate anxiety, defense mechanisms can be helpful. When overused, however, they become habits that give us the false illusion that we are coping. **If** psychological defense mechanisms are inadequate to diminish the threat and restore equilibrium, the person may develop an anxiety disorder.

Anger and Depression

Anger is a strong, uncomfortable feeling of animosity, hostility, extreme indignation, or displeasure. A person who cannot control stressors may become apprehensive (anxious about what may happen) and may respond with anger. Thus, moderate anger is often a first protective response against anxiety. As anxiety increases and the person recognizes fear, he feels more threatened

Table 24.2: Psychological Defense Mechanisms		
Ego defence mechanism	*Illustrations*	*Illustrations and consequences of overuse*
Avoidance–unconsciously staying away from events or situations that might open feelings of aggression or anxiety.	"I can't go to the class reunion tonight I'm too tired; I have to sleep."	The person becomes socially isolated because of the tension he feels when around other people.
Compensation–making up for a perceived inadequacy by developing or emphasizing some other desirable trait.	A small boy who wants to be on the football team instead becomes a great singer.	Use of drugs or alcohol to gain courage to enter a social situation.
Conversion–emotional conflict is changed into physical symptoms that have no physical basis. The symptoms often disappear after the threat is over.	Feeling back pain when it is difficult to continue carrying the pressures of life; developing nausea that causes the person to miss a major exam.	Laryngitis, inability to speak on the anniversary of father's death. Continued anxiety can lead to actual physical disorders, such as gastric ulcers.
Denial–transforming reality by refusing to acknowledge thoughts, feeling, desires, or impulses. This is unconscious; the person is *not* consciously lying. Denial is usually the first defense learned.	A student refuses to acknowledge that he is barely passing anatomy, does not withdraw from the class, and is now failing a nursing course. An alcoholic states, "I can quit any time I want to."	Overuse can lead to repression and dissociative disorders (e.g., dual personalities, selective amnesia).
Displacement–"kicking the dog." Transferring emotions, ideas, or wishes from one original object or situation to a substitute inappropriate person or object that is perceived to be less powerful or threatening.	Husband loses his job, goes home, and yells at his wife. (This mechanism is rarely adaptive.)	In extreme situations, this mechanism leads to verbal and physical abuse.

Contd...

Table 24.2: *Contd...*

Ego defence mechanism	Illustrations	Illustrations and consequences of overuse
Dissociation–painful events are separated or dissociated from the conscious mind.	A person who was sexually abused as a child describes the events as though they happened to a sibling.	May result in a dissociative disorder, such as multiple personality disorder.
Identification–a person takes on the ideas, personality, or characteristics of another person, especially someone that the person fears or respects.	Children play cowboy, police, fireman, or mommy.	Assumes mannerisms, wears clothing, and arranges hair and physical appearance to match those of the other person.
Intellectualization–cognitive reasoning is used to block or avoid feelings about a painful incident.	When her husband dies, the wife relieves her pain by thinking, "It's better this way; he was in so much pain." Person says, "I think" rather than, "I feel."	"My husband loves me, so he doesn't like it when another man talks to me; that's why he beats me."
Minimization–not acknowledging or accepting the significance of one's own behavior, making it less important.	"It doesn't matter how much I drink. I never drive when I'm drinking,"	Person engages in unhealthy or antisocial behavior; no motivation to change behavior.
Projection–Blaming others. Attributing one's own personality traits, mistakes, emotions, motives, and thoughts to another; "finger pointing."	The clinical instructor makes me nervous, so I cannot do well." "I forgot to bake cookies because you did not tell me that cookies were due at school today."	Person cannot see his own responsibility for a situation, so he cannot make adaptive behaviors. Person criticizes habits in others that are the same as one/s own bad habits.
Rationalization–use of a logical-sounding excuse to cover up or justify true ideas, actions, or feelings. An attempt to preserve self-respect or approval or to conceal a motive for some action by giving a socially acceptable reason. Similar to intellectualization, but uses faulty logic.	"It was God's will that this happened to me." "If I didn't have to work, I would be a better wife."	This mechanism can lead to self-deception.
Reaction formation–similar to compensation, except the person develops the exact opposite trait. The person is aware of her feelings but acts in ways opposite to what she is really feeling.	"It's OK that you forgot my birthday" (when it really is not O.K.)	Overuse can cause failure to resolve internal conflicts.
Regression–using behavior appropriate in an earlier stage of development to overcome feeling of insecurity in a present situation.	Cooks and eats a comfort food (e.g. hot fudge sundae). A 60-year-old divorcee dresses and acts like a teenager.	Can interfere with perception of reality.
Repression–unconscious "burying" or forgetting" of painful thoughts, feelings, memories, ideas; pushing them from consciousness to unconscious level. A step deeper than denial.	Having no memory of sexual abuse by sibling or father. An adolescent forgets to put out the trash because being "bossed" makes him angry, but he feels guilty if he consciously chooses not to do it.	Flashbacks, traumatic stress syndrome, and amnesia.
Restitution (undoing)–making amends for a behavior one thinks is unacceptable, to reduce guilt.	Giving a treat to a child who has been punished for wrongdoing.	May send double messages, Relieves the person of the responsibility for honesty about the situation.
Sublimation–unacceptable drives, traits, or behaviors (often sexual or aggressive) are unconsciously diverted to socially accepted traits.	Anger is expressed by aggression when playing sports. A person who chooses to not have children runs a day-care center.	The "acceptable" behavior might reinforce the negative tendencies, and the person may still show signs of the undesirable trait or behavior. For example, a person indulges in child pornography to obtain sexual gratification.

and may resort to bullying behavior to increase the personal feeling of power, control, and self-esteem.

Anger may be expressed in screaming or shouting, throwing things, or hitting, or more subtly with sarcastic, caustic remarks. Some people attempt to soften their hurtful remarks, or make them more socially acceptable, through the use of humor and joking. When anger involves destructive behaviors such as physical or verbal abuse, it is called **hostility.** When expressed appropriately and clearly (i.e. verbally), anger can be adaptive, because it temporarily releases the person's feelings of tension. When the anger is out in the open, both parties can deal with it. Nevertheless, even verbal expressions of anger can be destructive if the anger continues after the person expresses it.

Depression is sometimes associated with unresolved anger and may result from stress. It is normal to feel depression in response to any loss or a traumatic event, but long-term depression is a cause of concern.

Spiritual Responses to Stress

Spiritual responses to stress are multifaceted. Many people depend on a higher power or religious community for support when coping with stress. Some search for a larger meaning in the illness or other stressor. Others may view stress as a test, or a punishment, or a challenge.

Often, a first response during the alarm stage is to pray or ask for help. Prayer, meditation, and religious affiliation can also help during the second stage (adaptation). In the final stage, spiritual resources may be exhausted, leaving the person feeling abandoned, helpless, and hopeless. If your own spiritual life is healthy, you will be better equipped to support patients who are experiencing spiritual challenges.

Complication of Adaptation Failure

Living with continual stress strains adaptive mechanisms. This strain can lead to exhaustion and disease, which in turn can lead to more stress. Once established, this type of positive feedback loop is difficult to break. Three types of disorders that can develop when adaptation fails are stress-induced organic responses, somatoform disorders, and psychological disorders.

Stress-induced Organic Responses

As a result of repeated central nervous system stimulation and frequent elevation of certain hormones, continual stress brings about long-term changes in various body systems. People who use maladaptive coping strategies (e.g. overeating, substance abuse) create additional stress on the body, further contributing to disease.

- *Cardiovascular system:* Continued secretion of epinephrine may cause cardiovascular disorders including angina, myocardial infarction, cardiomegaly, and congestive heart failure, all of which lead to decreased cardiac output. As cardiac output decreases, less oxygen circulates to meet cellular metabolic demands, and the body experiences fatigue. Prolonged secretion of epinephrine and renin result in vasoconstriction, causing hypertension. ADH, aldosterone, ACTH, and cortisol create electrolyte imbalance and retention of sodium and water, thus promoting peripheral edema.
- *Endocrine system:* Continuing high levels of blood glucose and insulin can cause diabetes. Metabolic disorders of hyperthyroidism or hypothyroidism can result as persistent demands for thyroid hormone production cause a rebound failure of the gland.
- *Immune system:* Stress reduces the ability of the body's immune cells to differentiate between self and nonself. Thus, the immune cells begin to attack body tissues, producing autoimmune illness. Common auoimmune illnesses include rheumatoid arthritis, lupus, cancer, and allergies. In addition, studies of patients with HIV suggest that stress increases viral replication and suppresses the immune system.
- *Gastrointestinal system:* The gastrointestinal system may respond to central nervous system stimulation with constipation or diarrhea, gastroesophageal reflux, colitis, or irritable bowel syndrome. Continued secretion of hydrochloric acid produces gastric hyperacidity and erosion of the gastrointestinal tract.
- *Musculoskeletal system:* Constant readiness for fight or flight produces muscle tension and pain in various body sites. Tension headache and temporomandibular joint pain result from prolonged muscle tension in the head, neck, and spine.
- *Respiratory system:* Epinephrine and circulating hormones dilate the bronchial tubes and increase the rate of respiration. Hyperventilation can produce symptoms of alkalosis, including dizziness, tingling hands and feet, and anxiety. Distress in the respiratory system can exacerbate existing asthma, hay fever, and allergies.

Somatoform Disorders

Somatoform disorders are conditions characterized by the presence of physical symptoms with no known organic cause. They are believed to result from unconscious denial, repression, and displacement of anxiety. Certain people seem predisposed to somatoform disorders–for instance, those who do not handle anxiety well and those who are dependent, emotionally needy, frustrated, and resentful (Neeb, 2001). The physical symptoms allow the person to avoid a situation that, if confronted, would provoke extreme anxiety. The following are examples of somatoform disorders:

- **Hypochondriasis:** The person is preoccupied with the idea that he is or will become seriously ill. The person is abnormally concerned with his health and interprets his real or imagined symptoms unrealistically, fearing that they will get worse or become incurable.

- **Somatization:** In this disorder, anxiety and emotional turmoil are expressed in physical symptoms, loss of physical function, pain that changes location often, and depression. The patient is unable to control the symptoms and behaviors.
- **Somatoform pain disorder:** This is emotional pain that manifests physically. Pain is the patient's main concern. The level of pain the person states is inconsistent with the physical condition–that is, no physical cause can be found for the pain. The pain does not change location.
- **Malingering:** Malingering is different from the other disorders because it is a *conscious* effort to escape unpleasant situations. The patient merely pretends to have the symptoms.

Stress-Induced Psychological Responses

Even if coping mechanisms are effective initially, with long-term stress, exhaustion sets in, and the mechanisms begin to fail. The person may then try maladaptive ways to cope. As work and personal relationships deteriorate, the person loses self-esteem. Prolonged stress can eventually result in crisis and burnout. More severe responses include psychiatric illnesses, such as anxiety disorders, clinical depression, and post-traumatic disorder (PSTD). (Please read author's text on 'Psychiatric Mental Health Nursing' for more details).

Crisis

A crisis exists when (1) an event in a person's life drastically changes the person's routine and he perceives it as a threat to self, and (2) the person's usual coping methods are ineffective, resulting in high levels of anxiety and inability to function adequately. Such events are often sudden and unexpected (e.g. serious illness or death of a loved one, serious financial losses, an automobile accident, rape, and natural disasters).

Keep in mind that each person has a different tolerance for stress and that an event that creates a crisis for one may be just a minor nuisance for another. Nevertheless, most experts agree that people experiencing crisis go through five phases.

1. *Precrisis:* In response to the event and the anxiety, the person uses her usual coping strategies. The person has no symptoms, denies any stress, and may even report a feeling of well-being.
2. *Impact:* If the usual strategies are not effective, anxiety and confusion increase. The person may have trouble organizing her personal life. The person may feel the stress but minimize its severity.
3. *Crisis:* The person experiences more anxiety and tries new ways of coping, such as withdrawal, rationalization, and projection. The person recognizes the problem but denies that it is out of control.
4. *Adaptive:* The person redefines the threat and perceives the crisis in a realistic way. She begins to think rationally and does some positive problem solving, regains some self-esteem and is able to begin socializing again. Adaptation is more likely if the person can use effective coping strategies and if situational supports are available.

5. *Postcrisis:* The aftermath of a crisis may have both positive and negative effects on functioning. The person may have developed better ways of coping with stress. Or, she may be critical, hostile, and depressed, and she may use maladaptive strategies (e.g. overeating or substance abuse) to deal with what has happened.

People in crisis are at risk for physical and emotional harm, so intervention is essential.

Burnout

Burnout occurs when nurses and other professionals cannot cope effectively with the physical and emotional demands of the workplace. Examples of specific to nursing include the following:

- Dealing with difficult personalities (e.g. patient, supervisors, physicians)
- Working 12-hour shifts with minimal breaks for food, water, or rest
- Frequent rotating shifts that upset the circadian rhythm of the body and lower the immune system response
- Mandatory overtime
- Being "floated" to an unfamiliar unit (e.g. a maternity nurse may be "floated" to an orthopedic unit)
- Workload: low staffing ratio (one nurse to many patients)
- Frustration with patients (e.g. who do not follow therapeutic routines)
- Need to constantly anticipate patients' needs and cope with the unexpected
- Feeling helpless against patient's disease process or lack of healing
- Dealing with death and dying
- Lack of rewards (both intrinsic and extrinsic)
- Lack of participation in decision making
- Inability to delegate responsibilities
- Organizational philosophy that conflicts with personal philosophy.

Excessive demands by an employer serve as a catalyst for burnout. In some situations, the nurse receives no respect and little support from the employer or co-workers. Filled with feelings of injustice for treatment received, the nurse may respond with anger and frustration, feel overwhelmed and helpless, and suffer low self-esteem and depression. The nurse who burns out may develop a physical illness or a negative attitude or may use maladaptive coping techniques such as smoking, substance abuse, or distancing from patients–"going through the motions" but not really interacting with patients in a meaningful way. Many nurses in such situations give up and leave nursing. You will find suggestions for preventing burnout later in the chapter.

Post-traumatic Stress Disorder

Post-traumatic stress disorder (PTSD) is a specific response to a violent, traumatizing event, such as an earthquake or other natural disaster, or to physical or emotional abuse, such as rape, torture, or war experience. The victim experiences anxiety and flashbacks that may last for months or years. Other symptoms include social withdrawal, feelings of low self-esteem, changes in existing relationships, difficulty forming new relationships, irritability and outbursts of anger for no obvious reason, depression, and chemical abuse or dependence.

Counseling and special intervention are needed to help the person cope with and recover from the impact of the traumatic event.

Nursing Management

People under stress may not be thinking early, so it is important to intervene to relieve their immediate anxiety as much as possible, demonstrate empathy, and develop rapport before beginning an assessment. Focus the patient by asking short, direct questions and then proceeding to open-ended questions that will provide you with as much information as possible.

Assessment

Assessment should explore subjective and objective data about the person's stressors, risk factors, coping and adaptation, support systems, and stress responses.

- **Assess Stressors, Risk Factors, and Coping and Adaptation**
  Data about the patient's stressors and risk factors should help you to (1) determine whether the client has a realistic or an exaggerated perception of the stressors, (2) identify factors that increase risk for future stress, and (3) identify interventions to reduce current stress and to provide anticipatory guidance to prevent future stress. You might begin gathering this data by having the client complete a stress inventory, such as the Holmes-Rahe Scale.

- **Assess Responses to Stress**
  When assessing responses to stress, recall that stress responses are holistic. Therefore, you will need to assess physiological, emotional, cognitive, and behavioral indicators of stress.

- **Assessing Physiological Responses**
  Because the GAS is nonspecific, you must obtain data from all body systems. A check of vital signs for elevations in pulse, respiration, and blood pressure will indicate whether the fight-or-night response is present. In your general survey, or overview, of the patient, you should note hygiene, grooming, facial expression, and ability to make eye contact. If coping is successful, clinical signs and symptoms of stress may not be present.
  The physiological responses to stressors are as given below.
  - Dilated pupils
  - Muscle tension
  - Stiff neck
  - Headaches
  - Nail biting

- Skin pallor
- Skin lesions (e.g. eczema)
- Diaphoresis, sweaty palms
- Dry mouth
- Nausea
- Weight or appetite changes
- Increased blood glucose
- Increased heart rate
- Cardiac dysrhythmias
- Hyperventilation
- Chest pain
- Water retention
- Increased urinary frequency or decreased urinary output
- Diarrhea or constipation
- Flatulence

- **Assessing Emotional and Behavioral Responses**
  As the client answers questions, note posture, facial expression, body tension, and other nonverbal behaviors. Also note mood and affect. Does the client seem angry, anxious, or depressed? Check the client's records, observe for and ask the client about destructive behaviors (e.g. drug abuse, anger). The client mayor may not be aware that the feelings or behaviors are related to stress.

- **Assessing Cognitive Responses**
  You can assess the client's cognitive functioning as you assess other functional areas. Notice whether the person has difficulty focusing and responding to your questions. When you ask the client to describe and rate the intensity of the stressors, you can begin to assess whether he perceives the stressors realistically or in an exaggerated way. The client's responses concerning any coping strategies will give you an idea of his problem-solving abilities.

- **Assess Support Systems**
  Recall that support systems such as family, friends, and co-workers can be important to the success of a client's coping strategies. Conversely, these people may be affected by the same stressors or by the client's response to them. For these reasons, you should determine the supports available and their ability to assist the client–that is, do the significant others have the sensitivity and skills to be supportive?

- **Nursing Diagnosis**
  Stress is nonspecific, so there is almost no limit to the number of nursing diagnoses that could be stress-induced. It is important to correctly identify the etiology so that you can choose interventions to remove or modify the stressor. For example, if you believe a patient's diarrhea is being caused by stress, you would intervene by modifying the stressor, helping the patient to perceive the stressor differently, and so on. If, instead, the diarrhea were being caused by a gastrointestinal virus, your interventions would not have been helpful.

The nursing diagnoses associated with stress are as given below:

- *Physical Domain*
  - Constipation
  - Delayed growth and development
  - Diarrhea
  - Disturbed energy field
  - Disturbed sleep pattern
  - Fatigue
  - Imbalanced nutrition (can be more than or less than body requirements)
  - Nausea
  - Pain (e.g. backache)
  - Risk for imbalanced fluid volume risk for injury
  - Sleep deprivation

- *Behavioral Domain*
  - Ineffective health maintenance
  - Ineffective therapeutic regimen management

- *Cognitive Domain*
  - Disturbed thought processes
  - Impaired memory

- *Emotional Domain*
  - Anxiety decisional conflict defensive coping fear
  - Grieving (anticipatory or dysfunctional) impaired adjustment
  - Ineffective coping
  - Ineffective denial
  - Low self-esteem (chronic or situational)

- *Interpersonal Relationships Domain*
  - Caregiver role strain
  - Compromised or disabled family coping impaired parenting
  - Impaired social interaction
  - Ineffective community coping
  - Interrupted family processes
  - Post-trauma syndrome
  - Relocation stress syndrome
  - Social isolation

- *Spiritual Domain*
  - Hopelessness spiritual distress

Nursing Management of Stress According to Stages

Stage of Alarm Reaction: The first stage of the stress response is the alarm reaction of the GAS, in which the individual perceives a stressor physically or mentally and the "fight or flight" response is initiated. When the stressor is of sufficient intensity to threaten the steady state of the individual, it requires a reallocation of energy so that adaptation can occur. In this stage, the sympathetic fight or flight response is activated with release of adrenal-medullary hormones and the ACTH-adrenal cortical response begins. The alarm reaction is defensive and anti-inflammatory but self-limited. This temporarily decreases the individual's resistance and may even result in disease or death, if the stress is prolonged and severe, (because it is impossible to live in a continuous state of alarm).

The physical signs and symptoms of the alarm reactions are generally those of sympathetic nervous system stimulation. These signs include increased blood pressure, increased heart and respiratory rate, decreased gastrointestinal motility, pupil dilatation, and increased perspiration. The patient may complain of such symptoms as increased anxiety, nausea and anorexia.

Stage of Resistance: Since it is impossible to live in a continuous state of alarm, the person moves into the second stage, resistance. Ideally, the individual quickly moves from the alarm reaction to the stage of resistance, in which physiologic forces are mobilized to increase the resistance to stress. During this stage, adaptation to noxious stressors occurs. At this time, adaptation may occur, involving modification of the external and internal environment. Resistance is high at this time as compared to the normal state due to increased cortisol activity. The amount of resistance varies among individuals, depending on the level of physical functioning, coping abilities, and total number and intensity of stressors experienced. Although few overt physical symptoms and signs occur in this state as compared to the alarm stage, the person is expending energy in an attempt to adapt. This adaptive energy is limited by the resources of the individual.

Stage of Exhaustion: The stage of exhaustion occurs when all the energy for adaptation has expended. Exhaustion sets in and endocrine activity increases, producing deleterious effects on the body systems (especially circulatory, digestive and immune) that can lead to death. The physical symptoms of alarm reaction may briefly reappear in a final effort of the body to survive. This is exemplified by a terminally ill person who becomes alert and has stronger vital signs shortly, before death. The individual at this stage of exhaustion usually becomes ill and may die if assistance from outside sources is not available. This stage can often be reversed by external sources of adaptive energy such as medications, blood transfusion or psychotherapy. According to Selye, there is also a local adaptation syndrome (LAS). This syndrome includes inflammatory response and repair process that occur at the local site of tissue injury. The LAS occurs in small, topical injuries such as in contact dermatitis. If the local injury were severe enough, the GAS would be activated also.

The client faces an array of potential stressors, or demands that can have health consequences. The nurse needs to be aware of the situations that are likely to result in stress and also must assess the client's appraisal of the situations. The major areas that provide the nurse with useful guide in the assessment process include demands, human response to stressors and coping. It is always better to observe the following indices of stress, in which some are psychologic, some are physiologic, some-behavioral, and some reflect social behavior and thought process. Some of these reactions may be coping behaviors.

- General irritability, hyperexcitation or depression
- Dryness of the throat and mouth
- Overpowering urge to cry or run and hide
- Easily fatigued, loss of interest
- Floating anxiety–do not know what or why
- Easily started
- Stuttering or other speech difficulties
- Hypermobility, pacing, moving about, cannot look still
- GI symptoms–butterflies in the stomach, diarrhea, vomiting
- Change in menstrual cycle
- Loss or excessive appetite
- Increased use of legally prescribed drugs, e.g., tranquilizers
- Accident proneness
- Disturbed behavior
- Pounding of the heart
- Impulsive behavior, emotional instability
- Inability to concentrate
- Feelings of unreality, weakness or dizziness
- Tension, alertness
- Nervous laughter
- Grinding of teeth
- Insomnia
- Perspiring
- Increased frequency of urination
- Muscle tension and migraine, headache
- Pain in the neck and lower back
- Increased smoking
- Alcohol and drug addiction
- Nightmares

The probable nursing diagnosis in coping-tolerance pattern will be as follows:

- Impaired adjustment
- Caregiver role strain
- Ineffective individual coping; defensive coping/ ineffective denial
- Ineffective family coping; compromised
- Ineffective family coping; disabled
- Family coping; potential for growth
- Post-trauma response
- Relocation stress syndrome
- Risk for self harm
- Risk for violence

And plan the nursing interventions according to the situation or event and stress.

Nursing Interventions in Stress Management

The first step in managing stress is to become aware of its presence. This includes identifying and expressing stressful feelings (as stated above). The role of the nurse is to facilitate and enhance the coping and adaptation. Nursing interventions depend on the severity of the stress experience and demand. The nurse's efforts are directed to life-supporting interventions and to the inclusion of approaches aimed at the reduction of additional stressors to the client. The importance of cognitive appraisal in the stress experience should prompt the nurse to assess if changes in the way the client perceives and label particular events or situations (cognitive reappraisal) are possible. So the nurse should also consider the positive effects that result from successfully meeting, stressful demands. Greater emphasis should also be placed on the part of cultural values and beliefs enhancing or constraining various coping options.

An individual personal resource that aids in coping include health and energy. A health-promoting lifestyle provides these resources and buffers or cushions the impact of stressors. Lifestyle or habits that contributed to the risk of developing illness can be reduced or eliminated. Health risk appraisal is an assessment method designed to promote health by examining the individual personal habits and recommending change where health risk is identified. For example, smoking causes lung cancer and can be prevented by reducing or leaving the habit of smoking.

Coping Enhancement

Coping enhancement is a nursing intervention and defined as "assisting a patient to adapt to perceived stressors, changes, or threats which interfere with meeting life demands and roles" (McCloskey, Bulechek 1992). After completing a health risk approach, the nurse could use "coping enhancement" to assist the patient in an analysis of the appraisal and to explore methods to improve the person's coping abilities including appraisal of his or her own personal resources.

The activities of coping enhancement are as follows:
- Appraise the patient's adjustment to change in body image as indicated
- Appraise the impact of the patient's life situations on roles and relationships
- Encourage the patient to identify a realistic description of change in role
- Approve the patient's understanding of the disease process
- Approve and discuss alternative responses to situation
- Use a calm reassuring approach
- Provide an atmosphere of acceptance
- Assist patient in developing an objective appraisal of an event
- Help the client to identify the information he/she made interested in obtaining
- Provide factual information concerning diagnosis, treatment and prognosis
- Provide the patient with realistic choices about certain aspects of care
- Encourage an attitude to realistic hope as a way of dealings with feelings of helplessness
- Evaluate patient's decision-making ability
- Seek to understand the patient's perspective of a stressful situation

- Discourage decision-making when patient is under severe stress
- Encourage gradual mastery of the situation
- Encourage patience in developing relationships
- Encourage relationships with persons who have common interests and goals
- Encourage social and community activities
- Encourage the acceptance of limitation of others
- Acknowledge the patient's spiritual/ cultural background
- Encourage the use of spiritual resources if desired
- Explore the patient's previous achievement of success
- Explore patient's reason for self-criticism
- Confront patient's ambivalent (anger or depression) feelings
- Foster constructive outlets of anger and hostility
- Arrange situations that encourage patient's autonomy
- Assist patient in identifying positive responses from others
- Encourage the identification of specific life values
- Explore with the patient previous methods of dealing with life problems
- Introduce the patient to persons (or group) who have successfully undergone the same experience
- Support the use of appropriate defence mechanisms
- Encourage verbalization of feelings, perceptions and fears
- Discuss consequences not dealing with guilt and shame
- Encourage the patient to identify own strength and abilities
- Assist patient in identifying appropriate short- and long-term goals
- Assist the patient in breaking down complex goals into manageable steps
- Assist the patient in examining available resources to meet the goal
- Reduce stimuli in the environment that could be misinterpreted as threatening
- Appraise patient's needs/ desires for social support
- Assist the patient to identify available support systems
- Determine the risk of the patient's inflicting self-harm
- Encourage family involvement as appropriate as possible
- Encourage the family verbalize feelings about ill family member
- Provide appropriate social skills training
- Assist the patient to solve problem in a constructive manner
- Instruct the patient about the use of relaxation techniques as needed
- Assist the patient to grieve, and work through the losses of chronic illness and/ or disability if appropriate
- Assist the patient to clarify misconceptions
- Encourage the patient to evaluate his/her own behavior

Health Promotion Activities for Coping with Stress

People cannot always control the occurrence of a stressful event, and there are no high-tech treatments for coping with stress. However, a healthy lifestyle can prevent some stressors and improve the ability to cope with others. The following suggestions are a brief guide to a healthy lifestyle.

Nutrition

Nutrition is important for maintaining physical homeostasis and resisting stress. For example, adequate nutrition is essential to maintain the integrity of the immune system; and proteins are needed for tissue building and healing. In addition, overweight and malnutrition are stressors that may lead to illness. To summarize, you should advise clients to:

- Maintain a normal body weight.
- Limit the intake of fat (especially animal fat) to no more than 30% of daily calories.
- Limit the intake of sugar and salt.
- Eat more fish and poultry and less red meat.
- Eat smaller, more frequent meals to aid digestion.
- Consume 25 grams of fiber (fruits, vegetables, and whole grains) daily to promote bowel elimination.
- Consume no more than two alcoholic beverages per day.

Exercise

Regular exercise promotes physical homeostasis by improving muscle tone and controlling weight. It also improves the functioning of the heart and lungs and reduces the risk of cardiovascular disease. Exercise also improves emotional homeostasis by promoting relaxation and reducing tension. During exercise, endogenous opioids are released, creating a feeling of wellbeing.

- To achieve health benefits, the client needs to exercise for at least 30 minutes most, if not all days of the week (Thompson & Manore, 2004).
- Advise clients who are obese, chronically ill, or who have always been sedentary to consult a primary caregiver before beginning a new exercise program.
- Suggest that the client identify a variety of physical activities that he enjoys (e.g. swimming, bicycling, walking, sports) and, if possible, schedule regular sessions with one or more exercise "buddies." These strategies help the client adhere to the exercise routine.

Sleep and Rest

Sleep and rest restore energy levels, allow the body to repair itself, and promote mental relaxation. Most people need 7 or 8 hours of sleep a day; however, the amount of sleep varies among individuals. Stress, pain, and illness may interfere with the ability to sleep, so some clients may need help identifying and implementing techniques for relaxing and going to sleep.

Leisure Activities

As compared to exercise, which not everyone enjoys, leisure activities are any activities that provide joy and satisfaction. They may involve physical activity (after all, many people do enjoy exercising), or they may be sedentary activities, such as reading, painting, and even watching television. Leisure activities are a form of rest and, as such, are restorative.

Time Management

People who manage their time efficiently and organize their life routines feel more in control and, therefore, less stressed. If clients feel overwhelmed, you can help them to prioritize tasks and make "to do" lists. It is also important that they learn to delegate responsibilities and set boundaries on the use of time. A working couple with three children may need to assign each child mealtime tasks, such as setting the table, drying the dishes, and so forth. Or they may need to limit the amount of time they spend cooking, reserving elaborate meals for weekends.

Time management also includes saying no. Out of a need to be liked or a strong sense of responsibility to others, people sometimes try to make everyone happy by agreeing to all requests for assistance: from spouse, children, parents, friends, church, school, and the community. You can prompt clients to identify how much they can realistically accomplish–what is essential to do, and what would be "nice" to do. Help clients to work out a balance between their responsibilities to self and their responsibilities to others.

Avoiding Maladaptive Behaviors

Some people use maladaptive behaviors as a response to stress. For others, the behaviors themselves become stressors. Advise clients to avoid the following unhealthful behaviors:
- Drinking more than two alcoholic beverages per day
- Consuming excess caffeine (e.g. coffee, tea, colas)
- Eating large quantities of nutrient-poor food, such as sweets
- Smoking or chewing tobacco
- Using illegal street drugs
- Abusing over-the-counter medications
- Avoiding social interaction

Relieving Anxiety

Because anxiety is a common response to illness, medical tests, and treatments, you will use anxiety-relief interventions every day of your professional life. For example, when you tell clients what to expect before you perform a procedure or ask them to take deep breaths during a painful treatment, you lessen anxiety. If you have developed a therapeutic, trusting relationship, your very presence will help to ease the patient's anxiety.

Anger Management

Anger is a common response to stress. However, clients usually do not openly say, "I am angry." In fact, they may not even recognize that they are angry. Instead, they engage in angry behaviors. For example, they may become hypercritical of family members or caregivers, become verbally abusive, or become

demanding. By now you have probably heard stories from nurses about the client who is "on the call light constantly." Unfortunately, such behaviors often provoke anger in others–even nurses. Be aware *of* how you are responding *to* angry clients. Are you relieving your own stress, or are you relieving the client's stress? If you respond angrily to relieve your own stress, you may provoke further anger in the client and even escalate the situation to the point of violence.

Stress Management Techniques

It is important to teach your clients about relaxation and other stress management techniques. Most such techniques focus on discharging tension or simplifying one's life to modify stressors or control stress responses. Relaxation is a state of reduced physical and mental arousal. It is an important intervention because it generally reverses some stress responses. By elongating muscle fibers, relaxation reduces neural impulses sent to the brain. Other physical responses include increased peripheral skin temperatures and decreases in activity of the brain with alpha wave activity, activity in other body systems, blood pressure, heart rate, and respiratory rate and oxygen consumption.

- *Exercise* reduces stress because it releases tension held in muscles, improves muscle tone and posture, expresses emotions, and stimulates the secretion of endorphins, thus creating a feeling of well-being and relaxation.
- *Relaxation techniques* involve teaching the patient to relax individual muscle groups. Progressive relaxation in a quiet meditation state or lying in bed, relaxing and contracting muscle groups is much less traumatic and damaging to fragile joints and muscles than active exercise. Therefore, it may be used even by people who are not in good health. Passive relaxation, in which the person relaxes the muscle groups without first contracting them, is even less traumatic and requires even less energy.
- *Meditation* involves heightening one's attention or awareness. Regular meditation increases harmony between mind, body, and spirit, thereby reducing anxiety and giving the person control.
- *Visualization or imagery* techniques are often used *to* complement the effects of relaxation techniques.
- *Biofeedback techniques* use electronic instruments to measure neuromuscular and autonomic nervous system activity and provide information about those responses to the person. The immediate feedback helps the person become aware of and learn how to voluntarily control certain physiological responses, such as those produced by stress. Biofeedback practitioners require special training, and most are credentialed in biofeedback.
- *Acupuncture* involves insertion of a needle into "meridian points" to regulate the flow of energy or life force throughout the body. It can modify pain perception and restore normal physiological functions (e.g. decrease the heart rate). Special training is required to use this intervention.

- *Chiropractic adjustment* involves manual realignment of the vertebrae. Misalignment of the vertebrae is thought to lead to loss of function and to illness. Realignment is performed to free energy, release muscle tension, and improve body function and health. Chiropractors undergo special education and training before they are qualified to perform adjustments.
- *Reiki and therapeutic touch* are focused on energy modulation. Healing energy is channeled through a practitioner's hands to improve well-being.
- *Massage,* through manipulation of the soft tissues, relaxes muscles, releases body tension, improves circulation, and allows energy and blood to flow through muscles and soft tissues more readily.
- *Reflexology* is the application of pressure to specific points on the feet, hands, or ears, which are thought to correspond with certain organs of the body. The goal is to relieve blockage, promote the flow of energy, and reduce tension- thus, reflexology may be helpful in treating stress-related illnesses.

The following are simpler activities you can recommend to most clients to aid in relaxation and stress reduction:

- *Humor:* Reading and telling jokes, viewing funny movies or stand-up routines, and simply appreciating the humor of situations all help release tension and anger and increase coping abilities. Laughter releases endorphins and relieves feelings of stress.
- *Listening to music:* Music soothes and relaxes when its vibrations are in harmony with body frequencies. Listening to tranquil music can also relax the mind.
- *Engaging in art activities:* Painting, working with day, and engaging in other art activities help to express emotions and release endorphins.
- *Dance and sports,* like other forms of exercise, release pent-up physical tension and emotions.
- *Journal writing* helps the person to reflect on experiences and express emotions. The catharsis of journal writing often provides insights into causes of stress and ways to modify stressors.

Changing Perception of Stressors or Self

Recall that altering one's perception is one way to improve adaptation to stress. For clients who have an unrealistic perception of the stressor and can imagine only negative outcomes, a technique called *cognitive restructuring* may be helpful. Using this technique, you help the clients to recognize their negative focus and to restructure their thinking in more positive and realistic ways. For example, you might encourage a working mother with demanding parents to take a single positive step, such as saying no to someone at least once a day.

You can also help clients to identify positive aspects of themselves and their coping abilities. This promotes self-esteem and helps them to recognize and use the resources they have for coping with their stressors. *Positive self-talk* is another method for increasing self-esteem. Each time you hear negative self-talk, stop the client, and ask him to rephrase the statement so that it is positive.

Relaxation Techniques

Synder (1993) and Egan (1993) identified relaxation technique as the major method used to relieve stress, included in nursing interventions. Commonly used techniques cited were progressive muscle relaxation, relaxation with guided imagery, and Senson's relaxation response. The goal of relaxation training is to produce response that counter the stress response.

Progressive muscle relaxation: It involves tensing and releasing the muscles of the body in sequence and sensing the difference in feeling. It is best if the person lies on a soft cushion on the floor, in a quiet room, breathing easily. Self-taught or instructor-directed exercise that can involve learning to contract and relax muscles in a systematic way beginning with face and ending with feet. This exercise may be combined with breathing exercises that focus on inner self.

Relaxation with guided imagery: It is the purposeful use of imagination to achieve relaxation and/ or direct attention away from undesirable sensations. The nurse helps the person to select a pleasant scene or experience from his or her past. This image serves as the mental device in this technique. As the person sits comfortably and quietly the nurse guides him to review the scene; trying to feel and relieve the imagery with all of the senses. A tape recording can be made for description of science of experience for the pleasant one.

Benson's relaxation response: Benson and Proctor (1984) describe the following steps for this response which include:

Step 1   Pick a brief phrase or word that reflects your basic belief systems.
Step 2   Choose a comfortable position.
Step 3   Close your eyes.
Step 4   Relax your muscle.
Step 5   Become aware of your breathing and start using your selected focus word.
Step 6   Maintain a passive attitude.
Step 7   Continue for a set period of time.
Step 8   Practice the technique twice a day.

The response combines meditation with relaxation. The other techniques of stress management will also include the following.

Thought stopping: It is a self-directed behavioral approach used to gain control of self-defeating thoughts. When these thoughts occur the individual stops the thought process and focuses on conscious relaxation.

Exercise: Regular exercise, especially, aerobic movement, results in improved circulation, increased release of endorphins on an enhanced sense of well-being.

Humor: In the forms of laughter, cartoons, funny movies, riddles, audiocassettes, comic books and joke books, humor can be used for both the nurse and patient.

Assertive behavior: Open, honest, sharing feelings, desires and opinions in a controlled way. The individual who has control over one's own life is less subject to stress.

Social support: This may take the form of organized support and self-help groups, relationships with family and friends and professional help.

In addition, meditation, breathing techniques, therapeutic touch, music therapy, bio-feedback can be used as stress management technique.

Identifying and Using Support Systems

You can facilitate successful adaptation by helping clients to identify and contact people and groups who offer various supports (e.g. listening, encouragement, advice, problem solving, help with household tasks, financial support). Be aware of the groups available in your community (e.g. Weight Watchers, Alcoholics Anonymous, Parents Without Partners, Reach for Recovery). You may need to teach socialization skills to clients who are socially isolated so that they can begin to build a support system.

Providing Spiritual Support

In addition to helping clients obtain spiritual support from Church groups and clergy, you can help to strengthen the client spiritually. You may wish to:

- Pray for or with clients, if they desire. Prayer can help reduce their feelings of powerlessness and loneliness.
- Help clients to define their values and set boundaries that honor themselves and uphold those values.
- Teach clients to silently recite an affirming mantra (e.g. on inhalation, say, "I am free." Exhale and say, "Stress, leave me.")

Crisis Intervention

As an entry-level nurse in acute and ambulatory care settings, you are more likely to see patients in the first three phases of crisis and not be present for the adaptive and postcrisis stages. The goals of crisis intervention at an entry level of practice include the following:

- Assess the situation.
- Ensure safety.
- Defuse the situation.
- Decrease the person's anxiety.
- Determine the problem.
- Decide on the type of help needed.
- Return the person to precrisis level of functioning.
  Crisis centers often rely on telephone counseling ("hotlines"). If telephone counseling is not adequate, or if observations of the home environment are needed, home visits may be necessary.

Stress Management in the Workplace

You will need to pay attention to your feelings, your body, and your personal responses to stress. If you notice that you are eating constantly, yelling at your children, not sleeping well, and so on, check your body. Do you feel tired? Are the muscles in your face and shoulders tense? If so, you need to start managing your stress. You can manage workplace stress and help prevent burnout by following the advice you give your patients.

When stressors arise from the workplace, the following actions are especially important:

- Have realistic expectations of yourself and others. Don't be overcritical, most people, including you, are doing the best they can.
- Ask for help. Some nurses feel that they must know everything, but asking for help does not indicate weakness. It can even make others feel good by giving them the opportunity to practice collegiality.
- Support colleagues who need help with tasks or with their feelings. This adds to the overall good feeling on a unit.
- Accept the things that you cannot change. Complaining and negative talk add to your own stress and that of others. Get involved in constructive efforts to change policies (e.g. regarding staffing, overtime, safety practices, and so on). If you cannot effect the changes, and if you cannot accept things as they are, you may need to think about leaving the organization rather than subjecting yourself to continual stress.
- Join and support professional organizations, that address workplace issues.
- Obtain counseling for severe stress.

25

Perioperative Nursing and Bandaging

Introduction

Surgery became a medical specially, because often the treatment of a wide variety of illness and injuries include some types of surgical intervention. Surgery is an invasive method of treatment that may be planned or unplanned, major or minor, and that may involve any body part or system. Care for the client during all phases of the surgical experience needs to be continuous, and integrated surgical procedures require physical and psychosocial adaptations and are stressors for both the client and the family. The client's recovery from a surgical procedure requires skillful and knowledgeable nursing care whether the surgery is of outpatient or in the hospital setting. Nurses working in both settings must understand the principles of caring for surgical clients.

As stated earlier, a client faces variety of stressors when confronting surgery. Anticipatory surgery leads to fear and anxiety for clients who associate surgery with pain, possible disfigurement, dependence, and perhaps even loss of life. Family members often fear a disruption in lifestyle and experience a sense of powerlessness as the surgery approaches. The trauma sustained during surgery creates physical needs requiring close supervision and skilled intervention by the nurse and surgeon. Nurses use all phases of nursing process used perioperatively to make assessment and provide interventions necessary to promote the recovery of health, prevent further injury or illness, and facilitate coping with alterations in physical structure and function.

Definition

- **Perioperative nursing** refers to the role of the nurse during the preoperative, intraoperative and postoperative phases of a client's surgical experience. The concept of perioperative nursing stresses the importance of providing continuity of care.
- **A perioperative nurse** is defined as the registered nurse, who, using the nursing process, designs, coordinates and delivers care to meet the identified needs of the clients whose protective reflexes or self-care abilities are potentially compromised because they are under the influence of anesthesia during operative or other invasive procedures
- **Perioperative nurse,** possesses and applies knowledge of the procedure and the client's intraoperative experience throughout the client-care continuum. And also they assess, diagnose, plan, intervene and evaluate the outcome of interventions based on criteria and support of a standard care targeted towards the population
- **The perioperative nurse** addresses the changing physiological, pathophysiological, sociocultural and spiritual responses of the client that have been initiated by the prospect of performance of the invasive procedure.

Scope of Perioperative Nursing

The scope of perioperative nursing practice consists of three phases:
- Preoperative
- Intraoperative and
- Postoperative

Preoperative phase: It begins where the decision for surgical intervention is made and ends with transference of the client to the operative site. Nursing activities range from a baseline assessment of the client during the preoperative interview and continues with assessment in the pre-admission unit, client room, holding area, or induction room on the day of surgery. Before surgery, the nurse prepares the client and family for the surgery, performs diagnostic tests, and assesses the client in preparation for the operation.

Intraoperative phase: It begins where the client is transferred to the operating room bed and ends when the client is transferred to an area of recovery from anesthesia. In this phase, nursing interventions range from communicating the client's plan of care, identifying nursing activities, necessary for expected outcome and establishing priorities for nursing actions. During surgery, the nurse assists surgeons and other operating room nurses to ensure that the client receives optimal care. The nurse also coordinates client needs with team members and personnel's from other disciplines, coordinates the use of the supplies and equipment, controls the environment, prepares for potential emergencies, and communicates and documents the client's plan of care.

Postoperative phase: It begins with the client's transfer to an area for recovery and ends with client's recovery from surgery. Nursing activities range from communicating pertinent information about the client's surgery, to assist the client to be physical stability and wakefulness and institute measures to help the client achieve maximum recovery.

Classification of Surgical Procedure

Surgery can be defined as the art and science of treating diseases, injuries and deformities by operation and instrumentation. The surgical procedure involves the interaction of the patient, the surgeon, and the nurse. Surgical procedures usually are classified on the basis of urgency degree of risk, and purposes.

(i) Based on Urgency

Surgery may be classified as elective surgery, urgent surgery and emergency surgery.

Elective surgery: It is preplanned and performed on the basis of client's choice. It is not essential and may not be necessary for health and delay in surgery has no ill effects, can be scheduled in advance based on the choice of client.

The purposes of elective surgery are as follows:
- To remove or repair a body part
- To restore function
- To improve health
- To improve self-concept

For example, tonsillectomy, hernia repair, cataract extraction and lens implant, hip prosthesis, hemorrhoiditis, etc.

Urgent surgery: In which the surgery is the necessity for the client's health, but not an emergency. This is performed for the purposes as in elective surgery and to prevent further tissue damage. For example, removal of gallbladder, coronary artery, removal of tumor, etc.

Emergency surgery: When surgery must be done immediately to preserve the client's life, remove or repair body part, restore function, improve health and self concept. For example, perforated ulcer, intestinal obstruction, tracheostomy, cesarean section.

(ii) Based on Degree of Risk or Seriousness

Surgery has been classified as major or minor on the basis of risk for the client:

Major surgery: It involves extensive reconstruction or alteration in body parts poses great risks to wellbeing. It requires hospitalization usually belonged to wellbeing; has a high degree of risk; involves major body organs, life-threatening situations and potential postoperative complications. Major surgery may be elective, urgent, or emergency. For example, nephrectomy, cholecystectomy, colostomy, hysterectomy.

Minor surgery: It is primarily elective; it is usually a brief, carries low risk and results in few complications. It can be performed in clinics, outpatient clinic and minor operation theatres. For example, teeth extraction, removal of warts, skin biopsy, laparoscopy, dilatations and curettage.

(iii) Based on Purpose

Surgical procedures based on purpose include diagnostic, ablative, palliative, reconstructive, transplant, constructive.

Diagnostic: It is surgical exploration that allows physician to make or to confirm diagnosis, may involve removal of tissue for further diagnostic testing. For example, breast biopsy, laparoscopy, bronchoscopy, exploratory laparotomy (incision in peritoneal cavity to inspect abdominal organs).

Ablative: It is excision or removal of diseased body part. For example, appendicectomy, subtotal thyroidectomy, partial gastrectomy, colon resection, amputation, cholecystectomy, etc.

Palliative surgery: It is performed to relieve or reduce intensity of an illness or disease symptoms will not produce cure. For example, colostomy, nerve root resection (rhizotomy) debridement of necrotic tissue, balloon angioplasty, arthroscopy, etc.

Reconstructive surgery: It is performed to restore function to traumatized or malfunctioning tissues and to improve self-concept. For example, scar revision, plastic surgery, skin graft, internal fixation of fractures, breast reconstruction.

Table 25.1: Common Prefixes and Suffixes in Surgery

Prefixes		*Suffixes*	
Terms	*Definitions*	*Terms*	*Definitions*
Supra-	Above, beyond	-oma	Tumor, swelling
Artho-	Joint	-ectomy	Removal of organ
Chole-	Bile or gall	-rrhapy	The suturing or stitching of part of an organ
Cysto-	Bladder	-scopy	Looking into
Endocephalo-	Brain	-ostomy	Making an opening or stoma
Hystero-	Uterus	-otomy	Cutting into
Mast-	Breast	-plasty	To repair or restore
Menigo-	Membrane	-cele	Tumor, hernia, swelling
Myo-	Muscle	-itis	Inflammation of
Nephro-	Kidney		
Oophor-	Ovary		
Pneumo-	Lung		
Pyelo-	Pelvis, kidney		
Salpingo-	Fallopian tube		
Thoraco-	Chest		
Viscero-	Organ especially abdomen		

Transplant: It is performed to replace organs or structures that are diseased or malfunctioning. For example, kidney, cornea, liver, heart, joints, total hip replacement.

Constructive surgery: It is performed to restore function lost or reduced as a result of congenital anomalies. For example, repair of cleft palate, closure of a trial defect in heart.

Sometime combination of several surgery explained above also are performed as and when needed.

The common prefixes and suffixes used to explain the types of surgical procedures are described in Table 25.1.

Role of Nurse in Perioperative Care

General Care

Each surgical client responds differently in surgery, when he / she enters the healthcare setting in different stages of health. Many variables influence a person's physiologic and psychological responses to the surgical experience. These include physical and mental status, extent of disease, magnitude of the surgery, social and financial resources and psychological an physiological preparation for surgery. When considered effectively, these variables reveal the degree of risk for a client undergoing surgery.

While making physiological assessment before surgery, nurse elicits information about age; presence of pain; nutritional status; fluid and electrolyte balance; presence of infections; physical mobility, skin integrity, cardiovascular; pulmonary, renal, gastrointestinal, liver, endocrine, neurologic and hematologic function; sensory medication history, abnormalities, injuries and previous surgeries, health habits, and sociocultural history (see Health Assessment) and note any abnormalities and report to the concerned and take suitable measures to correct and sending the client to operating room.

The possible preoperative tests include the following and reasons for those tests and normal ranges stated are as follows:

- Complete blood count and picture should be tested
- Serum potassium (normal 3.5-5 mEq/L) to identify hyperkalemia or hypokalemia.
- Serum sodium (normal 136 to 145 mEq/L) to identify hypernatremia dehydration or overhydration
- Serum chloride (normal 96-100 mEq/L) to identify hyperchloremia, hypochloremia, or metabolic disorder.
- Glucose (normal 60-100 mg/dL) to identify hypoglycemia or hyperglycemia
- Creatinine (normal 0.7-1.4 mg/dL) to identify acute or chronic renal disease
- Blood urea nitrogen (BUN) (10-20 mg/dL) to identify impaired liver or kidney function or excessive protein or tissue catabolism
- Hemoglobin (Hb) (Female) (12 to 15 gm/dL; Male 13-17 gm) to identify the presence and extent of anemia
- Hematocrit (Hct) (Female 36%; Male 39-51%) to identify the presence and extent of anemia

- Prothorombin time (PT) or clotting time (CT) (11-18 seconds) to identify dysfunction of blood clotting (prothrombin level)
- Partial thromboplastin time (PTT) to identify deficiencies of coagulation factors
- Chest X-ray (No abnormal heart of lung lesion) to determine size and contour of heart, lungs, and major vessels
- Electrocardiogram (ECG) (Normal rate and rhythm) to determine the electrical activity of the heart
- Urine analysis to identify abnormalities

Any deviations from the normal, should be noted and reported to take precautions during surgery. And the common medical conditions that increase the high risk in surgery will include bleeding disorders, diabetes mellitus, heart diseases, upper respiratory infection, liver diseases, fever, chronic respiratory diseases, and immunological disorders. A special precaution should be taken on these cases before, during and after surgery.

Preoperative Nursing Care

Persons who require surgical intervention and nursing care enter the healthcare settings in a variety of situations, ranging from essentially healthy people who have planned elective procedure to emergency admissions for treatment of trauma.

Surgical client may be of any age and at any point on the health-illness continuum. It is the nurse's responsibility to identify factors that affect risk from a surgical procedure, assess physical and psychosocial needs of the client and family and establish a plan of care, based on appropriate nursing diagnoses, that includes interventions to meet needs and facilitate recovery as the client progresses through the perioperative period.

Preoperative Assessment and Teaching

The nurses make preoperative assessment by taking history, conducting physical examination, performing diagnostic tests as required preoperatively according to client's status/requirements, and takes informed consent in preoperative phase. Informed consent is very essential for anyone is undergoing any invasive procedure like surgery. A consent form is the legal document which signifies the client's informed consent for the procedure. The consent form guards the client against unwanted invasive procedure. It also protects the healthcare facility and healthcare professional.

In addition, preoperative teaching is an important component in the client's operative experience. Teaching about postoperative phase and is the nurse's responsibility. Clients and families need to know about surgical events, and sensations, how to perform physical activities necessary to decrease postoperative complications and facilitate recovery. The teaching-learning process is individualized to meet both specific and common client needs. Preoperative teaching allays anxiety and encourages clients to participate actively in their own care. The basic areas that must be covered in preoperative teaching are the following:

Deep breathing exercises and coughing exercises: These help expand collapsed lung and prevent postoperative pneumonia atelectasis. Coughing exercise help to guard the suture.

Turning exercises: These help prevent venous stasis, thrombophlebitis, decubitus ulcer formation, and respiratory complications.

Extremity exercises: These help prevent circulatory problems, such as thrombophlebitis, by facilitating venous return to the heart.

Ambulation: Early ambulation when appropriate, helps prevent postoperative complications.

Pain control: Regarding medication (IV or IM) or NPO (nothing per oral), relaxation technique are advisable. In addition, TENS and PCA are taught for pain control measure.

Postoperative equipments: Client may be instructed about equipments that may be used postoperatively. Depending upon the surgery, various tubes, drains, and IV lines are used.

Physical preparation: The physical preparation of the client for surgery may vary, depending on the client's physical status and special needs, type of surgery to be done and surgeon's order. Certain nursing interventions are appropriate for all surgical clients in the areas of hygiene and skin preparation, elimination, nutrition, and fluids and rest and sleep. The nurse is responsible for the preparation and safety of the client on the day of surgery.

(i) *Skin preparation:* The skin is cleaned by scrubbing the operative site one or more times with an antiseptic soap or solution to remove bacteria. This can be done by the client while taking a bath or shower. Ideally, a shower is taken in the evening before the morning of surgery. Shampooing the hair and the cleaning of the fingernails also help to reduce number of organism present. The incisional area usually is shaved before surgery because hair serves as a reservoir of bacteria. Usually the operative area is washed before surgery with an antiseptic such as povidoneiodine (Betadine) to clean and disinfect the skin.

(ii) *Elimination:* The gastrointestinal tract needs special preparation on the evening before surgery to:

- Reduce the possibility of vomiting and aspiration during anesthesia
- Reduce the possibility of a bowel obstruction, and
- Prevent contamination from fecal material during intestinal tract or bowel surgery.

Emptying the bowel of feces in no longer routine procedure before surgery, but the nurse should use preoperative assessment to determine the need for an order of bowel elimination. If the client is scheduled for surgery of the GI tract, cleansing enema usually ordered.

Insertion of an indwelling urinary catheter may be ordered before surgery, especially in clients having pelvic surgery, to prevent bladder distention or accidental injury. If an indwelling catheter is not in place, the client should void immediately before receiving premedication to ensure an empty bladder during surgery.

(iii) *Nutrition and fluids:* Preparation involves restricting food and fluid. If a client undergoing surgery is to receive a general anesthesia, foods and fluids are restricted 8 to 10 hours before the operation. This restriction significantly reduces the possibility of aspirations of gastric contents, which can cause aspiration pneumonia. Most clients have an NPO status after midnight.

(iv) *Rest and sleep:* These are important components in reducing stress before surgery and in healing and recovery after surgery. The nurse can facilitate rest and sleep in the immediate preoperative period by meeting psychological needs, carrying out teaching, providing a quiet environment, and administering prescribed bedtime sedative medication.

Preoperative Care on the Day of Surgery

Immediate preoperative preparations begin at least 1 to 2 hours before surgery in the hospital. The nurse's responsibility on the day of surgery will include the following:

- Note allergies according to institutional policy
- Take and record the vital signs, assess and report the abnormalities for elevated temperature
- Check the identification band to make sure it is legible, accurate and securely fastened to the client
- Be sure that informed consent has been obtained and is clearly documented
- If a skin preparation has been ordered, check that it has been completed accurately and thoroughly
- Check for the carry out any special orders, such as administering enema or starting on IV line, recurred previous records, inserting nasogastric tube, giving medications
- Verify that the client has not eaten for the last 8 hours. Check that fluids have been restricted although sometimes the physician will order clients to take their usual oral medication with a small sip of water
- Ask the client to void, measure and record the amount of urine (if indicated)
- Assist the client with oral hygiene if necessary
- Help the client to remove jewellery to prevent loss or injury from swelling, during or after surgery. Many facilities allow the client to keep wedding band or mangala suthra (tali) on as long as they are taped securely. If jewellery is removed, it should be stored according to policy or given to authorized member of their family
- Remove all hairpins or hairpieces. This prevents injury to the client during surgery as well as possible loss or hairpieces or wigs
- Remove colored nail polish from at least one nail for the pulse oximeter to allow intraoperative and postoperative assessment of skin and nailbeds for circulation and oxygenation of tissues
- If the client is wearing hearing aid, notify the operating room nurse. Leave it in place so that operating room personnel know it is there and can communicate with the client

- Remove all prosthesis, such as dentures, or partial plates, eye glasses, contact lenses and artificial limbs and store them safely (dentures may cause respiratory, distress)
- Give the preoperative medications that are prescribed, either at a scheduled time or "on call". The commonly ordered medications are:
    (i)   Sedatives and tranquilizers to alleviate anxiety and facilitate anesthesia induction, e.g. nembutol, chloropromozen, or diazopen
    (ii) Anticholenesterase to decrease pulmonary and oral secretions to prevent laryngospasm, e.g. atropine
    (iii) Narcotic analgesics to facilitate client's sedation and relaxation and to decrease the amount of anesthetic agent need, e.g. morphine
    (iv) Neurolephanalegiscs agents to cause a general state of calmness and sleepiness

To prevent omissions and preoperative nursing intervention, most facilities supply nurses with a preoperative checklist. As each intervention on the list is completed, the nurse initials it. Documents through checklists and narrative charting, the nursing intervention carried out.

- Assist in moving client from the bed to the operating room stretcher when it is time to transport the client to surgery, ensuring accurate identification.

Surgical Skills/Techniques/ Procedures

The condition of the hospitalized patient often requires an environment or procedures that are free from all microorganisms. This is called "surgical asepsis" or "sterile technique". Surgery, for example, is performed under strict surgical asepsis. Nurses use sterile technique daily in less dramatic skills such as changing sterile dressings, urinary catheterizations, and the preparation of intravenous medications. Because skills involving surgical asepsis are used daily by nurses, it is important that every nurse be competent in sterile technique. It is not necessary or even desirable for the nurse to memorize all of the steps in a sterile procedure. Rather, the nurse needs to understand the principles of sterile technique and be able to apply them in a variety of situations.

Several guidelines apply to every skill that requires sterile technique:

1. The purpose of sterile technique is to protect the patient from microorganisms which may be present on the patient's own body or which are transferred by caregivers. For example, during an operation only the patient's body is covered with sterile towels (called drapes) which serve to protect from microorganisms on the patient's own body.
2. If a sterile object touches an unsterile object, the sterile object may now have some microorganisms on it and must be considered unsterile or contaminated. This may occur with the nurse accidentally touches a sterile needle with a finger when drawing up an insulin injection.
3. Sterile objects that touch other sterile objects are still sterile. For example, the nurse wearing sterile gloves counts sterile bandages. Both the gloves and the bandages are sterile unless, of course, something else has contaminated either of them.
4. A sterile field is the area considered free from all microorganism. Frequently, a nurse sets up a sterile field on a table by opening a sterile drape over the table, much as table cloth is over a table. Sterile objects may then be placed on the sterile field and still be sterile.
5. The sterile field must be within the vision of the nurse at all times. This means that objects below the level of the waist (as in the operating room) are considered contaminated. The nurse does not walk away from a sterile field because, it is then impossible to determine whether it has been contaminated. The nurse also avoids reaching over a sterile field in order to decease the risk of contamination from microorganisms falling from the nurse on to the sterile field by gravity.

The following skills require knowledge and application of surgical asepsis.

Surgical Handwashing

Many patient care situations require a more thorough handwashing than the medical handwashing described above. Prior to entering a newborn nursery, assisting in the operating room, or performing sterile procedure, the nurse completes surgical handwashing. This is different from medical handwashing. This is different from medical handwashing in that here the elbows are considered most contaminated and the fingertips least contaminated. This handwashing also takes more time and may be required for as long as 10 minutes with three separate lather-and-rinse cycles. This will vary with institutional policy and the specific work area. This is described in Nursing Skill.

In order to determine whether medical or surgical handwashing is appropriate, the nurse questions who is "clean" and who is "dirty". In the above example, the nurse, physician, and other members of the surgical team are "dirty", that is, they have more microorganisms than the sterile field, in this case, the "dirty" nurse does a surgical handwashing. The closer one moves to the trunk of the nurse, the greater the number of microorganisms. For surgical handwashing, the hands are considered less contaminated with microorganisms than the elbows of the individual nurse.

If the nurse is considered "clean" compared to the patient, a medical handwashing is done. This is not often with the case in the general areas of the hospital. In medical handwashing, the elbows are considered to have fewer microorganisms than the hands which have been in direct contact with patients. Procedures of handwashing are given in Table 25.2.

Surgical Asepsis

Sterile means without life. If an object is sterile, it contains no life and therefore no infectious organisms. The exception is *prions,*

Table 25.2: Procedures for Surgical Handwashing

Supplies

- Soap as provided by the hospital
- Stick or brush for cleansing the fingernails
- Warm running water with foot or knee control
- Brush or sponge for cleaning the skin
- Towels (frequently sterile towels) are provided in the operating room

Preparation

Nurse must be in a short-sleeved uniform or scrub suit to perform this procedure since it involves scrubbing to the elbows

	Nursing actions		*Rationales*
1.	Remove all jewellery	1.	Jewellery harbors microorganisms and is difficult to clean
2.	Adjust water to comfortable temperature. Warm water enhances action of the soap	2.	Comfort of nurse. Excessively hot water opens pores to bacteria.
3.	Holding hands above the level of the elbow, wet hand thoroughly, apply soap.	3.	Water flows from area of least contamination of most contamination. Soap is mildly bacteriostatic
4.	Apply soap beginning at the fingertips lather and wash, using both circular and interlaced fingers technique. Move from fingertips to the elbows of one hand and repeat for the second hand. Use brush if available.	4.	Friction and lather raise microorganism. Wash from area of least contamination to area of most contamination. Use of brush maximizes friction
5.	Rinse each arm separately, fingertips first, holding hands above the level of elbows	5.	Do not let rinse water flow over clean area. Water should flow from area of least contamination to area of most contamination.
6.	Wash for the length of time and the number of times as required	6.	Different sterile procedures will require different handwashing times
7.	Using a separate towel for each hand. Wipe from the fingertips to the elbow, and then discard the towel	7.	Do not contaminate clean hand by using contaminated towel. Move from least to most contaminated during drying
8.	If donning sterile gloves and gown, hold hands above the level of the waist and do not touch anything. Immediately get into sterile garb.	8.	Contact with contaminated object renders clean object contaminated. Area below the level of the waist is considered contaminated
9.	If the nurse's hands touch "dirty" object during the procedure, steps 3 to 8 must be repeated	9.	Same as step 8

the protein particles that cause severe neurological degeneration in animals and humans. Researchers have not yet determined what types of antimicrobial techniques are successful in destroying prions. Inanimate objects, such as surgical equipment, gauze dressings, or wound irrigation fluid may be sterile. However, humans will always have pathogens in and on their bodies.

Surgical asepsis requires creation of a sterile environment and use of sterile equipment. It differs from medical asepsis in that it is more complex and it is not required for use with all patients. Sterilization can be accomplished through the use of special gases or high heat. Surgical equipment and implanted devices are examples of materials that must be sterilized (Table 25.3).

To create a sterile area, housekeeping personnel perform extensive cleaning using special solutions and procedures. All health personnel working in the area must wear appropriate surgical attire and perform a surgical hand scrub. A **surgical scrub** is a modification of the hand-washing procedure described

earlier. It involves an extended scrub of the hands using brush, nail cleaner, and a bactericidal scrubbing agent. Preparing and maintaining a sterile field is basic to many nursing procedures, such as inserting a urinary catheter and changing surgical dressings. It takes practice to develop a "sterile conscience, "a consistent awareness of what is sterile, and to maintain the sterility.

Before proceeding the nurse's should:

- Assess all packages to determine that they are dry and intact. Assesses the sterility of packages
- Assess the local environment for a dry, horizontal, stable area. A dry, flat workspace is best for a sterile field.

Equipment Needed

- Sterile kit as needed for procedure
- Sterile gloves (if not in kit)
- Sterile drape (if needed)
- Sterile solution (if needed)
- Other sterile items as required

Table 25.3: Surgical Asepsis: Preparing and Maintaining Sterile Field

	Nursing actions		Rationales
	Check clients identification band Explain procedure before beginning		To identity right patient To get cooperation and reduce anxiety
1.	Gather equipment for the type of procedure: • Select only clean, dry packages marked sterile and read listing of contents. • Check the package for integrity and expiration date.	1.	Prevents break in technique during procedure. If the package is moist or outdated, it is considered contaminated and cannot be used.
2.	Select a clean area in the client's environment to establish the sterile field	2.	Promotes access to the sterile field during the procedure.
3.	Explain procedure to the client; provide specific instructions if client assistance is required during the procedure.	3.	Gains client's understanding and cooperation during the procedure
4.	Inquire about and attend to the client's toileting needs	4.	Prevents break in technique during the procedure
5.	Hospital environment: If the procedure is to be performed at the client's bedside, the client should be in a private room or moved to a clean treatment room if available.	5.	Minimize microorganisms in the environment
6.	Home environment: Secure privacy and remove pots from the room	6.	Pots the client at case and promotes a clean environment
7.	Position client and attend to comfort measures: the client's position should provide easy access to the area and facilitate good body mechanics during the procedure	7.	Helps the client relax and prevents movement during the procedure: prevents reaching, decreasing the risk of contamination and back strain
8.	Cleanse hands	8.	Prevents transmission of microorganisms
9.	Place sterile package (drape or tray) in the center of the clean, dry work area.	9.	Prevents reaching over exposed sterile items when wrapper is removed
Drape			
10.	Open the wrapper, pulling away from the body first	10.	Prevents contamination
11.	Grasp the top edge with fingertips of one hand	11.	Edges are considered unsterile
12.	Remove the drape by lifting up and away from all objects while it unfolds: discard the outer wrapper with other hand	12.	If the drape touches an unsterile object, it is contaminated and musty be discarded
13.	With free hand, grasp the other drape corner, keeping it away from all objects	13.	Avoids contamination
14.	Lay the drape on the surface, with the drape bottom first touching the surface farthest from you: step back and allow the drape to cover the surface	14.	Prevents you from reaching over the sterile field: stepping back decreases risk that drape will touch your uniform
Tray			
15.	Remove outer wrapping the place the tray on the work surface so that the top flap of the sterile wrapper opens away from you	15.	Prevents reaching over the sterile items
16.	Reach around the tray, not over it. With thumb and index fingertips grasping the wrapper's top flap, gently pull up, then down to open over the surface	16.	Only the edges of the field can be contaminated, pulling up frees the top folded flap
17.	Repeat the same steps to open the side flaps	17.	Keeps the arm form reaching over the sterile field
18.	Grasp the corner of the bottom flap with fingertips, step back and pull flap down	18.	Creates a sterile work surface

Contd...

<table>
<tr><td colspan="2" align="center">Table 25.3: Contd...</td></tr>
<tr><td>Nursing actions</td><td>Rationales</td></tr>
<tr><td colspan="2">Adding Additional Sterile Items to Sterile Field</td></tr>
<tr><td>19.   While facing the sterile field, step back, remove the outer wrapper, and grasp the item in your nondominant hand so that the top flap will open away from you</td><td>19.   Keeps your dominant hand free, item remains sterile</td></tr>
<tr><td>20.   With your dominant hand, open the flaps as previously described</td><td>20.   Prevents reaching over the sterile item</td></tr>
<tr><td>21.   With your dominant hand, pull the wrapper back and away from the sterile field (toward your nondominant arm holding the item) and place the item onto the field</td><td>21.   Prevents the wrapper from touching the sterile field</td></tr>
<tr><td>22.   When adding additional gauze or dressings to the sterile field, open the package as directed, grasp</td><td>22.   Prevents contamination of item and sterile field</td></tr>
<tr><td colspan="2">Adding Solutions to Sterile Field</td></tr>
<tr><td>23.   Read the labels and strengths of all solutions three times before pouring</td><td>23.   Ensures proper solution and strength</td></tr>
<tr><td>24.   Remove the lid from the bottle of solution and invert the lid onto a clean surface</td><td>24.   Inverting the lid prevents contamination of the inner surface</td></tr>
<tr><td>25   Hold the bottle, label facing ceiling, 4 to 6 inches (10 to 15 cm) over the container on the sterile field: slowly pour the solution into the container to avoid splashing. Pour from the sterile field. Do not reach over it.</td><td>25   Prevents the label from getting wet. If the solution splashes onto the label, the field is contaminated because moisture conducts microorganisms from the non-sterile surface. Prevents contamination. If the solution splashes out of the container and the drape becomes wet, the field is contaminated</td></tr>
<tr><td>26.   Replace the lid on the container, label the container with the date and time, and initial the container</td><td>26.   Sterility of the solution will be lost if exposed to air for an extended period</td></tr>
<tr><td colspan="2">Using Sterile Gloves</td></tr>
<tr><td>27.   Cleanse hands and perform open gloving</td><td>27.   Prevents transmission of microorganisms</td></tr>
<tr><td>28.   Continue with procedure, keeping gloved hand above waist level at all times, touching only items on the sterile field</td><td>28.   Decreases chance of contamination</td></tr>
<tr><td>29.   If using a solution to cleanse a site, use the sterile forceps to prevent contamination of gloves; dispose of forceps after use or process instruments according to agency policy</td><td>29.   Prevents field contamination</td></tr>
<tr><td>30.   Post procedure, dispose of all contaminated items in colored plastic bag</td><td>30.   Decreases risk of transmission of microorganisms to all health care workers</td></tr>
<tr><td>31.   Remove gloves as shown in Procedure (Table 25.4)</td><td>31.   Minimizes risk of contact with infections wastes on the gloves.</td></tr>
<tr><td>32.   Reposition the client</td><td>32.   Promotes client comfort</td></tr>
<tr><td>33.   Clean the environment; cleanse hands</td><td>33.   Prevents transmission of microorganisms</td></tr>
</table>

Performing Open Gloving (Table 25.4)

Aspects, or sterile technique, consists of those practices that eliminate all microorganisms and spores from an object or area. The use of sterile gloves is at the heart of aseptic technique. The ability to manipulate sterile items without contaminating them is critical to many diagnostic and therapeutic interventions. Common nursing procedures that require sterile technique are:

- All invasive procedures, either intentional perforation of the skin (injection, insertion of IV needles or catheters) or entry into a body orifice (tracheobronchial suctioning, insertion of urinary catheter)
- Nursing measures for clients with disruption of skin surfaces (changing a surgical wound or IV site dressing) or destruction of skin layers (trauma and burns)

There are two methods for applying sterile gloves; open and closed. The open method is used most frequently when

<table>
<tr><td colspan="4" align="center">Table 25.4: Performing Open Gloving</td></tr>
<tr><td colspan="2">Nursing actions</td><td colspan="2">Rationales</td></tr>
<tr><td>1.</td><td>Cleanse hands</td><td>1.</td><td>Prevents transmission of microorganisms.</td></tr>
<tr><td>2.</td><td>Read the manufacturer's instructions on the package of sterile gloves; proceed as directed in removing the outer wrapper from the package, placing the inner wrapper onto a clean, dry surface. Open inner wrapper to expose gloves</td><td>2.</td><td>Different manufacturers package gloves differently; the instructions will tell you how to open properly to avoid contamination of the inner wrapper; any moisture on the surface will contaminate the gloves.</td></tr>
<tr><td>3.</td><td>Identify right and left hand; glove dominant hand first</td><td>3.</td><td>Dominant hand should facilitate motor dexterity during gloving</td></tr>
<tr><td>4.</td><td>Grasp the 2-inch (5 cm) wide cuff with thumb and first tow fingers of the nondominant hand, touching only the inside of the cuff</td><td>4.</td><td>Maintains sterility of the outer surfaces of the sterile glove</td></tr>
<tr><td>5.</td><td>Gently pull the glove over the dominant hand, making sure the thumb and fingers fit into the proper spaces of the glove</td><td>5.</td><td>Prevents tearing the glove material; guiding the fingers into proper facilitates gloving</td></tr>
<tr><td>6.</td><td>With the gloved dominant hand, slip your fingers under the cuff of the other gloved thumb abducted, making sure it does not touch any part on your nondominant hand</td><td>6.</td><td>Cuff protects gloved fingers, maintaining sterility</td></tr>
<tr><td>7.</td><td>Gently skip the glove onto your nondominant hand, making sure the fingers slip into the proper spaces</td><td>7.</td><td>Contact is made with two sterile gloves</td></tr>
<tr><td>8.</td><td>With gloved hands, interlock fingers to fit the gloves onto each finger. If the gloves are soiled, remove by turning inside out as follows</td><td>8.</td><td>Promotes proper fit over the fingers</td></tr>
<tr><td colspan="4">Removing Gloves</td></tr>
<tr><td>9.</td><td>Slip gloved fingers of the dominant hand under the cuff of the opposite hand or grasp the outer part of the glove at the wrist if there is no cuff</td><td>9.</td><td>Contact is made with two sterile gloves</td></tr>
<tr><td>10.</td><td>Pull the glove down to the fingers, exposing the thumb</td><td>10.</td><td>Frees the thumb for the next step</td></tr>
<tr><td>11.</td><td>Slip the uncovered thumb into the opposite glove at the wrist allowing only the glove-covered of the hand to touch the soiled glove</td><td>11.</td><td>Contact is made with two sterile gloves</td></tr>
<tr><td>12.</td><td>Pull the glove down over the dominant hand almost to the fingertips and slip the glove over the first glove</td><td>12.</td><td>Removes glove without contact with soiled surfaces</td></tr>
<tr><td>13.</td><td>With the dominant hand touching only the inside of the other glove, pull the glove over the dominant hand so that only the inside (clean surface) is exposed</td><td>13.</td><td>Exposes only the clean surface of the gloves</td></tr>
<tr><td>14.</td><td>Dispose of soiled gloves according to institutional policy and cleanse hands</td><td>14.</td><td>Prevents transfer of microorganisms</td></tr>
</table>

performing procedures that require the sterile technique, such as dressing changes, but that do not require donning a sterile gown.

Before performing the nurse should:

- Assess the glove package. If it intact? Is it wet or otherwise contaminated? Assesses the sterility of the glove.
- Assess the local environment. Is there an area suitable for opening the package and applying the gloves? Is it dry? Is it reasonably stable and horizontal? Are there obvious airborne contaminants? A flat, clear work space is necessary to successfully carry out the procedure

- Assess the correct glove size for proper fit. Gloves come in many sizes, and proper fit is conducive to maintaining asepsis and collect Package of proper-sized sterile gloves

Opening a Sterile Pack

All sterile supplies come wrapped in some types of pack, either paper or clothe, to protect the contents from environmental microorganisms. Many packs, such as the type that sterile gloves comes in contain an inner and an outer package. The outer package can be peeled apart using both hands. The inner pack

Table 25.5: Procedure for Opening a Sterile Pack

Supplies
- Sterile pack
- Clean table to surface to hold pack

	Nursing actions		*Rationales*
1.	Wash hands	1.	Decrease the transfer of microorganisms
2.	Set pack on clean dry surface. Position to the top flap of the wrapper is facing you. Remove type on pack	2.	Same as step 1. Wet surface under sterile field will contaminate it as solution is absorbed. Pack can be opened without reaching over a sterile field
3.	Pinching the top flap at the corner, open the pack away from yourself, bringing your arm back around the outside of the open pack	3.	Hands do not touch the inside of the wrapper which would contaminate it or cross sterile field
4.	Open side flaps one at a time	4.	Being able to watch each flap being opened decreases the risk of contamination
5.	Open flap nearest to you last	5.	Same as step 4
6.	Inside of wrapper is considered sterile and may be used as base for sterile field. Other sterile objects may now be added	6.	Sterility is maintained when sterile objects are placed within a sterile field

may then be added to a sterile field or opened to form the base of a sterile field. Cloth packs are sealed with a tape which indicates that the contents are sterile. These are opened in the manner described in nursing skill. Once opened, a sterile pack may not be reclosed and considered sterile for another use.

Procedure, see Table 25.5.

Putting on a Sterile Gown

The nurse wears a sterile gown under conditions of surgical asepsis when the purpose is to protect the patient from organisms which may be carried by the nurse. If protective cap, mask, and shoe coverings are required, they must be put on prior to donning the gown. These items are not sterile and may not be touched after handwashing is complete. Putting on a sterile gown must always be preceded by a surgical handwashing. Because the hands are never sterile, even after a surgical scrub, the sterile gown may be touched only at the neck and when put on. Thereafter, the nurse does not touch the neckband, which is now considered contaminated. Nursing skill describes one method of putting on a sterile gown (Table 25.6).

Putting on Sterile Gloves

The nurse wears sterile gloves not only in the operating room but anywhere a sterile procedure is performed (Table 25.7). It is the responsibility of nurse to ascertain the best fitting glove size for personal use, and then select gloves accordingly without the need to try on several pair. Gloves range from a small size 6 to a large size 8½. Gloves must be large enough to put on with ease, but small enough to fit snugly. Nursing skill lists this skill.

Pouring Sterile Liquids

The nurse may need to add sterile liquids to a sterile field, as when sterile normal saline is poured into a sterile container as part of a surgical procedure. The nurse is careful to pour the liquid without spilling on the sterile field, as well as not to reach over the sterile field. The outside of the bottle is not considered sterile so the nurse must not place the bottle on the field. Usually a second nurse who is not in sterile garb performs this task. Nursing skill describes this procedure (Table 25.8).

Sterile Dressing Change

Anytime the patient has a break in the skin, due either to surgical incisions or to trauma, the wound is covered with sterile dressings. Covering the wound results in faster wounds healing with less scarring than if the wound is left open (Strand, 1978). The disadvantage is that covered wounds have a greater danger of bacterial infection. The nurse uses techniques of surgical asepsis to change sterile dressings. Although sterile gloves are always worn, a face mask may be optional. Some institutions require that face masks be worn to protect the wound from droplet infection from the nurse's respiratory tract. For some patients, a dressing change is a painful procedure. The nurse assesses the patient's pain and attempts to make the patient more comfortable before starting the dressing change.

The decision when to change a sterile dressing depends upon several factors. If the patient has had surgery, the physician may wish to change the dressing the first time. If the incision is draining, the nurse may leave the original surgical dressing in place and apply additional dressings on top of the original. This is called reinforcing the dressing. The nurse documents the type

Table 25.6: Procedures for Putting on a Sterile Gown

Supplies

- If required: Shoe covers, face mask, protective cap
- Sterile gown

	Nursing actions		*Rationales*
1.	Wash hands	1.	Decrease transfer of microorganisms
2. (a) (b)	If required put on: Protective cap Face mask-secure mask with four ties, above the ears, and at the nape of the neck. Paper masks are adjusted by bending a flexible nosepiece and by elastic straps	2.	Putting on cap, mask and shoe covers is intended to cover parts of the nurse's body that are sources of contamination. These are not sterile. Proceed from area of least contamination to most contamination: hair, face, shoe covers
3.	Complete surgical handwashing	3.	This is a sterile procedure
4.	Open sterile pack containing gown (see Nursing skill) grasp gown by the neck band and hold away from the body and at shoulder level to unfold	4.	Pack containing gown is sterile. Neckband of gown is considered sterile
5.	While holding neckband, slide one arm into sleeve	5.	Neckband is considered unsterile
6.	With the first arm encased in the sleeve and holding the gown slide second arm into the gown. Do not touch the outside of the gown with hands	6.	The gown acts as a sterile "mitt" which assists in movement into the gown. Hands are not sterile and touching would contaminate the gown
7.	A second person who is not in sterile garb will now, touching only the inside surface of the gown, pull the gown into place and tie the neckties. The gowned nurse then bends forward to make the waist ties (located waist level of side of gown) fall away from gown. These are then tied by the second person who is careful not to touch the front of the gown. If the waist ties are on the back of the gown, they are simply tied by the second nurse (Figs 25.1A to D)	7.	The inside of the gown is considered red contaminated and thus may be touched by the unsterile person. Care must be taken not to permit neckties to fall forward to the front of the gown as this would contaminate the gown. Waist ties are sterile until touched by the second person.
8.	If the gown is contaminated at any point, it is discarded and steps 3 to 7 are repeated	8.	Contact with any unsterile object makes the gown unsterile

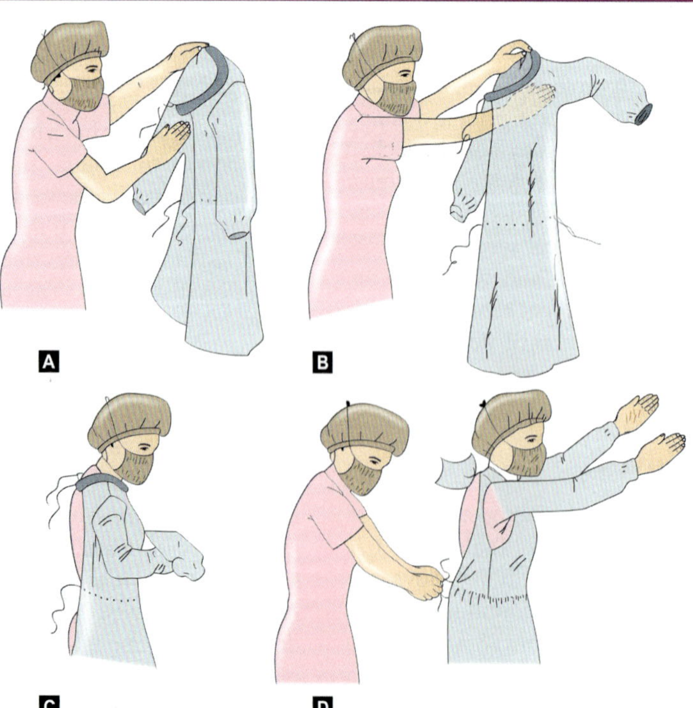

Figures 25.1A to D: Putting on a sterile gown

Table 25.7: Procedure for Putting on Sterile Gloves

Supplies

- Package of sterile gloves in correct size
- Clean table or surface to hold open glove package

	Nursing actions		*Rationales*
1.	Remove all jewellery and wash hands	1.	Decreases transfer of microorganism
2.	Open glove package without contaminating and lay on flat surface. Open inner wrapper and touching only the outside, secure both flaps in open position	2.	The outside of inner wrapper is contaminated. The inside of the inner wrapper is sterile
3.	Remove first glove from the package by grasping the inside fold of the cuff. Lift the glove, holding away from the body, above the waist, fingers of the glove down	3.	The inside of the first glove is now contaminated because it has been in contact with the nurse's hand. The outside of the glove remains sterile
4.	Slide glove on first hand, still touching only the inside fold of the cuff. Lift the glove, holding away from the body, above the waist, fingers of the glove down	4.	Same as step 3
5.	Remove second glove from the package by sliding three fingers of the first hand, now gloved, under the cuff of the second glove. Lift the glove away from the body, above the level of the waist. Slide the second hand into the second glove, touching only the inside of the glove with the second hand (Figs 25.2A to F)	5.	Same as step 3
6.	Pull glove over wrist with first hand which is gloved without touching second arm	6.	Both outside surfaces of the gloves remain sterile
7.	Adjust fingers of both gloves using opposite gloved hand	7.	If a sterile object (first gloved hand) touches a second sterile object (second gloved hand), both objects remain sterile
8.	If contamination occurs at any point in steps 1 to 7, again rinse the gloves and begin disinfect the gloves	8.	Use of any nonsterile object in a sterile procedure introduces microorganisms and is potentially dangerous

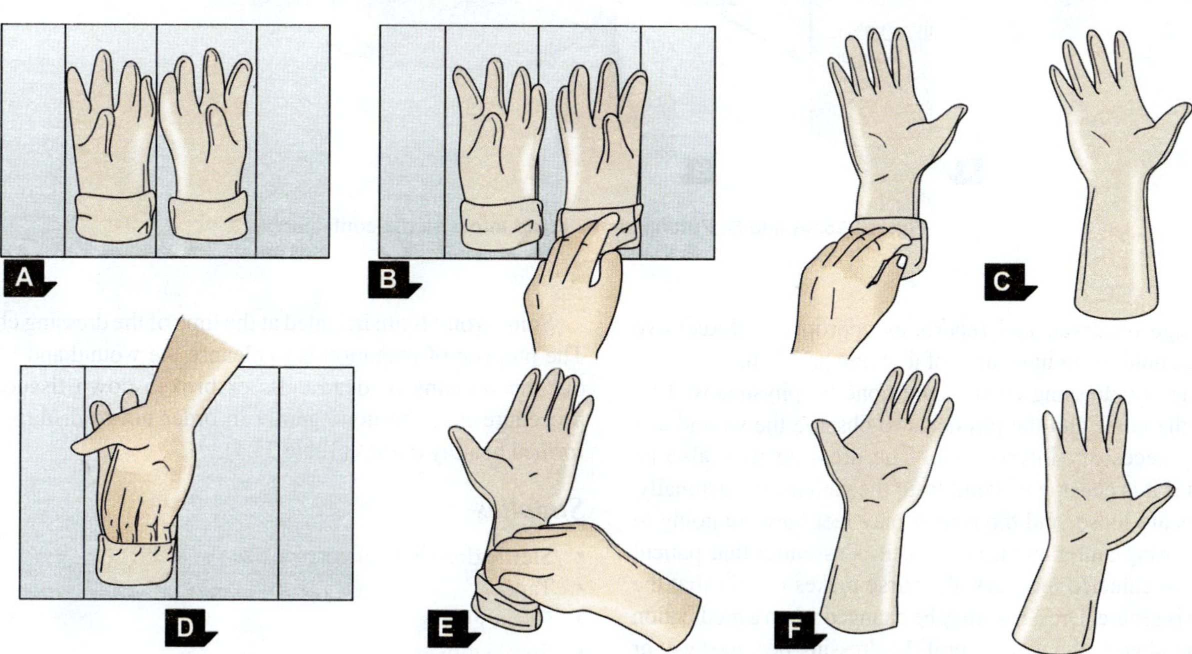

Figures 25.2A to F: Putting on a sterile gloves

Table 25.8: Procedure for Pouring Sterile Liquids

Supplies

- Sterile liquid
- Sterile container in which to pour

	Nursing actions		*Rationales*
1.	Wash hands	1.	Decreases the transfer of microorganisms
2.	Carefully read and check the label on the bottle	2.	Safety prevents errors of using of using wrong solution
3.	Remove the cap from the bottle without touching the inside of the cap. Set the cap, top down, on a clean surface	3.	Outside of the cap is unsterile. Inside of the cap is sterile
4.	If this is a previously unopened bottle; pouring away from the label, pour the required amount into the sterile container without touching bottle to container (Figs 25.3A and B)	4.	Lip of the bottle is sterile. Outside the bottle is considered contaminated. Prevents solution from running over label, making reading difficult
5.	If the bottle had been previously opened, pour a small amount of the liquid away from the label into a waste receptacle without permitting the bottle to touch the receptacle. Pouring away from the label, pour the required amount into the sterile container	5.	Cleanses the tip of the bottle. Keeps the label of the bottle clean and readable. Same as step 4
6.	Replace the cap tightly on the container, being careful not to touch the sterile inside surface. Label the bottle with the date it was opened.	6.	Maintain sterility of the bottle. The next person using the bottle if it can be used. Opened sterile solutions are usually kept for only 24 hours

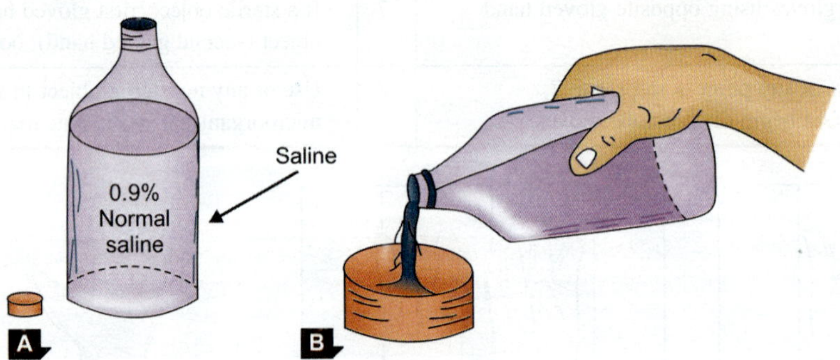

Figures 25.3A and B: Putting sterile liquid into a sterile container

of drainage observed and reports as appropriate. Excessive drainage could be an indication of a severe problem.

Frequently, dressing changes are done by physicians. This permits the nurse and the physician to observe the wound and take any necessary intervention. The dressing may also be changed if it is causing discomfort to the patient. Occasionally, dressings are loose, and the patient may feel they are going to fall off during ambulation. Because it is essential that patient exercise to enhance recovery, the nurse makes certain that the dressing is secure. Dressings may be changed when a medication is to be applied to the wound, or if the dressing becomes wet or soiled. The nurse uses judgment in selecting the amount and size of the dressings necessary.

Some wounds are irrigated at the time of the dressing change. The purpose of irrigation is to cleanse the wound and to flush out the remains of dead cells or broken-down tissue. This procedure must be done gently in order not to disturb newly formed healthy tissues (Table 25.9).

Supplies

- Sterile dressings of correct size
- Tape
- Clean gloves
- Sterile gloves
- Sterile basin, sterile cleansing solution (sterile forceps optional) if irrigating the wound

Table 25.9: Procedures for Sterile Dressing Change

	Nursing actions		*Rationales*
1.	Put on mask, if necessary. Wash hand.	1.	Limit the transfer of microorganisms
2.	Position bag for soiled dressings, open and convenient contaminating anything else in the environment	2.	Nurse will need to place soiled dressing into the bag without
3.	Loosen tape holding dressing, pulling tape towards the wound. If Montgomery ties are used, untie the straps and open	3.	Montgomery tapes remain in place and secure dressings without the use of tape
4.	Put on clean gloves and remove soiled dressings. If dressings adhere to the wound, it may be necessary to moisten with sterile saline in order to loosen. If pouring solution for another to use, repeat name and concentration of solution to verify correctness	4.	Prevents the transfer of microorganisms from the wound to the nurse's hands. Moistening the dressing permits the dressing to be removed without disturbing healing process. Prevention of medication error.
5.	Cleanse the wound, using swabs moistened in sterile cleansing solution. Wipe only once with each swab, moving in outward direction from the center of the wound. Discard swabs in bag. If no wound irrigation is to follow, gloves may be removed by peeling off inside out and placing in bag.	5.	Cleanse moving from cleanest to least clean area. Even if the wound is not contaminated, this direction prevents microbes present on the skin from entering the wound Gloves are considered soiled and are not used for sterile procedure
6. a. b. c. d.	Wound irrigation if ordered: Place waterproof pad to protect the bed and the patient Position sterile basin to catch the solution Using sterile syringe, draw up irrigating solution and release over the wound with gentle pressure, so that solution flows from the cleanest area to the least clean area Dry the area with sterile gauze for each wipe, and moving out from the center of the wound (Figs 25.4A to C)	6. a. b. c. d.	Wound irrigation: Keeps bed and patient dry As above Water flow must be at gentle pressure to avoid disrupting the healing process. Direction of water flow decreases the spread of microorganisms. Limit the spread of microorganisms. Same as step 5.
7.	Put on sterile gloves	7.	Use sterile gloves to keep the procedure as clean as possible
8.	Apply sterile dressings to the wound, using sterile forceps or sterile gloved hand. Cover with large dressing or abdominal	8.	Maintain sterility of dressings. Large dressing helps to secure smaller dressings and closes off the dressing from the environment
9.	Secure dressing with tape or ties. Remove gloves	9.	Patient will be ambulating and moving in bed so dressings must be secure
10.	Assist patient to be comfortable position	10.	Demonstrates concern for the patient

Contd...

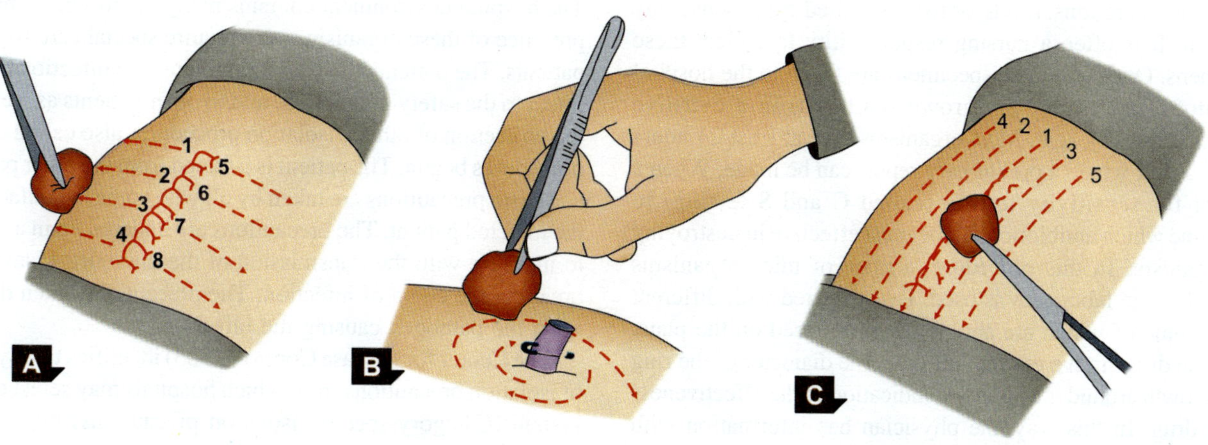

Figures 25.4A to C: Cleaning wound

Table 25.9: *Contd...*

	Nursing actions		Rationales
11.	Remove soiled equipment	11.	Decrease microorganisms in the patient's environment
12.	Document the procedure:	12.	Continued data collection for patient care plan. Fulfill legal requirements
(a)	Time and date of dressing change		
(b)	Amount and type of drainage on soiled dressing		
(c)	Appearance of wound—size, shape, depth, odor.		
(d)	Type of replacement dressing		
(e)	Condition of the patient during procedure—pain, nausea, movement, response to teaching.		

- Sterile syringe (at least 30 ml size)
- Sterile basin, irrigating solution (90-95°F)
- Waterproof pad
- Prepackaged irrigation tray may be available to which the nurse needs only add irrigating solution
- Face mask if required
- Plastic or lined bag for soiled dressings.

Preparation

Explain the procedure to the patient. If the patient is experiencing pain, it may be necessary to relieve the pain before proceeding. Many methods of pain relief are available to the nurse. Provide privacy for patient, closing the door and pulling the curtains around the bed. Position the patient comfortably and expose as necessary to permit access to the wound.

Infection Preventive Measures

Determination of the Presence of Infection

In order to determine the presence of an infection, as well as the specific pathogen causing the infection, samples of body secretions, excretions, fluids, or tissues (called specimens) may be taken. It is often a nursing responsibility to collect these specimens. Once obtained, specimens are taken to the hospital laboratory where they are grown (cultured) in a nutritive substance, usually agar. Most organisms take at least 24 hours to grow, after which a preliminary report can be made. When a request for sensitivity testing (called C and S testing) to determine which antibiotics will be most effective in destroying the organism. In this procedure, a plate of microorganisms cultured in the laboratory is used. Disks treated with different agents some of which are antibiotics, are placed on the plate. Since the drugs move out into the agar, the diameter of the ring of no growth around the disk is an indication of the effectiveness of the drug. In this way, the physician has information with which to select appropriate medications.

To collect a specimen, the nurse first completes handwashing, then selects the correct container for the specimens and determines if any needs to be added to the container before it is used. Some specimen require the addition of preservatives or fixative to the container. The nurse then explains the procedure to the patient, indicating what the patient is to do. In collecting the sample the nurse is care full not to touch the inside of the container for this would contaminate the sample. The container is then closed securely. The outside of the container is cleaned. After handwashing, the nurse labels the container with the patient's name, room number, date, time and contents. The specimen is then sent directly to the laboratory. The nurse documents specimen collection in the patient's record.

The nurse may be required to secure cultures such as wound, throat, and nose cultures. The procedure involves using a sterile swab to wipe the suspected area on the patient's body. Then, the swab is placed directly in a sterile, sealed container and taken to the laboratory. When a wound culture is taken, the nurse uses sterile technique to avoid contaminating the specimen.

While awaiting the results of the culture, the physician may decide to initiate isolation precautions. These can later be initiate isolation the results indicate an absence of pathogen, isolation begun for an identified pathogen, isolation precautions are usually continued until a later culture is negative for the organism.

Protection from Infection

The hospital environment contains many microorganisms. The presence of these organisms may require special care for some patients. The patient who has a communicable infection poses a threat to the safety of the nurse and to other patients as well. For the protection of others, isolation procedures also called barrier procedures begun. The patient is isolated from the other patients and extra precautions are taken by all who come in contact with the infected patient. The precautions are undertaken in an effort to interfere with the transmission of the microorganisms, thus breaking the chain of infection. The precautions taken depend upon the pathogen causing the infection.

The Center for Disease Control (1983) identifies two systems of isolation precautions from which hospitals may select one. In system (Category-specific isolation precautions) diseases for which similar precautions are required are grouped together. There are seven such groupings. Each disease within the group is treated by the same set of precautions. Although this system has the advantage of being simple and easy to teach to hospital personnel, more precautions are applied to certain patients than are required by the specific disease. Other diseases within the group require the full range of precautions of the group designation. This system is summarized in Table 25.10. Category-specific isolation precaution cards which may be placed on the patient's chart and door.

In system B (Disease-specific isolation precautions) each infections disease is treated separately and only those precautions that are required to interrupt transmission of the disease are applied. This system saves time, supplies, and expense since only the measures actually needed are begun. However, since isolation precautions are often begun before a specific diagnosis is confirmed, it may be necessary to use the category-specific isolation precautions. A card may be placed both on the door and on the chart of the patient in disease-specific isolation. The necessary precautions would be indicated.

Patients with certain conditions, such as those receiving total body irradiation prior to organ transplant, cancer, leukemia, or steroid therapy, are very susceptible to infection. At times a procedure known as protective isolation (or reverse isolation) may be instituted in an attempt to protect the patient from microorganisms in the environment. Nurses caring for a patient in protective isolation use surgical aseptic technique. Hair covering and mask are required. A surgical handwashing is completed prior to donning sterile gown and gloves. The nurse may then enter the room and give care to the patient. The protective isolation procedure is no longer included in the Center for Disease Control Guidelines. The publication states that protective isolation does not appear to reduce the risk of infection any more than strong emphasis on appropriate handwashing during patient care. Moreover these highly susceptible patients are often infected by their own microorganisms or by nonsterile items such as food, air, or water used in protective isolation. The CDC Guidelines state that the care of these patients requires frequent and appropriate handwashing before, during, and after patient care.

When isolation procedures are begun, the nurse must explain the procedure to the patient both in terms of what will be done and why it is done. The patient in isolation may feel very lonely

Table 25.10: Category-specific Isolation Precautions

	Category	Private	Mask	Gown	Gloves	Handwahing	Examples
1.	Strict	Yes-door	Yes	Yes	Yes	After touching patient or contaminated articles before caring for another patient	Diphtheria, plague, chickenpox
2.	Contact isolation	Yes	Yes likely	Yes-if soiling is	For touching infective material	Same as above	Acute respiratory infections in infant, Impetigo Scables
3.	Respiratory isolation	Yes	Yes	No	No	Same as above	Measles meningitis mumps
4.	Tuberculosis isolation	Yes	Only if patient is coughing	Only if needed to prevent contamination of clothing	No	Same as above	Pulmonary tuberculosis
	• Enteric precautions	If patient hygiene is poor	No	Yes-if soiling is likely	For touching infective material	Same as above	Amebic dysentery, cholera, poliomyelitis
	• Drainage secretion precautions	No	No	Yes-if soiling is likely	For touching infective material	Same as above	Wound infection infected decubitus ulcer conjunctivitis
	• Body/fluid precautions	If patient hygiene is poor	No	Yes-if soiling is likely	For touching blood or body fluids	Must be washed immediately if they are potentially contaminated with blood or body and before taking care of another patient	Acquired immune deficiency syndrome (AIDS) hepatitis B malaria

and rejected. Teenagers may feel the separation especially keenly. Very young children may feel that isolation is a punishment. Nursing intervention includes meeting the patient's needs for social contact. This is done by instructing visitors about how to enter and exit the room. The nurse also tries to spend time with this patient beyond the time required for physical care. This may even include playing a game of cards or a board game with the patient as a form of recreation.

Isolation procedures are expensive, inconvenient, time-consuming, and often complex. Nurses must complete multiple handwahing in the course of a day, may be in exclusive contact for long periods of time with a patient who may be irritable and may have to wait for assistance to complete procedures. The nurse caring for a patient in strict isolation may also experience real concern about personal safety. This may create additional stress for the nurse at a time when patient care demands are already high. The nurse caring for patients in isolation needs the support of colleagues. It is also important for the nurse to take regularly scheduled rest and meal breaks in order to meet personal needs for refreshment and human contact. These provide relief from stress for the nurse.

Strict Isolation (Table 25.11)

The patient in strict isolation must be placed in a private room. Signs on the patient's door clearly indicate the precaution and the measures which must be carried out. Visitors are directed not to enter the room without contacting the nurse for assistance. All persons entering the room must wear protective haircovers, masks, shoe covers, gown and gloves. Depending on hospital

Table 25.11: Procedures for Strict Isolation Technique			
	Nursing actions		*Rationales*
To enter the isolation room			
1.	Remove watch and rings	1.	Jewellery traps microorganisms and is difficult to clean jewellery effectively
2.	Put on clean mask. Wash hands	2.	Limit the transfer of microorganisms
3.	Put on gown • If gown is reusable, pick up gown from the inside slide arms into sleeves, tie gown at neck and over-lapping the gown at the back, tie the gown at the waist • If gown is disposable there is no special way to get into the gown • The inside of the gown and the neckband and ties are considered clean from the patient's microorganisms • The entire gown is clean at this point. The purpose of the gown is to protect the clean uniform of the nurse	3.	The purpose of this is to protect the nurse from the microorganisms of the patient
4.	Put on gloves	4.	Gloves protect the hands of the nurse and limit transfer to other patients
5.	Upon entering room, identify yourself for the patient	5.	Garb conceals identity of nurse
To double-bag soiled linen			
1.	The gowned nurse places all linen bag inside the room	1.	All contaminated linen is handled within the room to decrease the transfer of microorganisms
2.	Ungowned assistant outside the room holds second linen bag, cuffing hands with the bag	2.	Outside of first linen bag is contaminated. The second nurse's hands are protected by the cuff of the clean bag
3.	Gowned nurse comes to the doorway of the isolation room and places first bag into the second	3.	—
4.	Assistant seals the bag and dispose of it according to institutional policy	4.	Bag must be sealed in such a manner as not to transfer the microorganism to the environment and be identified as contaminated to protect laundry workers
All soiled linen must be double bagged, to protect the laundry workers from contamination. Gowns worn by the nurse and visitors must also be discarded			

Contd...

Table 25.11: *Contd...*

	Nursing actions			Rationales
To exit isolation room				
1.	Remove gloves by peeling off inside out and disposing of properly Remove mask (only touching ties)		1.	The contaminated outside surface of the glove is contained within the glove Removing mask with clean hands limits the transfer of microbes to the face
2. (a) (b) (c) (d) (e)	If gown is to be reused: Untie waist ties Wash hands if waist ties are in front of gown Untie neck ties Place fingers of one hand under the cuff of the opposite sleeve and pull the sleeve over the opposite hand. With the second hand covered by the sleeve, pull the outside of the opposite sleeve down over arm and off, being careful not to let the neck ties fall forward to the front of the gown Fold the gown with the inside in and hang gown contaminated side out		2. (a) (b) (c) (d) (e)	___ The waist ties are contaminated but not as much as the gloved hands Hands were contaminated by the waist ties if near patient contacts Neck ties are clean Inside of the gown is clean. Neck ties are clean and touching the contaminate front side of the gown would contaminate them Protect the clean inside of the gown.
3. (a) (b) (c)	If gown is disposable: Untie waist ties Place clean hands under the neckband and peel off the gown over the shoulders Touching only the inside of the gown. Roll the gown up inside out and dispose of it		3. (a) (b) (c)	___ Waist ties are considered less contaminated than gloved hands The inside of the gown is clean Same as above
4.	Wash hands		4.	Wash hands upon leaving isolation room because contamination may have occurred without your awareness. This will also decrease the possibility of spreading the microorganisms to the next patient of the nurse

policy, some of these items may be omitted. Some hospitals use disposable gowns. Although this is expensive, it gives maximum protection. Reusable gowns may be used, if necessary, but this is a less desirable technique because of a greater chance of microorganisms transfer.

All times in contact with the patient must be sterilized or thrown away. For this reason, patients in strict isolation usually receive meals with paper or plastic supplies.

Supplies

- Disposable gown (preferably) or reusable gown
- Mask
- Clean gloves
- Double bag for soiled linen

Preparation

Prior to entering the isolation room, the nurse gathers all the equipment which will be needed to provide care for the patient. Once in the room, the nurse may not leave the room without removing all garb and washing hands. In order to maximize efficiency, the nurse attempts to anticipate needs for equipment and supplies. The patient in isolation must be prepared for the initiation of the procedure since all persons coming into the room will be wearing gowns, gloves, and masks. Signs must be pasted on the door to the patient's room which state that the patient is on isolation precautions and anyone entering the room must first check with the nurse for assistance.

Preoperative Nursing (Table 25.12)

Intraoperative phase begins when the client enters the surgical site and ends with admission to the recovery area. Nursing care during this phase focuses on the client's emotional wellbeing, as well as on physical factors such as safety positioning, maintaining asepsis and controlling the surgical environment. The nurses are the client's advocates upon induction of anesthesia.

In the surgical holding area, the nurse is responsible for reviewing the record for completeness, ensuring proper identification of the client, client's safety and providing emotional support. It is important to deal with the fears and concerns of a frightened or agitated client. A relaxed client undergoes anesthetic induction easier than who is anxious. If the client still seems anxious despite sedation and reassurance, notify the surgeon or anesthesia personnel. Here the anesthesiologist sees

Table 25.12: Procedure for Preoperative Client Care: Hospitalized Client

Nursing actions		*Rationales*	
General			
1.	Identify clients for whom surgery is a greater risk:	1.	This allows for recognition of clients who may be prone to complications after surgery
(a)	Very young and elderly clients		
(b)	Obese or malnourished clients		
(c)	Clients with fluid and electrolyte imbalances		
(d)	Clients in poor general health from chronic diseases and infectious processes		
(e)	Clients taking certain medications (e.g. anticoagulants, antibiotics, diuretics, depressants, steroids).		
(f)	Clients who are extremely anxious		
2.	Reviewing nursing data base, history and physical examination. Check that baseline data are recorded	2.	Review identifies clients who are at surgical risks
3.	Check that diagnostic testing has been completed and results are available	3.	The check may influence type of surgery and anesthetic as well as timing of surgery or need for additional consultation
4.	Promote optimal nutrition and hydration status	4.	This promotes wound healing
5.	Identify learning needs of client. Conduct preoperative teaching regarding the following:	5.	This minimizes surgical risk and allays anxiety by preparing clients for postoperative period
(a)	Coughing and deep-breathing exercises		
(b)	Management of pain after surgery		
(c)	Leg exercises and ambulation		
(d)	Postoperative equipment and monitoring devices		
Day before surgery			
6.	Provide emotional support. Answer questions realistically. Provide spiritual assistance if requested	6.	This allays client's misconceptions and fears
7.	Follow preoperative dietary restrictions	7.	This reduces risk of vomiting and aspiration during surgery. Anesthetic agents temporarily depress gastrointestinal function and processes
8.	Prepare for elimination needs during and after surgery	8.	Anesthetic agents and abdominal surgery interfere with normal elimination function. A urinary catheter inserted preoperatively minimizes risk of inadvertent trauma to bladder during surgery
9.	Attend to client's special hygiene needs (e.g. use of antiseptic cleaning agents)	9.	This decreases potential for infection
10	Provide for adequate rest	10	Rest minimizes stress before surgery
Day of surgery			
11.	Check that proper identification band is on client	11.	Double-checking ensures identify of client
12.	Check that preoperative consent form are signed and medical record is in order	12.	This fulfills legal requirement related to informed consent
13.	Check vital signs. Notify physician of any pertinent changes (i.e. rise or drop in blood pressure, elevated temperature, cough, symptoms of infection)	13.	This provides baseline data for comparison
14.	Provide hygiene and oral care. Remind client not to swallow water if NPO for surgery	14.	This promotes comfort
15.	Continue nutritional and hydration preparation	15.	This prepares client for operative procedure
16.	Remove cosmetics and prostheses (e.g. contact lenses, false eyelashes, dentures, and so forth). Asses for loose teeth	16.	These interfere with assessment during surgery

Contd...

	Table 25.12: *Contd...*		
	Nursing actions		*Rationales*
17.	Have client empty bladder and bowel prior to surgery complications during and after surgery	17.	An empty bladder and bowel minimize risk of injury or
18.	Place valuables in appropriate area. Hospital is safe and most appropriate place for valuables. They should not be placed in narcotics drawer	18.	This ensures safety of valuables and personal possessions
19.	Attend to any special preoperative orders	19.	This prepares client for operative procedure
20.	Complete preoperative checklist and record of client's preoperative preparation	20.	This ensures accurate documentation
21.	Administer preoperative medication as ordered by physician	21.	Medication reduces anxiety, provides sedation and diminishes salivary and bronchial secretions

the client, IV fluids starts time him or her nurse anesthetist. Nurse-anesthetist also can administer medication needed during surgery. The procedures vary among institutions of health care.

Introduction to Anesthesia

Anesthesia means the absence of pain (Greek: an = without + aesthesis = feeling). Anesthesia is an artificially-induced state of partial or total loss of sensation, with or without loss of consciousness. Anesthesia produces muscle relaxation, blocks transmission of nerve impulses and suppresses reflexes.
There are two types of anesthesia, i.e. general anesthesia and regional anesthesia.

General Anesthesia

General anesthesia is a drug-induced depression of the central nervous system (CNS) that is reverted either by metabolic elimination in the body or by pharmocologic means. General anesthetic agents produces analgesia, amnesia and unconsciousness, characterized by loss of reflexes and muscle tone.

There are four stages of anesthesia. Brief explanation and nursing intervention in these stages are as follows:

Onset: Starts from anesthetic administration to loss of consciousness. In this stage, client may bedrowsy or dizzy and may experience auditory or visual hallucinations. Nursing action in this stage will include, close operating room doors, keeping room quiet, and stand by to assist client.

Excitement: Starts from loss of consciousness to loss of eyelid reflexes. Here there will be increase in automatic activity, irregular breathing. In such a case client may struggle. In this stage, nurse has to remain quietly as client's side, assist anesthetists if needed.

Surgical anesthesia: This stage starts with loss of eyelid reflexes, to loss of motor reflexes and depression of vital functions. Here client is unconscious, muscles are relaxed and no blink or gag

reflexes. In this stage, begins preparation (if indicated) only when anesthetists indicate stage III has been reached and client is under good control.

Danger (death) stage: Vital functions too depressed may lead to respiratory and circulatory failure. In this stage, client is not breathing and he may or may not have a heartbeat. If arrest occurs, nurse responses immediately to assist establishing airway, provides cardiac arrest tray, drugs, syringes, long needles, assist surgeon with closed or open cardiac massage.

General anesthesia can be administered by inhalation or intravenously. An inhalation agent will include nitrous oxide, halothane (Fluothene), enflurase (Enthrane) and isofluorane (Porane) and the intravenous drugs are thiopental sodium (Penthathol), fentanyl citratedroperidol (Innovar) and ketamine hydrochloride. The selections of anesthetic agents are according to decision of the anesthesiologist. But continuous monitoring of side effects of the drugs, vital are essential.

Regional Anesthesia

Regional anesthesia blocks the pain stimulus at the origin and along afferent neurons of along the spinal cord. Regional anesthesia produces a loss of painful sensation in only one region of the body and does not result in unconsciousness. The client may receive sedative that produces drowsiness. The regional anesthetic agents block the conduction of impulses in nerve fiber without depolarizing the cell membrane are: Local agents and topical agents. An example of local agents are Bupivacaine HCL (Marcaine HCL) (Xylocaine) and examples of topical agents will include benzocaine, ethylchloride spray, tetracain HCL. All these agents have their own side effects. Contraindication for children. Test dose can be given prior to use, of these agents to know any allergies to these agents.

The types of regional anesthesia are as follows:
- Topical anesthesia
- Local infiltration anesthesia
- Field block anesthesia
- Peripheral nerve block anesthesia

- Spinal anesthesia
- Epidural anesthesia
- Caudal anesthesia.

The other types of anesthesia are used in modern drugs acupuncture, cryothermia and hypnoanesthesia. The type of anesthesia chosen depends on the surgery performed and level of unconsciousness desired.

Nursing Care during Surgery

Nursing care during surgery will include providing emotional care, assisting the client with positioning (as required – for type of surgery). Maintaining safety, maintaining surgical asepsis, prevent client's heat loss, monitoring malignant hyperthermia, assisting with surgeon to perform surgery by providing proper equipments and supplies, assisting with wound closure, assessing drainage, and transferring client to recovery room.

Postoperative Nursing

The postoperative phase of surgery is final phase of the surgical experience. Nursing plays a critical role in returning the client to an optimal level of functioning. The postoperative period can be divided into two phases, i.e. immediate postanesthesia and postoperative period, and later in postoperative phase.

Immediate Postoperative Phase

Immediate postoperative phase is the first few hours after surgery when the client is recovering from the effect of anesthesia. Here the nurse has to keep all emergency equipment and drugs, etc. for the use of patient's recovery from anesthesia and on admission to postoperative unit, the nurse performs the following:

- Assess airway patency and support as needed, cramp, strider, wheezes or decreased breath sounds
- Applies humidified oxygen via nasal cannula or facemask (unless otherwise ordered)
- Records vital signs (blood pressure, heart rate, strength and regularity, respiratory rate and depth, oxygen saturation, skin color, and temperature)
- Assess the client's level of consciousness, muscle strength and ability to follow commands
- Observe the client's IV infusions, dressings, drains and special equipment
- Remain at the client's bedside, continuing close observations of the client's conditions

After the client has been positioned safely and baseline vital signs status has been ascertained, the nurse receives verbal report regarding surgery in detail, i.e. type of surgery, time of incision, patient's condition during surgery, type of anesthesia, sedative, all untoward incident happened and everything about surgery and documents the reliable and retainable information for further care that follow surgeon's and anesthetist's instructions for patient's recovery.

It is very important that nursing intervention associated with immediate recovery (ABCs) are as follows:

Airway (A)

- Maintain Patency, keep head tilted up and back may position on side with the face down and neck slightly extended
- Note presence or absence of gag/swallowing reflex
- Suction until awake and alert
- Provide oxygen if necessary.

Breathing (B)

- Evaluate depth, rate, sounds, rhythm and chest movement
- Assess color of mucous membrane
- Place hand above nose to detect respirations if shallow
- Initiate coughing and deep breathing as soon as able to respond
- Chart time oxygen is discontinued.

Consciousness (C)

- Able to extubate airway
- Responds to commands
- Verbalizes responses
- Reacts to stimuli.

Circulation (C)

- Monitor IPR every 15 minutes; to take axillary or rectal temperature, if necessary
- Assess rate, rhythm, quality of pulse
- Evaluate color and warmth of skin and nailbeds
- Check peripheral pulse if indicated
- Monitor IVS solution, rate, site.

System Review (S)

- Assess neurological functions
- Monitor drains, tubes, color and amount of output
- Evaluate pain response, may need to give analgesics
- Observe for allergic reactions
- Assess urinary output, if Foley's catheter is in place.

For remaining postoperative period, nurse has to take following measures to (Table 25.13):

- Continuous assessment of respiratory and circulatory assessment
- Ensure optimal respiratory function—deep breath and coughing exercises
- Relieving postoperative discomforts by relieving pain, restlessness nausea and vomiting, abdominal distention, hiccups, etc.
- Maintaining normal body temperature
- Avoid injury by providing proper positioning in bed
- Maintaining normal nutritional status by IV fluids, total parenteral nutrition
- Promoting normal urinary functions

Table 25.13: Procedures for Postoperative Care when Client Returns to Room	
Nursing actions	*Rationales*
Immediate	
1. Place client in safe position on side with face down and neck slightly extended. Note level of consciousness.	1. This prevents aspiration of vomitus data are obstruction
2. Monitor and record vital signs frequently. Assessment order may vary, but usual frequency includes taking vital signs every 15 minutes the first hour, every 30 minutes the next two hours, every hour for four hours, and, finally, every 4 hours	2. Comparison with baseline preoperative vital signs may indicate impending shock or hemorrhage
3. Provide for warmth, assess skin color and condition	3. Depressed level of functioning results in fall in body temperature
4. Check dressing s for color, odor, and amount of drainage and feel under client for bleeding.	4. Hemorrhage and shock are life-threatening complications of surgery
5. Verify that all tubes are patent and equipment if operative	5. This ensures maintenance of vital functions
6. Maintain intravenous infusion at correct rate	6. This provides nutrition and prevents dehydration
7. Provide for a safe environment. Keep bed in low position with side rails up. I have call bell within client's reach. Have "No smoking" sign pasted if client is receiving oxygen	7. This prevents accidental injury
8. Record assessments and interventions on chart	8. This provides for accurate documentation
9. Relieve pain by administering medications ordered by physician. Check record to verify if analgesic mediation was administered in recovery room.	9. Analgesics are used for relief of postoperative pain
General	
10. Promote optimal respiratory function: (a) Coughing and deep breathing (b) Incentive spirometry (c) Early ambulation (d) Frequent position change (e) Administration of oxygen as ordered	10. Anesthetic agents may depress respiratory function: Clients who have existing respiratory or cardiovascular disease or abdominal or chest incisions or who are obese or elderly or in a poor state of nutrition are at greater risk of developing respiratory complications
11. Maintain adequate circulation: (a) Maintenance of intravenous therapy (b) Early ambulation (c) Application of antiembolic stockings if ordered by physician (d) Leg and range-of-motion exercises if not contraindicated	11. Preventive measures can improve venous return and circulatory status
12. Assess urinary elimination status: (a) Promote voiding by offering bedpan at regular intervals (b) Monitor catheter drainage if present (c) Measure intake and output	12. Anesthetic agents may temporarily depress bladder tone and response
13. Promote optimal nutrition status and return of gastrointestinal function: (a) Assess for return of peristalsis (b) Assist with diet progression (c) Encourage fluid intake (d) Monitor intake (e) Medicate for nausea and vomiting as ordered by physician	13. Anesthetic agents depress peristalsis and normal functioning of gastrointestinal tract
14. Promote wound healing: (a) Use surgical asepsis (b) Assess condition of wound (c) Assess any drainage	14. Alterations in nutrition, circulatory and metabolic status may predispose clients to infection and delayed healing
15. Provide for rest and comfort	15. This shortens recovery period and facilitates return to normal function
16. Provide emotional and spiritual support	16. This facilitates individualized care and client's return to normal health.

- Promoting bowel elimination—preventing paralytic ileus, and constipation
- Restoring mobility by proper positioning
- Early ambulation—bed exercises
- Prevent and treatment of complication like shock, hemorrhage, deep venous thrombosis (DVT), pulmonary embolism, respiratory complication like undetected hypoxemia, atelectasis, bronchitis, bronchopneumonia and lobar pneumonia, hypostatic pulmonary congestion, pleuracy, etc. and gastric complication like nutritional anemia, intestinal obstruction and postoperative psychosis.

Care of the Surgical Wound

A wound may be described as a disruption in the continuity of cells; it follows, then, that wound healing is the restoration of that continuity.

When wounds occur, a variety of effects may result: (i) immediate loss of all or part of organ functioning, (ii) sympathetic stress response, (iii) hemorrhage and blood clotting, (iv) bacterial contamination, and (v) death of cells. Careful asepsis is the most important factor in keeping these effects to a minimum and promoting the successful care of wounds.

Wound Classification

Wounds may be classified in two different ways, i.e. according to the mechanism of injury and the degree of wound contamination at the time of surgery.

Mechanism of Injury

Wounds may be described as incised, contused, lacerated, or puncture.

Incised wounds: These are made by a clean cut with a sharp instrument, for example, those made by the surgeon in every surgical procedure. Clean wounds (those made aseptically) are usually closed by sutures after all bleeding vessels have been ligated carefully.

Contused wounds: These are made by blunt force and are characterized by considerable injury of the soft part, hemorrhage and swelling.

Lacerated wounds: These are with jagged, irregular edges, such as would be made by glass or barbed wire.

Puncture wounds: These result in small openings in the skin, for example, those made by bullets or knife steps.

Degree of Contamination

Wounds may be described as clean, clean-contaminated, contaminated, or dirty or infected.

Clean wounds: These are uninfected surgical wounds in which there is no inflammation and the respiratory, alimentary, genital, or uninfected urinary tracts are not entered. Clean wounds are usually sutured closed; if necessary, a closed drainage system (e.g. Jackson Pratt) is inserted. The relative probability of wound infection is 1 to 5 percent.

Clean-contaminated wounds: These are surgical wounds in which the respiratory, alimentary, genital and urinary tract are entered under controlled conditions; there is no unusual contamination. The relative probability of wound infection is 3 to 11 percent.

Contaminated wounds: Theses include open, fresh, accidental wounds, and surgical procedures with major breaks in aseptic technique or gross spillage from the gastrointestinal tract; included in this category are incisions in which there is acute, non-purulent inflammation. The relative probability of wound infection is 10 to 17 percent.

Dirty infected wounds: These are those in which the organisms that caused postoperative infection were present in the operative field before surgery. These include old traumatic wounds with retained devitalized tissue and those that involve existing clinical infections or perforated viscera. The relative probability of wound infection is over 27 percent.

Treatment

Prophylactic antibiotics are administered when bacterial contamination is expected, or when a prosthetic device is being inserted into a clean wound. Infected wounds are not closed until every effort has been made to remove all devitalized and infected tissue a procedure called "debridement". Often a small drain is inserted before the wound is sutured to prevent lymph and blood from collecting and retarding the healing process.

Physiology of Wound Healing

Various continuous and overlapping cellular processes contribute to the restoration of a wound; cell regeneration, cell proliferation, and collagen production. The response of tissue to injury goes through several phases, i.e. inflammatory, proliferative and maturation (Table 15.14).

Inflammatory Phase

Vascular and cellular responses occur immediately when tissue is cut or injured. Vasoconstriction of vessels occurs and a fibrinoplatelet clot forms in an attempt to control bleeding. This reaction lasts from 5 to 10 minutes and is followed by vasodilation of the venules. Microcirculation loses its vasoconstriction ability because norepinephrine is destroyed by the intracellular enzymes. Also histamine is released, which increases capillary permeability.

When the microcirculation is damaged, blood elements such as antibodies, plasma proteins, electrolytes, complement and water permeate the vascular space for 2 to 3 days. Neutrophils are the first leukocytes to move into damaged tissue. Monocytes that

Table 25.14: Phases of Wound Healing		
Phases	*Length of time*	*Events*
Inflammatory (also called lag or exudative phase)	1 to 4 days	Blood clot forms wound and it becomes edematous Debris of damaged tissue and blood clot are phagocytized
Proliferative (also called fibroblastic or connective tissue phase)	5 to 20 days	Collagen produced granulation tissue forms, Wound tensile strength increases
Maturation (also called differentiation, resorptive, remodeling or plateau phase)	21 days to months or even years	Fibroblasts leave wound, tensile strength increases Collagen fibers reorganize and tighten to reduce scar size

transform to macrophages engulf the debris and transport it from the area. Antigen-antibodies also appear. Basal cells at the wound edges undergo mitosis, and the resulting daughter cells migrate.

With this activity, proteolytic enzymes are secreted and dissolve the base of blood clots. The gap between both sides eventually meet in 24 to 48 hours. At this point, cell migration is enhanced by hyperplastic bone marrow activity.

Proliferative Phase

Fibroblasts multiply and form a lattice framework for migrating cells. Epithelial cells from buds at the edges of the wound; these buds develop into capillaries, the nutritional source for the new granulation tissue.

Collagen is the primary component of replaced connective tissue. Fibroblasts initiate the synthesis of collagen and mucopolysaccharides. In a period of 2 to 4 weeks, amino acid chains form into fibers of increasing length and diameter; these fibers become a well-structured pattern of packed bundles. The synthesis of collagen causes capillaries to decrease in number. Thereafter, collagen synthesis decrease in an attempt to balance the amount of collagen that is destroyed. Such synthesis and lysis result in increased tensile strength.

After 2 weeks, the wound has only 3 to 5 percent of the original skin strength. By the end strength. By the end of a month, only 35 to 59 percent of wound strength has been reached. Never more than 70 to 80 percent of strength is regained. Many vitamins, particularly vitamin C, aid in the metabolic process involved in wound healing.

Maturation Phase

About 3 weeks after injury, fibroblasts begin to leave the wound. The scar appears large, until collagen fibrils reorganize into tighter positions. This, along with dehydration, reduces the scar but increases its strength. Such tissue maturation or 12 weeks, but it never reaches the original strength of the prewound tissue.

Forms of Healing

In the surgical management of wound healing, wounds are described by first, second, or third intention.

Healing by First intention (Primary Union)

Wounds made aseptically, with a minimum of tissue destruction, and properly closed, as with sutures heal with little tissue reaction by first intention.

When wounds heal by first intention, granulation tissue is not visible and scar formation is minimal.

Healing by Second Intention (Granulation)

In wounds in which pus formation (suppuration) has occurred or in which the edges have not been approximated, the process of repair is less simple and takes longer.

When an abscess is incised it collapses partly, but the dead and the dying cells forming its walls are still being released into the cavity. For this reason, drainage tubes or gauze packing is often inserted into the abscess pocket to allow drainage to escape easily. Gradually, the necrotic material disintegrates and escape easily and the abscess cavity fills with a red, soft, sensitive tissue that bleeds very easily. This tissue is composed of minute, thin-walled capillaries and buds that later form connective tissue. The cells surrounding the capillaries change their round shape to become long, thin and intertwined with each other to form a scar or cicatrix. Healing is complete when skin cells (epithelium) grow over these granulations. This method of repair is called healing by granulation, and it takes place whenever pus is formed or when loss of tissue has occurred for any reason

Healing by Third Intention (Secondary Suture)

If a deep wound either has not been sutured early or breaks down and then is resutured later, two opposing granulation surfaces are brought together. This results in a deeper and wider scar.

Nursing Management in Wound Healing

As a wound undergoes the phases of healing many elements, such as adequate nutrition, cleanliness, rest and position determine how quickly the process occurs. These factors are influenced by nursing interventions. Specific nursing assessments and interventions that address these factors and help to promote wound healing are presented in Table 25.15.

Methods for reducing the incidence of wound infection are described in Table 25.16.

Goals Reduce risks that inhibit wound healing, lower incidence of wound infections.

Dressing

A dressing is a protective covering applied to a wound. The goal of a wound care is to promote tissue repair and regeneration, so that skin integrity is restored. Dressing is used as a protective cover over the wound which helps meet the goal of wound care. Most dressings especially for the surgical wounds, consist of three layers. The dressings applied directly over the wound called contact layer, allows drainage to pass into the middle layer. This layer should be able to be removed without causing further tissue damage. This middle layer dressings absorbs the drainage and the outer layer keeps the two inner layers in place.

Purposes of Dressings

There are many different types of dressings, but all have essentially the same purposes as follows:
- Remove necrotic tissue
- Prevent, eliminate, or control infection
- Absorb drainage of discharge
- Control bleeding
- Apply medication
- Maintain a moist wound environment
- Promote quick healing
- Provide comfort
- Protect the wound from further injury
- Protect the skin surrounding the wound.

Advantages of Dressings

Dressings have advantages and disadvantages. The advantages of wound dressing are as follows:
- Dressings absorb drainage to help promote wound healing
- Dressings protect the wound from mechanical injury
- Dressings when used as a pressure dressings or with elastic bandages promote homeostasis, help prevent hemorrhage, and aid in wound edge approximation
- Dressings when used as a pressure dressing or with elastic bandages promote homeostasis, help prevent hemorrhage, and aid in wound edge approximation
- Dressing splint or immobilize the wound, facilitating healing and preventing further trauma
- Dressings prevent contamination from the external environment
- Dressings provide physical, psychological and aesthetic comfort

The nurse prepares the client for the dressing change by explaining what will be done before starting the procedure. Proper screening is used to provide privacy. The client is assisted to a position that is comfortable and also convenient for the person changing the dressing. The area is exposed while maintaining proper draping. It is important to use appropriate aseptic techniques when changing the dressings to prevent nosocomial infections. The wound is cleaned and dressing accordingly the procedures as described in Table 25.17.

Purposes of an Effective Dressing

As stated earlier, a dressing is applied to a wound for one or more of the following reasons:
1. To provide a proper environment for wound healing
2. To absorb drainage
3. To splint or immobilize the wound
4. To protect the wound and new epithelial tissue from mechanical injury
5. To protect the wound from bacterial contamination and from soiling by feces, vomitus, and urine
6. To promote hemostasis, as in a pressure dressing, and
7. To provide mental and physical comfort for the patient.

In some instances, dressings are eliminated during the immediate postoperative period. Examples, of circumstances in which dressings are not necessary, are facial lacerations, pedicle flaps, or skin grafts on a smooth surface.

When the initial dressings on a clean, dry incision is removed, often it is not replaced. Generally, initial dressings on clean, dry incisions are left in place until the wound edges are sealed and the wound is healing (usually 24 hours).

The advantage of not using any dressings include the following:
1. The conditions that promote growth of organisms (warmth, moisture and darkness) are eliminated
2. The wound can be readily observed
3. Bathing is easier
4. Reactions to tape are avoided
5. Patient's comfort and activity are increased
6. Costs for dressings are reduced, and
7. Psychologic impact of the surgical incision is reduced.

Age considerations: To keep a dressing intact or to prevent contamination of wound and supplies on an infant or young child, it may be necessary to restrain the child's hand. An old stocking or piece of stockinette may be sued to encircle child's hand and then may be secured to the bed or crib with a tie or safety pin. Care must be taken not to compromise circulation to that extremity.

Home care considerations: Reinforce need for thorough handwashing before and after dressing change. Heave plastic bag available for safe disposal of soiled dressings and equipment. Boil any nondisposable equipment (e.g. forceps) for 10 minutes to ensure sterility inform client about availability of disposable wound care supplies.

Table 25.15: Factors Affecting Wound Healing

Factors	Rationales	Nursing Assessment/Interventions
Age of patient Handling of tissues Hemorrhage	The older the patient, the lesser resilient the tissues. Rough handling causes injury and delayed healing Accumulation of blood creates dead spaces as dead cells that must be removed. The area becomes a growth medium for infection.	Handle all tissues gently Handle tissues carefully and evenly Monitor vital signs observe incision site for evidence of bleeding and infection
Hypovolemia	Insufficient blood volume leads to vasoconstriction and reduced oxygen and nutrients available for wound healing	Monitor for volume deficit (circulatory impairment). Correct by fluid replacement as prescribed.
Local factors edema	Reduces blood supply by exerting increased interstitial pressure on vessels	Elevate part; apply cool compresses
In adequate dressing technique		
Too small	Permits bacteria invasion and contamination	Follow guidelines for proper dressing technique
Too tight	Reduces blood supply carrying nutrients and oxygen	Follow guidelines for proper dressing technique
Nutritional deficits	Insulin secretion may be inhibited, causing blood glucose to rise Protein-calorie depletion may occur	Monitor blood glucose levels. Administer vitamin A and C supplements as prescribed Correct deficit: This may require parenteral nutritional therapy
Foreign bodies	Foreign bodies retard healing	Keep wounds free of dressing threads, talcum and power from gloves
Oxygen deficit tissue oxygenation insufficient	Insufficient oxygen may be due to inadequate lung and cardiovascular function as well as localized vasoconstriction	Encourage deep breathing, turning controlled coughing
Drainage collection	Accumulated secretions hamper healing process Institute measures to remove accumulated	Monitor portable and other closed drainage system for proper functioning secretions
Medications Steroids	May mask presence of infection by impairing normal inflammatory response	Be aware of action / effect of medications patient is receiving
Anticoagulants	May cause hemorrhage	
Broad-spectrum/ specific antibiotics	Effective if administered immediately before surgery for specific pathology or bacterial contamination. If administered after wound is closed ineffective because of intravascular coagulation.	
Patient overactivity	Prevents approximation of wound edges Resting favors healing	Utilizes measures to keep wound edges approximated: taping, bandaging, splints Encourage rest.
Systemic disorders Hemorrhagic shock	These are depressants of cell function that directly affect wound healing	Be familiar with the nature of the specific disorder
Acidosis	—	Administer prescribed treatment
Hypoxia Renal failure Hepatitie disease, Sepsis	—	Cultures may be indicated to determine appropriate antibiotics
Immunosuppressed state	Patient is more vulnerable to bacterial / viral invasion. Defence mechanisms are impaired	Provide maximum protection to prevent infection. Restrict visitors with cold, institute mandatory hand washing for all staff.
Wound stressors vomiting Valsalva maneuver Heavy coughing Straining	Produce tension on wounds, particularly of the torso	Encourage frequent turning and ambulation, and administer antiemetic medications as prescribed.

Table 25.16: Effective Methods of Lowering Incidence of Wound Infection

Nursing interventions	Rationales
Preoperative	
Short preoperative hospitalization. Treatment of coexistent infections	Reduces exposure of patient to nosocomial infections Infections, such as respiratory can initiate pulmonary complications
Avoid shaving of hair; if necessary, remove hair with clippers or depilatories rather than a razor	The fewer nicks and cuts in the skin, the less opportunity for infection
If shaving is requested, it is performed immediately before the surgical procedure	The longer the time between shaving and the operation, the greater the incidence of infection
Thorough cleansing of operative site with-povidone-iodine (betadine) the evening before the repeated preoperative cleansing with antiseptic detergents Prophylactic antibiotics with contaminated cases	Resident bacteria and skin contaminants are reduced to a minimum
Intraopeative	
Thorough cleansing of operative site to remove superficial flora soil and debris	Reduces risk of contaminating the wound with patients skin flora
Flawless aseptic technique	Any breaks in technique can initiate infection by introducing contaminants
Powder or talcum washed off sterile gloves	Foreign particles in a wound, such as talcum or starch, will adversely affect the healing process
Bleeding controlled with meticulous hemostasis	A clean wound heals without infection
Drains eliminated in clean wounds	Drains are associated with higher wound infection rates
Closure delayed in contaminated wounds	Permits healing from base of wound to exterior-otherwise, pocket of infection may develop
Postoperative	
Meticulous aseptic technique during dressing changes Thoroughly cleanse the area around drainage tube	Help prevent microorganisms from entering the wound
Easy discharge	Reduces exposure of patient to nosocomial infection

Table 25.17: Procedures for Cleaning a Wound and Applying a Clean Dressing

Equipment

- Sterile gloves
- Gauze dressings or squares
- Sterile dressings set or suture set (contains scissors and forceps)
- Cleaning solution
- Clean disposable gloves
- Sterile basin (optional)
- Sterile drape (optional)
- Plastic bag for soiled dressings
- Waterproof pad
- Bath blanket
- Tape or ties
- Surgical pads or ABDs (optional)
- Additional dressing supplies as needed or ordered (antiseptic ointments, extra dressings)
- Acetone or adhesive remover (optional)
- Sterile normal saline

	Nursing actions		Rationales
1.	Explain procedure to client	1.	An explanation encourages client cooperation and reduces apprehension
2.	Gather equipment	2.	This provides for organized approach to task
3.	Wash your hands	3.	Handwashing deters spread of microorganisms
4.	Check physician's order for dressing change Not if drain is present	4.	This clarifies type of dressing
5.	Close door or curtain. Use bath blanket as needed when exposing area to be redressed. Position water proof pad under client if desired	5.	This provides for privacy and warmth

Contd...

		Table 25.17: *Contd...*		
	Nursing actions			*Rationales*
6.	Assist client to be in comfortable position that provides easy access to wound area		6.	This provides for comfort
7.	Place opened, cuffed plastic bag near working area		7.	Soiled dressings may be placed in disposal bag without contaminating outside surfaces of bag
8.	Loosen tape on dressing. Use adhesive remover is necessary. If tape is soiled, don gloves.		8.	It is easier to loosen tape before putting on gloves
9.	Don clean disposable gloves, and remove soiled dressings carefully in a clean to less clean direction. Do not reach over wound. Check position of drains before removing dressing. If dressing is not wet-to-dry application and is adhering to skin surface, it may be moistened by pouring a small amount of sterile saline onto it. Keep soiled side of dressing away from client's view.		9.	This protects the nurse from handling contaminated dressings. Cautious removal of dressing is more comfortable for client and ensures that drain is not removed if one is present. Saline provides for easier removal of dressing
10.	Assess amount, type, and order of drainage		10.	Wound healing process or presence of infection should be documented
11.	Discard dressings in plastic disposal bag. Pull off glove inside out and drop it in bag		11.	This prevents spread of microorganisms by contaminated dressings
12.	Using aseptic technique, open sterile dressings and supply on work area		12.	Supplies are within easy reach, and sterility is maintained
13.	Open sterile cleaning solution, and pour over gauze sponges in plastic container or over sponges placed in sterile basin		13.	Sterility of dressings and solution is maintained
14.	Don sterile gloves		14.	Maintains surgical asepsis
15.	Clean wound or surgical incision. Use sterile forceps if desired as shown in		15.	—
(a)	Clean from top to bottom or from center outward		(a)	Clean from least to most contaminated area
(b)	Use one gauze square for each wipe, discarding each square by dropping into plastic bag.		(b)	Previously cleaned area is not recontaminated
(c)	Do not touch bag with forceps		(c)	Move from least to most contaminated area
(d)	Clean around drain, if present, moving from center outward in a circular motion. Use one gauze square for each circular motion.		(d)	Moisture provides medium for growth of microorganisms
(e)	Dry wound using gauze sponge and same motion		(e)	Growth of microorganisms may be retarded and healing process improved
(f)	Apply antiseptic ointment if ordered			
16.	Apply a layer of dry, sterile dressings over wound. Use sterile forceps if desired		16.	Primary dressing serves as a wick for drainage
17.	Use sterile scissors to cut sterile 4 x 4 gauze square to place under and around drain if one is present or use precut sterile gauze		17.	Drainage is absorbed and surrounding skin area is protected
18.	Apply second gauze layer to wound site		18.	This provides for increased absorption of drainage
19.	Place surgical-pad or ABD dressing over wound as outermost layer		19.	Wound is protected from microorganism in environment
20.	Remove gloves from inside out, and discard them in plastic waster bag. Apply tape or the existing tapes to secure comfortable		20.	Tape is easier to apply after gloves have been removed
21.	Wash hands. Remove all equipment, and make client comfortable		21.	This prevents spread of microorganisms
22.	Check dressing and wound site every shift. Record dressing change and appearance of wound, and describe any drainage in chart		22.	This provides accurate documentation of procedure

Table 25.18: Procedures for Irrigating a Sterile Wound

Equipment

- Sterile irrigation set (basin, container for irrigant, irrigating syringe)
- Clean disposable gloves
- Water proof pad
- Sterile gauze and surgical pads or ABDs (for dressing change)
- Packing gauze (as specified by physician)
- Goggles (optional)
- Tape

- Sterile gloves
- Sterile dressing set or suture set (contains scissors and forceps)
- Plastic bag for soiled dressings
- Gown (optional)
- Bath blanket

	Nursing actions		*Rationales*
1.	Explain procedure to client. Check physician's order for irrigation	1.	Explanation facilitates client cooperation. Clarifies procedure and type of supplies required
2.	Gather equipment	2.	This provides for organized approach to task
3.	Wash your hands	3.	Handwahing deters the spread of microorganisms
4.	Close door or curtain. Use bath blanket at needed when exposing wound site	4.	This provides for privacy and warmth
5.	Position client so irrigating solution will flow from upper end of wound towards lower end. Place waterproof pad under client.	5.	Gravity directs flow of liquid from least contaminated to most contaminated area. Waterproof pad protects client and bed linens
6.	Warm sterile irrigating solution body temperature	6.	Warmed solution is more comfortable for client and promotes vasodilation
7.	Place opened, cuffed plastic bag near working area. Don gown and goggles if recommended	7.	Soiled dressings and packing may be placed in disposal bag without contaminating outside surfaces of bag. Gown protects uniform from contamination if splashing should occur. Goggles protect mucous membranes of eyes from contact with irrigant fluid
8.	Loosen tape on dressing and put on clean gloves to remove soiled dressings	8.	Nurse is protected from handling contaminated dressings
9.	Assess amount, type and odor of drainage. Observe condition of wound	9.	This provides information about wound healing process or presence of infection
10.	Discard dressings in plastic disposal bag. Remove gloves inside out and drop in bag	10.	Spread of microorganisms by way of contaminated dressings is prevented
11.	Using aseptic technique, open sterile dressings and supplies on work area	11.	Supplies are within easy reach and sterility is maintained
12.	Pour warmed sterile irrigating solution into sterile container. Amount may vary from 200 to 500 mL depending on size of wound	12.	This facilitates wound irrigation
13.	Put on sterile gloves	13.	This maintains surgical asepsis
14.	Position the sterile basin below the wound to collect irrigation fluid with nondominant hand	14.	Irrigation if facilitates and, client and bed linens are protected form contaminated fluid
15.	Use dominant hand to fill syringe with irrigant. Gently direct a stream of solution into wound. Keeping tip of syringe 1 inch (2.5 cm) above upper insert it gently into wound to point of resistance	15.	Debris and contaminated solution flow from least contaminated to most contaminated area. Catheter allows introduction of irrigant into wound with small opening or one that is deep
16.	Continue irrigation until solution returns clear. Try to maintain a steady flow of solution	16.	Irrigation removes exudates and debris
17.	Dry area around wound with a sterile gauze sponge	17.	Moisture provides medium for growth of microorganisms

Contd...

Table 25.18: *Contd...*

	Nursing actions		Rationales
18.	Apply layers of sterile dressing	18.	Drainage is absorbed and surrounding skin area is protected
19.	Remove gloves and discard them in plastic waste bag. Apply tape to secure dressings	19.	Tape is easier to apply after gloves have been removed
20.	Wash hands. Remove all equipment and make client comfortable	20.	This prevents spread of microorganisms
21.	Check dressing and wound site every shift. Record dressing change, appearance of wound and describe any drainage in chart.	21.	This provides for accurate documentation of procedure

Special considerations: If insertion of packing is ordered:
- Use sterile forceps to gently insert sterile packing into wound
- Be careful not to pack wound excessively because this may impede blood flow and delay healing
- Cut packing with sterile scissors, if necessary
- Allow a small strip of packing to protrude from small and deep wound to facilitate removal

Special considerations: Client must be instructed that any break or interruption in the suture line may require immediate intervention and the surgeon should be notified immediately. Instruct client and family about significant changes that need to be reported to the nurse or physician.

Encourage splinting or wound during activity (coughing, sneezing, sudden movement, or change of position).

Surgical Dressings – Nursing Interventions

Although all initial postoperative dressings are changed by the surgeon, subsequent dressings in the immediate postoperative period are usually changed by the nurse. If necessary, the nurse can determine the dressing needs to be reinforced before the first dressing change. Reinforcement keeps the outer dressing layer dry and clean, thus reducing contamination. The condition of surgical dressings and wounds is documented.

Preparation of the Patient

The patient is told that the dressing is to be changed and that changing the dressing is a simple procedure associated with little discomfort. The dressing change is scheduled for a suitable time (dressings should not be changed at mealtime). If the patient is in an open unit, the curtains are drawn to ensure privacy; the patient should be unduly exposed. The incision should not be referred to as a "scar", because for some patients the term has negative connotations. Assurance is given that the incision will shrink as it heals and the redness will fade.

Removal of Adhesive Dressings

Disposable gloves are worn. The adhesive is remove by pulling it parallel with the skin surface and in the direction of hair gown, rather than at right angles. Alcohol wipes or non irritating solvents aid in removing adhesive painlessly and quickly. The old dressing is removed and then deposited in a plastic bag designated for biomedical waste disposal. In accordance with universal precautions, dressings are never touched by ungloved hands because of the danger of transmitting pathogenic organisms, including viruses such as HIV and hepatitis B. after instruments are used in the changing of dressings, they are placed in a bag or covered receptacle, on surfaces where they might contaminate clean areas. Disposable instruments are discarded in the proper receptacle.

Simple Dressing

The tray for a routine dressing change includes gloves, cotton balls, a packet of antiseptic solution, dressings and forceps. When the sterile tray has been properly opened, the nurse places additional dressings on the field, if needed, and moistens the cotton balls with the antiseptic. Forceps are used in cleansing the wound and surrounding skin with the moistened cotton balls.

The new dressings are then applied.
- Soiled dressings must not be removed with ungloved hands
- All wound dressings are applied with sterile gloves
- If there is any doubt about the sterility of an instrument or a dressing, it is considered unsterile (Table 25.18).

Completion of a Dressing

Dressings are held in place with tape that comes in many types and widths. If the patient is sensitive to adhesive material, hypoallergenic tape is used. Many tapes are porous to permit ventilation and prevent maceration of the skin.

The correct way to apply tape is to place the tape at the center of the dressing and then press the tape down on both sides, applying tension evenly away from the midline. The wrong method of applying tape—fixing one end of the tape to the skin and pulling it tight over the dressing—often wrinkles and pulls the skin is the process. The resulting continuous and forceful traction produces a shearing effect, causing the epidermal layer to slip sideways and become prematurely separated from the deeper dermal layers.

A commercial silicone aerosol is available that can be sprayed over the adhesive used to hold dressings in place; the silicon water proofs the dressing so that the patient can bathe or swim, and it isolates the area from contamination. The spray is odorless, colorless, nonstaining, noninflammatory, heat stable and hypoallergenic.

Elastic adhesive bandage (Elastoplast, Micro-foam – 3M) is preferable for holding dressings is place over mobile areas, such as the neck or the extremities, or where pressure is required.

When the dressing is completed, the soiled dressings are placed in a waterproof bag and deposited in a biochemical waste can for disposal.

Dressing of Draining Wounds

The risk of wound infection is reduced if there is adequate drainage. The wound needs to drainage freely to release accumulated blood (clots), body fluids, pus, and necrotic material that otherwise would collect in the wound and provide a rich growth medium for microorganisms. If a wound is draining, the skin is not completely closed, so a pathway exists for microorganisms to enter and cause infection. Therefore, closed drainage is preferred to open drainage.

The drainage from an infected wound is frequently irritating to the surrounding skin. Often this situation can be avoided by using a protective ointment or dressing. Petrolatum gauze and zinc oxide care effective preparations. The drainage is excessive, an enterostomal therapies (ET) or wound care nurse specialist may be consulted about strategies to contain the drainage and protect the skin.

Portable Wound Suction

The principle involved in portable wound suction is the use of gentle, constant suction to enhance drainage of serosanguineous fluid and to collapse the skin flaps against the underlying tissue. The Hermovac apparatus is a spring diaphragm evacuator for closed suction equipped with multiple small, perforated intert polyethylene tubed. The tubes are inserted in the drainage areas in the operating room, and the wound is completely closed. The Surgivac is a bellow-shaped evacuatory for thicker drainage. These devices come in different sizes. The Jackson-Pratt is small and shaped like a grenade. Portable suction has several advantages; it is disposable, light weight, inexpensive, silent and space saving.

Patient Education

While changing the dressing, the nurse has an opportunity to teach the patient how to care for the incision and change the dressings at home. The nurse observes for clues to the patent's readiness to learn, such as looking at the incision, expressing interest, or assisting in the dressing change. Information on self-care activities and possible signs of infection is summarized as given below:

1. Keep the wound dry and clean
   (a) If there is no dressing, ask your nurse or physician, if you can bathe or shower.
   (b) If a dressing or splint is in place, do not remove it unless it is wet or soiled
   (c) If wet or soiled, change dressing yourself if you have been taught to do so; otherwise call your nurse or physician for guidance
   (d) If you have been taught, instruction might be as follows:
       (i) Cleanse area gently with 70 percent isopropyl alcohol once or twice daily
       (ii) Cover with a sterile Telfa pad or gauze—sufficiently large to cover wound
       (iii) Apply hypoallergenic Dermacel or paper tape (adhesive is not recommended because it is difficult to remove without possible injury to incision site).
2. Report immediately if any of these signs of infection occur:
   (a) Redness, marked swelling (beyond 2.5 cm (1½ in) from incision site). Tenderness, increased warmth around wound.
   (b) Ed streaks in skin near wound
   (c) Pus or discharge, foul odor
   (d) Chills or fever (over 37.7° C (100°F)
3. If soreness or pain is causing discomfort, apply a dry cool pack (containing ice or cold water) or take prescribed acetaminophen tablets (2) every 4 to 6 hours. Avoid aspirin without direction or instruction because bleeding may be enhanced with its use.
4. Swelling following a surgery is common. To help reduce swelling, elevate the affected part to the level of the heart
   (a) Hand or arm:
       (i) Sleep—elevate arm on pillow at side
       (ii) Sitting—place arm on pillow on adjacent table
       (iii) Standing—rest affected hand on opposite shoulder support elbow with unaffected hand=
   (b) Leg or foot:
       (i) Sitting—place a pillow on a facing chair, provide support underneath the knee
       (ii) Lying—place a pillow under affected leg.

After Sutures are Removed

Although the wound appears to be healed when sutures are removed, it is still tender and will continue to heal and strengthen for several weeks:

1. Follow directives of physician or nurses as to extent of activity
2. Keep suture line clean do not rub vigorously; pat dry. Wound edges may look red and may be slightly raised. This is normal.
3. Massage around wound gently using a bland baby oil, petroleum, or moisturizing cream (twice a day)
4. Report to the healthcare provider if after eight weeks the site continues to be red, thick, painful to pressure (This may be due to excessive collagen formation and should be checked).

Wound Complications

Hematoma (Hemorrhage)

The dressings are inspected for hemorrhage at frequent intervals during the first 24 hours after surgery. Any undue amount of bleeding is reported. At times, concealed bleeding occurs in the wound, beneath the skin. This hemorrhage usually stops spontaneously but results in clot formation within the wound. If the clot is small, it will be absorbed and need not to be treated. When the clot is large, the wound usually bulges somewhat, and healing will be delayed unless it is removed. After several sutures are removed by the physician, the clot is evacuated and the wound is packed lightly with gauze. Healing occurs usually by granulation, or a secondary closure may be performed.

Infection (Wound Sepsis)

Surgical wound infections: Theses are the second most frequent nosocomial infection in hospitals. Risk factors for wound infections are listed in Table 16.18.

The most important area of prevention lies in meticulous wound management and surgical technique. In addition, cleanliness and environmental disinfections are important.

Staphylococcus aureus accounts for many postoperative wound infections. Other infections may result from *Eischerichia coli, proteus vulgans, Aerobacter aerogenes, Pseudomonas aeruginosa,* and other organisms.

The risk factors contributing to wound sepsis as follows:

Clinical factors
- Wound contamination
- Foreign body
- Faulty suturing technique
- Devitalized issue
- Hematoma
- Dead space

General factors
- Debilitation
  - (a) Dehydration
  - (b) Malnutrition
  - (c) Anemia
- Advanced age
- Extreme obesity
- Shock
- Length of preoperative hospitalization
- Duration of surgical procedure
- Associated disorders (e.g. diabetes mellitus; immuno-suppression)

When the inflammatory process occurs, it usually causes symptoms in 36 to 48 hours. The patient's pulse rate and temperature increase, the WBC count rises, and the wound usually become swollen, warm and tender with incisional pain. Local signs may be absent when the infection is deep. When a diagnosis of wound infection in a postoperative wound is made, the surgeon usually removes one or more sutures and, under aseptic precautions, separates the wound edges with a pair of blunt scissors or a hemostat. Once the incision is opened, a drain is inserted.

Cellulitis: It is a bacterial infection that spreads into tissue planes. All the manifestations of inflammation are evident; *streptococcus* is frequently the responsible organism. Systemic antibiotics are usually effective. If an extremity is the site of the infection, elevation reduces dependent edema and the application of heat promotes local blood circulation. Rest decreases muscular contractions that could introduce the offending organisms into the circulatory system.

Abscess: If is a localized bacterial infection characterized by a collection of pus (bacteria, necrotic tissue, and WBCs). Usually a "point" develops that is tender. Because the area is under pressure, there is a tendency for the infection to seed bacteria that may invade adjacent tissues (cellulites) or vascular spaces (bacteremia, sepsis). Treatment is surgical drainage or excision and the administration of antibiotics. Recurrence is prevented by allowing the treated wound to drain. Rest, elevation of the part and heat are helpful.

Lymphangitis: It is a spread of infection from a cellulites or abscess to the lymphatic system. This is created by rest and antibiotics.

Dehiscence and Evisceration

The complications of dehiscence (disruption of surgical incision of wound) and evisceration (protrusion of wound contents) are especially serious when they involve abdominal incisions or wounds. These complications result from sutures giving way, from infection, and, more frequently, after marked distention or strenuous cough. They may also occur because of increasing age, poor nutritional status, and the presence of pulmonary or cardiovascular disease in patients who undergo abdominal surgery.

When the wound edges separate slowly, the intestines may protrude gradually, or not at all, and the earliest sign may be a push of bloody (serosanguineous) peritoneal fluid from the wound. When the rupture of a wound occurs suddenly coils of intestine may push out of the abdomen. Frequently, the patient may say that "something gave way". The evisceration causes pain and can be associated with vomiting.

When disruption of a wound occurs, the surgeon is notified at once. The protruding coils of intestine are covered with sterile dressings moistened with sterile saline.

An abdominal binder, properly applied, is an excellent prophylactic measure against an evisceration of this kind, and often it is used along with the primary dressing, especially for surgery on patients with weak or pendulous abdominal walls, or when rupture of a wound has occurred. Vitamin deficiency or lowered serum protein or chloride may require correction.

Applying Abdominal, T- and Breast Binders (Table 25.19)

In the past, abdominal binders were primarily used to provide support and comfort for an incision following abdominal surgical procedures. Today binders are most often used to hold dressings in place, to support soft tissue, or to suppress lactation. Single and double T-binders hold rectal or perineal dressings to place. Abdominal binders support the abdomen and hold abdominal dressings in place. Stretch net binders are not designed for support, but simply to hold dressings in place.

A breast binder or a tight bra is used as a nonpharmacologic device to aid in lactation suppression. In addition, a breast binder may be used after reduction surgery a mastectomy or breast reconstruction surgery. The binder is placed over the breast to prevent breast and nipple stimulation. Ice packs are used in conjunction with breast binders to relieve discomfort associated with breast engorgement.

Proper placement of any binder is essential comfort and effect. The binder must be smooth, the right size for the client, not interfere with circulation or put too much pressure on the bound area.

Before applying binders nurse should:
- Assess the reason the binder is needed to determine the correct binder and correct placement
- Assess the client's skin condition for rashes, inflammation, open areas, or dressings to provide a baseline for future assessment
- Assess and measure the client to determine what size binder will be needed.
- Assess for any special circumstances that may affect the placement of the binder, such as dressings, tubing, catheters or IV lines to determine a plan for binder placement.
- Assess the client's understanding of the reasons for the binder and the method of placing the binder to determine what types of client teaching will be needed.

Equipment Needed for Binders include:
- Correct binder for intended purpose (latex-free if indicated)
- Safety pins or fasteners

Abdominal binder application may be performed by ancillary personnel after the nurse has assessed the client's tolerance of the binder. The client should be able to breathe effectively and move adequately. In addition, ancillary personnel should be instructed to ensure that the client's skin is intact and to report any breakdown for nurse evaluation.

After application of binders nurse should evaluate:
- For breast binder, lactation is suppressed
- Binder provides support for dressings or soft tissue
- Binder is not too tight and does not compress the skin
- T-binder on a male client does not compress the testicles
- Client assists in placement of the binder as much as possible

Application of binders should be note in nurse notes as given below:
- Time, date and type of binder
- Difficulty the client experienced with the procedure

Bandages and Slings

Bandages are made from flannel, calico elastic net or special paper, they can be improvised by any of the above material, one from stockings or ties.

Bandages are used to
- Maintain direct pressure over a dressing to control bleeding.
- Retain dressing and slings in position
- Prevent or reduce swelling.
- Provide support for a limb or joint
- Restrict movement
- Assists in lifting and carrying casualty.

Table 25.19: Applying Binders

Nursing actions		Rationales	
	Check clients identification band Explain procedure before beginning		To identity right patient To get cooperation and reduce anxiety
Abdominal Binders			
1.	Cleanse hands	1.	Reduces transmission of microorganisms
2.	Choose correct binder. If a stretch net binder is being used, select the correct circumference and cut length to fit.	2.	Select the correct binder for the job. The correct size will make the binder most effective.
3.	Help the client into the proper position to place the binder. • For abdominal binders, the client should lie supine and lift the hips, or, alternatively, position the client on one side, and roll the client onto the binder. For stretch net binders, slide the net over the head and neck, or slide the net up from the feet, depending on which is easier for the client. • Place the scultetus binder with the upper border no higher than the waist.	3.	Applying binders can be awkward if the client is not positioned correctly. If binders are too high, they interfere with breathing.

Contd...

Table 25.19: *Contd...*

	Nursing actions		Rationales
4.	Wrap the straight abdominal binder, starting form the lower abdomen and working upward. • Stretch net binders should be adjusted to cover the dressings they will be holding place • Bring the tails of the scultetus binder across the center of the abdomen, one at a time, alternating sides, starting at the bottom (For a postpartum client, work from the top down). Each tail should overlap the next lower one by about half the width of tail for maximal support. Secure only the last tail.	4.	Supports the abdomen and, if needed, secures dressings.
5.	Secure binders fasteners. If the binder does not have Velcro fasteners, secure with safety pins. Stretch net binders cling and stretch over the body part and do not need additional fastening. Check for snug fit.	5.	Fasteners will keep binder in place. Be sure that all fasteners are closed securely to prevent possible client injury.
6.	Adjust if necessary. Be sure that binders are not restricting breathing or circulation. Be sure that binders are knot restricting are in place between the binder and any wound	6.	Binders that are too tight may make breathing difficult and may contribute to skin irritation or breakdown.
7.	Cleanse hands	7.	Reduces transmission of microorganisms
T-Blinders			
8.	Cleanse hands	8.	Reduces transmission of microorganisms
9.	Select a single-tall binder for a female, a double-tail binder for a male. Have the client lift the hips or, alternatively, position the client on one side and roll the client onto the binder. Place the waistband at the waist, with the single or double tails pointing downward along the spine	9.	Proper binder keeps dressing in place
10.	Wrap waistband around the waist and secure • Bring the tall (s) of the T-binder up between the client's legs. For the male, one tail should be placed on each side of the testicles. Join tails to the waistband and secure.	10.	Secures dressings and promotes client comfort
11.	Cleanse hands	11.	Reduces transmission of microorganisms
Breast Binders			
12.	Cleanse hands	12.	Reduces transmission of microorganisms
13.	Assist the client to sitting position	13.	Sitting will allow ease in placement of the binder. If not possible, turn client side-to-side while applying binder.
14.	Apply binder, adjusting for a snug fit	14.	The tightness of the binder will be instrumental in adequate lactation suppression.
15.	Adjust if necessary. Be sure that breast binder is not restricting breathing or causing skin irritation	15.	Breast binders that are too tight may make breathing difficult and/or may contribute to skin irritation or breakdown
16.	Add use of adjunctive treatments (e.g. ice packs, analgesics) for additional comfort, if needed.	16.	If breasts are engorged, adjunctive treatment may be required to increases client's level of comfort
17	Cleanse hands	17	Reduces transmission of microorganisms

Bandages should be applied firm enough to keep dressing and splints in position. But not so tight as to cause injury to the part or to impede the circulation of the blood. A bluish tinge of the finger or nails may be a danger sign that the bandages are too tight. Loss of sensation is another sign.

Bandages and Binders: A single gauze dressing is often not enough to immobilize or provide support to wound. Bandages and binders are used to secure dressings, apply pressure and support the wound; they are especially useful in injuries of the extremities. Bandages are strips of cloth, gauze (e.g. roller gauze) of elasticized material (e.g. ace bandages) to wrap a body part. They come packed in rolls and vary in width from 1 to 6 inches. Binders are designed for a specific body part and including slings, abdominal binders, chest binders, and T-binders. They may be made of cloth (flannel, muslin) or of an elasticized material that fastens together with Velcro.

Functions of Bandages and Binders

Bandages and binders applied over or around dressing can provide extra protection and therapeutic benefits by the following:
- Creating pressure over the body part (e.g. an elastic bandage applied over an arterial puncture site)
- Supporting a wound (e.g. an abdominal binder applied over a large abdominal incision and dressing)
- Immobilizing a body part (e.g. an elastic bandage applied around a sprained ankle)
- Reducing or preventing edema (e.g. a breast binder used to minimize swelling between skin and tissue layers after masectomy)
- Securing a splint (e.g. a bandage applied around hand splints for correction of deformities)
- Securing dressings (e.g. elastic webbing applied around leg dressings after a vein strapping)

Bandaging Materials

A bandage is a length of material applied to fit smaller parts of the body. Bandages are available in various materials, lengths, and widths. They are soft and conform to body areas. Most bandages are used to provide pressure and hold dressings in place.

Materials used for bandages include straight weave and knit weave cotton gauze (Kling, Kerlix), flannel, muslin, elasticized knit, rubberized self-adhering material (Elastoplast, Coban), elastic net webbing (Surgifix, Surgiflex), ribbed tubular cotton (stockinette), and knit tubular cotton (Tube-gauze).

Gauze is commonly used. It is absorbent yet porous, allowing air to circulate. Gauze frays when laundered, so it is usually not recycled. Flannel is sturdier, withstands repeated washings, and keeps the part warm. Muslin and flannel are less flexible than gauze. They are used to immobilize or create pressure.

Elasticized net bandages come in various sizes and shapes. Some are tubular, others are shaped like a shirt or pants. Some of these bandages are designed to keep dressings in place. Others are more constricting and apply pressure.

Caution: Frequently assess areas distal to bandages. Bandages may become too tight (from edema) and must be loosened or removed and replaced to prevent tissue death or gangrene. Bandages that are too tight are uncomfortable, are dangerous, and may cause permanent damage.

Principles of Bandages and Binder Application

1. Position the body part to be bandaged in comfortable position of normal anatomical alignments.
2. Bandages cause restriction in movement. Immobilization in normal functioning position reduces risks of deformity or injury. Placing and supporting the body part to be bandaged in the normal functioning position prevents deformity and discomfort.
3. Prevent friction between and against skin surfaces by applying gauze or padding. Skin surfaces in contact with other (e.g. between toes, under breasts) can rub against each other to cause abrasion or chafing. Bandaged over bony prominences may rub against skin to cause breakdown.
4. Apply bandages securely to prevent slippage during movement. Friction between bandage and skin can cause skin breakdown
5. When bandaging extremities apply bandage first at distal-end and progress toward trunk, gradual application of pressure from distal toward proximal portion of extremity promotes venous return and minimizes risk of edema or circulatory impairment.
6. Apply bandages firmly with equal tension exerted over each turn or layer; Avoid excess overlapping of bandage layers. Application prevents unequal pressure distribution over bandaged body part. Localized pressure causes circulatory impairment. The tension of each bandage turn shall be equal and unnecessary and uneven overlapping of turns should be avoided.
7. Position pins, knots, or ties away from wound or sensitive skin areas. Materials can exert localized pressure and irritation. They also cause discomfort for the client if located incorrectly.
8. When removing bandage, it is best to cut the bandage with a bandage scissors to prevent excessive manipulation of the part.
9. Avoid using unclean bandages and binders, because these may cause infection if applied over a wound or skin abrasion.
10. An unnecessarily thick or extensive bandage should be avoided. It causes heat and moisture. Prolonged heat and moisture on the skin may cause skin breakdown.

In addition to keeping above principles, in mind, prior to bandage or binders is applied, the nurse's responsibilities include the following:
- Inspecting the skin for abrasions, edema, discoloration or exposed wound edges
- Covering the exposed wounds or open abrasions with sterile dressings

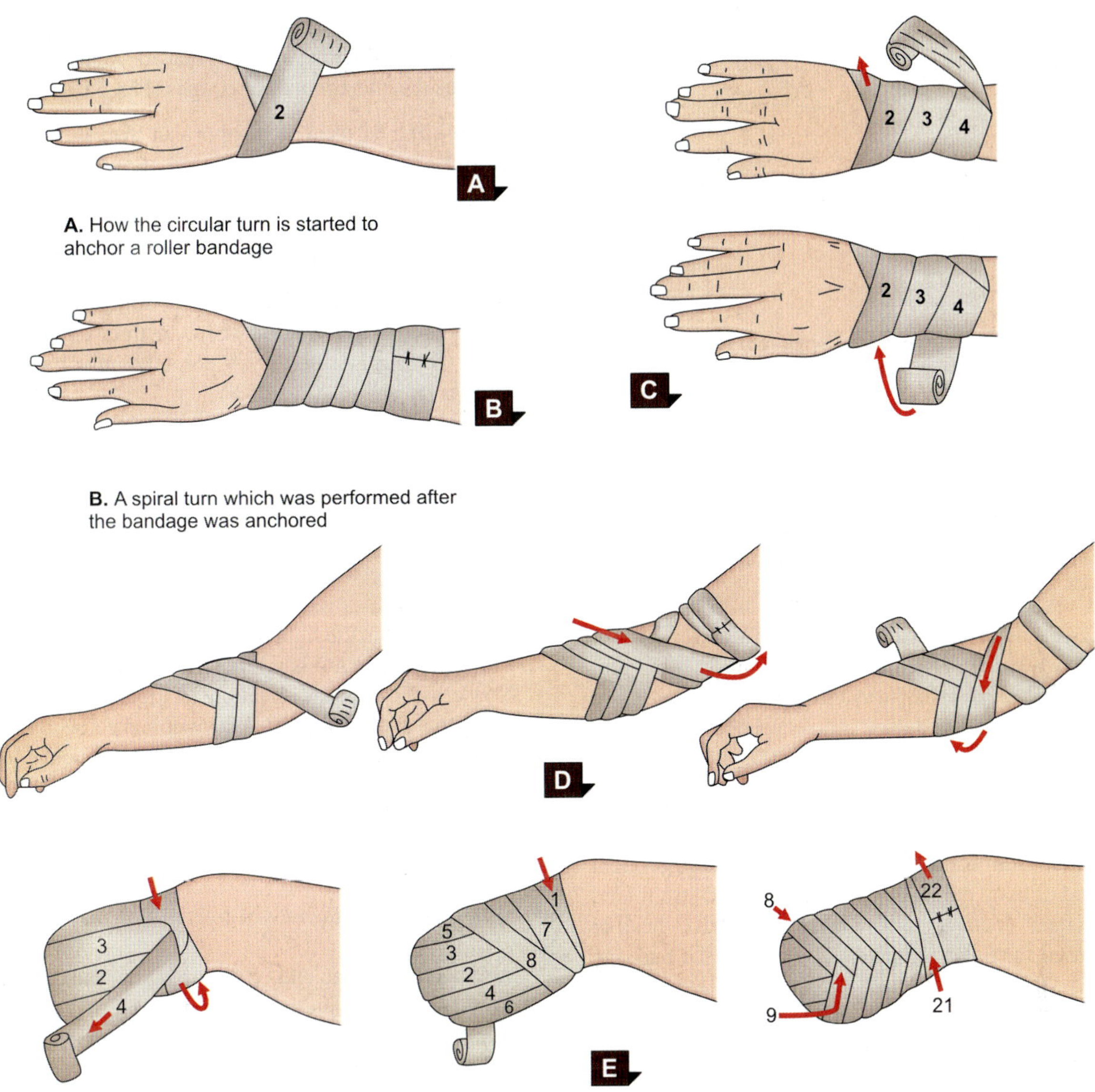

Figures 25.5A to E: Techniques for applying various types of roller bandages: (A) Circular turn, (B) Spiral turn, (C) Spiral-reverse turn, (D) Figure of eight turn, (E) Recurrent-stump bandage

- Assessing the condition of underlying dressings and changing them, if soiled
- Assessing the skin of underlying body parts and the parts that will be distal to the bandage for signs of circulatory impairment (coolness, pallor, numbness, and tingling) to provide a means for comparing changes in circulation after bandage application.

Applying Roller Bandages

A roller bandage is a continuous strip of material wound on itself to form a cylinder or roll (Figs. 25.5A to E).

Plain gauge, elastic webbing, and stretchable roller bandages are made in various widths and lengths. When the bandaging in begun, the free end is held in place with one hand while the other hand passes the roll around the body part. After the bandage is anchored, the roll is passed or rolled around the body part, taking care that equal tension is exerted with each turn. It is easier to keep tension equal by unwinding the bandage gradually and only as it is requested.

The basic turns for roller bandages are as follows:

Circular turn: In this bandage turn overlapping previous turn completely. It anchors at the first and final turn covers small part. When using this turn, the bandage is wrapped around the body part with complete overlapping of the previous bandage turn. It is used primarily for anchoring a bandage where it is begun and where it is terminated (Fig. 25.6).

Spiral turn: In this stage, ascending body part wrapped with each turn overlapping previous one by one-half or two-thirds

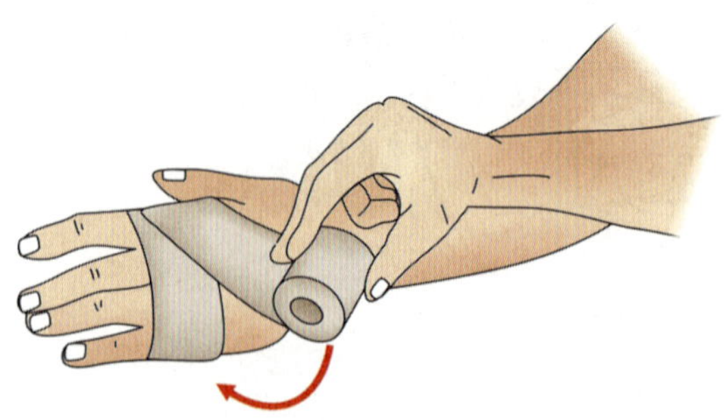

Figure 25.6: Complete overlapping of the previous bandage turn

width of bandage. When using this turn, the bandage ascends in a spiral manner so that each turn overlaps the preceding one by one-half or two-thirds of the width of bandage. The spiral turn is useful when the body part being bandaged is cylindrical, such as the area round the wrist, the fingers and the trunk (Fig. 25.5B).

Spiral-reverse turn: This turn requiring twist or reversal of bandage half-way through each turn. Actually it is a spiral turn in which reverses are made half-way through each reverse turns particularly effective for bandaging cone-shaped body part such as the thigh, the leg or the forearm (Fig. 25.5C).

Recurrent turn: Here, bandage is first secured with two circular turns around the proximal end of body part; half turn made perpendicular up from bandage edge; body of bandage brought over distal end of body part to be covered with each turn folded back over on itself. It covers uneven body parts such as head or stump. It is used for finger, amputated limb and head bandage (Fig. 25.5E).

Applying Binders

Binders are especially designed for the body part to be supported. The most common type of binders are as follows (Figs. 25.7A and B).

T-binders: T binders look like the letter 'T' and is used to secure rectal or perineal dressings and in the groin. The single T-binder is used for female clients and the double T-blinder is used for male clients. The belt is passed around the waist and secured with safety pains. The single or double tails are passed between the legs and pinned to the belt (Fig. 25.7A)

Breast binder: A breast binder looks like a tight-fitting sleeveless vest. It conforms to the shape of the chest wall and is available in different sizes. Breast binders can provide supports after breast surgery or exert pressure to reduce lactation in a woman after childbirth. It is essential that excess pressure should be avoided to prevent chest expansion impairment.

Abdominal binder: A many-tailed binder or scultetus binder, consists of a rectangular piece of fabric, with tails that are about 5 cm (2") wide attached to its sides. The binder supports abdomen

or holds dressings on it or on the chest. An abdominal binder supports large abdominal incisions that are vulnerable to tension or stress as the client moves or coughs (Fig. 25.7B).

Sling: A sling is used to support an arm with sprains or fractures.

Triangular Bandage

Triangular bandage has three borders. Longest is called base and the other two as the sides. There are three corners. The one opposite the base is called as 'A' point the other two are called the ends as 'B' and 'C' (Fig. 25.8).

Applying of Knot

The knot should be applied where it does not hurt the skin or where it does not become a source of discomfort and friction.

For a firm bandage Reef knot should be used:
- Catch the ends of the bandage separately in each hand
- Cross the end in the right hand from below and then over and above the end in left hand thus making a turn
- Now cross in opposite direction, i.e. right hand over and then under the end in left hand. This will make a second turn Application of granny knot will keep the bandage loose.

Slings

Slings are used to support arms and to prevent pulls.

Arm sling: It is used in cases of fractures of wrists, hands, ribs, etc.

We have to put one end of the triangular bandage over the uninjured shoulder with the point on the injured side, pass the end around the neck and bring it over the injured shoulder. The other free end will now be handing down over the chest. Place the forearm horizontally across the chest and cover the forearm by bringing the end up. Tie two ends in such a way that the forearm is horizontal or slightly tilted upward and now remains at the collar bone. Loose part of the sling may be tucked at the elbow.

Triangular sling: It is used in fracture of the collar bone in keeping the hand raised high. Ask the patient to place the forearm across the chest towards the opposite shoulder and palm over the breast.

Place the open bandage over the chest, with one end over the hand and the point beyond the elbow. Tuck the base of the bandage under the forearm and hand.

Fold the lower end around the elbow and tie it with the other free end over the uninjured shoulder.

Collar and cuff sling: This is used to support the wrist. Ask the patient to keep the hand on the opposite shoulder. A cleve hitch is passed around the wrist and the ends tied in the hollow above the collar bone on the injured side. Improvised slings can be made of mufflers, ties and other soft cloth.

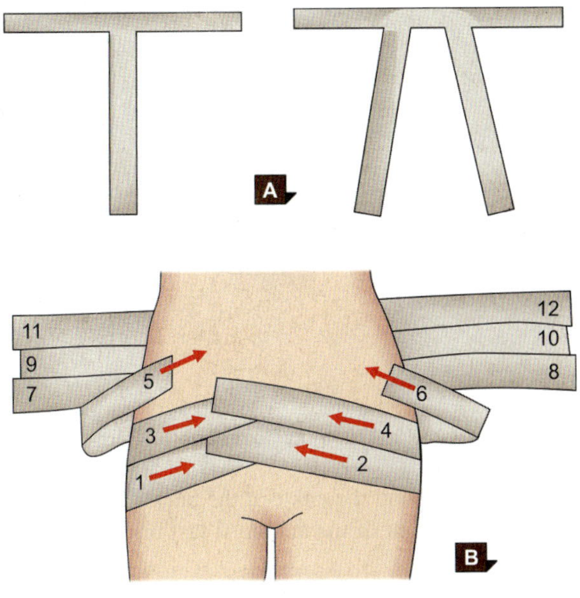

Figures 25.7A and B: Binders: (A) T-binders, (B) Many tailed binders

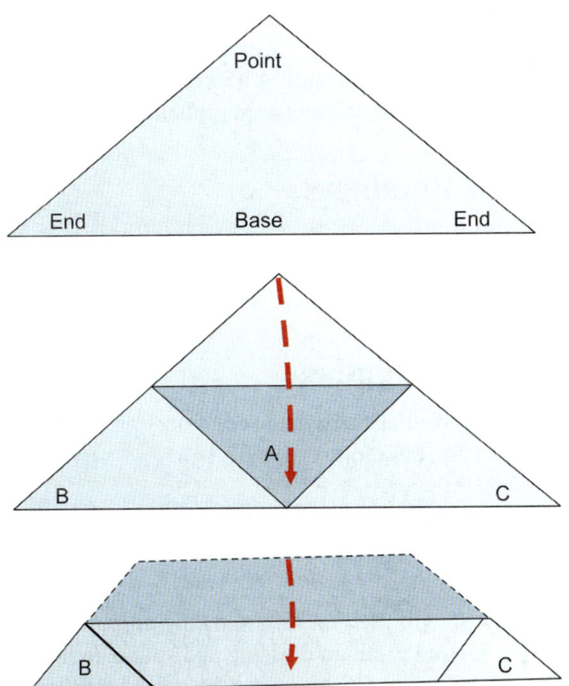

Figure 25.8: Folding of triangular bandage

Bandaging with Triangular Bandage

For scalp: Place the folded bandage on the forehead of the level of eyebrows. Take the two ends backwards (Fig. 25.9).

After placing the body of the bandage over the head, the point of the bandage will be over the nape of the neck.

Cross the two ends and bring these forward over the ears to meet on the forehead, where finally those are tied. Now bring the free point upwards and tuck it.

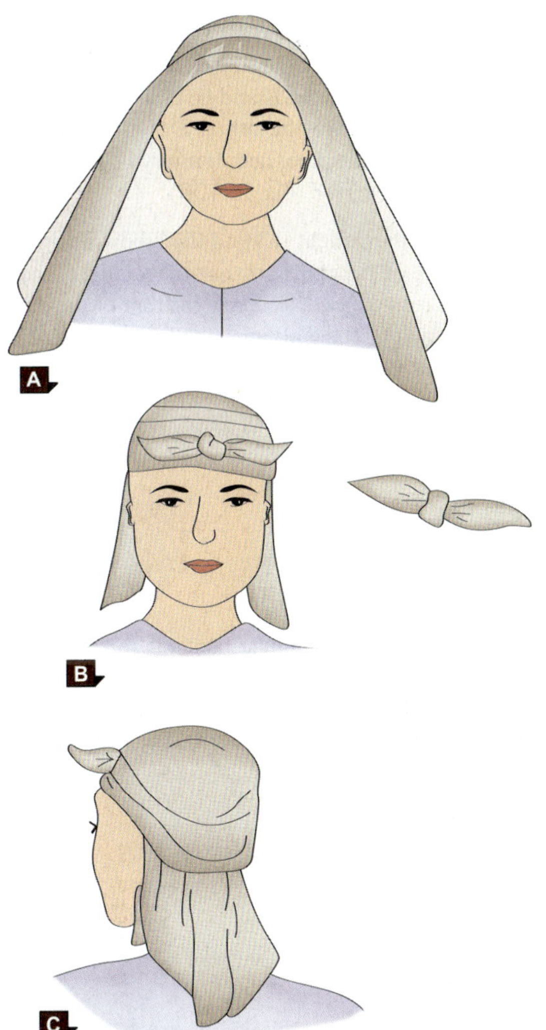

Figure 25.9: Use of triangular bandage for head

For hand: Place the open bandage and put hand over it. Turn the point toward the fingers and base across the wrist. Cross over and tie it up over the point. Now pin the point over the knot (Fig. 25.10A).

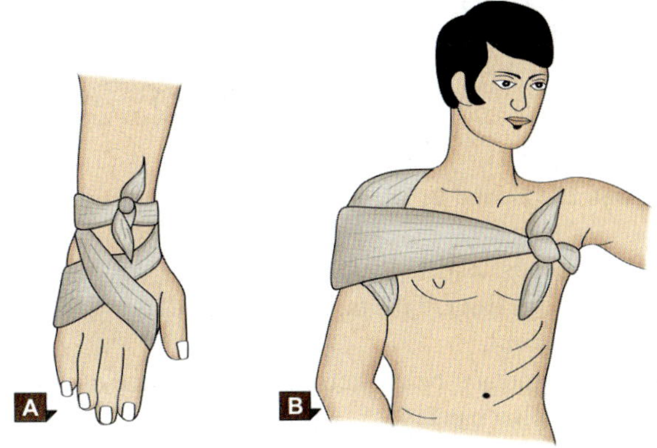

Figures 25.10A and B: Triangular bandage over wrist and shoulder

For chest: Place the center of the open bandage over the dressing and point 'A' over the sound shoulder. Carry the ends of the bandages round the body and tie it in such a way that one end remains longer than the other. Draw the point A over shoulder and tie it to the other end. If injury is over the back the procedure may be reversed (Fig. 25.10B).

For elbow: Ask the patient to bend the elbow at right angles. Lay the point 'A' on the upper arm and the middle of the base on the forearm. Cross the ends B and C in front of the elbow, and round the arm and tie the ends above the elbow (Fig. 25.11).

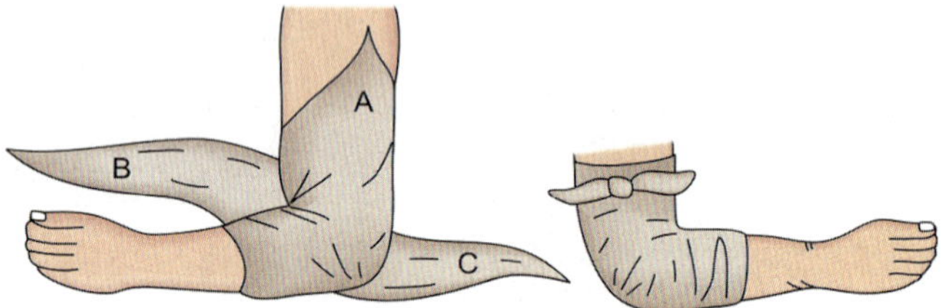

Figure 25.11: Triangular bandage for elbow

For knee: Ask the patient to keep the at right angle. Place the open bandage in front of the knee with a point 'A' open the thigh (Figs 25.12A and B).

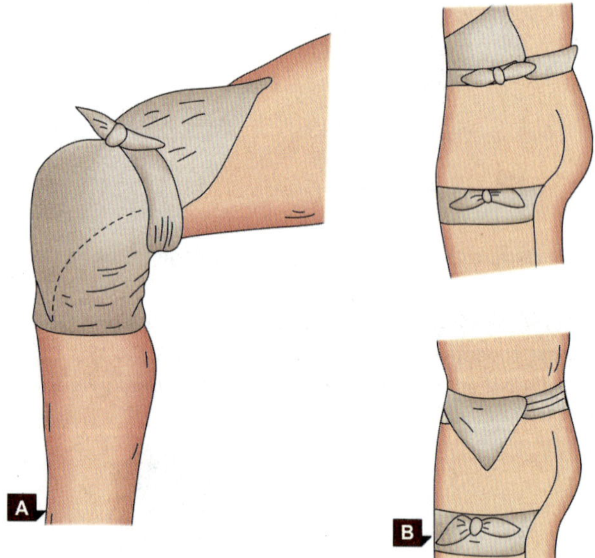

Figures 25.12A and B: Triangular bandage for knee and hip

Cross the ends, take them upward and from back of the thigh bring them to the front of the thigh and tie up. Later on bring the flap 'A' downward.

If knee cannot be bent, then figure of 8 bandage may be applied with roller bandage.

For foot: Ask the patient to put the foot in the center of an open bandage with a point. A beyond the toes. Now draw the point over the foot toward ankle (Fig. 25.13).

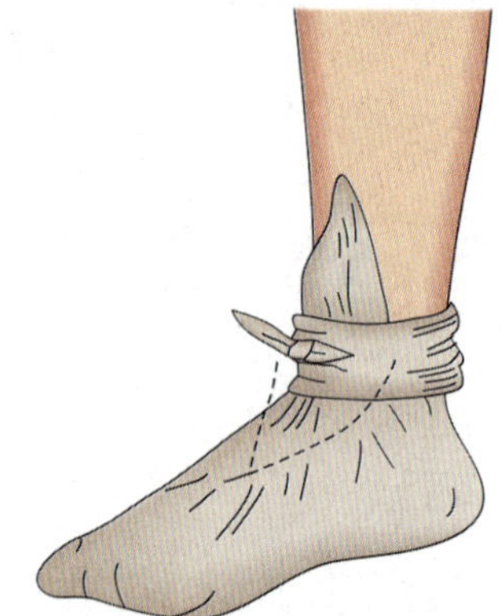

Figure 25.13: Triangular bandage for foot

Cover the ends round the ankle at the back. Bring the ends forward and tie in front of the ankle. At last bring the point A downward and pin up.

Stump Bandaging

After an amputation stump is bandaged in a definite manner to prevent edema to encourage venous return, to accustom the stamp to become constantly covered in future. Usually crepe bandage provides better result. A 15 cm width is used above-knee stamp and 10 cm width is used for below-knee stump.

Types of Bandages

1. Triangular
2. Roller
3. Special-such as, many tail or 'T' bandages

Triangular Bandage

The triangular bandage may be used in nursing and for slings, to support an arm after injury (Fig. 25.14).

Roller Bandages

Uses

Roller bandages are used for the following purposes.
1. To cover and to retain dressing and splints in position.
2. To exercise pressure on a part in order to prevent or to reduce swelling.
3. To provide support for a part, as a sprained or dislocated joint.
4. To prevent and control haemorrhage, and to drive blood from the part, bandaged, in cases of extreme collapse due to haemorrhage.
5. To restrict movement.
6. To correct deformity.

Materials

Roller bandages are made from strips of different material of varying lengths and widths, according to the part to which they

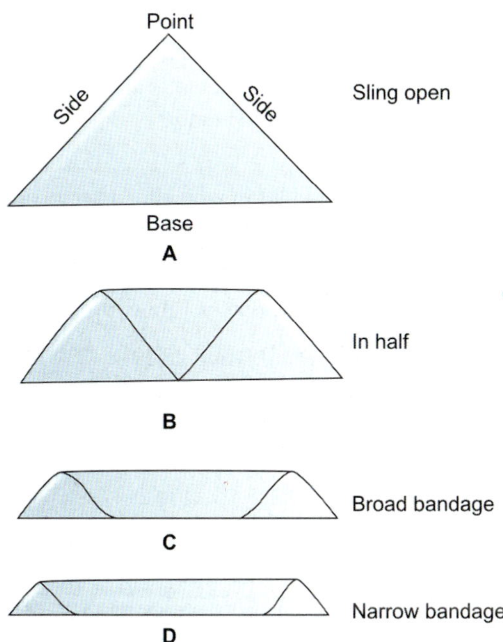

Figure 25.14: Triangular bandage

are applied. Materials commonly used include, flannel, open wove cotton, fast edge cotton, calico, crepe or elastic net.

Before use, the bandage should be firmly and evenly rolled, either by hand or by machine. If two people are available, it may be found helpful to run the bandage over the back of a chair.

The parts of the bandage are referred to as the head and the free end or tail. Usually, a single roller bandage is used, but for, some certain parts, a double headed roller bandage is required. In this, the free ends of two roller bandages are sew together leaving the heads to close together, on the same side of the bandage.

Most roller bandages are 6 yards long, except the very narrow ones, which are, usually, short. The width lay according to the part of the body to be bandaged. The usual width of the bandages are, 1 inch to 4 to 6 inches.

Part Bandage	Width
Fingers	1 inch
Arm	2 to 2 inches
Leg	3 to 3 inches
Trunk	4 to 6 inches
Head	2 inches

Rules for the application of roller bandages

1. Use a tightly rolled bandage of the correct width.
2. Support the part to be bandaged through out, for the forearm, the hand should be prone.
3. Always stand in front of the patient, except, when applying a cape line bandage.
4. Bandage a limb in the position in which it is to remain.
5. Hold the bandage with the head uppermost and apply the outer surface of the bandage to the part, never unroll more than a few inches of bandage at a time.

6. Bandage from within outwards and from below upwards, maintaining even pressure throughout.
7. Begin the bandage with a firm oblique turn to fix it and allow each successive turn to cover two thirds of the previous one, with the free edges lying parallel.
8. Make any reverses or crossing a line on the outer side of the limb, except, when this brings them over a wound or prominence of bone, in which case, they must be on the front of the limb.
9. Pad the axilla or groin when bandaging these parts, so that, two of the surfaces of skin do not touch beneath the bandage.
10. Finish off with a straight turn above the part, hold in the end and fasten with a safety pin.

Points to be observed

1. The comfort of the patient is the first consideration, except, when arresting haemorrhage or correcting a deformity
2. Neatness and economy must be considered, but, the bandages must fulfill its purpose and must cover the dressing completely.
3. The bandages should be firm and applied with even pressure throughout, but the extremities must be carefully watched for any signs of swelling or blueness due to interferences with circulation by a bandage that is too light.

Turns used in roller bandaging

1. Simple spiral
2. Reverse spiral
3. Figure of eight
4. Spica

Simple spiral

Is used for parts which are of uniform thickness, such as, a finger, a wrist. The bandage is applied obliquely round the part, each turn cover tow thirds (2/3) of the proceeding one, and the edges being kept parallel (Fig. 25.15).

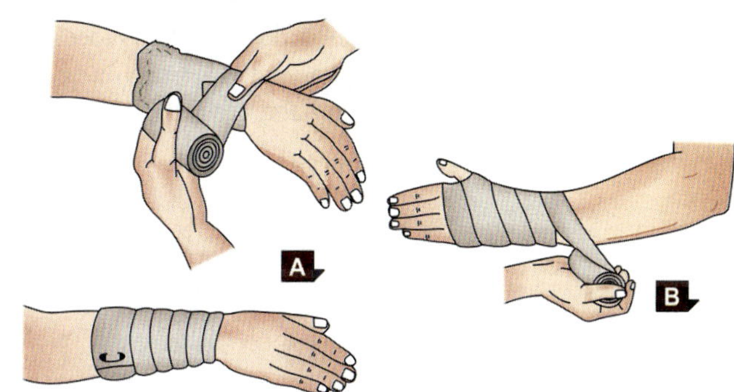

Figures 25.15A and B: Simple spiral

Reverse spiral

It is used for parts which vary in thickness and upon which the bandage of circular turns cannot be tied properly like leg and forearms. One or two simple spiral turns are usually made to carry the bandages to the point at which the spiral can no longer be employed, and then the lower edge of its last spiral is fixed with the thumb about halfway between the mid line and outer surface of the limb. The bandage is then reversed and brought down and carried round the limb, when another reverse is made immediately above the former one. These reverses are repeated as far as necessary and the bandage completed with one or tow spiral turns straight round the limb. Care should be taken and that, each reverse occurs immediately above the previous one, so that, the pattern is even. Each turn should cover two thirds of the preceding one, as in the simple spiral (Fig. 25.16).

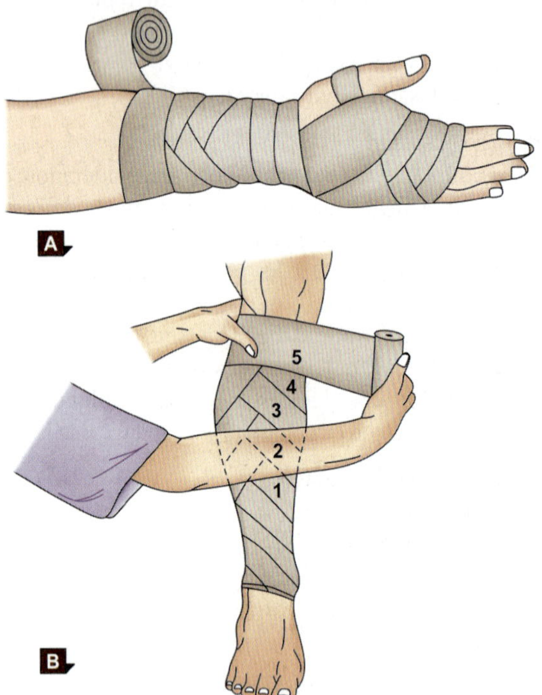

Figures 25.16A and B: Reverse spiral

Figure of Eight

Is used for bandaging limb and for covering joints. It consists of series of loops, encircling the part in the form of a figure of eight. The upper loops being completely hidden by the successive turns end the lower loops forming the pattern. Each one cover the two thirds of the preceding loop and crossing in the same line (Fig. 25.17).

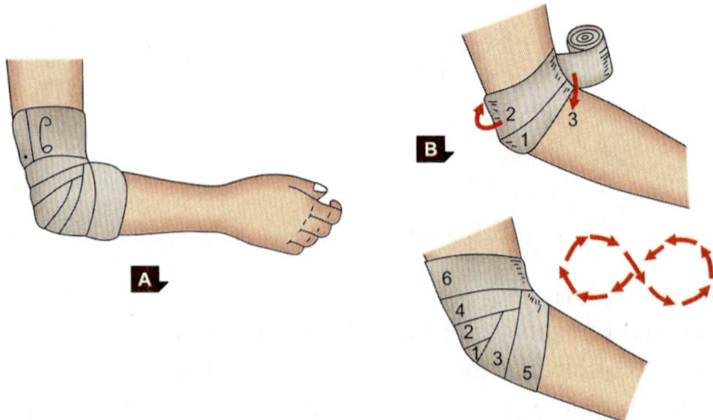

Figures 25.17A and B: Figure of eight bandage

The Spica

Is a form of the figure of eight in which one turn is very much larger than the other. It is used for joints at right angles to the body. E.g.: Shoulder, Groin and Thumb.

The Divergent Spica

Is a form of the figure of eight in which the turn go alternately above and below a fixed starting turn ending above, and is used for bent joints, as the elbow or heel.

Bandages for Hand, Wrist, Forearm, Elbow and Arm

Hand Bandage (Figs 25.18A&B and 25.19)

With the pronated, that is, the pain held down wards fix the bandage by a turning round the wrist and carry the roll obliquely

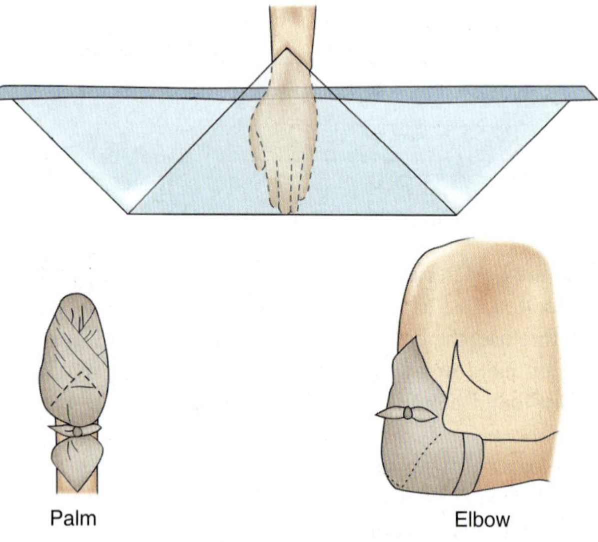

Figure 25.18A: Hand bandage

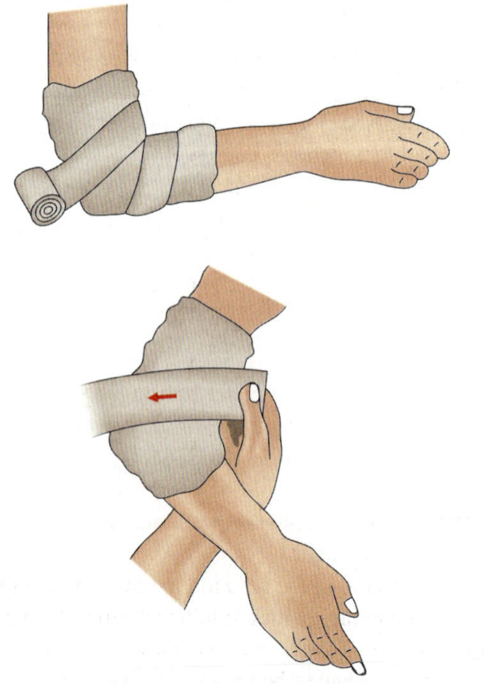

Figure 25.18B: Elbow bandage

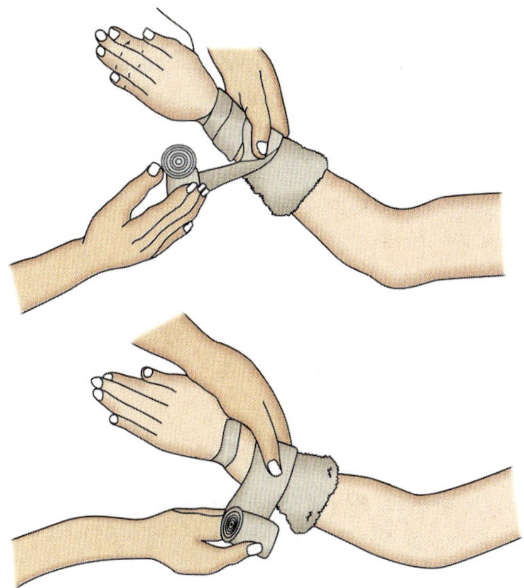

Figure 25.19: Wrist bandage

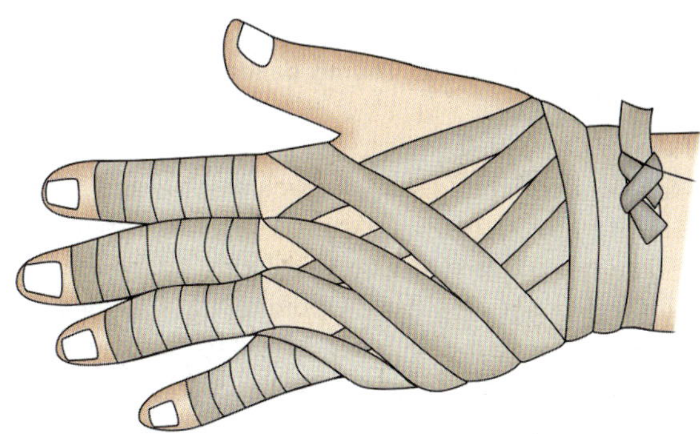

Figure 25.20: Finger bandages

the little finger side. Take on spiral turn to the base of the finger nail and then cover the finger by simple spiral turns. Then carry the bandage a cross the back of the hand to the wrist. Secure the bandage by a safety pin or by tying two ends of the bandage together. If more than one finger as to be bandaged, take a turn round the wrist between each two fingers and continue as above until the bandage is complete.

over the back of the hand to the side of the little finger. Carry the bandage round the palm, encircling the finger with one horizontal turn, so that the lower boarder of the bandage, just touches the root of the nail of the little finger. Carry the bandage one more round the palm and then return obliquely to the wrist. The figure of eight turn round the wrist and hand are repeated until the hand is covered and the bandage is then finished with a spiral turn round the wrist.

Wrist, Forearm, and Upper arm Bandage

The wrist and forearm are bandaged by use of the simple and reverse spiral until the elbow is reached. The figure of eight turn can be so used, as the limb enlarges as an alternative to the reverse spiral turn, if preferred (Figs 25.28A&B and 25.19).

To Cover the Elbow

Bend the elbow at right angles, lay the outer side of the bandage on the inner side of the joint and take one straight turn carrying the bandage over the elbow tip and round the limb of the elbow. The second turn is made to encircle forearm and the third arm. Each of these turns being made to cover the margins of the first turn. Continue the turns alternately, below and above the first turn, allowing each to cover a little more than two thirds of the previous turn, and finishing about the elbow.

The Upper Arm

The bandages, as in the forearm, by a succession of reverse spirals or figure of eight turns, and the bandages may be carried on from the forearm, or elbow or started independently, as most conveniently.

Finger Bandages (Figs 25.20 and 25.21)

With the hand pronated, fix the bandage by two circular turns a round the wrist leaving the end free from tying off. Afterwards, carry the bandage obliquely over the back of hand to the base of the finger to be bandaged. Taking the fingers is order, start form

To cover the finger tip

A recurrent bandage is used. Commence as before, but take the bandage straight up to the back of the finger and over the middle of the tip and down the front to the level of the second joint. Holding the turns back and front with the fingers of the other hand, make two more turns over the tip of the finger, one on either side of the first turn. Fix the loop with a straight circular turn as near to the tip as possible and then cover the finger by simple spiral turns as before. Being careful to make them form within outwards. Take a straight turn round the wrist and either finish off as before or continue the next finger.

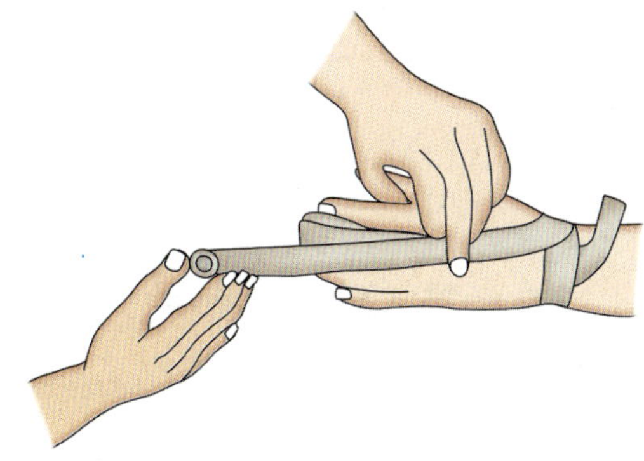

Figure 25.21: To cover the finger tip

Spica of Thumb Bandage (Fig. 25.22)

With the hand held, so that, the back of the thumb is upper most, take two turns round the wrist and carry the bandage over the back of the thumb. Encircle the thumb with one or two straight turns, so that, the lower border of the bandage is level with the root of the nail. Carry the bandage back, over the back of the hand, round the wrist and repeat the figure of eight turns round thumb and wrist, until the wall of the thumb is completely covered. Complete the bandages with one straight, round the wrist.

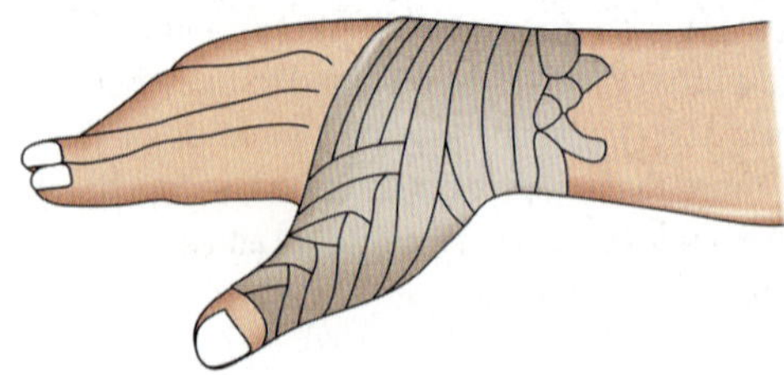

Figure 25.22: Thumb bandage

Spica of shoulder bandage

Place a small pad of cotton wool in each axilla. Take 3-4 inch bandage and fix it with two spiral turns round the upper part of the arm. Take two or three reverse spiral turns round the upper arms until the bandages reaches the point of the shoulder. Then carry the bandage over the shoulder, across the back and under the opposite armpit. Bring it back across the chest and arm round under the armpit an cover the shoulder again, covering two-thirds of the previous turn (Fig. 25.23).

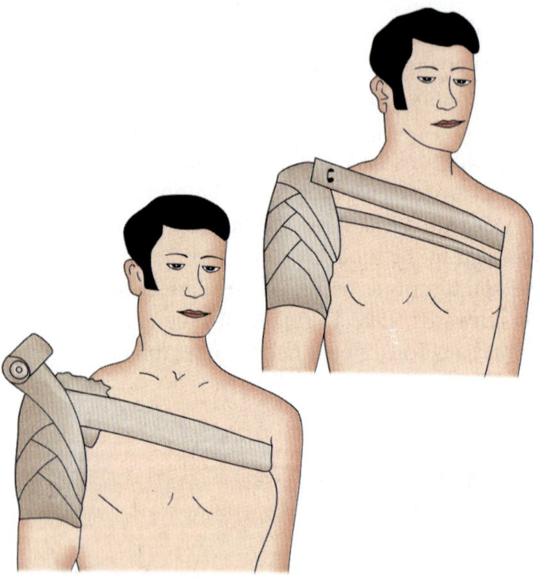

Figure 25.23: Shoulder bandage

This forms a figure of eight round the arm and the body and the turns are repeated until the whole shoulder is covered. The bandage should be secured by a pin immediately over the injured shoulder.

Bandages for the foot, ankle and leg

If the patient is in bed, the heel should be elevated on a support, about 6 inches high. If he is up and about, he should be seated in a chair with the foot supported on a stool or another chair. To avoid stooping, the nurse may, if she prefers, sit opposite to the patient and take his foot on her knee.

Foot and ankle bandage

Take one or two turns round the ankle to fix the bandage and then take it on obliquely across the foot to the root of the little

toe. Make one horizontal turn right round the foot at his level and then carry the bandage back over the back over the foot and take a turn round the ankle just above the heel. Figure of eight turns are then repeated round the foot and ankle, each turn over lapping the preceding turn by two third of its width, until the whole foot is covered (Fig. 25.24).

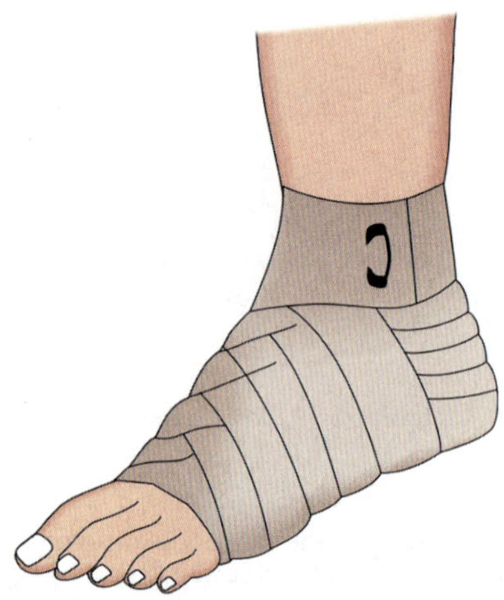

Figure 25.24: Foot and ankle bandage

Leg

If the bandage is to be continued up the leg, the reverse spiral or figure of eight turns may be used as for the arm (Fig. 25.25).

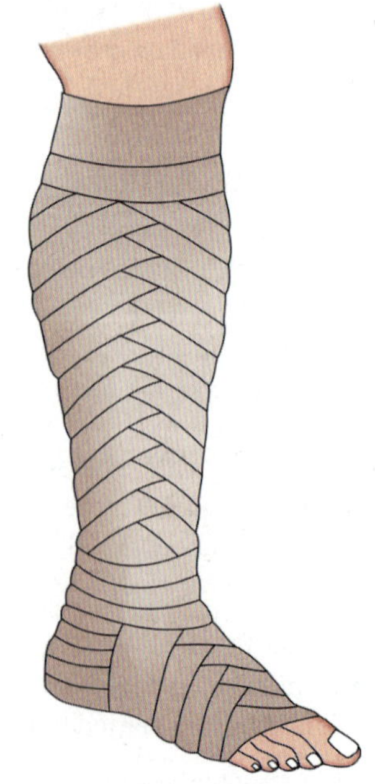

Figure 25.25: Leg bandage

To cover the heel

The leg should be supported, so that, the heel projects well over the edge of the chair, stool or cushion on which it is placed. The foot should be kept at right angles to the leg (Fig. 25.26).

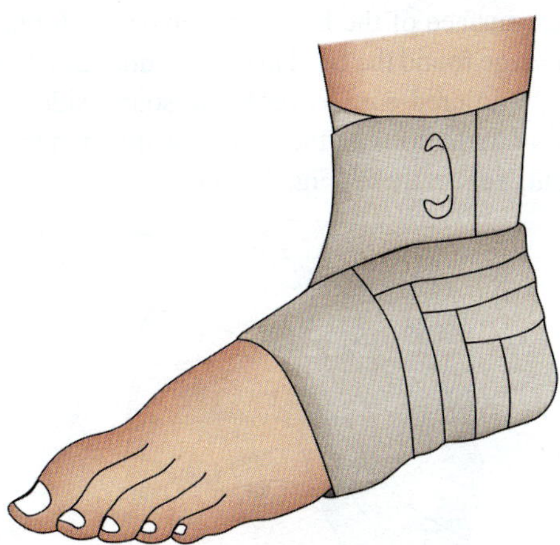

Figure 25.26: Heel bandage

Commence the bandage by a turn over the tip of the heel. The bandage is then carried round the foot just below the tip of the heel, so that, the margin of the bandage covering the tip of the heal is well covered. It is then brought over the ankle and taken round the leg, just above the tip of the heel, so that the other margin of the bandage covering the heel tip is now also covered. The turns are repeated. Each turn being made just below and above the preceding one, until the heel is well covered and the bandage so extends from halfway along the foot to well above the ankle.

Bandage for the knee

Flex the knee, lay the outer side of the bandage against the inner side of the knee and take one straight turn over the knee cap. The bandage is thus brought round the knee, just below and then just above. Note that the margins of the bandage covering the knee cap are covered as in the elbow and heel bandages.

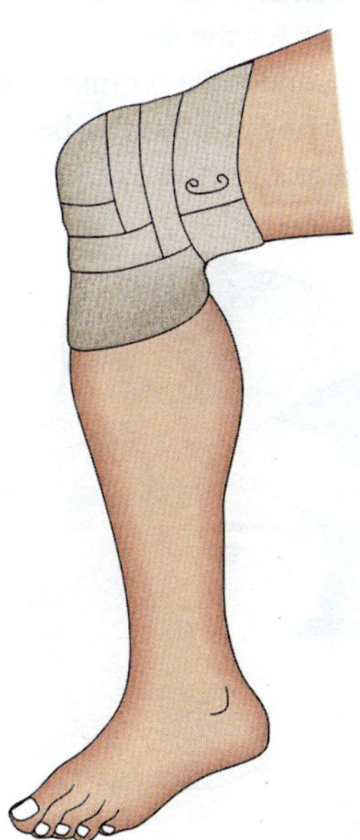

Figure 25.27: Knee bandage

The turns are repeated below and above the joint until the whole knee is covered and the bandage is then secured by one straight turn round the thigh (Fig. 25.27).

Spica of hip bandage

Place the outside of the bandage on the inner side of the thigh about 6 inches below the groin. Carry the bandage horizontally round the limb and make three or four ascending reverse spiral turns round the thigh. Carry the bandages from within outwards over the front of the groin and up round the hip and back, passing over the prominence of the hip bone on the opposite side. Bring the bandage down, over the abdomen to the outer side of the thigh and repeat the figure of eight round the body and the thigh until the hip is covered (Fig. 25.28).

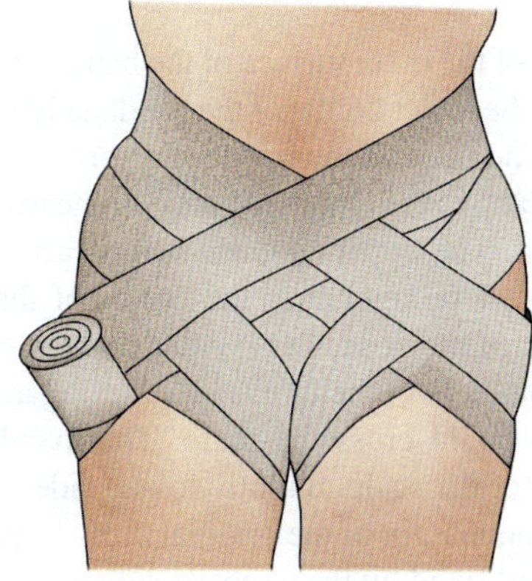

Figure 25.28: Hip bandage

Spica of groin bandage

This is applied in the same way as the spica for the hip, except that the bandage is started higher up. The reverse spiral and omitted and the crossings are made over the front of the groin instead of on the outer side of the front of the thigh.

Double spica of groin bandage

Lay the outer surface of the bandage over the right groin from without inwards and pass the bandage round the thigh, carrying it up over the front of the right groin to the left hip. Round the back and right hip and over the lower part of the abdomen to the outer side of the thigh. Pass the bandage under the thigh, up to the left groin round the back and right hip and down again to the inner side of the right thigh. Theses turns, which really form of double figure of eight, round left thigh, are repeated until both groins as covered each turn being slightly higher than the covering two-thirds of the preceding one (Fig. 25.29).

Head and other bandage

Capeline bandage

This bandage is, sometimes used when the whole scalp is to be covered. A double headed roller bandage is used. The patient should be seated and the nurse should stand behind the patient.

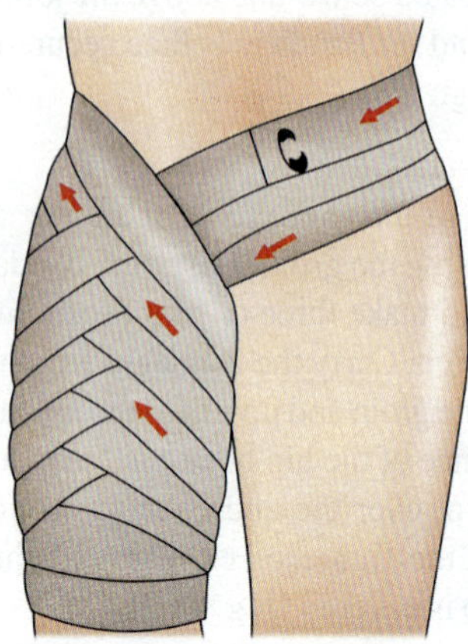

Figure 25.29: Groin bandage

Place the center of the outer surface of the bandage in the center of the forehead, the lower border of the bandage lying just above the eyebrows. The head of the bandage as brought round over the temples and above the ears to the nape of the neck where the ends are crossed. The upper bandage being carried on, round the head and other brought over the center of the top of the scalp to the root of the nose. The bandage which encircles the head is now brought over the forehead, covering and fixing the bandage which could cross the scalp. This bandage is then brought back over the scalp. Slightly to one side of the center, thus covering one margin of the original turn. At the back, it is again crossed and fixed by the opposite side of the center line, now covering the other margin of its original turn. These backward and forward turns are repeated to alternate side of the center, each one being, in turn, fixed by the encircling bandage until the whole scalp is covered. The bandages is completed by a circular turn round the head and pinned in the center of the forehead (Fig. 25.30).

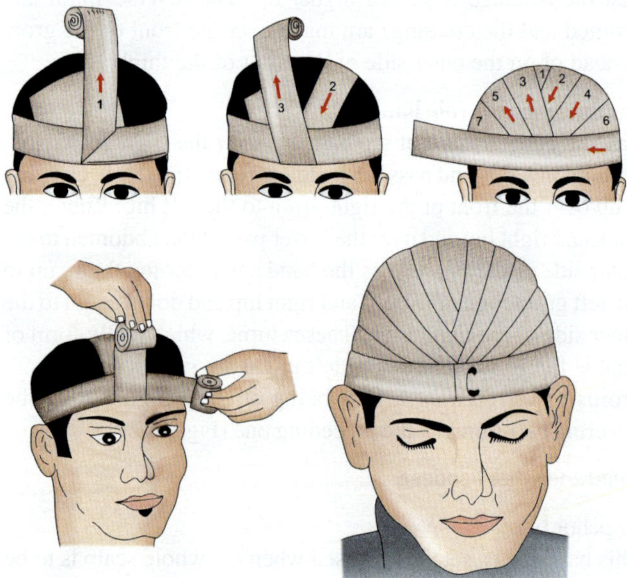

Figure 25.30: Capeline bandages

Ear bandage

Lay the outer surface of the bandage against the forehead and carry the bandage round the head in one circular turn, bandaging away from the injured ear. Towards the sound side, carry the bandage round to the back of the head, low down in the nape of the neck again, repeat these (Fig. 25.31).

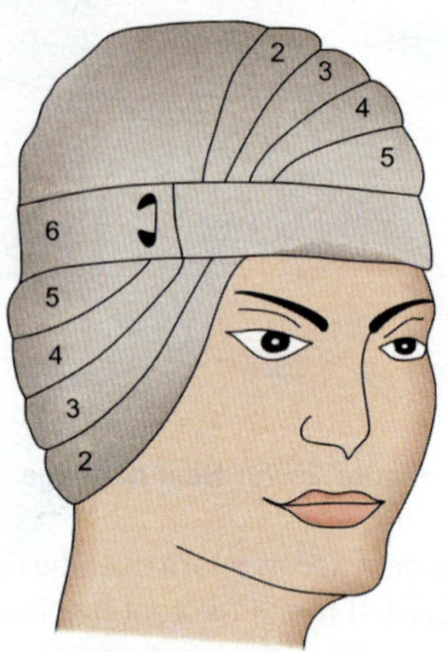

Figure 25.31: Ear bandage

Each turn being slightly higher than the previous one as it cover the dressing, but slightly lower as it covers the hair. Continue until the whole is covered and complete the bandage by one straight turn around the forehead, pinning where all the turns cross one another. Some people prefer to take the bandage round the forehead between each turn covering the dressing, but this makes a heavy bulk around the head which is not really necessary.

Eye bandage

Lay the outer surface of the bandage against the forehead and take the circular turn round the head, bandaging away from the injured eye. Carry the bandage on, round the head until it reaches the ear on the round side for the second time. Take it obliquely to the back of the head, under the prominence at the back of the skull and from there bring it upwards beneath the ear of the affected side, over the pad of the eye to the circular turn and

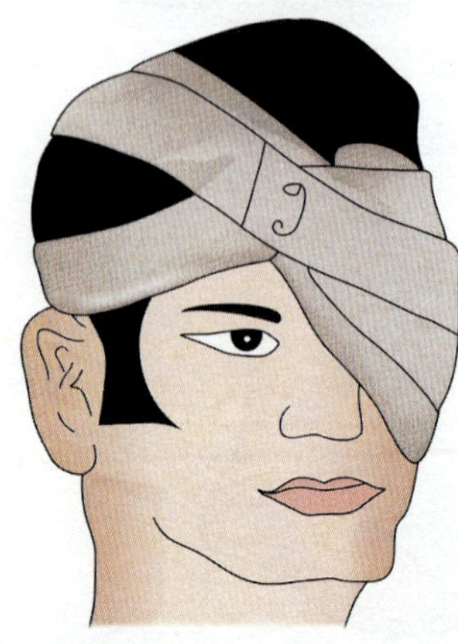

Figure 25.32: Eye bandage

continue over the head to the starting point. Repeat this turn tow or three times until the dressing is covered, finishing with a safety pin just above the good eye. The pattern resembles that of the ear bandage, but there are fewer turns. The bandage should be light in weight and should not obstruct the view of the good eye (Fig. 25.32).

Breast bandages to support one breast
Take a 3 inch bandage and starting below the breast to be covered and working away from it towards the sound side, carry the bandage twice round the waist. Bring the bandage up, under the breast to be supported over the opposite shoulder obliquely down across the back or under the arm and once more round the waist, on covering two-third of the previous turns (Fig. 25.33).

These turns are repeated until the breast is sufficiently covered.

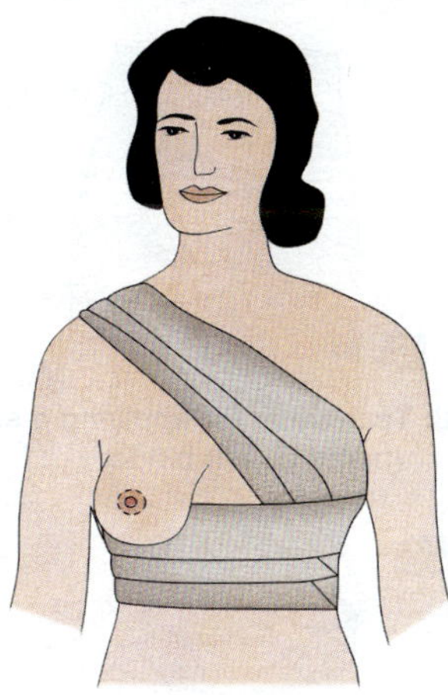

Figure 25.33: Breast bandage to support one breast

To support both breasts
Start with two circular turns round the waist as for the single breast, starting under the right breast and bring the bandage up,

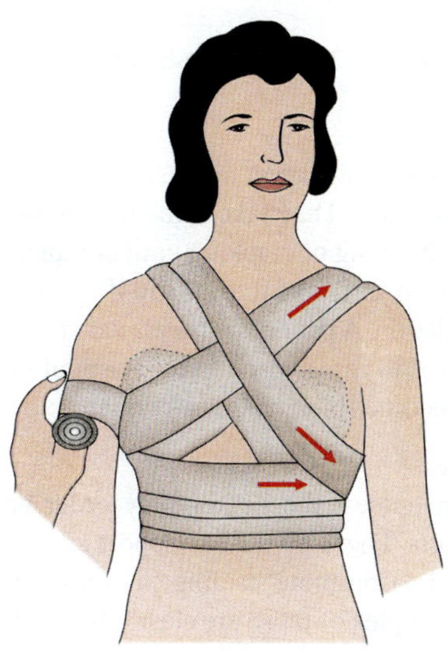

Figure 25.34: Breast bandage to support both breasts

under the right breast, over the left shoulder, obliquely down across the back, under the right arm and across the front of the waist, horizontally. Carry the bandage under the left arm, up across the back to the right shoulder and down across the chest, under the left breast, form here, it is passed under the left arm and turns horizontally across the back to beneath the right breast again. These turns are repeated until both breast are covered (Fig. 25.34).

Stump bandage
Using a 4-inch bandage, place the end of the bandage in the center of the upper side of the limb and carry the bandage, over the center of the stump to the same level behind, holding the turns back and front with the thumb and fingers of the other hand. Repeat the recurrent turns over the end of the stump first and on the stump on the left and on the right side of the original turn until the whole of the dressing is covered. Fix the loops with a straight turn around the stump until the dressing is completely covered and secure it with a safety pin. In an amputation of the leg above the knee, special care in bandaging is necessary to produce stump upon such an artificial limb can be worn on. To do this as soon as the dressing has been removed, a 6 inch crepe bandage should be applied firmly from below upward. The pressure around the stumps is gradually eased as the bandage is carried upwards as high as possible. The object being to produce a conical stump owing to stretching. The bandage may require re-application several times daily and the patient should never be allowed to go about on crutches when such a bandage is worn (Fig. 25.35).

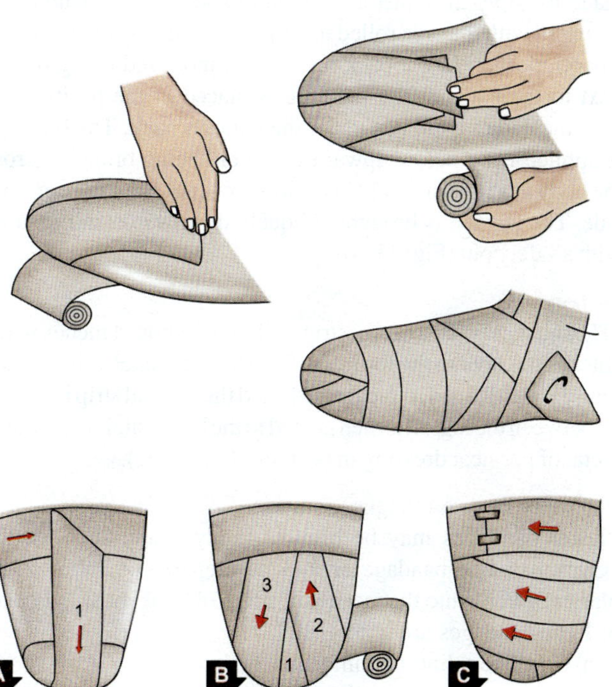

Figure 25.35: Stump bandage

Special Bandages

Many tail bandages

Many tail bandages are used for abdominal wound, certain chest dressing and fro any part where the use of a roller bandage would entail a great amount of movement and exertion for the patient. It consists of a number of strips or tails of flannel domette or cotton material, 4-6 inches wide and of sufficient length to encircle the part and overlap atleast 8 inches. Each strip overlies the one above by two thirds of its width and the whole is secured in the center by a piece of the same material. All seems must be sewen with herring bone and no turning made anywhere, so that, there are no hard ridges to hurt the patient. Bandages for the chest are sometimes provided with two tails, stitched to the top of the back piece and slanting slightly outwards, which pass over the shoulder and are pinned to the front of the bandage when the other tails are folded over to keep the bandage form slipping down. Similarly, abdominal bandages are sometimes provided with two tails stitched to the bottom of back piece and are called groin straps which are passed between the legs and secured to the front of the bandage to prevent it from slipping up. Smaller many tail bandages may sometimes be used to keep a dressing on a limb. The advantages of the many tail bandage are that, it is easily applied and adjusted and a wound can be inspected without any disturbance to the patient. The disadvantages are that, it is given little. If any support it tends to slip and become displaced and can easily be undone by the patient.

The application of an abdominal many tail bandage

For the bandage to be comfortably and efficiently applied, two people are required, although in an emergency one can manage. The patient should be lying quite flat before any attempts is made to apply or adjust a many tail bandage. The bandage is prepared with the tails rolled into the center, from either end, the smooth portion of the back being uppermost and being placed next to the patient. The bandage is placed in the position, so that, the center band lies under the patients back. The bandage is applied from below upwards. One tail being brought across the body at a time and held in position by a tail from the opposite side. The last tail is brought obliquely downwards and secured with a safety pin (Fig. 25.36).

'T' bandages

'T' bandages consist of two strips of flannel, about 4 inches wide, stitches together in the form of a 'T'. The horizontal strip is made long enough to pass round the body and the vertical strip is passed up between the legs. It is then pinned to the horizontal strip to keep rectal of perineal dressing in position (Fig. 25.37).

Plaster of Paris bandages

Plaster bandages may be brought ready-made, such as, the "Gypsona" tape bandage or may be prepared by rubbing dry plaster of Paris into the meshes of strips of book muslin. Plaster of Paris bandages are used,

(a) To make splints to immobilize fractures.
(b) To protect the wound or to immobilize a part to relieve a pain and promote healing.
(c) To make plaster beds and jackets.

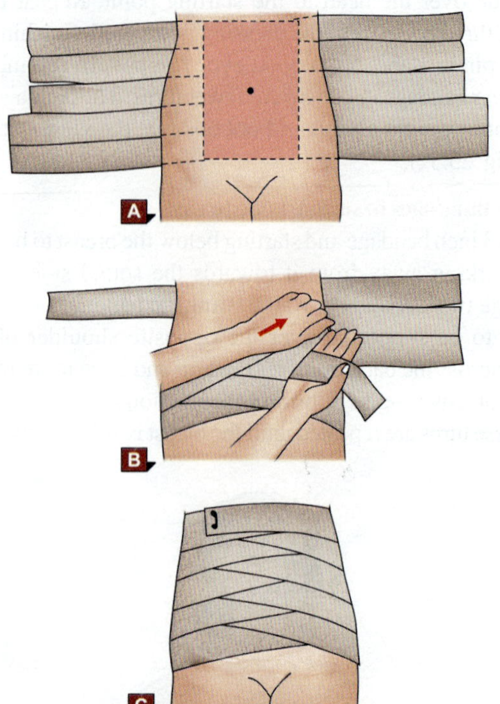

Figure 25.36: Technique for applying a scultetus (many tailed) binder

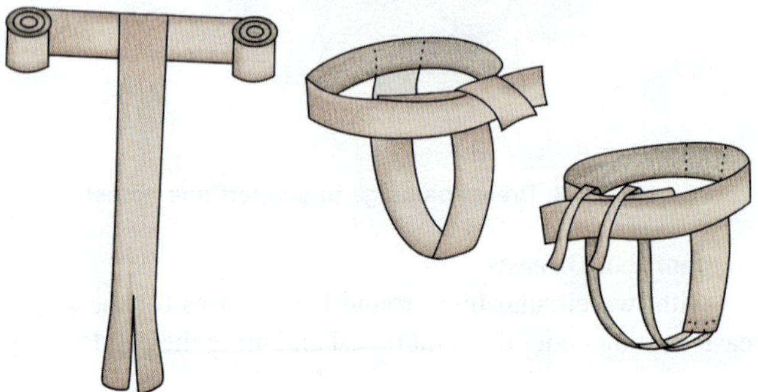

Figure 25.37: 'T' bandages

The bandages are applied wet and as they dry, they form a hard protective covering. They take some time to dry and must be protected from bending or cracking until completely dry and set. A plaster tends to shrink as it dries and if it gets too light, it may impede circulation. A patient with a plaster applied to a limb should be instructed to report back to the hospital immediately if the extremely becomes blue, cold, or swollen.

Adhesive bandage

In certain circumstances, the doctor may order an adhesive bandage to be worn. These give fine support and may be used for protection and to promote healing in condition. Such as, varicose ulcer. Examples of those are elastoplast and viscopaste bandages. These are supplied according to similar rules to those relating to roller bandages. But great care must be taken skin and that, there are no folds or wrinkles in the bandage.

Tabular gauze bandage

This is a special form of tubular bandage, which can be applied with an applicator to any part of the body. It is ideal for small dressing on hands and limbs.

Bandage for the jaw

Take a narrow strip of material, about 4 feet long or a narrow fold triangular bandage and place the center of it, under the chin. Carry one end upwards over the top of the head and cross with the other end above the ear. Carry the shorter end low down across the front of the forehead and the larger end in to opposite direction round the back of the head and tie off close, above the other ear.

Slings

Uses of Slings

(a) To support injured arms
(b) To prevent pull by upper limb of injuries to chest, shoulder and the neck
Different types of slings:

The arm slings

The arm sling is used in cases of fractured ribs, injuries of upper limbs and in cases of fracture in the forearm, wrist and hands after the application of splints or plaster casts and bandaging (Fig. 25.38).

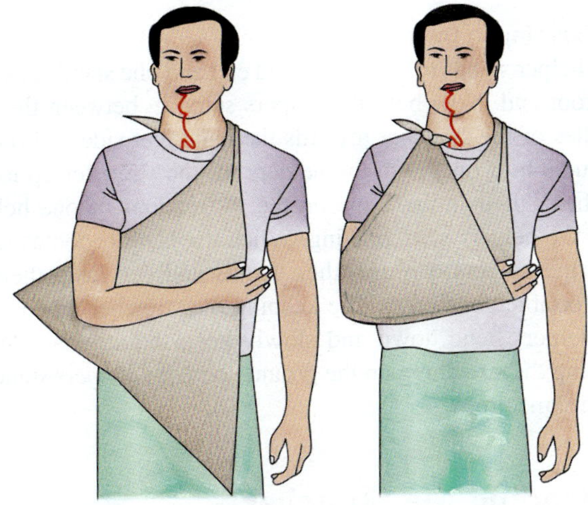

Figure 25.38: Arm sling

Applying the sling

1. Face the casualty, put one end of the spread triangular bandage over the uninjured shoulder with the point on the injured side.
2. Pass the end around the neck and bring it over the injured shoulder. The other end will, now, be hanging down over the chest.
3. Place the forearm horizontally across the chest and bring the hanging end up. The forearm is now covered by the bandage.

4. Tie the two ends in such a way that the forearm is horizontally or slightly tilted upwards and the knot is placed in the pit, above the collar bone.
5. Tuck the part of sling which is loose at the elbow, behind the elbow and bring the fold to the front and pin it up to the front of the bandage.
6. Place the free base of the bandage in such a way that its margin is just at the base of the nail of the little finger. The nails of all the finger should be exposed
7. Inspect the nails to see, if there is any bluish colour. A bluish colour shows that there is a dangerous tightening of splints or plasters and, therefore, free flow of blood is not possible.
8. If the casualty is not wearing a coat, place a soft pad under the neck portion of the sling to prevent rubbing of the skin in that place.

Collar and cuff sling (Fig. 25.39)

This sling is used to support the wrist only.
1. The elbow is bent and the forearm is placed across the chest in such a way that the fingers touch the opposite shoulder. in this position, the sling is applied.
2. A clove hitch is passed round the wrist and the ends tied in the hollow above the collar bone on the injured side.

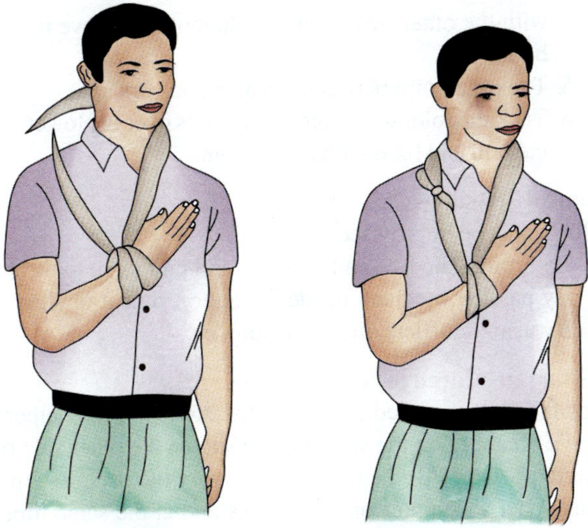

Figure 25.39: Collar and cuff sling

Triangular sling

A triangular sling is used in treating a fracture of the collar bone. It helps to keep the hand raised high up, giving relief from pain due to the fracture (Fig. 25.40).
1. Place the forearm across the chest with the fingers pointing towards the opposite shoulder and the palm over the breast bone.
2. Place an open bandage over the chest, with one end over the hand and the point beyond the elbow.
3. Tuck the base of the bandage comfortably, under the forearm and hand
4. Fold the lower end, also round the elbow and take it up and cross the back over the uninjured shoulder and tie it

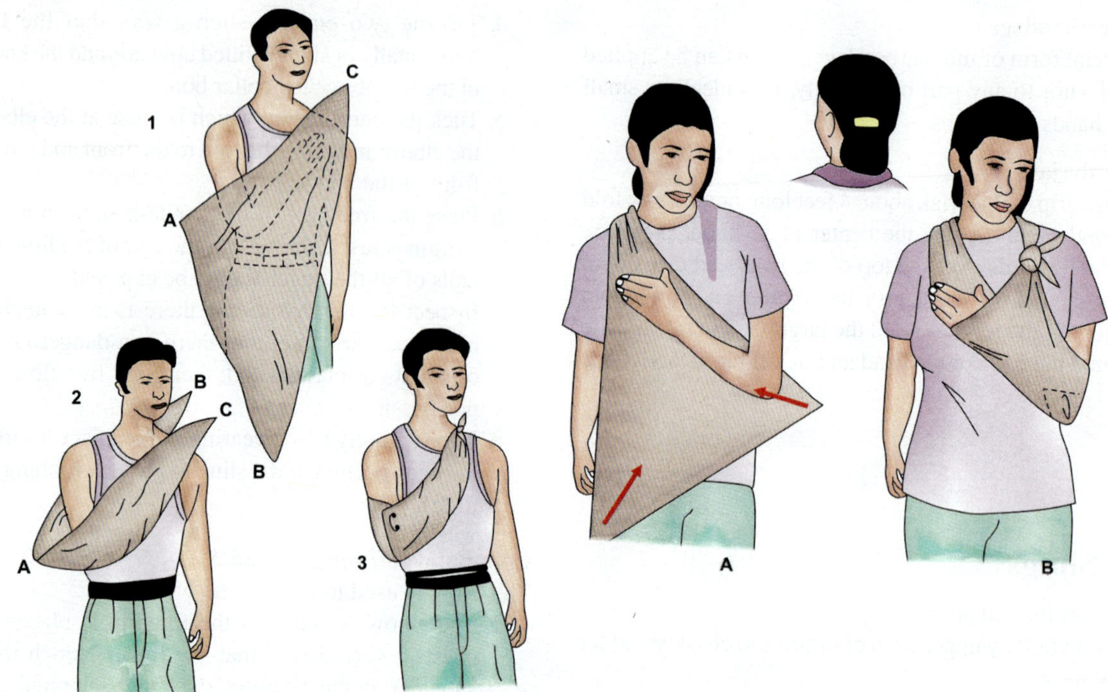

Figure 25.40: Triangular sling

with the other free hand into the hollow, above the collar bone.

5. Tuck the point between forearm and bandage
6. Tuck the fold, so formed, backwards over the lower half of the arm and fix it with a safety pin.

Improvised slings

Slings may be improvised.

1. By turning the free end of a coat and pinning it to the sleeve
2. By passing the hand inside the buttoned coat or shirt
3. By using mufflers, ties, soft cloth, etc.

Lifting an injured person

For lifting the injured person on the stretcher, the helpers lay down on knees on the side and one sits on the other side of the injured person. All the helpers than carry the person with their hands and so support on their knees and at the same time one other helper keeps the stretchers in position at once. Now the helper keeps the person on the stretcher, slowly. The head is supported by blanket or bed sheets. Now, the stretcher is ready for carrying.

Carrying a Loaded Stretcher

1. Carrying by four helpers

On this indication from one helpers lift the stretcher with their inner hand up to the length of their arms. All the four helpers proceed stepping first with their inner legs. These helpers should walk comfortably. If the helpers become tired, then the hand can be kept in comfortable position on the instruction of the other helper. Remember, do not carry the stretcher with the other hand while keeping the stretcher, gradually bending yourselves. On the instruction of one of the helper and all other helpers stand up, at the same time.

2. Carrying by two helpers

One helper stands towards the head end and one stands towards the foot end. Now both the helpers stand in between the two handles of the stretcher towards the hand feet side and on the instruction of one, both the helpers lift the stretcher up to the height of their limbs. Now on the instructions of one helper, both the helpers start walking. When the hand becomes tired, both the helpers can turn their hands and can keep them in comfortable position. While keeping the stretcher down, both the helpers bend down and slowly keep the stretcher. After keeping the stretching on the ground, both the helpers stand up at the same time.

Unloading the Stretcher

The injured person is unloaded form the stretcher after being brought to the hospital or house. The methods applied for the unloading are same as loading patient on the stretcher described earlier. If the injured person is lying in bed sheet or blanket, then he is picked up by the four corners with the help of four persons and is made to lie on the bed, then the sheet is drawn out. If the person is not lying on the blanket, then the helpers sit around the person in all sides, then they rest their hands below the head, waist, chest, hips and legs of the injured person and lift him up from the stretcher.

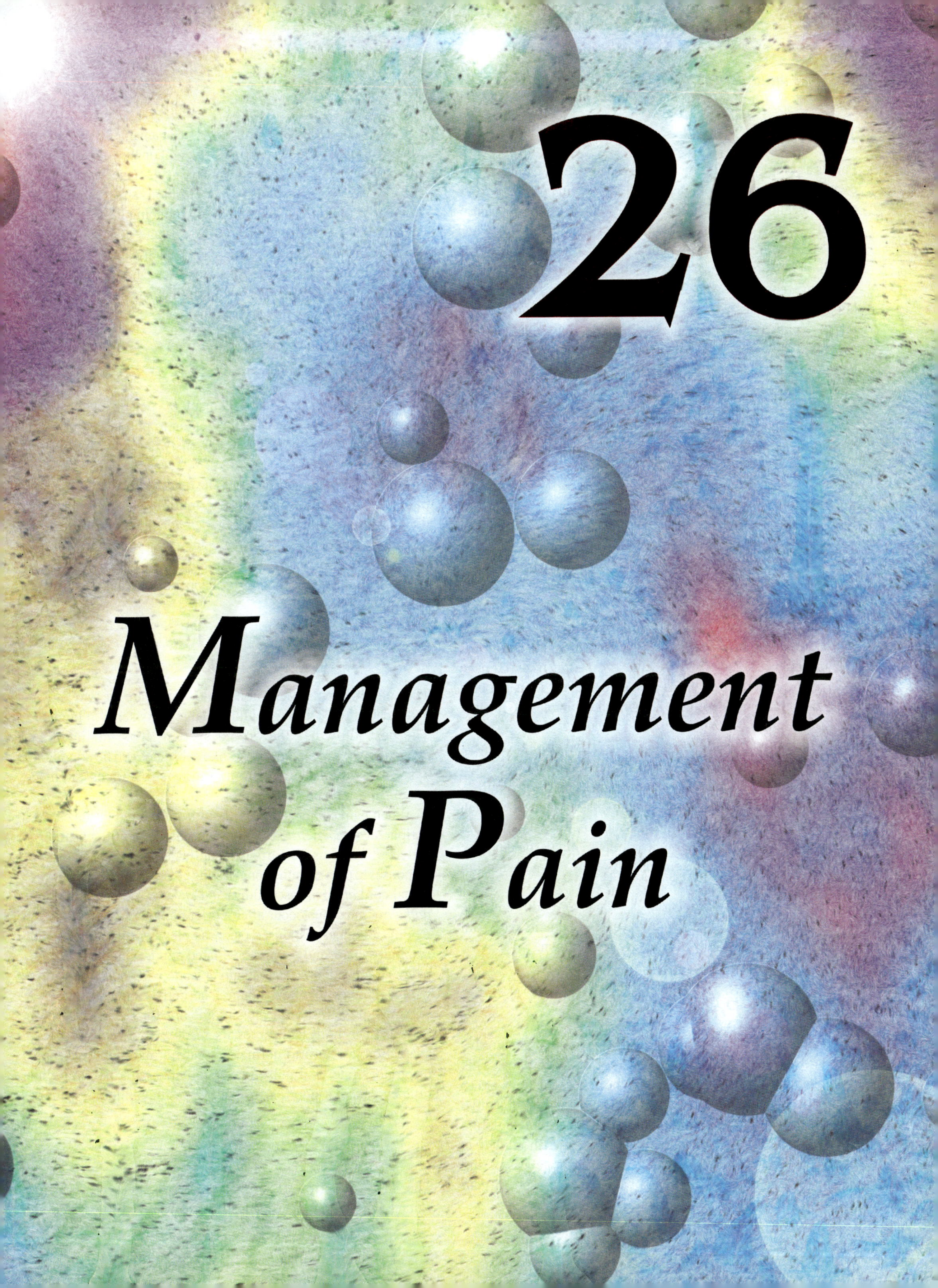

26
Management
of Pain

Introduction

Pain is a complex, multidimensional phenomenon. Everyone has experienced some types or degrees of pain. Pain prompts people to seek healthcare more often than any other problem. Pain is one of the most common problems being faced by nurses when they are dealing with the patients. And also nurses are in an excellent position to work with the client in pain and to help the client overcome the pain. For which nurse has to gain more knowledge about pain and its management. The nurse has a responsibility to understand the experience of pain and to initiate measures that provide relief or help the client learn to cope. Because, the nurse spends more time with the patient in pain than any other healthcare professionals and has the opportunity to help relieve pain and its harmful effects. Some of the definitions enhance the nurse's ability to assess the client who is in pain by focusing on specific aspects of the pain experience.

Definitions of Pain

1. Pain is defined by McCaffery as "whatever the person experiencing the pain says it is, existing whenever the person says it does". It is subjective experience with no objective measurement.
2. The International Association for the Study of Pain (IASP) defined, "pain is an unpleasant sensory and emotional experience associated with actual or potential tissue damage or it is described in terms of such damage". Pain can be a major factor inhibiting the ability and willingness to recover from illness.
3. Mount Castle defined pain as "that sensory experiences evoked by stimuli that injure or threaten to destroy tissue, defined introspectively by every man as that which hurts".
4. Sternbach defined pain as "(i) an abstract concept which refers to a personal, private sensation of hurt; (ii) a harmful stimulus that signals current or impending tissue damage; and (iii) a pattern of responses to protect the organism from harm".

The nursing definition of pain is "whatever bodily hurt, he says it does". The cardinal rule in the care of patients with pain is that all pain is real, even if its cause is unknown.

Nature of Pain

As stated earlier pain is whatever the experiencing person says it is and existing whenever the person says or does. This statement/definition makes the client the expert about his or her own pain. Because clinical pain is subjective and no objective measures of it exists, the only people who can accurately define their own pain are experiencing that pain. Although it is subjective in nature, the nurse charged with accurately assessing and helping to relieve the client's pain. To help a client gain relief, that nurse must believe that the pain exists.

Pain is a protective physiological mechanism. A person with a sprained ankle avoids bearing full weight on the foot to prevent further injury. Pain is a warning that tissue damage has occurred. The client who is unable to feel sensation, such as one with spinal cord tumor, is unaware of pain inducing injuries. Pain is a leading cause of disability. As the average lifespan increase more people have chronic diseases in which pain is a common symptom. Additional medical advances have resulted in diagnostic and therapeutic measures that are uncomfortable. Nurses care daily for clients in pain.

Purpose of Pain

Pain serves as a protective mechanism. If a person touches a hot stove, the pain signal causes the person to pull the hand away immediately. The skin would be seriously burned if this did not happen.

Pain can be a diagnostic tool. The quality and duration of the pain give important dues in determining a client's medical diagnosis. For example, in acute appendicitis, the clinician looks for rebound tenderness (the pain increases when pressure is released) when palpating the abdomen. This particular type of pain helps confirm the diagnosis of appendicitis rather than other gastrointestinal disorders.

Physiology of Pain

The opioid system and the nonopioid system are the two known endogenous (developing within) analgesia systems in humans. The best known is the opioid system. It is mediated by *endorphins* (endogenous opiate-like substances). The nonopioid system is mediated by monoamine substances such as norepinephrine and serotonin.

When pain occurs, sensory input from injured tissue causes peripheral *nociceptors* (receptive neurons for painful sensations) and central nervous system (CNS) pain pathways to enhance future responses to pain stimuli. Long-lasting changes in cells within the spinal cord *afferent* (ascending) and *efferent* (descending) *pain pathways* may thus occur after a brief noxious stimulus.

Physiological responses (such as elevated blood pressure, respiratory rate, and pulse rate; dilated pupils; perspiration; and pallor) to even a brief acute pain episode will show adaptation within minutes to a few hours. The body cannot sustain the extreme stress response physiologically for more than short periods. The body conserves its resources by physiological adaptation: a return to normal or near normal blood pressure, respiratory rate, and pulse rate; pupil size; and dry skin with little evidence of poor perfusion, even with continuing pain of *the same intensity.*

Stimulation of Pain

The specific action of pain depends on the type of pain. Cutaneous pain rapidly travels through a simple reflex arc from the nerve ending (point of pain) to the spinal cord at approximately 300 feet per second, with a reflex response evoking an almost immediate reaction. This is why, when a hot stove is touched, the person's hand jerks back *before* there is conscious awareness of damage (Fig. 26.1). After a hot stove is touched, a sensory nerve ending in the finger skin initiates nerve transmission that travels through the dorsal root ganglion to the dorsal horn in the gray matter of the spinal cord. The impulse then travels though an interneuron that synapses with a motor neuron at the same level in the spinal cord. This motor neuron stimulating the muscle is responsible for the swift movement of the hand away from the hut stove.

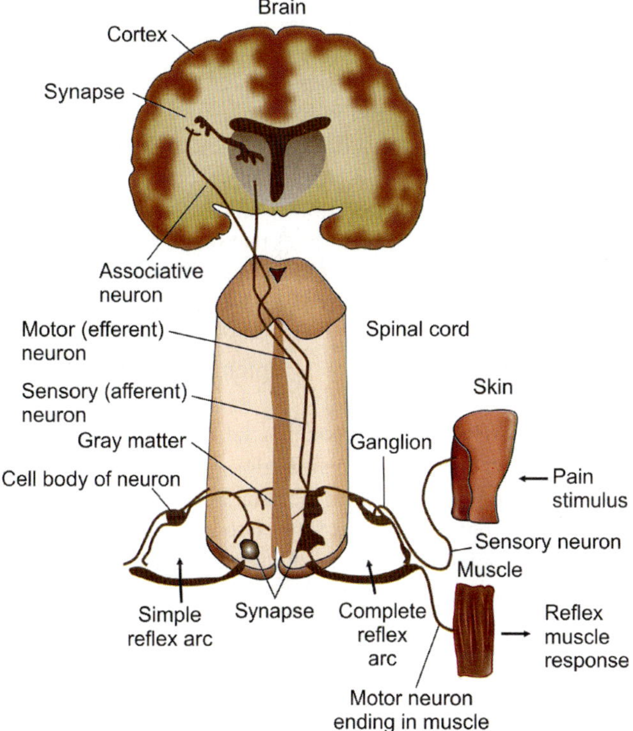

Figure 26.1: Reflex arcs

In the case of the hot stove, the sensory neuron also synapses with an afferent sensory neuron. The impulse travels up the spinal cord to the thalamus, where a synapse sends the impulse to the brain cortex. Once the impulse is interpreted, the information is consciously available. Then the person is aware of the location, intensity, and quality of pain. Previous experience adds the affective feature to the pain experience. Descending or efferent motor neuron response moves from the brain through the spinal cord, synapsing with a motor neuron in the spinal cord, and innervates the muscle.

The transmission of visceral pain impulses is slower and less localized than cutaneous pain. Internal organs (including the gastrointestinal tract) have few nociceptors, which is why visceral pain is poorly localized and is felt as a throbbing sensation or dull ache: however, internal organs are very sensitive to distension. The cramping pain of *colic* (acute abdominal pain) results when:

Constipation or flatus distends the stomach or intestines. There is hyperperistalsis, as in gastroenteritis. Something tries to pass through an opening that is too small.

The physiology of *ischemic pain*, or pain occurring when the blood supply to an area is restricted or cut off completely, also differs. Blood flow restriction causes inadequate oxygenation of the tissue supplied by those vessels and inadequate removal of metabolic wastes. The onset of ischemic pain is most rapid in an active muscle and much slower in a passive muscle. Examples of ischemic pain are muscle cramps, myocardial infarction, angina pectoris, and sickle cell crisis. When ischemic pain occurs in a muscle that continues to work, a muscle spasm (cramp) occurs. If the blood supply to the heart is completely cut off or severely restricted and not restored quickly, a myocardial infarction occurs.

Substances released from injured tissue in acute pain episodes lead to stress hormone responses. There is an increase in metabolic rate, enhanced breakdown of body tissue, increased blood clotting, impaired immune function, and water retention. The light-or-flight reaction is triggered, leading to tachycardia and negative emotions.

The Gate Control Theory: Pain transmission and interpretation theories try to describe and explain the pain experience. Early pain theorists focused on the neuroanatomical and neurophysiological mechanisms.

In 1965, Melzack and Wall proposed the *gate control pain theory*, which was the first one recognizing that psychological aspects of pain are as important as physiological aspects. The gale control theory combined cognitive, sensory, and emotional components–in addition to the physiological aspects–and proposed that they can act on a gate control system to block the individual's perception of pain. The basic premise is that transmission of potentially painful nerve impulses to the cortex is modulated by a spinal cord gating mechanism and by CNS activity. As a result, the level of conscious awareness of painful sensation is altered.

The theory suggests that nerve fibers that contribute to pain transmission converge at a site in the dorsal horn of the spinal cord. This site is thought to act as a gating mechanism that determines which impulses will be blocked and which will be transmitted to the thalamus. The image of a gate is useful in teaching clients and their families about pain relief measures. If the "gate" is closed, the signal is stopped before it reaches the brain, where *perception* (being aware of) of pain occurs. If the gate is open, the signal will continue on through the spinothalamic tract to the cortex, and the client will feel the pain. Whether the gate is opened or closed is influenced by impulses from peripheral nerves (the sensory components) and nerve signals that descend from the brain (motivational-affective and cognitive components). For example, stimulation of some types of peripheral nerves by cutaneous stimulation such as massage can close the gate, whereas stimulation of the nociceptors will open the gate.

If a person is anxious, the gate can be opened by signals sent from the brain down to the mechanism in the dorsal horn of the spinal cord. On the other hand, if the person has had positive experiences with pain control in the past, the cognitive influence can send signals down to the gating mechanism and close it. The gate theory offered a great benefit by suggesting new approaches to relieving both acute and chronic pain. Pain could be relieved by blocking the transmission of pain impulses to the brain by both physical modalities and by altering the individual's thought processes, emotions, or other behaviors.

Conduction of Pain Impulses

Conduction of pain impulses refers to the physiologic processes that occur from the initiation of the pain signal to the realization of pain by the individual. Four processes are involved in the conduction of this signed. The first, *transduction*, is when a noxious stimulus triggers electrical activity in the endings or afferent nerve fibers (nociceptors). Once the signal is triggered, *transmission* occurs. The impulse travels from the receiving nociceptors to the spinal cord. Projection neurons then carry the message continues to the somatusensory cortex. Then the third step, perception of pain, occurs. Here neural messages are converted into the subjective experience. The fourth process, *modulation*, is a CNS pathway that selectively inhibits pain transmission by sending blocking signals back down to the dorsal horn of the spinal cord (Fig. 26.2).

The client is the only authority about the existence and nature of his or her pain. Age, previous experience with pain, drug abuse, and cultural norms account for the differences in clients' individual responses to pain.

Age can greatly influence clients' perception of pain. They may continue pain behaviors learned as children and may be reluctant to admit pain or seek medical care because they fear the unknown or fear how treatment may impact their lifestyle. Older adults may ignore their pain, believing it is a consequence of aging. Family and health care members may thoughtlessly support this idea and be less responsive to an older client's complaints of pain.

Previous experience with pain often influences clients' reactions. Past coping mechanisms may affect clients' judgments about how pain will affect their lives and which measures they can use to successfully manage the pain on their own. Teaching clients about pain expectations and management methods can often allay their fears and lead to successful pain management.

A drug abuser is likely to be *less* tolerant of pain than someone who does not use drugs. Drug abuse may cause changes in the central nervous system, resulting in an exaggerated neuro-physiologic response to painful stimuli. To keep a drug abuser comfortable, withdrawal must be prevented.

Cultural Norms

Cultural differences in pain responses can lead to pain management problems. Studies on subjects of various cultures found no significant difference among the groups in the intensity level at which pain becomes perceptible. The same studies showed that the intensity level or duration of pain the client was willing to endure differed significantly. Cultural values guide the expression of pain. Some cultures tolerate pain and "suffering in silence," whereas others fully express pain, including physical and emotional responses. Be careful not to equate the level of pain expression with the level of actual pain experienced, but consider cultural and other influences that affect the expression of pain.

Pain management standards were included as given below. The health care organizations arc expected to:

- Recognize the right or patients to appropriate assessment and management of pain.
- Assess the existence and, if so, the nature and intensity or pain in all patients.
- Record the results of the assessment in a way that facilitates regular reassessment and follow-up.
- Determine and assure staff competency in pain assessment and management and address pain assessment and management in the orientation of all new staff.
- Establish policies and procedures that support the appropriate prescription or ordering or effective pain medications.
- Educate patients and their families about effective pain management.
- Address patient needs for symptom management in the discharge planning process.

Pain consists of five components, i.e. affective, behavioral, cognitive, sensory, and physiologic. Affective component includes the emotions related to the pain. Behavioral components includes the behavioral responses to the pain. Cognitive components include the beliefs, attitudes, evaluation and goals about the pain, and sensor components include the control how pain is perceived by altering transmission of nociceptive stimuli to the brain, that is, physiologic components of pain. These components are also called as dimensions of pain which help in assessment and management of pain. Pain results from complex interactions among these dimensions and can be understood by considering first the physiologic and thereafter the sensory, affective, behavioral and cognitive dimensions.

Pain Process

Pain is a complex phenomenon. It is a mixture of physical, emotional and behavioral reactions. One way to gain the understanding of the pain experience is to conceptualize pain as a process made up of three physiological steps, i.e. reception, perception and reaction. Examining these steps of the process helps the nurse better understand the pain experience and better treat the client in pain.

Reception of Pain

Reception components involves three major steps: Transduction, transmission and modulation.

Pain Transduction

The strain of events that leads to pain begins where pain fibers are excited by a variety of stimuli. The stimuli consist of mechanical events such as stretching of organs or pressures, extremes of temperature, i.e., heat or cold, and chemical changes such as ischemia. Specific fibers that react to these stimuli are classified as mechanical, thermal or chemical nociceptors. Fast pain is usually elicited by mechanical and thermal type of receptors (A-delta fibers) whereas slow pain can be elicited by all receptors (C-fibers). Together these fibers referred to as primary afferent nociceptors–PAN fibers.

Fast pain: It is the pain that occurs in about 0.1 second when painful stimuli are applied. It is often referred to as sharp, prickling, acute or electric pain. It is transmitted through a A–delta fibers. Fast pain is mostly caused by a more superficial stimulus.

Slow pain: It is pain that begins one second or more after stimulation and increases slowly over seconds or minutes. This pain is also known as burning, aching, throbbing or chronic pain. It is often associated with tissue distraction and is felt in both superficial and deep tissues. It is transmitted through the more primitive type of fibers. A wide variety of chemical substances, including bradykinin, serotinin, histamine, substances of potassium, iron, acids, proteolytic enzymes, prostaglandins, and acetylcholine are significant in slow pain that often follows tissue injury.

Pain Transmission

Once the PAN (primary afferent nociceptors) are stimulated, the impulse they discharge travel as electrical activity to the spinal cord and on to the brain. This electrical activity becomes the experience of pain when it is reached the brain. There will

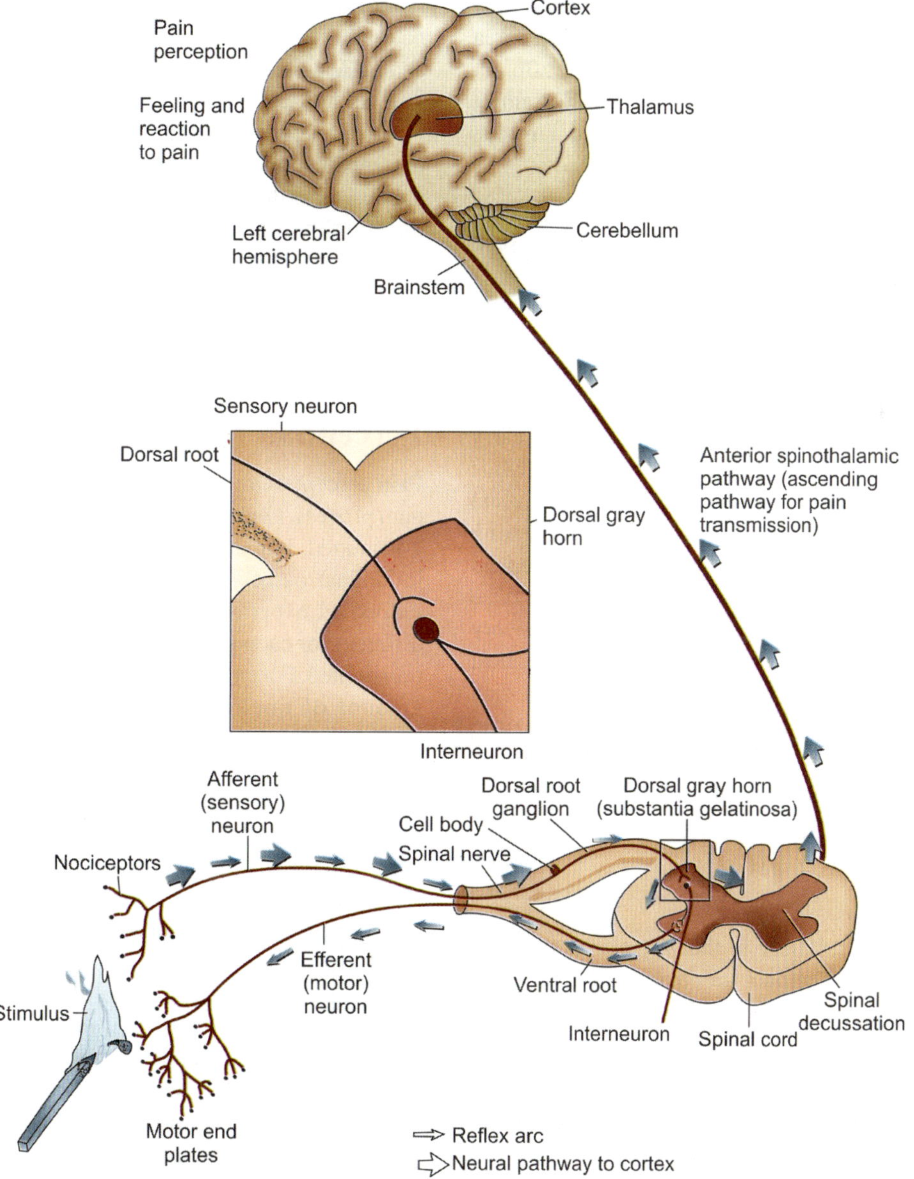

Figure 26.2: The nociceptive pathway and pain modulation

be no experience of pain, when/if the neural pathway for these impulses is blocked by surgical cutting or medications which inhibit the activity of pathways fibers or natural methods (endogenous) that block portion/the pain pathways (Fig. 26.2).

Nerve fibers that carry somatosensory information from the body periphery to the spinal cord include A beta, A delta, and C fibers. A-type fibers have a myelin sheath that speeds up information transmission. A-delta fibers transmit pain stimuli, A-beta fibers are larger and carry other sensory information such as touch. C-fibers transmit pain stimuli more slowly because they have no myelin sheath. C-fibers also conduct thermal, chemical and strong mechanical impulses. Pain sensation following stimulation of A-delta fibers differs from that following C-fiber stimulation. A-delta fiber activity is felt more slowly after painful stimulation but the sensation is more constant and continuous. It is persistent, dull and acting and is difficult to localize. These different fibers enter the dorsal root of the spinal cord, which transmits the pain impulses. The fibers separate as they enter the cord and then reform in the dorsal horn. This area receives, transmits and processes sensory impulses. The afferent nociceptors end at the level of the first, second and fifth laminae. The substation gelatinosa is found in the second laminae hypothezed to be gating mechanism (Gate control theory).

Gate control theory: A pain proposed by Melzack and Wall (1965) suggests that pain impulse can be regulated or even blocked by gating mechanisms along with central nervous system. The proposed location of the gates is in the dorsal horn of the spinal cord. Further findings suggested other gates exist (Melzact, Denis 1978). When gates are open, pain impulses flow freely. When gates are closed, pain impulses become blocked. Partial opening of the gates may also occur. Small fibers carry most potentially painful impulses. Excitation of C-fibers inhibits gating mechanisms so that pain stimuli flow easily to cortical controls of brain. Large A-fibers pass through the same gating mechanisms. Whether the gates remain open or closed depend on whether competing passages from larger nerve fibers stimulate the gating mechanism. A bombardment of a large fiber sensory imp uses such as those from the pressure of the back sub or heat of a warm compress closes the gates to pain stimuli. Transmission of pain impulses from the spinal cord to the cerebral cortex can be inhibited or facilitated thus altering perception. This gate control theory gives the nurse a conceptual basis for pain relief measures to some extent.

Pain Modulation

There is a great deal of variations in the way clients perceive similar to painful stimuli. The pain modulation system is one reason, thus occurrence of variance. There are variety of mechanisms that contributes modulation as follows.

Modulation via the dorsal horn: The dorsal horn was once considered a simple relay for impulses, but is now known to contain extremely complex circulatory and multiple biochemical agents that both transmit and modulate nociceptive input. The dorsal horn is now thought to modulate the nociceptive impulses rather than simply receive and transmit these impulses. A high degree of processing of the sensory impulses occurs at this level.

Modulation via descending pathways: The descending serotoninergic inhibitory fibers originate in the peraquaductual gray matter (PAG) of the midbrain and descend downward into the nuclear raphe magnus. Neurons from the P AG project downward to the dorsal horn at the first and fifty lamae levels. The neurotransmitters serotonin and substance P are released into these areas, contributing modulation of pain.

Modulation via endogenous chemicals: Some chemical compounds released by injury or inflammation stimulate nociceptors, for example, histamine, bradykinin, serotonin, substance P and prostaglandin E. Pain may be reduced by medication that block these agents such as steroids, aspirin and other nonsteroidal anti-inflammatory drugs (NSAIDs) that reduce inflammation and block prostaglandins. There is also a naturally occurring system within the nervous system called the" analgesia systems".

This analgesia system described by Guyton and Hall has three parts: (i) neurons from the periadaductal gray area of the mesencephalon and upper pons surrounding the adequate of sylvius send their signals to (ii) the raphe magnus nucleus, a thin midline nucleous located in the lower pons and upper medulla. Where the signals are sent down the dorsolateral columns in the spinal cord to (iii) a pain inhibitory complex located in the dorsal horns of the spinal cord. At this point in the system, pain can be blocked.

Perception of Pain

Pain perception refers to interpretation of the next phase of the pain process. Once the nociceptive input has been received and transmitted, it must be perceived or interpreted. Because every individual perceives and interprets pain based on his or her individual experience, this one point at which pain becomes different for each person. Pain modulation occurs as it is being transmitted. For example other sensory input will help reduce the amount of nociceptive information that is transmitting supraspinally.

Pain perception does not depend solely on the degree of physical damage. It is generally agreed both physical stimuli and psychosocial factors influence a person's experience of pain. Although there is little consensus on the specific effects of these factors, it is known that anxiety, experience, attention, expectation and measuring of the situation in which injury occurs affect pain perception. Brain activities such as distraction or anxiety may also affect the severity and quality of the pain experience.

In the past, pain was viewed as a primary sensation and motivational and cognitive processes were believed to influence only our reaction to pain, it now seems apparent that there are mechanisms within the body that can modify pain-related neural impulses even before they are transmitted to the brain. Thus, pain is likely to be determined by a relative balance between the sensory peripheral input and mechanisms of central control (brain) input to gating mechanisms in the spinal cord.

The first point the nurse needs to consider is the client's pain threshold. This is defined as the lowest intensity of a painful stimulus that is perceived by the client as pain. The pain threshold may vary based on physiologic factors such as inflammation or injury near pain receptors, but essentially it is similar for all people if the central and peripheral nervous system are intact. The second part of pain pertains to the individual's tolerance of pain. Tolerance is different for each person who experiences pain. This may vary within each person based on many subjective factors, such as meaning of pain and the setting. It really refers to the amount of pain the client willing to endure. Some individuals have high tolerance, they can tolerate any extend of pain without distress, whereas others have a very low tolerance. This tolerance will also vary for a given individual depending on a variety of factors that influence pain such as nausea, fatigue and other sensory input. Only the client not the healthcare team can tell the tolerance level. The nurse must remember that pain tolerance can vary from situation to situation or from event to event.

Another aspect that will alter a person's perception of pain is his or her experience with pain. This may be the reason that people incorrectly assume that infants do not have pain. When infants feels pain, it is simply that the infant has no experience with pain and therefore, is unable to interpret it, and cannot communicate what is being felt. The reverse is also true. When a person has a bad experience with pain, the anticipation that future pain may be bad can make any work. There is also a physiologic reason if the pain is in the same area, that is persons with recurrent low back pain actually have a lower pain threshold and that area than persons who have not had low back pain.

Reaction to Pain

The reaction to pain is the physiological and behavioral responses that occur after pain is perceived. In physiological responses; as pain impulses ascend the spinal cord toward the brain system and thalamus, the automatic nervous system becomes stimulated as part of the stress response. Pain of low to moderate intensity and superficial pain elicits the flight or flight reaction of the general adaptation syndrome. Stimulation of the sympathetic branch of the autonomic nervous system results in physiological responses. If the pain is unrelenting, reverse or deep, typically originating from involvement of the visceral organs (such as with myocardial infarction, and colic from gallbladder or renal stones). The parasympathetic nervous system goes into action. Sustained physiological responses to pain could cause serious harm to an individual. Except in case of severe traumatic pain, which may send a person into shock, most people reach a level of adaptation in which physical signs return to normal. Thus, a client in pain will not always exhibit physical signs.

The behavioral responses of pain may be described in three phases of a pain experience which include anticipation, sensation and aftermath (Mein Hart and McCaffery 1983). Usually anticipation phases occur before pain received except some unforeseen painful situations. Anticipation of pain often allows a person to learn about pain and its relief. With adequate instruction and support, client learns to understand pain and control anxiety before it occurs. Nurses play an important role in helping clients during the anticipatory phases with proper guidance, which help clients make aware of unknown and they cope with their discomfort. Sensations of pain occurs when pain is felt. The ways that people choose to react to discomfort vary widely. A person's tolerance of pain is the point at which there is an unwillingness to accept pain of greater severity, or duration. The extent to which a person tolerates pain depends on attitudes, motivation and value. Pain threatens physical and psychological wellbeing. Typical body movements and facial expressions that indicate pain include holding the painful part, bent posture and grimaces. A client may cry moan. Often the client expresses discomfort through restlessness and frequent requests to the nurse. The nurse soon learns to recognize patterns of behavior that reflect pain. Aftermath phase of pain occurs when it is reduced or stopped. Even though the source of discomfort is controlled, a client may still require the nurse's attention. Pain is a crisis. After painful experience client may experience physical symptoms such as chills, nausea, vomiting, anger or depression. If there are repeat episodes of pain, aftermath responses can become serious health problems. The nurse helps clients gain control and self-esteem to minimize fear over potential pain experience.

The individual reaction to pain adds even more variation to the pain process. There are many variable factors in this part of the process, including situation, culture, age, sex, cause of pain, tolerance, value and meaning of pain and various psychological factors such as fear, anxiety and depression.

Factors Influencing Pain

Situation

The situation associated with the pain influence the person's response to it. A person's responses to pain experienced in a formal crowded situations may differ greatly from the responses were he or she alone or in a hospital.

Culture

Culture influences how people learn to react to expressing pain. People respond to pain in different ways. The nurse must never assume to know how clients will respond. However, an understanding of cultural background, socioeconomic status, and personal attitudes help the nurse more accurately assess pain and its meaning for clients. A young girl in a stoic culture may be allowed to cry because of pain whereas boys are not allowed to cry in some cultures.

Age

Age is an important variable that influences pain, particularly in children and older adults. Age may release a client from culturally imposed norms in relation to pain expression. Developmental differences found among these age groups can influence how children and older react to the pain experience. Young children have difficulty in understanding pain and the procedures nurses administer that may cause pain. Young children who have not developed vocabularies also have difficulty verbally describing an expressing pain to parents/caregivers. Cognitively toddlers are unable to recall explanations about pain or associate pain as experiences that can occur in various situation. Older people may assign different meanings to that pain. Pain is often thought by the elderly as natural manifestation of aging.

Sex

Gender may be an important influence in pain. In most cultures boys are expected to show less expression of pain than girls. As they grow older men are also expected to express less pain than women.

Meaning of Pain

The meaning of a person's pain is a factor that influences his or her responses to pain. A person will perceive pain differently if it suggests a threat, loss, punishment, or challenges. For example a woman in labor perceives pain differently from women expressing pain from a recent back injury or pain caused by childbirth may be responded differently from pain caused by surgery. If the cause is unknown, more negative psychological factors use such as fear, anxiety, etc. come into play and the pain may be misinterpreted resulting in an inappropriate response. A client copes differently with pain, depending on its meaning.

Anxiety

The degree of anxiety the client is experiencing also may influence the client's response to pain. It is not possible to separate the mind from the body, so pain is always has both physiologic and psychological components. When anxiety is high pain is felt greater. Emotionally healthy persons are usually able to tolerate moderate or even severe pain than those whole emotions are less stable.

Fatigue

Fatigue heightens perceptions of pain. This intensifies pain and decreases coping abilities. Pain is often experienced less after a restful sleep than at the end of a long day.

Attention

The degree at which a client focuses on pain can influence pain perception. Increased attention has been associated with increased pain, whereas distraction has been associated with a diminished pain response. This concept is one that nurses apply in various pain relief measures such as relaxation, guided emergency and massage.

Previous Experience

Each person learns from painful experiences. Previous experience does not necessarily mean that a person will accept pain more easily in the future. If a person has had frequent episodes of pain without relief or bouts of severe pain, anxiety or even fear may occur. In contrast if a person had repeated experience of pain, may be better prepared to tolerate or take necessary actions to relieve pain to some extent.

Coping Style

The experience of pain can be lonely, when client experiences pain in healthcare setting such as hospitals, the loneliness can be unbearable. Frequently client feels a loss of central pain and an inability to control their environments or the outcome of events coping style thus influences the ability to deal with pain.

Family and Social Support

Parents and attitudes of significant others also affect pain response. People in pain often depend on family members for support, assistance or protection. An absence of family members or friends can often make the pain more stressful. For children presence of parents is very essential.

Types of Pain

There are different ways to define types of pain, which include according to onset, duration, severity, modes of transmission, location, causation and causative force. The examples of which are as follows:

- Onset or time of occurrence, e.g. postoperative pain
- Duration, e.g. chronic pain or acute pain
- Severity or intensity, e.g. severe, mild or scored (0 to 10 on a scale)
- Location or source, e.g. superficial, deep or central pain
- Causation, e.g. pain due to receptor stimulation or nerve damage, or psychophysiologic pain
- Causative force or agent, e.g. spontaneous, self inflicted or other pain

  The common terms used to classify pain are as follows.

Acute Pain

Acute pain is usually of recent onset and is most commonly associated with a specific injury. It is time limited and generally has a defined cause and purpose. It may be mild, moderate or severe in nature and is usually sudden in onset. It occurs abruptly after an injury or disease, persists until healing occurs, and often intensified by anxiety or fear. Acute pain consistently increases during wound care, ambulation, coughing and deep breathing. It is described in sensory terms such as sharp, stabbing and shooting. Acute pain indicates that damage or injury has occurred. It draws the attention to the fact that it is occurring and teaches us to avoid similar potentially painful situation. So acute pain is seen as a useful and limiting pain in that indicates injury and motivates the person to get relief by treatment of the pain and usually the cause. Acute pain is usually reversible or controllable with adequate treatment. If no lasting damage occurs or systematic disease exists, acute pain usually decreases as healing occurs; this generally occurs in less than six months and usually less than one month. Acute pain can be described as lasting from a few seconds to 6 months, e.g. prick of finger in a second and fracture for 6 months.

Usually the acute pain leads to discomfort, uncomfortable and disturbs the individual in many aspects according to the nature and extent of pain. An unrelieved acute pain can affect the pulmonary, cardiovascular, gastrointestinal, endocrine and immunologic system. It leads to autonomic response that is considered with sympathetic stress response. The significant negative effects are increased heart rate, increased stroke volume, increased blood pressure, increased papillary dilation, increased muscle tension, decreased gastrointestinal motility, decreased salivary flow (dry mouth). The stress response may increase the patient risk for physiologic disorder (MI, pulmonary infection, thromboembolism, prolonged panalyticileus) and the psychologic disorders which include anxiety and persists. If acute pain is not effectively managed, it may progress to a chronic pain.

Chronic Pain

Chronic pain is a complex physiological and psychological phenomenon that causes varying degrees of disability in a large portion of the population. Chronic pain is constant or intermittent in nature that persists over a period of time. It lasts beyond the expected time and often cannot be attributed to a specific cause or injury. Chronic pain is often defined as pain that lasts for six months or larger. It may begin as acute pain but it persists over an extended period of time. The pain may be mild, moderate or severe and may be intermittent or continuous.

Chronic pain is classified as malignant or nonmalignant.

Nonmalignant Pain

Chronic pain is usually considered pain that lasts more than six months or one month beyond the normal end of the condition causing pain and has no forserable and except very slow healing, as with bums, or death. It is continuous or persistent and recurrent. Chronic pain may have an identifiable cause although the cause may be difficult to determine; and is often described using effective terms, such as 'hateful' or 'sickening' and is often much more difficulty to treat than acute pain. It is considered useless pain because it is not usually a manifestation of impending damage. For example, severe rheumatic arthritic chronic pain is often frustrating and difficult for a person to live with. It gives no clues about how to lessen it. Clients experiencing continuous and continually recurring chronic pain often become increasingly engrossed by their illness. They may seem fearful, tense, fatigued and depressed. Many persons with an unending chronic pain become withdrawn and isolated. Their pain often exhausts them and their families physically and emotionally.

Malignant Pain

Malignant pain is considered to have qualities of both acute and chronic pain. It can be of different types. An individual mental response to pain depends on the duration and possibility and the intensity of the pain. Pain that is constant, continuous and moderate is often described by the client (patient as far more difficult to bear that pain than paraxysmal and intense). The duration of chronic pain includes months and years of pain, not minutes or hours. It is associated with withdrawal and despaired. Anxiety may give way to depression. Some chronic pain patients/clients learn to adapt and cope with the pain, adjusting their lives.

The sympathetic arousal that may be associated with acute pain diminishes over weeks or months even though the pain itself persists. Sympathetic adaptation occurs over time. The nurse must remember, however, that the absence of expected expression of severe pain does not mean that the pain is gone. The nurse must depend on the client's description, not the manifestation are expected to find in the clients. Most clients have major effective and behavioral changes when experiencing pain for prolonged period. Such changes may be compounded and chronic pain syndrome can develop. The following are the characteristics of chronic pain syndrome:

- Depressed mood
- Increased or decreased appetite and weight, decreased libido capacity, poor physical tone and increased depression
- Social withdrawal–withdrawal from outside interests and relationship
- Preoccupation with physical manifestation
- Poor sleep and chronic fatigue, leads to inactivity, analgesics, depression

For example, in cases of cancer pain, arthritis, trigeminal neuralgia, etc. some clients with chronic pain may not exhibit any of the above mentioned manifestations or they may exhibit only a few. However, once these changes take place, they may become more significant to treatment than the pain's original physical source. Unfortunately, psychosocial implications about pain sometimes reinforce the idea that clients may make too much fuse over that pain.

Superficial Pain

Superficial pain occurs when the receptors in surface tissues are stimulated. Superficial or cutaneous pain is classified into two types:

(i) Pain with an abrupt onset and a sharp or stinging quality, and

(ii) Pain with a slower onset and burning quality.

Superficial pain may be delineated by having the client point to the painful area. It may occur along each segment representing a portion of the body surface innervated by one dorsal root, a dermatome or skin segment in an area of skin supplied by one dorsal root. Each spinal nerve has dorsal and sensory root. The boundaries of dermatome may appear to be distinct in anatomic drawings, but nerve distribution actually overlaps. Irritation of one posterior root produces pain in adjacent dermatomes. A spinal nerve attaches the spinal cord with two roots anterior and posterior. The anterior root contains efferent nerve fibers that carry impulses from the CNS to the periphery of the body. The posterior root contains afferent nerve fibers that carry impulses from the body's periphery towards CNS. Cutaneous pain is relatively uncomplicated because it is readily localized, that is, which client can indicate exactly where it hurts.

Deep Pain

Deep pain arises from deeper tissues. Deep pain is divided automatically into splanchnic which refers to pain in the viscera and deep somatic referring to pain in deep structures other than the viscera, such as muscle, tendons, joints and periosteum.

Splanchnic Pain

Viscera refers to abdominal viscera. Actually, a viscus (plural viscera) in any of the large interior body organs occupies any body cavity such as the cranial, thoracic, abdominal or pelvic cavities. Visceral pain tends to be diffuse, poorly localized, vague, dull pain. Nerve fibers innervating body organs follow the sympathetic nerves to the spinal cord. This may be the reason why autonomic manifestations (e.g. diarrhhea, cramps, sweating, hypertension) frequently accompany visceral pain. Typical visceral pain includes acute appendicitis, cholecystitis, inflammation of the biliary and pancreatic tract, gastroduodenal disease, cardiovascular disease, pleurisy and renal and ureteral colic. Visceral pain is transmitted through the sympathetic and parasympathetic fibers of autonomous nervous system, with the pain being referred to the body surface, often in sites at a distance. Visceral pain also may be sent through the nerve fibers in the parictal pleura, pericardium, or peritoneum and is called parictal pain. Parictal pain is transmitted directly to the spinal nerves, with the pain being felt directly over the painful area. Parictal tissue is well supplied with spinal nerve instead of sympathetic nerves. Pain starting in the parictal tissue is often very sharp.

Deep Somatic Pain

Somatic structures are those of the body wall, such as muscles and bones. Pain in the somatic structures is complicated phenomenon. The main difference between superficial pain and deep pain is difference between cutaneous and deep sensitivity (i.e. the capacity to receive stimulus and respond to them is the difference in nature) of the pain evoked by noxious or harmful stimuli. For example, unlike cutaneous pain, deep pain is poorly localised, may produce nausea, and is frequently associated with sweating and changes in the blood pressure. Deep somatic pain

is generally diffuse, less localizable than cutaneous pain. This is because the area supplied by one posterior nerve root (sclerotome) is less well defined than in dermatome and does not correspond with a dermal segment. Also pain from deep structures frequently radiates/spreads from primary site, e.g. pain from lumber disc is felt along the sciatic nerve.

Somatic structures vary in their sensitivity to pain. Highly sensitive structures include tendons, deep fascia, ligaments, joints, bone periosteum, blood vessels and nerve. Skeletal muscle is sensitive only in stretching and ischemia. Bone and cartilage respond to extreme pressure and chemical stimulation, for example, Rh arthritis, osteomyelitis.

Localised Pain

Localised pain arises directly from the site of the disturbance.

Referred Pain

Referred pain is one which is felt in a part of the body which is remote from the actual point of stimulation. The impulses usually arise in an organ, but the pain is projected to a surface area of the body. Both visceral and somatic pains are usually referred to as segment of skin because visceral fibrosynapse at the level of the spinal cord close to fibers innervating some subcutaneous tissue. A classical example of referred pain is that associated with 'angina pectoris', the pain originates in the heart muscle as a result of ischemia, but it may be experienced in the midsternal region, the base of the neck and down the left arm. Similarly in myocardial infarction, pain is not felt in the heart, but it is felt at left arm shoulder or jaw pain. It may be due to the fibers innervating these areas are close to those innervating the myocardium resulting in the referred pain. Similarity in pain of appendicitis is often reported by the patient as being in the midline of the abdomen, above the umbilicus whilst the appendix is usually located deep in the abdomen, close by the appendix, on the right side.

Identification of the segment of the spinal cord that is involved, is transmitting referred pain is diagnostically helpful. Pain arising from a deep structure, whether a deep somatic structure or a viscus, has a referred segmental distribution, or a pattern of pain, determined according to the spinal cord segment supplying to this structure.

Intractable Pain

Persistent, severe pain that cannot be effectively controlled by the usual medication is referred to as "intractable pain". Intractable chronic pain states, producing prolonged and intense bombardment of the central nervous system, are very difficult to bear. The client may become suicidal or at least take no steps to prolong life.

Headache

Headache is the most common type of pain, frequently discomfort experienced by many people, and applies to the pain sensation that is perceived as being in the cranial vault (excluding facial pain, toothache and earache). There are many causes of headache involving both intracranial and extra cranial structures. The brain itself is almost insensitive to pain, although the venous sinuses, tentorium, dura, some of the cranial nerves and associated vasculature are pain sensitive. One of the most sensitive areas in the brain is middle meningeal artery. Changes in intracranial pressure, either decrease or increase, may lead to headache, because the pressure changes cause the pain sensitive structures in the head to shift.

There are many types of headache of intracranial origin. Vascular headache is common type of intracranial headache. This headache can be caused by a variety of problems such as hypertension, sepsis, hypoxia, and various medications. Other causes of intracranial headache include infection, hemorrhage, and changes in intracranial structures. Migraine is also a type of headache of intracranial origin but cause is unknown.

There are many types of headaches of extracranial original which are common and have many causes. Many extracranial structures are sensitive to nociceptive stimuli. These structures include the skin, subcutaneous tissues, muscles, arteries and periosteum of the skull. Problem in the eyes, sinuses, ears, teeth, nose, and jaws also may lead to headache. The mechanisms of these headaches are similar to headaches of intracranial origin. Stimuli such as traction, distention, dilation and spasms of vessels, irritation of nerves and inflammation of various structures can cause them. The common types of extracranial headache are muscle tension, temporomandibular joint syndrome, ocular sinus, dental and otic.

Headaches can be best treated by first identifying the cause and if possible treating it.

Psychogenic Pain

Psychogenic pain is that experience when there is no detectable organic lesion. However, pathology may still be present. Psychogenic pain refers to pain that believed primarily due to emotional factor rather than physiologic dysfunctions. Clients experiencing psychogenic pain have a real pain experience. Psychogenic pain is different from pretended pain. Although psychogenic pain starts without a physical basis, repeated severe stress probably alters the complex physiology of pain transmission, modulation, and perception. The pain the client feels is real to that client and the tension and/ or stress the client is feeling may lead to pronounced physiologic changes. When the psychogenic effect of stress, anxiety, feat and anger produces painful alteration in physiology, these can be called "psychophysiologic pain". Psychogenic pain requires that the cause may be found and treated.

Nursing Management of Pain

In the management of pain, nursing has an important role in anticipating and preventing pain, and in supporting clients who have been thorough physically painful experience. Appropriate information effectively communicated can do much to help provide a sense of control and minimizing anxiety. Advance knowledge of the physiological and psychological dimensions of plan provides a challenge for the nurse critically to examine nursing practices in pain assessment and management.

Assessment

Assessment is essential for diagnosis and for planning of pain control measures. Pain is difficult to measure because pain is a subjective experience or phenomena. One of the priorities for adequate treatment of pain is an accurate assessment. The goal of pain assessment is to identify the etiology of the pain; to understand the patient's sensory, affective, behavioral and cognitive pain experience for the purpose of implementing pain management techniques; and to identify the patient's goal for therapy and resources for self-management of the pain. It is the nurse often who is responsible for gathering and documenting assessment data.

Assessment, however, is highly influenced by the client's ability to delineate aspects of the pain experience accurately. If the client cannot communicate clearly (e.g. child, unconscious patient) then this aspect of the pain assessment is altered. Without the subjective information, it is difficult to intervene effectively except by trial and error. Ongoing assessment of pain is useful. This ongoing assessment should include subjective and objective assessment, that is, the individuals' verbal description of the pain and observation of person's behavior.

Each person has a basic human need to be free of pain and discomfort. Humans are motivated to avoid pain. Pain can occur as a result of inadequate satisfaction of other basic human needs. For example, need to eliminate urine not met because urinary stones block the bladder outlet, pain occurs. Part of the nursing assessment is to identify any unmet needs that may contribute to person's pain.

Each person experiences and expresses uniquely, and attaches personal meaning or explanations to pain experiences. The personal meanings nurses attach to pain may interfere with the assessment. The personal meanings attached to pain result from personal pain experience throughout life and may arise from a person's individual experience and sociocultural experiences. The cultural and familial role modeling a person exposed to as a child teaches the following:

- What pains are appropriate or inappropriate to talk about?
- Behavior that is appropriate or inappropriate when one experiences pain
- Circumstances likely to produce pain, which should therefore be avoided
- Various methods to avoid pain
- Reasons, why one may experience pain such as punishment, testing by supernatural or divine powers, or bad thoughts
- Possible consequence of pain, such as attention or lack of attention from others, imminent death

A pain experience is also affected by personal factors:
- Pain expectancy (The anticipation of pain)
- Pain experience (Willingness to experience pain)
- Pain apprehension (Generalized desire to avoid pain)
- Pain anxiety (The anxiety of pain provokes because of its associated mystery, loneliness, helplessness, threat).

Since the pain evokes emotional responses, observation of behavior of the client/patient provide a nurse with understanding of a person's feelings and of what pain means to a particular person. By accepting behaviors and trying to understand their origins, nurses can help individuals experiencing pain. To do this, well, nurses must:
- Accurately observe client's behavior
- Listen to all that clients say
- Never judge clients or jump to conclusions.

Perception pain is influenced by number of factors, which include integrity of the nervous system, state of consciousness, age, physical states (fatigue, debility, lack of sleep, and prolonged suffering all reduce a client's ability to tolerate pain) and emotional states (worry, fear, and anxiety reduce a person's ability to tolerate pain).

Assessment Process

The assessment process should provide the nurse with understanding of the patient's/client's pain, as well as establishing the nurse as a partner in the patient's search for pain relief. Patient teaching is an integral part of assessment, as information is provided clarifying the nurse questions or responding to the patient's concern. As the patient's discomfort is a source of stress to the family, it is important to involve the family and other members of the patient's network in the pain assessment. If the patient's ability to speak for himself or herself is limited, it is imperative to involve the family.

An accurate history is essential to assess a client's/patient's experience of pain. A detailed system analysis is performed using the following guidelines, to find out various aspects of pain.

Location The location should be identified as specifically as possible. To determine the location of the patient's pain ask the following questions:
- Where in the body is pain
- Is the pain internal or on the surface (external)
- Is the pain always in these areas
- If the pain is in more than one spot, are the pains equal, or does one trigger the others
- Is the pain on both sides of your body? If so, is it the same on each side.

The site may be well-defined or diffuse or the pain may radiate, involving wider area. To determine the extension and radiation of patient's pain ask the following questions:
- Does the pain extend from where it started? Does it cover a wider area, or can you point to where it is
- Is there a pattern in which the pain spreads
- Is the pain on the surface or deep inside.

Observing the pain locations on the patient's body will help localize the sites of pain as well as identify any physical changes at the site such as swelling/or discoloration.

Onset and duration When the pain first began and how the pain has changed over time should be determined. To determine the onset and pattern of the patient's pain ask the following questions:
- When did the pain begin? Is it a regular pain or does it vary? Does it occur in cycles? e.g. sometimes, every day, every month or every spring
- What triggers the pain? Are there specific things that always trigger it? Can you identify particular patterns?
- Does the pain begin suddenly or gradually over time? Is it continuous, or does it vary? Are there separate episodes of pain? If, so, does the pain go away completely between episodes or does it just get better?
- Has the pain pattern changed at all since it began?
- Has your lifestyle changed since the pain began?

To determine the duration of the patient's pain, ask the following questions:
- How long does the pain last? Are you free of pain between episodes?
- Is the pain constant, intermittent or rhythmic?

Character or quality A description of the pain, using patient's own words is helpful in determining the origin of pain and possible pain relief measures. To determine the character or quality of the patient's pain, ask the client the following question to describe it.
- Is the pain, dull, sharp, throbbing, burning, electric or shooting?

If the patient is unable to provide such descriptions the descriptors used in the McGillMelzack pain questionnaire can be used.

Exacerbating factors Often patients may be comfortable at rest, but have difficulty in morning due to pain. Activities which exacerbate the pain should be identified. To determine the factors, that precipitate, aggravate and alleviate the patient's pain ask the following questions:
- What seems to trigger pain? Can you identify a specific cause or event that always or sometime precedes the pain
- Does anything alter the pain? Does anything make it worse, such as smoking, drinking alcohol, eating, heat or tension? Is there anything that makes the pain better, such as rest, activity–heat or cold or medications.

Associated manifestations The impact of pain on the person's physical functioning should be explored. To determine whether there are any manifestations associated with client's pain, ask the following questions:
- Are there any other problems caused by your pain?
- Do you have any nausea/vomiting, restlessness, insomnia, excessive sleeping, or loss of appetite?

Associated manifestations also include profuse perspiration, fainting, inability to perform usual functions, dulling of senses, apathy, clouding of consciousness, disorientation and inability to rest and sleep.

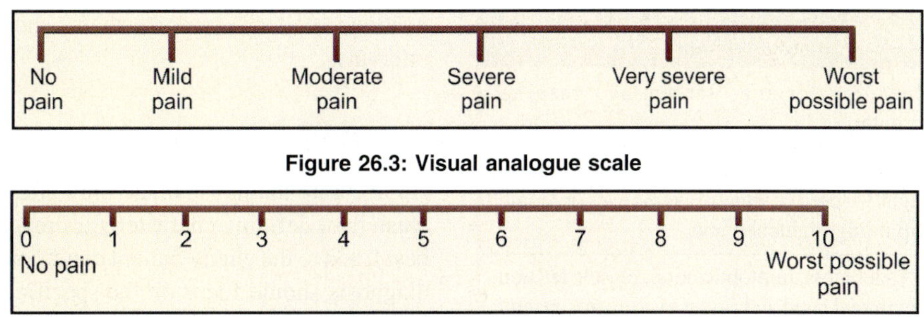

Figure 26.3: Visual analogue scale

Figure 26.4: Numerical rating scale

Effect on activities of daily living To determine how the client's pain affects activities of daily living, ask the following questions:
- Does the pain interfere with work, sleep, driving, eating, school work, sexual relations, housework, social activity or other activity?
- Has the pain caused any changes in your lifestyle?
- When did you last have a good night's sleep?

Intensity A new pathogenic condition must be ruled out when there is sudden increase in pain intensity, the intensity of the pain can be measured in several ways which are summarized as follows:
- *Visual analogue scale (VAS)*–consists of a 10 cm line vertical or horizontal with one end marked 'no pain' and other 'worst possible pain' (Fig. 26.3).
  The patient marks the line to show where the pain lies. This approach works well for acute pain. It is not useful in chronic pain. Some patients have difficulty in understanding the basic concept involved in it, and may not be able to use the scale at all.
- *Numerical rating scale (NRS)*–typically runs from 0 (no pain) to 10 (unbearable) although 0-5 or 0-7 may be used. Here the patient simply gives a score to indicate that pain level (Fig. 26.4).
- *Verbal descriptor scale (VDS)*–here, a range of words are used to describe the potential spectrum of pain and the patient states which word most accurately reflects how they feel.
- *McGill pain questionnaire*–is complex but reliable and sensitive tool which involves multidimentional measurements of pain with time, the effect it has on the patient, location and intensity of pain.

To determine the intensity of patient's pain the following should be done:
- Ask, on a scale of 0-10 with '0' being 'no pain' and '10' being 'the worst pain you can imagine' how would you rate your pain now? How would you rate it worst? How would you rate it with activity?
- Note what nonverbal manifestation of pain the client exhibits–grimacing, crying, moaning, sleeping, appearing exhausted, or remaining immobile.

Relief measures The efficacy of measures used by the patient to relieve pain should be identified. To determine how the patient obtains pain relief, ask the following questions:

- What do you do to relieve the pain (Ask about both invasive and noninvasive pain relief measures)?
- What has not worked to relieve your pain?
  This includes both those activities suggested by the medical and nursing staff such as the use of analgesic, as well as measures employed by the patient himself, such as distraction, visualization, rubbing, etc. All drugs used by the patients and their dose.

Physical examination Start the examination by having the patient show where the pain is and describe how it feels. Pain is subjective and the patient himself is an expert about his/her pain, but objective manifestations that observed by nurse and other healthcare providers give clue to its cause. Objective manifestations of pain can be divided into three categories which include sympathetic responses, parasympathetic responses and behavioral responses.

Sympathetic responses are often associated with minimal to moderate pain intensity or superficial pain. They signify the other body defenses are mobilized and that the fight-or-flight response has begun. Objective manifestations include pallor, increased pulse, increased blood pressure, increased respiration, skeletal muscle tension, dilated pupils and diaphoresis.

Parasympathetic responses are often associated with pain of severe intensity or with deep pain. In this, body defenses may collapse in an attempt to lessen the effects of external threat. Manifestations of parasympathetic response include decreased blood pressure, decreased pulse, nausea and vomiting, weakness, prostration, pallor and loss of consciousness.

The patient may exhibit the behavioral responses in the acute pain as follows (Table 26.1).
- Assume a posture that minimizes pain such as lying rigidly, guarding drawing up the legs, or assuming the fetal position
- Moan, sign, grimace, clench the jaws or fist, become quiet, or withdraw from others
- Blink rapidly
- Cry, appear frightened, exhibit restlessness
- Have a drawn facial expression
- Have twitching muscles
- Withdraw when touched
- Hold or protect the painful area or remain motionless

Although it is unreasonable to think that the nurse would be performing the detailed assessment constantly with a patient,

Table 26.1: Behavioral Indications of Effects of Pain

Vocalization	Meaning, crying, screaming, gasping, grunting.
Facial expression	Grimace, clenched teeth, wrinkled forehead, tightly closed or widely opened eyes or mouth, lip biting, tightened jaw.
Body movement	Restlessness, immobilization, muscle tension, increased hand and finger movements, pacing activities, rhythmic or rubbing motions, protective movement of body parts.
Social interaction	Avoidance of conversation, focus only on activities for pain relief, avoidance of social contact, reduced attention span.

portions of it are important and should be done at regular intervals.

Nursing Diagnosis

An accurate diagnosis made only after a complete assessment clusters of defining characteristics reveal the nursing diagnosis best fitted to the client/ patient condition and needs. The nursing diagnosis should focus on the specific nature of these pains to help the nurse identify the most useful types of interventions for alleviating pain and minimizing its effect on the client's lifestyle and function.

The nursing diagnoses are directly associated with care of patients with pain, i.e. chronic pain. The other nursing diagnoses that may be appropriate because of the effects of pain on other aspects of a patient's life include the following (Table 26.2):

Table 26.2: Simple Nursing Care for Pain Relief

Problems	Reasons	Objectives	Nursing Interventions
Pain related to (R/T) abdominal incision movement	c/o sharp, localized pain over lower abdominal incisions worsening during coughing and movement. Guards abdomen rigidly while turning and breathing deeply.	1. Client will achieve control of pain within 24 hours after surgery. 2. Patient will initiate movement in bed without painful behavioral cues. 3. Client will express relief during PCA infusion.	1. Position client anatomically on side with knee flexed and small pillow below legs. 2. Have colleagues available to lift client in bed for repositioning. Encourage client to ask for assistance. 3. Explain the purpose of PCA device, method for initiating device and expected response. 4. Demonstrate and coach client through relaxation exercise.
Improved physical mobility R/T musculoskeletal pain	c/o pain, edema manifested by painful movement, decreased range of motions. Loss of muscle strength.	Patient will demonstrate increase in mobility of joints.	Place the patient in position of comfort, suggests joints anatomically with pillow or pads and change position every hour: • Assist in ROM exercise • Avoid restrictive clothing • Assist to ambulate as tolerated • Maintain save environment
Self-care deficit R/T pain	Not dressed Not groomed	Patient's independence in selfcare activities will increase within the parameters of disability.	• Teach self-care activities • Establish and teach routine plan of ADLs • Set goals with patient, encourage short-term easily accomplished goal • Discuss the use of snaps on clothing and slip-on shoes
Chronic low-self-esteem R/T inability to work	Preoccupation with body changes and verbalization of powerlessness	Patient will verbalize understanding of changes in body image caused by disease process and will begin to exhibit increased confidence in dealing with self-esteem.	• Encourage verbalization about fears and anxiety of disease process • Deal with behavioral change denial, powerlessness, etc. • Be supportive and kind in setting goals setting goals • Encourage independence • Modify environment
Knowledge deficit R/T home cure management	Having misconception about medication regimen, exercise program and diet		

- Anxiety
- Knowledge deficit (specify)
- Body image disturbance
- Altered nutrition
- Colonic constipation
- Impaired physical mobility
- Ineffective family coping, disabling
- Ineffective individual coping
- Powerlessness
- Altered family processes
- Altered role performance
- Fatigue
- Selfcare deficit (specify)
- Fear
- Sexual dysfunction
- Anticipatory grieving
- Sleep pattern disturbance
- Social isolation
- Altered thought process

Following are the examples of nursing diagnoses for pain:

1. Anxiety related to (R/T) unrelieved pain.
2. Pain R/T physical injury/reduced blood supply to tissue/ natural child birth process.
3. Chronic pain R/T chronic physical disability/psychosocial disability/inadequate pain control.
4. Hopelessness R/T chronic malignant pain.
5. Ineffective individual coping R/T chronic pain.
6. Impaired physical mobility R/T musculoskeletal pain/ incisional pain.
7. Risk for injury, R/T reduced pain reception.
8. Self care deficit (specify) R/T musculoskeletal pain.
9. Sexual dysfunction R/T arthritic hip pain.
10. Sleep pattern disturbance R/T low back pain.

Planning

For each nursing diagnosis identified, the nurse develops a care plan for the client/ patient needs. Together the nurse and patient discuss realistic expectation for pain-relief measures and the degree of pain relief to expect. Objectives of the care are selected on the basis of the nursing diagnosis and client condition. Appropriate measures and therapies are chosen on the basis of the related factor contributing to the patient's pain or health problem.

A critical element in the management of a patient with a pain syndrome is the establishment of a trusting relationship and good rapport with the patient and the family. The patient and the family need to know that the nurse considers the pain significant and understands that pain may totally disrupt a person's life. The nurse's goal is to help the patient cope with the pain by using medications and techniques to help with relaxation, comfort, sense of aloneness and isolation, and protection from depersonalizations and the nurse will help the patient maintain or regain control over the environment. A priority for the nurse caring for a patient with pain is to let it be known that the nurse

believes the person has pain and to explain some of the physiologic mechanisms of pain.

Nursing actions that promote the establishment of an effective relationship with the person who is experiencing pain and with the family should include the following.

Believe the patient: The patient needs to be able to trust the nurse to believe in the pain's existence. This message can be conveyed verbally to the patient by saying "I know you are in pain". The nurse may need to help the family believe the patient.

Clarify responsibilities in pain relief: Discuss what the nurse is going to do, and what the patient and the family are expected to do.

Respect the patient's response to pain: The nurse should accept the right of the patient to respond to the pain in the necessary manner. The family also needs help in this area. The patient may need help to accept the reasons of pain; the behavior may be less than is expected by the patient and the family.

Collaborate with the patient: The patient should be encouraged to use coping techniques that have been effective in the past. The patient and the family should be helped to participate actively in setting goals for pain relief.

Explore the pain with the patient: The nurse needs to find out the meaning of the pain to the person enduring the pain and to the family.

Be with the patient often: The nurse should act as buffer for the patient and the family during difficult times. The nurse's physical presence may reassure or distract the patient or it may offer variety, thus relieving the pain.

Pain relief is a complex phenomenon requiring input from various members of the health care team. The nurse's role is pivotal in managing a client's pain. The physician also plays a key role, diagnosing and treating the medical cause of the pain, which includes prescribing appropriate medications. In complex cases, other professionals, such as physical therapists, psychologists, social workers, or chaplains, may be needed. The multidisciplinary team approach is the most successful way to manage chronic pain and improve the quality of a client's life.

Pharmacologic and nonpharmacologic interventions can both be effective in caring for clients in pain. Nonpharmacologic techniques may be the primary intervention in some cases of mild pain, with medication available as "backup." Cases of moderate to severe pain may use nonpharmacologic techniques as effective adjunctive, or complementary, treatment.

There are three categories of pain control interventions: pharmacological, noninvasive, and invasive. Each category is discussed separately, but these methods are often used in combination.

Combining analgesics and the use of adjuvant medication provides effective pharmacologic intervention for clients with pain. *Adjuvant medications* are those drugs used to enhance the analgesic efficacy of opioids, to treat concurrent symptoms that exacerbate pain, and to provide independent analgesia for specific types of pain. The ladder recommends that the analgesic, plus or minus an adjuvant, is chosen based on the level of pain the client is experiencing. For mild pain, the ladder recommends a nonopioid. If the pain persists or if the client has moderate pain to begin with, WHO recommends a weak opioid, plus or minus the nonopioid, plus or minus an adjuvant. If pain persists, a strong opioid is used. The nonopiod should be continued, and an adjuvant medication should be considered. This ladder gives health care workers guidelines in determining if the drug regimen is appropriate for the client with cancer pain.

Nurses' Role in Administration of Analgesics: The nurse spends the most time with the client in pain and is the team member who most often assesses the effectiveness of pain control interventions. When analgesics are prescribed, the nurse often has choices of drug, route, and interval. For example, the postoperative client may have the following orders:

- Morphine 10–15 mg IM or IV q2-4h prn severe pain
- Vicodin i–ii tabs q3-4h pm moderate pain

When this client complains of pain, which analgesic should the nurse administer? Which route? Which dose? How frequently? The nurse has a large responsibility in making these decisions but also has autonomy in making these decisions. Each nurse may make a different decision, often based on the nurse's own biases.

The responsibilities of the nurse in administering analgesics includes:

- Determine whether to give the analgesic, and if more than one is ordered, which one.
- Assess the client's response to the analgesic, including assessing the effectiveness in pain relief and occurrence of any side effects.
- Report to the physician when a change is needed, including making suggestions for changes based on the nurse's knowledge of the client and pharmacology.
- Teach the client and family regarding the use *of* analgesics.

Invasive Intervention

The drugs used to relieve pain work by altering pain sensation, depressing pain perception or modifying the patient's response to pain as the nurse has considerable control over .and responsibility for the effective use of medicines to reduce pain, knowledge of the drugs used in pain control, their routes of administration and side effects are needed. Examples of analgesic are of four types as follows:

1. Non-narcotic analgesics
   - Acetanililophen (Tylenol, Datnol)
   - Acetyl salycyclic acid (Asprin)
   - Choline magenesium trisalycylate (tritisate)
2. NSAIDs
   - Ibuprofen (Brufen)
   - Naproxen (Naprosyn)
   - Indomethacin
   - Tolmetin
   - Piroxicam

3. Narcotic analgesics
   - Meperidine
   - Methylmorphine (Codiene)
   - Morphine sulfate (Morphine)
   - Fentany (Sublimzae)
   - Butorphanol (Butarin)
   - Hydormorphene HCL
4. Adjuvants
   - Amitriptyline
   - Dydroxyzine
   - Caffeine
   - Chloropromozine
   - Diazepam

There are four types of analgesic as mentioned below which include (i) non-narcotic analgesics (ii) NSAIDs (iii) opiods and (iv) adjuvants or coanalgesics. Non-narcotic and NSAIDs provide relief for mild and moderate pain.

Principles of Administering Analgesics: Principles should be applied in the administration of analgesics, no matter which one is given.

Establishing and maintaining a therapeutic serum level is important. Peaks and valleys often occur when analgesics are administered in the traditional PRN (as needed) manner. When the dose is administered on an intermittent schedule, a larger dose is often required, causing the client to have a peak serum drug level in the sedation range. The client must wait for the return of pain before requesting the next dose of analgesic. Depending on the length or time it takes to obtain the medication and, once taken, to reestablish an adequate blood level, there could be a period of up to an hour or so without adequate pain control.

Preventive Approach: Pain is much easier control if treated when it is anticipated or at a mild intensity. Once pain becomes severe, the analgesics ordered may not be effective enough to relieve it. Many clinicians still teach their clients to wait to take medication until they are sure they really need it. This practice leads to uncontrolled pain. There are two ways the preventive approach may be implemented:

- ATC (around the clock). When pain is predictable, for example, the first few days following surgery or with chronic cancer pain, the medication is administered on a scheduled basis. This prevents the peaks and valleys of serum drug level that can lead to oversedation or toxicity and recurrence of pain, respectively. If the analgesics are ordered by the physician to be given PRN, it can still be a nursing measure to administer the drugs ATC, as long as they are given within the time constraints of the order.
- PRN (Latin for *pro re nata,* which means "as required"). Pain is not always predictable: therefore PRN dosing may be required. For some clients this may be used in addition to scheduled dosing for "breakthrough" pain (pain that surpasses the level of *analgesia,* or pain relief without anesthesia, that the steady level of analgesics is providing). Examples of this include a cancer client on prolonged-release morphine who

needs extra analgesics to participate in activities such as shopping or receiving visitors. Another example would be the orthopedic client who is receiving regularly scheduled analgesics for postoperative pain who needs additional pain relief for therapy sessions. In order to implement the preventive approach with PEN dosing, the medications should be given as soon as the pain appears, or when it is anticipated to begin.

Titrate to Effect: Because of the pain experience, the analgesic regimen needs to be titrated until the desired effect is achieved. This involves adjusting the following:

* *Dosage:* Some clients may require more or less than the standard dose. Many factors may influence the pharmaco-kinetics in an individual client. The individual's response is assessed, and the dosage or the analgesic is regulated accordingly. In clients with chronic cancer pain, opioid analgesics are recommended to be increased until pain relief is obtained or unacceptable side effects occur. This may be done because of the lack of a *ceiling effect* (the dosage beyond which no further analgesia occurs) in pure opioids. The lack of a ceiling effect means there is no limit to the dose that can be given. For example, cancer clients have been known to receive more than gram per hour intravenously. Because the dosage is gradually increased, the client develops a *tolerance* (requiring larger and larger doses or an analgesic to achieve the same level of pain relief) to the sick effects or the opioid.
* *Interval:* Some clients metabolize the analgesics faster than others. For example, young adults tend to metabolize opioids faster; therefore, they may need more frequent doses. Older clients tend to metabolize them slower, so they require a longer interval between doses.
* *Route:* The appropriate route is chosen depending on how rapidly pain relief is required, the client's ability to take medications orally, the client's diagnosis, and assessment or the client's response to the current route. Intravenous administration provides the most rapid onset of pain relief. All other routes require a lag time for absorption or the analgesic into the circulation. In postoperation pain, IV is the preferred route for opioids when the oral route is not appropriate. If IV access is not available, sublingual, rectal, or transdermal routes should be considered.

With cancer pain, the oral route is preferred. If the client is unable to take oral medications, rectal and transdermal routes are preferred because they are less invasive than other routes. In addition, tolerance develops at a slower rate with the oral route compared to the more invasive routes.

* *Choice of drug:* If one drug is not providing relief or has unacceptable side effects, another analgesic may be tried.

It is import to take or request pain medication before the pain becomes severe and more difficult to control. Numerous nonpharmacologic approaches can be used to augment pharmacologic pain management. Pain management is individual. (The client may be taking different medications or dosages than other individuals)

The key to administering an analgesic is to monitor the client's response to it. This includes assessing the effectiveness of pain relief and t he occurrence of side effects.

Classes of Analgesics: Three classes of drugs are used for pain relief: (1) nonopioid analgesics: (2) opioid analgesic's; and (3) analgesic adjuvants.

Nonopioids: The medications in this category are useful for a variety of painful conditions, including surgery, trauma, and cancer (American Pain Society, 1999). The indications include mild to moderate pain, and they are used in conjunction with opioids. These drugs differ from opioids in several ways in that they:

* Are subject to the ceiling effect.
* Do not produce the effect of tolerance or physical dependence.
* Are antipyretic and should not be given in cases where they may mask an infection.

Ketorolac is the only nonsteroidal anti-inflammatory drug (NSAID) available in parenteral form and has proven useful in clients on NPO status who would benefit from a NSAID. Even when administered intramuscularly or intravenously, ketorolac produces significant gastric irritation and the potential for gastric bleeding. The most frequent use of ketorolac is orally or intramuscularly in adults, but some pediatric centers have used it intravenously under strict supervision for a limited course (less than 5 days) in children and adolescents with great success.

Action: Action or these drugs is thought to inhibit prostaglandin formation. If prostaglandins are inhibited, the sensory neurons are less likely to receive the pain signal. Thus this class or analgesics works in the peripheral nervous system.

Opioids: The opioid analgesics fall into three classes: pure opioid agonists, partial agonists, and mixed agonist-antagonists (a compound that blocks opioid effects on one receptor type while producing opioid effects on a second receptor type). Pure agonists produce a maximal response from cells when they bind to the cells' opioid receptor sites. Morphine (the gold standard against which all other opioids are measured), fentanyl, methadone (Dolophine), hydromorphone hydrochloride (Dilaudid), and codeine are pure agonists. Meperidine (Demerol), although classified as a pure agonist, is not recommended except in clients with a true allergy to all other narcotics, because of its neurotoxicity. Meperidine produces clinical analgesia for only 2.5 to 3.5 hours when given intramuscularly in adults.

Unlike the NSAIDs, pure agonist opioids are not subject to the ceiling effect. As the dosage is increased, pain relief increases.

Types of Nonopioid Drugs

* *Salicylates.* These include aspirin and other salicylate salts. Common side effects of aspirin include gastric disturbances and bleeding caused by the antiplatelet effect. Some of the salicylate salts, such as choline magnesium trisalicylate (Trilisate) and salsalate (Salgesic) have fewer gastrointestinal and bleeding effects than aspirin.

- *Acetaminophen*: This nonsalicylate is similar to aspirin in its analgesic action but has no anti-inflammatory effect. Its mechanism of action for pain relief is not known.
- *NSAIDs*: The effectiveness of these drugs varies, with some being close to the effectiveness of aspirin and acetaminophen, whereas others are much stronger. Clients tend to vary in response, so once the maximum recommended dose has been tried with ineffective results. It would be worth trying another NSAID. The drugs in this group inhibit platelet aggregation and are contraindicated in clients with coagulation disorders or on anticoagulation therapy.

Action: Opioids act in the CNS by binding to opiate receptor sites on afferent neurons. The pain signal is stopped at the spinal cord level and does not reach the cortex where pain is perceived.

Side Effects: The only limiting factor in the use of pure agonist opioids is the degree of side effects, particularly respiratory depression and constipation. Other side effects include pruritus and nausea, but the degree to which they are present from each medication varies among individuals. Clients must be instructed regarding these normal responses to opioids and informed that it does not mean that they are allergic to them. A true allergy to opioids would be indicated by a rash or hives that starts after receiving the opioid, a local histamine release at the site of infusion, or anaphylaxis. Clients also need to know that the pruritus and nausea generally subside after 4 to 5 days of opioid therapy. In the meantime, an antihistamine such as diphenhydramine hydrochloride (Benadryl) or hydroxyzine hydrochloride (Atarax, Vistaril) may be used for pruritus, and an antiemetic such as metoclopromide hydrochloride (Clopra) or trimethobenzamide hydrochloride can be used to treat the nausea.

Almost all medications used to treat side effects have their own side effect of sedation. Thus there is the possibility of a cumulative effect of severe sedation. These medications must be used with caution and appropriate monitoring until the client's response is determined. Ondansetron hydrochloride is one antiemetic on the market with little, if any, sedative effect. It has recently received approval for use with postoperative nausea and has been effective in clients with refractory nausea and vomiting unresponsive to other antimetics.

Mixed agonist-antagonist opioids are believed to be subject to the ceiling effect for pain relief, as well as a ceiling effect for respiratory depression. Mixed agonist-antagonist opioids activate one opioid receptor type while simultaneously blocking another type. Butorphanol tartrate, pentazocine hydrochloride, and nalbuphine hydrochloride are the most frequently used in pain management.

Opioid antagonists include naloxone and naltrexone, with the most commonly used being naloxone. They work by blocking opioid stimulation of receptor sites. Naloxone effectively reverses opioid side effects of sedation, respiratory depression, and nausea and it completely reverses any pain control.

Effects of Meperidine (Demerol)

- In the elderly, most of whom show decreased glomerular filtration rates, there is generally a higher peak and longer duration of action because it takes longer to excrete the opioid as well as its toxic metabolite, normeperidine.
- In pediatric clients receiving intravenous meperidine, analgesia may last for only 1.5 to 2 hours.

Opioid Analgesia in the Elderly

- Cheyne-Stokes respiratory patterns are not unusual during sleep in the elderly and should not be used as a reason to restrict appropriate opioid pain relief unless accompanied by unacceptable degrees of arterial desaturation (less than 85%).
- The elderly are more sensitive to sedation and respiratory depressant effects and experience a higher peak and longer duration of effect from opioid medications.
- Opioid dose titration must be based on analgesic effects and degree of side effects, such as sedation, urinary retention, constipation, respiratory depression, or exacerbation of Parkinson's disease.

Constipation and Opioids

Clients who are expected to require opioid analgesics for more than 1 or 2 days should be administered a stool softener as soon as they are taking fluids orally. While they are still NPO, a glycerin or bisacodyl (Dulcolax) suppository should be administered if the client has not had a bowel movement in 1 or 2 days.

Alternative Delivery Systems: Opioids are administered in more than just the traditional oral, subcutaneous, intramuscular, intravenous, and rectal routes.

Patient-Controlled Analgesia: Patient-controlled analgesia (PCA) is most often delivered by a device that allows the client to control the delivery of intravenous, epidural, or subcutaneous pain medication in a safe, effective manner through a programmable pump. This system helps eliminate the time required for the nurse to draw up the medication and allows the client to fed some control over the pain. The pump has the safely feature of locking out once a maximum dose has been reached. This prevents the client from overdosing. Requirements for the use of PCA are the cognitive ability to understand how to use the pump and the physical ability to push the button. The PCA has been successfully used with many types of pain and in many settings, including pediatrics and home health.

Oral PCA is relatively new in hospitals and is becoming increasingly popular. Client teaching is the key for success. The client must understand how pain, pain medication, and pain relief are related and how to maintain a pain-relief diary. A Velcro sealed wrist pouch is applied to the client with one or two doses of the prescribed oral analgesic, even controlled substances, in the pouch. The client notifies the nurse when a dose is taken, so it can be replaced. If the client does not comply with the oral PCA policy, it is discontinued.

Epidural/Intrathecal Analgesia: Epidural analgesia refers to administering the opioid via a catheter that terminates in the epidural space, the space outside the dura matter that protects the spinal cord. Intrathecal analgesia refers to administering the drug directly into the subarachnoid space. These may be administered as a one-time injection by the anesthesiologist or via a catheter that has been placed. Both of these routes are occasionally referred to as *intraspinal anasthesia*. Because the opioid is delivered close to the site of action, these routes require much lower doses of opioid (usually morphine or fentanyl are used) for pain relief. The incidence of systemic side effects is also much lower with these routes. Duration is longer than systemic routes (e.g., the duration of one dose of intrathecal morphine can last 24 hours).

Transdermal Analgesia: Another route of opioid administration is the transdermal patch. The only opioid drug currently available via this route is fentanyl (Duragesic). This medication is on an adhesive patch that attaches to the skin. [t is available in 25, 50,75, and 100 mcg/hour dosages. The fentanyl transdermal patch allows slow infusion of the drug through the skill. The fentanyl patch is indicated for continuous pain with high dosage requirements. The advantage of this route is that it is simple to apply and effective for 72 hours. The disadvantage is that dosage adjustments are difficult to make because of the slow infusion rate. In addition, side effects may not be reversed as rapidly as when opiates are administered via the oral route.

Local Anesthesia: Local anesthetics are effective for pain management in a variety of settings. Topical anesthetics are available for teething, sore throats, denture pain, laceration repair, and intravenous catheter insertions. One topical anesthetic, EMLA cream, is a mixture of local anesthetics, combining prilocaine and lidocaine (Xylocaine). It produces complete anesthesia for at least 60 minutes when topically applied on intact skin. Another topical anesthetic, TAC, is available for anesthesia during closure of lacerations. It is a combination of tetracaine hydrochloride (Pontocaine) 0.5%, adrenaline (epinephrine) 1:2000, and cocaine 11.8% in a normal saline solution that can be applied directly to the open wound surface in place of local anesthetic infiltration with a needle. This allows pain-free cleansing of the laceration as well as suturing. Because both adrenaline (epinephrine) and cocaine cause vasoconstriction, TAC cannot be used in areas supplied by end-arteriolar blood supply such as digits, the ear, or the nose. It also is contraindicated on burned or abraded skin because this could lead to increased systemic absorption of cocaine and tetracaine, thus placing the client at risk for seizures.

Noninvasive Interventions

Noninvasive relief measures consist of cognitive behavioral strategies and physical modalities that use cutaneous stimulation.

These treatments can be used to supplement pharmacological therapy and other modalities to control pain. Clients and their families can also be instructed to utilize these treatments at home and in inpatient settings.

Cognitive-Behavioral Interventions: The cognitive-behavioral interventions influence the cognitive and the motivational-affective components of pain perception. These methods can not only help influence the level of pain, but also help the client gain a sense of self-control.

Trusting Nurse-Client Relationship: Establishing a therapeutic relationship is the foundation for effective nursing care. The clients most likely to be comfortable are those who trust their nurses to be there, to listen, and to act.

Relaxation: Relaxation techniques (a variety of methods used to decrease anxiety and muscle tension) result in decreased heart rate and respiratory rate, and decreased muscle tension. The body's response to pain is almost "tricked" into reversing itself when relaxation exercises are implemented.

Relaxation exercises help reduce pain by decreasing anxiety and decreasing reflex muscular contraction. There are a wide variety of relaxation techniques, including focused breathing, progressive muscle relaxation, and meditation. Simple techniques should be used during episodes of brief pain (e.g., during procedures) or when pain is so severe that the client is unable to concentrate on complicated instructions.

To teach simple relaxation techniques, the nurse can instruct the client to (i) take a deep breath and hold it; (ii) exhale slowly and concentrate on going limp; and (iii) start yawning. The yawning triggers a conditioned response in the client (i.e., the body associates yawning with relaxation and will relax when the client yawns). The technique can be enhanced if the nurse starts yawning. It is so contagious that even the client compromised by severe pain will usually start yawning with the nurse.

A more complex technique is *progressive muscle relaxation*, a strategy in which muscles are alternately tensed and relaxed. This type of technique is especially useful for clients who do not know what muscle relaxation feels like. By purposely contracting and releasing the muscle groups, the client is able to compare the difference and identify feelings of relaxation. Meditative relaxation techniques are also available, including audiotapes sold inmost bookstores.

Relaxation is a learned response. The more frequently the client practices these techniques, the more skilled the body will be in learning to relax. Ideally, the best time to teach the client these methods is when pain is controlled or before the pain occurs (e.g., in the preoperative period).

Reframing is a technique that teaches clients to monitor their negative thoughts and replace them with more positive ones. For example, teach a client to replace an expression such as, "I can't stand this pain, it's never going away," with one such as, "I've had similar pain before, and it's gotten better,"

Distraction: Distraction focuses one's attention on something other than the pain, therefore placing pain on the periphery of awareness. Successful or distraction does not eliminate the pain; it makes it less troublesome. The main disadvantage of distraction is that as soon as the distractive stimuli stop, the pain returns in full force. For this reason, the most appropriate use of distraction techniques is for the relief of brief, episodic pain. It can be effective for procedural pain or the period between administration of an analgesic and the onset of the drug. Examples of distraction include the following:

- Active listening to recorded music (have the client tap fingers in rhythm to the beat)
- Reciting a poem or rhyme (children do this well)
- Describe a plot of a novel or movie
- Describe a series of pictures

Guided Imagery: Guided imagery uses one's imagination to provide a pleasant substitute for the pain. It incorporates features of both relaxation and distraction. The client imagines a pleasant experience, such as going to the beach or the mountains. The experience should use all five senses to fully involve the client in the image.

The images chosen need to be ones that are pleasant for the client. Describing an ocean cruise would not be appropriate for a person who becomes seasick.

Humor: The old saying, "Laughter is the best medicine," carries some truth to it. Although there is nothing very funny about pain, laughing has been shown to provide pain relief. The act or laughing can cause distraction from the pain, induce relaxation by taking deep breaths and releasing tension, release endorphins, and provide a pleasant substitute for pain. This technique can be implemented by encouraging the client to watch humorous movies, read funny books, or listen to comedy routines. Because different people see humor in different types of situations, be sensitive to what the client views as funny.

Biofeedback: Biofeedback is a method that may help the client in pain to relax and relieve tension. Individuals learn to influence their physiological responses to stimuli and thus alter their pain experience.

Cutaneous Stimulation: The technique of cutaneous stimulation involves stimulating the skin to control pain. It is theorized that this technique provides relief by stimulating nerve fibers that send signals to the dorsal horn of the spinal cord to "close the gate." The main advantage of these therapies is that many techniques are easy for the nurse to implement and easy to teach the client and family to perform. They are not usually meant to replace analgesic therapy, but to complement it.

Hot and Cold Application: In addition to stimulating nerves that can block pain transmission, superficial heat application increases circulation to the area, which promotes oxygenation and nutrient delivery to the injured tissues. It also decreases joint and muscle stiffness. Heat is contraindicated in cases of acute injury because it can increase the initial response of edema.

It is also contraindicated in rheumatoid arthritis flare-ups and over topical applications of mentholated ointments. Heat treatments should be limited to 20- to 30-minute intervals because maximum vasodilatation occurs in that time.

Teach the client or family that hot or cold applications:
- Must have at least one layer of towel between the heating or cooling device and the skin.
- Should be placed on the skin only for short periods.
- Should not be applied to tissue that has been exposed to radiation therapy.

Cryotherapy (cold applications) induces local vasoconstriction and numbness, therefore altering the pain sensations. It is contraindicated in any condition where vasoconstriction might increase symptoms (e.g., peripheral vascular disease). For best results, cold therapy should be limited to 20- to 30-minute intervals. Either heat or cold can be used as cutaneous stimulation unless one is specifically contraindicated. Cold often provides faster relief. If the client has used heat or cold before, incorporate the modality that the client believes will be the most effective. Combining the two might provide better relief. An example of this would be to apply a hot pack for 4 minutes, followed by an ice pack for 2 minutes, repeated four times. In a hospital setting, a physician order is required for this therapy.

Acupressure and Massage: One of the first responses to pain is to rub the painful part. People seem to instinctively understand the pain-relieving aspects of this intervention. In addition to blocking the pain transmission through nerve stimulation, massage can also promote relaxation. Acupressure is a type of massage that consists of continuous pressure on or the rubbing of acupuncture points. It is based on the same principles as acupuncture, but needles are not used. Massage also provides a form of nonverbal communication that can be therapeutic on its own.

Mentholated Rubs: Ointments or lotions containing menthol are thought to provide relief by providing a counterirritation to the skin. The menthol gives the client the perception that the temperature of the skin has changed (becoming either warmer or cooler). This alters the sensation of pain or provides a distraction from the pain. Client response varies to mentholated rubs: some gain effective relief, but others have poor results. Their use is contraindicated on broken skin, on mucous membranes, or if pain increases.

Transcutaneous Electrical Nerve Stimulation: Transcutaneous Electrical Nerve Stimulation (TENS) is the process of applying a low-voltage electrical current to the skin through cutaneous electrodes. This modulates pain transmission, as do other cutaneous stimulation methods, but also distracts the client from pain. Research supports the effectiveness of using TENS for the relief of postoperative pain. It has also been used successfully in many pain syndromes (e.g., chronic low-back pain, menstrual cramps, temporomandibular joint (TMJ) syndrome, phantom limb pain, and others). It is administered by specially trained health professionals, usually a physical therapist. Other modalities of pain management should not be abandoned while a trial of TENS occurs.

TENS Contraindications

- No electrodes should be placed in the area over or surrounding demand cardiac pacemakers.
- No electrodes can be placed over the uterus of a pregnant woman.

Exercise: Exercise is an important treatment for chronic pain because it helps mobilize joints, strengthens weak muscles, and helps restore balance and coordination. Do not use passive range of motion if it increases discomfort or pain. Immobilization is frequently used to stabilize fractures or for clients with episodes of acute pain. Prolonged immobilization can lead to muscle atrophy and cardiovascular conditioning.

Psychotherapy: Psychotherapy may be beneficial to some clients, particularly those:
- Who are clinically depressed
- Who have a history of psychiatric problems
- Whose pain is difficult to control

Some psychotherapists use *hypnosis* (altered state of consciousness when a person is more receptive to suggestion) to help clients alter pain perception. Hypnosis can be effective but should be used only by specially trained professionals.

Positioning: The final noninvasive technique is proper positioning and body alignment. Moving the client with the least possible stress on joints and skin will minimize exposure to painful stimuli. This includes supporting joints appropriately and maintaining wrinkle-free sheets.

Invasive Interventions

Invasive Interventions are meant to complement behavioral, physical, and pharmacological therapies in those clients who do not obtain relief from those measures alone (AHCPR, 1994). Invasive measures are indicated primarily for chronic cancer pain and in some cases of chronic benign pain. These procedures are usually tried only when noninvasive measures have been attempted first with poor results.

Nerve Block: Neural blockade is the process of injecting a local anesthetic or neurologic agent into the nerve. An anesthetic agent may be injected to act as a diagnostic tool in order to identify the nerves involved in a pain syndrome. A neurolytic agent is a chemical agent that causes destruction of the nerve and, therefore, creates an interruption in the pain signal.

Neurosurgery: Neurosurgical measures for pain control include neurostimulation procedures and destructive or ablative procedures, Neurostimulation procedures involve the implantation of electrical stimulation devices that send impulses to different parts of the nervous system. Some of these devices stimulate areas of the brain: others stimulate the spinal cord. Relief is thought to be provided by blocking the afferent fiber input at the spinal cord level or by stimulating release of endorphins using the body's ability to modulate pain.

Destructive or ablative procedures are used to destroy part of the nervous system that conducts pain. By interrupting the pain signal, it is prevented from reaching the cortex where realization of pain occurs. These procedures are reserved for clients with terminal illness.

Radiation Therapy: Radiation can be used as a palliative measure for pain relief in clients with cancer. It can relieve both metastatic pain and pain caused by tumors at the primary cancer site. It enhances other pain management strategies, such as analgesic therapy, because it is aimed specifically at the cause of the client's pain. When administered for pain relief, the smallest dose of radiation is utilized to minimize side effects.

Acupuncture: Acupuncture is the insertion of small needles into the skin at specific (hoku) sites. The sites are chosen after the practitioner takes a detailed history and uses traditional Asian diagnostic techniques. The needles used for acupuncture have rounded ends that enter the skin without cutting the tissue. The practitioner may twirl or vibrate the needles manually or electrically. It is important that the nurse keep an open mind when the client chooses this therapy, or the client may be reluctant to discuss its use.

Evaluating pain management interventions is ongoing, focusing primarily on the client's subjective reports. Objective data to evaluate pain management include the following:
- Continuing use of pain assessment tools
- Client's facial expression and posture
- Presence (or absence) of restlessness
- Vital sign monitoring

Pain may be defined as "an unpleasant sensory and emotional experience associated with actual or potential tissue damage," and "whatever the client says it is, existing whenever the client says it does."

The gate control theory proposes that several processes (sensory, motivational-affective, and cognitive) combine to determine how a person perceives pain.

Assessment of pain helps establish a baseline of data and helps evaluate the effectiveness of the interventions.

Factors influencing pain perception include age, previous experience with pain, and cultural norms.

The subjective data to gather include location of pain, onset and duration, quality, intensity (on a scale of 0 to 10), aggravating and relieving factors, and how pain affects the activities of daily living.

Guidelines for Individualizing Pain Therapy

When providing pain relief measures, the nurse chooses therapies suited to the client's unique pain experience, McCaffer (1979) suggests nine useful guidelines for pain therapy. The following guidelines are eleven which include nine.

Establish a relationship of mutual trust: Always believe the client and try to convey concern. An adversial relationship between nurse and client lessens the effectiveness of pain therapies.

Use different types of pain relief measures: Using more than one therapy has an additive effective reducing pain. In addition, the character of pain may change throughout the day, requiring several different therapies.

Provide pain relief measures before pain becomes severe: It is easier to prevent severe pain than to relieve it after it exists. Giving analgesics half an hour before, client must walk or perform an activity is an example of controlling pain early.

Consider the client's ability or willingness to participate in pain relief measures: Some client cannot actively assist with pain therapy because of fatigue, sedation or altered level of consciousness. However, there are variations of pain-relief measures that require little effort, such as relaxation exercises in bed or listening to music as a distraction. The nurse will not relieve pain by forcing an unwilling patient to participate in therapy.

Choose pain-relief measures on the basis of the client's behavior reflecting the severity of pain: It would be a poor judgment to administer a patient narcotic if a client has only mild pain. The nurse carefully assesses the client's comments and behavior before choosing pain therapy. Some clients acquire relief from severe pain after using only mild analgesics. Only the client can determine the potency of an effective therapy.

Use measures that the client believes are effective: The client is the expert of pain. The client may have ideas about measures to use (e.g. rubbing lotion on a swollen finger) and times to use them will make pain therapy successful.

If a therapy is ineffective at first, encourage client to try again before abandoning it: Often, anxiety or doubt prevents a therapy from relieving pain, or the measure may require adjustment or practice to become effective. The nurse should be patient and understanding in helping the client learn to use measures that do not afford immediate relief.

Keep an open mind about what may relieve pain: New ways are often found to control pain. There is still much to be learned about the pain experience. Rejecting nonconventional therapies leads to mistrust. The nurse should se to it that sure all therapies are safe.

Keep trying: The nurse can easily become frustrated when efforts at pain relief fail. The nurse should not abandon the client when pain persists but reassess the situation and consider alternative therapies.

Protect the client: A pain therapy should not cause more distress than the pain itself. The nurse always observes the efforts response to therapy. The nurse's aim is to relieve pain without disabling the client mentally, emotionally or physically.

Educate the client about the pain: When possible, the nurse should explain the cause of the pain, time of occurrence, duration and quality and ways to gain relief. Education promotes the prevention of pain.

The basic nursing responsibility is protecting the client from harm. One simple way to promote comfort is by removing or preventing painful stimuli. The following measures can be performed by the nurse to assist in pain control:

- Tighten and smooth wrinkled bed linen
- Reposition drainage tubes/ other objects on which patient is lying
- Place warm bath blankets for coolness
- Loosen constricting bandages (unless specifically applied as a pressure dressing)
- Change wet dressings
- Position the client in an anatomical alignment
- Check temperature of hot or cold applications including bath water
- Lift client on bed–do not pull. Patient up in bed; handle gently
- Position patient correctly on bed pain
- Avoid exposing skin or mucous membrane to irritants (e.g. diarrheal stool, wound drainage)
- Prevent urinary retention by keeping Foley's catheters patent and free-flowing
- Prevent constipation with fluids, diet and exercises.

Nursing Intervention

Nursing interventions for pain relief can be grouped and discussed in two broad categories:

1. Noninvasive or nonpharmocological intervention/ pain relief strategy.
2. Invasive interventions/pain relief strategies.

Noninvasive Interventions

The noninvasive techniques which may be offered by the nurses often used as adjuncts to the analgesic regimen, not alternatives.

Trusting relationship: Develop good trusting relationship as already explained.

Alleviate anxiety: For alleviating anxiety, stay with the client for a while. Allow the client to talk and express feelings and fears. Communicate empathy and willingness to listen. Take measures to relieve anxiety in positive direction according to experience of nurses. With patient with pain, for example, self-directed pain prevention/reduction techniques such as meditation, using therapeutic touch, backrub, applying cool cloth, etc.

Distraction or diversion: It is one of the measures used to pain relief. Distraction helps to focus attention away from the pain and to some extent, any contact the nurse with the patient which is not focused on pain *per se*. Distraction which reduces the conscious awareness of pain usually works with mild pain than severe pain. Distraction may take many forms, viz. occupational therapy, conversation, reading, watching television, listening to radio, meditation, self-hypnosis, biofeedback, and auto-suggestion, etc. Distractions serve to increase pain tolerance, that is, it makes the pain more bearable.

Combating anticipatory fears: Anticipatory fears are those fears that occur prior to an experience of pain-producing stimuli. These help prepare clients to meet pain realistically by talking with them about the pain they fear.

Providing physical care: Effective physical nursing care for clients experiencing pain is directed at reducing mechanical, chemical and thermal stressors that lower pain tolerance. This includes protecting patient from local irritations or inflammation such as infection or thrombosis, muscle spasm or muscle strain, interference with local blood supply and venous and lymphatic drainage, distention of hollow visceral organs such as the bowel and bladder and further damage to traumatised tissue.

There are several important principles of physical nursing care as follows:

- Identify the source of pain and eliminate or reduce the pain
- Handle sensitive or injured tissue carefully
- Always perform painful procedures when pain-relieving medications are producing their maximal effect
- Check drainage tubes frequently to ensure that they are not caught, stretched, pulled, kinked, or looped and that they are positioned correctly
- Protect the client from fatigue and helping the client to get a good night's sleep
- Be alert to inflammation and ischemia caused by immobilization–take suitable measure to reduce it
- Change the position to relieve muscle spasms, maintain good body alignment of the client
- Use gentle massage, and application of heat or cold if needed
- Use dormal stimulation, i.e. application of pressure, acupressure, massage. TENS (transcutaneous electric nerve stimulation), ice massage (massaging area with ice).

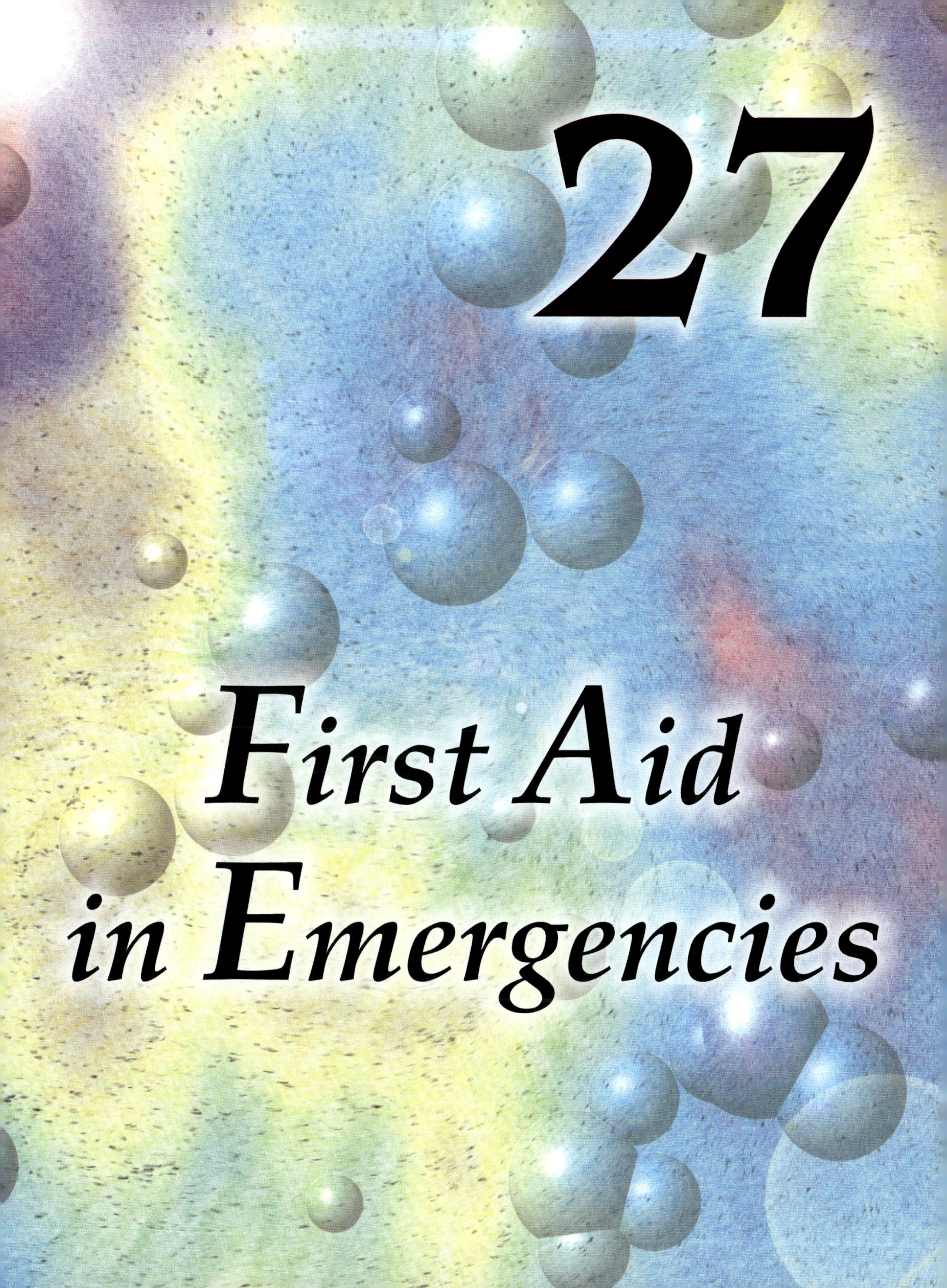

27
First Aid
in Emergencies

An emergency is the unforeseen events which calls for prompt and quick action to save the life of a person or to prevent from further severe damage. When nurses are happened to be at the site when an emergency arises, nurse may have to deal with it promptly with knowledge and skill and also use confidentiality. The main aims of providing prompt and proper first aid in an emergency are as follows.

Meaning of First Aid

First aid is an immediate temporary assistance given to a person who is injured or as suddenly become ill, using facilities or materials available at that time before regular medical help is imparted.

First aid includes assessing the victim for life threatening conditions, performing appropriate interventions to sustain life and keeping the person in the best possible physical and mental conditions until she/he can enter the emergency or causality unit in the hospital.

Objectives of First Aid

The objectives of the first aid will include the following:
- To preserve life
- To prevent further injury and deterioration of the condition
- To prevent complications related to injury or illness or conditions
- To make the victim as comfortable as possible to conserve the strength
- To put the injured person under professional medical care at the earliest

Principles of First Aid

When any person comes across another seriously injured person he should follow the following principles:
- Make sure that victim's airway is not blocked by the tongue, secretions or some foreign body – restore respiration
- Make sure that the person is breathing, if not administer artificial respiration – restore respiration
- Make sure that the patient has a pulse or no pulse if no pulse is felt, administer cardiopulmonary resuscitation (CPR) – restoration of circulation
- Check for bleeding – take measures to control bleeding
- Act fast if the victim is bleeding severely or if he has swallowed poison or if his heart or breathing has stopped every second counts for his survival
- Arrange without delay for shifting of the victim to hospital for medical attention, although most injured persons can be safely moved. It is vitally important not to move a person with serious neck and/or back injuries unless taking proper measure to ensure and have to save him from further danger
- Keep the victim/patient lying down and quieten. If he has vomited and there is no danger that his neck is broken – turn him on his side to prevent choking. Keep him warm with blankets or coats

- Have someone called for medical assistance while applying first aid. The persons who summons help should explain the nature of the emergency and ask what should be done if the arrival of the ambulance is pending
- Examining the victim gently, cut clothing, if necessary to avoid abrupt movements if added pain. Do not pull clothing away from burns unless it is still smouldering
- Reassure the victim, try to remain clam yourself. Your calmness can allay his fear and panic
- Do not give fluids to an unconscious or semiconscious victim
- Do not try to arouse an unconscious persons by slapping or shaking
- Look for an emergency identification card for medical information related to victim. Check your progress.

Life-saving Technique/Resuscitation Technique

Artificial Respiration

When any person approach the victim, his breathing has stopped please do these in rapid succession

Step 1
- Open the airway. Unless you suspected a broken neck, place the victim on his back.
- Wipe any foreign substance – solid or liquid – out of his mouth with the cloth.
- Place the palm of one hand on the forehead and tilt the head back, place the fingers of the other hand under the chin and lift to bring it forward (Fig. 27.1). This position prevents obstruction of airway by the tongue.
- Opening the airway may start the persons breathing again. Watch the chest for rise and fall listen for the sound of breathing place your cheek close to the victim's mouth and nose to feel any exhaled air (Fig. 27.2) if there is none, take step 2 at once.

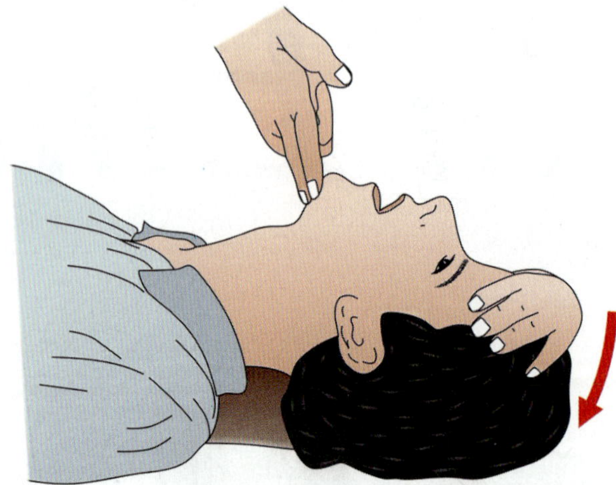

Figure 27.1: With one hand on forehead and the other under the chin, tilt head partially back

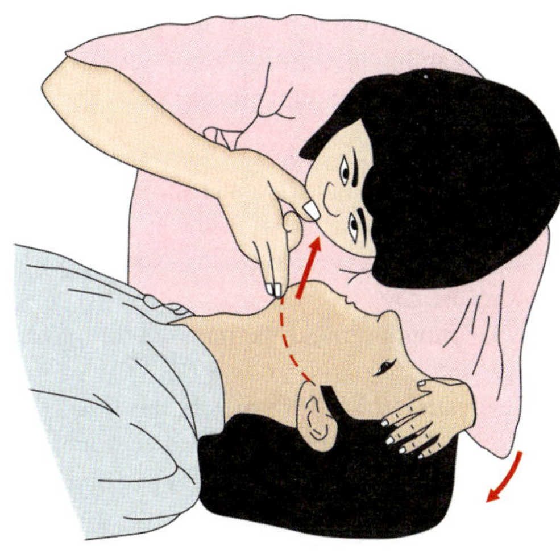

Figure 27.2: Listen for breathing, watch chest, feel any exhaled air

Step 2

- Pinch the nostril closed. Used the thumb and index finger of the hand that is on the victim's head to do this to maneuver hand so that it continues to exert the necessary pressure and the head to maintain the proper tilt (Fig. 27.3).
- Place your mouth over the victim's mouth, and give two full breaths, taking a deep gulp of air in between the two. Each ventilation should cause the victim's chest to rise and fall.
- If this fails to happen, try adjusting the victims response and repeat rescue breathing
- If this too fails to ventilate, suspect an obstruction of the airway (Treat chocking).
- When you are able to ventilate the victim quickly take step 3.

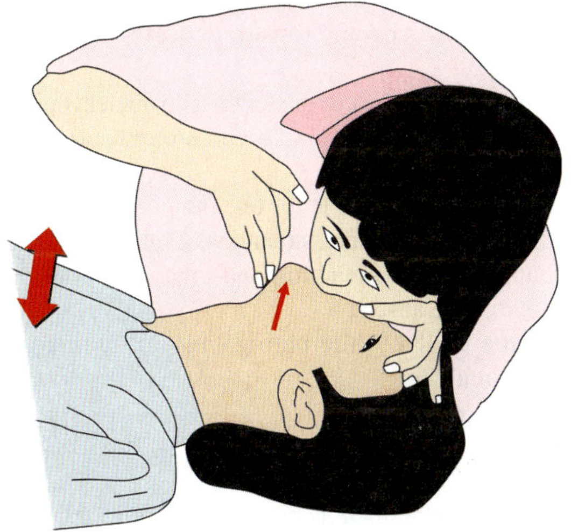

Figure 27.3: Pinch nostrils and blow into open mouth

Step 3

- Feel the carotid pulse in the neck between 5 and 10 seconds (Fig. 27.4) if there is no pulse, go to CPR (see CPR). If there is pulse but still no breathing, begin step 4 – steady mouth to mouth breathing.

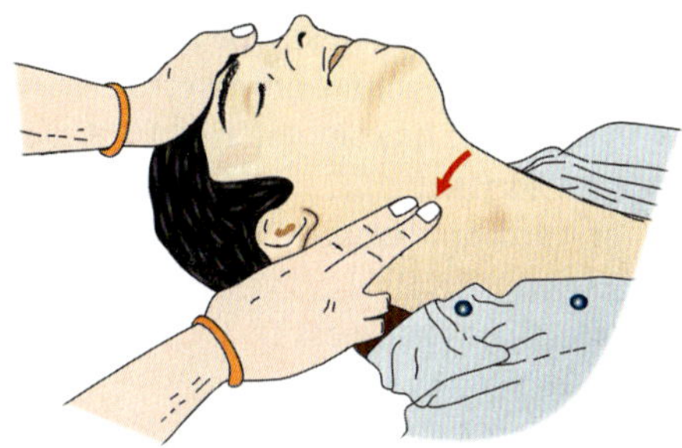

Figure 27.4: To feel carotid pulse, locate Adam's apple and slide tips of fingers into groove beside it

Step 4

- With victims head tilted as in step 1, and his nose pinched shut: Place your mouth over the victims and blow hard.
- Remove your mouth and allow the victim to exhale and you take another deep breath (Fig. 27.5).
- Watch for the rise and fall of the chest and listen for the sound of inhaled air.
- Then blow again. Repeat the procedurc, giving one vigorous breath every second until the victim starts to breathe spontaneously or help arrives.

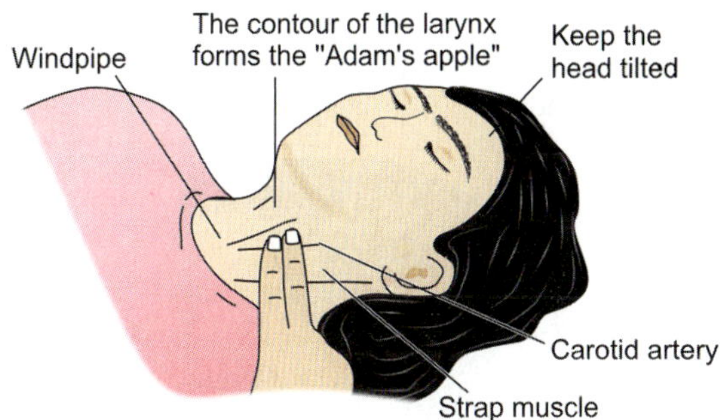

Figure 27.5: Allow the victim exhale

For small children and infants the above procedure is modified, as follows,

- To open the airway, avoid overextension of child's head.
- Lift the chin slightly, using one or two fingers.
- Leave the other hand on the forehead and keep the head in proper positions.
- Do not pinch the nose but cover the mouth and nose with your mouth.
- Gently give slow breaths. Use only light puffs of air to inflate child's lungs.
- Feel the pulse inside the upper arm between the elbow and shoulder for infants (Brachial pulsation).
- If there is pulse, give one gentle puff of air once every 3 seconds for an infant, every 4 seconds for a child.

Cardiopulmonary Resuscitation (CPR)

Cardiopulmonary resuscitation is a life-saving technique to be performed with skill and practice. When you come across a victim with cardiopulmonary arrest, you are expected to have quick assessment of cardiopulmonary arrest because, it is the critical factor in time. The quicker you start CPR the better the victim's chances of survival.

The signs of cardiopulmonary arrest will include the following:

- Immediate loss of consciousness
- Absence of pulse
- Cessation of perceptible respirations and after 45 seconds arrest
- Dilatation of pupils

(i) Resuscitation for Adults

When the victim appears unconscious, or lifeless the ABC of resuscitation needs to be performed in order to assess his/her most urgent needs. Once you are sure that there is no danger carry out assessment on the basis of ABC rules. This should be done as quickly as possible following these 4 steps:

- Check for consciousness – by shaking shoulders and asking him
- Open the airway (A) – by removing blockages and lifting chin as shown in Figures 27.6 A to C.
- Check the breathing (B) – by looking for chest movements, listening for sounds of breathing and feeling for breath for 5 seconds
- Check for circulation (C) – by feeling for the carotid pulse for five seconds.

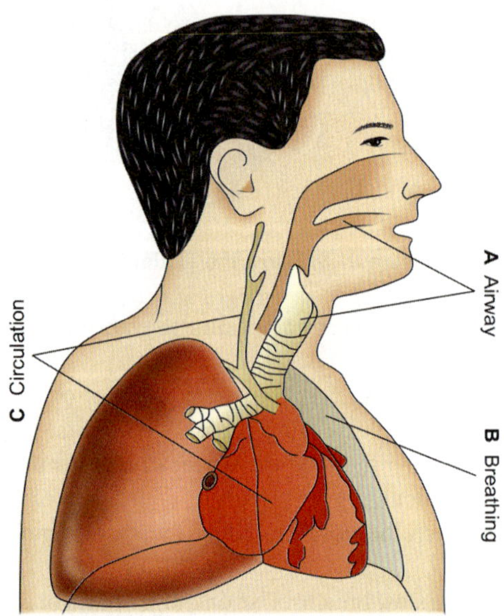

Figure 27.6: ABC of life support

A. Airway

To clear the airway you have to remove obstructing substance from the mouth with finger.

- Use first finger as a hook to dislodge any material causing obstruction
- Hyperextend the neck to open the airway
- Place one hand under nape of neck
- Place other hand on forehead and tilt head back

- Lift chip up gently without closing mouth
- Check if breathing is restored
- If not, start mouth to mouth breathing

B. Breathing

You are expected to act quickly and restore breathing by giving mouth-to-mouth resuscitation as follows:

- Pinch and compress nose to close nostrils
- Take deep breathe
- Place your mouth around victims mouth, make an airtight seal
- Quickly breath into victim's mouth four times
- Refill your lungs by inhaling deep after stopping breath
- Watch victim's chest movements for rise and fall of chest
- Allow patient to exhale

C. Circulation

You are expected to act quickly and restore circulation by pericardial thump and/or external cardiac compression.

First you try pericardial thump by striking upper left-chest forcibly midsternum region with closed fist (except MI cases). This may result in resuscitation of normal heartbeat. If you are succeeding to get good results start external cardiac compression by following steps given below:

- Place the victim on hard surface and kneel at victim's side
- Locate the xiphoid process, measuring 1-2″ above xiphoid process (Fig. 27.7A)
- Place heel of one hand at this point on the sternum
- Place the other hand on top of it (Fig. 27.7B)
- Interlock fingers to keep them off the victim's ribs
- Keep elbows straight and lean forward
- Make dull use of your body weight when delivering downward compression (Fig. 27.7C)
- Apply steady smooth pressure to depress victim's sternum 1.5 to 2″
- Then relax pressure completely but do not let your hand leave victims chest or you may loose correct hand position (Fig. 27.7D)
- Repeat or perform CPR for one minute as follows
- After 15 chest compressions give 2 quick lung inflation by mouth to mouth breathing and then two more inflation if carotid pulse absent
- Resume CPR by alternating lung inflations with chest depression

Principles of Resuscitation

Resuscitation is defined as restoration to life or consciousness of the person whose respirations have ceased. It is an emergency technique used in cardiac disorders to re-establish heart and lung functions, until more advanced life support is available. It is vital to maintain a constant supply of oxygen to the brain. Tissue get oxygen by the blood circulation. Heart maintains this circulation acting as a "pump". If the heart stops functioning, death will result, unless an urgent action is taken. The flow of oxygenated blood is rapidly restored to the brain by means of

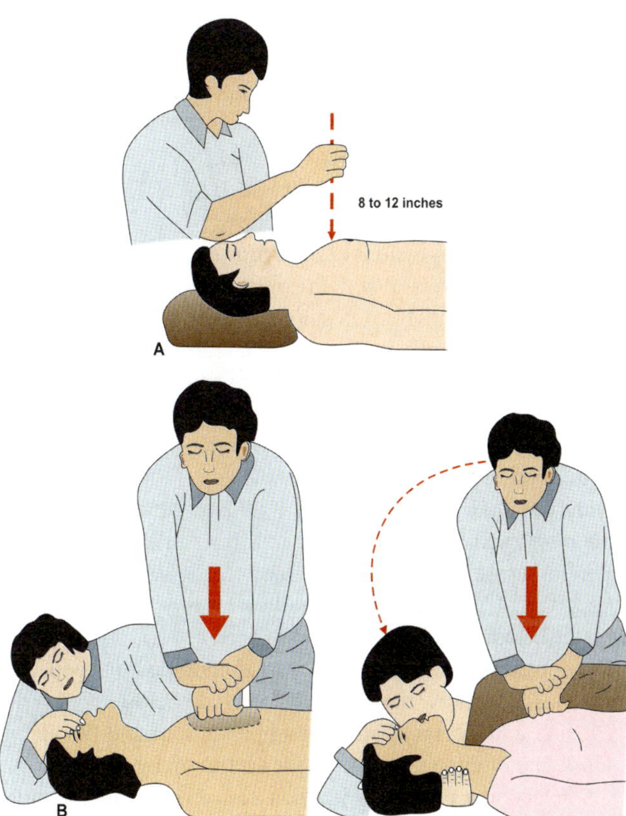

Figures 27.7A to C: External cardiac massage

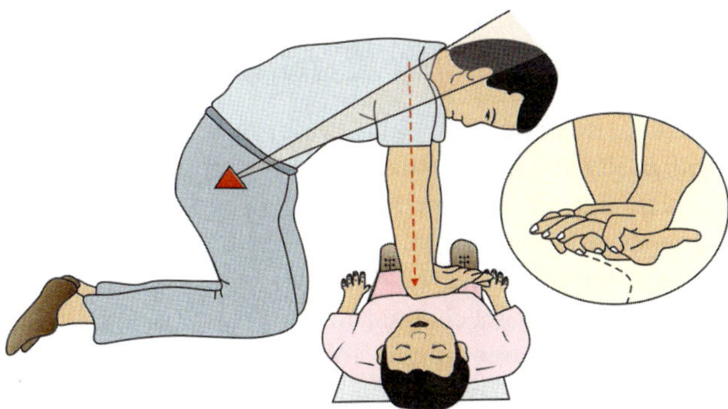

Figure 27.7D: Rescuer's position for external compression

artificial ventilation and chest compression (cardio-pulmonary resuscitation, or CPR).

Defibrillation is carried out immediately.
The victim is rushed to hospital for further care. The CPR bridges the gap between arrival of ambulance and casualty's collapse.

The principles of resuscitation includes:

(i) clear airway
(ii) review breathing
(iii) restore circulation.

Clear Airway

When you want to clear airway of an unconscious casualty's airway may be blocked, making breathing difficult and noisy.

The main reason for this is, that muscular control in the throat is lost which allows the tongue to sag back and block the throat. The ways of clear the airway includes the following:

- Remove obstructing substance from the mouth with finger.
- Use the first finger as a hook to dislodge any material causing obstruction (Fig. 27.8)

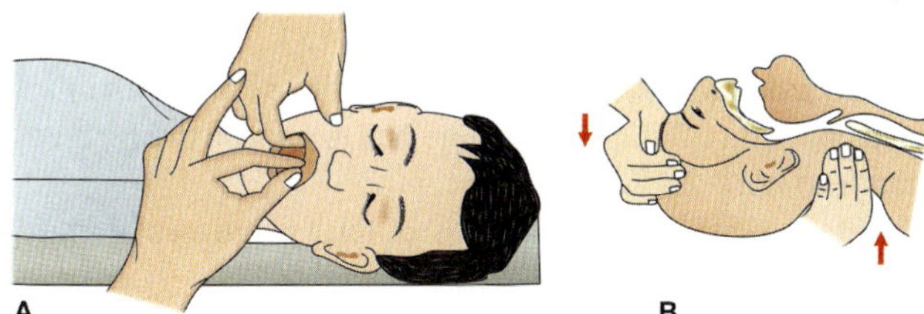

Figures 27.8A and B: A—Use finger to remove obstructing material from mouth, B—Opening the airway

- Hyperextend neck to open the airway
  (a) Place one hand under nape of neck
  (b) Place the other hand on forehead and tilt head back
  (c) Lift chin up gently without closing mouth
  (d) Check if breathing is restored
  (e) If not, start mouth-to-mouth breathing

Review Breathing

To review breathing of an unconscious victim put your face close to the casualty's mouth and look, listen and feel for breathing for five seconds, before you take further course of action.

If the heart is beating it will generate a pulse in the neck (the carotid pulse) where the main arteries pass up to the head. With the head tilted back feel for the Adam's apple with two fingers. Slide your fingers back towards you into the gap between the Adam's apple and the strap muscle (Fig. 27.4).

Restore breathing by giving mouth-to-mouth resuscitation: to start mouth-to-mouth breathing (Fig. 27.9).

- Pinch and compress nose to close nostrils
- Take deep breath
- Place your mouth around victim's mouth; make an airtight seal,
- Quickly breathe into victim's mouth for times
- Refill your lungs by inhaling deep after each breath
- Watch victim's chest movement for rise and fall of chest and
- Allow patient to exhale.

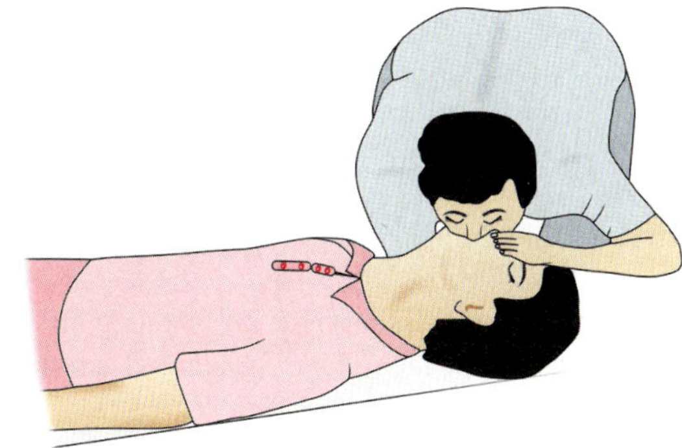

Figure 27.9: Mouth-to-mouth breathing

If the chest does not rise, check that
- the head is tilted sufficiently far back
- you have a firm seal around the casualty's mouth
- you have closed the nostrils completely
- airway is not obstructed by vomit, blood or foreign body.

Mouth to Nose Ventilation

In situations such as rescue from water, or where mouth injuries make a good seal impossible, one has to choose the method of mouth-to-nose artificial ventilation.
- With the casualty's mouth closed, form a tight seal with your lips around the casualty's nose and blow.
- Open the mouth to let the breath out continue at the normal rate.

Restore Circulation

Restore circulation by Precordial Thump and/or External Cardiac Compression.

Precordial Thump

First try precordial thump in following manner:
- Strike upper left chest forcibly in mid-sternum region with closed feast (except for patients known to have myocardial disease), and
- This may result in resumption of normal heartbeat e.g., in electric shock cases.
  External Cardiac Compression, also known as external cardiac massage, can be carried out by one or two individuals. Use technique suitable for single individual, if you are alone:
- Place victim on hard surface, and
- Kneel at victim's side.
- Locate xiphoid process
- Measure 1-2" above xiphoid process
- Place heel of one hand at this point on the sternum
- Place the other hand on top of it
- Interlock fingers to keep them off the victim's ribs
- Keep elbows straight and lean forward
- Make full use of your body weight when delivering downward compression
- Apply steady smooth pressure to depress victim's sternum 1½" to 2"
- Relax pressure completely but don't let your hand leave victim's chest or you may lose correct hand position
- Repeat
  Perform Cardio-Pulmonary Resuscitation (CPR) for 1 minute as follows:
- After 15 chest compressions give 2 quick lung inflations by mouth-to-mouth and then 2 more inflations if carotid pulse is absent
- Resume CPR by alternating lung inflations with chest depressions

The steps of Cardio-Pulmonary Resuscitation are:
- Clear airway
- Breathe into victim's mouth from times quickly
- Compress chest 15 times
- Give 2 quick lung inflations
- Alternate 15 chest compressions with 2 quick lung inflations
- In a minute, the victim should receive
  - 60 chest compressions (15 at a time multiplied by 4 times)
  - 8 lung inflations (2 at a time multiplied by 4 times)
  After Breathing has been Restored treat the victims as follows:
- To promote warmth and circulation, start rubbing the limbs upwards, with firm grasping pressure and energy. This must be continued under the blanket or over the dry clothing.
- Promote the warmth of the body by the application of hot water bottles
- If the patient has been carried to a house after respiration has been restored, let there be free and fresh air in the room
- On the restoration of life, a teaspoonful of swarm water can be given. If the power of swallowing has returned, small quantities of tea or coffee can be given
- Patient should be kept in bed, and encouraged to sleep
  And also Cautions may be taken as given below:
- Prevent unnecessary gathering of persons around the victim
- Under no circumstances hold the victim up by the feet
- On no account place the victim in a warm bath, unless under doctor's directions

Resuscitation for Children

Fortunately, it is rare for a child's heart to stop, but there are dangers in airway blockage and inadequate breathing. Artificial ventilation and chest compression can be performed on older children just as for adults, but they must be done slightly faster, and with lighter pressure. The techniques require some modifications for small children and babies.

Check Baby's Breathing as follows:
- Open the airway by gently lifting the chin and tilting the head. It helps to support the head slightly. Look, listen, and feel for breathing. (Fig. 27.10)

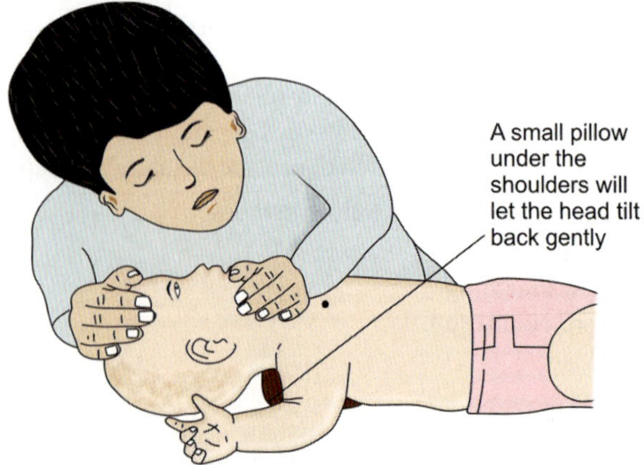

Figure 27.10: Checking for a baby's circulation

- DO NOT, if clearing an obstruction with a finger, touch the back of a young child's throat. If the child is suffering from an infection of the airway, this can cause swelling and, possibly, total blockage. (Fig. 27.11)

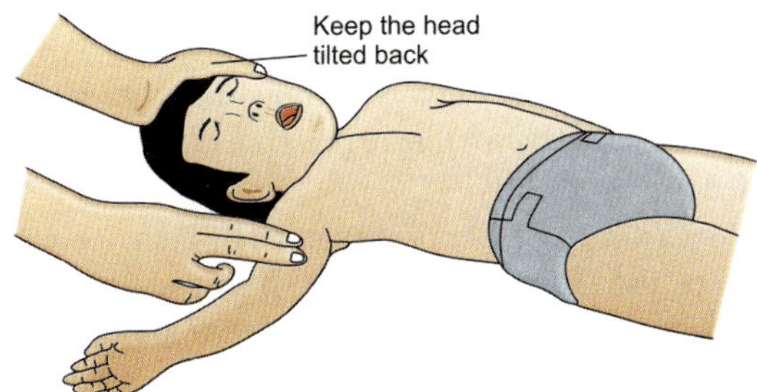

Figure 27.11: Checking for a baby's circulation

- It is difficult to feel the carotid pulse in an infant so, instead, use the brachial pulse. This is located on the inside of the upper arm, midway between shoulder and elbow.
- Place your index and middle fingers on the inside of the arm, and press lightly towards the bone. It may help to place your thumb on the outside of the arm. Feel the 5 seconds before deciding there is no pulse. (Fig. 27.12)

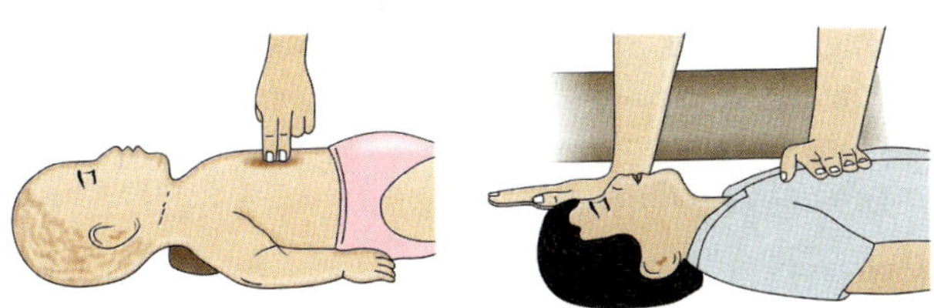

Figure 27.12: Artificial ventilation for a baby

- Babies should be given artificial ventilation at twice the rate used for adults and children, using the mouth-to-mouth-and-nose technique.
- Make a tight seal around the baby's mouth and nose with your mouth, and breathe into the lungs until the chest rises.
- Let the chest fall. Continue giving breathe at a rate of 20 per minute.

Chest Compression

- If you cannot detect a pulse or, in infants, if it is very slow (less than 60 beats per minute), apply chest compressions to the lower half of the breastbone. Use the adult technique for a child of school age; for *babies and small children,* modify the technique and rate as below.
- Remember that, in the absence of a pulse, chest compression must be combined with artificial ventilation.
- Lay the baby on a firm surface. To locate the correct position, imagine a line joining the baby's nipples. Place the tips of two fingers just below the mid-point of this line, and press at a rate of 100 compressions per minute, to a depth of 1.5 – 2.5 cm (½ – 1 in).

- Combine with artificial ventilation, giving five compressions to one breath. Find the correct position on the chest as you would for an adult.
- Using one hand only, press at a rate of 100 compressions per minute, depressing the chest by 2.5 – 3.5 cm (1-1 ½ in).
- Combine with artificial ventilation, giving five compressions to one breath.

Procedure for Recovery Position

Any unconscious victim should be placed in the recovery position. This position prevents the tongue form blocking the throat, and, because the head is slightly lower than the rest of the body, it allows liquids to drain from the mouth, reducing the risk of the casualty inhaling stomach contents. The head, neck and back are kept in a straight line, while the bent limbs keep the body propped in a secure and comfortable position. If you must leave an unconscious casualty unattended, he or she can safely be left in the recovery position while you get help.

The technique for turning shown assumes that the victim is lying on her back from the start. Not all the steps will be necessary if a victim is found lying on his or her side or front.

Before turning a victim, remove his or her spectacles, if worn, and any bulky objects from pockets.

1. Kneeling beside the victim, open her or his airway by tilting the head and lifting the chin. Straighten her or his legs. Place the arm nearest you out at right-angles to her or his body, elbow bent and with the hand palm uppermost (Fig. 27.13).

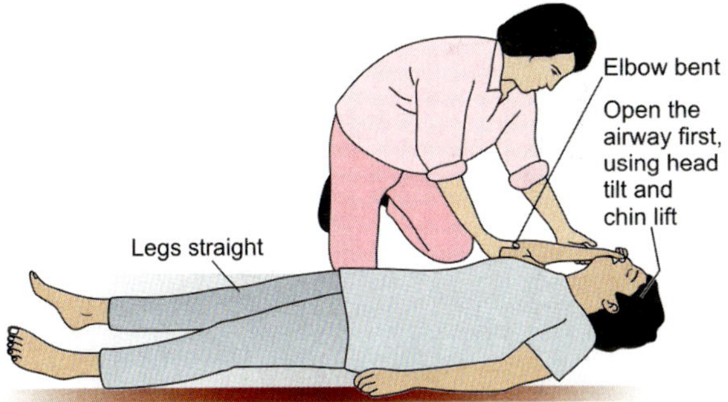

Figure 27.13: Step 1

2. Bring the arm furthest from you across the chest, and hold the hand, palm outwards, against the victim's nearer cheek (Fig. 27.14).

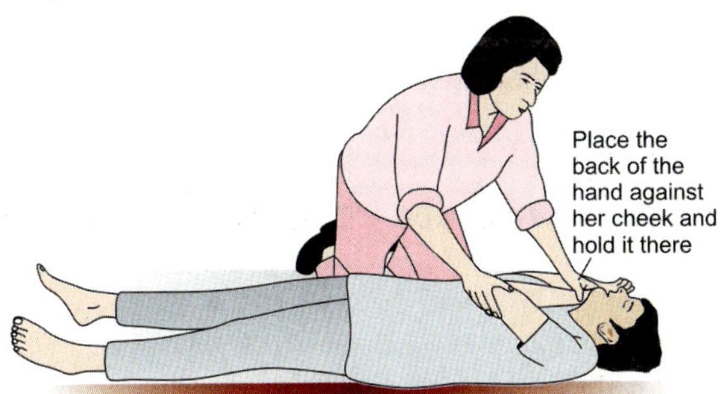

Figure 27.14: Step 2

3. With your other hand, grasp the thigh further from you and pull the knee up, keeping the foot flat on the ground. (Fig. 27.15)
4. Keeping her or his hand pressed against her or his cheek, pull, at the thigh to roll the victim towards you and on to her side.
5. Tilt the head back to make sure the airway remains open. Adjust the hand under the cheek, if necessary, so that the head stays in this tilted position.
6. Adjust the upper leg, if necessary, so that both the hip and the knee are bent at right-angles.
7. Dial for an ambulance. Check breathing and pulse frequently while waiting for help to arrive.

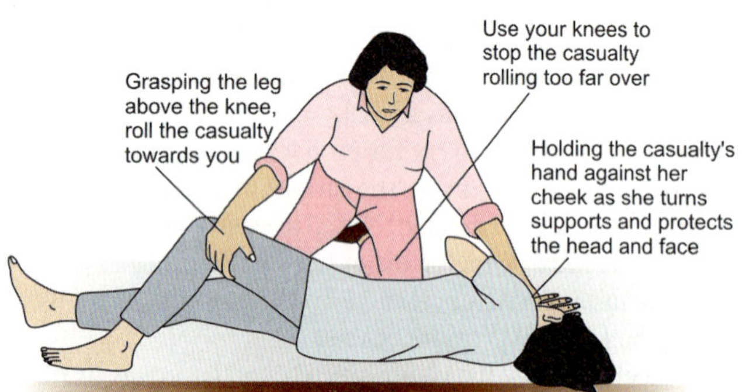

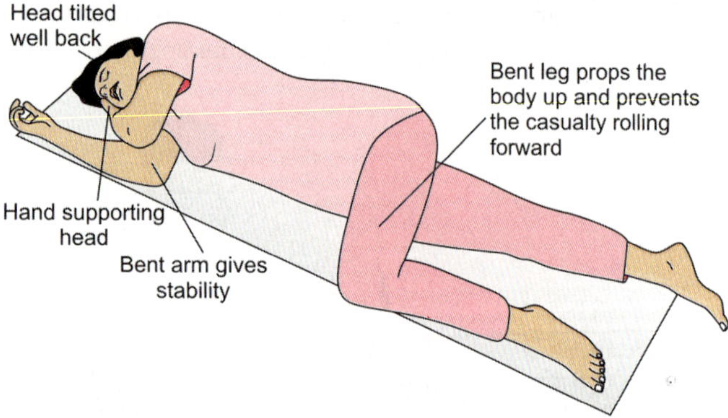

Figure 27.15: Step 3

Depending on the victim's condition, you may have to modify the recovery position to avoid making injuries worse. For example, an unconscious victim with a spinal injury needs extra support at the head and neck during turning, and in the final position, to keep the head and trunk aligned at all times. If limbs are injured and cannot be bent, use extra helpers or place rolled blankets against the victim's body to prevent it toppling forward.

Wounds and its First Aid Measures

1. Concepts of Wounds

A wound is an injury in which the skin is cut or penetrated. For instance a knife, bullet, ice pick or wood splinter may inflict a wound. If the wound is deep, severe bleeding may occur or there may be serious damage to structures within the body, such as the stomach, lungs or brain. Depending on how they are caused e.g., by blunt force, sharp weapon or firearm, they are classified as follows:

- *Abrasion (scratches, grazed or pressure marks)* An abrasion is a superficial injury involving only the outer layers of the skin. It is caused by friction or pressure of some rough object. It bleeds very slightly.
- *Bruise (contusions)* A bruise is caused by blunt force i.e. stick, stone or fist. There is infiltration of blood into the tissues following rupture of vessels and hence it appears red.
- *Lacerated Wound* These are wounds in which the skin and underlying tissues are torn as a result of application of blunt force. These wounds have irregular and torn edges and bleed less. They are usually caused by industrial accidents, falling over of houses, roofs or walls, fall on rough surfaces, pieces of shells and by claws of animals etc.
- *Incised Wound* An incised wound is an injury caused by a weapon with a sharp cutting edge e.g., knife, razor etc. The edges of the wound are clean cut. All the tissues are cleanly divided including the blood vessels so they bleed much.
- *Punctured Wound (stab wound)* A punctured wound is an injury caused by a pointed weapon, when it is driven in through the skin. Such wounds are caused by knife, dagger, needle, spear, arrow, scissors, ice pick etc. They have small openings but may be very deep. The vital organs of body may be injured through them.

2. Concepts of Hemmorhage

Hemmorhage or Bleeding means the escape of blood from the blood vessels. It is a common cause of death in accidents. Because of bleeding the total blood volume of the body decreases and so does the blood pressure. These two together lead to circulatory failure and then to death.

Hemmorhage can be classified as: External Hemmorhage and Internal Hemmorhage

A. External Hemmorhage

- **Arterial bleeding:** The blood, richly oxygenated is bright red and under pressure from the pumping heart, *spurts* from the wound in time with the heart beat. A severed artery may provide a jet of blood several feet high, and can rapidly empty the circulation of blood.
- **Venous bleeding:** Venous blood, having given up it oxygen, is dark red in colour. It is under less pressure than arterial blood, but since the vein walls are capable of great distension, blood may "pool" within them; this blood from a severed major vein may gush profusely.
- **Capillary bleeding:** This type of bleeding characterized as oozing, occurs at the site of all wounds. Although capillary bleeding may at first be brisk, blood loss is generally negligible. A blunt blow may rupture capillaries beneath the skin, causing bleeding into the tissues (a bruise).

- **Melena:** Bleeding from rectum or presence of blood in the stool. It may be present in large quantities or it may be just a trace.
- **Epistaxis:** Bleeding from the nose.
- **Hemetemesis:** Vomiting of blood usually coming from the stomach, resembles coffee grounds.
- **Hemoptysis:** This is bleeding from the lungs. Blood is coughed out, often it is mixed with air, usually bright red in colour. It may be mixed with sputum. Found in pulmonary tuberculosis.

The principles of first aid management of wounds always the same: that is, *Control Bleeding* and *Prevent Infection*

Control of bleeding: It is important to appreciate that the bleeding from most wounds will stop spontaneously even though no treatment whatever is given. Nature has two highly effective methods of minimizing blood loss: Retraction of vessels and Clotting of blood

There are some simple measures than can help nature to stop, which includes:

- **Rest:** If the casualty is encouraged to lie down quickly and particularly to keep the wounded part still, his blood pressure will drop, his pulse will become slow, and the amount of blood flowing into the wounded area will diminish. All of these factors will help to minimize the loss of blood from the wound.
- **Elevation:** Blood, like water, does not readily run uphill. If it is possible to elevate the wounded arm, or leg, or head, above the level of the heart, bleeding will be diminished and will stop more quickly.
- **Direct pressure:** The application of firm pressure directly on the wound is by far the most important method of controlling bleeding. Ordinarily, pressure is applied through a dressing which is bandaged firmly on the wound. The dressing should be thick and compressible to facilitate the application of even pressure over the whole wound area.

It is easy to understand how the pressure of a firm dressing reduces bleeding:

- It compresses all blood vessels leading into the wound and so lessens blood flow
- It retains shed blood in the wound until clotting occurs

If bleeding is not quickly controlled by a properly applied dressing, put on more pressure by:

- Adding a further dressing on the outer side and bandaging more tightly (i.e., reinforcing the dressing) or
- Pressing on the dressing with the palm of the hand

Rarely, in cases of profuse bleeding, when a dressing is not immediately available, it is permissible to press with the bare hand directly on the bleeding point. The exact site of maximum pressure can be altered until the effective position is found. If such pressure is maintained for ten minutes by the clock it will almost be found possible to replace the hand with a snugly applied dressing.

Very occasionally, in a wound of arm or leg involving a large artery, bleeding is so rapid and forceful that it can be controlled only by a constant pressure with the hand over the cut vessel. For such cases the first aider must move with the casualty to the hospital so that the vital pressure may be maintained without interruption.

The tourniquet is NOT recommended as a first aid measure. It is often ineffective and frequently harmful. Bleeding can always be stopped by the safe, simple methods described above.

- **Indirect pressure:** If direct pressure is not possible to apply or bleeding is not stopped after its application, then indirect pressure may be applied to a "pressure point", where a main artery runs close to a bone. Pressure at these points will cut off the blood supply to the limb. It must not be applied for longer than 10 minutes. Various Pressure Points to Control Bleeding, includes the following (Fig. 27.16),
- For a wound of the scalp or temple, compress the temporal artery.
- For a wound of the lower face (below the eyes), apply pressure to the facial artery along the lower border of the mandible.
- For a neck wound, compress the wound site. Do not compress the carotid artery, as this could cause stroke.

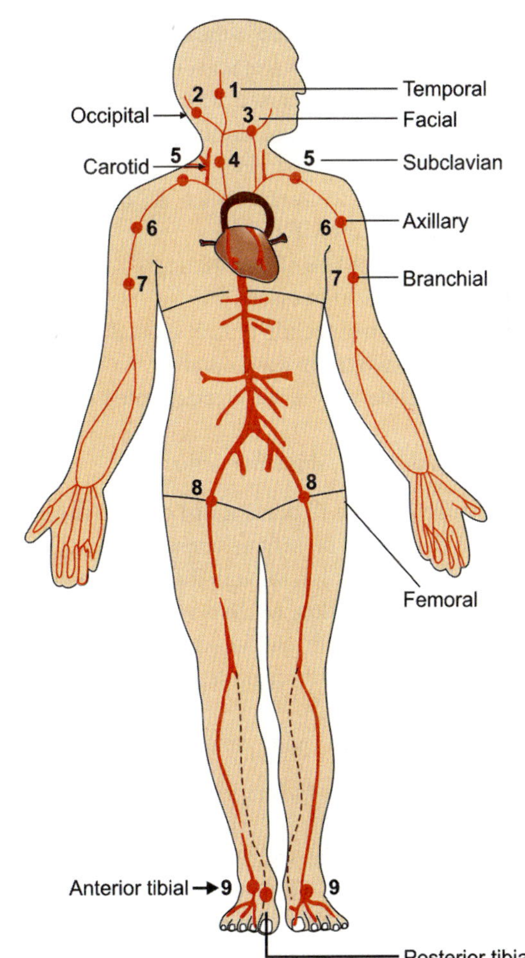

Figure 27.16: Arteries pressure points

- For a shoulder wound or hemorrhage of the upper arm, compress the sub clavian artery against the clavicle.
- For a wound of the lower part of the upper arm or of the elbow, press the brachial artery against the humerus.
- For foot wounds, compress the entire network of arteries in the ankle.
- For a wound of the lower arm, press the ulnar and radial arteries at the antefubital fossa.
- For thigh wounds, apply great pressure to the femoral artery against the femur.
- For wounds of the lower leg, apply pressure to the popliteal artery, behind the knee.

The loss of large amount of blood will lead to pallor, weakness, collapse, unconsciousness and head. In such cases, after control of haemorrhage, it is necessary at the earliest opportunity to replace by transfusion the blood which has been lost. Immediately the victim should be shifted where facilities are available to save victim.

Prevention of Wounds Infection

There are two ways by which germs can enter wounds:
- Some germs may be embedded in the wound by the knife, bullet, rusty nail or other object which causes the injury
- Some germs may be implanted in the wound after the original injury. These come from two main sources:
  (a) The nose and throat of person who breath, talk, cough or sneeze into the wound (i.e. 'droplet infection')
  (b) The skin of careless first aiders, nurses or doctors who allow their fingers to enter or touch the wound
  The Signs of Infection will includes:
- Wound which do not heal within 48 hours
- Increasing pain and soreness
- Swelling, redness and feeling of heat around the injury
- Pus within or oozing from the wound
- Swelling and tenderness of the glands in the neck, armpit or groin
- Fever, sweating, thirst, shivering, lethargy.

Dangers of Infection: It will occur if dirt or dead tissue remain in the wound there may be serious consequences. Germs can multiply and spread infection through the body (septicemia) or tetanus infection may develop, which is very dangerous. Tetanus germs are carried in the air and in soil as spores. They may release a toxin that spreads through the nervous system causing muscle spasms and paralysis.

Prevention of Infection can be obtained by:

1. *Removal of germs embedded in wound at the time of injury:* Complete removal of these embedded germs can be accomplished only by the surgeon, who with the help of anesthesia opens the wound widely and washes it out thoroughly. However, when circumstances permit it to be done promptly, as in many peace-time accidents, the first aider may help by washing out the wound with a large quantity of sterile water.

2. *Protection of wound against germs implanted after the injury:* This is the main objective of first aid in relation to wound infection. Cover the wound as quickly as possible with a sterile or clean dressing and keep it covered.

Before applying the dressing
 (i) If possible, wash your hands carefully
 (ii) It is also advisable, under ideal circumstances, to wash off the skin around the wound with soap and warm water.

While applying the dressing
 (i) Do not breathe, talk, cough or sneeze into or over the wound. Either cover your mouth and nose with a 'mask' (e.g. clean handkerchief), or keep your face turned slightly away from the wound until the dressing is in place.
 (ii) Keep fingers out of the wound
 (iii) Do not touch the surface of the dressing which will be placed next to the wound

3. *Giving Tetanus toxoid:* Tetanus is difficult to treat, but can be prevented by immunization, which is a part of baby's vaccination programme. Adults should receive boosters every ten years. Always ask a casualty when he or she last had a tetanus injection and accordingly seek medical advice, it has to be given after injury.

Comfort of the victim can be provided in following manner:
- After bandaging, keep the injured part in a position of comfort
- If the head is injured, make the patient lie down with his head resting upon a pillow or cushion covered with a clean towel.
- If the forearm is injured, bring it across in front of the chest and support it in a sling
- If the leg be wounded, it may be supported upon a cushion or blanket
- In wounds of the chest, raise the head and shoulders until the patient is able to breathe comfortably
- If the abdomen be wounded, place the patient on his back with his knees drawn up.

B. Internal Hemorrhage

This is the bleeding within one of the cavities of the body, which is not visible, such as cerebral haemorrhage, or bleeding in peritoneal or chest cavity. This is usually due to head injuries or injuries to chest and abdomen in traffic accidents, falls, collapse of building or houses. Initially there are no signs of internal bleeding but slowly a large amount of blood may be lost from the circulation ultimately resulting into a serious situation, like shock and damaging pressure on lungs or brain. Internal bleeding is indicative, when shock develops without obvious blood loss. There may be blood at body orifices, either fresh or mixed with the contents of injured organs.

Generally Signs and Symptoms of internal haemmorrhage will be:
- The skin is cold and clammy
- Face pale and pinched
- Subnormal temperature
- Eyes sunken

Table 27.1: Sites, Appearance and Causes of Haemmorrhage

Site	Appearance	Cause
Mouth	Bright red, frothy, coughed-up blood (haemoptysis). Vomited blood (haematemesis), possibly dark reddish-brown and resembling coffee grounds	Bleeding in the lungs Bleeding within the digestive system
Ear	Fresh, bright-red blood Thin, watery blood	Injury to the inner ear; perforated ear drum Leakage of cerebrospinal fluid following head injury
Nose	Fresh, bright-red blood Thin, watery blood	Ruptured blood vessel in the nostril Leakage of cerebrospinal fluid following head injury
Anus	Fresh, bright-red blood Black, tarry offensive-smelling stool (melaena).	Injury to the anus or lower bowel. Injury to the upper bowel
Urethra	Urine with a red or smoky appearance (haematuria)	Bleeding from the bladder or kidneys
Vagina	Either fresh or dark blood	Menstruation, miscarriage, disease of, or injury to the vagina or womb

- Breathing deep and sighing
- Pulse rapid, weak and irregular
- Blood pressure is low
- Patient feels thirsty, anxious, worried
- Fainting and dizziness occurs

In addition the sites, appearance and possible causes of hemorrhage are shown in Table 27.1.

The following first aid measures should be taken for internal hemmorrhage:

- Reassure the patient
- Place the casualty in flat position with feet raised
- Keep the casualty warm and at complete rest
- Check and record breathing, pulse and level of response every 10 minutes
- Do not give food or drinks by mouth
- Transport the casualty to hosptal as quickly as possible

First Aid Measures in Minor Wounds

Minor bleeding is easily controlled by pressure and elevation. A small adhesive dressing is normally adequate. If bleeding does not stop, then seek medical help.

- Wash your hands thoroughly in soap and warm water
- Avoid touching the wound with your fingers. (Use disposable gloves, if possible).
- Don't talk, cough, sneeze over the wound or dressing
- If the wound is dirty, clean it by rinsing lightly under running water from tap
- Pat gently dry with a sterile swab
- Temporarily cover the wound with sterile gauze. Clean the skin around it with soap and water. Use new swab for each stroke
- Pat dry, then cover the wound with an adhesive dressing (plaster)

Large foreign bodies, such as fragments of glass or metal, if projecting from the wound, may be gently removed, provided this can be done without putting fingers into the wound. If the foreign body is deeply embedded or there is any difficulty in removing it, leave this alone. Put a sterile gauze, cotton pad and bandage lightly. Send the patient to a doctor.

It should be emphasized that 'antiseptics' are almost completely ineffective in killing or removing germs embedded in a wound. The chief result of introducing these strong chemicals into or on a wound.

For a small household scratch, antibiotic creams like Soframycin, Furacin or antiseptic solutions like Dettol or Savlon can be used but not for large wounds.

Contusion is wound in which the deep tissues are torn without the overlying skin being broken. Bleeding beneath the skin leads to the 'black and blue' colour changes. A dressing is not necessary as germs cannot penetrate the intact skin. Ice packs or cold compresses, if promptly applied, may diminish the amount of bleeding and relieve the pain.

First Aid Measures in Major Wounds

Many serious and major wounds do not bleed profusely, e.g. chest wounds, wounds to the abdomen, eye wounds, etc. but may cause considerable internal damage.

(i) Chest wound: The heart and lungs and the major blood vessels around them, lie within the chest. A penetrating wound may cause severe internal damage. The lungs are subject to injury as the air may enter the pleural space and exert pressure on the lungs for its subsequent collapse.

The Signs and Symptoms

- Breathing difficult and painful
- Signs of shock
- Frothy blood on coughing
- Mouth, nails and skin appears blue
- Blood bubbles out of the wound

The first aid measures for chest wound includes the following:

- Cover the open wound by palm of your hand
- Cover the wound by sterile dressing or pad, then cover the pad by plastic wrap, which should be non porous. Aluminium foil or plastic covering of a cigarette pack are also useful

- The covering is sealed along the edges by adhesive tapes. If a gauze dressing is used, it is covered with petroleum jelly to make it air tight
- Support a conscious casualty in a comfortable position, inclined towards the injured side
- If the casualty becomes unconscious, check pulse, breathing and place him in the recovery position lying on the injured side.
- Send for doctor or ambulance or arrange stretcher for transportation

(ii) Abdominal wound: Wounds which penetrate the abdominal wall may damage stomach or bowels. Hence, give *nothing to eat or drink*. In such cases. Dress the wound and adjust the patients position so that the wound does not gape e.g., if the wound is horizontal, place him on his back with heads and shoulders raised and a pillow under his knees. Send to hospital on stretcher.

If the intestines have come out:
- Cover with clean pads
- Don't give anything to eat or drink
- Obtain medical aid; till then give casualty rest in bed
- He has to be transported to a hospital. There may be severer haemorrhage when patients pulse becomes feeble and he goes in shock. In that case he should be sent to hospital as a priority case.

If there is an open abdominal wound, evisceration of abdominal organs may occur, with resultant drying and subsequent necrosis of the organs. Any abdominal organs lying outside the abdominal cavity must therefore be kept moist. If sterile dressings and sterile water are not available, it is preferable to cover the organs with a clean moist cloth and risk infection than to risk necrosis and loss of tissue.

(iii) Eye injuries: These are frequently a bit of dust or a speck of material lodges on the eye surface. In such cases. Do not rub either eyes. Never attempt to remove the material with a toothpick, match or any other instrument and Never attempt the eye until you have washed your hands thoroughly.

It is better to send the injured person to the doctor by keeping sterile pads over both the eyes and putting a bandage tightly. The uninjured eye is also to be covered, for its movement also moves the other eye even though that may be bandaged and hence aggravates the injury in the other eye.

If you are careful and knowledgeable, you may succeed in removing a speck of material by using the *following method:*
- Pull down the lower eyelid to see whether the body lies on the undersurface if the lid. If it does, it can be lifted off gently by touching it with the corner of a clean cloth.
- Grasp the lashes of the upper eyelid gently between thumb and forefinger. Have the patient look upward, and pull the upper eyelid forward and downward over the lower lid. If this measure does not help, do not persist in trying it.
- In case of falling of harmful chemical, or hot oil or floating grit, lay the casualty in her back supporting her head. Irrigate

the eye with water. Tilt the head to drain water away from the face.
- *Do not irrigate an eye with a wound or a foreign body lodged or sticked to the eyeball.*
- Red eyes sometimes indicate that a bit of material has been present in the eye, or it may mean that an infection is present. In either case the first aider should not try to treat the eye.

(iv) Amputation: An injury may cause a part of limb or a limb partially or completely severed. Now-a-days it is possible to "re-plant" the amputated part. So, the sooner the casualty and amputated part reach hospital it is better. The objects of first aider must be to minimize blood loss and preservation of amputated part and *Care of the victim includes the* Control bleeding and raise the injured part and Apply a sterile dressing or clean pad secured with a bandage

Care of the Amputated Part includes the following:
- Wrap the severed part in kitchen film or a polythene bag
- Wrap again in gauze or soft fabric, then place the package in another container filled with crushed ice. Chilling will help preservation
- Do not wash severed part nor allow its direct contact with ice
- Do not use a tourniquet
- Mark the time of injury and casualty's name to be handed personally to the doctor

First Aid Measures for Bleeding from Special Parts
(i) Skull: As a result of head injury, blood and blood mixed brain fluid (cerebrospinal fluid) may flow out of the nose, ear or mouth. In this condition please do the following:
- Lay the patient on the affected side
- Do not pack ear or nose, but clean them dry and put a dressing lightly
- Arrange for transportation to a hospital

(ii) Scalp: The scalp has a rich blood supply and when it is damaged, it bleeds profusely. It often makes injury appear more serious than it really is. However examine the casualty carefully, as sometimes injury may be serious due to skull fracture or head injury. In such situation do the following:
- Press down directly upon the scalp near the edge of the wound, on the side from which the bleeding proceeds.
- A large pad and bandage will control bleeding till the patient is sent to a hospital
- Secure the dressing using a triangular bandage. If bleeding persists, re-apply pressure on pad.

(iii) Nose: Nose bleeds appears unpleasant but can sometimes be dangerous, if blood loss is excessive. If nosebleed follows a head injury, the blood may appear thin and watery. This is serious, as it indicates that cerebrospinal fluid is leading from around the brain. *The Causes of bleeding from nose may be:*
- Picking out crusts and hair
- Blowing the nose
- High blood pressure
- Bleeding disorders

- In summer – usually no cause
- Injury to the bones of the nose
- Injury to front of the head
- Common cold and other infections

If the bleeding from the nose is not because of fracture of bones nose or skull, then proper first aid will control the bleeding in 10-15 minutes. In such condition following action is needed.

- Let the patient sit up, with head slightly bent forwards
- Press the nostrils together, holding the pressure for several minutes
- Apply a towel, wet with cold water or cracked ice, over the nose, face, forehead, and at the back of the neck
- Loosen clothing at neck
- Do not let the patient talk, cough, laugh, walk about, or blow the nose. Activity and excitement may increase the bleeding or cause it to restart.
- Immediately take a narrow strim of gauze and crowd a small portion at a time into a nostril, pushing well into nose with a pencil or penholder until a tight plug is produced. Keep plug in nose for several hours, and when bleeding has stopped, remove it carefully so as not to renew bleeding.
- Call a physician, if bleeding is excessive or continuous.

Nose care after a nose bleed includes

- Do not pick your nose or insert anything into it, (such as cotton swabs, handkerchiefs). Do not blow your nose forcefully.
- If you must sneeze, expel the sneeze through your open mouth
- Do not stop or exert. When you lie down, elevate your head using two or three pillows
- On the second day put a little petroleum jelly inside your nostrils to soften the crusts that form after a nose bleed. Continue it for 7 days
- Avoid hot drinks and alcoholic beverages for 4 days
- If you are constipated, take a laxative. Avoid straining.
- Do not smoke or take aspirin for 5 days

(iv) Ears: Bleeding from the ears is mainly because of cuts or injury to external ear as this is very vascular. Bleeding from inside the ear is usually because of fracture of skull, injury to ear drum or ear canal or infection inside. The casualty may experience a sharp pain as the eardrum ruptures, followed by earache and deafness. If bleeding follows a head injury the blood may appear thin and watery which is very serious condition. The *Causes of bleeding from ears may be,*

- Foreign body in the ear
- A blow to the side of the head
- Explosion

In such condition following actions are needed.

- If the bleeding is from external ear, apply pressure with a sterile gauze over the wound for 10 minutes. This will usually stop the bleeding. Apply bandage.
- If the bleeding is from inside, never pack the ear. This will collect the blood inside, which later on may get infected.
- Do not put any medicine in the ear, unless under supervision of a doctor.

- Lay the patient on the side of the bleeding ear, so that blood comes out easily and does not collect inside.

(v) Mouth: Cuts to the tongue, lips or lining of the mouth range from minor injuries to more serious wounds. The cause is usually the casualty's own teeth, following a blow or fall. Bleeding may be profuse and appear alarming. Bleeding from a tooth socket may be the result of accidental loss of a tooth, or dental extraction. The following action is needed in such condition.

- Sit the casualty down, with her head forward and inclined towards the injured side, to allow blood to drain.
- To control the bleeding, place a gauze dressing pad over the wound and ask the casualty to squeeze it between her finger and thumb, maintaining the pressure for 10 minutes.
- If the bleeding is from a tooth socket, place a pad of gauze, thick enough to prevent the casualty's teeth from meeting when he bites across the socket and tell him to bite on it.
- If bleeding persists, replace the pad with a fresh one. Tell the casualty to let any escaping blood dribble; if swallowed, it may induce vomiting.
- Advise the casualty to avoid hot drinks for 12 hours.

If the wound is large, or if bleeding persists beyond 30 minutes or recurs seek medical or dental advice.

(vi) Gums: After tooth extraction, bleeding from tooth socket may occur immediately or after a few hours. It needs following actions.

- Rinse mouth with water or saline
- Place a thick cotton wool ball in the socket and ask him to bite on it
- Send the patient to a dentist or doctor.

(vii) Temple: Press with the thumb upon the bone just in front of the ear to compress the artery. Make a permanent compress by means of a piece of plain gauze folded in the form of a pad, and hold it in place with a roller or triangular bandage.

(viii) Face: Press firmly against the jaw bone with thumb. Control bleeding of the check and lips by passing the thumb into the patients mouth and grasping the cheek, just below the wound, between the thumb and the fingers, thus compressing the artery leading to the wound. Bind a folded piece of gauze as a permanent pad compress.

(ix) Neck: Stab wounds, cut throat or other wounds of this region require prompt attention. Without an instants delay, grasp the patient neck. Put the thumb into the wound and press the wounded vessels straight back against the spine and not against the wind pipe. Continue the thumb pressure until assistance arrives.

(x) Palm: There is usually severe bleeding from injures to the palm, as there are many blood vessels present. It needs following methods.

- Raise the arm above the head or support it in a triangular sling.
- Grasp the wrist with your hand tightly for 10 to 15 minutes

- Have the patient grasp some small, hard object like a ball, covered with sterile gauze. The pressure may be made permanent by binding the hand firmly while in this position.

(xi) Fingers: Raise the arm above the head. Apply pressure to the hand or wrist binding with a pad and bandage. No violent pressure.

(xii) Lungs: When bleeding occurs from lungs, blood is bright red, sometimes light coffee colour. It needs following measures.
- Lay the patient down with head and shoulders raised.
- Summon a physician immediately.
- Keep patient absolutely quiet, cool, applying cold, wet clothes to the chest.
- Give finely chopped ice.

(xiii) Stomach: The colour of blood is dark coffee colour. It needs following measures.
- Give ice water or broken ice with a teaspoonful of vinegar repeating the dose at intervals
- Summon a physician at once.

(xiv) Tongue: If severe, apply pressure as for bleeding of the arteries of the neck.
- Let the patient suck ice or sip very hot water

(xv) Thigh: Thigh wounds require prompt attention needs following measures.

Exert pressure upon the inner surface of the thigh just below the groin, or where the artery of the thigh (femoral artery) comes out of the body, about two-thirds of the way from the knee to the hip joint.

To control the artery, place a knotted cloth or a large round stone in the groin doubling the leg back on the thigh; press the thigh up against the abdomen; finally hold it there with a bandage.

A piece of elastic tubing (inner tube of an automobile tyre) or a pair of suspenders passed around the limb several times, stretched at each turning and made tight, is often effective. Draw only tight enough to control bleeding. Loosen every 20 minutes and retighten if bleeding is not checked.

(xvi) Varicose veins: Veins in the legs keep the blood flowing towards the heart. If these deteriorate, blood collects behind them, causing distension. It can burst by gentle knock and bleed profusely. If bleeding is not controlled, shock may develop. It needs following measures.

Lay the casualty on her back and raise the injured leg as high as possible. This may reduce or stop the bleeding.

Expose the site of the bleeding and apply firm direct pressure over a sterile dressing or clean pad, or with your fingers, until bleeding is controlled.

Remove garters or stockings that may be obstructing blood flow back to the heart.

Shock and its First Aid Measures

Shock results from the failure of the cardiovascular system to provide sufficient blood circulation, (oxygen) to all parts of the body. To maintain circulatory homeostasis the following mechanisms must be present.
- A functioning of heart to circulate blood
- A sufficient amount of blood volume
- The capability of the vascular system, accommodating blood flow to the capillaries and returning to the right side of the heart, inability of the body to compensate for failure of one or more of these mechanism results in shock.

Causes of Shock

The most common causes of shock are as follows:
- Severe loss of blood
- Intense pain
- Extensive trauma
- Burns
- Poisoning
- Emotional stress or intense emotion
- Extreme heat and cold
- Electrical shock
- Allergic reactions
- A sudden or severe illness

Types of Shock

Shock is classified according to cause as given below:

Hypovolemic shock: It is also known as hemorrhagic shock. It is caused by decrease in fluid volume from bleeding, prolonged vomiting or diarrhea, or loss of fluid surgery or trauma.

Cardiogenic shock: It results from poor heart function and is caused by various cardiovascular abnormalities. The heart is unable to maintain sufficient blood pressure to all parts of the body.

Neurogenic shock: It is caused by failure of the nervous system to maintain a normal contraction of the blood vessels.

Septic shock: It results from the severe infection. The microorganism causes loss of fluid through the blood vessel wall.

Psychogenic shock: It is caused by nervous system reactions to an emotional stimulus. The blood vessels dilate temporarily, decreasing blood flow to the brain which result in unconsciousness or syncope.

Anaphylactic shock: Anaphylactic results from a sudden severe, allergic body reaction to a foreign substance.

The nurse must be aware of the following points when assessing the victims of shock.

Level of consciousness: The victim may experience changes in behavior, restlessness, anxiety, confusion, syncope and agitation. As the condition worsens, the victim becomes more lethargic, unconscious and death can result.

Skin changes: The skin becomes cool, pale. As shock progresses cynosis develops over the lips and nailbeds.

Cardiovascular blood pressure: Initially the blood pressure may be normal, but as shock progresses there is steady decrease in blood pressure.

Pulse: The pulse rate usually increases in all types of shock. It also becomes weak and thready in character.

Respiration: Respiratory rate increases, respiration may also be shallow, rapid, labored or irregular as result of vasoconstriction in the lungs, causing fluid accumulation.

Urinary output: With decreased circulation of fluid volume the amount of urinary output is decreased (oliguria).

Neuromuscular changes: Decreased oxygen to the tissues results in weakness and /or tremors of the arms and legs. Eyelids close and pupils dilate.

Gastrointestinal changes: Because of loss of fluid and fluids shift, the victim will complain of thirst, nausea, vomiting and dry mucous membranes may also be present.

The nurse must immediately treat the cause of shock.
- Take measures to establish an airway
- Take steps to control bleeding if it is present
- Take steps to reduce pain
- Appropriate positioning of victim in shock determined by the type and extent of injuries as follows:
  - The victim should lie flat with the head slightly lower than the rest of the body, unless the victim is sustained head and chest injuries,
  - If the victim is unconscious, with vomiting and bleeding around the nose and mouth he should be positioned on the side to allow the airway to clear and encourage drainage.
  - The head and shoulder should be elevated if the victim is having difficulty in breathing
  - If neck or spinal injuries suspected, the victim just not be moved unless it is necessary to prevent further injury.
  - Maintain the victims body temperature keeping him and dry by placing blankets or other coverings under the victim to prevent heat loss on surfaces
  - The victim should be covered with available material. Overblanket covering should be avoided.
  - The victim should not be given anything to eat or drink because internal injuries may be present and needs urgent surgical intervention and the patient may aspirate the fluid.
  - A moistened cloth will relieve dry mouth or mucous membrane (IV fluids may be given if he is in serious condition).
- Take measures to relieve pain
- Give emotional support and reassurance
- Give medication as per standing instructions or prescribed by the physician

When a person is badly injured, he may develop a serious condition called shock. In shock cases, the blood flow in the body is disturbed, even in parts, distant from the injury. The brain does not get enough blood. Thinking is difficult, digestion of food is slowed, and all body processes are at a low level.

Unless, the injured person receives proper care, he may die of shock, or his recovery may be greatly delayed.

True shock will be seen in following conditions:
 (i) Severe bleeding
  - Shock is produced with loss of blood
  - It may develop at once or be delayed
  - Bleeding may be seen outside when coming out of a cut artery or the tear of a varicose vein; or it may be inside, for example, bleeding into the chest or abdominal cavity
  - The faster the loss of blood, faster will be onset of shock. But beware of slow loss of blood, which will appear to be simple at first but later may become very serious.
 (ii) *Severe burn:* When extensive i.e., when more than half the skin surface is affected
 (iii) *Heart attacks:* When the blood supply to the heart is obstructed
 (iv) *Abdominal emergencies:* Like burst appendix, perforated peptic ulcer, intestinal obstruction etc.
 (v) *Crush injuries:* As in collapsed buildings, explosion etc.
 (vi) *Loss of body fluid:* Due to excess of vomiting, diarrhea, dysentery etc.
 (vii) *Bacterial infections:* Discharge of toxins (poisons) into the blood caused by bacteria.
 (viii) *Electric current:* By touching open electric wires
  The Signs and Symptoms of Shock will includes the following:
- Cool, clammy skin
- Face and limbs – pale.
- Weak, rapid pulse
- Vomiting and retching
- Sighing or irregular breathing
- Perspiration with pale skin
- Half opened eyelids
- Dilated pupils
- Dullness of mind, apathy, lethargy
- Blurring of vision
- Oliguria or anuria

Whenever you get an opportunity to give first aid to a seriously injured person, always try t o prevent shock. Act immediately. Do not wait for shock to appear.
- *Make the victim lie down at once* with his head level with or lower than the rest of his body. However, it his breathing in this position is difficult because of chest injuries, raise the head and shoulders by placing pillows under them
- *Cover him properly:* Carefully place a blanket under him. If the weather is not hot, place a coat or blanket over him. If the weather is very cold, use several blankets. But do not make him sweat; too much covering is undesirable. Use bottles of hot water, rubber water bags, hot bricks, blankets etc., in fact anything hot and convenient. Be careful that applications are not too hot. Apply heat along inner sides of arms and legs. Do not apply heat to the head. Do not give hot drinks in brain injuries nor in severe bleeding. Do not give whisky, brandy or other liquors. If patient is able to swallow, one hold

teaspoonful of aromatic spirit of ammonia in ½ cup of water every 15 minutes for not more than 4 doses be given. In summer cold water may be given. Ordinarily hot water bottles or electric heating pads should not be used on accident victims. However, they may be used if the weather is very cold and there are not enough blankets. The best places to use them are under the armpits or about the chest. To prevent burning the skin, they should be only slightly warmer than body temperature.

- *Look for any serious bleeding or cause of severe pain:* Try to control bleeding a described previously. Do not disturb the injured person unnecessarily. Try to avoid measures that would cause more pain.
- *Loosen tight clothing, but do not remove them.*
- *In cases of injuries to abdomen and chest,* give nothing by mouth for he may require an operation later on
- *Under no circumstances* fluids be given by mouth to an unconscious casualty
- Do not let a crows gather round the patient
- Do not let him see his own injuries
- Reassure the casualty if he is conscious
- Arrange for transportation to a hospital or institution on a priority basis.

Anaphylactic Shock

This is a severe body response to allergic substance or protein. Allergic substance on its introduction into the body causes sudden release of histamine into the blood stream and allows blood plasma to flow through capillary walls, thus decreasing blood flow to the heart, giving rise to circulatory failure. Its onset is sudden. A person under such shock stands good chances of survival if he receives treatment within 20 minutes of its onset or else he dies. The *Causes of anaphylactic shock may be:*

- Pollen
- Particular food
- Wasp sting, bee sting
- Drugs like penicillin, sulpha, iron, serum etc.

The Signs and Symptoms of anaphylactic shock will be:

- Nausea and vomiting
- Diarrhea, coughing
- Anxiety
- Widespread red, blotchy skin eruption
- Swelling of the face and neck
- Rapid pulse
- Wheezing and gasping for air

The victim urgently needs oxygen and a life saving injection of adrenaline. There is no particular first aid measure, except assisting in breathing and minimizing shock till the doctor arrives. Help a conscious victim sit up in the position which relieves any breathing difficulty. If he becomes unconscious, check breathing and pulse and resuscitate if necessary.

Burns and its First Aid Measures

Burns are due to dry heat (including friction), where as scalds are due to wet heat. Burns and scalds are considered together as burns as they produce the severe type of injury. It is more important that burns and scalds are treated correctly so as to limit the effects of the injury and to prevent possible long-term scarring.

Causes of Burns and Scalds

(i) *Burns* are caused by the following:

- Fire, explosions of pressure stoves, petrol burns, hot metals, etc.
- Electricity
- Corrosive chemicals, e.g. strong acids and strong alkalis

Burns are wounds caused by excessive exposure of the body to heat, such as by flame, hot liquids, chemicals, electricity or radiation. Flame and scalding water are the two most common causes of burns. The person who has sustained a major burn is critically ill. The body systems are threatened not only from physiologic and psychologic effects of the burn, but also from other physical trauma that may occur simultaneously. Recovery is a slow progress. However the principles of burn care remain the same regardless of causes.

The Causes of Burns also classified as given below:

Dry heat: Direct contact with a flame or hot object

Scalds: Moist heat such as boiling water, steam or hot tea and coffee

Friction: Contact with a moving wheel, rope, wire or asphalt

Chemical: Acids and alkalies

Electrical: Overexposure to sun and radiant heat sources

(ii) *Scalds* are caused by the following:

- Boiling water, steam, hot oil, etc.

  The extent of injury caused by burns and scalds depends on the following two factors:

- The duration of contact between the skin and the substance causing injury
- The strength of the substance. This is particularly important when chemicals and electric current are the causes of injury

  Certain areas of the body are of special concern when burns occur, due to high potential for loss of function. Burns of the face, eyes, ears, neck, hands or feet and genitals are major. Damage to the tracheobronchial tree through heat and smoke inhalation is also a major problem.

Characteristics of Burn Injuries

Severity of a burn injury is determined by five factors:

1. Surface area of body burned
2. Depth of tissue damage

3. Age of casualty
4. Past medical history
5. Part of body burned

Surface Area of the Body Burned (Fig. 27.17)

A quick approximate estimate of the percentage of body surface burned may be made using the Rule of Nines. The rule of Nines, is useful for adult patients only and should not be used for children under age of 15 years. The body is divided into areas, each of which represents 9%. The apportionment is as follows: the whole of the upper limb is 9%, a thigh 9%, a leg (below the knee) 9%, the posterior chest 9%, the abdomen 9%, the lower half of the back (lumbar and sacral regions) 9%, the head and neck 9%, and the perineum 1%. If the burns are scattered, the palm of the patients hand may be taken to represent 1% of his or her total body surface area.

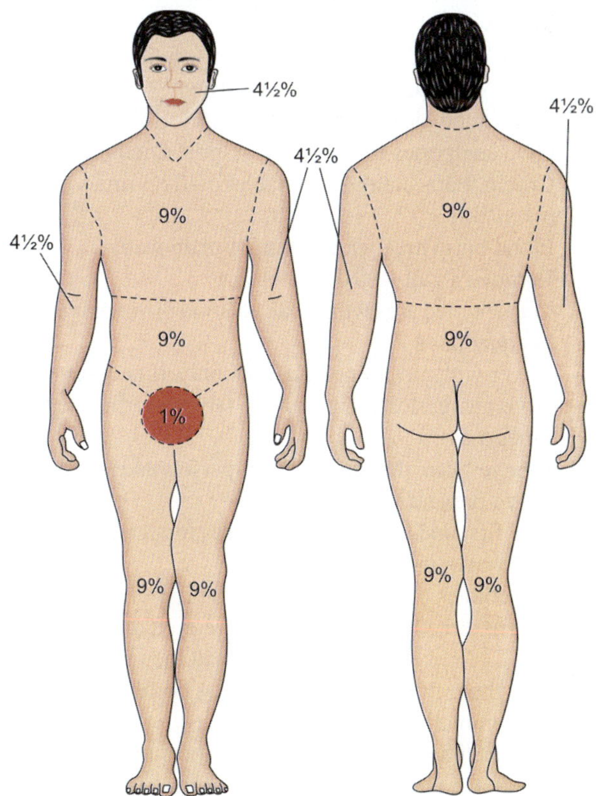

Figure 27.17: Rule of nines, used for estimating the percentage of body surface burned

If approximately 10% or more of the body surface of a child or 15% or more of that of an adult is burned, the injury is considered to be major burn. The patient requires hospitalization and fluid replacement to prevent shock.

Classification of Burns

The depth of burn is the result of two factors:
1. Temperature of burning agent
2. Duration of exposure.
   It is classified as:
1. First-degree or superficial partial thickness burn

2. Second degree or deep partial thickness burn
3. Third degree or full thickness burn

A *superficial partial-thickness* burn involves total destruction of the epidermis and very minor involvement of the dermal layers and appendages. Healing usually occurs within 7-10 days.

A *deep partial-thickness* burn involves total destruction of the epidermis and major involvement of upper dermal layers only. Lower dermal layers remain intact. Healing usually occurs within 14-21 days.

A *full-thickness* burn involves total damage to the epidermis and major damage to both upper and lower dermal layers. Subcutaneous tissue, muscle and bone may also be involved. Healing by the formation of normal epithelial tissue cannot occur, given the extensive damage to the body's skin reproducing cells; skin grafting therefore is required (Table 27.2).

Table 27.2: Characteristics of Partial-thickness and Full-thickness Burns		
Factor	*Partial-thickness burn*	*Full-thickness burn*
Sensation	Normal or increased sensitivity to pain	Anesthetic to pain and temperature
Blisters	Large, thick-walled will usually increase in size	None or, if present, thin-walled and will not increase in size
Color	Red, will blanch with pressure and refill	White, brown, black or red. If red, will not blanch with pressure
Texture	Normal or firm	Firm and leathery

Person younger than 2 years and older than 50 have the highest incidence of morbidity and mortality. The severity of the burn increases with age. A person of 20 withstands a burn better than a 40 year old, and the patient of 40 has a much better chance of survival than a 60 years old, even though the percentage of body surface burned and the depth are the same. Infants and young children also tolerate burns less well than young adults.

Management of the Burns

The Management of the Burns has following Goals
- Stopping the burning process
- Reduce pain
- Providing life support (oxygenation, fluids nutrients)
- Preventing complications e.g., respiratory damage, infection, etc.
- Restoration of functions.

When we saw the Victim, first try to Stop the burning process. With flame burns the words "Stop – Drop – Roll – Cool" apply. Do not allow the person to run about, as it increases the severity. Lay him flat on the ground. Put any thick clothing which is available at that moment like a woolen coat, blanket, carpet, shawl etc., over him to extinguish flames. Do not try to remove the burning clothes or move the person unnecessarily for it will only increase the fire.

Immediately cool the burn wound. The burned area must be held or immersed under cool, running water or cool moistened towels or compresses can be applied. Cooling reduces pain and decrease the effect of heat-transmission through the tissues. Ice is avoided.

Burn blisters should be left untouched as they protect the wound from contamination.

All articles like, bangles, belt and boots which may become constricting agents after edema develops, should be removed.

Following cooling procedures, the burns should be covered with a clean sheet over which a blanket can be placed to maintain body heat, to avoid hypothermia.

Oils, ointments, lotions and other preparations should not be applied, and adherent clothing is not removed.

The burnt area is covered with a moist, sterile or clean material to exclude air. Cling film is an excellent first-aid dressing. Face burns may be covered with clean handkerchief.

Non-burn areas are covered with warm dry covers.

While awaiting transportation, the patient is kept at rest.

Give warm fluids to drink if casualty can take it, and restrict the movement and handling

In case of extensive burns if the person goes into shock then the fir st aid for shock be given and person rushed to a nearby hospital as fast as possible.

The resulting injuries range from mild to fatal. Major burns simply make outer layer of skin red and painful, but severe burns penetrate more deeply and can damage nerves, blood vessels, glands and even muscle and bone.

They can also cause life-threatening metabolic abnormalities and disrupt immune system.

Generally burns are classified as follows:

First degree: Which causes both pain and redness but no blisters and the damage are confined to the epidermis, the skin's tough outer layer. The skin is reddened, and may be swollen. This type of burn scalds painful superficial burns.

Second degree: Which produces blisters and damages both epidermis and the dermis, the inner layer of the skin. These can be quite painful but usually are not serious unless they cover large part of the body or blisters becomes infected.

Third degree: Which looks charred, white or blackened and extends to the tissue below the skin. The skin is burnt away and the damage ends into the muscle and fatty layers. There is a pale, waxy look to the burn with charred areas also possible. Because the nerve endings have been damaged, these types of burns/scalds involve little or no pain.

The severity of burns is determined by the percentage of the body surface they cover. To calculate the extent, usually you can use the "rule of line", which divides the front and back of the body into roughly equal segments, each representing 9 percent of the total body surface. Exceptions to the rule are the face and arms, which represent 4.5 percent and the groin which represents 1 percent.

1. *Burns, thermal*
   - Stop burning process, by extinguish flames
   - Cool burned area immediately with stream of cold water
   - Assess airway, breathing circulation and intervene with basic life support measured (see Subsection on Basic Life Support Techniques)
   - Remove clothing and cover burned area with sterile material or clean linen
   - Treat for shock
   - Advise immediate hospitalization
2. *Burns, acid*
   - Cool area with stream of plain water
   - Remove acid-soaked clothing
   - Bathe affected part with alkaline solution (1 tablespoon of baking soda and 1 liter of water)
   - Cover with clean linen material only, if necessary
   - Give analgesics for pain, e.g. Asprin, Diclophen, Brufen, Crocin, Paracetamol (one tablet orally 3 times a day)
3. *Burns, alkali*
   - Flood burnt area with stream of plain water
   - Remove alkali – soaked clothing
   - Wash burned area with weak solution of vinegar and water in equal parts
   - Cover with clean linen material only, if necessary
   - Give analgesics for pain, e.g. tablet asprin one tablet 3 times a day

For above burn, the nurse or any person take the following measures to prevent further damages

- For the first and second degree burns immerse the burn part in cool water, if possible.
- Apply cold packs to reduce pain and swelling but do not apply ice directly to the skin. Leave a cold pack on for 20 minutes, remove it for 10 minutes and then reapply it.
- Advice them to take tablets asprin or brufen to reduce pain and inflammation
- Allow the blisters to develop, do not puncture them, this increases the risk of infection.
- If blisters open on it s own wash the area gently with soap and water. Apply an antibiotic ointment and cover with sterile dressing
- Change the dressing at least once a day
- If any sign of infection or inflammation, refer to health center

For Third Degree Burns

The main effects of burns and scalds are shock, pain and sepsis, your efforts must be directed to deal with these conditions:
- Make the patient to lie down comfortably
- If possible gently remove any rings, watches or constricting clothing from the injured area before it starts to swell
- Keep him warm, give hot drinks, e.g. strong tea with plenty of swell

- Cover the burns area with an antibiotic ointment and sterile dressing and apply bandage
- Treat shock
- Transfer the patient to nearest healthcare center or hospital, where facilities are available to treat such cases as early as possible with fluids, electrolytes, antibiotics etc.

Wound Care in Burns

Initial burn wound care should be carried out in only those persons whose burns are of such limited extent that they do not require in-hospital care. Extensive burns are not to be cleaned. These are covered with dry dressing or cloth and sent to hospital. Any clothing which is sticking to the burnt area is gently removed after it has been cut with a clean sterile scissors from its surroundings. The burnt areas should be cleansed gently using a surgical soap or detergent, following which loose non-viable skin should be excised. Blisters less than 2 cm in diameter can be left intact, but larger ones commonly rupture, are easily infected and should be excised.

A topical antibiotic cream like silver-sulfa, soframycin, furacin or betadine can be applied in thin layer, and then dressed with gauze, over which are applied cotton pads. The burnt parts should be elevated with the help of a pillow sling to minimize edema formation, both before and during transportation.

- In case of minor burns and scalds at home which may occur while working in kitchen by hot oil, steam or flame, clean the area gently with clean water. Apply any antibiotic cream which is available at home and cover with dry dressing. Give warm drinks like tea or coffee.
- Sometimes drinking very hot tea, coffee or milk or swallowing very hot food in a hurry may burn the mucosa of mouth and throat. This leads to swelling of the tissues of the mouth and throat, which if very extensive may lead to obstruction of respiratory passage. In this take following measures:
- Ask the patient to sip ice cold water slowly or he can suck small piece of ice.
- Keep wet sponges (ice-cold) around the neck.
- If the condition does not improve, call a physician.

Inhalation of hot gases burn: The respiratory tract. These are serious burns with high rate of mortality. A mild case of respiratory tract burns will lead to sore throat, hoarseness, coughing. The severe cases of respiratory tract burn will be dysponic, with presence of gloss in chest and cyanosis. Such conscious patient are also overanxious due to fear of suffocation. First 24 hours are very critical in such cases. In such conditions following measures to be taken:

Remove the victim from source, allow fresh air circulation around the victim, release any tight clothing around the neck, apply cold compress to neck, give cold soothing drinks in mild cases. Severe burn cases, after initial assessment and first aid, are safely to the hospital at the earliest possible moment. These cases will require tracheotomy to out exudates. Postural drainage may be done if there is no other injury. Carefully administration of fluids is important, as such cases are likely to develop pulmonary edema.

Chemical Burns

Chemical burns produce localized irritations and tissue damage. Various acid and alkali preparations used in our daily life e.g., turpentine, petroleum products, strong antiseptics, detergents, etc. have first aid directions written on the container. The severity of burns caused by strong acids and alkalis depend on concentration amount and duration of contact of such chemical agents with the tissue. In such cases the following measures to be taken:

The very aim of our first-aid treatment is to wash the site with copious amount of plain water. In an acid burn, sodium bicarbonate is added to plain water. In case of whit e phosphorous the burnt part is totally submerged in water. Phosphorous particles are removed by forceps from the wound.

Contrary to the case in all other burn patients, immediate wound care takes priority in persons with chemical burns. Initial management consist of removal of the offending material from further Contact with body. The first thing to be done is to remove all clothing contaminated by the chemical agent (including under clothing, shoes and gloves). Then wash the burnt areas with plenty of water to dilute the agent and to reduce the heat content of injured tissue.

The application of neutralizing agents has no advantage over washing with plenty of plain water. It may even be harmful, since time may be lost in attempting to locate a specific neutralizing agent and the heat of reaction between the chemical agent and the neutralizing solution may increase tissue damage.

There are several chemical agents and the burns caused by them need more specific treatment. The common ones with their neutralizing solution are given below:

Agent	*Specific treatment*
• Hydrofluoric acid burn usually occurs in glass	• Irrigation of the wound with benzalkonium chloride solution
• Burns caused by phenol, which is a household commodity fro cleaning, widely used in hospitals	• After initial water lawage, wash with-polyethylene glycol/propylene glycol/glycerol
• White phosphorous	• A dilute solution of copper sulphate (0.5 to 1 percent)
• Anhydrous ammonia, mustard gas and chlorine	• Monitor the respiratory passages for they cause inhalation injuries

Chemical Burns of Eye: Burns by hot water or steam, hot ashes, exploding powder, caustics such as lime from white wash, or strong acids and alkalis may harm the eye considerably. Acid injuries in the eye are non-progressive, whereas alkali injuries are progressive.

First aid for chemical burn of the eye should be given as quickly as possible by thoroughly washing the face, eyelids and the eye for atleast 10-15 minutes. If the person is lying down, turn his head to the side, hold the eyelids open and pour water from the inner corner of the eye outwards. Make sure that chemical does not wash into the other eye. Cover the eye with a dry, clean protective dressing and bandage. Send the person to an eye specialist for further management.

Fires: If any person are caught amidst fire in a house or building, do not loose patience. Take decisions calmly and quickly. Try to find and emergency exit which is usually present in all modern constructions. Before opening any door or window make sure that it does not feel very hot on touch. For on opening it, hot smoke and vapours from other side harm his/her eyes and face may produce respiratory problems. Do not jump down from windows but try to seek help from the persons standing below. If person have to cross fire, wrap a blanket or a thick wet cloth around his/her face, hands and other exposed parts. In most cases of fire, carbon monoxide is produced which is higher than air and hence it rises and spreads upwards. Never walk erect but crawl along the floor.

- The victim must be prevented form panicking and rushing outside; any movement or breeze will aggravate the flames.
- Lay the victim down with the burning side uppermost, and extinguish the flames by dousing the victim with water or other non-flammable liquid. Alternatively, wrap the casualty tightly in a coat, curtain, blanket rug or other heavy fabric and lay him on the ground. This stops the flames.
- Over accidental fires of ghee, oil and petroleum substances do not pour water. It only aggravates the fire. Such fires can only be extinguished by sand, mud or soda. All petrol pumps should have provision of sand filled buckets for any such emergency.

Electrical Burns

The passage of electrical current through the body may stun the casualty and cause breathing and even the heart to stop. The current may cause burns both where it enters the body and where it leaves the body to "earth". It also causes muscle spasms that often prevent the casualty from letting go of an electric cable.

A person while indoors may receive an electric shock, perhaps fatal, by touching a bare electric wire, a wire of which the covering is worn, or an electric socket, especially if at the same time some part of his body touches a grounded metal object that is an object that directly, or by an extension, touches the ground. The dangers are greater if the floor or one's body is wet.

Out of doors one may be electrocuted by touching an electric wire or by flying a kite having a damp or metal string that touches an electric wire. Contact with high-voltage current found in power lines and overhead high-tension cables, is usually immediately fatal. Severe burns always result. The power must be cut off before casualty is approached.

Signs and Symptoms

There may be burns, either superficial or deep. It depend on the strength of the electric current causing the injuries.

There may be fatal paralysis of heart.

There may be sudden stoppage of breathing due to paralysis of muscles used in breathing.

Heart may continue to beat, while breathing has stopped. In this condition the face appear blue.

The following measures should be initiated:

1. Free the victim from the circuit immediately

Shut of the current if you can quickly do so. You can pull the main switch, or you can grasp the electric cord where it is not bare or wet and pull it form the socket. At the same time avoid grounded objects.

If you cannot use either method, try to remove the victim from contact with the wire by taking a dry wooden stick, dry towel, or the like, encircling the wire with it – do not touch the wire – and pull the wire from the victim or – less safe – use the cloth to pull the victim from the wire, being careful not to touch him directly until his contact with the wire is broken. The wire may cling to him; therefore, you may have to pull his body for some distance to break the contact.

Stand on dry insulating material such as a wooden box, a rubber or plastic mat, or thick pile of newspapers. Use a wooden chair or stool to push the casualty's limbs away from the source.

Out of doors the danger in rescue is very great. Even the ground near a fallen electric wire may be dangerous to walk on. Do not risk a rescue yourself. Call the electricity or the police or fire department instead.

2. Start artificial respiration

As soon as the victim is clear of live conductor, quickly feel with your finger in his mouth and throat and remove any foreign body (tobacco, false teeth etc.). Then begin artificial respiration. Do not delay to loosen the patients clothing; every moment of delay is serious.

Begin artificial respiration at once.

If possible, avoid laying the subject so that burned places are pressed.

Do not permit bystanders as they crowd about and shut off fresh air.

While this is being done, an assistant should loosen any tight clothing around the subjects neck, or waist.

Continue artificial respiration without interruption, until natural breathing is restored.

3. Other Measures

Clean and cover with a sterile dressing the burnt part and carry out other first aid measures as in burn.

There may be fracture of bones because of electric current itself or a person may fall down from a height after sustaining electric shock and have fractures. Give first aid as follows.

If a number of persons have been injured by electric shock, give priority to those breathing has stopped or pulse has disappeared. Take help of bystanders in all such cases.

Preventive Measures of Electrical Burns

Accidents due to electricity are of frequent occurrence. In handling electrical apparatus everyone should have before him the caution-safety first. The avoidance of electrical accidents is fairly easy to accomplish burnt the restoration of the injured patient is not easy.

- Rubber gloves should be worn by all workers handling the cables and wires, whether they are 'live' or not. The workman should satisfy himself before beginning work that the gloves are in good condition. Working on 'live' circuits especially alternating current, should be avoided as far as is practicable. A man should not work on wire or conductors of any kind with sleeves rolled up or arms exposed, nor should wires ever be handled while sitting or standing in a wet place.
- In handling any circuit over 11.5 volts known to be 'live', it is best if possible, to use only one hand. Keep the other in the pocket or behind the back. If the power has been cut off by opening a switch located at some distance from where the work is being done, a sign should be always placed on the switch stating that men are working on the line.
- No examinations, repairs or alterations of cables, wires, machines or other apparatus under high voltage, should be made. In any case such work should be done only by a trained electrician.

Lightning and its Protective Measures

During rains we often hear thunder and see lightning. This can lead to shock and death, if a person or an animal comes in contact with it. Although a first aider comes across such cases very rarely, but in case he has to face such a situation, then the management is same as for electric shock. In such cases following preventive measures helpful:

- Take shelter under those buildings and houses only; where there is an antenna or metal frame for earthing the lightning.
- During rains if you are in a jungle, away from a town or village, never take shelter under a tree, near an electricity pole or near a hillock. Do not stand in open or near fenced wiring.
- At such times take shelter in a ditch, under thickly grouped trees or near base of a hill, or inside a motor vehicle.

  The following points to be kept in mind to prevent Electric burns:
- Too many lamps or appliances on a single circuit may cause a fuse to blow; this is a danger signal. The cause (usually overloading) should always be corrected before you replace you replace the fuse.
- While correcting any fault, or changing wires, switch off the mains or take off fuse plugs
- An electric appliance, radio, or light switch should not be touched if your hands are wet or if you are standing on a wet floor (toilet).
- Electric cords should not run in door jambs or under rags. Constant closing of the door will damage the insulation, as will walking on the cord – when it is under a rug. Such damage will not be seen.
- An electric iron should never be left connected and unwatched even for a few minutes.
- Plugs should not be pulled out of sockets by the cord, but by pulling on the plug itself

- Cords with damaged insulation should be replaced immediately. Sharp corners of furniture; twisting or pulling on cords can cause protective insulation to wear out.
- Repairs or additions to wiring require services of a qualified electrician. Electrical jobs do not constitute "do-it-yourself" project.
- Electric appliances like washing machine, air conditioner, hot plate, power motor etc. should have earthing wire.

Back Pain and its First Aid Measures

The lower back and neck are the most common sites of muscle strain or ligament sprain. Back and neck strain can be caused by prolonged bending by lifting heavy weights, by strenuous exercise or by an awkward fall. Neck sprain may be caused by the *"whiplash"* effect produced in a car accident. Other causes of backache include kidney disease, pregnancy and menstruation. The Signs and Symptoms of back pain includes:-

- Dull or severe pain in the back or neck, increased by movement.
- Pain travels down any of the limbs possibly with tingling and numbness.
- Spasm of the muscles, causing the neck or back to be held rigid or bent.
- Tenderness in the muscles.
  The first aid measures are to be taken in such pain:
- Make the casualty lie down in the most comfortable position, either on the ground or on a firm mattress
- Advise the casualty to rest until the pain eases and send for doctor if pain persist
- If the pain is in the neck a "collar" may provide relief (Refer chapter of bandaging to learn "making of a collar").

  If back pain is complicated by muscle spasms, fever, headache, nausea, vomiting, impaired consciousness, incontinence or loss of sensation, the casualty needs urgent hospital treatment.

Fractures and their First Aid Measures

A fracture is a break o crack in a bone. Generally, considerable force is required to break a bone, except old or diseased bones which become brittle and can easily break.

Any type of fracture may be associated with an open wound, injury to adjoining muscles, blood vessels, nerves and organs.

Direct injury: The bone break at the application of force e.g., fracture of leg (Tibia) if the bumper of a motor car strikes the bone, fracture of heel bone (Calcaneum) on jumping from a height, fracture of skull bones on falling over head.

Indirect injury: The bone breaks away from the place of application of force e.g., collar bone fracture when the fall is on outstretched hand, thigh bone fracture on jumping from a height.

Forceful muscular contraction: When there is a forceful and violent contraction of a group of muscles it may lead to fracture of the bone on which they are acting. This occurs very rarely i.e. fracture of limb bones in athletes and fracture of ribs on violent coughing.

Spontaneous or pathological fracture: Bone may be the seat of a number of diseases, which weaken it, and make it liable to break even on very minor injuries. Such fractures are known as spontaneous or pathological fractures.

Types of Fracture (Fig. 27.18)

Simple or closed fracture: This is simply, a clean break or crack in a bone. The broken ends of the bone do not cut open the skin nor are visible outside.

Compound or open fracture: This is accompanied by a wound, the skin is broken and the bone may be exposed to contamination from the skin surface and the air.

Comminuted fracture: The bone is broken into several small pieces, which surrounds the main break.

Impacted fracture: Broken ends of the bone are driven or forcibly embedded into one another.

Depressed fracture: Broken parts of the none are driven inward e.g., in cases of a fracture of upper skull.

Green stick fracture: Bone is partially broken or bent. Common in children due to incomplete calcification of bone.

Pathological fracture: The pathological changes or carcinoma of the bone make the bone weak and brittle; it breaks spontaneously without or with a little force. Common in old age.

Complicated fracture: Along with the fracture there is associated injury to some internal structure like brain, spinal cord, liver, lungs, spleen, kidney, etc.

Signs and Symptoms of Fractures

- Pain and tenderness at the point of a fracture especially on movement
- Deformity of the part; alternation in its shape, length
- Irregularity of the bone often felt by passing of the hand over the skin, specially when it is near the skin
- Limitation of loss of power or function of the part and unnatural mobility

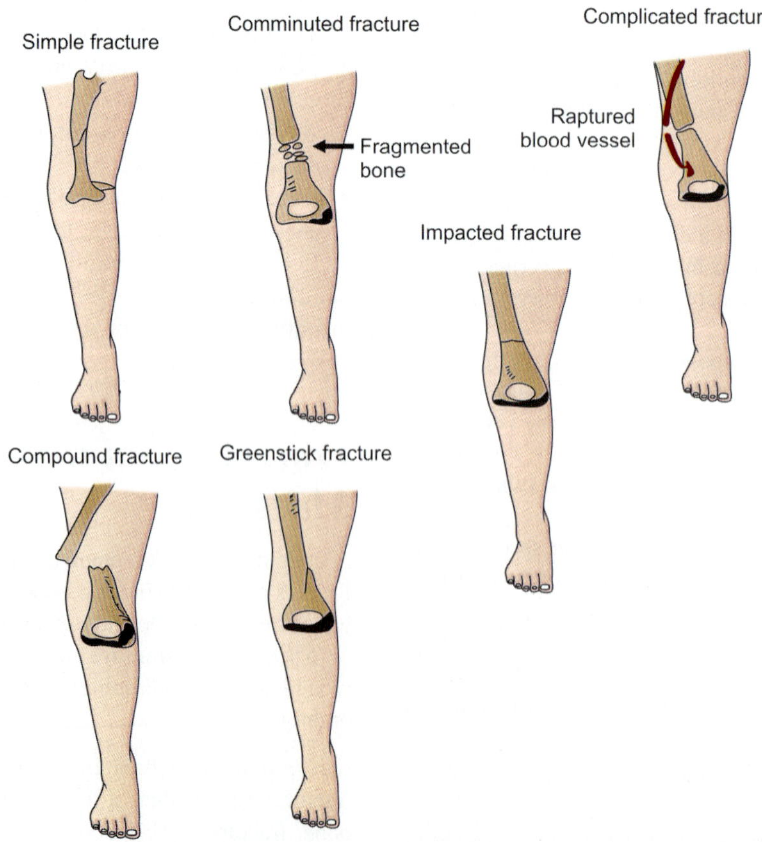

Figure 27.18: Types of fractures

- Crepitus – a crackling sound is heard or a sensation of grating is felt when the ends of broken bone are moved against each other. *But the sign should not be tried.*
- Ecchymosis

However the presence of the these signs vary with the site of fracture and the bone broken e.g., pain may be absent in simple fracture of small bones. Toes can be moved in case of fracture of tibia and fingers in the case of Colle's fracture. Fracture of bones like fibula will hardly impair function of the leg if it is broken.

First Aid Measures for the Fractures

When bones are broken, a good rule to follow is *"Do not permit motion of the broken ends or of the joints near the injury. This prevents pain and further damage."* The person wants help victim should keep in mind the following:

- For a closed or simple fracture place the limb in as natural a position as possible without causing discomfort to the victim. Handle very gently; avoid all unnecessary movements of the injured part.
- Since the danger of infection is very great in broken bones that break through skin (compound fractures), it is always better to get help from a doctor in caring for the injury. Clean the wound and the exposed bone and apply dressing.
- If there is an excessive bleeding from an open fracture, apply pressure dressing to control it. Give first aid for shock if it results from excessive bleeding.
- Never try to bring the bones to normal position or reduce the fracture.
- Before trying to move or carry a person with a broken bone, immobilize the broken ends with splints, strips of bark, or a sleeve of cardboard, pole or metal rod etc.
- Send for a qualified doctor or an ambulance as quickly as possible. Also inform victim's relatives.

Immobilization of the Fractured Part

First aid for broken bones should not extend beyond preventing pain and further injury. Immobilization of fractured part will achieve both objectives. The important thing to remember is immobilize the fracture site and the joints on both sides of fracture e.g., above and below the fracture site. This can be done by using bandages and/or by using splints where available. Here, the other uninjured limb or body of the patient is used as a splint. In cases of upper limb fractures the body is used as a splint; while in lower limb fractures the other uninjured limb is used as a splint. Keeping the injured part steady and avoiding all unnecessary movements, bandaging should be done with broad bandages, towels or a big size cloth. The bandage should be fairly firm so that there is no movement of the broken ends. Never apply bandage over the area of fracture. Apply knots on the sound side.

Splints must be long enough to extend well beyond the joints above and below the fracture site. Wide splints are always better than narrow ones. Any firm material can be used, board, pole, metal rod, walking stick, a book or an umbrella or even a thick magazine or thick folded newspaper. Use clothing or other soft material to pad splints to prevent skin injury. Fasten splints with bandages or cloth at minimum three sites, *below joint below break; above joint above break; and the level of break.* The bandaging should be fairly firm but not too tight to stop the circulation of blood in the area. Always place padding material like cotton, socks, handkerchief or small towel between the natural hollows like ankles and knees, if a splint is to be tied over them. After the fracture ends have been stabilized, do not waste time and arrange for a quick transportation to a nearby hospital or doctor.

Facial Fractures: Common injuries to the face include a broken nose, cheekbone or jaw. The main danger is obstruction of the airway, either by swollen, displaced or lacerated tissue, by loose teeth or by blood and saliva. There may be damage to brain, skull or neck. The injuries may appear horrifying with distortion of the eye sockets, nose, upper teeth and palate. There may be bleeding from the nose or mouth.

Cheekbone and Nose Fractures: These are common. The associated swelling is uncomfortable and may block the air passages in the nose. Apply a cold compress and treat an associated nosehold if necessary. These injuries should always be checked at hospital.

Lower Jaw Fractures: Jaw fractures are usually the result of direct force, such as a heavy blow. A blow to one side of the jaw can sometimes cause a fracture on the other side. A fall on to the point of the chin can fracture both sides.

Signs and Symptoms

- Pain of ten sickening, increased by jaw movement and swallowing
- Distortion of the teeth and dribbling
- Swelling, tenderness and bruising
- A wound or bruising inside the mouth

In the following measures to be taken:
- Ensure an open airway
- Ask the patient not to speak
- For a conscious casualty who is not seriously injured, help him to sit up with head well forward, to allow any blood, mucus, and saliva to drain away.
- If the casualty vomits, support his jaw and head and gently clean out his mouth
- Ask the casualty to hold a soft pad firmly in place to support the jaw
- If the patient is conscious, send him to hospital with his face leaning forward and downward in sitting position. If the patient is unconscious, and the fracture of jaw is too complicated, send the patient to hospital in a stretcher with his face placed downwards.

Collar bone fracture: The two collar bones (clavices) form struts between the breast bone and the shoulder blades, giving support to the arms. They are commonly broken by indirect force, such as fall on to the outstretched hand or impact at the shoulder.

Signs and Symptoms
- Pain and tenderness at the site of the injury increased by movement
- Attempts to relax muscles and relieve pain
- Casualty may support the arm at the elbow, and incline the head to the injured side.

In such condition following measures to be taken:
- Sit the casualty down. Place the arm on his injured side across her chest.
- Support the arm in an elevation sling
- Secure the arm to her chest with a broad-fold bandage over the sling
- Send casualty to hospital in sitting position

Upper arm fracture: The long bone of the upper arm may be fractured across its shaft by a direct blow, but it is much more common, especially in the elderly. Because this is a stable injury, casualties may walk around for sometime with the fracture unprotected and without seeking medical advice.

Signs and Symptoms
- Pain, increased by movement
- Tenderness over the fracture site
- Rapid swelling
- Bruising which may develop more slowly

In such case following measures to be taken:
- Sit the casualty down. Gently place the injured arm across his chest in the position that is most comfortable. Ask him to support his arm, if possible.
- Support the arm in arm sling, and secure the limb to his chest; place soft padding the arm and chest, and tie a broad-fold bandage around the chest over the sling (Fig. 27.19).
- Transport the casualty to hospital in sitting position.

Elbow fracture: Fractures at the elbow joint are fairly common, of ten resulting from a fall on to the hand. A fracture to the head of the radius is characterized by a stiff elbow that cannot be fully straightened.

In children, fracture of the humerus just above the elbow is fairly common. This is an unstable injury; the broken bone ends may move and damage surrounding blood vessels and nerves. It is important to make frequent checks on the circulation at the wrist pulse.

Signs and Symptoms
- Pain, increased by movement
- Tenderness over the fracture site.
- Possible swelling and bruising
- If the head of the radius if fractured, a stiff elbow.
  The following measures to be initiated:
  For an elbow that cannot be bent

- Lay the casualty down, and place the injured limb on his trunk
- Do not attempt to forcibly bend or straighten the elbow
- Insert soft padding between the injured limb and his body to ensure that bandaging will not displace the broken bones
- Bandage the injured limb to the trunk, first at the wrist and hips, then above and below the elbow
- Check the pulse at the wrist every 10 minutes

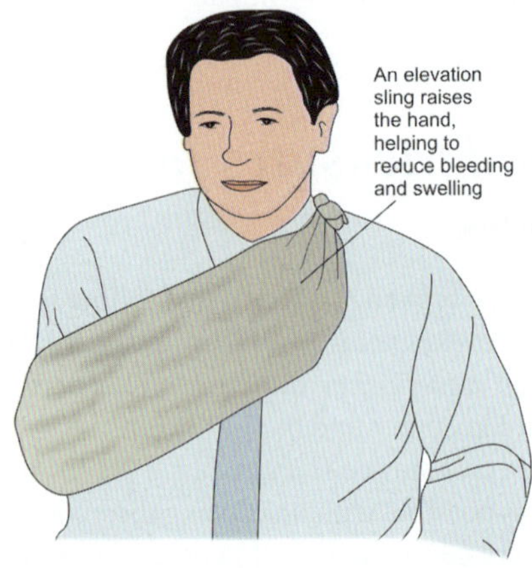

Figure 27.19: First aid for fracture elbow

For an injured elbow that can be bent
Treat as for a fracture of the upper arm. Check for the pulse at the affected wrist every 10 minutes. If it is not present, gently straighten the elbow until the pulse returns and support it in that position.

Fracture of the forearm and wrist: The bones of the forearm (the radius and ulna) may be fractured across their shafts by a heavy blow. Because the bones have little fleshy covering these factures are often open-associated with a wound.

The most common fracture around the wrist is a Colles' fracture, usually sustained by older women who fall on to an outstretched hand. In a young adult this may break one of the small bones in the wrist.

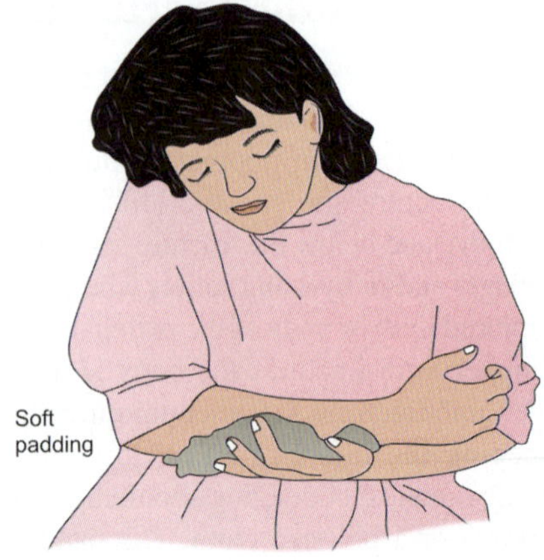

Figure 27.20: First aid for fracture—forearm and wrist

In such cases following measures to be initiated:

- Sit the casualty down. Gently steady and support the injured forearm across her chest. If necessary, carefully expose and treat any wound.
- Gently surround and cradle the forearm in folds of soft padding (Fig. 27.20).
- Support the arm in an arm sling. You may, if necessary secure the limb to her chest using a broad-fold bandage tied over the sling close to the elbow. Tie the knot in front, on the uninjured side.
- Take or send the casualty to hospital, transporting in the sitting position

Fractures of the hand and fingers: The hand is made up of many small bones with movable joints, any one of which may be injured by direct or indirect force.

Multiple fractures affecting all of the hand are usually caused by crushing injuries, and there may be severe bleeding and swelling. Minor fractures are usually caused by direct force. The most common injury is a fracture of the knuckle between the little finger and the hand, which often results from a misplaced punch.

Dislocations and sprains may affect any of the fingers. The thumb is particularly prone to dislocation caused by a fall on to the hand. The following measures to be initiated.

- Protect the injured hand by surrounding it in folds of soft padding
- Gently support the affected arm in an elevation sling
- You may, if necessary, secure the arm to the chest by applying a broad-fold bandage over the sling. Tie the knot in front on the uninjured side.
- Take or send the casualty to hospital, transporting in the sitting position

Fracture of the ribcage: Rib fractures may be caused by direct force (a blow to, or fall on to, the chest), or by indirect force produced in crush injury. If the fracture is complicated by a penetrating wound or a "flail chest" injury, breathing may be seriously impaired.

Flail Chest Injuries

If multiple rib fractures isolate a portion of the chest wall, this portion will move in when the casualty breathes in, and out when the casualty breathes in, and out when the casualty breathes out – the opposite of the normal chest movement. This state of "paradoxical breathing" produces severe respiratory difficulties.

Signs and Symptoms

Depending on severity, there may be:

- Sharp pain at the site of the fracture
- Pain on taking a deep breath; the casualty's breathing may be shallow.
- Paradoxical breathing
- An open wound over the fracture, through which you might hear air being "sucked" into the chest cavity
- Features of internal bleeding and shock

In such cases the following measures to be taken:

- In case of fractured rib, support the limb on the injured in an arm sling and send casualty to the hospital
- In case of open or multiple fractures, immediately cover and seal any wound to the chest wall
- Lay the casualty down. He may be most comfortable in a half-sitting position, with head and shoulders turned and body inclined towards the injured side (Fig 27.21). Support the limb on the injured side in an elevation sling.
- Call ambulance

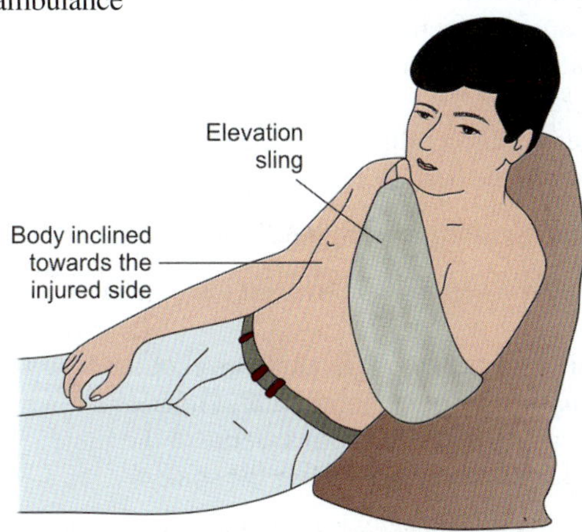

Figure 27.21: First aid for fracture ribcage

If the casualty becomes unconscious, or breathing becomes difficult and/or noisy, place him in the recovery position, uninjured side uppermost.

Fracture of Backbone/Spine

Injuries to the back include fractures of the bones of the spine, a displaced intervertebral disc ("aliped disc"), muscle strains and ligament sprains. The chief danger with any back injury, but particularly fractures and disc injuries, is that the spinal cord or nerves may be damaged.

The spine, or backbone, is actually made up of a column of small bones, each of which is called a *vertebra*. The spine supports the trunk and head and surrounds and protects the spinal cord. The spinal column is supported by many strong ligaments and the muscles of the trunk. The danger of any spinal injury is that the spinal cord may be affected. The spinal cord is delicate and if damaged, loss of power or sensation can occur in parts of the body below the injured area. Temporary damage can be caused if the cord or peripheral nerves are pinched by displaced disc or bone fragments; permanent damage will result if the cord is partially or completely severed. Although the spinal cord may be injured without any damage to the bones, spinal fracture vastly increases the risk. Fractures of the vertebrae can be caused by both direct and indirect force. The most vulnerable parts of the spine are the bones in the neck and in the lower back. Always suspect spinal injury when unusual or abnormal forces have been exerted on the back or neck, and particularly if the casualty complains of any disturbance of feeling or movement.

The history or the injury is the most important indicator. If the casualty or witness tells that the accident involved a violent forward bending, a backward bending, or a twisting injury of the spine, you must treat as for a fractured spine.

Causes of Spinal Injury

- Falling from a height
- Falling awkwardly at gymnastics
- Diving into a shallow pool
- Being thrown from a horse or from a motorbike
- Collapse of a serum at rugby
- Sudden deceleration in a motor vehicle (for example, a head-on crash).
- A heavy object falling across the back
- Injury to the head or face

Signs and Symptoms of Spined Injury includes the following.

When only the spinal column is damaged, there may be (Fig. 27.22):
- Pain in the neck or back at the level of the injury. This may be masked by other, more painful injuries
- A step or twist in the normal curve of the spine
- Tenderness on gently feeling the spine

When the spinal cord has also been damaged, there may be:
- Loss of control over limbs. Movement may be weak or absent
- Loss of sensation
- Abnormal sensations – for example, burning or tingling. The casualty may tell you that limbs feel stiff, heavy, or clumsy.
- Difficulty with breathing

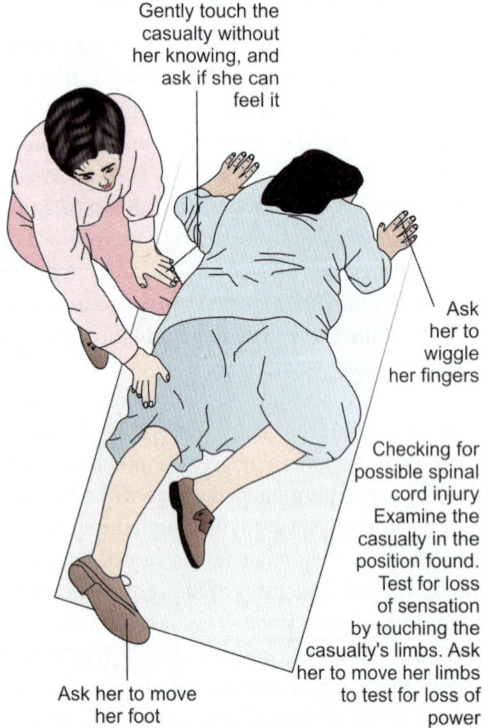

Figure 27.22: First aid for spinal injury

The measures of First Aid are as follows for Conscious victim
- Do not move the casualty from the position found unless she is in danger or unconscious
- Reassure the casualty and tell her not to move
- Steady and support her head in the neutral position by placing your hands over her ears (Fig. 27.23). Maintain this support
- If you suspect neck injury, get a helper to place rolled blankets or other articles around the casualty's neck and shoulders
- If arrival of the ambulance is imminent, maintain support with your hands until it arrives
- If removal is delayed you may, if the neck is injured, apply a collar

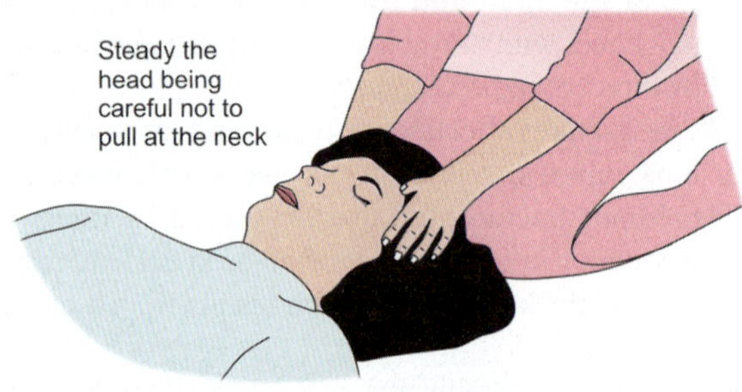

Figure 27.23: First aid for conscious victim

You must continue to hold the head and neck while, and after, the collar is fitted.

For an Unconscious victim
- Check breathing pulse. If it is present, place the casualty in a recovery position
- Open and, if necessary clear the airway. Tilt the head and lift the chin more gently than usual so that the head and neck remain the neutral position (Fig. 27.24).

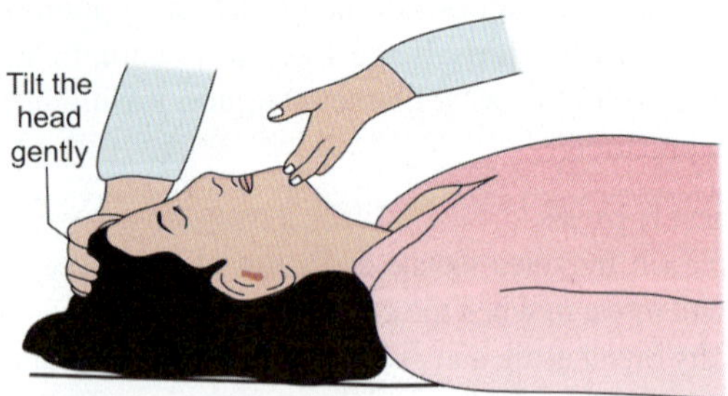

Figure 27.24: First aid for unconscious victim

- Check breathing and pulse again. If they have not returned, combine artificial ventilation with chest compressions until help arrives.
- If you have to turn the casualty on to her back to resuscitate, you should keep head, trunk and toes in a straight line. While you maintain support at the neck, ask helpers (ideally five) to gently straighten the casualty's limbs, and "log-roll" her over. You can use the same technique to roll the casualty on to a stretcher.

If the victim is unconscious with breathing and pulse present, you must place him in the recovery position. With spinal injuries, you should ideally modify the position in order to keep the casualty's head and trunk aligned at all times. You will need atleast one helper to do this successfully (as shown below); use more if you have them, but remember that even if you are alone with the casualty, he must be turned in order to protect the airway.

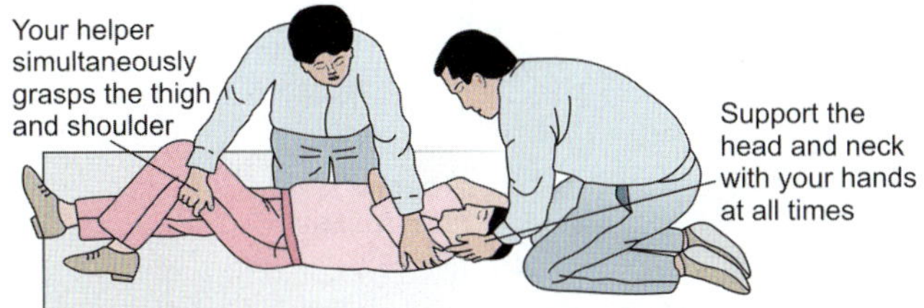

Figure 27.25: Drawing up the knee, then bringing the casualty's other arm across his chest

- Steady and support the casualty's head by placing your hands over his ears. Be prepared to maintain this support throughout, until help arrives
- Ask your helper to straighten the casualty's legs and bring the arm nearest to him out, elbow bent, palm uppermost, at right-angles to the body
- Your helper grasps the casualty's thigh, drawing up the knee; then, bringing the casualty's other arm across his chest, grasps the far shoulder (Fig. 27.25)
- As he pulls the casualty towards him, you control the neutral position of the head and neck (Fig. 27.26)
- Do not pull the neck
- Once the casualty is fully turned on to his side, both you and, if possible, your helper should support the casualty in this position until help arrives

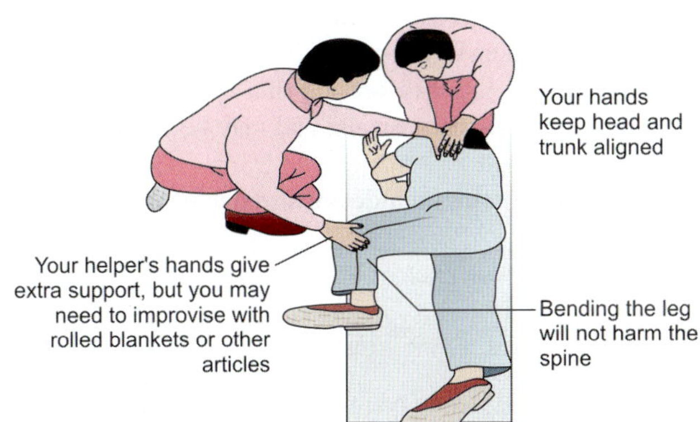

Figure 27.26: Neutral position of the head and neck

If you have to send your helper to summon aid, rolled blankets, costs, or other articles may be placed alongside the casualty to keep him steady.

If the injury is to the neck, a collar may be applied for further support. This is not a substitute for support by the hands.

Fracture of Pelvis: Injuries to the pelvis are usually caused by crushing, or by indirect force, such as might occur in a car crash. The impact of a car dashboard on a knee can force the head thigh bone through the hip socket. Pelvic injuries may be complicated by injury to internal tissues and organs, particularly the bladder and urinary passages, which the pelvis protects. Because of the bulk of body tissue surrounding the pelvis, internal bleeding may be severe, and shock often develops.

Signs and Symptoms

- Inability to walk or even stand, although the legs appear sound
- Pain and tenderness in the region of the hip, groin or back, increased when the casualty moves.
- Blood at the urinary orifice, especially in male casualty. The casualty may not be able to pass urine, or may find this painful
- Signs of internal bleeding and shock

The following measures to be taken as such cases:
- Help the casualty to lie on her back with her legs straight – or, if it is more comfortable for her, bend her knees slightly and support them
- Immobilize her legs by bandaging them together; placing padding between bony points
- Dial for an ambulance. Treat the casualty for shock
- Do not bandage the legs together, if this causes intolerable pain

Fracture of Hip and Thigh: Fractures of the neck of the thigh bone (femur) at the hip joint are common in the elderly, and more frequent in women, whose become more porous and brittle as they age. This can be a stable injury; the casualty may be able to walk around for some time before the fracture is discovered. The hip may also, more rarely, be dislocated.

It takes considerable force (such as in road accidents, or falls from heights) to fracture the shaft of the thigh bone. This is a serious injury because, in most cases, a large volume of blood is lost into the tissues. This may cause shock to develop.

Signs and Symptoms

- Pain at the site of the injury
- Inability to walk
- Signs of shock
- Shortening of the thigh, s powerful muscles pull broken bone ends together
- A turning outwards of the knee and foot

The following measures to be initiated:
- Lay the casualty down. Ask a helper to steady and support the limb by holding it above and below the injury.
- Gently straighten the lower leg and apply traction at the ankle, pulling steadily in the line of the limb
- Call for an ambulance. If the ambulance will arrive quickly, support the leg with your hands until it arrives.
- Take any steps possible to treat the casualty for shock; insulate him from the cold, but do not raise his legs

If the ambulance will be delayed, immobilize the limb by splinting it to the uninjured limb, as explained:
- Gently bring the casualty's sound limb alongside the injured one

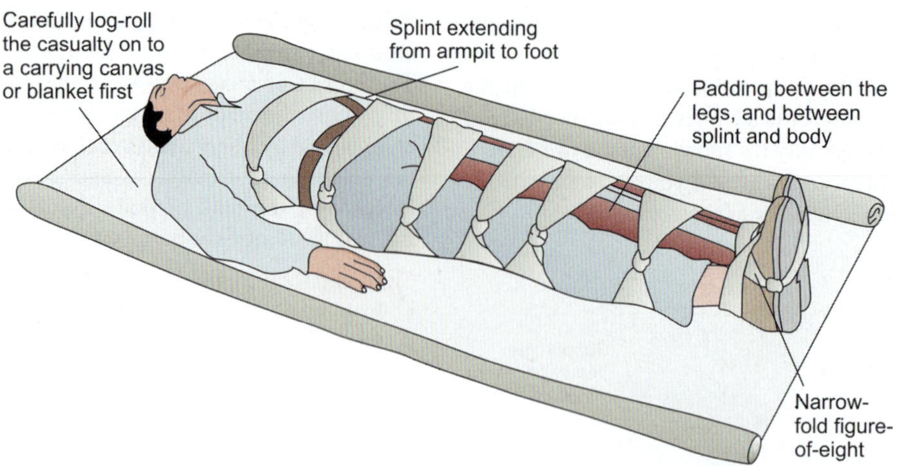

Figure 27.27:: Method of transporting the casualty over a distance

- Maintaining traction at the ankle, gently slide two bandages under the knees. Ease them into position above and below the fracture by sliding them backwards and forwards. Position another bandage at the knees and one at the ankles.
- Insert padding between the thighs, knees, and ankles, to prevent bandage-typing displacing the broken bone
- Tie the bandages around his ankles and knees. Then tie the bandages above and below the fracture site.

To Transport the Casualty over a Distance

If you have to carry casualty on a stretcher to reach help (for example, across a moor), sturdier support for the leg will be needed. A purpose made femoral traction splint is ideal, but can only be used by trained personnel. As an alternative, place a wooden leg splint, reaching from the armpit to the foot, against the injured side. Pad between the legs, and between the splint and the body. Secure the splint with broad-fold bandages, at the chest and pelvis, and then at the legs (Fig. 27.27). Do not bandage directly over the fracture. During transport, keep the foot of the stretcher raised to minimize swelling and shock.

Fracture of The Knee Joint: The knee is the strong hinge joint between the thigh bone (femur) and shin bone (tibia). It is capable of bending, straightening, and, in the bent position, slight rotation. The knee joint is supported by strong muscles and ligaments, and protected in front by a disc of bone, the kneecap (patella). Any of these structures may be damaged by direct elbows, violent twists or strains.

Signs and Symptoms
- History of a recent twist or blow to the knee
- Pain, spreading from the injury to become deep-seated in the joint
- If the bent knee has "locked", acute pain on attempting to straighten the leg
- Rapid swelling at the knee joint

The following measures to be initiated:
- Help the casualty to lie down, supporting her leg and knee in the most comfortable position
- Wrap soft padding around the joint, and bandage it carefully in place
- Take or send the casualty to hospital, transporting as a stretcher case

Please note that:
- DO NOT attempt to force the knee straight. Displaced cartilage or internal bleeding may make the joint impossible to straighten safely.
- DO NOT give the casualty anything to eat or drink; she may need to be given an anesthetic.
- DO NOT let the casualty walk.

Fracture of the Lower Leg: The study shin bone (tibia) of the lower leg usually requires a heavy blow to break it (for example, form the bumper of a moving vehicle). The thinner splint bone (fibula) can be broken by the type of twisting injury that sprains the ankle. Because the load-bearing shin bone remains intact, the casualty may be able to walk, and may be unaware that a fracture has occurred.

Signs and symptoms includes localized pain and there may be:
- A recent blow or wrench of the foot
- An open wound
- Inability to walk

The following measures to be initiated as a First Aid
- Help the casualty to lie down, and carefully steady and support the
- Straighten the leg using traction, pulling gently in the line of the shin.
- Call an ambulance. If the ambulance will arrive quickly, support the leg with your hands until it arrives.

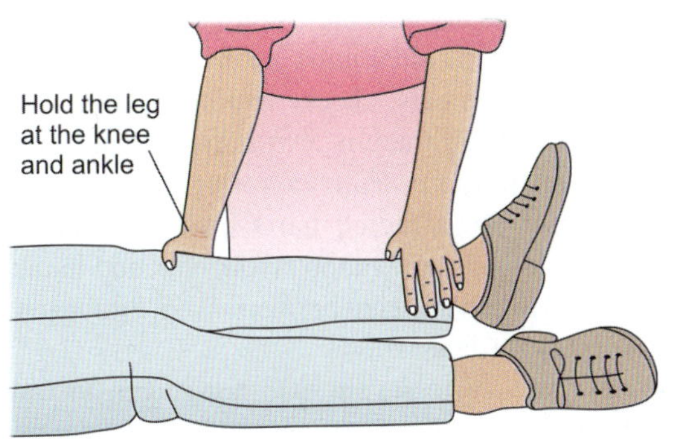

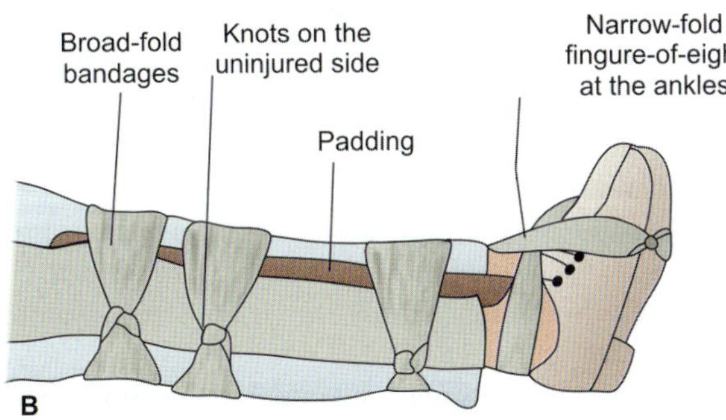

Figures 27.28A and B: First aid for fracture of lower legs

If the ambulance will be delayed, splint the injured limb to the sound one.

- Gently bring the sound limb alongside the injured one (Fig. 27.28A).
- Maintaining support at the ankle, gently slide bandages under the knees and ankles. Position them above and below the fracture, and at knees and ankles, avoiding the fracture if it is close to a joint.
- Insert padding between the knees and ankles, and between the calves (Fig. 27.28B).
- Tie the bandages around ankles and knees, then above and below the fracture. Bandage firmly, but avoid jerky movements

If you have to transport the casualty on a stretcher, place extra padding (for example, rolled blankets) on either side of the legs, from the upper thigh to the foot. Secure with broad-fold bandages at the thigh and knee, and above and below the fracture. Tie a figure-of-eight around the feet and ankles with a narrow-fold bandage.

Extremes of Heat and Cold Heat and First Aid Measures

Some groups of people can be identified as high risk in relation to heat and heat related problems. Athletes and military personnel who are undergoing rigorous training and conditioning in hot, humid either are particularly vulnerable. Farmers are a high risk group. Infants and elderly people are also at high risk. Individuals with such health problems as cardiovascular disease, obesity, diabetes mellitus, malnutrition or alcoholism are vulnerable to heat related problems.

Poorly insulated and ventilated homes, sedentary life styles, congested neighbourhoods are all sociocultural factors that increase the risk of heat related problems, especially for the poor and elderly.

There are *three* of heat related problems: which includes Heatstroke, Heat exhaustion, Heat cramps.

(i) Heatstroke: Both these conditions are similar and can prove to be dangerous. Sunstroke is caused by too high a temperature in atmosphere by the sun rays. While heatstroke may be caused by high temperatures in factories, boilers or furnaces or illness involving a very high fever (e.g., malaria). In both conditions the heat regulating mechanism of the body fails & body rapidly becomes dangerously overheated. The *Signs and Symptoms of heat stroke includes*

- Headache, dizziness and discomfort
- Restlessness and confusion
- Hot, flushed, dry skin
- Slow and rapid pulse
- Rapid unconsciousness
- The body temperature rises up to 104° F even higher.

The following measures are taken for heatstroke

- Remove the patient to a dry and shady place, loosening his collar and any other tight clothing
- Raise the head the upper part of the body
- Sprinkle cool water on his body or wrap him in a thin-wet sheet and fan him
- Use fan freely
- Keep on taking body temperature every 10 minutes
- Do not let the body temperature of patient fall below 103° F by the above method
- After this stage is reached, wrap him in a dry sheet and keep fanning so that the temperature does not rise up again
- If the patient is conscious, cool water mixed with salt and glucose can be given to him for drinking
- Remove to the hospital

Heat Exhaustion: It is used caused by too high a temperature in the atmosphere directly by the sun, or due to hard work and confinement in a close, hot atmosphere like factories etc. Excessive sweating with loss of body water and slats result in this condition. The Signs and Symptoms includes.

- Headache, dizziness, nausea, vomiting and sometimes abdominal cramps or cramps in the limbs
- Face is pale with cold sweat
- Pulse is weak
- Shallow breathing
- Temperature is normal or slightly raised
- Sometimes there is unconsciousness
- There may be shock
- Loss of appetite

The following measures to be taken in this condition; which includes.

- Remove the casualty to a cool place

- Place him flat on his back
- Loosen his clothing
- Give him plenty of salted water (1/4 liter every ½ hourly) or fruit juice
- Observe that he does not develop heat stroke

Heat Cramps: These are intermittent, painful contraction of skeletal muscles. These cramps often occur in individuals who replace the fluid lost in sweat by drinking water, but do not replace sodium. The sodium depletion is believed to be responsible for the cramps. Heat cramps usually occur in muscles that have been involved in strenuous activity – most often those of the legs. The cramps last a few minutes and generally disappear spontaneously. With heat cramps, the body temperature is normal and the serum sodium may be normal or low.

The treatment is to replace sodium with salt tablets or an electrolyte solution. In severe cases, effected cases, effected person is referred to hospital or physician for intravenous salt solutions which may be required. Adding more salt to the diet will usually prevent heat cramps.

Preventive Measures of Extreme Heat

To prevent the Problems of Extreme Heat the following points to be kept in mind:
- Limiting the strenuous activities in the hot weather to the cooler times of the day
- Gradually expose yourself to hot weather (it takes 10-20 days to become acclimatized to extreme heat)
- Stay indoors and wear a minimum of clothing during heat waves
- When temperature are unusually high, strenuous outdoor activities should be cancelled, and use a parasol or a wide brimmed hat and stay in the shade if you must go out.
- Wear clothes that are loose fitting, light in colour, and that cover as much of the body as possible when outdoors
- Loose weight if you are obese, but avoid heavy exercises for weight reduction
- Use measures to improve ventilation and reduce heat by shades and drapes to cut direct sunlight
- Cooking should be done in the early morning or late evening to avoid heating up the house during the hot part of the day
- Fans and vents over stoves and ovens should be used to help remove heat from the house
- Eating more salts, but must be accompanied by an increased amount of fluids
- Drink lot of water, even the person with cardiovascular disease who might otherwise be limiting fluids

Cold

Effects of excessive cold are common in persons who live or work in a climate where temperature falls below 32° F or are in high altitudes. Extent of the injury caused depends on the degree of the temperature and the period to which exposed to cold.

(i) Frost Bite: Skin is the first tissue to become cooled. Muscles, nerves and vessels are also highly susceptible. The parts most frequently subject to cold trauma are the hands, feet, facial skin and particularly the ears, cheeks and nose. During very cold weather, especially if there is also a strong wind, frost bite is liable to occur on nose, chin, ears, fingers, toes. After being painfully cold the affected parts become waxy white in appearance and feel quite numb. Whiteness and numbness are danger signals which must not be overlooked. Prolonged freezing will do irreparable damage.

Persons exposed to severe cold must learn to watch each other's faces for the tell-tale changes of colour, a white patch on a red face. At the same time the development of numbness in hands or feet must be recognized as an emergency requiring urgent treatment. The Signs and Symptoms of frostbite includes:-
- The exposed part becomes cold, painful and ultimately numb.
- Colour first is red then becomes white which may later lead to gangrene
- The part feels waxy and has no feeling while it is frozen
  In such condition following measures are needed:
- General warming by body heat is the safest way to relieve frost bite
- Remove all wet or tight clothing from the frost bitten area
- Carry the patient to a closed room without a fire and undress him carefully
- Remove tight gloves, boots, socks, rings etc. from the body
- Do not rub the frozen part with snow or anything else
- Put him to bed and cover him snugly with a dry cloth
- Give him warm drinks
- If face or ear is affected, cover the frozen patch with a gloved hand until normal colour and sensation return.
  In the case of frozen fingers or toes, remove tight gloves and boots. The hand may be placed under the clothing in the armpit. The feet may be wrapped in a warm blanket or under a companion's jacket.
- Send for a physician immediately
- All cases of severe frost bite resulting from prolonged exposure to cold in persons who have been lost or immobilized by other injuries, must be recognized as "serious" injuries necessitating evacuation by stretcher for urgent medical care.
- Do not rub frost bitten parts. Do not use hot water bottles or a heat lamp. Do not place victim near a hot stove. Do not allow the victim to walk, if the feet are affected. Do not allow the victim to smoke because the nicotine in tobacco may further constrict the blood vessels.

Preventive Measures for Extreme Cold

To prevent Cold Injury following points to be kept in mind:
- Plan activities carefully to minimize exposure
- Always let someone know where you are and when to expect you back
- Dress for the weather. Protection is more important than fashion

- Avoid vigorous washing of the face and shaving the beard until after the day's outing
- Apply protective cream to the face prior to exposure
- Wear several layers of loose, warm clothing (rather than a single, fitted layer)
- Use hand protection. Mittens are generally more effective than gloves
- Avoid alcohol and cigarettes
- Avoid becoming unduly fatigue
- Do not use snow, ice, cold water or excessive heat to thaw frozen tissues
- If freezing does occur, avoid thawing the part until refreezing is eliminated as a threat

Asphyxia

Asphyxia is a deficiency of oxygen in the blood and an increase of carbon dioxide in the blood and tissues. It occurs due to an interruption in the normal exchange of oxygen and carbon dioxide between the lungs and outside air. Lungs do not get sufficient supply of oxygen for breathing. If this condition continues for some minutes, breathing and heart action stops and death occurs. The cause of asphyxia will be as follows: Drowning, Electric shock, Foreign body in the air passages (choking), Inhalation of smoke and poisonous gases, Suffocation under bed, earth, etc, Hanging, strangulation by tight rope

The Signs and Symptoms of Asphysia in stage wise as given below

First stage
- Rate of breathing increases
- Breath gets shorter
- Veins of the neck becomes swollen
- Face lips, nails, fingers and toes turn blue
- Pulse gets faster and feebler

Second stage
- Consciousness is lost totally or partially
- Froth may appear at the mouth and nostrils
- Fits may occur
  In such conditions following measures to be taken:
- Remove the cause if possible
- Very quickly, make sure that the air passage is not obstructed:
  - Loosen his collar
  - Put finger down the throat to scoop out seaweed or any foreign material
  - Remove false teeth
  - Null tongue forward
- Place the individual on his back. Support the nape of the neck on your palm and press the head backwards. Then press the angle of the jaw forward form behind. This will extend the head on the neck and lift the tongue to clear off the airway. If airway is opened by this method the individual starts to breathe. Give three inflations to the lungs to facilitate breathing mouth-to-mouth method. If the heart is beating, carotid pulse can be felt in the neck.

- Apply artificial respiration to ensure prompt ventilation of the lungs, and, if necessary do external cardiac massage.
- During artificial respiration ask helpers to
  - Call doctor and ambulance
  - Cover casualty with blankets
- Continue artificial respiration rhythmically and without interruption until natural breathing is resumed. A few casualties have been revived after several hours of such efforts
- If the victim begins to breathe on his own, adjust your timing to assist him. Do not fight the victim's attempts to breathe. Synchronize with his efforts.
- After breathing is restored, keep the victim at rest and arrange for medical care.

Here we are dealing with asphyxia due to drowning and choking.

(i) Drowning

Accidental fall into a well, pond, canal or river and inability to swim, results in *drowning*. There is complete immersion of nose and mouth in water. Water enters the respiratory passage and cause *asphyxia,* with cold. Usually only a small amount of water enters the lungs. The water that often gushes out of a casualty's mouth is from stomach, and should be allowed to drain naturally.

One should not swim out to rescue anyone unless he has had life saving training.

- Most drowning occur only a few feet from shore, from a dock or float, or from water of standing depth. If the victim is near enough, extend a pole, branch, or oar to him. Wade through the shore if necessary, but do not wade too far.
- If you cannot extend an object to the victim, throw to him something that will float. If possible, use a lifebuoy or a plank of oar size or larger. Smaller objects may help, but unfortunately most victims become panic-stricken, thrash about and do not get as much benefit from a floating object as they should. Therefore use a large object if possible. The victim should clasp it close to him and try to keep his face above water.
- A good way to aid a drowning person is to use a boat if one is handy. The rescuer should know how to row and manage the boat. If waves are high or there is a swift current, or if the boat is small and unstable no attempt at rescue by this means should be made because of the danger of being overturned.
- The best way to approach a drowning person is to back the stern (rear) of the boat within his reach and allow to climb in from there is he can, or to hold on while you row him to shore. Do not allow him to climb in from the side. Sometimes the person may be gone so far that he is in danger of going down before the boat can be turned. In this case, row the boat alongside the victim and push the blade of an oar within his grasp; then swing him around to the stern and let him hang on.
- Do not wade out if the condition of the bottom is unknown for a sudden drop off, a hole, bed of quick sand of mud may cost your life as well as that of the victim.

The aim of first aid is to drain out water from the body.
- Very quickly put the victim in the prone position (face down) and make sure that his air passage is not obstructed.
  - Loosen his collar

- Put finger down the throat to scoop out seaweed or other foreign material
- Remove false teeth
- Pull tongue forward
• Raise the middle part of the body with your hands round the belly. This is to cause water to drain out of the lungs.
• Do not attempt to force water out from the stomach
• Give artificial respiration until breathing comes back to normal. This may have to go on for as long as two hours.
• Remove wet clothing. Keep the body warm, cover with blankets, provide hot drinks
• Do not allow him to sit up
• During artificial respiration ask helpers to send for doctor and ambulance
• The casualty should always receive medical attention, even if he appears to recover rapidly

(ii) Choking

Choking occurs due to blockage of the throat by foreign object. In adults if any happen while taking food and in children it may happen accidentally. There is difficulty in speaking and breathing.

The following measures to be taken for an Adult (Fig. 27.29):
• Reassure the casualty. Bend her forwards so that her head is lower than her chest.

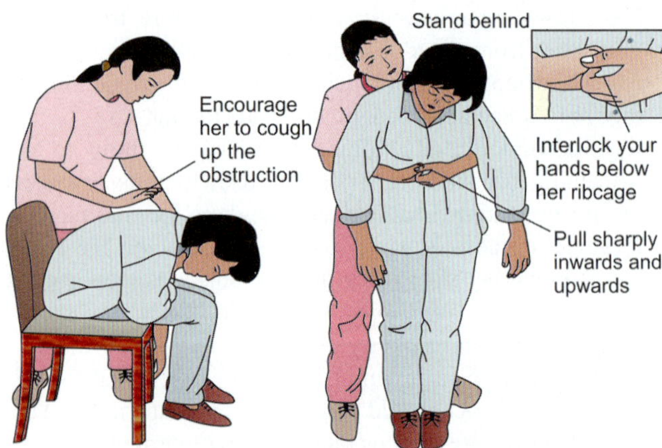

Figure 27.29: Choking measures: In Adult

• Give up to five sharp blows to her back, between the shoulder blades, with the flat of your hand.
• If backslaps fail, try abdominal thrusts. The sudden pull up against the diaphragm compress the chest, and may expel the obstruction.

If this does not free the blockage, try again four times, then alternate five back blows with five thrusts. Abdominal Thrusts
• Stand behind the victim
• Wrap your arms around the waist
• Make a first, clasp fist with free hand
• Press in with a quick inward and upward thrust

In case of Child the following measures to be taken (Fig. 27.30):
• Place the child over your knee, head down. Slap him between the shoulder-blades using less force than for an adult.

• If back blows fail, use the abdominal thrust only if you have been trained to do so on a child. Otherwise, begin resuscitation.

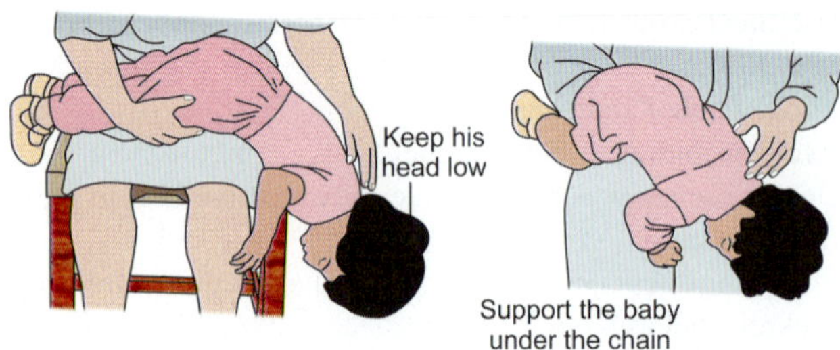

Figure 27.30: Choking measures: In child

In case of Baby

Lay the baby along your forearm. Slap her between the shoulder blades, using less force than for a child. If the baby becomes unconscious, begin resuscitation. DO NOT use the abdominal thrust.

For a Casualty who Becomes Unconscious

• Loss of consciousness may relieve muscle spasm, so check first to see if the casualty can now breathe. If not, turn her on her side and give 4-5 blows between her shoulder blades
• If back blows fail, kneel astride the casualty, and perform abdominal thrusts.

If she starts to breathe normally, place her in the recovery position and call an ambulance. Check and record breathing and pulse rate every 10 minutes.

Inhalation of Fumes and Gases

The inhalation of smoke, gases or toxic fumes can be dangerous and saving efforts should not be attempted if you are at risk.

Usually it is caused by two types of gases:
(1) *Carbon monoxide* (lighter than air)
(2) *Carbon dioxide* (heavier than air)

Carbon monoxide is lighter than air and is present in car-exhaust fumes, in gas from burning coal, coal mines, during fire etc. Carbon dioxide is heavier than air and is found I in coal mines, deep unused mines and sewerage.

In such cases following measures are necessary:
• Before attempting to rescue a person from a room filled with harmful gas, always open the doors and windows, or break the windows, to ventilate the room first
• There may also be danger that an explosion will occur
• Stay away from the room fro sometime while it ventilates. It is the only safe procedure for first aider
• A victim can be rescued from a small room at once after opening the door if you can pull him out quickly while holding your breathe
• Crawl along the floor if the poisonous gas is lighter than air i.e. carbon monoxide
• Enter in upright position if the gas is heavier than air
• Artificial respiration is given if there is breathing difficulty

Unconsciousness

Any interference with the normal functioning of the brain and the nerves brings about unconsciousness. An unconscious state indicates not only that there might be some disease or injury of the brain but serious injuries and diseases elsewhere in the body. In many instances the cause of unconsciousness will not be readily apparent. From time to time the first aider may be called upon to deal with a person who is found unconsciousness.

Types of Unconsciousness

- **Stupor:** It is the state of semi-unconsciousness in which casualty responds to external stimuli or loud noise. Pupils of the eyes contact if exposed to bright light.
- **Fainting:** It is the temporary loss of consciousness and the casualty recovers spontaneously
- **Somnolent:** It is a state when person feels drowsy or sleepy
- **Coma:** It is complete loss of consciousness. Person is not aware of himself and the environment, and cannot be aroused, if he is in deep coma. Characterized by an absence of eye movements and response to painful stimuli. Pupils do not respond to light

Causes of Unconsciousness

- Brain injuries
- Head injuries
- Fainting
- Convulsions
- Apoplexy
- Heat stroke or exhaustion
- Diabetes or overdose of insulin
- Heart attacks
- Hysteria
- Epilepsy
- Shock
- Haemorrhage
- Acute fever
- Alcohol consumption
- Poisons
- Severe loss of body fluids
- Metabolic disturbances
- Anesthesia
  In such condition following first aid measures are to be taken:
- You should not try to arouse an unconscious person. Just let him lie quiet. There is no reason to pour water on an unconscious patient unless he is overcome by heat.
- Do not move the casualty unnecessarily, because of the possibility of spinal injury. Never attempt to make an unconscious person sit or stand upright.
- 'Give him air'. Do not let people gather around for they interfere with the examination and obstruct fresh air. If you are indoors, open the doors and windows.
- Loosen clothing's at neck, chest and waist.

- Provide covering for the patient both above and below
- Never give water or anything else to an unconscious patient to drink. It might get into his windpipe.
- Apply specific treatment for the cause of unconsciousness
- Let him lie undisturbed while you summon help

Is he breathing well? If he is not breathing, give artificial respiration, provided the victim's condition was caused by drowning or some other type of accident for which artificial respiration is recommended. Cases of stroke and of concussion are, in general, not helped by artificial respiration, even though the person has stopped breathing.

It is important to remember that all unconscious persons are in danger of suffocation if they are left lying on their back. In this position the tongue falls back into the throat and saliva collects there, thus obstructing the entrance of air into the lungs. Moreover, if for any reason, vomiting occurs, the vomitus coming into the throat is almost sure to be sucked back into the lungs causing death or serious damage.

As evidence of this danger of suffocation, it may be noted that many unconscious persons while lying on their back appear to be choking or struggling for breath, and often their skin looks bluish because of lack of oxygen. Breathing will often become easier and colour promptly improve when they are turned into the prone position. Many lives have been unnecessarily lost because such cases were left lying on their back.

All Unconscious Persons Must Immediately be Placed in the Prone (Face Down) or Semi Prone (On side with face turned towards ground) Position.

In this position the tongue will fall forward and vomitus and saliva will run out of the mouth rather than back into the lungs.

To further facilitate breathing, it is often helpful to bend the neck slightly backwards and hold the chin forward with thumb and fingers.

Fainting: This occurs most frequently in healthy young people, especially during hot weather, and while standing for long periods as in crowds or amongst soldiers "on parade". People who are hungry, tired, emotionally upset, fearful or see blood may faint even though they are in good health. As soon as immediate cause is an insufficient supply of blood to the brain. As soon as they lie flat, they recover consciousness, because then the brain gets enough blood.

The Signs and Symptoms of fainting includes:
- The person who is about to faint feels giddy, looks pale and collapse on the ground
- Pulse is weak and slow
- Skin is cold and clammy
- Breathing becomes less deep than normal

The following measures needed for fainting victim:
- Keep the victim lying flat, and raise and support his legs. Raising the legs improves the blood flow to the brain
- Loosen tight clothing at neck
- Do not let a crowd gather around, let there be plenty of fresh air

- Consciousness will return in one or two minutes
- After he recovers consciousness, a cup of tea or coffee may bring further relief
- If he does not recover very soon, the case is not of simple fainting and a doctor should be consulted.

Prevention

If a person feels giddy and about to faint, he should bend forward at the waist, bringing the head down between the knees, or better yet, he should lie down.

Convulsion (Epilepsy)

A convulsion, or fit, is an involuntary contraction of many of the body's muscles, caused by disturbance in the function of the brain. Convulsions are usually accompanied by loss of consciousness. The Causes of convulsion will include:

- Head injury
- Brain damaging disease
- Less oxygen supply to brain
- Intake of poison
- High temperature (in children)
- Condition epilepsy
  The Signs and Symptoms of Convulsion will be:

The usual sequence for the person affected is, utter a cry, stiffen out his limbs, then jerk arms and legs about haphazardly (convulsion), and finally subside into a deep sleep. During the attack, which usually lasts only a few minutes, it is not uncommon, for the victim to exhibit "frothing at the mouth" and there may be involuntary passage of urine or stools. Person may also make odd noises.

The victim is completely unconscious from an instant before the onset of the attack, and afterwards has not memory of the event.

The following measures needed during convulsion:

- Just keep the casualty under control; do not use force to stop the convulsions. Remove objects that may cause injuries. Protect his head. Make space around him.
- If a person has an epileptic attack, he may bite his tongue. Prevent biting of tongue by inserting a folded cloth or a strong stick or a spoon wrapped in a handkerchief between the teeth
- After the attack, do not question the victim unless absolutely necessary
- Wipe out froth from the mouth
- He should be lied down undisturbed
- Advise him to consult a doctor undisturbed

Convulsions in Young Children

Although young children can have epileptic fits just like adults, they may, more commonly, develop convulsions at the onset of an infectious disease or a throat or ear infection associated with a greatly raised body temperature (Fever).

These *febrile* convulsions can be alarming, but they are rarely dangerous if properly managed. However, for safety's sake the child should be seen at a hospital to eliminate any serious condition.

The Signs and Symptoms of Convulsion in young children will includes:

- Clear signs of fever : hot, flushed skin and perhaps sweating
- Violent muscle twitching, with clenched fists and an arched back
- Breath-holding, with congestion of the face and neck
- Drooling at the mouth
  The measures to be taken during this condition are:
- Remove any cloth or covering bedclothes. Ensure good supply of cool, fresh air (though be careful not to overcool the child)
- Sponge the child with tepid water; start at the head and work down
- Position pillows or soft padding so that even violent movement will not result in injury
- Keep the airway open, by using the recovery position if possible

Hysteria

It is a psycho-neurotic problem in which the individual converts his anxiety created by emotional stress and mental tensions into physical symptoms, e.g., tics, mutism, paralysis of arm or leg etc. It has no organic basis, but there is temporary loss of consciousness over the emotions.

Signs and Symptoms

- Patient may fake unconsciousness but on examination, signs will not be present
- Convulsions. But these are not typical
- Excessive crying, tearing hair
- Patient falls down deliberately, so that no injury is caused to any part of the body
  The first aider or nurse may have difficulty in diagnosing a hysterical attack. If sure of hysteria then:
- Ignore the attack
- Be firm but kind in dealing
- Try to find out the family environment and personal background so the basic problem can be dealt with.

Apoplexy (Stroke)

It is a condition in which the blood supply to part of the brain is suddenly and seriously impaired by a blood clot, or a ruptured artery.

Strokes are more common in later life, and in those who suffer from high blood pressure or other circulatory disorder. The effect of a stroke depends on how much, and much, and which part, of the brain is affected. Major strokes can be fatal, but many people make successful recoveries from minor stroke.

Signs and Symptoms
- A sudden, severe headache.
- A confused, emotional mental state that could be mistaken for drunkenness
- Sudden or progressive loss of consciousness
- Signs of weakness or paralysis, possibly (but not always) confined to one side of the body. Slurred or impaired speech; loss of power or movement in the limbs; inequality of the pupils; loss of bladder or bowel control.
  In such condition following first and measures are helpful:
- If the casualty is conscious, lay him down with his head and shoulders slightly raised and supported. Incline his head to one side, and place a towel or cloth so that it will absorb any dribbling
- Loosen any constricting clothing that might interfere with breathing. DO NOT give the casualty anything to eat or drink. If the casualty becomes unconscious, check breathing, pulse, and level of response and be prepared to resuscitate if necessary. Place him in the recovery position
- Dial for an ambulance/doctor

Hypoglycemia

It is a condition in which the blood-sugar level falls below the normal, affecting the brain. It is most often found in people suffering from *diabetes mellitus*. If the hypo attack is advanced, consciousness is lost. Diabetes is a condition in which the body fails to regulate the concentration of sugar in the blood.

Insulin – a hormone, produced by pancreas controls blood sugar levels. Without insulin, sugar accumulates in the blood causing *hyperglycemia*. Too much insulin and too little sugar causes *hypoglycemia*.

Causes
- Insulin overdose
- Delay in eating
- Rapid combustion of carbohydrates due to over exertion

Signs and Symptoms
- Weakness, faintness, hunger
- Palpitations and muscle tremor
- Strange action and behavior
- Sweating
- Cold and clammy skin
- Strong pulse
  In such condition following measures to be taken:
- If casualty is unconscious, open the airway and record vital signs.
- Resuscitate if required
- If casualty is conscious, give him a sugary drink, sugar lumps, chocolate, sweets etc.
- If condition do not improve send for doctor
- In hyperglycaemia, skin becomes dry, pulse is rapid and smell of acetone is felt on the casualty's breath. Urgent hospitalization is needed

Head Injuries

All injuries to the head are potentially dangerous, and always require medical attention, particularly if severe enough to cause impaired consciousness. This may indicate damage to the brain, blood vessels inside the skull, or skull fracture.

Conversely, impaired consciousness may mask the presence of other injuries: examine the casualty closely.

Concussion

The brain move a little within the skull, and can thus be, "shaken" by a violent blow. This may cause concussion, a condition of temporary disturbance of the brain. The period of unconsciousness is short and followed by complete recovery.

Signs and Symptoms
- Brief or partial loss of consciousness following a blow to the head
- Dizziness or nausea on recovery
- Loss of memory of events at the time of, or immediately preceding, the injury
- A mild, generalized headache

In such condition following measures needed:
- If the casualty remains unconscious after three minutes, dial for an ambulance. Place him or her in the recovery position. Monitor and record breathing, pulse, and level of response
- For a casualty who swiftly regains consciousness, watch closely for any deterioration in the level of response, even after apparent recovery
- Advise the casualty to see his or her own doctor

Skull Fracture

The skull is a domed vault with an irregular and complex base. It surrounds and protects the brain. Fractures of skull are thus potentially very serious injuries, because there may be associated brain damage. The brain can be bruised (cerebral contusion), or there may be bleeding within the skull that accumulates and exerts pressure on the brain (cerebral compression).

Cerebral compression invariably requires surgery.

A wound may alert you to the possibility of fracture, and also presents the danger that germs, and hence infection, can enter the brain. There may be cerebro-spinal fluid leading from the ear or nose, as clear fluid or watery blood, which indicates another entry point for germs.

Suspect a fractured skull in any casualty who has received a head injury resulting in unconsciousness that lasts for more than three minutes. Note, however, that it is violent head movement (especially "fore-and-aft") that causes unconsciousness. Some injuries (for example, crushing) can fracture the skull without causing loss of consciousness.

The skull may be fractured in several different ways, by both direct force (a blow to the head) and indirect force a fall from a height, landing heavily on the feet). Fractures caused by indirect force commonly occur at the base of the skull, and these injuries may be accompanied by damage to the spinal column.

Many types of skull fracture, particularly linear fractures (cracks) in the domed vault and fracture to the base of the skull, can only be diagnosed by X-ray or other imaging methods in hospital. Severe injuries may cause multiple cracking (an "eggshell" fracture), which may extend to the base of the skull. A "depressed" fracture may cause bone fragments to be driven in to injure, and exert damaging pressure on, the brain.

Signs and Symptoms
- A wound or bruise on the head
- A soft, boggy area or depression of the scalp
- Impairment of consciousness
- A progressive deterioration in the level or response
- A flow of clear fluid or watery blood from the nose of ear
- Blood in the white of the eye
- Distortion or lack of symmetry of the head or face

In such condition following measures necessary (Fig. 27.31):
- If the casualty is unconscious, check breathing and pulse , and place her in the recovery position
- Help a conscious casualty lie down, with the head and shoulders raised and comfortably supported

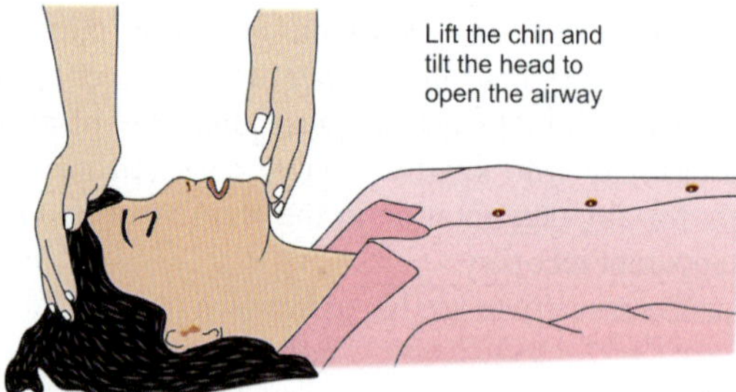

**Figure 27.31: Placing the patient with skull fracture
in recovery position**

If there is discharge from an ear, position the casualty so that the affected ear is lower. Cover the ear with a sterile dressing or clean pad, lightly secured with a bandage. Do not plug the ear.
- Control any bleeding from the scalp. Look for, and treat, other injuries.
- Dial for an ambulance. Check and record breathing and pulse rate, and level of response, at 10 minute intervals and accompany the casualty to hospital

Bites and Stings

Animal bites, always require some degree of medical attention, because germs are harboured in the mouths of all animals. Bites from sharp, pointed teeth cause deep puncture wounds that carry germs into the tissues. Serious wounds require hospital care; any bite, bite, breaking the skin needs prompt first aid, followed by medical attention.

Snake Bite

There are about 2500 to 3000 species of snakes. But amongst these, approximately 250-300 only are poisonous, therefore in the cases of snake bite if the snake can be seen in nearby place it should be confirmed whether it is poisonous or not. If the snake is not seen then idea can be drawn by seeing the prints of fangs of the snake on the bitten area.

Commonly two types of snakes are found in our country: (1) *Colubrine* and (2) *Viper.* Colubrine snakes are quite long and very poisonous, and their teeth have no holes. These types of snakes are mainly found in the form of King Kobra, Common Kobra, Common Krait and Common Striped Krait. The vipers type are found in the form of Pit Viper and Russell's Viper. The snakes living in water are also poisonous.

Signs and Symptoms
- The poison of the Cobra bite very quickly affects the nervous system. So in such cases there is severe pain on the bitten area. Uneasiness, giddiness and sometimes vomiting occur. Because of the nervous system getting affected, the muscles of the body start getting affected with the result that there is weakness of hands and legs, loss of sensation, watering of mouth, slow respiration and weak pulse rate. The pupils of the eye look contracted. In cases of snakebite, generally death occurs due to fear itself but if first aid is not given in time on bite of Kobra species then death occurs very soon.
- The blood vessels of the bitten area get affected by Viper bite. The blood clotting process is disturbed due to the effect of poison of Viper snakes. So there is excessive bleeding from the bitten area and the wounded part looks swollen. With the absorption of poison in the body there is uneasiness, giddiness, vomiting, weakness, slow pulse rate and expansion of eyelids.

Snakes are chiefly found in two places, one living in water and the other on the earth. The tail of the snakes living on earth is round and in the shape of a roller and the tail of the snakes living in water is flat. The difference between the poisonous and non poisonous is as following (Table 27.3).

The confirmation of snake bite can be done by the presence of teeth prints on the affected area. Make the person lie down comfortably and give him physical and mental rest and try to build his courage. If the snake was really not poisonous then person should be made to understand that he will soon become alright. But if the snake was really poisonous and has bitten on hand or foot (These are the common places of snake bite) then tie with some rope, handkerchief or tourniquet at a distance away form the bitten area to avoid the venous blood flow towards the heart. Tourniquet should not be tied so tight that the blood flow to that organ is inhibited. Now put an inch long cut overt the snake bitten area and start sucking and spitting out the blood mixed liquid coming out from the wound. If the medical help is not available then after half an hour's suction, make the arrangement to send the patient to the doctor.

Table 27.3: Difference between Poisonous and Non-poisonous Snakes

Specific things	Poisonous snakes	Non-poisonous snakes
Example	Sea snakes, Koral snake, Krait and Viper (simple and Pit Viper)	Snakes living in river and nalas, Dhamin snakes etc.
Ventral scales or scales of lower surface	Ventral scales are so broad and long that they seem to touch the costal margins around.	Ventral scales are either small or sometime big so they do not touch the nearby costal margins
Head's scales	• If there are very small scales on the head then it can be a Viper snake. (A) If there is a hole between eye and nostril then it is 'Pit viper' snake. (B) If this hole is not present then it is pitless viper. • If the third scale of the lips touches the scales of eyes and nose then 'Nagraj snake'. If there is no sign on the head then 'Fandhar' snake. • If the vertebral are big and the scales are under the tail and straps on their back then it is Krait snake.	There are no such peculiarities.
Teeth prints	On the upper jaws instead of teeth there are fangs which are hollow. These are related to poison gland. Common types of types are found on the lower jaw. These teeth are bent towards back so that the prey escape their grip.	Teeth are found on both the jaws. In most nonpoisonous snakes four rows of teeth are found on the upper jaw. These teeth are also bent on the back side so that the prey is not lost out of their reach.

Common care: If the patient is unconscious then do not give him any liquid by mouth and keep him awakened if he is getting sleep. If the patient is in consciousness then tea or coffee can be given. If the patient is in condition of shock then the first aid of shock should be given and arrangement should be made to send the patient to the hospital. In children the snake bite creates a serious condition because the amount of poison is more in proportion to the body size. So the child should be sent to the hospital without wasting time.

Local care: Wash the wound with soap and water and apply some antibiotic cream, keep some sterilized gauze and cotton properly. Tie the bandage.

SCORPION BITE: Generally scorpion can be seen in the moist dark places and in rainy season. Though scorpions are not seriously poisonous but sometimes person can become unconscious with their bite. Scorpion bite rarely leads to a serious condition but there is severe burning, intolerable increasing pain in the bitten area. Sometimes person complains of giddiness, vomiting and can become unconscious.

If the symptoms are not severe and are restricted to the bitten area, the patient should be made to lie comfortably and soothing cream should be applied. This pain should subside in one hour and if it does not and the patient complains a feeling of unconsciousness, send him to doctor or hospital. Sometimes a big blister is seen after 6 to 12 hours and it bursts by itself. In such condition do the dressing with antibiotic cream.

DOG BITE: Domestic dogs which are not immunized against rabies and which comes in contact with stray dogs/wild animals have a chance to contract the rabies virus and become rabid. Rabies is a filterable virus that affects brain. It is commonly found in dog but can be carried by any animal like cats, rats, foxes, wolves, bats & monkeys. Saliva of infected animal can get injected into human being even by licking if there is a break in the skin of the licked part. Rabies or hydrophobia is a fatal infection.

Rabis dog can be restless, barking, biting or it is quiet like babies and stay close to the master as if it is unwell. Master may try to open his mouth to find out the cause of his quietness. In the process if he has break in his skin he will get infected from dog's saliva. Thus quiet dogs are more dangerous than those that are restless. Incubation period ranges from 10 days to more than a year or so.

Untreated victims are likely to develop rabies. The Signs and Symptoms of rabies includes: Headache, Malaise, Fever,

1. Hydrophobia
2. Aerophobia

In such cases following actions is necessary:

- Thorough washing of the bitten area with soap and water or detergent solution for 5 to 10 minutes under running water. Wound is dressed with clean sterile gauze or cloth. Apply antibiotic cream
- In cases of suspected rabid dog bite the wound should be bled
- Victim should be immediately referred to a doctor
- The dog should be dept under observation for ten days. If the dog remains healthy then there is no risk, but if the dog gets mad, then it should be killed by any measure

Other measures

- As preventive measure the cases of rabid dog bites are immediately notified. All pets should be registered and vaccinated. Stray dogs are eliminated

- Rabid patients die of respiratory failure due to paralysis. These require emergency admission. In hospital such patients are nursed in a separate, darkened and quiet room on a well-padded railed bed, in hollow position and suction done to drain out excessive saliva
- Nurse looking after such cases should use gloves and take antirabies serum as prophylaxis.

CAT BITE: Generally the cats keep roaming around the houses but if they are disturbed and touched they become violent and can attack, causing two types of wounds (1) On biting with teeth (2) Scratches by the nails. Sometimes the cats attack the sleeping child. The condition does not become serious by cat bite but sometimes there is infection in the wound, therefore such wounds should be washed and dressing is done properly.

RAT BITE: Rats are not only enemies of grains in the godowns but harm the human beings in different ways. (1) The flea found on their body spread a dangerous disease called Plague. (2) Sometimes they scrap the palm of hand or foot of sleeping person.

Generally rats live in dirty places so the places scraped by them get easily infected and the person starts getting fever. So in such cases the wound should be washed and dressed properly, and the person should be sent to the hospital.

BEES AND WASP BITES: The most harmful amongst the insects are the bees and wasps and other insects of same type. Their sting causes local pain, itching and severe swelling because their stings have one type of poison which is little in quantity. Some people are very sensitive to this poison and therefore certain reactions like histamine, local pain and swelling, respiratory inhibition because of throat swelling, and low blood pressure because of the contraction of the air pipe occur. The patient becomes unconscious and if the first aid is not given in time then death can occur due anaphylactic shock.

If the sting is present then, instead of pulling it by force it should be taken out by slightly scrubbing the skin, so that a hole is formed from which the poison can come out easily. If the swelling and pain is severe then keep wet bandage or ammonia bandage. Keep the place cool by applying alcohol, spirit or ice. After thins, apply antibiotic cream and do the dressing. If the patients condition is serious or he is in a condition of shock then send him immediately to the hospital.

TICKS AND MITES BITES: Tick is a small insect like bed bug. It is about ½ or 1 cm long. It has a terrible capacity to stick to the body. It sticks itself to the body and keeps sucking the blood. During this period it spreads germs of certain diseases in the body which Tuloraemia, Rocky mountain spotted fever and other such conditions can arise.

As these are generally found in animals, wood, camps in open grounds etc., care should be taken while going to these places. Mites are generally found in wood and stored grains. Their bite can cause typhus fever.

If tick or mite has bitten and it is sticked than it should be immediately removed. It should not be pulled forcefully otherwise some part of their body will be left in the wound and if it gets crushed then the disease causing germs will enter the body. Therefore these should be taken out either by the forceps or they will fall themselves by applying burning cigarette on their dorsal surface. These also come out by applying some oil, turpentine or kerosene. The wound should be washed with soap and water they are taken out. An antibiotic cream should be applied and bandaged.

SPIDER BITE: Generally two types of spiders are found: (1) Black spider (2) Tarantula (3) Black spider is more poisonous whereas tarantula is big hairy and less poisonous. These spiders are generally found in the gaps of wood, hollow places, corners of the house and dark places.

Signs and Symptoms

It causes redness, severe pain and local swelling. After the absorption of the poison from the bitten area, the affected person suffers from stomach cramps and muscles become hard. the face, hands and legs look swollen. There is breathlessness and condition of shock can arise. There can be cramps in small children. Death rarely occurs by their bite. Small localized blisters arise due to their poison.

The patient should be made to lie in a comfortable position and should be covered with blanket or bed sheet. A cloth or rope should be tied at a distance from the bitten area so that blood is not absorbed in other parts of the body. If the patient is conscious then he should be given tea or coffee to drink. Rest should be given to the affected area by keeping cold bandage and the bitten area should be cleaned and bandaged. If the doctor is not available and the patient is serious then send him to the hospital immediately.

LEECH BITE: Leech is generally found in tanks, rivers, moist and muddy places. Though a serious condition does not arise with their bite but these suck quite a large amount of blood. It is not to take them out by pulling because these are very delicate and flexible and therefore can break. On applying a burning stick or cigarette on their dorsal surface they come out easily. After taking them out, the wound should be washed and bandaged.

FISH STINGS: Two breads of thorny fish, viz. sting ray fish and jelly fish generally harm the human beings by stinging. The stings of both these fishes can cause severe pain but death can never occur. The sting of sting ray fish is situated on the lower border of its tail.

Its stings breaks on the local spot and the affected area starts looking blue or black. There can be local blood poisoning. The jelly fish generally stings on the hand or feet. The patient starts having the feeling of uneasiness and there is local pain.

If the sting is seen on the surface then take it out by scratching the skin. Wash the wound and do the dressing. To get relief from the burning sensation, apply cold bandages of ammonia and water. Medical aid is generally not required in such condition but if the pain is really severe and sustains for long time then get the medical aid.

Foreign Bodies in the Skin

Small foreign bodies (wood splinters, shards of glass) usually cause minor puncture wounds with little or no bleeding. If a portion of the object protrudes from the skin, you may attempt to draw it out. Foreign bodies deeply embedded in a wound should not be removed by a first aider; you may cause further injury. Foreign bodies are often contaminated with dirt and bacteria. Ensure that the wound is clean, and that the casualty's tetanus immunization is up to date.

Splinters: Small splinters of wood, metal, or glass in the skin, particularly of the hands, feet, and knees, are common injuries. The splinter can usually be successfully drawn out using tweezers. However, if the splinter is deeply embedded, lies over a joint or proves difficult to remove, it is better left alone until seen by a doctor. For which

- Clean area around the splinter with soap and warm water. Sterilize a pair of tweezers by passing them through a flame
- Grasp the splinter as close to the skin as possible, and draw it out along the track of its entry
- Squeeze the wound to encourage a little bleeding. Clean the area and apply an adhesive dressing "plaster"

Foreign Bodies in the Eye: Sand particles, small pieces of glass, coal, emery stone, metal, usually enter the eye, as foreign bodies. These particles usually get situated under the eyelids or eyeball.

Signs and Symptoms

- If any foreign body enters the eye then one feels uneasy. There is pain and irritation. Water starts coming out of the eyes and it becomes difficult to open the eye in the light (Photophobia).
- The first aider should try to take out only those foreign bodies which are lying only on the surface area of the eyes because the untrained trial to take out the deep seated particles lead to serious damage and blindness.
- In no condition the untrained person should be allowed to try to take out the foreign bodies from the eyes. If in emergency condition it becomes necessary to take out the foreign body then the hands should be washed properly and cotton piece or soft handkerchief should be made wet with a corner made pointed and then the foreign body should be taken out with the help of pointed end.
- If the foreign body gets sticked on the middle portion of cornea then do not try to take it out because this can lead to great harm. The eye then should be closed, padded and the person should be sent to the hospital.
- If the foreign body is sticked on the inner portion of the feeling of lower eyelid an is not seen on the round portion of the eye and if the feeling of irritation sustains then slide the lower eyelid under the upper one and then open the eye. The foreign body sometimes comes out when the hairs of the lower eyelid get rubbed with the upper under part of the eye. But even if it does not come out and the medical help is not available then make the patient sit in the light. Stand at the back of his head. Keep a knitting needle on the upper lid. Turn the hair of the upper lid upwards with the support of the knitting needle and

see whether the foreign body is sticked or not on the inner surface (Generally it is sticked) and if it is sticked then take it out with the cotton or corner of a clean handkerchief.
- Now put some drop or ointment. Keep a pad on the eye and do the dressing. Send the person to the hospital.

Remember the following points to avoid severe loss by the foreign bodies:

(1) Do not rub the eyes vigorously because by doing this the soft tissues of the eye get scratched
(2) Until the hands are washed do not examine the eyes because there can be an infection if hands are dirty
(3) Examine the eye carefully with soft hands
(4) Do not try to take out the foreign bodies with toothpaste, knife, match stick etc.
(5) Do not try to take out the embedded foreign body in any condition. In such cases the patient should be sent to the doctor

Foreign Bodies in the Ear: The cases of foreign bodies in the ear occur generally in children. Solid substances like peas, buttons can enter the ear. Among these, some substances like peas and other seeds absorb moisture, swell up and obstruct the ear and then it becomes difficult to take things out. Flies, mosquitoes or bed bugs can also enter the ear.

Never use pin or piece of wire to take out foreign bodies from the ear because by using them ear drum may get ruptured. Mosquitoes, bed bugs or flies die by putting olive oil or soda bicarb in lukewarm water into the ears. Then murmuring sound of these insects stops. Now send the person to the hospital.

Foreign Bodies in the Nose: Certain foreign bodies like pieces of betel nut, grains or peas and other seeds enter the nose. Generally this happens mostly in children. By putting olive oil in the nose the foreign body comes out or the irritation of the nose subside.

Do not sneeze forcefully in effort to take out the foreign body or do not close the unaffected nostril and try to sneeze out with the affected nostril because by doing so there is fear cessation of respiration. Though there is no immediate risk but the person should be sent to the hospital as soon as possible.

Foreign Bodies in the Throat: Generally in the throat or upper part of the respiratory tract some pieces of food, small bones of fishes, coins or artificial teeth or other things can enter. Though these rarely cause total obstruction of the respiratory tract, but due to spasm in the throat, symptoms of suffocation can arise. The person's become blue, he starts coughing and the respiration stops.

If the respiration is normal and the colour of his face is also normal, assure him and get the first aid immediately. Generally the foreign body is not seen in the throat and even if it is seen then do not try to take it out by finger or by other measures.

If the respiration rate is slow and the face becomes blue then by bending that person down and by patting on the shoulder the thing comes out. But if the foreign body not come out and the respiration slows down then start giving artificial respiration and obtain medical help or arrange to send the patient to the hospital.

Foreign Bodies in the Stomach: The cases of introduction of foreign bodies into the stomach are generally found in children. The things which can enter are buttons, seeds of fruits, coins, safety pins etc. though there is no immediate risk and the foreign bodies get eliminated during evacuation with the normal movements of the intestines. There is no need to give (as Bananas are commonly given) laxatives or other substances.

Fish Hook in the Skin: While catching the fishes the hook fixed in the tool of catching fishes can enter the skin sometimes. It has a specific structure and it is difficult to take it out from the skin. To take out the fish hook form the skin, first wash the surrounding area with antiseptic lotion (dettol) and cut the raised pointed head of the hook after slightly raising up from the skin and take out the hook by turning it towards back. Remember do not try to take it out by pulling forcefully because there will be more harm on the skin by doing this. Now do the dressing on the wound and send the person to the hospital.

Emergency Childbirth

Most babies are born in hospitals or other institutions where professional medical care is available. However, when time is miscalculated, babies may be born at home, buses, planes, ambulances, rails or ships. The shorter the period of child birth (labor), the more chance there is that the mother may not make it to the hospital. In addition to miscalculation of time, storms, accidents or local or national disaster may make it impossible to get the mother to a doctor or professional help, or vice-versa. The first aider rarely comes across such emergencies.

If the mother is having labor pains and no part of the baby is seen at the opening of the birth canal, call a doctor or midwife immediately or send the mother to a nearby hospital. Sometimes no such help can be obtained and the first aider will have to manage the childbirth alone.

There are two situations in which you may need to administer first aid to a pregnant woman: *Miscarriage and Childbirth.*

Miscarriage is a common but critical and dangerous event and needs medical attention.

Miscarriage: A miscarriage is the loss of the embryo or fetus at any time before the 28th week of pregnancy.

Some women experience a "threatened miscarriage" with only slight vaginal bleeding. Complete miscarriages carry the danger of severe bleeding and shock. Any woman who is, or appears to be, miscarrying must be seen by a doctor.

Remember that the woman may be frightened and very distressed. Though your efforts may be rejected., try and offer as much help as you can without being intrusive. A woman who suspects that she is miscarrying may be reluctant to confide in a stranger, particularly if that person is a man.

Signs and Symptoms
- Cramp-like pains in lower abdomen or pelvic area
- Vaginal bleeding, possibly sudden and profuse
- Signs of shock
- Passage of the foetus and other products of conception

In such condition take following measures:
- Reassure the woman. Help her to lie down in a semi-reclining position.
- Give her a sanitary pad or clean towel
- Check and record pulse and breathing rate
- Keep any expelled material (out of the woman's sight, if possible) for medical inspection
- If the bleeding and/or pains are only slight, call a doctor.

Childbirth: The majority of births do not threaten the lives of either mother or baby. Nevertheless, a woman who goes into labour unexpectedly may become very anxious, and you must do your best to reassure and clam her. Labour usually lasts several hours, an there is normally plenty of time to arrange transport to hospital, or for the assistance of a midwife or doctor.

Never try to delay a birth in anyway. Allow the delivery to proceed without interfering until the baby's head in emerging. Rarely, the baby's position is reversed and it emerges bottom first (a breech delivery). This requires urgent medical attention.

The stages of Childbirth
Labour is divided into three stages:
- *First stage* (often around 12-14 hours) – dilation of the neck of the womb
- *Second stage* (up to 2 hours) – descent of the baby from the womb to the vaginal entrance, and delivery
- *Third stage* (up to 30 minutes) – delivery of the afterbirth

NOTE
- If the baby's is DOWN, his birth is likely to go well.
- If the baby's head is UP, the birth may be difficult, and it is safer for the mother to give birth in hospital or near it.
- If the baby is SIDEWAYS, the mother should have her baby in a hospital. She and the baby are in danger.

Things to be kept Ready at the Time of Delivery
1. A lot of very clean clothes or rags
2. An antiseptic soap (or any soap)
3. A clean scrub brush for cleaning the hands and finger nails
4. Alcohol for rubbing hands after washing them
5. Clean cotton
6. A new razor blade (Do not unwrap until you are ready to cut the umbilical cord)
7. If you do not have a new razor blade, have clean rust free scissors ready. Boil them before cutting the cord
8. Sterile gauze or patches of thoroughly cleaned cloth for covering the navel.
9. Two ribbons or strips of clean cloth for typing the cord. Both patches and ribbons should be wrapped and sealed in paper packets and then baked in an oven or ironed

Additional Supplies for the Well prepared Birth Attendant

1. Torch or flashlight
2. Suction bulb for sucking mucus out of the baby's nose and mouth
3. Sterile syringe and needles
4. Several injections of ergonovine or ergometrine
5. Two bowls – 1 for washing hands and 1 for catching and examining the afterbirth
6. Fetoscope or fetal stethoscope for listening to the baby's heartbeat though the mother's belly
7. Two clamps (hemostats) for clamping the umbilical cord or clamping bleeding veins from tears of the birth opening
8. Sterile needle and gut thread for sewing tears in the birth opening
9. Silver nitrate drops for the baby's eyes

Prevention of Infection

When preparing for, and during the delivery it is extremely important to pay strict attention to hygiene.

- Keep anyone with a cold, sore throat, or septic spots on the hands well away
- Wear a facemask. You can improvise one from a clean handkerchief or a folded triangular bandage.
- Remove outer clothing and roll up you sleeves. If possible, wear a plastic apron
- Wash your hands and scrub your nails thoroughly for about five minutes. Wear disposable gloves if available
- After the delivery, wash your hands thoroughly again.

Procedure (Figs 27.32A to E)

1. Cover the bed, sofa, or floor with plastic sheeting, towels, or newspaper and make the woman comfortable.
2. Ask her to remove any clothing that will interfere with the delivery. During the early second stage, keep her covered with blankets for as long as possible.
3. Put cotton, lint, or sheeting under her buttock, for warmth and to absorb mess. Place a clean pad over the anus, as involuntary bowel movements may occur
4. Tell the mother to grasp her knees or the back of her thighs. This will help her push with the contractions, which by now may be coming every 2-3 minutes
5. DO NOT give the mother anything to eat or drink. If she is thirsty moisten her lips with water.
6. If there is soiling, clean the area form front to back to protect against infection.
7. Inspect the vaginal area. When the *perineum* (between the vagina and the anus) bulges, the baby's head should become visible. Support it as it emerges.
8. When the widest part or crown, of the head is through, tell the mother to stop pushing and pant during the contraction. This will enable you to swiftly the head.

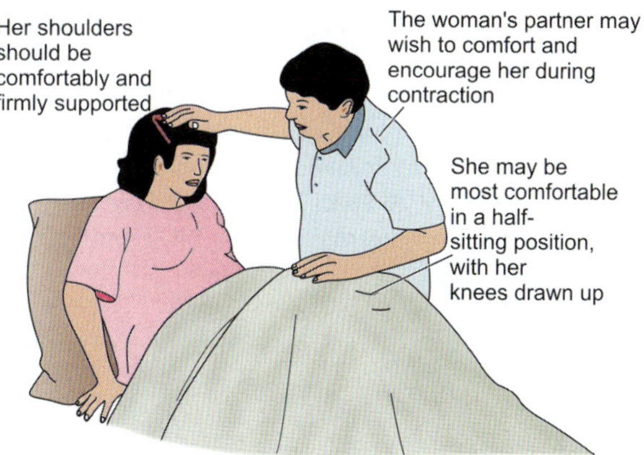

Figure 27.32A

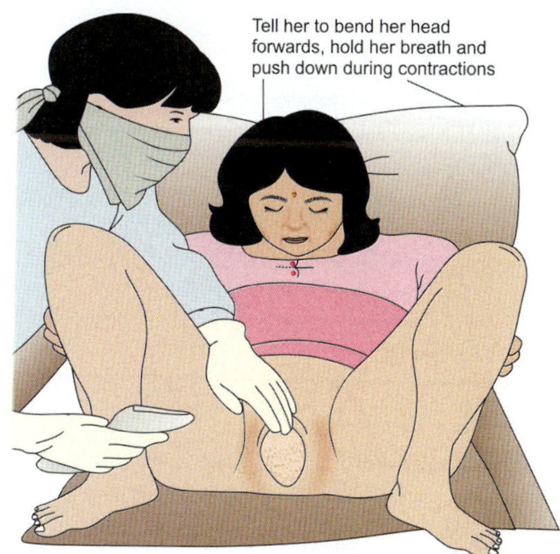

Figure 27.32B

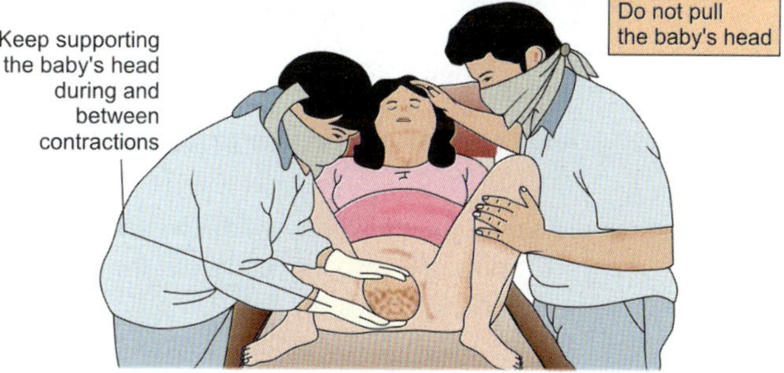

Figure 27.32C

9. Check that there is no membrane covering the baby's face if there is, tear it away.
10. Check that the umbilical cord in not around the baby's neck. If it is, pull it over the over baby's head.
11. The baby's head will turn to face to the side. Allow this to happen naturally while supporting the head.
12. Continuing support, lower the baby's head until the uppermost shoulder appears at the birth canal.

13. Once the first shoulder is clear, lift the head upwards towards the mothers abdomen to free the second shoulder from the birth canal; the rest of the baby will be expelled rapidly. DO NOT pull at the shoulders
14. Lift the baby away from the birth canal. Newborn babies are very slippery, and need to be handled carefully. Gently lay the baby on the mother. DO NOT pull or cut the umbilical cord.

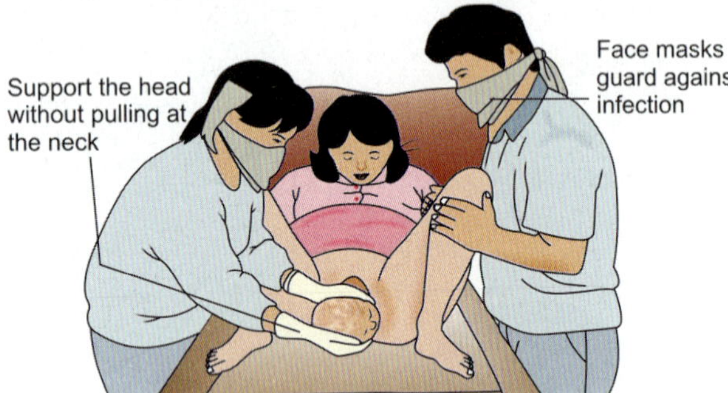

Figure 27.32D

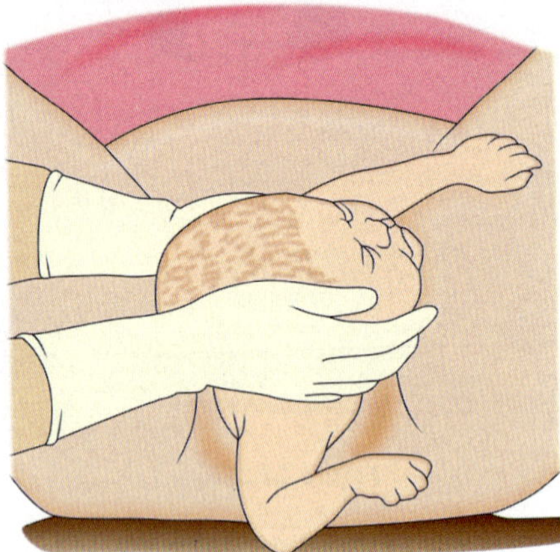

Figure 27.32E

Figures 27.32A to E: Procedures for emergency childbirth

15. Clean out the baby's mouth with a swab. The baby should start to cry; if it does not respond, carry out the ABC of resuscitation. DO NOT Smack the baby.
16. Wrap the baby and put it in the mother's arms while you attend to the afterbirth. Make sure the baby is lying on its side with the head low, so that fluid or mucus can drain from the nose and mouth.

The Delivery of the Placenta (Afterbirth)

1. Normally, the placenta comes out 5 minutes to an hour, after the baby is born, but sometime it is delayed.
2. When the afterbirth comes out, pick it up and examine it to see if it is complete. If it is torn and there seem to be pieces missing, get medical help. A piece of placenta left inside the womb can cause continued bleeding or infection.

3. In the end, clean the external genitals of the mother with a hot sponge or a clean cloth. Put one or two cotton pads there. Give hot tea or coffee to the mother.
4. Wrap placenta in paper or place in mud pot and bury it three feet or burn it, if custom permits.

Controlling Bleeding

When the placenta comes out, there is always a brief flow of blood. It normally lasts only a few minutes and not more than 1 cup of blood is lost. Sometimes a woman may be bleeding severely inside, without much blood coming out. Feel her belly from time to time. If it seems to be getting bigger, it may be filling with blood. Check her pulse often and watch for signs of shock.

If heavy bleeding continues, or if the mother is losing a great deal of blood through a steady trickle, do the following:
1. Get medical help fast
2. Clean the mother, apply clean pads, and ask her to lie flat with the legs close together.
3. The mother should drink lot of liquids. If she goes faint or has a fast, weak pulse or shows signs of shock, put her legs up and her head down.

If the mother is losing a lot of blood and is in danger of bleeding to death, try to stop bleeding like this:

Using all of your weight, press down with both hands, one over the other on the belly. Just below the navel. You should continue pressing down for a long time after the bleeding stops.

If the bleeding is still not under control:
Grasp the womb between your hands and squeeze hard. keep squeezing it firmly until the bleeding has stopped for several minutes or until you get medical help.

Danger signs that make it important that a doctor or skilled midwife attend the birth
- If the woman begins to bleed before labor
- If there are signs of toxemia before pregnancy
- If a woman is suffering from a chronic or acute illness
- If the woman is very anemic or if her blood does not clot normally
- If she has had serious trouble or severe bleeding with other births
- If it looks like she will have twins
- I fit seems the baby is not in a normal position in the womb
- If the bag of water breaks and labor does not begin within a few hours (The danger is even greater if there is fever)
- If she has a hernia

Care of the Baby at Birth

Immediately after the baby comes out:
1. Put the baby's head down so that mucus comes out of his mouth and throat. Keep it this way until he begins to breathe
2. Keep the baby below the level of the mother until the cord is tied. (This way, the baby gets more blood and will be stronger

3. If the baby does not begin to breathe right away, rub his back with a towel or a cloth
4. If the baby has not begun to breathe within one minute after birth, start mouth to mouth breathing at once
5. Wrap the baby in a clean cloth. It is very important not to let him get cold. Maintain body temperature. Receive in warm blanket lined with soft cloth.
6. Do not bathe for 12 hours. Vernix is a valuable skin protection. Remove blood and excess vernix with moist cotton swap. Give warm pour bath, if customs demands.
7. Put baby to breast soon after delivery if mother's condition allows, or else allow to nurse one breast for five minutes at the end of 12 hrs, then alternate breasts every 3 hrs. for 15 minutes until nursing schedule is established.
8. Inspect the newborn for any abnormality
9. Change position from side to side frequently to prevent pressure on any one part.

Cutting the Cord

1. When the child is born, the cord pulsates and is fat and blue
2. After a while, the cord becomes thin and white. It stops pulsating. Now, tie it in two places with very clean, dry strips of cloth, string or ribbon. These should have been recently ironed or heated in an oven.
3. Cut the cord with a clean, unused razor blade (Fig. 27.33). Before unwrapping it, wash your hands very well. If you do not have a new razor blade, use freshly boiled scissors. Always cut the cord close to the body of the newborn baby. Leave only about 2 cms attached to the baby. These precautions help prevent tetanus.
4. The most important way to protect the freshly cut cord from infection is to keep it dry. To help it dry out, the air must get to it. If the home is very clean and there are no fires, leave the cut cord uncovered and open to air. If there are dust and files, cover the cord lightly. It is best to use sterile gauze.

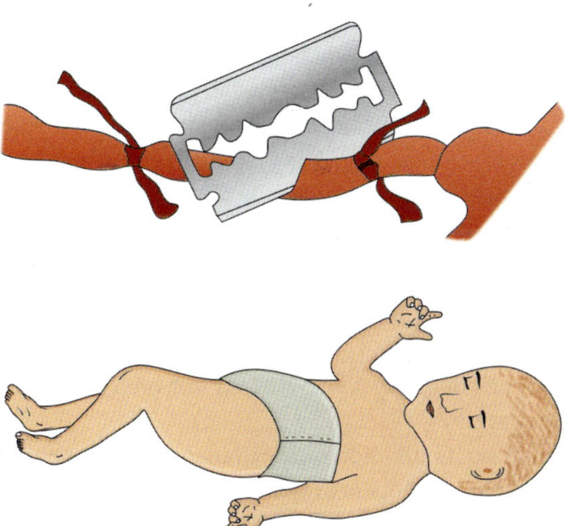

Figure 27.33: **Cutting of umbilical cord**

Minor Ailments of Illness

(i) Common cold: Cold and flu are common virus infections that may cause runny nose, cough, sore throat and sometimes fever or pain in the joints. There may be mild dirarrhoea, especially in young children.

It is unfortunate that many people think this illness as trivial. Colds of ten pave the way for more serious disease. Germs in the body that previously could not get a foothold sometimes grow rapidly when the body is weakened by a cold. Then such disease as pneumonia, sinus infection and ear infection may develop. The following measures to be take in such condition.

- Drink plenty of water and get enough rest.
- Inhale steam; this helps to clear a stuffy nose
- No special diet is needed. However, fruit juices especially orange juice or lemonade, are helpful.
- Colds and flu almost always go away without medicine
- Aspirin helps lower fever and relieve body aches and headaches. More expensive cold tablets are no better than aspirin. So why waste your money?

Prevention

- Keep away from those with colds. If you cannot keep entirely away, stay as far as you can.
- Getting enough sleep and eating will help prevent colds. Eating oranges, tomatoes and other fruit containing vitamin C may also help.
- Wash your hands before eating
- Wear clothing that is sufficiently warm
- Guard against chilling, particularly after active play or hard work
- After washing the hair, dry it thoroughly and stay indoors several hours

(ii) Fever: When body temperature is above 98.6° F (36.9°) taken by mouth or 99°F by rectum, the patient is said to have a fever. The temperature of the mouth and rectum is generally at least half a degree higher than that of groin or axilla.

There are three classical types of fever:

- *The Continuous Fever:* When fever does not fluctuate more than 1°C (or 1.5°F) during the twenty four hours, but at not time touches the normal, is known as continuous fever.
- *The Remittent Fever:* When the daily fluctuations exceed 2°, it is known as remittent
- *The Intermittent Fever:* When fever is present only for several hours during the day, it is intermittent fever.

Fever itself is not a sickness, but a sign of many different sicknesses. High fever, and fever which persists for more than 24 hours, indicate involvement more severe than the body can handle without professional help. Low fever which persist over periods of days or weeks may indicate a chronic infection, such as tuberculosis, rheumatic fever, mononucleosis, or one of many other causes. Infections, diseases of gastro-intestinal system, chronic illness, malaria and malignancies, all give rise to fever.

Signs and Symptoms

A rigor, or shivering attack is common at the beginning of many fevers. Tachycardia is usual. The appearance of the patient is characteristic. The face is flushed and the skin hot and dry, though sweating is characteristics of some fevers and occurs in most when the temperature falls. The appetite is diminished, but thirst is great. The tongue is dry and furred. The bowels are usually constipated, though diarrhea may occur in intestinal infections. Urine is dark colored and less in amount. Headache, bodyache and vomiting may be associated with above signs and symptoms.

The following measures to be initiated:

- Small children with fever should be undressed completely and left naked until the fever comes down. Never wrap a child with fever in clothing or blankets
- Anyone who has fever should drink lots of water, juices or other liquids. For small children, especially babies, give boiled and cooled drinking water.
- When fever goes very high, it must be lowered at once. Pour cool water over him, or soak some pieces of cloth in cool water. Place these wet cloths on his forehead, arms and legs. Fan the cloths and change them often, to keep them cool. Continue to do this until the fever goes down below 100.4°F or 38°C.
- Fresh air or a breeze will not harm a person with fever. On the contrary, a fresh breeze helps lower the fever
- If a person has fever, he loses lots of energy. Give him plenty of cool water with a little sugar or jaggery to drink, to keep up his strength.
- Give aspire to lower the fever
- If a high fever does not go down soon or if fits (convulsions) begin, continue cooling with water and seek medical help.

(iii) Headache: Headache is one of the most common complaints of 20th century man. Headache, to be quickly recognized, is not a disease by itself, but rather a symptom of a disease or a functional disturbance. The causes of many headaches are relatively simple to discover; others may tax the brain of top notch specialists.

Tension headaches and headaches of emotional origin are extremely common, probably constituting the most usual cause of headache observed by physicians. Headaches due to eye strain can be corrected by using proper glasses. Still others are caused by glaucoma, migraine, infections of the ear, nose, throat and sinuses. In addition, headache is common with any sickness that causes fever i.e. meningitis, influenza, pneumonia etc. high or low blood pressure, brain tumors may also cause headache. Overwork less sleep and dark surroundings are other causes.

The following first aid measures are follows:

- Simple headache can be helped by rest and aspirin
- Lie down in a dark, quiet place. Do you best to relax. Try not to think about your problems
- It is important to eat well and get enough sleep
- It often helps to put a cloth soaked in hot water on the back of the neck and to massage the neck and shoulders gently
- Seek medical help if the headache do not go away

(iv) Backache: Like headache, backache is also a common ailment

Causes

- Standing or sitting in wrong posture, with the shoulders dropped is a common cause of backache
- In older people, chronic backache is due to arthritis
- Low back pain that is worse the day after heavy lifting or straining may be a sprain
- Severe low back pain that first comes suddenly when lifting or twisting may be a slipped disc
- Pain in the middle of the back may be due to kidney diseases
- Low backache is normal for some women during menstrual periods or pregnancy
- Very low back pain sometimes comes from problems in the uterus, ovaries or rectum

The following first aid measures required:
- Simple backache, including that of pregnancy, can often be prevented or made better by:
    - Always standing erect
    - Sleeping on a firm flat surface or on the floor
    - Back bending exercises
- Aspirin helps calm most kings of backaches
- Sitting in a hot water tub may also help
- If pain does not get better, seek medical advise

(v) Toothache: Toothache usually is, though not always, the result of dental neglect. In the majority of cases toothache is the reaction of irritated nerve endings within the tooth occurring because of decay or accident. In this type of ache the patient can usually locate the tooth because it hurts when a particle of food or hot or cold water enters the cavity. When the pain is caused by inflammation at the root end of the tooth, the offending tooth is more difficult to locate.

The following measures are initiated:
- If the aching tooth is obviously decayed, the pain may be relived by slightly, dampening a small pledged of cotton with oil of clove and inserting it into the cavity
- Taking one or two aspirin tablets may lessen the pain
- Never place an aspirin tablet on the gum tissue surrounding the offending tooth; that will seriously irritate the gums and will not relieve the pain
- Hot or cold clothes applied to the cheek will give some relief
- Go to a dentist if pain does not get better

Prevention

Fortunate is the family that observes the four basic dental health rules:

- Follow an adequate, well balanced in which sweets are kept at a minimum
- Cleanse the mouth thoroughly immediately after eating
- Have early and frequent examinations and care by your dentist
- Drink fluorinated water or have fluoride solution applied by the dentist directly to the children's teeth

(vi) Earache: Earache occurs due to exposure to cold, an infection in a part of the ear called middle ear or a foreign body in the ear.

There is a passage way between the nose, throat and middle ear so that in case of colds, germs sometimes reach the middle ear. The danger is greater if one blow the nose vigorously, particularly if he shuts one nostril and closes the mouth at the same time.

- Go to bed and care for the cold
- Do not blow the nose improperly
- Apply a hot water bottle or an electric pad to the ear
- If the heat so applied does not give relief, use cold applications instead
- Do not try to remove foreign body but seek medical help
- Ear infection should always be treated by a physician. Otherwise more serious disease may develop and partial deafness may result.

(vii) Vomiting: Many people, especially children, have an occasional 'stomach upset' with vomiting. Often no cause can be found. There may be mild stomachache or abdominal colic or fever. This kind of simple vomiting usually is not serious and clears up by itself.

Vomiting is one of the signs of many different problems, some minor and some quite serious, so it is important to examine the person carefully. Vomiting often comes from a problem in the stomach or guts, such as : an infection (diarrhea, poisoning from spoiled food, or acute abdomen (for example, appendicitis of something blocking the gut). Also, almost any sickness with high fever or severe pain may cause vomiting, especially malaria, hepatitis, tonsillitis, earache, meningitis, urinary infection, gall bladder pain or migraine headache.

Danger Signs with Vomiting Seek Medical Help Quickly

- Dehydration that increases and that you cannot control
- Severe vomiting that lasts more than 24 hours
- Violent vomiting especially if vomit is dark green, brown or smells like faeces
- Constant pain in the abdomen, especially if the person cannot defecate
- Vomiting of blood

In such condition:

- Do not let patient eat anything while the vomiting is severe
- Sips of tea with sugar but without any milk can be given afterwards. Adding sugar or lime juice may also help
- For dehydration, because of loss of fluid and electrolytes in vomiting, give small frequent sips of water, tea or rehydration drink

(viii) Diarrhea: When a person has loose or watery stools, her has diarrhea. If mucus and blood can be seen in the stools, he has dysentery. Diarrhea can be mild or serious. It can be acute (sudden and severe) or chronic (lasting many days).

Diarrhea is more common and more dangerous in young children, especially those who are poorly nourished. Diarrhea has many causes. Sometimes special treatment is needed. However, most diarrhea can be treated successful in the home, even if you can not sure of the exact cause of causes.

Causes

- Poor nutrition. This weakens the child and makes diarrhea from other causes more frequently
- Virus infection
- An infection of the gut caused by bacteria, amoebas or giardia
- Worm infections
- Infections outside the gut (ear infections, tonsillitis, measles, urinary infections)
- Food poisoning
- Inability to digest milk
- Side effects produced by certain medicines, such as ampicillin or tetracycline
- Laxatives, purges, irritating or poisonous plants, certain poisons
- Eating too much unripe fruit or heavy greasy foods

In such condition following measures needed:

- For most cases of diarrhea no medicine is needed
- If the diarrhea is severe the biggest danger is dehydration. A person with watery diarrhea must drink large amounts of liquids. If diarrhea is severe or there are signs of dehydration give him rehydration drink. Even he does not want to drink, gently insist that he does so. Have him take several swallows every few minutes.
- *Rehydration drink:* In 1 liter of boiled water put 2 tablespoons of sugar or honey and ¼ teaspoon bicarbonate of soda. If available, add half a cup of orange juice or a little lemon juice to the drink
- A person with diarrhea needs food as soon as he will eat. This is especially important in small children or persons who are already poorly nourished
- When the person is vomiting or feels too sick to eat, he should drink:
  - Tea
  - Rice water
  - Chicken, meat, egg or bean broth
  - Rehydration drink
  - Sweetened drink
  - Breast milk (in infants)
- As soon as the person is able to eat, in addition to the above drinks he should be eat a balanced nutritional diet free of chillies and spices.
- Seek medical help if needed

Prevention

- Although diarrhea has many different causes, the most common are infection and poor nutrition
- With good hygiene and good food, most diarrhea could be prevented
- Use of latrines, clean water and protection of foods from dirt and flies are the key points of cleanliness

(ix) Acute Abdominal Pain: Abdominal pain should not be dismissed lightly for it may be caused by a serious disease, such as appendicitis. The other conditions producing abdominal pain are peptic ulcer, diseases of liver and gall bladder, diseases of small and large gut and diseases of kidneys. Indigestion, constipation and diarrhea may also cause abdominal pain.

In such cases:

- Put the victim to bed in a comfortable position
- Withhold all food
- A laxative should not be given
- Always play the safe in case of abdominal pain
- Seek medical help immediately. Too often, in case of abdominal pain, people postpone calling a doctor and give extremely harmful first aid by administering a laxative. Then, if the trouble is appendicitis, the appendix may rupture, and even more serious illness or death may follow

(x) Asthma: A person with asthma has fits or attacks of difficult breathing. It often begins in childhood and may be a problem for life. It is not contagious, but is more common in children with relatives who have asthma. It is generally worse during certain months of the year or at night. Persons who have had asthma for years may develop emphysema. An asthma attack may be caused by eating or breathing things to which the person is allergic. In children, asthma often starts with a common cold. In some person nervousness or worry also plays a part in bringing on an asthma attack. In an asthma attack, a hissing or wheezing is heard, especially when patient breaths out. If the person cannot get enough air, his nails and lips may turn blue, and his neck veins may swell. Usually there is no fever. There may be cough with a little white thick mucous.

In such cases:

- Remain calm and be gentle with the person. Reassure him
- If asthma gets worse inside the house, the person should be taken out where the air is cleanest
- Divert the attention of patient by giving him something to read or see, this will reduce the tension
- Most of the patients feel relieved in a sitting position. Make the person sit comfortably with a back rest
- Give a lot of liquids. This loosens mucous and makes breathing easier. Breathing water vapour may also help.
- Usually patients of asthma keeps medicines with themselves. Ask him to take it
- If the person does not get better, seek medical help

Prevention

- A person with asthma should avoid eating or breathing things that bring on attacks
- The house or work place should be kept clean
- Do not let chickens or other animals inside
- Put bedding out to air in sunshine
- Sometimes it helps to sleep outside in the open air
- Persons with asthma may improve when they move to a different area, where the air does not contain substance that cause allergy.
- If you have asthma, do not smoke – smoking damages your lungs even more

(xi) Allergic reactions: An allergy is a disturbance or reaction that affects only certain persons, when things to which they are sensitive or allergic to are:

- Breathed in
- Eaten
- Injected
- Or has touched the skin
  Allergic reactions, which can be mild or very serious, include:
- Itching rashes, patches or hives
- Runny nose and itching or burning eyes
- Irritation in the throat, difficulty in breathing or asthma
- Allergic shock
- Diarrhea (in children)

An allergy is not an infection and cannot be passed from one person to another, however, children of allergic parents also tend to have allergies.

Often allergic persons suffer more in certain seasons – or whenever they come in contact with the substances that bother them.

Causes

- Pollen of certain flowers and grasses
- Chicken feathers
- Dust
- Feather pillows
- Moldy blankets or clothes
- Hair of cats and other animals
- Certain medicines, especially injections or penicillin or horse serum.
- Specific foods – fish, shell fish, beer etc.

In such cases:

- Immediately stop the use of specific substance, medicine, clothes etc., which give rise to allergic reactions
- In cases of severe skin itching and burning, apply cold sponges, calamine lotion or a solution of sodabicarb locally
- Keep the nails of children trimmed so they do not keep on scratching the rashes over skin. Gloves or a cloth may be tied over their fists
- Seek medical help.

Prevention

Preventive measures are the same as described for prevention of Asthma.

(xii) Hiccups: Hiccups occur due to spasms of the muscle dividing the abdomen from the chest. They are commonly due to eating or drinking too much or too fast, and they ordinarily recover by themselves, which explains why there are so many hiccup remedies. They all work when the hiccups are ready to stop anyhow. Hiccupping which lasts for days, however, is exhausting and can indicate disease. This symptom should therefore have medical attention if it does not stop within a few hours to home remedies.

In such cases:

- One of the best ways to stop hiccup is to lie down and rest
- Sometimes the hiccup stops if you drink water slowly
- Take a deep breath and hold it as long as you can, releasing it slowly

- Try breathing in and out of a paper bag that fits tightly over the mouth
- Or take half a teaspoonful of baking soda in water, drinking it slowly

(xiii) Constipation: A person who has hard stools and have not had a bowel movement for 2 or more days is said to be constipated. Constipation is often caused by a poor diet (especially not eating enough fruits, green vegetables or foods with natural fibre) or by lack of exercises. Acute fevers and diseases of intestines may also cause constipation. Simple constipation is usually not a serious condition.

In such condition:
- Drinking more water and eating more fruits, vegetables and food with natural fibre like tapioca or wheat bran is better than using laxatives.
- Older people may need to walk or exercise more to milk of regular bowel movements
- A person who has not had a bowel movement and he does not have pain in his abdomen can take a mild salt laxative like milk of magnesia. But do not take laxatives often
- Never use strong purgatives or laxatives – especially if there is abdominal pain
- A glycerine suppository or an anema of soap or liver oil may also be used
- If there is acute abdominal pain with constipation, seek medical help immediately.

(xiv) Indigestion: Indigestion and 'heart burn' often come from eating too heavy or greasy food or from drinking too much alcohol. Tension and excitement may also lead to indigestion. These make the stomach produce extra acid, which causes discomfort or a 'burning' feeling in the stomach or midchest. Some people mistake the chest pain called 'heartburn' for a heart problem rather than indigestion. Ulcer in stomach may also lead to signs and symptoms of indigestion.

In such condition:
- Make the patient lie comfortably in bed. Gentle massage over upper abdomen may help
- Milk is one of the best medicines for indigestion
- Antacids, such as milk of magnesia or magnesium and aluminium hydroxide relieves discomfort and pain
- Stop all solid foods by mouth
- Seek medical help if:
  - person starts vomiting blood
  - the stools become black like tar
  - pain persists

(xv) Hernia: A hernia is an opening or tear in the muscles covering the belly. This permits a loop of gut to push through and form under the skin. Some babies are born with a hernia. In men, hernias are common in the groin. If the hernia suddenly becomes large or painful, does not reduce, causes vomiting and person cannot have a bowel movement, this can be very dangerous. Seek medical help fast, surgery may be necessary.

In such cases:
- Let the patient lie in bed, covered up comfortably
- Do not try to make it go back
- Stoop everything by mouth
- Seek medical help fast

(xvi) Piles (Hemorrhoids): Piles or haemorrhoids are varicose veins of the anus or rectum, which feel like lumps or walls. They may be painful but not dangerous. They frequently appear during pregnancy and may go away afterwards. If a haemorrhoid begins to bleed, the person will have signs of anaemia.

In such cases do the following:
- Piles may be caused in part due to constipation. It helps to eat plenty of fruits or food with a lot of fibre and drink water in sufficient quantity to relieve constipation
- *Sitz bath:* To get relief from pain, fill a tub with warm water. Add some potassium permanganate. Soak your buttocks in this hot water for half an hour. Do this two or three times a day
- Seek medical help if:
  - Very large haemorrhoids
  - Severe pain
  - Non stop bleeding of haemorrhoids

(xvii) Retention of Urine: When the collected urine in the bladder is not passed out because of some disease or operation, it is called *retention of urine*. This usually occurs in older people. The causes are enlarged prostate gland, stones in bladder, diseases of bladder, lying in the bed for a long time, and operations around and over lower part of abdomen, penis or anus. Patient feels a dull ache over lower abdomen and he may pass a little urine drop-by-drop with great difficulty.

In such case following measures to be taken:
- Keeping hot water bags over lower part of abdomen on bladder
- Sitting in a hot water tub
- In some instances walking over a cold wet floor or dashing cold water on the legs and thighs, will cause a discharge and bring relief
- Going to toilet and opening the tap to run water may also help in urination
- If none of these help then seek medical help

(xviii) Motion Sickness: Motion sickness is a sensitivity to movement, acceleration, or deceleration. It can ruin an otherwise enjoyable trip by ship, plane, train, car or bus. The person has severe nausea and vomiting during the journey. Some people are susceptible to this because of disturbance in the 'equilibrium centrre' of the body. Excitement and nervousness may also result into this.

In such case following measures initiated:
- Most of the time this miserable experience can be avoided if susceptibility is known.

To Prevent the Spread of Disease
- Call a physician when the first symptom appear
- Keep the sick away from contact with the well (Isolation)

- Cleanse and disinfect all things that have come in contact with the sick
- When the physician shall advice, use vaccination, injection of serums etc
- Keep flies and insects away from the sick room
- Disinfect the bodily discharges of the sick, especially the sputum
- In waterborne diseases use boiled and cool drinking water
- Do not neglect colds. Colds are communicable. They are often the beginning of serious diseases
- Watch mild cases of diphtheria, measles, scarlet fever, and like malady. They may produce virulent cases in others
- Consider the period of recovery dangerous. In many diseases the apparently well may still convey the disease
- Keep sick children away from school until the doctor advises their return. After recovery, cleanse and disinfect clothing and premises.

(xix) Angina Pectoris: It is a cardiac pain which occurs on exertion, due to insufficient blood supply to the heart muscle. Coronary arteries are unable to deliver sufficient blood to the heart muscle to meet the increased demand, of exertion, excitement etc. The causes of angina pectoris may be to:
- Strenuous exercises e.g., walking uphill or upstairs
- Much exertion
- After heavy meals
- Exposure to cold weather
- Emotional upsets

The duration of pain: Usually between 2-5 minutes and the *signs and symptoms includes the following* (Table 27.4).
- The pain is crushing or squeezing in nature spreading to the left arm and jaw
- Feeling of tingling in the arms
- The pain may radiate up to elbow, wrist or even fingers
- Weakness, often sudden and extreme
- Person may look pale and anxious with rapid pulse

In such condition:
- The pain usually disappears after taking rest for a while or after taking nitroglycerine or a puff of aerosol
- Help the casualty sit down. Reassure him and make him comfortable

Prevention of such condition includes the following:
- Heavy physical activities to be curtailed
- Avoid smoking and fatty foods
- Good sleep and mental rest necessary
- Avoid exposure to cold weather
- Warm climate is beneficial
- Avoid excessive tea or coffee
- Physical strain with loaded stomach to be avoided

(xx) Heart Attack: A heart attack commonly occurs when the blood supply to part of the heart muscle is suddenly obstructed, e.g., a clot in one of the coronary artery (Coronary thrombosis). The seriousness largely depends on how much of the heart muscle is affected. The Signs and Symptoms of heart attack include:
- The onset is acute and occur usually during the rest

Table 27.4: Comparison of Angina Pectoris and Myocardial Infarction

	Angina Pectoris	*Myocardial Infarction*
• Onset	After effort	At rest
• Attitude of patient after onset	Still and motionless	Restless
• Duration of pain	Minutes	Hours and days
• Blood Pressure	May be little elevated	Progressively declines
• Features of shock and collapse	Absent	May be present
• Cardiac findings	S4 sometimes audible	S3 and S4 with typical gallop rhythm; pericardial rub, muffling of heart sounds may be present
• Pulmonary basal crepitations and dyspnoea	Usually absent	Usually present
• Fever	Absent	Present
• Relief of pain	By nitroglycerin	By stronger sedatives like Morphine and Pethidine

- The pain is crushing often radiating from heart but unlike anginal pain, it does not ease with rest, conversely may occur at rest, and persist longer.
- Breathlessness and restlessness
- Discomfort in abdomen like severe indigestion
- Blueness at the lips
- Rapid pulse
- Cold limbs, excessive sweating

In this condition:
- Help the casualty into a relaxed position to ease strain on the heart.
- A half sitting position with head and shoulders supported and knees bent is comfortable
- Give ordinary aspirin tablet and tell him to chew it slowly. *Thrombolytics* are the drugs which aid recovery by dissolving the clot.
- While sending for a doctor, keep constant observation on pulse, breathing, etc., and be ready to resuscitate.

(xxi) Cardiac Arrest: The sudden stoppage of heart beat is cardiac arrest.

Causes of cardiac arrest will be:
- Heart attack
- Severe blood loss

Table 27.5: Common Toxic Substances and their First Aid

Toxic	Sources	First aid
Acetyl salisylic acid	A.P.C and Aspirin containing tablets	Induce vomiting. Give one teaspoon of soda bicarb in one glass of water
Concentrated acid	Hospitals, laboratories motor workshops, some factories	Do not induce vomiting. Give excess water to weaken the acid. Give one tablespoon of milk of magnesia, chalk or soda bicarb in one glass of water
Concentrated alkali	Hospital, laboratory and some factories	Do not induce vomiting. Give excess water to weaken the alkali. One tablespoon of vinegar, orange, lemon
Arsenic	Rat killing medicine, insecticides	Induce vomiting. Give sweet beverages like milk, egg white or solution of wheat flour in water
Atropine or Belladona	Eye ointment, eye drops	Induce vomiting. Give tea or coffee to drink
Carbon monoxide	Gas burner smoke, smokes of motors	Give artificial respiration. Give oxygen if available (available in some garages and factories)
Hypnotics (Barbiturates group)	Hypnotics and tablets and powder to get relief from pain	Give a tablespoon of Epsum salt in a glass of water. Give hot tea or coffee. Keep the person awakened. Give artificial respiration, if necessary
Disinfectants like cresol, Lysol, dettol etc.	Hospital and house	Do not induce vomiting. Give epsum salt in one glass of water or paraffin
Lead	Some colors and hair dyes	Induce vomiting. Give one spoon of epsum salt in a glass of water.
Mercury	Mercury	Give milk after giving egg white mixed with water. After this induce vomiting
Morphine	Hospitals, house and agricultural fields	Induce vomiting. Give some grains of potassium permanganate in one glass of water to drink. Give hot tea or coffee to drink. Keep the person awakened. Keep him covered.
Paraffin and petrol kerosene	House, garages and factories	Induce immediately. give water to drink in excess amount. If a person had drunk kerosene then liquid paraffin in one glass of water can be given.
Phosphorous	Rat killing medicine	Induce vomiting. Give some grains of potassium in a glass of water to drink
Prussic acid	Photography and electroplating. Bitter almond oil	Get to induced vomiting immediately. give artificial respiration
Strychnine	Some insecticides	Get to induced vomiting before the cramps are started. Keep the patient peaceful. Do not try to control his severe movements by hand. If the respiration is stopped then give artificial respiration.

- Suffocation
- Electric shock
- Drug overdose
- Hypothermia

The Signs and Symptoms of cardiac arrest will be:
Absence of pulse and breathing

In such condition do the following:
- Resuscitate immediately
- Call for doctor/ambulance
- Many ambulances carry, defibrillators, which is an instrument by which normal rhythm is restored in ventricular or atrial fibrillation by the application of a high-voltage electric current

- The role of first aider is to keep the brain supplied with oxygen by cardiopulmonary resuscitation until a debrillator is brought to the casualty and used by a trained operator.

Poisoning

Poisoning is a condition caused by introduction to harmful substances or chemicals into the body either by injection, inhalation or ingestion. A poison (or toxin) is a substance which, if taken into the body in sufficient quantity, can cause temporary or permanent damage (Table 27.5). Poisons may be swallowed, inhaled through the skin, instilled at the eye, or injected. Once in the body, poisons may work their way into the bloodstream, and be swiftly carried to all the tissues. Signs and symptoms vary depending on the poison and its method of entry, though vomiting is common to many cases, with the risk to the casualty that stomach contents may be inhaled.

(i) Household Poisoning

Almost every household contains poisonous substances, such as bleach, paint stripper, glue, paraffin, insecticides, pesticides, alcohol, petroleum products, acids, alkalis, sedatives etc. household poisoning may be due to chemical burn or by swallowing. Children are at more risk from accidental household poisoning. The signs and symptoms of severe poisoning depend on the types and time spent after the ingestion of poison. The symptoms of poisoning appear suddenly and intensify gradually and can take a serious form if the first aid is not provided in time. The ingestion of certain poisons can lead to severe stomach ache, vomiting, muscular cramps or spasms. Certain other substances like sleeping pills can cause unconsciousness. The ingestion of concentrated acid or alkali may cause tongue to appear stained, spotted or burnt.

In such cases following first aid measures are helpful:

The first aider or nurse should always be ready to look after the poisoning case at once because this is such a crucial condition in which the life of the affected person can be saved by giving immediate help. Poisoning is a serious problem so the patient should at once be taken to the hospital or someone should be sent to call the doctor. If the appearing symptoms an signs can be noticed, then the name of the poisonous substance should be noted. The empty packets or bottle of the suspected poisonous substance and the vomit of the patient should be preserved and brought to the notice of the doctor.

- **Dilute or weaken the poisonous substances:** Excess water should be given to the known cases of poisoning because many substances cannot produce dangerous effects when weakened by water, as they in their concentrated state like strong acid or strong alkalies.
- **Taking out of poisonous substances by inducing vomiting:** The poisonous substances can be taken out of the body by inducing vomiting. This can be done by mixing two tablespoons of salt in one glass of water or two teaspoons of soda bicarb in a glass of water or by mixing one teaspoon of mustard powder in lukewarm water. If the above substances are not available then lukewarm alone is alone useful.

If it is known that the ingested poison is concentrated acid or alkali then efforts should not be made to make the person vomit out because these poisonous substances come in contact with the soft tissues and cause irritation. One tablespoon of Epsom salt mixed in a glass is beneficial after the stomach is empty.

General Care: Due to the effects of the poisonous substances or in effort to take these substances out, a person can become unconscious. In such cases give the first aid as is given in shock. If the respiration is not normal then give artificial respiration. The possibility of cessation of respiration is due to poisoning caused by sleeping pills. A person can die in shock caused by poisoning. In such cases first aid should be given immediately.

- **In all cases of poisoning seek the medical help or call the doctor immediately:** During the period, if the first aider can note the initial symptoms and signs, the things lying around the casualty can be of much help to the doctor. Any empty bottle or medicine packet and other things lying around the person should be handed over to the doctor or the police.

If the ingested substance is in the form of concentrated acid or alkali then in such cases water mixed with magnesium or milk should be given. If it is concentrated alkali then one gets relief by giving vinegar or lemon juice in water. And in this way vomiting can be induced after giving 4-6 glasses of water because then these substances get weakened in water. Now give milk, cream or egg white to the casualty for drinking.

Hypnotics: Like Morphine, heroines and barbiturates can lead to sleep, deep coma by which the respiration is slowed down. In such cases if the patient is conscious then try to take out the poisonous medicines by including vomiting or weaken those substances by giving more water to drink. Though some medicines get absorbed through the stomach still if these are diluted then there poisonous effect can be lessened.

Keep the person awakened who is sleeping with the effect of sleeping pills: Keep him awakened by piercing pin, tickling or if he is conscious then keep him awakened by giving tea or coffee. If respiration is very slow then give artificial respiration immediately and get the first aid quickly.

(ii) Gas Poisoning

Severe symptoms can arise with the inhalation of poisonous gases. These gases are carbon monoxide (coal gas), carbon dioxide, inflammable gases, stema of ammonia etc. thus this poisoning can occur due to engines running on petroleum products or gases evolved from gas burners or stove, refrigeration plant or cold storage. These poisonous gases (1) Reduce the amount of oxygen in inhaled air. (2) Affects the oxygen carrying capacity of blood. (3) Damage the mucous membrane of the respiratory tract, not allowing the oxygen to be absorbed in the blood from the lungs.

The places or sites and sources of carbon monoxide are given below:

	Source
Automobile	Incomplete combustion of gasoline
	Faculty exhaust pipes
	Faulty muffler
	Heater drawing in exhaust fumes from car ahead congested traffic yielding high concentration of CO into surrounding air
Enclosed Buildings	Car engine running in garage
	Incomplete combustion of heating fuels: gas, coal, oil, wood
	Clogged chimney flue in heated building
	Lit charcoal frill moved indoors
	Paint stripper containing methylene chloride which metabolizes to CO

Industry	Industrial plants
	Kilns
	Mines
	Mills
	Workshops

The signs and symptoms of gas poisoning are:
- Dizziness
- Tightening of chest
- Loss of consciousness
- Meiosis
- Respiratory failure
- Fall in blood pressure and pulse rate
- Twitching and convulsions
- Asphyxia
- Cyanosis
- Circulatory collapse

In such cases following aid measures are helpful:
Remove the patient immediately from the accidental spot and bring him in the open air. The first aider in such cases should not stay longer in gas afflicted area, as he may also come under such attack. If the respiratory process is stopped then start giving artificial respiration. Keep the patient warm under blanket or bed sheet. Continue giving artificial respiration unless the respiratory process comes to normal and regular. If there is no quick improvement in the patient's condition then make an arrangement to send him to hospital.

(iii) Food Poisoning

Food poisoning generally occurs in summer. It is commonly due to contaminated water, food substances, unboiled and uncleaned vegetables, contaminated kulfi, milk and cream products. This poisoning is due to toxins produced by bacteria present in these foods. Such cases mostly occur in groups in marriages or dinners due to consumption of contaminated food.

Signs and Symptoms
- Nausea and vomiting
- Cramping abdominal pains
- Diarrhea (possibly bloodstained)
- Headache
- Fever
- Features of shock
- Collapse

In such cases the following first aid measures are helpful:
The main aim of first is to eliminate the poison, to avoid their absorption or to make them less harmful. The care after this is to be handled by the doctor. Give bland fluids such as water, diluted fruit juice or weak tea. Help and encourage the casualty to take plenty of fluid. If much time has not lapsed to the intake of poisonous substance the its effect can be weakened by inducing vomiting but if lot of time has passed then inducing vomiting is useful. Sometimes with constant vomiting and diarrhea the water an electrolyte balance of the body gets disturbed which results in to the weakens and condition of shock arises. In such case an arrangement to send the patient to the doctor and hospital should be made immediately.

Sometimes people fell sick in groups because of eating in marriage ceremonies etc. such condition can be lead to uneasiness, cramps, vomiting and diarrhea. With loss of body water there is severe thirst and weakness. Such cases should be immediately sent to the hospital.

(iv) Alcohol Poisoning

Alcohol (ethanol) is a drug that depresses the activity of the central nervous system. Small quantities generally produce only a slight change of mood. Prolonged intake can result in all physical and mental abilities becoming severely impaired, and deep unconsciousness can ensure. The Dangers of alcohol poisoning includes the following:
- An unconscious casualty is in danger of inhaling and choking on vomit
- Because alcohol dilates the blood vessels, hypothermia may develop if the casualty is exposed to the cold.
- A casualty with head injuries who smells of alcohol may be misdiagnosed

Signs and Symptoms
- A strong smell of alcohol
- Unconsciousness. The casualty may be rousable, but will quickly relapse
- A flushed and moist face
- Deep, noisy breathing
- A full, bounding pulse

In the later stages of unconsciousness
- A dry, bloated appearance to the face
- Shallow breathing
- Dilated pupils that react poorly to light
- A weak, rapid pulse

If a person is in intoxication of liquor the he should be made to sit and vomit. After this give him strong tea or coffee. If the patient is unconscious and the symptoms of head injury are seen, then arrange to send him to the hospital immediately.

(v) Dhatura Poisoning

This poisoning is due to consumption of seeds of tree 'Dhatura' which may be eaten unknowingly or accidentally or may be due to consumption of Belladona alkaloids containing medicine. In this condition there is fever and the skin looks shiny, red patched and dry. The eye balls are expanded and there is difficulty in swallowing. The respiration can slow down. In later condition there is spasm and unconsciousness.

In such cases the following measures are helpful:
Keep the patient in cool, dark and silent room and control the severe movements patiently. If more time has not gone in appearance of the symptoms then some poisonous substances

come out by inducing vomiting. But vomiting should be not induced in conditions of unconsciousness and cramps. Cold bandages on the body and on the head gives relief in high fever. In the condition of respiratory feebleness, artificial respiration can be given. Hot tea or coffee can be given. If there is no improvement in the condition then immediately receive the medical help or arrange to send him to the hospital.

Protective Measures of Accidental Poisoning

In children the accidental poisoning occurs generally due to the intake of attractive substances. In anxiety or ignorance and in adults it occurs due to carelessness. The toxic effects of various types of medicines and intoxicating substances if taken in excessive amount can be seen. The normal dose given to adult person can be toxic to children. The normal dose given to adult person can be toxic to children. Therefore, following rules should be observed:

- Medicine bottles and packets should be clearly labeled. Medicines of unlabelled bottles should not be used and should be destroyed.
- Write the word 'poison' on the toxic medicines and household insecticides. Keep them in locked almirah
- Never take medicines from the unclearly labeled bottles. Do not take them in dark room
- The label on the bottle should be read before taking the medicine, during measuring the dose and while keeping the bottle back to the place
- Caustic soda or potash solution used for cleaning the floor appear like water and by mistake it is drunk as water when one feels thirsty. Therefore clear label should be put on the bottle.
- Empty bottles are filled with some acids, like acid used in the batteries, acids used in cleaning sink, wash basins, toilet etc., and are sold in the market, in which sometimes the original label should be removed and the new label of the filled substance should be put and the bottles should be kept beyond the reach of the children
- To avoid food poisoning food should be prepared with cleanliness and kept covered. Flies should be prevented to sit on the cooked food. Vegetables should be washed and boiled properly, and in suspected case boiled water must be consumed.

28

Rehabilitation/ Rehabilitative Nursing

Definitions

1. Rehabilitation means the restoration of one's physical, mental, social, vocational and economic capacity to the fullest extent to which one is capable—NCR

2. Rehabilitation is a creative procedure which includes the cooperative efforts of various medical specialists and their associates in other health fields to improve the mental, physical, social and vocational aptitudes of persons who are handicapped with the objective of prescribing their ability to live happily and productively on the same level and with the same opportunities as their neighbors—Frank Krusen

3. Rehabilitation as a treatment process designed to help physically handicapped individual to make maximal use of residual capacities and to enable them to obtain optimal satisfaction and usefulness in terms of themselves, their families and their communities—Helen J Yesner

4. Rehabilitation is concerned typically with the people who have disabilities with enduring and pervasive effect. The essence of the rehabilitation is recognition that what has happened to the patient affects and will continue to affect many aspects of his life extending beyond limits of bodily functions—Dr William Fordyce

5. Rehabilitation is a transient episode during which, a human being with a physical, psychological impairment is given the opportunity to realize himself latent potentialities for improved independence of action and of personal care—Dr Sedwick Mead

6. Rehabilitation is a program designed to enable the individual who is physically disabled, chronically ill or convalescing to live and to work to the utmost of his capacity. It is an integral part of clinical non-institutional and community responsibility in meeting the problems of chronic illness—Dr Howard Rusk

7. Rehabilitation is spinning or bridging gap between uselessness and usefulness, between hopelessness and hopefulness, between despair and happiness—Miss Mary Switzer

8. Rehabilitation is creative process that begins with immediate preventive care in the first degree of an accident or illness. It is continued through the restorative phase of care and involves adaptation of the whole being to a new life.

9. Rehabilitation is a creative process that allows maximal use of existing abilities. It is basically an optimistic process which concedes that despite continuing and even catastrophic disability a better way of life for the patient is possible.

10. Rehabilitation is the process of maximising an individual's abilities and resources to promote optimum growth and focusing on the individual's decision-making ability. This begins with preventive care in the initial stage of accident and/or illness, it continues through the restorative phase and it involves adaptation of new life.

Philosophy of Rehabilitation

Rehabilitation is a dynamic, health-oriented process that assists an ill or disabled individual to achieve the greatest possible level of physical, mental, spiritual, social and economic functioning. The rehabilitation process helps the person to achieve an acceptable quality of life with dignity, self-respect and independence.

Rehabilitation programs are designed for individuals with physical, mental and emotional disabilities. During rehabilitation, the individual is assisted to adjust to the disability by learning how to use resources and to focus on existing abilities, are emphasized.

Rehabilitation is an integral part of nursing. Rehabilitation efforts should begin during the initial contact with the patient. Every major illness or injury carries with it the threat of disability. The principles of rehabilitation are basic to the care of all patients. The emphasis of rehabilitation is to restore the patient to independence or to the pre-illness or pre-injury level of function in as short a time as possible. If this is not possible, the aims of rehabilitation are maximal independence and quality of life acceptable to the patient. Realistic goals based on individual patient assessment are established with the patient to guide the rehabilitation program.

Rehabilitation services are required by more people than ever before, because of advances in technology that saves the lives of the seriously ill, injured and disabled. Increasing numbers of patients who are recovering from serious illness or injuries are returning to their homes and communities with ongoing needs for rehabilitation. Every patient regardless of age, socioeconomic status, or diagnosis, has a right to rehabilitative services.

The economic advantage of rehabilitation is readily apparent. Instead of being unemployed, the person is rehabilitated into employment. Instead of being dependent on society, the person contributes to it.

Rehabilitation Team

Rehabilitation is a creative and dynamic process that requires a team of professionals working together with patients and family. The team members represent a variety of disciplines, with each health professional making a unique contribution. Each health professional assesses the patient's needs within the discipline domain. Rehabilitative goals are set. Team members meet in group sessions at frequent intervals to collaborate, to evaluate progress, and to modify goals as needed to facilitate rehabilitation.

The patient is the key member of the rehabilitation team. Patient is the focus of the team effort and that one who determines the final outcomes of the process. The patient participates in goal setting in learning to function using remaining abilities, and in adjusting to living with disabilities. The rehabilitation team promotes independence, self-respect and an acceptable quality of life.

The patient's family is incorporated into the team. The family is a dynamic system. Disability of the one member affects other family members. Only by incorporating the family into the rehabilitation process can make the family adapt to the change in one of its members. The family provides ongoing support, participates in problem solving and learns to provide necessary ongoing care.

The rehabilitation nurse develops a therapeutic and supportive relationship with the patient and the family. The nurse always emphasizes the patient's assets and strengths. During nurse-patient interactions, the nurse actively listens, encourages and shares the patient's triumph. The patient is praised for efforts to improve self-concept and self-care abilities. Through application of the nursing process, the nurse develops a plan of care designed to facilitate rehabilitation, to restore and maintain optimum health, and to prevent complication. The nurse helps the patient to identify strengths and past successes and to develop new goals. Frequently, coping with the disability, self-care, mobility, skin care, and bowel and bladder managements are areas of nursing intervention.

The nurse assumes role of caregiver, teacher, counselor, patient's advocate and consultant. Frequently, the nurse if the case manager responsible for coordinating the total rehabilitative plan. The nurse collaborates with and co-ordinates the services provided by all members of the healthcare team including the home health nurse who is responsible for directing the patient's care after return to the home.

The rehabilitation team also may include a physician, surgeon, psychiatrist, physical therapist, occupational therapist, speech-language pathologist, psychologist, social worker, vocational counselor, orthotist/prosthetist, and rehabilitation engineer.

Basic Aims of Rehabilitation

In order for patients to receive the greatest benefit from a rehabilitation program, it is imperative that nurse perceive rehabilitation as a process that begins when a patient first suffers acute disease or trauma. The elements of rehabilitation nursing need to be viewed as a part of basic nursing rather than as a speciality. Those who work at rehabilitation centers where patients are severely disabled naturally have additional knowledge in this field of nursing. However, this is a matter of degree and depth of knowledge rather than a matter of a completely new body of knowledge. Both early care during the acute phase of a condition and continued care after a rehabilitation program are essential to the patient's ultimate and continued adjustment. With this in mind, it becomes evident that at least some degree of knowledge of rehabilitation nursing is required by all nurses. The nurse who is convinced of this need will translate her knowledge into actions that go beyond feeding and turning patients.

Three basic aims of rehabilitation are considered in the care given by all members of the health team. It will be useful to understand the nurse's responsibility in each of these areas before discussing them further in the following.

Prevent Further Impairment

While the prevention of further impairment must be considered throughout the rehabilitation process and long afterward, it is helpful to consider it first. Unfortunately preventive measures are never noticed unless they were not used. A pressure sore is visible but the lack of one is not. Basically, prevention must be future-minded.

Examples of preventive measures will illustrate the variety of ways this aim is accomplished. When there is an automobile accident, the ambulance driver is probably the first person to handle the patient. The way he moves and lifts the person from the street into the ambulance prevent further injury. The emergency room nurse also prevents further impairment by her knowledge of body mechanics, body alignment and first aid. If we visit the patient throughout his hospital stay, we will see measures taken to prevent contractures, foot drop, pressure sores, dependency and so forth.

It is nursing which can and must see that fewer and fewer patients endure treatment or what is worse, hospitalization for preventable conditions. Too many patients have prolonged or postponed rehabilitation programs because of the need to correct or minimize a problem that never should have been allowed to occur.

Maintain Existing Abilities

There is a gray area between preventing further disability and maintaining existing ability. Certain methods used to prevent arm contractures and to maintain its existing ability are similar. However there also needs to be emphasis on the maintenance of the ability of non-injured parts. For example, why should someone with a fractured hip develop hypostatic pneumonia? Why should a young child develop a pressure sore from wearing a leg brace? Why should an amputee develop a hip flexion contracture?

Maintaining existing abilities actually entails preventing additional injury or deterioration of uninvolved parts. Once again, nursing can make sure that no additional treatment of hospitalization is required because of a lack of knowledge on the part of those caring for the patient. As with preventive measures, efforts to maintain existing abilities are continued long after the formal rehabilitation program.

Restore as much Function as Possible

The third aim of rehabilitation is to restore as much function as possible in the injured or diseased part. This is the era of rehabilitation in which the nurse working in a rehabilitation center will have a greater depth of knowledge than the nurse in a nursing home, extended care facility, public health agency or general medical surgical area of a hospital. However, some nurses in the other areas require the same degree of specialized knowledge as those in the rehabilitation center.

The nurse works with the health team to help the patient to regain strength, to restore speech, to walk, to re-learn activities of daily living and to gain new ways to handle bowel and bladder problems. While prevention of further impairment and maintenance of existing ability continue throughout a patient's rehabilitation program, restoration takes procedure at this time. It is the area of restoration that is often responsible for the tendency to isolate rehabilitation as a speciality. It is hoped that there will be a greater awareness of the interrelatedness of these different areas of the total process of rehabilitation, a great many of which occur simultaneously, rather than separately. The result of this awareness will be a higher level of total patient care.

Even where nurses have acquired a greater degree of rehabilitation knowledge, we find varying degrees of this. A nurse may have attained increased knowledge and insight through self-study, in-service education, seminars or short courses, or by attending a formal postgraduate program at a college or university.

Role of the Rehabilitation Nurse

At least some rehabilitation knowledge is required whether the nurse works in the emergency room, the intensive care unit, the extended care facility, the medical service, the geriatric service, the surgical service or the psychiatric service. Prevention of further damage or disabilities and intenancee of existing abilities are particularly vital, no matter where the patient is. We often forget about the physical disabilities that accompany mental diseases. If a person with schizophrenia is allowed to sit in a chair throughout the day, he can develop hip flexion contractures just as easily as someone who is allowed to remain in Fowler's position too long. Problems with ambulation are often severe in mental hospitals. Conversely, we frequently do not use appropriate psychiatric knowledge in our care of patients with physical problems.

In other words, basic rehabilitation knowledge can be used whether the patient has hemophilia, cancer, arthritis, multiple sclerosis, mental illness or cerebral palsy, whether he has had a stroke, a spinal cord injury or a burn. It is up to the nurse to apply the appropriate concepts and techniques to the patients under her care.

Knowledge, Skills and Attitudes

Certain knowledge, skills and attitudes, while pertinent to many areas of nursing, are required in greater depth by the nurse who works with patients having a chronic illness or in a rehabilitation program. First of all, the nurse needs a good understanding of the psychological effects of long-term illness in order to respond appropriately to patient needs during the various stages of adjustment to advisability. Also, she/he needs during the various stages of adjustment to a disability. Also, she/he needs to increase her/his knowledge of anatomy, physiology, and pathophysiology, especially of the nervous system, the musculoskeletal system and the urinary system. The patient also needs to know something about kinesiology—the science of body movement. She will have to be able to communicate with persons who have difficulty in expressing themselves and understanding others. She will need to know how to plan ways in which a patient can achieve bowel and bladder control.

The nurse must also be aware of the interrelatedness of psychosocial and economic problems. What radical changes are occurring to the family as a result of the disease? Is this the breadwinner who has been struck down by some accident or illness? Is this the housewife who must be replaced in the family? Is it a child? What social and vocational obstacles lie ahead? How do individual perceptions of the condition affect planning? What environmental alterations will be needed? Lastly, age must know and use community resources. In the community, the public health nurse will both find rehabilitation candidates and follow those who have completed a program. Public health nursing follow-up is a key factor in maintaining rehabilitation gains in many instances.

In addition to specialized knowledge, the rehabilitation nurse needs to be expert in certain skills. While these skills are used in hospitals treating acute disease, a greater number of variations are required when dealing with the disabled. Each of these skills will be discussed later.

Position changes are essential to maintain body alignment, to prevent skeletal deformities and to prevent pressure sores. If a patient comes to a long-term care facility with a contracture or one or more pressure sores, nursing ingenuity will be vital.

Another necessary skill is the performance of transfer techniques. How has the patient been taught to transfer himself? What kind of technique does he use? What kind of equipment does he use? What kind of wheel chair does he have? Can he transfer independently? How much assistance if any is needed? Can these techniques be used at home?

Skill in performing range of motion exercises vary with the age and condition of the patient. Range of motion exercises will be applied to the disabled part as well as the nondisabled parts to prevent additional problems resulting from disuse.

Finally, the rehabilitation nurse needs to possess special attitudes. All of us have observed the difference in temperament between the operating room nurse and those in slower moving areas of the hospital. Operating room problems are immediate, often a matter of life and death, and the pace is quick. Rehabilitation problems are long-term, a matter of future adjustment, and the pace is slow by comparison. It is important that we know ourselves as well as what will be required of us personally when we select a field of work. Consequently we can suggest that the nurse who prefers quick results works where the pace is more compatible with her temperament.

The rehabilitation nurse needs to be slightly slow-geared. She must have patience and understanding in order to be sensitive to her patient and to adjust her actions accordingly. At certain times, the patient may need a lot of encouragement, at other times pressure is required and on occasion a person may need to be slowed down in his efforts.

The nurse must encourage the patient and praise him not only for achievement but also for effort. The latter is important since results may not be evident for weeks or even months.

Patients need time to perform their tasks, not only when they are first learning but also, perhaps, permanently. No one learns to perform an act from observation. Practice is essential. No one learns to play the piano by watching somebody else playing it. This is equally true in relearning or learning new ways to eat, dress, walk and so forth. We want to allow the patient time. This means allowing ourselves time to let patients do things for themselves.

Some nurses find it difficult to retrain from assisting patients during periods of learning. The helping role of the nurse in rehabilitation differs from that of in acute care. The emphasis is not to help the patient but to help him to help himself. When a nurse first works with patients who have a disability or a chronic disease, she must be especially cognizant of the ultimate goal—patients must become independent in every way allowed by the disability.

Nursing Functions

In many respects the functions of the rehabilitation nurse are similar to those of nurses in other settings. However, there are certain areas of priority and emphasis to which a rehabilitation nurse must address herself.

The nurse will encourage progress from simple to complex procedures, she will proceed from providing much assistance to providing as little as necessary; and she will help the patient to make the adjustment from hospital living to home living. She will need to be constantly vigilant for the many small things that can make the difference between dependent and independent living. She will be aware of the needs that lie ahead, so that returning home presents the least number of unexpected obstacles.

Planning Patient Care

This role includes the integration of objective data from the patient's history and physical examination, careful observation of the patient, application of nursing knowledge and finally, patient participation. These tools and data will help the nurse to assess patient's problems, more accurately and ultimately to assist him to a greater degree. The areas of concern include the physical, psychological, social and environmental spheres of the patient's life. Patient care planning will be discussed in greater detail later on.

Implementing Preventive Nursing Measures

Some nurses have somewhat narrow awareness of what nursing care encompasses. A most unfortunate practice is to limit the activities of the nurse to these ordered by a physician. This is only one function—the dependent on the physical function of the nurse. Even more regrettable, and frequently disastrous, is that the nurse sometimes waits for the physician to order nursing care.

The use of footboards, turning schedules, positioning techniques, range of motion exercises (in most cases), transfer belts, comfort measures and so forth should be initiated by the nurse, not the physician. Her assessment of patient needs takes place over a 24-hour period and is more current than that of any other health professional, including the physician. Therefore, our aim must be to enhance patient care though the initiation of independent nursing measures.

The nursing home is a growing area of practice. In a few homes, where a highly skilled multi-professional staff exists, an unusual situation exists because patients who were thought to be lifetime residents are frequently discharged. This becomes a problem of readjustment for both patients and families who often experienced great conflict about the decision to enter a nursing home. Discharge from a nursing home may imply a poor initial decision. As all personnel begin to study the results of their care, they are finding that new ways of care bring new and unexpected results.

Coordination of a Multidisciplinary Approach

Coordination is a key role of the nurse who cares for patients receiving attention from a variety of health workers. This does not refer to the administrative function of coordinating appointments, request and other activities. It refers to the coordination of the learning from various therapies into the patient's activities throughout his day.

For example, if a patient spends 30 minutes with the speech therapist two or three times a week, he will need to use what he learns between appointments. In order to do this, the nurse must know what the speech therapist would like the patient to practice. Such information must be incorporated to the plan of care. This same concept of coordination holds true of other departments such as physical therapy and occupational therapy. If a patient learns a transfer method of 10.00 A.M. and is allowed to transfer carelessly the other 23/2 hours of the day, his learning will obviously be slow and difficult. In addition, he will become discouraged, and it will negatively affect his motivation for further learning.

In order to coordinate patient learning, the nurse must have open channels of communication between departments. This is sometimes done informally at lunch, during coffee or through telephone calls. However, such informal methods do not guarantee a systematic information flow for each patient. Most rehabilitation centers find that interdisciplinary patient conferences provide an excellent avenue for sharing information. Such meetings are mutually helpful because therapists become more aware of problems encountered outside the confines of their treatment areas. Ultimately, of course, the patient benefits from a treatment team whose members view his problems together. In this way, no therapy works is in isolation.

Teaching

A major role of the rehabilitation nurse is that of patient and family teaching. The patient usually has much to learn. He may need to learn new ways of performing activities of daily livings (ADLs) such as dressing, bathing, eating and toileting. He may need to learn to walk again, to use a wheel-chair or a variety of other new living adaptations.

In order to accomplish the goal of successful patient and family teaching, the nurse must know as much about learning as she does about teaching.

Support

The nurse has her more traditional role in the area of support. It is in this role that she uses her communication skills—listening, in particular. She will need to help both patients and families to visualize a new life, altered though it may be. Her assistance in interpreting the differences between short-term and long-term goals will prevent misunderstanding at various stages of a rehabilitation program. Listening, realising encouragement, helping to clarify misunderstanding, and acceptance of patient's feeling will provide support for the patient and his family at a time when both confusion and fear are most acute.

The nurse's role in rehabilitation has been discussed. The aims of rehabilitation, and the necessary knowledge, skills and attitudes and the major functions of the nurse have been introduced.

Restorative Care of Physically Handicapped

Care of physically handicap or restorative care or restorative nursing synonymous with the more traditional terms rehabilitation care or rehabilitation nursing. In nursing literature the word restoration represents the positive focus of the nurse to assist the client in the acute and the restorative aspects of care and it gradually replaces the word rehabilitation. Likewise, the terms "residual functional deficit" and the "residual functional capacity" are being used instead of "handicap" or "disability" and the term "restorative client" is being used in the place of the terms the "disabled" and the handicapped". Restorative care is an effort by a health care team including the nurse to assist the client to return to the maximal functioning capacity. In other words restorative care is devoted to minimizing the residual functional deficit and maximizing the residual functional capacity.

Clients have a baseline level of functioning which is referred to as their functional capacity. Many health problems affect the clients and result in one or more problems that limit his capacity.

Classifications of common health problems that limit functioning and necessitate restorative care are:

- Disease conditions such as heart disease, pulmonary diseases, neurological and vascular diseases
- Congenital conditional such as cystic fibrosis, club feet, heart defects, e.g. arteriovenous malformations
- Traumatic conditions such as motor vehicle accidents, falls or other injuries especially involving the spinal cord
- Mental an cognitive conditions such as drug induced psychosis. Mood disorders (depression), memory loss and dementia (e.g. Alzheimer's disease).

The reduced functional capacity created by one or more health problems is referred to as residual functional capacity which is the level of functioning remaining after the health problem occurred. The difference in functioning between the original functional capacity (before the health problem occurred) and the residual functional capacity is referred to as the residual functional deficit.

The overall goals of nursing care are to promote, maintain and restore the clients health. Although many definitions of health exist, the advanced definition by WHO is applicable for clients in all health care settings including the restorative care area. Nurse assist client to achieve their maximum level of health and function by intervening at the primary level to promote health, at the secondary level to maintain health or at the tertiary level to restore health.

Restorative care settings: Restorative care settings are numerous. They include but are not necessarily limited to inpatient and outpatient rehabilitation facilities, sub acute care facilities, clinics, and home health care agencies. The services provided in the restorative care settings are those designed to bring the client to the maximal level of health and function: In some instances restorative services are used to assist the family in providing for a terminally ill family member in the home care settings.

Historical perceptive: Since the opening of the first rehabilitation facility in 1893 restorative care has become an increasingly vital component of health care delivery system. Initially restorative services were primarily needed for young persons who were the victims of traumatic injuries or accidents or for certain debilitating diseases such as polio, however 20th century advances in the control of infectious diseases, treatment of life-threatening conditions, nutrition technology and other aspects of health care widen the expanse of restorative care and continue to increase it into the twenty first century. At present restorative care is rapidly expanding. A most important event in the development of restorative care in the United States occurred with the passage of the rehabilitation act of 1973 which was designed to increase awareness of the need for restorative service and to extend these resource throughout the community. The goals of restorative care were to return clients to the community and to increase their control of and participation in their care.

Before the end of the IInd world war restorative services were increasing as a segment of the health care delivery system. These services were primarily available in association with military service. The social security Act of 1935 was the first attempt to extend the restorative services to the American public. Also, during that era restoration was viewed solely as a medical specialty and physicians were virtually the only restorative care professionals.

Initially the inclusion of these restorative care team was limited. In 1965 American Nurses Association realized the need of including nurses in rehabilitation team and published its guidelines for the practice of Nursing on the rehabilitation team as an answer to the growing need and to keep standards of care for the nurse to work in the restorative care team. The disability Act of 1990 in America consider that physical barriers and discrimination trials against the "disabled" were illegal. As a result further advanced changes became important and prevalent for restorative care in the community setting. The current wide spread availability of structural modifications such as wheel chain, access ramps in public institutions especially in hospital, raised toilet seating in public resting rooms, widened "handicap" parking places are notable examples of such physical enhancement.

With the rehabilitation Act of 1973 the role of nursing in restorative care is expanded rapidly. Increasingly nurses assisted the clients as restorative care managers, care givers and advocates. The nurse became a dominant member and with the client, a co-leader of the restorative care team. In 1974 the Association of Rehabilitations Nurses are formed. Ten years later that association began to grant credentials to specialists in rehabilitation nursing.

Restorative health care team: Supports the client's effort to maximize independence within the constraints of the residual functional capacity and as soon as possible to reintegrate the client in the community in the previous or modified role and setting. Ideally the nurses try to eliminate the residual functional deficit, thereby restoring the client to the original functional capacity. It may not be possible in all clients. Usually there will be some residual functional deficit after function compromising health problem such as a cerebrovascular accident. The nurses realistic role is to minimize the effects of deficit, which includes preventing complications and further deterioration, in order the client to the highest level of functional and health possible.

Goal of restorative care: The overall goal of restorative care is to assist the individual to regain maximal functional status there by enhancing the individual's quality of life. Although health care professionals including nurse and various health institutions are involved in restorative care the purpose is to promote client independence and self-care, thus facilitating the clients resumption of a place in the community.

The most important ideas to restorative care are the client's adaptations to the problems necessitating restorative care and fulfillment of all needs in Maslow's hierarchy (Review the Maslow's hierarchy needs). The restorative health care team supports the client's adaptations to or adjustment of the loss of function, maximization of the residual functional capacity and return of the client to the community.

Restorative health care team: Restorative health care requires an interdisciplinary team approach to ensure the delivery of comprehensive, cost effective, non-fragmental quality care. This team is composed of a variety of health care professionals, the client and the clients family and significant others.

The care members of the health care team members are the client, clients family and significant others, the nurse and the physician. Besides the nurse and physician, other health care professionals may be on the team on an as needed base. Some other persons also may be included in the team less frequently and for a shorter period.

The restorative care team functions as a unit to assist the client to achiever the maximal possible level of functioning and to reintegrate into the community. As a whole the team engages in clinical decision making involving assessment, diagnosis, planning implementation and evaluation. Although the health care professionals work together as a team, members participate and contribute from the specific focus of their own respective disciplines. For example, if the team is concerned with a functional problem related to mobility, the physical therapist focuses on foods and feeding schedules to increase activity tolerance during mobility, or for a client with bathing self care deficit, the nurse assistive with the bathing while supervising and reinforcing the clients use of transfer techniques taught by the physical therapist and assistive devices provided by the occupational therapist. For the effective functioning of the restoration care team the following points should observed:

- Leadership should be determined. Ultimately the client is the leader of the team. When counting the interaction between the client and the nurse, she has the responsibility of co-coordinating the activities of the restorative care team and managing the care of the client and in fact nurse is the team leader. The nurse also ensures proper use of resources and facilitates timely on discharge of clients.
- Communication has to be effective frequent and documented. Case conferences involving as many members of the team as possible especially the client and family or significant others and shared written reports are central to this communication.
- Collaboration among team members must be complete and genuine. All areas of experts of the team are used in the plan of care.
- Conflict resolution among disciplines must be quick. Conflicts are best resolved by mutual respect among team members.

Other Possible Members of the Restorative Care Team and their Functions

- Volunteers – Visit or call clients and run errands.
- Clergy – Meeting spiritual needs of the client-support and counsel clients and their significant others
- Psychologist – Meeting mental health needs-support and counsel clients and their significant others
- Respiratory therapist – Meeting oxygenation needs-technical support for oxygen therapist

- Audiologist – Meeting auditory and balance needs-diagnose and counsel concerning hearing aids and other assist devices
- Biomedical engineer – Design and manufactures various prosthetic and adaptive devices to meet particular client needs
- Prosthetist or orthotist – Design and manufacture various prosthetic and adaptive devices to meet particular client needs such as artificial limb.

Restorative Care

Functional problems of Restorative Care

Various illness or injuries create the need for restorative care to maximize the functional capacity of the client. Mostly functional limitation or impairment exists that decreases the client's ability to perform tasks. Trauma, illness and the client's functional limitations are the important considerations in restorative care. If the interdisciplinary team is to assist a client to effectively adapt to limitations, the overall focus of care is directed to all of the clients needs.

In some instances the client's functional deficit will remain. However the client an family are taught how to adapt so that the clients maximal level of health and independence is achieved. When one working in a restorative care team the following points must be taken into account: the client's willingness to participate in care, family structure and relationship, environmental situation and living arrangements and resources availability. As the emphasis for early discharge continues, there are many clients receiving their restorative care in home settings.

Home health care: Home health care is the profession of the medically related professional and Para-professional services and equipment to clients and families in their places of resident for health maintenance, education, illness prevention, diagnosis and treatment of disease palliation and rehabilitation. The most common services include nursing, medical and social work, physical, occupational, speech and respiratory therapy, nutritional therapy and physical care. Of these services, nursing is used most often as a result of client needs.

Para-professional services include home health care aids, housekeepers and companions. Many of these caregivers provide personal care and household support services that prevent the need for costly hospitalization or care in a skilled nursing facility.

Home health care equipment is any medically related products adapted for home use, including highly technical items such as mechanical ventilators, intravenous infusion pumps and non technical items such as hospital beds and walkers.

Home health agencies have extended almost every type of health care services into the clients residence. Health promotion and education are traditionally the primary objectives of home health care with the intension of encouraging the client and family independence through teaching of self-care. Problems related to lifestyle, safety, environment, family dynamics and health care practices can be readily identified in home situation from the client and family members. Clients who need home health care have a variety of physical, socio-economic and psychological problems. Some of the clients are in medically unstable conditions and may heave an acute problem such as wound infection or a chronic condition like lung disease. They usually require home treatment, professional assessment, education and changes in therapy. Some clients may be medically stable condition such as chronic insulin dependent diabetes, but they require long-term care to prevent exacerbations and hospitalization. Insurance reimbursement for medically unstable clients has improved. But government policies do not reimburse to clients of long-term diseases.

To meet client needs for home health care services and equipment and to ensure adequate reimbursement, nurses must understand the services available and the way clients are reimbursed. Home health care services are reimbursed by three mechanisms such as government funds, private insurance and private pay.

Home heath care agencies are private duty agencies and durable medical equipment companies

Geriatrics Principles for Restorative Care: As persons get order the process of meeting their restorative needs involves a longer and more involved intervention because in comparison with younger persons to older persons are:

- More prone to injuries such as hip fracture and illness such as cardiovascular accidents requiring prolonged, complex restoration.
- Have more chronic conditions (diabetes mellitus, Parkinsonism, etc.) with unknown origins, extensive therapeutic regimens and multiple complications of their own, which complicate and slow any recovery or restoration.
- Heal or recover more slowly because of functional decrements in perfusion, oxygenation, nutrition, skin integrity and tissue integrity. The quantity and efficiently of delivery of oxygen, glucose, and other nutrients to affected areas is decreased.
- Respond less quickly because of sensory deficits (decreased vision, hearing, etc.) and slower transmission of both sensory and motor neurological impulses. Clients perception, comprehension and mobility are limited and safety and self care are at risk. Client learning and active participation in the restoration may be impaired.
- Have less resources available (social, financial, etc) to support or aid restoration.

Nursing Roles in the Restorative Care

Nurse assumes many roles, from nurse to agency, owner and director. Home health care provides a great deal of autonomy and flexibility and offers opportunities for independent clinical practice, management, marketing, teaching, clinical specialization, and research. The nurse continuously assist the client in restoration and co-ordinates the restorative care team as given below.

Home health care nurses provide creative, adaptive care to clients in the home. A holistic, nonjudgmental and family centered philosophy is essential for the nurse in the home.

Home Health Care Management: Most home health care agency directors, managers and field supervisors are nurses who possess advanced training in administration and experience in home health care practice. They provide a vital link among caregivers, clients, physicians, community resources, advisory board members, and regulatory and reimbursement agencies. In addition to clinical and personal management they are responsible for financial management, quality assurance and program development. Home health care nursing management requires a strong ability to promote staff excellence while containing costs and complying with reimbursement and regulatory guidelines.

Teaching and Research Activities: Most nurses in home health care agencies are involved in many educational activities. In fact, the primary focus of home health care nursing is client and family education to establish self care and independence. Nurses determine client and family learning abilities and needs, develop and implement individualized teaching plans and evaluate the success of the client in meeting learning objectives. Frequent visits to homes allow the nurse to evaluate whether clients are successfully applying new knowledge to health care practices.

Legal and Ethical Responsibilities: Nurses are legally able to perform independent nursing activities based on educational preparation and experience. Nurses can evaluate clients for home health care services without a medical order but must provide care under the direction of a written plan of treatment signed by a physician. Home health care nurses often establish the plan care and collaborate with the physician for medical treatment plans. The most controversial legal issues in home health clinical practice include the following:

- Risks associated with providing highly technical procedures such as administration of I.V. medication and blood products in the home.
- Legal aspects of client teaching such as liability for errors made by family care givers based on misuse of information provided by the nurse
- Compliance with medicare or other government home health care regulations.

Because of limited highly fragmented funding for home health care, home health care nurses must determine whether to continue providing services when there is risk of inadequate reimbursement.

Discharge Planning: Discharge planning is a major function of most home health care agencies, especially those affiliated with hospitals. Nurses attend discharge planning rounds and consult with medical, nursing and social work staffs in hospitals and clinics. Nurses facilitate access to all home health care equipment and services during a clients discharge from the hospital or clinic. Through assessment and data collection by the co-ordinator before hospital discharge, facilitates continuity of care and in many cases can speed the discharge process.

Nursing Procedure which the Nurse can do in Homes

- **Wound care:** Sterile dressings, debridement and irrigation of wounds, packing assessment of drainage, assessment and culture of wounds, and instructing clients and families in wound care.
- **Respiratory care:** Management of oxygen therapy, mechanical ventilation and suctioning and care of tracheotomy
- **Vital signs:** Monitoring blood pressure, cardiopulmonary status and instructing clients and families in pulse taking
- **Elimination:** Clients with new ostomy appliances often need assistance with irrigation and skin care procedures, as well as with learning to use specialized equipment. Assessment and teaching, insertion of urinary catheters, irrigation, observation for injection and instruction of family in intermittent catheterization are also provided.
- **Nutrition:** Assessment of nutrition and hydration status instruction on prescribed diet, administration of tube feedings and instructing family in tube feedings
- **Intravenous therapy:** Instructing clients and families on medication, action, and side effects, monitoring compliance and effectiveness of prescribed medications.
- **Intravenous therapy:** Assessment and management of dehydration, giving antibiotic medications, parental nutrition, blood products and analysis and chemotherapeutic agents.
- **Selected laboratory studies:** Drawing blood for related to disease processes or medications.

29

Management of Unconscious Patient

Conscious means aware of an responding to ones surroundings consciousness refer to the state of being conscious. The fact of awareness by the mind of itself and the world. The words related to consciousness are as follows:

- Normal consciousness is an awareness of the self and the environment
- Sleep is a state of physical and apparent mental inactivity from which the patient can be aroused to normal consciousness.
- Clouding of consciousness is a state of reduced awareness, inattention, and sensory perception and difficulty in following detachment. There is impaired spoken words
- Delirium is characterized by irrelevant talks, disorientation, fear, irritability and misperception of stimuli
- Stupor is the state of minimal mental and physical activity, the response to spoken words is either absent or slow. The patient responds inadequately only by vigorous and repeated stimuli
- Coma is a state of total unresponsiveness. There is complete absence of response to the external environment, needs and even to repeated nervous stimuli
- *Unconsciousness* is an abnormal state resulting from disturbance of sensory perception to the extent that the patient is not aware of what is happening around him. It may be momentary or prolonged to days or even months. Clinically the patient who does not respond to the spoken word is unconscious. But the degree varies.

Unconscious Patient

The comatose condition of the patient can be distinguished from lighter states of impaired consciousness or the semi comatose state, in that, in the latter the patient makes some response to spoken word. There are many degrees of coma.

(i) *Light coma:* This is spontaneous and evoked movement.
(ii) *Deep coma:* The heart rate is slow. But the respiratory rate is fast and the depth increased.
(iii) *Premoribund:* The rhythm is periodic. There is tracheal tug. Pulse is irregular. Blood pressure is rising.
(iv) *Moribund:* Apnoeic respiration, pupils dilated and fixed, pulse fast, blood pressure falling.

The degree of unconsciousness or level of unconsciousness includes

(i) *Excitatory type:* Patient does not respond to but disturbed by sensory stimuli i.e., bright light, noise and sudden movement.
(ii) *Somnolent:* Patient is extremely drowsy and will respond only if spoken to directly
(iii) *Stuporous:* Responds only to painful stimuli i.e., pricking or pinching
(iv) *Deep coma:* Does not respond to any type of stimulus and his reflexes are gone.

Management of unconsciousness is a lack of awareness of one's environment and the inability to respond to external stimuli. Therefore observation of the patients condition and care to prevent any complications are particularly important. If possible a nurse should be assigned "special" to the patient or alternatively he could be nursed to intensive care ward.

Etiology of Unconsciousness

Common causes of unconsciousness includes the following

(i) *Ineffective:* (i) Meningitis (ii) Cerebral abscess (from middle ear infection).
(ii) *Traumatic:* (i) Head injury (ii) Operation on the brain
(iii) *Neo-plastic:* Innocent or malignant growth of brain
(iv) *Metabolic:* (i) Uraemia (ii) Diabetic coma (iii) Insulin coma (iv) Overdose of certain drugs
(v) *Degenerative:* Cerebral arteriosclerosis causing – Thrombosis, Haemorrhage or Hypertensive Encephalopathy.
(vi) *Poisoning:* (i) By anaesthesia (ii) Snake bite (iii) Drugs – Opium poisoning, Alcohol poisoning, Barbiturate poisoning.
(vii) *Cerebral Anemia:* (i) Due to shock (ii) Due to Haemorrhage (iii) Due to embolus (including air and fat embolus).
(viii) *Anaphylactic shock*
(ix) *Hypopituitarism*
(x) *Stokes Adams syndrome*
(xi) *Cholemia*
(xii) *Eclampsia*

The Common causes of unconsciousness (in Children) includes the following

(i) Purulent Meningitis
(ii) TB Meningitis
(iii) Head injury
(iv) Hyperpyrexia
(v) Foreign body in respiratory tract
(vi) Cerebral hemorrhage
(vii) Intracranial tumor

Nursing Management of Unconscious Patient

1. *Aim:* The primary objective is preservation and prolongation of life. Treatment of airway obstruction, shock, or cardio-respiratory failure should be started before going into details of the cause of these disorders.
   (a) Maintenance of airway:
2. Signs and airway obstruction: Stridor, respiration with effort, wheezing or cyanosis. A finger is to be swept deep into the oropharynx to remove clotted blood, mucus, vomitus, any loose teeth or dentures or any foreign body.
3. The patient is kept in semi prone position and should not lie or be restrained flat on his back in spread-eagle fashion. Spinal injury requires special consideration:
   (a) To maintain normal body function
   (b) To prevent complications

Generally Nursing management of unconscious includes the following:

• **Positioning of the patient:** The patient is nursed in the prone, lateral or Sim's position. An unconscious patient is not nursed on his back because there is a risk that he may inhale vomitus or secretions from his mouth and pharynx.

• **Airway:** An adequate airway must be maintained at all times. It may be necessary to hold the patients jaw forward

Garments must be loose to allow free movements of the chest and abdomen. Frequent suction is sometimes required to prevent the pooling of secretions in the patients pharynx. Sufficient ventilation should be provided.

• **Observation and Charting:** A chart may be kept to note the patients level of consciousness, reaction to vocal stimulation, the size of pupils and their reaction to light. These observations if required, may be taken every half-hour or hour.

Temperature, pulse and respiration may be recorded every two or four hours and sometimes more frequently, particularly when the patient has a head injury.

A blood pressure chart is usually kept, the frequency depending upon the cause of unconsciousness.

The occurrence of muscular spasms is recorded. The nurse should note the area affected and the duration of the fits.

A urine analysis chart will be commenced for patients suffering from diabetes mellitus or renal failure.

• **Hygiene**

A mosquito net, provided the mesh is fine enough to observe the patients colour, is used to protect the patient from flies and mosquitoes.

Sponging is performed as frequently as necessary. Tepid sponging may be required if the patient becomes febrile. When sponging the patient and giving pressure care, the limbs should be put through a full range of movements (passive physiotherapy). Passive physiotherapy for patients who remain unconscious for a long period helps to prevent stiffening of joints, muscular contractions and venous stasis.

Mouth toilets are performed to prevent drying of the mucous membrane and formation of sordes.

Eye toilets may be necessary to keep the lid margins free form discharge. The eyes must be kept closed to prevent drying of the conjunctiva and corneal ulceration

The doctor may order the instillation of sterile oily eye drops.

• **Care of Pressure Areas and the Prevention of Foot Drop**

The patient should, if possible, be nursed on a ripple mattress. The bed linen must be kept taut and dry.

A bed cradle may be used to take the weight of the bedclothes.

Pillows protected by plastic covers may be used to separate the bony prominences between the knees and ankles.

The patients position should be changed every hour and pressure areas massaged every two hours. Any sign of reddening or injury to the skin must be reported and the treatment intensified.

Foot drop occurring during hospitalization can be prevented by careful nursing. The feet should be kept at right ankles to the legs. Foot drop is liable to occur if the bedclothes are tucked in, tightly, causing constant pressure over the toes and feet.

A foot board or pillow at the bottom of the bed may be used to prevent the pressure and weight of clothes on the feet.

Passive physiotherapy will help to keep the ankles and feet in good condition. Padded splints may be used to maintain the correct position. If splints are used they must be removed for pressure area, sponging and physiotherapy and then carefully replaced. The hands and wrists may also need splinting to prevent wrist drop.

• **Nutrition:** The diet must certain adequate supply of all the nutrients required for life. These may be supplied as intravenous fluids or gastric tube feedings. If gastric tube feedings are commenced, care is taken that a variety of fluids are given, e.g. high protein milk, drinks, fruit juices and also water. The patient must be well nourished and hydrated.

• **Elimination:** The patient is observed for any signs of urinary retention and constipation. Any signs or symptoms of either condition will, be reported, e.g. the abdomen may be distended if there is urinary retention and frequently the patient becomes very restless.

If the patient is constipated, a glycerine suppository may be ordered. However a patient having a fluid diet will have very little faecal residue.

Incontinence of urine may occur in which case a bedpan or divided mattress may be used for a female patient and for a male patient a padded urinal or other suitable appliances may be used. These must be inspected at least every two hours.

If the patient has retention of urine, gentle pressure over the bladder region will be helpful in partially emptying the bladder. However catheterization is generally necessary.

Accurate recordings must be on the patients fluid balance chart and the patient must be closely observed.

• **Relatives:** The relatives and friends must be given special consideration as they may be distressed at the patients condition. The ward sister usually arranges an appointment for them with the medical officer so that they may be informed of the patients progress. The nurse may assist the relatives as follows:
  1. Check the room and remove any unnecessary equipment before the visitors arrive
  2. Explain to the visitors any new piece of equipment there may be to prevent undue alarm
  3. Arrange for a member or the clergy to visit the patient, if the relatives request this.

• **Routine care of unconscious patient**

1. *Maintenance of an adequate airway:*
  (a) The unconscious patient must be nursed on one side – semiprone position to avoid any tendency of the tongue to fall back on the throat and to encourage secretions from the mouth, respiratory tract and oesophagus to drain

outward by gravity. Extension of the head and elevation of the jaw will raise the tongue out of the posterior oropharynx.

(b) If the patient is lightly comatose an indwelling airway tube may stimulate vomiting or an endotracheal tube may produce coughing. But in deeply comatose patient, a rubber or metal airway should remain in the mouth until the cough reflex returns. If this is insufficient an endotracheal tube should be inserted, or positive pressure ventilation should be started where applicable.

(c) Cleansing the air passage with an electric sucker or gauze piece

(d) Patient is to be kept in steam tent to make the secretions less which should be cleaned off and on

(e) Tracheotomy may have to be done to provide an adequate airway (assisting doctor if needed). Proper care of tracheotomy tube and of the wound has to be taken as a routine

If there is cardiac arrest mouth to mouth ventilation and closed chest massage should be started immediately. Ventilation with an oral airway and a mask if available is very effective.

2. *Control of hemorrhage:* From the scalp or other parts of the body is the next most important step. This can usually be done by a suitable piece of gauze placed over the wound and secured by firm bandage. This should immediately be followed up by examination of the rest of the body for injury and management.

3. *Maintenance of circulation:*
(a) Circulation of blood is enhanced by muscle movement. The patient must not be left in a position that hampers circulation to any part of the body.
(b) Position is to be changed every 2 hours.
(c) Reddened area should be massaged gently.
(d) Air pressure mattress is helpful in preventing the development of decubitus ulcer.

4. *Moving and position:*
(a) Turning sheet should be used in moving an unconscious patient.
(b) To prevent foot drop – the foot is to be kept straightened in position against foot blocks.
(c) Both hands are to be kept in position, the fingers are to be rested on the pillow.
(d) The wrist is to be supported on the pillow to prevent wrist drop.
(e) If the patient does not move, all extremities should be put through the complete range of joint motion at least twice every day.
(f) Massage of extremities is essential to promote circulation and to prevent venous thrombosis.

5. *Anticonvulsants:* During comatose condition a single convulsion may endanger patient's life. A nonhypnotic anticonvulsant like diphenyl hydration is useful.

6. *Antibiotics:* Are necessary depending on infectious condition, injury etc. Any suitable one should immediately be started with.

- **Immediate care after admission**

Complications arise from loss of sensation, from paralysis and from general lowering of metabolic activity. For these reasons during nursing management a close watch is to be kept on the above mentioned points. Observation should be every 15 minutes at first till condition shows signs of improvement.

(a) The unconsciousness patient is placed in a clean railed cot.
(b) The patient is kept in flat position, at first head turned to one side and neck is to be extended for better salivation and oxygenation
(c) Oxygen inhalation should be started immediately
(d) Pulse rate respiration rate and body temperature should be noted carefully
(e) A call book is to be send immediately to the house physician concerned indicating name, bed no., age, sex, time of admission, pulse, respiration, temperature, state of the patient and if possible the cause. Whether patient has passed urine and stool or has vomited etc. and any treatment received outside or not should be noted.
(f) After sending call book emergency tray is to be kept nearby which includes:
   (i)   Physical examination set
   (ii) Sterile Ryle's tube with syringe and specimen tube.
   (iii) Catheterization set
   (iv) Infusion set
   (v)   Lumbar puncture set
   (vi) Tracheostomy set
   (vii) Sucker machine with sterile catheter
   (viii) Injection tray with emergency drugs
(g) If temperature is high – ice cap is to be applied over the head. If subnormal – patient is to be kept warm wrapped with blanket
(h) Close observation and individual nursing care is essential for such patient
(i) Assisting doctor during physical examination and treatment e.g., lumbar puncture or gastric lavage or during catheterization

- **Skin care**
(a) Thorough bath with warm water is to be given daily
(b) The skin should be dried properly to stimulate circulation
(c) If the skin is too dry – lanoline or cold cream to lubricate
(d) Proper hair wash is to be given once in a week

- **Mouth care or oral hygiene**
(a) Proper mouth care is to be given at every two hours interval
(b) Artificial dentures should be removed and safely stored until the patient is fully conscious
(c) Mouth gag is to be used during mouth care
(d) Glycerine is to be applied over the tongue and lips because it has hygroscopic action
(e) Painting of gum with 2% Mercurochrome

- **Eye care**
(a) Eyes should be carefully inspected several times a day
(b) If corneal reflex is absent or if the lids are not completely closed they should be covered with an eye shield

(c) Sterile paraffin or 0.5 to 1% Methyl solution should be dropped in each eye to protect the cornea from drying up by providing moisture and lubrication. Negligency may cause drying of the cornea followed by ulceration which may lead to blindness.

- **Food and fluids**

Nutrition is not a serious matter unless the state of unconsciousness lasts for more than three or four days. Metabolic activity is depressed in these patients and caloric requirement is therefore very low. On the other hand loss of consciousness may be associated with injury or other disorders which may themselves require administration of glucose, electrolytes, water, plasma or even blood.

(a) Protein and carbohydrate should be administered by I.V. infusion but not fat

(b) To maintain all his nutritional needs nasogastric tube is used an small amount of liquid containing all essential foods are usually given 100 to 200 cc, 2-3 hourly

(c) Electric sucker is to be kept ready before feeding as there is chance of aspiration

(d) Before starting feeding, one should be sure that the tube is in position

(e) Before and after feeding water should be given gently. Medicine may also be given slowly through the Ryle's tube

(f) Proper intake and output chart must be maintained.

- **Hyperthermia**

(a) If heat regulating center (Hypothalamus) is disturbed patients temperature will suddenly rise

(b) Elevation of temperature is a sign of complication i.e., pneumonia, wound infection, dehydration, uremia, etc.

(c) If temperature is 38.4°C (101°F) bed clothes should be removed and antipyretics as advised should be given through tube or by injection

(d) Tepid sponge may be given according to doctors order.

(e) If temperature is due to increased intracranial pressure lumbar puncture is also done several times.

- **Hypothermia**

The unconscious patient may have a temperature that is too low (due to depressed vital center).

(a) This type of patient needs extra cover

(b) Room heater may be used for such patient

- **Problems of elimination**

The unconscious patient often has both urinary and faecal incontinence.

(a) *Regarding bladder:* Foley's type of catheter should be introduced and left indwelled to control urinary incontinence, to prevent bed soiling and to keep intake-output chart. Proper aseptic technique has to be maintained to prevent complications.

Continuous drainage is to be given.

Proper care of the tube is to be taken.

Bladder wash with acriffin soln. 1: 10,000 with proper aseptic care.

Urine has to be examined for sugar, acetone and albumin at every four interval when indicated.

Report is to be given to doctor and to treat accordingly.

Proper output is to be maintained.

(b) *Regarding bowel:* (i) The unconscious patient usually is given an enema two or three days interval to help to prevent faecal incontinence

If nasogastric tube is present mild laxative such as Milk of Magnesia may be given.

(c) *Care of vaginal discharge:* If patient has vaginal discharge it should be reported to the doctor. Sometimes cleansing douche is ordered.

The patient who is menstruating will need private care every four hour.

- **Prevention of further accident or injury**

(a) Precautions are to be taken to prevent accidents.

(b) No external heat is to be used, e.g. hot water bag.

(c) Padded side rails should be kept on both sides since patient might have convulsions.

(d) The unconscious patient should be observed half hourly. If condition is critical he needs observation at every 15 min. interval.

(e) Paraldehyde 5 cc or sodium phenobarbitone 30 to 60 mg. may be ordered. After sedation observation is essential for signs of depression of vital function.

(f) Patient should not be kept isolated in a room.

- **Observation**

(a) Pupillary reaction

(b) Level of consciousness

(c) Stiffness of neck

(d) Condition of limb-flaccidity etc

(e) Convulsion etc

These will help doctor for proper diagnosis and treatment.

A rising blood pressure with slowing of pulse rate indicates increased intracranial pressure and it should be reported immediately

Any marked change of pulse, respiration or any increase or decrease of level of consciousness should be reported immediately.

- **Convalescence**

(a) Patient may completely recover after being unconscious for several weeks

(b) Effort should not be made to arouse him until the level of consciousness has lightened.

(c) During convalescence – definite rest periods should be planned each day

(d) Patient needs encouragement and security of knowing that family and friends are concern and interested in his/her recovery

(e) Observation should be made for development of any complication which should properly be dealt with

Patient will also need to be reoriented since the memory is usually failing for the time immediately before, during and after the period of unconsciousness.

30

Management of Patient with Fever

Fever is an abnormally high body temperature, usually accompanied by shivering, headache and in severe instances, delirium.

The normal temperature in the closed mouth lies between 36.0°C to 37.5°C (98.8-99.5°F) when the body is at rest. Skin temperature is usually lower than that of deeper structures of the body. The rectal temperature is higher by 0.3 – 0.6°C (0.6–1.2°F) and the axillary temperature is 0.5 - 1°C lower than the oral temperature.

Pyrexia or fever is an elevation of body temperature above normal.

Low pyrexia 99°F - 101°F or 37.2°C – 38.3°C.

Moderate pyrexia 101°F - 103°F or 38.3°C – 39.4°C.

High pyrexia 103°F - 105°F or 39.4°C – 40.5°C.

Hyper-pyrexia 105°F – 40.6°F and above.

Fever is a disturbed condition of the body which accompanies a rise in temperature. Fever or pyrexia present when the body temperature is raised above normal. In healthy persons the body temperature remain very constant around 98.4°F (36.9°) although a slight swing of 0.5°F (0.3°C) above or below this figure may be normal in some people.

The temperature of the body is the balance between the heat production by means of the general metabolism of various bodily functions and heat loss through skin, lungs and exertion. The heat regulating center in the brain is responsible for the constant level of the body temperature in health.

In infection, fever is one of the most constant and reliable signs. It is probably caused by the toxic products produced by the infecting organisms.

Acute diseases, particularly infections may result in a rise of temperature. Such a condition is called pyrexia. Psychological upset such as fear or anger and hot atmospheric conditions may produce slight rise of temperature. A lowered body temperature is called hypothermia. This condition is commonly seen in elderly people in the winter season and may be caused by cold, damp accommodation, poor diet, inadequate clothing and too little exercise. Newborn babies are also susceptible to hypothermia.

Etiology

Common Causes of Pyrexia

- Bacterial or virus infections, e.g. diseases such as typhoid fever, lobar pneumonia
- Foreign protein, e.g. inoculations with serum or vaccine
- Injury of any type and inflammation
- Sunstroke
- Cerebral haemorrhage
- Any acute infectious disease, e.g. typhoid, broncho-pneumonia, viral pneumonitis, encephalitis, tonsilitis
- Malaria
- Measles
- Severe dehydration
- Severe salt depletion
- Rheumatic heart disease

- Diarrhea
- Head injury
- Alcohol intoxication.

Clinical Manifestations

- Skin is hot and dry, urine scanty and highly colored and often contains albumen
- Pulse is bounding and full at first and later becomes weak and rate increased
- respiration rate is increased in proportion to the increase in temperature and pulse
- Mouth is dry, the tongue coated and there may be nausea and vomiting
- Loss of appetite and the patient may be usually constipated
- There may be headache, irritations, restlessness and in high pyrexia, delerium and coma may occur.

Signs and Symptoms of Pyrexia

- Onset of fever is sudden or gradual according to cause
- Loss of appetite, often nausea and vomiting are associated symptoms
- Headache accompanied by restlessness and delirium
- Malaise and sometimes pain all over the body
- Constipation or diarrhoea
- Photophobia
- Convulsion
- The skin is red, hot and dry
- Pulse and respiration rate is increased. In a few cases, like Typhoid pulse rate is not increased
- The output of urine is decreased.

Although fever is an essential part of the defence mechanism, most Doctors advise that a patient with a temperature over 38°C (100.4°F) should stay in bed since his respiratory and pulse rate are increased. Because headache and irritability often accompany severe systemic infection with high fever, the room should be kept quiet and glaring light dimmed. The patient should be encouraged to sleep. A warm sponge bath, back rub and a smooth bed may help to induce sleep. Bath is needed since more body waste may be excreted through increased perspiration. To prevent drying of the mucous membrane of the mouth and nose, vegetable oil may be used to lubricate the lips and nose, patient is encouraged to clean the mouth and to take generous amount of fluids.

In fever associated with infection, toxins are often excreted through kidneys, more fluid than usual is evaporated by perspiration from the skin and by rapid respiration, more fluids are needed for accelerated metabolism. Therefore an adult patient is urged to take 2500 to 3000 ml of fluid per day. In addition to water, fluids high in calories and containing vit. C, protein, salts and potassium, if not contraindicated by the disease, should be taken by the patient because they help to supply the body's metabolic an electrolyte needs. Solid food usually are not palatable to the patient with fever, but may be given if desired.

At any cost, adequate rest and additional fluid intake are inevitable for the patient with fever.

Nursing Management:

The nursing management (Table 30.1) of the patient with fever includes the following:

• **Isolation:** Isolation procedure is necessary only if the fever is due to some infections diseases. The fundamental aim of isolation is to prevent the spread of infection to others including nurse herself. The patient is nursed in a separate isolation cubicle. In some cases barrier nursing is implemented in a general ward selecting a corner bed near a window and separated by a screen with all precautions to prevent the spread of infection.

• **Rest:** In all cases of fever except in very mildest the patient is kept in bed because making a person to lie on bed is the only possible way of ensuring rest. The room should be well ventilated without draught. Proper ventilation prevents the risk of infection as well as add comfort to the patient. Temperature of the room most comfortable (5° to 19°C).

Clothes should be loose garments. Position depends upon the nature of illness. If the lungs are likely to be affected upright position and if the heart is likely to be involved semi recumbent position is used. The urgency of further rest depends on the cause of the fever. Any special reason for adoption of specific position and the wishes and comfort of the patient should be considered and the congestion of the lungs by the sameness of position should be prevented.

Rest both physical and mental is essential for the patients. So quietness with minimum disturbances is provided. Frequent disturbing of patients for doing nursing procedures and other various medications are disturbing and preventing rest to patient. As these are all essential for the cure of disease, it should be carried out in proper times but the maximum amount of rest and quietness should be provided and especially during sleep.

• **Sleep:** Sleeplessness or insomnia is frequently present in fever or illness. Anxiety or worry about his illness, stay in the somewhat frightening surroundings of the hospital, or many other such feelings will be the cause for insomnia. Every word or actions of the nurse or doctor near the patient will be observed suspiciously. So a cheerful countenance, sympathy and reassurance of the nurse may allay the anxiety and ensure mental rest and sleep.

Nursing measures to induce sleep such as wiping the perspiration, changing the dress, straightening the bed linen, offering bedpan or urinal, providing additional blankets, giving the drinks at bed time, shading the bright light, meeting spiritual need, carrying out the treatment before sleep, using comfort devices, proper ventilation, avoiding draughts, relieving pain if any, solving problems before night, reducing fever by nursing measures, etc. should be adopted.

In addition to the above measures to relieve the physical causes of insomnia, symptoms such as cough and dyspnea in respiratory and circulatory diseases, indigestion, constipation or hunger pains in gastrointestinal diseases, pruritus in jaundice or skin disease may all interfere with sleep. These symptoms may be relieved by specific measure. Or, sedatives may be ordered for simple reasons of insomnia after trying the nursing measures.

• **Diet:** A suitable diet in fever is most important because such patient will have little or no appetite and yet adequate nourishment should be given to supply the bodily needs and to replace the wear and tear and to compensate the fluid loss through sweating. In the first few days of fever, fluids or semisolid foods, at least 4 to 5 pints of fluid should be given daily such as fruit juices, weak tea, cocoa, etc. milk is the most valuable food and easily assimilated. Pure milk, Custards, Bournvita, Horlicks, Ovaltines, etc. with or without milk are suitable. If pure milk is difficult to digest, citrated milk (60 mg of sodium citrate to each ounce of milk) is useful. Carbohydrate in the form of glucose, ordinary cane sugar, syrup, honey or as chocolate is of particular value in fever as it supply energy and easily digested.

As soon as possible, after acute stage, the patient should be given egg, fish, meat and fruits in palatable form to maintain adequate nutrition. Particularly in long-term illness, proteins should not be withheld for long, as they are essential to replace the wear and tear.

The type of food needed to fever patients is important. So also, a suitable type of food, even should be served as frequent small feeds. Otherwise over loading digestion may give rise to flatulence, epigastric pain and abdominal distension, producing respiratory and cardiac embarrassment and such abdominal distension, will interfere with his rest and sleep. The patients own appetite is a good guide to the amount of food required.

Also, the food should be served in an attractive manner to help the patient to increase the appetite, not to waste the food and to take and digest sufficient nourishment. In fever caused by certain particular illness, specific diets are essential with special items.

• **Skin and Pressure Areas:** In case of high fever, usually there is severe sweating which needs frequent change of clothes. As sweating is very distressing and produce insomnia, tepid sponging with water at a temperature of 70° to 80°F (21° to 27°) is good and conductive to sleep and help to reduce temperature.

Particular attention to the pressure areas of patients with prolonged confinement to bed especially with elderly people and frequent change of position is important because they are prone to develop pressure sores. Avoiding creases in bed-sheet and providing comfortable mattress are essential details. Rubber mattress is very useful. The presence of any paralysis or incontinence calls for extra-attention to prevent developing pressure sores.

• **Attention to the Mouth:** With fever of any degree, the mouth is usually dry and liable to become infected resulting stomatitis. So careful routine cleansing of the mouth is done at specific times during day and swabbing with suitable solutions is best. But swabbing should be done gently as too vigorous swabbing will only do more damage. Suitable solutions for cleansing the mouth are soda bicarbonate, dilute lemon juice or glycothymoline. Adequate administration of fluid is one essential way of ensuring a clean mouth. Juices or citrus fruits will increase the salivary secretions and keep the mouth clean and prevent drying of mucous membranes of the mouth.

- **Incontinence:** In long term illness especially in elderly people, incontinence of urine an stool needs special attention to prevent the development of pressure sores. Again, incontinence may be caused by an overflow resulting from retention of urine. So a distended bladder should be watched for and catheterization with strict aseptic precaution should be done if the nursing measures fail to make the patient void. In persistent incontinence, a retention catheter may be provided with drainage bottle or with frequent releasing of the same.

- **Constipation:** Constipation is a constant feature in acute feverish illness. It will cause distension and discomfort to the patient. It must be treated and prevented. Purgatives like senokot and cascera or glycerine suppositories or an enema may be ordered according to the condition of the patient. If a patient is on fluid diet, bowel is not be opened daily and excessive purgation will be distressing to fever patients. Some patients are prone to constipation and used to regular purgatives. The nurse must ascertain form the patient the name of the usual purgative he takes and it should be given in consultation with the doctor.

- **Prevention of Venous Thrombosis:** In patients with prolonged confinement to bed, thrombosis in the deep veins of the legs and pelvis is a danger due to sluggish circulations and trauma. In deep venous thrombosis a clot may break off, travel to the lungs, and cause pulmonary embolism which is fatal. So the limbs are moved actively and passively at intervals to prevent thrombosis and embolism and to prevent the joints becoming fixed with prolonged recombency especially in elderly people.

- **Rigors:** A rigor in the course of an illness is most frightening to the patient. So reassurance is important. The patient should be kept warm and adequately covered. Additional warmth may be given by the careful application of hot water bottle before sweating starts. When perspiring, tepid sponging will be necessary. Special nursing care of patient with rigor should be implemented.

- **Delirium:** Constant and skilled attention is necessary in all delirious patients. These patients are extremely restless and often try to get out of bed which may have serious effect. The nurse must try to restrain him with minimum force and extreme tact. In febrile delirium, cold compress to the forehead is often useful and soothing. Bed boards suitably padded to prevent injury may be needed. In most cases sedatives such as chloral hydrate, paraldehyde, compose or barbiturates may be ordered. In severe cases hyocine or morphine by inspection may be given.

In all cases of delirium, utmost skill of the nurse is required to ensure the adequate fluid intake of the patients. Elderly patients who are liable to become delirious when seriously ill require special care in the matter of fluid intakes. But delirium developed due to high fever is relieved when the fever is reduced. So measures to reduce the fever should be resorted in such occasions.

- **Administering of Antipyretic Drugs:** Antipyretic drugs such as salicylates in the form of aspirin, crossin, etc. are given to patients with fever to reduce the temperature owing to their action on heat regulating center. They relieve pain in the muscles and joints. But in strong concentrated form it is irritating to the mucous membrane of the stomach.

Whatever is the antipyretic drugs ordered, it should be given properly and the nurse should know the dose, effects and toxic reaction of the same when it is administered. Most of the drugs have good and bad effects. These should be realized by the nurse and nursing action should be directed accordingly. Salicylates in different names with different trademarks are used as antipyretics for the patient with fever. Different types of cold applications are also useful in reducing fever.

To sum up nursing measures of patient with pyrexia includes the following:

- A patient with high temperature should be kept in bed as long as fever persists. He may be permitted to get up to toilet only
- The room should be quiet and well ventilated, bright light should be avoided and the temperature is best kept between 60°F to 65°F
- An infant or young child should be placed in railed cot
- Clothing should be light and loose
- The attendants must wash their hands in an antiseptic solution before and after nursing care of the patient
- Careful observation and nursing measure should be taken to relieve discomfort. The mouth and tongue should be cleansed with sodi-bi-carb and glycerin before and after each meal. Frequent cold bath may be needed as body wastes are excreted through increased perspiration
- To prevent drying of the mucous membranes of the mouth and nose, glycerin should be applied to lubricate anterior nasal passage and lips
- Back care with methylated spirit and powder and special attention for pressure points
- Four hourly temperature, pulse and respiration should be taken and recorded on the chart
- If constipation is troublesome, the bowel should be moved by simple enema or mild laxative if there is no contraindication. If urine becomes concentrated or less than 100 ml. Daily in an adult, plenty of fluids by mouth is to be given
- Hyperpyrexia is best treated by cold and tepid sponging, cold compress to the forehead, ice cap on the head or ice packing on the body when needed. Sometimes ice-cold rectal saline is also used as retention enema to reduce body temperature

  (N.B. Hypothermia is now used widely for variety of illness when extremely high temperature occurs. Precaution should be taken for sudden lowering of temperature which may lead to shock. Hypothermia decreases the body's metabolic needs, lowers body temperature and inhibits growth of infection).

- A suitable diet in acute febrile condition is most important.

Table 30.1: Nursing Care Plan of Patient with Fever

Problem	Reason	Objective	Nursing intervention (rationale)	Evaluation
1. Altered comfort R/T increased body temperature (infection)	Due to infection • Temperature↑ • Malaise + • Heart rate ↑ • ↑Respiratory rate • ↑WBC count	Have body temperature below 100°F (37.8°)	• Assess the patient, temperature 4th hourly (to monitor temperature) • Administer antipyretic drugs 4th hourly if ordered (to reduce temperature) • Keep environmental temperature at 70°F (21.1°C) • Avoid heavy layers of clothing or bed covers (to aid in lowering body temperature) • Give tepid sponge bath, after antipyretic therapy (to reduce temperature through evaporation rapidly) • Use skin lotions (to prevent drying) • Change the linen frequently if patient is diaphoretic (to prevent chilling and subsequent rise in body temperature from muscular activity) • Implement appropriate measure (to treat causes of fever) (PI response to be written in the column)	
2. Risk for fluid volume deficit	• Metabolic rate • Diaphoresis • Decreased oral intake	Have no signs of dehydration	• Assess for rapid respiration and pulse • Assess damp skin, clothing and bed clothing • Assess unwillingness or inability to ingest fluids • Assess signs of dehydration (to determine risk for fluid deficit) • Encourage fluid intake to 3-4 2/day (to replace fluids loss due to fever) • Monitor TPR and BP 4th hourly (to know any indication of hypovolemia) • Administer IV fluids if necessary • Monitor intake and output accurately • Give careful estimate of insensible losses (to evaluate need for replacement)	
3. Risk for altered nutrition: less than body requirement R/T increased. Caloric need.	• Metabolic rate↓ • Oral intake↓	Have no weight loss	• Assess intake and monitor weight daily (to know the risk) • Give high caloric, high proteins, easily digested food and fluidity (to maximize intake and minimize energy expanse) • Help patient balance activity and rest to conserve energy (to ensure preferred activity) • Monitor alternate method of nutritional intake, i.e. enteral, parenteral.	

↑ = Increased, ↓ = Decreased, + = Present

Patient is seriously ill and inclined to take little food or has no appetite at all but adequate nourishment must be given to maintain the nutrition. In addition, owing to the excessive loss of fluid through the skin by evaporation and due to rapid respiration more fluid are needed for maintaining the metabolic processes. The adult therefore is usually urged to take 2500 to 3000 ml of fluid a day. Infant and children should be given smaller amount. In addition to water fluids with some caloric values and containing Vit. C., protein, salt and potassium is preferred. If not contraindicated by the disease fluid should be taken by the disease fluid should be taken by the patient because they help to supply the body's metabolic and electrolyte needs. Solid food usually is not palatable to the patient with a fever but may be allowed if desired. The main diet is milk, but if there is any abdominal distention it is better to give skimmed milk or diluted milk. Water and sweetened fruit juice may be given freely. In addition to fluid and milk, carbohydrate is given to supply energy for the body in the form of glucose, honey, syrup or chocolate. As soon as possible further addition of semisolid diet must be made such as chicken broth, custard, cornflower, half boiled egg, soji, bread etc. Solid food should not be added until the temperature has returned to normal

Treatment of fever includes the following:
- Antipyretic drugs may be given for lowering the temperature orally or IM or rectally, e.g. Aspirin, Paracetamol
- Anti-histaminic drugs sometimes give relief to symptoms of "Cold" which is usually accompanied by fever
- Hypnotics and tranquilizers may be required to prevent restlessness or convulsion
- If nausea and vomiting accompany a generalized infection, food and fluid should be withheld for the time. Ant-emetics are often useful in relieving nausea. If fever is high and vomiting is frequent fluid may be given parenterally. Infants need fluid replacement much sooner than adults. Tea, broth and soda, biscuits and dry toast are usually retained best as nausea subsides
- Other specific drugs are used according to cause.

After the episode of high fever the patient usually should stay in bed until the temperature has been normal for twenty four hours. After a high and prolonged fever most adults feel weak, perspire on physical exertion and become tired easily for several days and weak. The patient of any age should have extra rest and should eat food rich in protein and high in calories. Children and young adults usually recover much more rapidly than elderly persons. During recovery the patient of any age needs quiet recreational activities such as reading to help pass the time and visitors.

31

Management of Patient with Shock

Shock is a clinical syndrome indicating inadequate circulation that results from a variety of causes. Inadequate circulation leads to tissue hypoxia. Prolonged shock is incompatible with life. The faster the shock state can be reversed, the greater is the chance of uncomplicated recovery for the patient. In the care of patients careful attention to nursing assessment and intervention is as important to recovery as in management of patient in shock. "Shock is a state of generalized inadequate circulation, which causes decreased perfusion of the body tissues with blood and produces a wide range of systemic effects."

Physiology of Shock

Shock is the condition is an abnormal physiologic state in which there is disproportion between the circulating blood volume and the area of the vascular bed resulting in circulatory failure and anoxia. Circulatory integrity can be viewed as a resultant of three basic components:

- The pump (heart)
- The blood volume
- The vascular bed, consisting of
  - Resistance vessels – Arteries and arterioles containing about 20% of normal blood volume
  - Exchange vessels – The capillary net work containing about 5% of normal blood volume
  - Capacitance vessels – Veins and venules containing about 76% of total blood volume

In a state of shock there is, insufficient tissue blood flow (perfusion) results from a depressed cardiac output due either to–

- Factors that interfere with the ability of the heart to pump blood. This can be called "Cardiogenic shock" or "Pump failure". It can result from:
  - Factors that interfere with cardiac filling, such as pericardial tamponade, severe mitral stenosis, tachyarrhythmias
  - Factors that interfere with cardiac filing, such as myocardial infraction, myocarditis, heart block, severe aortic stenosis
- Factors that cause inadequate venous return
  - Decreased blood volume
    - Ø From external loss – hemothorax, dehydration, burns, vomiting, diarrhea
    - Ø From internal loss – hemothorax, retroperitoneal hemorrhage, peritonitis, intestinal obstruction, fractures, angioneurotic edema
  - Increased vascular bed-vasodilatation and pooling
    - Ø Gram-negative bacteremia
    - Ø Anaphylaxis
    - Ø Central nervous system depressants such as anesthesia, barbiturates
    - Ø Spinal cord transaction
- Impediments to blood – viz. massive pulmonary embolism or vena – caval obstruction. In any patient there may be certain elements of each of these with the haemodynamic state representing a resultant of several related factors.

Classification of Shock

- *Hypovolemic shock (oligemic shock):* Due to a reduction in the circulating blood volume (in haemorrhage, burns, trauma, etc). The volume of blood filling the vascular channels is low. This may be internal or external.
- *Cardiogenic shock:* In which the circulatory failure involves faulty pumping of the heart when more than 50% of the wall of ventricle is damaged by acute myocardial infraction. The circulatory failure is central rather than of peripheral origin.
- *Vasovagal shock:* There is diffuse vasodilation resulting in an increase in the size of the vascular bed. The dilated vessels afford so much room for blood that it does not easily move along. While remaining in the vessels this blood is just unavailable to the circulatory effort as if it had been lost through hemorrhage. When blood becomes trapped in small vessels and in viscera it is lost temporarily to the mainstream of circulating fluid. The skeletal muscles and viscera may be engorged with blood, but volume of circulating blood is reduced. The reduced cerebral perfusion causes cerebral hypoxia and unconsciousness
- *Neurogenic shock:* Involves loss of sympathetic control of vessels. This produce vasodilatation, reduces systemic blood pressure and effective circulatory blood volume. The type of shock may be caused by brain damage spinal injury or spinal anesthesis
- *Psychogenic shock:* Follow sudden fright of sudden pain
- *Septic shock:* Occurs in gram-negative infection viz. strangulated hernia, leaking intestinal anastomosis
- *Anaphylactic shock:* Occurs due to anaphylaxis caused by essentially certain drugs and measures viz. injection of penicillin anaesthetics, serum injections, dextran, etc. there is release of large amounts of histamine and SRS-A (Slow Release Substance Anaphylaxia) which cause bronchospasm, laryngenal oedema, edema, hypoxia, hypotension and shock.
- *Other shocks:* e.g. insulin shock due to hypoglycemia, transfusion reactions, electric shock.

Stages of Shock

Shock is a dynamic condition in which a patient's status is constantly changing. The patho-physiology can be divided into following stages.

(i) *Initial stage:* The cardiac output is insufficient to supply the normal nutritional needs of the tissues but not low enough to cause serious symptoms.

(ii) *Compensatory stage:* The cardiac output is reduced further but due to compensatory vaso-construction the BP tends to remain within normal range. Blood flow to the skin and kidneys decreases while blood flow to central nervous system and myocardium is maintained.

(iii) *Progressive stage:* The unfavorable changes become more and more apparent – falling blood pressure, increased vasoconstriction increased heart rate, oliguria. If the compensatory mechanisms are unable to cope with the reduced cardiac output shock becomes progressively more severe and passes on to next stage.

(iv) *Irreversible stage:* In this stage of shock no type of therapy can save the patients life. Blood pressure decreases further and respiration is depressed. Blood volume can be normal in this stage though irreversible damage has already taken place. Fluid transfusions may restore BP only temporarily. Blood pressure declines until death occurs.

Signs and Symptoms

- The patient presents an anxious, tired expression. The restlessness and anxiety may later be replaced by a picture of apathy or exhaustion
- Skin feels cool and is pale and mottled and there is evidence of decreased capillary flow exhibited by easy blanching of the skin particularly the nail beds
- In neurogenic shock pulse rate is normal, low blood pressure and a warm dry skin. Rapid pulse may not be evident until the patient is moved or elevated to a sitting position
- Patients having wound or haemorrhagic shock will appear to be restless, anxious and give appearance of great fear. Restlessness will give way to apathy and patient will appear sleepy. When aroused may complain of weakness or of a chilly sensation. If blood loss is unchecked patients apathy and sleepiness will rapidly progress into coma
- Nausea and vomiting due to hypovolaemia and excessive thirst

Management of Shock

For first aid measure in shock please read chapter 27.

The aim of treatment of all forms of shock are directed towards improving and maintaining tissue perfusion. Clinical care of shock varies according to the specific etiology of the type of shock.

The main objective in shock is to maintain or restore cellular metabolism. This can be achieved through following measures:

- *Maintenance of respiratory function:* An adequate supply of O_2 and removal CO_2 are essential to biochemical homeostasis. The first step in treatment of shock is to be certain that airway is open and functioning. In severe respiratory failure patient may need ventilatory support from a respirator. An endotracheal tube inserted or tracheostomy may be performed that will maintain an arterial PO_2 of 80 mm of Hg or higher.
- *Maintenance of adequate blood pressure:* Despite a loss of as much as 25-35% in the blood volume and if it is not too rapid there may be moderate drop in BP. With loss of 50% or more shock is very severe or lethal.
- *Fluid replacement:* When enough fluid is lost sufficient fluid has to be infused to produce an adequate cardiac output. The best gauge for measuring the adequacy of fluid replacement is the response of the CVP to the administered fluid.

In general if patient is hypovolemic he will have low CVP. The kind and amount of shock depends on the nature and quantity of fluid lost, urgency of the situation and type of fluid available.

In general three types of fluids are used (a) Blood and plasma (b) Plasma expander and (c) Crystalloid solutions.

In emergency Ringers lactate or isotonic solution with bicarbonate may be used to expand blood volume.

- *Support of the heart:* Some estimation of the condition of the heart can be made by monitoring the ECG and noting the character of the pulse. Any arrhythmia has to be corrected because it tends to reduce cardiac efficiency.

  Quinidine and procainamide are used to treat various arrhythmias but they tend to reduce myocardial contractility.

  Digitalis is often very useful.

  Isoproterenol is a sympathomimetic amide that acts primarily on beta receptors.
- *Regulation of the size of the vascular chamber:* If vasoconstriction is insufficient to maintain blood flow especially to the heart and brain vasopressors viz. metaraminol (Aramine) and norepinephrine (Levophed) may be used.

  Norepinephrine is also a very powerful vasoconstricor. Although theses drugs may initially be beneficial by maintaining perfusion of heart or brain prolonged use may cause death or irreversible damage. Therefore vasopressor therapy should be used for a shortest possible period.
- *Maintenance of renal function:* Correction of metabolic acidosis is essential as severe metabolic acidosis is injurious to the kidney and other organs.

  Mannitol an osmotic diuretic is used. By promoting diuresis it helps to prevent accumulation of hemolyzed cells and other debris in the renal tubules. This action is most beneficial when hypotension is temporary. It is also useful in identifying the patient who has suffered renal damage in shock.
- *Specific therapeutic techniques:* Adrenal steroids stabilize lysosomal membrane and prevent intracellular release of enzymes. They also increase blood volume by increasing sodium retention.

  Hypothermia: Reducing the metabolic requirements of cells, increase patients chance for survival. With a 10°C reduction of the body temperature needs of cells can be reduced by about 50%.

  Antibiotics: Are important adjunct to treatment in any type of shock especially when caused by sepsis.

Nursing Management

The aims of nursing management will include the following:

(i) To improve the circulation in order to increase the oxygen supply to the tissues throughout the body.

(ii) To correct the specific cause.

(iii) Making and reporting observations on the state of the patient.

(iv) Regulating the environment in relation to the needs of the patient.

(v) Carrying out treatments, such as those directed towards circulatory and respiratory disturbances

To accomplish the aims following nursing measures are needed:

- ***Observation***
  (a) The patient in shock must be under systemic observation. The pulse, blood pressure and respirations are recorded every 15 minutes and the interval only as the patients condition improves.
  (b) Blood pressure and pulse are considered to be the best indexes of the degree of shock. A rapid weak pulse and a systolic blood pressure below 90 mm of Hg signify danger. The lower the diastolic blood pressure the more serious is the shock as this points to a failure of compensation.
  (c) The temperature is recorded and the skin is checked for colour and moisture, patient's level of response, anxiety and worry are to be noted.
  (d) Mouth and mucous membrane are observed for dryness.
  (e) Accurate record of intake and output chart. The amount of urine excreted is an important indication of the degree of shock and response to treatment. Output of 15 ml or less per hour is of ominous sign.
  (f) Continuous monitoring and observation of the patient is imperative since changes in cardiovascular and respiratory function can occur rapidly and treatment must be adjusted accordingly.
- ***Rest:*** Physical and mental rest are essential to reduce his metabolism and thus needs for O_2 and nutrients.

  Patient is kept at absolute rest. Sufficient assistance is given when patient is to be moved for treatment. The environment is kept as quiet and free of stimuli as possible.
- ***Positioning:*** The patient in shock is kept in recumbent position with elevation of lower limbs to increase venous return
- ***Warmth:*** Loss of body heat is prevented by application of a cover but sweating has to be avoided. Heat applications are not used to prevent fluid loss through perspiration and because heat increases metabolism in the tissues making a greater demand on the already depleted O_2 supply.
- ***Pain:*** Adequate pain relief is necessary since pain intensifies shock. Narcotics and sedatives are not unnecessary. Restlessness may be due to lack of O_2 to the brain rather than pain.
- ***Fluids:*** With intravenous infusion frequent observation is made to determine if the desired rate of flow and supply of solution are being maintained and to see that solution is not leaking into the subcutaneous tissues.

Fluids may be given by mouth to relieve patients thirst if tolerated and when no gastrointestinal tract lesion is there or surgery is anticipated. Frequent rinsing of mouth provide some comfort an help to prevent possible parotitis.

Preventive Measures of Shock

Shock can be prevented as follows:
- Careful preoperative preparation – both physical and mental are important in the prevention of shock.
- Estimation of patients blood volume and its replacement preoperatively.
- Surgery necessary to save patients life is undertaken while patient is in shock in arterial haemorrhage. To prevent blood loss surgery is a mandatory step to reach bleeding vessel. Nurse should become expert at estimating fluid loss both in and out of operating room. A health adult can lose upto 500-ml. of blood, without need for replacement. The ill, elderly or poorly nourished need replacement therapy for less blood loss.
- The ability of an individual to avoid shock cannot be predicted. All accident victims and patients with acute M.I. should be treated as if shock imminent. All post operative patients belong to this category. Nurse must watch for signs that are evident on major defensive mechanism to maintain blood pressure.

32

Management of Patient with HIV/AIDS

HIV infection is one of the most dreadful diseases. Individuals infected with HIV has thus far eventually developed' Acquired Immune Deficiency Syndrome (AIDS)'. AIDS severely compromises the body's ability to fight various infections and some forms of cancer. The incidence of HIV infections and AIDS continue to increase steadily worldwide. Therefore, nurses must understand the critical concepts related to this problem. AIDS was considered to be universally fatal until quite recently. Advances in drug treatment however, are delaying the onset of AIDS for selected persons infected with HIV and are providing new hope to infected persons.

Etiology

AIDS is an acquired viral disease. The virus integrates itself into CD4 (T4 helper) cells, causing immune dysfunction and rendering the infected person unusually susceptible to life threatening infections and malignancies. The causative agent of AIDS is infection with HIV, a human retrovirus that belongs to the Lentivirus subfamily. Several human retroviruses have been identified. Two of them, HIV-1 and HIV-2 have been associated with T4 helper cell depletion, resulting in loss of cellular immunity characterized by AIDS.

The routes for transmission of HIV are well documented, which includes:

1. Directly from person to person by sexual contact.
2. Direct inoculation with contaminated blood products, needles, or syringes and
3. From infected mothers to her fetus or newborn.

HIV is a fragile virus that can only be transmitted under specific conditions that allow contact with infected body fluids, including blood, semen, vaginal secretions, cerebrospinal fluid, saliva, tears and breast milk. However, blood, semen and vaginal secretions are the primary routes of infection. Epidemiological studies indicate that transmission through body fluids such as saliva, tears and breast milk is inefficient and likely to produce infection.

HIV is not transmitted by casual contacts, including sneezing, coughing, spitting, handshakes, contact with potential secretions on toilets seats, bath tubs, showers, swimming pools, utensils, dishes or linens used by infected persons. Mosquito bites are not a source of infection.

HIV is a blood-borne STD. During any form of sexual intercourse, (anal, vaginal or oral), the risk of infection is considerably greater for the partner who received the semen, although infection, can also be transmitted to an inserting partner. The increased risk occurs because the receiver has prolonged contact with the semen; this helps to explain why women are more easily infected than men during heterosexual intercourse. The risk factors for HIV infection are summarized as follows:

1. Sexual practices
   - Unprotected sex (without condom use)
   - Multiple sexual partners
   - Anal or oral sexual activity
   - Improper condom use or condom breakage
   - Open sore, lesions or irritation in the genital area
2. Contaminated blood
3. Contaminated needle (SC or IM or IV, etc.)
4. Occupational exposure
   - All healthcare workers-acute care
   - Long term care, and home care (Doctors, Nurses and others)
   - Dental workers
   - Correction officers and law enforcement personnel (Police and others)
5. Perinatal exposure (During pregnancy, birth or breastfeeding)
   Approximately 25 percent children of HIV-positive mother are infected with HIV.

Pathophysiology

The natural history of HIV infection is associated with unpredictable course of disease progression. Many patients undergo a prolonged period of clinically silent infection, often lasting more than 10 years. Although the virus is consistently detectable throughout this time, patients typically have only subtle immunological alterations. Once the patient becomes symptomatic, however, decreases in the number of T4 helper cells can be detected and viral replication increases.

The life cycle of HIV is similar to that of the other retroviruses. Mature virions interact with specific host receptors and then use the host cell for viral replication. HIV interacts with the CD4 glycoprotein, which occurs on the membrane of the specific cells, primarily the CD4 + (T4) helper lymphocytes. The CD4 protein may also be found on the surface of several other cells as well, including some monocytes, macrophages, glial cells and gastrointestinal cells (GI). Presence of the CD4, glycoprotein allows the virus fuse to the host cell. The viral core is subsequently injected into the cell cytoplasm, where the viral ribonucleic acid (RNA). Genome is translated into deoxyribonucleic acid (DNA) by a retroviral enzyme called reverse transcriptase. Infection and subsequent viral replication eventually depletes the hosts T4 helper cells, resulting in a dramatic loss of the protective immune response against invading microorganism.

Many potential cofactors may be associated with HIV disease progression. These cofactors which may be viral, host, or environmental are thought to directly influence the replication of HIV or the severity of its pathogenic effects.

Viral cofactors: That may influence the progression of the disease include herpes simplex virus (HSV) cytomegalovirus (CMV), Epstein-Barr virus (EBV).

Host cofactors may include variety of cytokines and intracellular mediators.

Environmental cofactors may induce hyperactivation of the immune system, resulting in an expansion of the pool of HI V, replicating cells. As viral 1 replication increases, depleting the body of T4 lymphocytes, the body's defense mechanism are progressively weakened. Infections that were once disarmed by the healthy immune system are eventually able to cause serious and potentially life-threatening disease. The spectrum of HIV infection ranges from asymptomatic to potentially life-threatening opportunistic infection.

Clinical Manifestation

The early phases of infection with HIV varies from person to person. Some individuals experience symptoms similar to flu or mononucleosis, consisting of fever, fatigue, nausea, vomiting, headache, rash or lymphadenopathy; symptoms may be mild or serious enough to warrant hospitalization. It is during this time that the viral load (amount of HIV present) is very high, CD4 helper cells drop dramatically and the person converts to seropositive HIV status. The initial phase of infection may be followed by a period of latency that may last from several months to 10 years or more. During this time, the persons may be completely asymptomatic or experience only mild symptoms such as fatigue. As the immune system becomes further compromised, the symptoms of AIDS develop. Clinical manifestations associated with AIDS are primarily those of opportunistic infections. The common symptoms include the following:

- Chills and fever
- Malaise
- Night sweats
- Fatigue
- Dry productive
- Oral lesions
- Cough
- Skin rash
- Dyspnea
- Abdominal discomfort
- Lethargy
- Diarrhea
- Confusion
- Weight loss
- Stiff neck
- Lymphadenopathy
- Seizures
- Progressive genera
- Headachelized edema

The complications of HIV disease present a complex picture of opportunistic infections, neoplasms or condition related to immunodeficiency. If not treated in time, symptoms of opportunistic infection also develop. The common AIDS-related opportunistic infection includes the following:

- *Bacterial infections: Mycobacterium avium* complex (MAC), Mycobacterium tuberculosis causes fever, diarrhea, profound wasting.
- *Fungal infections:* Candidiasis (thrush or vaginal infection), Cryptococcosis (coccosis causes meningitis), histoplasmosis (associated with fever and weight loss).
- *Protozoal infection: Cryptosporidium* (causes fulminant diarrhea), *Pneumocystis carinii* (ac. resp. failure), *Toxoplasma gondii* (causes encephalitis).

- *Viral infections:* HSV, CMV, (cause retinitis, blindness).
- *HIV related cancer:* Kaposi's sarcoma, non-Hodgkins lymphomas, cervical cancer.

HIV can cross the blood-brain barrier, attach to microglial cells and cause encephalopathy or motor dysfunction.

Management

HIV infection or AIDS is diagnosed when an individual with HIV has at least one of these additional conditions.

1. CD4 + T cell count drops below 200/ MI
2. Development of one of the following opportunistic infections (OIs).
   - *Fungal:* Candidiasis of bronchi, trachea, lungs or esophagus; *Pneumocystis carinii* Penumonia (PCP), disseminated or extra pulmonary hissopharmosis.
   - *Viral:* Cytomegalovirus (CMV) disease other than liver, spleen or nodes CMV retinitis (with loss of vision); herpes simplex with chronic ulcer or bronchitis, pneumonitis, or esophagitis, progressive multifocal leucoencephalopathy (PML), extra pulmonary cryptococcosis.
   - *Protozoal:* Disseminated or extra pulmonary coccidio-mycosis, toxoplasmosis of the brain; chronic intestinal isosporiasis; chronic intestinal cryptosporidiasis.
   - *Bacterial: Mycobacterium tuberculosis* (any site); any disseminated or extrapulmonary; *Mycobacterium* including MAC or *M. kansacii*, recurrent pneumonia; recurrent *Salmonella septicemia.*
3. Development of one of the following opportunistic cancer; Invasive cervical cancer, Kaposi's sarcoma (KS). Burkitt's lymphoma, immunoblastic lymphoma, or primary lymphoma of the brain.
4. *Wasting syndrome occurs:* Wasting syndrome defined as a loss of 10 percent or more of ideal body mass.
5. *Dementia develops:* The most useful screening test for HIV are those that detect HIV specific antibodies. The most commonly used test is the Enzyme-linked-immunosorbent assay (ELISA). A positive ELISA must be confirmed by the Western blot technique. Both depend on antibody formation. The following steps are used in the process of testing blood for antibodies to HIV:
   - A highly sensitive enzyme immunoassay (EIA, ELISA) is done to detect serum antibodies that bind to HIV antigens on test plates; blood samples that are negative on this test are reported as negative.
   - If the blood is EIA reactive, the test is repeated.
   - If the blood is repeatedly EIA reactive, a more specific confirmatory test, such as the Western blot (WB) or immunofluorescence assay (IFA) is done.
     - Western blot (WB) testing used purified HIV antigens electrophoresed on gels. These are incubated with serum samples of antibody in the serum, its prevention can be detected.
     - IFA is used to identify HIV in injected cells. Blood is located with a fluorescent antibody against ph or p24

antigen and then examined using a fluorescent microscope.

- Blood that is reactive in all of the first three steps is reported as HIV antibody positive.
- If the results are indeterminant, testing should be repeated within 6 months. Consistently indeterminant tests results require the use of polymerase chain reaction (PCR), viral culture, and other diagnostic measures.
  - PCR analysis DNA extracted from lymphocytes and/ or HIV from serum using an *in vitro* amplification procedure.
  - A cell culture system can be used to grow viruses from infected lymphocytes. Since these tests are expensive and difficult to do, they are usually not used for screening purposes, but may be done in situations where the index of suspicion is high and antibodies are negative. HIV can be classified as laboratory categories as follows: (CDC 1993)
    - Ø Category I: Greater than or equal to 500 CD 4 + Cells
    - Ø Category II: 200 to 499 CD4 + Cells
    - Ø Category III: Less than 200 CD4 + Cells.

HIV classification for adolescents and adults according revised Centers for Disease Control and Prevention (CDC 1993) as *Clinical Categories* are as follows:

Category A: One or more of the following conditions occurring in an adolescent or adult with documented HIV infection. Conditions listed in categories Band C must not have occurred.
- Asymptomatic HIV infection.
- Persistent generalized lymphadenopathy.
- Acute (Primary) HIV infection with accompanying illness or history of acute, HIV infection.

Category B: Symptomatic conditions occurring in an HIV infected adolescent or adult that are not included among conditions listed in category C and that meet atleast one of the following criteria:
- The conditions are attributed to HIV infection or are indicative of a defect in cell-mediated immunity.
- The conditions are considered by physicians to have a clinical course or management that is complicated by HIV infection. Examples of conditions in clinical category B include but are not limited to:
- Bacterial endocarditis, meningitis, pneumonia or sepsis.
- Candidiasis, oropharyngeal (thrush).
- Cervical dysplasia, severe or carcinoma.
- Constitutional symptoms such as fever (greater than 38.5°C) or diarrhea lasting more than a month.
- Hairy leukoplakia, oral.
- Herpes zoster (shingles), involving atleast two distinct episodes or more than one dermatome.
- Idiopathic thrombocytopenic purpura.
- Listeriosis.
- *Mycobacterium tuberculosis* infection, pulmonary.
- Nocardiosis
- Pelvic inflammatory disease.
- Peripheral neuropathy.

Category C: Any condition that has occurred, the person will remain in category C, i.e.
- The conditions clinical category C are strongly associated with severe immunodeficiency, occur frequently in HIV infected patients and cause serious morbidity or mortality.
- According to proposed classification system, HIV-infected patient would be classified on the basis of both:
  - The lowest accurate (not necessarily the most recent) CD4 + lymphocyte determination and
  - The most severe clinical condition diagnosed regardless of the patient current clinical condition.

Treatment

There are no specific treatment in the early stages of HIV infections. Respiratory treatment may become necessary as the patient's disease progresses. Standard precautions are necessary when the patient is hospitalized or being treated at home. Treatment associated with maintenance and improvement of nutritional status also usually become necessary. Specific treatment related to opportunistic infections are briefly discussed as given below:

1. *Respiratory System*

- *Pneumocystis carinii* Pneumonia *(PCP):* There will be non-productive cough, hypoxemia, progressive shortness of breath, fever, night sweat and fatigue. This is diagnosed by chest X-ray, induced sputum culture and bronchoalveolar lavage. It can be treated by Bactrim, Cleocin, Mepron and Corticosteroids.
- *Histoplasma capsulatum:* In this, there will be pneumonia, fever, cough weight loss, disseminated disease. Diagnosis made by sputum culture, serum or urine antigen assay. This is treated by using Amphotericin-B, Itraconazole (Sporanox) Fluconazole (Diflucon).
- *Coccidioides immitis:* There will be fever, weight loss, cough, test includes sputum culture, serology, treatment as in *Histoplasma capsulatum.*
- *Mycobacteria TB:* There will be a productive cough, fever, night sweats weight loss, diagnosis by chest X-ray, sputum for AFB and culture. Treated by antituberculosis drugs INH, Streptomycin, Rifampicin
- *Kaposi's sarcoma:* There is dyspnea, respiratory failure, chest X-ray and biopsy all helps to diagnose. Cancer chemotherapy radiations are the treatment.

2. *Integumentary System*

- *HSV1 & HSV2*: Orolabial mucocutaneous ulcerative lesions (type 1) genital and perineal mucocutaneous ulcerative lesion (type 2). Do viral culture and treat with Acyclovir, Famuclovir, Valacyclovir. (Valtrex)
- *Varicella zoster virus (VZV):* Shingles, erythematous maculopapular rash and treat with Acyclovir, Famuclovir (Famvir) Valtrax and Foscarnet (Foscavir).

- *Kaposi's sarcoma:* Firm, flat, raised nodular, hyperpigmented, multicentric lesions found in skin. Do biopsy lesions. Treat with cancer chemotherapy, alpha interferon, radiation of lesions.
- *Bacillary angiomatosis:* Erythematous vasccular papules, subcutaneous nodules are seen on skin. Do biopsy and treatment with Erythromycin, Doxycycline.

3. Eye

- *CMV retinitis:* Lesions on the retina, blurred vision, loss of vision, do ophthalmoscopic exam and treat with Canciclovir (Cytovene) Foscarnet or Cidofovir (Vistide).
- *HSV1:* Blurred vision; corneal lesions, acute retinal necrosis or ophthalmoscopy exam. Treat with Acyclovir, Famuclovir, etc.
- *VZV:* Occular lesions, acute retinal necrosis. Do ophthalmoscopy and treat with antiviral drugs.

4. GI System

- *Cryptosporidium muris:* Watery diarrhea, abdominal pain, weight loss, nausea are seen. Do stool examination. Small bowel or colon biopsy. Treat with antidiarrheals, Flaramomycin, Azithromycin, Asovaquone, Sandostatin (Octreotide)
- *CMV:* Stomatitis, esophagitis, gastritis, colitis, diarrhea, bloody diarrhea, pain, weight loss. Do endoscopic visualization, culture, biopsy for ruling out the causes, and treat with Ganciclovir and antiviral drugs.
- *HSV:* Vesiular eruption on tongue, buccal, pharyngeal or perioral esophage 1 mucosa seen. Do viral culture, administer antiviral drugs.
- *Candida albicans:* There will be whitish-yellow patches in mouth esophagus, GI tract. Do microscopic examination for scraping from lesion, culture. Administration of Fluconazole, Mystatin, Clotrimazol (Lotrimin), itraconazole, Amphotericin-B are helpful.
- *Mycobacterium avium complex (MAC):* There will be watery diarrhea, weight loss. Do small bowel biopsy with AFB stain and culture. Administer Clarithromycin (Biaxin) Rifampin, Ciprofloxacin, Azithromycin, according to culture.
- *Isospora belli:* Diarrhea, weight loss, nausea, abdominal pain are seen. Do stool exam. Small bowel colon biopsy. Treat with Trimethoprim + Sulfamethoxazole, Pyrimethamine + Folinic acid.
- *Salmonella:* Gastroenteritis, fever, diarrhea, Do stool and blood culture. Administer Ciprofloxacin, Ampicillin, Amoxycillin, – Sep.
- *Kaposi's sarcoma:* There will be diarrhea, hyperpigmented lesions of mouth and GI tract. Do GI series and biopsy. Treat with cancer chemotherapy, alpha-interferon and radiation.
- *Non-Hodgkins lymphoma:* There will be abdominal pain, fever, night sweats, weight loss, Do lymph node biopsy and treatment with chemotherapy.

5. Neurologic System

- *Toxoplasma gondii:* There is cognitive dysfunction, motor impairment, fever, altered mental status, headache, seizures, sensory abnormalities. Diagnosis by MRI, CT scan, toxoplasma serology, brain biopsy. Treat with Pyrimethamine + Folinic acid + Sulfadiazine, Clindamycin Azithromycin, Clarithromycin.
- *JC Papovirus:* Progressive multifocal leukoencephalopathy (PML), mental and motor declines. Diagnosis by MRI, CT scan-brain biopsy. Effective antiretroviral therapy may help.
- *Cryptococcal meningitis* There is cognitive impairment, motor dysfunction, fever, seizures, headache, CT scan, serum, antigen test, CSF analysis help to diagnosis. Treatment with Amphotericin-B, Flucystosine, Fluconazale, helps.
- *CNS lymphomas:* Cognitive dysfunction, motor impairment, aphasia, seizures, personality charges, headache. Do MRI, CT scan. Treat with radiation and chemotherapy.
- *AIDS-dementia complex (ADC)* There is insidious onset of progressive dementia. Do CT scan. Effective antiretroviral therapy may help.

Nursing Management

Health assessment of all patients should include an appraisal of potential risk factors for HIV infection. Obtaining complete, accurate sexual history including past and present sexual activities, requires skillful interviewing techniques and professional relationship based on trust. Nurses need to be able to explain the need for information on intimate sexual activities and phrase questions in appropriate but comprehensive terms.

A major goal of health promotions is to prevent disease. HIV infection is preventable. Until a vaccine is available; education and behavior changes are the only effective tools. Educational messages should be specific to the patients' need, culturally sensitive, language appropriate and age specific. Nurses are excellent resources for this type of education, but nurses must be comfortable with and knowledgeable about sensitive topics such as sexuality and drug use. Risk reducing sexual activities decrease the risk of contact with HIV through the use of barriers. Barrier should be used when engaging in insertive sexual activity (oral, vaginal or anal) with partner who is known to HIV infected or with partner whose HIV status is not known. The most commonly used barriers is the *male condom*. The major points for correct use of *male condom* are as follows:

- Use only condoms (rubber) that are made out of latex or polyurethane. - Natural skin. Condoms have pores that are large enough for HIV to penetrate.
- Store condom in a cool, dry place and protect them from trauma. The friction caused by carrying them in back pocket, for instance can wear down the latex.
- Do not use condom if the expiration date has passed or if the package looks worn or punctured.
- Lubricants used in conjunction with condoms must be water soluble.

- Oil based lubricants can weaken latex and increase the risk of tearing or breaking.
- Non-lubricated, flavoured condom can provide protection during oral intercourse.
- The condom must be placed on the erect penis before any contact is made with the partner's mouth, vagina or rectum to prevent exposure to pre-ejaculatory secretions that may contain HIV.
- Remove the penis and condom from the partner's body immediately after ejaculation and before the erection is lost. Hold the condom at the base of the penis and remove both at the same time. This keeps semen from leaking around the condom as the penis becomes flaccid. Remove the condom after use. Wrap in tissue and discard. Do not flush down the toilet as this can cause plumbing problem.
- Condoms are not reusable. A new condom must be used for every act of intercourse.

Now female condoms are also available. Use can be complicated. So careful instructions and practice are required as given below:

- Female condom consists of a polyurethane sheath with two springs from rings.
- The small ring is inserted into the vagina and holds the condom in place, internally. This ring can be removed if the condom is to be used anal intercourse. It should not be removed by the condom, is to be used for vaginal intercourse.
- The larger ring surrounds the opening the condom. It functions to keep the condom in place externally while protecting the external genitalia.
- Use only water-soluble lubricants with female condoms.
- Female condoms come prelubricated and with a tube of additional lubricant.
- Lubrication is needed to protect the condom from tearing during sexual intercourse and can also decrease the noise that results from friction of the penis against the condom.
- Some men have reported that female condom feels better than the male condom. Other men like male condoms better. The only way to find out which type of condom works best is to try them both.
- Practice inserting the female condom. Lubrication makes the condom slippery, but do not get discouraged. Just keep trying.
- During sexual intercourse, ensure that the penis is inserted into the female condom through the outer ring. It is possible for the penis to miss the opening, thus making contact with the vagina and defeating the purpose of the condom.
- Do not use a male condom at the same time as female condom.
- After intercourse, remove the condom before standing up.
- Twist the outer ring to keep the semen inside. Gently pull the condom out of the vagina and discard.
- Do not flush down the toilet, as this can cause plumbing problem.
- Do not reuse female condom.

Cleansing the equipment before use is a risk-reducing activity. It decreases the risk for those who share equipment.

The patient should be taught to recognize clinical manifestation that may indicate progression of the disease so that prompt medical care can be initiated. An overview of the symptoms that the patient should report includes the following:

1. Report the following signs and symptoms immediately.
   - Any change in level of consciousness, lethargy, hard to arouse, unable to arouse, unresponsive, unconscious.
   - Headache accompanied by nausea and vomiting, changes in vision, changes in ability to perform coordinated activities, or after any head trauma.
   - Vision changes; blurry or black areas in vision field, new floaters.
   - Persistent shortness of breath related to activity and not relieved by a short rest period.
   - Nausea and vomiting accompanied by abdominal pain.
   - Dehydration, unable to eat or drink, because of nausea, diarrhea, or mouth lesions; severe diarrhea or vomiting, dizziness when standing.
   - Yellow discoloration of the skin.
   - Any bleeding from the rectum that is not related to hemorrhoids.
   - Pain in the flank with fever and unable to urinate for more than 6 hours.
   - New onset of weakness in any part of the body, new onset of numbness that is not obviously related to pressure, new onset of difficulty in speaking.
   - Chest pain not obviously related to cough.
   - Seizures.
   - New rash accompanied by fever.
   - New oral lesions accompanied by fever.
   - Severe depression, anxiety, hallucinations, delusions or possible danger to self or others.

2. Report the following signs and symptoms within 24 hours.
   - New or different headache, constant headache not relieved by Aspirins or Acetominophen.
   - Headache accompanied by fever, nasal congestion or cough.
   - Burning, itching or discharge from the eyes.
   - New or productive cough
   - Vomiting 2 to 3 times a day.
   - Vomiting accompanied by fever.
   - New, significant or watery diarrhea (more than 6 times a day)
   - Painful urination, bloody urine, urethral discharge.
   - New significant rash (widespread, painful, itchy, or following a path down the leg or arm, around the chest or on the face) difficulty in eating because of lesions.
   - Vaginal discharge, pain or inching.

In addition all nurses have the responsibilities to take special precautions to protect themselves from HIV infections, because certain pathogenic microorganisms can be found in the blood and other body fluids of infected individuals. These pathogens can be transmitted to uninfected individuals from infected individuals. OSHA has developed standards and guidelines for employees who are at risk for exposure to blood and other infectious materials. All potentially infectious material are to be considered infectious regardless of the perceived status of the source client. The most significant pathogens that require preventive measures are the hepatitis B virus (HBV) and human immunodeficiency virus (HIV). OSHA standards require that universal precautions guidelines, developed by the Centers for Disease Control (CDC) in Atlanta, Georgia, be observed at all facilities.

Basic Rules of Universal Precautions

- The purpose of universal precautions is to prevent or minimize exposure to blood-borne pathogens.
- Approach *all* clients as if they are HIV or HBV-infectious.
- Universal precautions apply to tissues, blood, and other body fluids containing visible blood.
- Approach *all* blood, body fluids, and tissues as if they are HIV or HBV-contaminated
- Approach *all* needles and sharps as if they have been contaminated HIV or HBV.
- Blood is the single most important source of HIV, HBV, and other blood-borne pathogens in the workplace.
- Universal precautions also apply to tissues, semen, vaginal secretions, cerebrospinal fluid, synovial fluid, pleural fluid pericardial fluid, and amniotic fluid.
- Universal precautions do not apply to feces, nasal secretions, breastmilk, sputum, sweat, tears, urine, and vomitus unless they contain visible blood.
- Precautions do not apply to saliva, except in dentistry.
- Anticipate the kind of client contact and use appropriate personal protective equipment.
- Know the limitations of the personal protective equipment being used, when it can protect and when it cannot.
- Do not recap needles.
- Do not break or otherwise manipulate needles.
- Place contaminated sharps in puncture-resistant containers.
- Wash hands immediately after contamination or removing gloves.
- Universal precautions do not eliminate the need for other category-specific or disease-specific isolation precautions, such as enteric precautions for infectious diarrhea.

Hand Protection

- Wash hands before and after contact with any client whether gloves are worn or not.
- Wash hands before and after a procedure is performed whether gloves are worn or not.
- Always wear gloves when obtaining, handling, or testing specimens (body fluids, excretions, secretions) or touching any items or articles exposed to substances with contamination potential.
- Change gloves between clients or when soiled or torn.

- Wash hands or any skin or mucous membrane area immediately following contact with blood, body fluids, or any potentially infectious material; flush with water or wash with soap and water as soon as is feasible following the contact.
- Gloves are not to be washed or decontaminated for reuse.

Personal Protection

- Anticipate splashing of blood or body fluids, and attempt to eliminate or minimize spills or splashes.
- Wear disposable gown, apron, or lab coat when in contact or potentially in contact with blood or other infectious materials.
- Wear mask, eye protection (goggles with solid side shield) or chin-length face shield, as indicated, to protect skin, eyes, and mouth from contact with splashes, sprays, splattering, or droplets or potentially infectious body fluids.
- All garments contaminated by blood should be removed immediately; garments and protective equipment that are worn should be removed and disposed of properly prior to leaving work.
- Wearing apparel that is contaminated with blood or body fluids should be placed in a waterproof labeled bag in a designated area.

Needles and Sharps

- Contaminated needles and other sharps should not be bent, recapped, removed, sheared, or purposely broken; in cases where there is no alternative to removal or recapping a needle, a mechanical device or one-handed technique should be used.
- In cases where a needle puncture accidentally occurs, report immediately for further evaluation and counseling.
- Discard used disposable needles, syringes, and other sharps in puncture and leakproof containers marked with a biohazard label; the articles should be discarded as soon as feasible following use:
  - Discard reusable sharps in a color-coded, labeled container for decontamination.
  - Never reach into the container of used needles or sharps.
  - Replace containers when they are three-quarters full; close the full container and place in a designated area.

Specimens

- Gloves should *always* be worn when collecting, handling, and testing specimens that are or have a potential to be contaminated with infectious microorganisms.
- Gloves should *always* be worn when collecting blood specimens, as all specimens are assumed to contain potentially infectious material.
- Avoid accidental sticks from needles when obtaining blood samples.
- Mouth pipetting of blood or other potentially infectious materials is prohibited.
- Always use disposable supplies to collect specimens when possible.

- Specimens of blood or other potentially infectious materials should be placed in a container and then in a biohazard bag that prevents leakage during the collection, handling, processing, storage and transport of the specimens.
- Containers should be labeled or color-coded. If the outside of the primary container is contaminated, it should be placed in a secondary container that is puncture-resistant.
- Specimens that are to be transported outside of the facility are to be labeled with a biohazard sticker on the container.

- All microbiologic waste such as cultures and stocks of etiologic agents must be steam sterilized in the lab prior to transport.
- All anatomic pathology wastes are placed in a color-coded bag or lined box prior to transport by housekeeping.
- All blood product containers are placed in a bag within a biohazard-labeled container.
- Cleanse any spills of body fluids during collection or handling by wiping with paper toweling first, then washing with soap and water and then washing with a disinfectant solution.

33

Management of Loss, Grief and Death

"Unique function of the nurse is to assess the individual sickness or wellness, in the performance of these activities contributing to health or its recovery (or peaceful death)...." The aspect of activity in relation to peaceful death also is counted very important, because taking care of dying patients and their families can be one of the most challenging aspects of nursing care because dying is the final stage of human growth and development; it is essential that nurse be as knowledgeable about the process of dying as they are about the process of birth. When nurses dealing with grieving families and dying patients, they are confronted with their own mortality and other discomforting issues that accompany loss. Such factors can influence quality of care. All losses have the possibility of triggering the grief process. Understanding loss, the grief process and the task of dying can assist the nurse in delivering quality care to those patients and families experiencing death.

Loss, Grief and Death

Life is a series of losses and gains. Everyone experiences losses at various points in the life continuum. Birth, loss and death are universal and individually unique events of the human experience. At any stage of one's life, there is the potential for loss, grief and death.

The goals of nursing focuses on health maintenance and health restoration, with an emphasis on facilitating maximum potentials in wellness. One of the function of the nurse is, however, to facilitate coping with the disabilities and death. The nurse is the key person in providing support and care when loss or death occurs. To provide effective care the nurse must have accepted his or her own feeling about death and understand the stages of grieving and dying. Nurses need to understand loss and grief. Because death is a frequent reality in many nursing care settings. Most nurses interact daily with client's and family's experiencing loss and grief. We will examine these one by one as given below.

Loss

A person experiences loss in the absence of an object, person's body part or function, or emotion that was formerly present.

Five Categories of Loss

Loss of External Object

It involves any possession that is worn-out, misplaced, stolen or ruined by disaster, e.g. jewellery, to money, etc.

Loss of a Known Environment

It is a loss associated with separation from a known environment, includes familiar setting for a period or relocating permanently and transfer from place to place, hospitalization.

Loss of Significant Others

It includes loss of parents, spouses, children, siblings, teachers, friends, neighbors and colleagues. And also entertainment figures, and well known persons like cine actors, athletes, cricketers, popular figures of a particular field.

Loss of an Aspect of Life

It includes loss of a body part, physiological function, or psychological function, e.g. loss of limb, eye, hair teeth, breast, etc., loss of urinary or bowel control, loss of memory, humor of self-esteem, of self-confidence, of power, of respect, of love, self-concept, self-identity, of job.

Loss of Life

Each person responds differently to death. Some will welcome death as a relief, some will have fear of separations, abandonment, loneliness, or mutilation, etc.

Other Classifications of Loss

Actual Loss

It is easily identified and can be recognized by others as well as person sustaining the loss, loss of a limb, of a spouse, of a object and of a job.

Perceived Loss

It is felt by the person but is intangible or less intangible to others. For example:
  (a) Makirational loss, i.e. loss resulting from normal life transitions (loss of youth, of financial independence).
  (b) Situational loss, i.e. loss occurring suddenly in reference to a specific external event (sudden death of loved one).

Other example of actual or perceived loss are physical loss, and psychological loss, e.g. losing limb from accident, losing limb leads to loss of self-image.

Anticipatory Loss

Anticipatory loss in which a person displays loss and grief behavior for a loss that has yet to take place, e.g. sickness or death.

Grief

Grief is a normal response to any loss, grieving is the emotional reaction to loss. It occurs with loss caused by separation as well as with loss caused by death. Sometimes the terms, grief, mourning and bereavement are often used interchangeable.
• Grief—is a form of sorrow that follows the perception or anticipation, loss of one or more valued or significant objects.

These responses often include helplessness, loneliness, hopelessness sadness, guilt and anger.

- Bereavement—is the state of grieving during which a person goes through grief reaction. It is the state of thought, feeling, and activity that follows loss, or includes grief and mourning. It is the experience of having lost something or someone by death.
- Mourning—is the period of acceptance of loss and grief during which the person learns to deal with loss. It is the process that follows, a loss and includes working through grief. The process of grief and mourning are intense, internal, painful and lengthy. Mourning refers to culturally defined patterns of expressions of grief. Mourning patterns include funerals, wakes, memorials, black dress and defined time of social withdrawal.

Grief Process (Reactions to Grief and Death)

Grief is the emotional pain caused by a loss. Reactions to both grief and dying are similar. The stages of these reactions overlap and vary among individuals. Engel (1954) proposed that grieving process has six phases as given below.

Shock and disbelief: Here the person usually refuses to accept the fact of loss, followed by a stunned or numb responses; 'No' 'not me' etc.

Developing awareness: It is characterized by physical and emotional responses such as anger, feeling empty, and crying: 'why me?'

Restitution: It involves the rituals surrounding loss and with death includes religious, cultural, and social expressions of mourning such as funeral service.

Resolving the loss: It is dealing with the void left by the loss.

Idealization: It is the exaggeration of the good qualities of the person or object lost, followed by acceptance of loss and lessened need to focus on it.

Outcome: It is the final resolution of the grief process, including dealing with loss as a common life occurrence.

Kubler Ross (1969) considered a pioneer in the study of grief and death reactions defined five stages of reactions similar to those of Engel.

Denial and isolation: In this stage, the client denies that he or she will die, may repress that is discussed, and may isolate self from reality. The person may think "they made a mistake in the diagnosis", "they may not come to hospital" etc.

Anger: The client expresses rage and hostility in the anger stage and adopts a "why me?" attitude. Hostility may be directed towards care givers or loved ones.

Bargaining: The client tries to barter for more time. "If I can live up to my son's graduation, I will be satisfied. Just let me live until then". Many clients put their personal affairs in order, make wills and fulfill last wishes.

Depression In this stage, the client goes through a period of grief before death. The grief is characterized by crying and not speaking much. "I waited all these years to see my son to get married, I will die before he gets married, etc."

Acceptance When the stage of acceptance is reached, the client feels tranquil. She or he has accepted the death and prepared to die. He may think, "I have tied up all the loose ends, made all arrangement to my son to lead a happy life."

In 1985, Martocchio, described five stages of grief, similar to the above Table 33.1.

	Table 33.1: Five Stages of Grief of Martocchio	
	Stages	*Response*
i.	Shock and disbelief	Denial
ii.	Yearning and protest	Anger and bargaining
iii.	Anguish, disorganization and despair	Depression
iv.	Identification in bereavement	
v.	Reorganization and restitution	Acceptance

Nursing Role in Grief

Nursing interventions and details of behavior during phases of grief reactions are as follows:

Denial

As stated earlier, denial is immediate response to news of loss or impending loss. The client's physiological responses may include muscular-weakness, tremors, deep signs, flushed or cold and clammy skin, diaphoresis, anorexia and discomfort. Usually individuals avoid accepting reality of situations by making decisions; they may attempt activities that they are no longer able to do, fail to comply with treatment, search for evidence that loss has not occurred or will not occur and appear artificially happy. Mood swings are common. Individuals isolate themselves from sources of accurate information or reject offers of comfort and support. He serves as a buffer to the patient to shield himself/herself until the individual is able to mobilize alternate defenses.

In this stage, nurses should follow the following:
- Support emotional needs without supporting denial
- Offer to remain with clients, without discussing, reasons for behavior or need to cope, unless they bring it up
- Offer regressive care such as food, drink and safety.

Anger

In this stage, individuals may express anger and retaliate against family, staff, physicians, or supreme being; bereaved may express anger toward deceased. Individual becomes demanding and accusing. Anger may precipitate guilt and lead to anxiety and lowered self-esteem. He may feel resentful and jealous of others who still have lost object or loved one and may be reluctant to share feelings and thoughts. Hostility may be directed toward caregivers or loved ones.

In this stage, nurses should follow the following:
- Provide anticipatory guidance about feelings and their intensity experienced as a part of grief. Focus especially on anger.
- Do not take anger personally
- Meet needs that cause angry response.

Bargaining

Here, individuals are willing to do anything to avoid loss or change prognosis or fate. They make bargains with supreme being and also accept new forms of therapy. Bargaining is often made with God. It is an attempt to postpone death and is a positive way to maintain hope.

In this stage nurses provide information needed for decision-making.

Depression

In this stage person shows reality, and permanence of loss becomes recognized. And confusion, disinterest, indecision and crying are common; withdrawal from relationships and activities occurs. Individuals may become quiet and non-communicative and show loneliness surface, reminiscence about past and lost object begins. Individuals may lose interest in appearance and may become suicidal or cope by beginning unhealthy behaviors such as excess drug use, sadness and grief. Time of introspection, usually request only significant others to be with them. The patient struggles with painful realities of life and preparing for death.

In this stage, the nurses should follow the following:
- Provide support and empathy
- Support crying by offering touch that communicates caring
- Listen absently
- Assess risk of harm to self and refer to mental health professional, if needed.

Acceptance

In this stage, individuals accept terms of loss and death and begin plans for it. Individuals can share feelings about loss and reminiscence about past occurrences. Good times begin to outweigh bad. Life begins to stabilize. Resolved the fact that the death is imminent. Peaceful acceptance and positive feeling are often present.

In this stage nurses should follow the following:
- Offer opportunities to share feelings verbally in writing or art, or by tape recording
- Allow and encourage review as often as clients want to talk
- Show acceptance of liability of feeling
- Assist in discussing future plans.

Death

Death is present when an individual has sustained either irreversible cessation of circulatory and respiratory functions or irreversible cessation of all functions of the entire brain, including the brain stem. The supportive nursing care during death are as follows:

To give compassionate nursing care and support to the family and patient during both the grieving and dying process, the nurse should consider the five aspects of human functioning. By using the nursing process, the nurse does an assessment of each aspect; physical, emotional, intellectual, sociocultural, and spiritual to fully understand and adequately provide interventions in these areas.

Physical

While interviewing and observing the patient, the nurse should assess such areas as sleeping patterns, body image, activities of daily living. (ADLs) mobility, general health, medications and pain. The nurse also should address the basic needs of nutrition, elimination oxygenation, activity, rest, sleep and safety.

Goals for interventions should be: (i) energy conservation, (ii) pain reduction techniques, (iii) comfort measures, (iv) promotion of sleep and rest, and (v) increasing self-esteem through body image acceptance.

Emotional

Preparing for one's death is a personal endeavor filled with anxiety and fear. Assessing the patient and family's anxiety level, guilt, anger, level of acceptance, and identification is important. Major fears of the dying patient include fears of abandonment, loss of control, pain and discomfort, and the fear of the unknown.

The nurses can intervene appropriately when they are able to accept the patient's family's individual feelings, offer encouragement and support, and give the patient's "permission to die" by assisting the patient in saying "good-bye".

Intellectual

Intellectual assessment includes an evaluation of the patient and family's educational level, their knowledge and abilities, and expectations they have in regard to how and when death will occurs. Some aspects of the intellectual dimension can be altered during the dying process because of physiological changes, medications the patient's emotional state, or the disease process. Being alert, to these changes will avert problems if the patient's memory or sensations are decreased.

Intervention is directed toward patient/family education and support. Keeping all people informed of procedures, changes in condition of the patient, and hospital policies contributes to well-informed decisions being made when necessary.

Social

Assessing the patient and family's support systems is valuable. Ascertaining if family members desire to assist in the patient's daily care will not only lessen the family's sense of loss of control but also will clarify what tasks the family will do and what will be done by nursing staff. Not making these needs and desires can result in distrust and hostility between family and nursing staff. Each family and each individual member are unique in what they wish to do. The nurse should never assume that families want to deliver daily care. Many do, but others do not, and they need the opportunity to make that choice.

During the social assessment, it is necessary to learn whom the patient considers significant others. Although families are considered important, it is crucial to learn whom the patient considers the most supportive person in his or her life. It may be a friend, coworker, or church member. This person should become a part of the patient's supportive network and be included in planning the patient's care. The nurse encourages these social support persons to become involved and at the same time maintains and promotes the patient's independence whenever possible.

Spiritual

The nurse assesses the spiritual dimension by gaining insight into the patient's philosophy of life, his religious resources, and how the rituals of his faith group have significance in dealing with his death.

Interventions in this area can come from clergy, friends, family, healthcare providers, and significant others. Supporting the patient and family belief system and values is important. By completing the nursing process of assessment, diagnosis, planning, implementation, and evaluation, the nurse can develop a nursing care plan.

Special Supportive Care

Often death occurs outside the realm of serious illness, injury or aging. Perinatal, pediatric, suicidal, and geriatric deaths are some examples that warrant special consideration.

Perinatal Death

The death of a child is often viewed as one of the most devastating losses that can occur in a family. If the death of the child occurs before, during, or shortly after birth, it is called perinatal death.

Special considerations by healthcare providers should be addressed so that the parents and family can grieve adequately. Because there are no or few memories that loved ones can share about the child, "acting as though it never happened" place parents in jeopardy of living with unresolved grief. When possible, the parents should see, touch and hold the infant, so that the reality of the situation can be faced and resolution of the grief can occur. Listening attentively and allowing the parents to express their feelings over their losses beneficial. Referring

to the baby as "your baby, "your son, "your daughter," or using the given name can reinforce that the baby was indeed a unique individual who was loved and will be missed. The usual cultural rituals after death should take place for the baby, such as a funeral or memorial service.

Pediatric Death

Children faced with death present a need for special nursing skills. Nurses should be aware of how children view or understand death, both for themselves and for others (Table 33.2).

Table 33.2: Children's Beliefs about Death	
Age (Years)	*Belief system*
3	: See death as a separation. Unable to comprehend permanent
3 to 5	: Fear death but see it as reversible. View death as a loss of an object.
6 to 10	: Generally see death as permanent. Often have morbid feelings about death. Fear pain and mutilation.
11 to 18	: Recognize death as permanent and irreversible. Attitudes and beliefs greatly influenced by parents. Often act as if they are invincible.

Children facing death are usually aware that they are going to die. They often try to protect their parents. They need to be told the truth in language they can understand and be allowed to share their fears, feelings, and opinions.

Parents and loved ones have much difficulty in accepting the reality of a child's impending death. Death of a child is an "out of sequence" death and therefore is often more difficult to accept. Parents often harbor extreme guilt. They may express hostility and anger toward health care providers, God, or the world in general. When a grandchild is dying, the grandparents suffer a double grief—for themselves and for their son or daughter. Siblings also extremely affected and need much support at this time. Supporting group thereby is often beneficial for the survivors after a child's death, as well as during the dying process.

Suicide

Survivors of suicide suffer all the emotions of grief in addition to profound guilt or shame. Because of this, they are at high risk for suicide themselves, and a grief counselor may be very helpful. Because suicide is usually not considered acceptable, many families of suicide victims are not given the same support from the church, community, or workplace as those whose loved ones have died from other causes. Because of the family's anger, fear, and shame, others do not reach out to help them.

Geriatric Death

It is often assumed that the elderly will display some understanding and acceptance toward the death process. This is not always true. The elderly patient must be treated as an individual and the nurse should assess the patient's needs in the same way for any patient facing a terminal illness. It is important to include the elderly person in his or her own care and in decisions to undergo or refuse extensive therapeutic or resuscitative measures. Even when aggressive technological options are rejected, patients still need to have intensive nursing care and pain control. Families who suffer the loss of an elderly person may accept the death but nonetheless must experience the grieving process.

Other considerations in caring for dying patients include such issues as euthanasia, DNR, organ donations, fradulent treatment methods, and the dying person's bill of rights.

Role of Nurses in the Stages of Dying (Table 33.3)

Issues of Dying in Death

Euthanasia

Easy death in relatively painless killing or permitted of death of a terminally ill reasons of mercy, sometimes referred to as mercy killing.

Nurses face legal or ethical issues when dealing with the terminally ill patient in regards to prolonging life by artificial means.

Euthanasia is sometimes considered when death is inevitable and there is no chance of returning to a functioning life situation. Active euthanasia is considered a crime and is illegal in the United States.

Do not Resuscitate

Patients and families should control any decisions related to any conditions that withhold or withdraw treatment. Death with dignity remains a concern for all. A do not resuscitate (DNR) decision should be a joint decision of the patient, family, and healthcare providers. All facts regarding the patient's condition should be explained to the patient and family, as well as all treatment options. DNR means only not to resuscitate, it does not mean to withhold any other care, such as hygiene, nutrition, fluids or medications. All DNR order and the discussion with

Table 33.3: Stages of Death and Nursing Care	
Stages	*Nursing care*
Stage 1: Denial This is a stage of disbelief. When common people first learn they are dying May last until death or person may move on to next stage Patient may talk about future plans, incorrect tests or diagnosis, or denial of symptoms Patient may use denial in presence of family in an effort to protect them; may only be honest with the nurse about seriousness of illness "No, not me" reaction.	Try to avoid directly contradicting the patient; find out what the patient and family were told Maintain an open communication with the patient. Try not to avoid the patient. If the patient begins to talk in realistic terms about an illness, take time to listen. Reassuring the patient that everything will be all right is not helpful.
Stage 2: Anger Patients may be angry at God, at physician, at the nurses and at family, or at themselves. The reaction here is "why me!" Patient may revert to denial periodically,	Try not to take the patient's outbursts or criticism personally. The patient is angry about dying, not at you as a person or as a nurse. Try to maintain contact with patients rather than avoiding them.
Stage 3: Bargaining Patients realise that they are going to die but try to make a bargain for more time. Bargaining often done with God. Usually done privately and not discussed with others. Reaction is "Yes, me but...."	The nurse cannot give the person the promise, of extra-time no matter how much this is wanted for the person. If the person shares the bargain with the nurse, listen without judging or falsely reassuring.
Stage 4: Depression Reaction is "Yes, me." Recognizes and accepts the closeness of own death. Patient often withdrawn and may be inappropriate.	Trying to cheer patients with comments, about the good things in their lives or in the environment is usually grieving the loss of loved ones, and of own existence. Let the patient be upset. The dying person is about to lose all that has been important and loved. Try to be there if the patient needs to talk or cry.
Stage 5: Acceptance Reaction is "Yes, me and that's OK" Described as neither happy or sad, but separate from feelings. Often wants one other loved person to stay until death occurs—some one who is able to accept death for the other. the patient and maintain physical contact until	The patient has accepted death as inevitable, and the nurse who can do the same will be the one who can comfort the patient during the final moments. The nurse will also be supporting family members who may then be able to sit quietly with death.

the patient and family should be thoroughly documented in the patient's chart.

Legal Issues

Characteristics of acceptable do not resuscitate (DNR) orders

A medical order not to resuscitate a patient is an acceptable order when the order is documented in the written medical record. The order specifies the exact nature of the treatment to be withheld. Patients, when they are able and families participate in the decision. The decision not to resuscitate is discussed with caregivers, including the nurses.

The order is periodically reviewed. Staff realize the order is not equivalent to medical or psychological abandonment of patients.

Do not resuscitate (DNR) orders are commonly understood to mean the withholding of CPR, which is used to treat cardiac arrest. It involves external chest compression and some forms of artificial respiration. Because of potential misunderstanding of what the DNR order specifically means, it is advisable that the DNR order be written identifying the exact condition not to be treated and the specific intervention to be withheld. The practice of not writing the DNR order is unacceptable. In fact, the medical record, read as a whole, should reveal the clear responsibility for the DNR order, the rationale for it, and the process used in its formulation, some hospitals and nursing homes may have more specific requirements in their policies that the medical/surgical nurse should follow.

Every competent adult has the right to refuse treatment, even life-sustaining procedures, such as CPR. The patient's informed consent should be obtained by the physician who will write the order, and should be documented in the medical record. Or, if unable to consent, the patient's family participation should be sought and documented. The patient's incapacity to participate must also be documented to reflect the rationale for involving the family. In some states the law may be that when it is two physicians' opinion that a patient lacks capacity to consent, a surrogate is sought from a list provided in the law. That surrogate must consent to the DNR order.

DNR orders must be reviewed periodically, because the patient's status may change or new knowledge may come to light about the patient's condition. Continual review of the DNR order helps reassure staff that they are not abandoning the patient; it will also ensure that the "hopeless" patient is still cared for.

Some patients request or have a living will, which describes their wishes regarding their medical care. This document can assist the family and healthcare providers in carrying out an individual's wishes. In some states the living will is legally binding. Courts in some states where living wills are not recognized as legal documents have upheld treatment decisions that a competent, rational adult has made for himself.

Organ Donations

Patients and families also have the right to give permission before the patient's death for organ donations upon death. Nurses often are present when such requests are given. Organs cannot be bought or sold, and all donations must be voluntary. These donations can include the following:

- Body organs
- Kidney
- Heart
- Lung
- Heart-lung
- Heart valve
- Liver
- Pancreas
- Body tissues
- Cornea
- Bone
- Skin

Fraudulent Methods of Treatment

Often patient and family seek the unconventional methods of treatment to prolong the patient's life. Such treatments may include special diets, enemas unproven drugs, and machines or devices. Nurses may assist patients and families in sorting out which treatments are real and which are fraudulent. Fraudulent treatments are those that are misrepresented, whether by concealment or nondisclosure of facts, for the purpose of inducing another to use the product. Any treatment that does not offer the patient informed consent with information regarding options, results, and approvals from federal agencies should be suspect.

Rights of Dying Patients

- Death with dignity is the goal in caring for the dying patient.
- I have the right to be treated as a living human being until I die.
- I have the right to maintain a sense of hopefulness however changing focus may be.
- I have the right to be cared for by those who can maintain a sense of hopefulness, however changing this might be.
- I have the right to express my feelings and emotions about my approaching death in my own way.
- I have the right to participate in decisions concerning my care.
- I have the right to expect continuing medical and nursing attention even though "cure" goals must be changed to "comfort" goals.
- I have the right not to die alone.
- I have the right to be free from pain.
- I have the right to have my questions answered honestly.
- I have the right not to be deceived.
- I have the right to have help from and for my family in accepting my death.
- I have the right to die in peace and dignity.
- I have the right to retain my individuality and not be judged for my decisions which may be contrary to beliefs of others.
- I have the right to discuss and enlarge my religious and/or spiritual experiences, whatever these may mean to others.

- I have the right to expect that the sanctity of the human body will be respected after death.
- I have the right to be cared for by caring, sensitive, knowledgeable people who will attempt to understand my needs and will be able to gain some satisfaction in helping me to face my death.

The Dying Patient

Assisting the Patient in Saying Good-bye

Many terminally ill-patients are fully aware that they are dying. One of their most difficult tasks is in the "saying of good-byes" to their loved ones. Saying good-bye acknowledges leaving and may be expressed in verbal, nonverbal, concrete, and symbolic ways. By working through these tasks, the family members are moving toward the completion of unfinished business with the patient. Unfinished business will complete the transition through the grieving process. This is an area where nurse can assist the dying person and the family.

Therapeutic Dialogue

Family Support

Family member: I can't go back in that room. He just lies there and stares. I don't know what to do or say.
Nurse: Being near someone who is dying can be uncomfortable.
Family member: It makes me so sad to see him like that. Do you think he knows I'm there?
Nurse: It's very possible that he does. Would you like me to go in with you?
Family member: Yes, please, I wonder if he can hear me.
Nurse: It must be very difficult for you not to be certain that he is hearing you. If there is something you want to say to him, get close, take his hand, and speak directly to him. Most people in this condition can hear but are very weak and may not have the strength to respond.
Family member: I just feel like I am not able to do anything for him anymore.
Nurse: Just being there is letting him know that you care. That's something very important to any person.

Family member: I suppose you're right. I guess I'm ready to go in now. You will stay close, won't you?
Nurse: Yes, I'll be right here next to you.

First, the nurse can provide a private, comfortable environment. The patient may request that the nurse or another healthcare provider be present or very nearby to be of assistance if emotional expression becomes overwhelming. Patients can be assisted in saying their goodbyes through role playing, letter writing, or audio or video recording. Helping patients focus on what they want to say can be facilitated by asking them to talk to their loved ones as if they were going to be separated for a long time. They should be encouraged to express those feelings and thoughts and they would most want their loved ones to know in their absence. Asking a dying person what he would want to say to his 6-year-old when the child is 12 and help the patient formulate appropriate letters or tape recordings. Often dying patients become depressed because they do not have a purpose in life. Working on tasks, such as poems, letters, and recordings, affords patient's feelings of control and productivity in their last days.

Physical Care

The nurse has an important responsibility in assisting patients to meet their physical needs. Providing adequate nutrition and maintaining elimination patterns are priorities in providing for the dying patient's physical needs. Keeping the patient clean, dry, well-groomed, odor free and comfortable decreases the chances of skin breakdown and also provides the patient with feelings of self-esteem and self-worth.

Adjusting the environment to increase comfort and safety is paramount. Side-rails should be used for both safety and assisting weak patients to adjust their own positions when possible.

Assessments and Interventions for the Dying Patient (Fig. 33.4)

Care of the dying patient has many facets. The core of nursing interventions in the care of the dying focuses on communication, relief of symptoms and pain, knowledge of available resources, facilitation of problem solving, and fostering involvement in and control of decisions affecting the patient's care.

Table 33.4: Nursing Interventions for the Patient Near Death

	Physical needs		Nursing intervention
1.	Decreased sensation and reflexes.	1.	Good skin care and range-of-motion exercises.
2.	Decreased circulation.	2.	Frequent positioning.
3.	Decreased sphincter control (urinary and bowel incontinence).	3.	Meticulous hygiene and skin care.
4.	Decreased hearing and sight.	4.	Clear and slow verbal communication stand within patient's vision.
5.	Decreased need for pain medication.	5.	Evaluate and differentiate between pain and anxiety.
6.	Increased need for touch	6.	Touch gently.
7.	Usually conscious.	7.	Involve patient in care; explain all actions.

Table 33.5: Postmortem Care of the Body	
Preparations	*Rationales*
1. Rearrange work load as needed	1. The nurse caring for the dead patient will have added time commitments with the patient's family, care of the body, and documentation in the chart, before transporting to the morgue. Other patients under this nurse's care may be neglected unless some of the work assignment is delegated to other capable people
2. Notify appropriate people: Incharge nurse Physician Clergy Morgue Family	2. Notification of the nurse in charge of the medical area, the physician, and the morgue is important so hospital personnel can do their jobs effectively. The charge nurse can help with reassigning the nurse's work load and assuring hospital policy is followed. The physician will pronounce the patient dead and identify whether an autopsy is desired. Care and notification of the family may be shared by the nurse, and the physician.
3. Review the institution's policy on postmortem care.	3. Each institution may have slightly different ways of caring for the body; there may be differences within the institution, depending on the age of the patient and cause of death.
4. Talk with the family about their wishes to spend time with the deceased or help in preparing the body. Find out if the family wants any religious activities before transporting the patient to the morgue.	4. Some family may want to see, touch and help in giving the final physical care. Offering the family some choices may help meet their needs. If the family feels the patient's religious needs were omitted, it can be a further source for distress.
5. Follow institutional policy for handling the patient's possessions. Have relatives sign for any possessions they take with them.	5. Possessions are very important to the family even when actual value may be minimal. Giving the patient's belongings to identified relatives and having them sign for what they received will eliminate confusion and provide documentation for the institution.
6. Consider any necessary precautions because of patient contamination if there was infection or isolation.	6. If the patient was infected, the organisms are still present and could infect other people coming in contact with the body.
7. Assemble equipment; clean gown, envelope for valuables, container for personal possession, wash basin, towels body wrap, masking tape, identification tags, and dressings for draining wounds left when and if tubes are removed.	7. Organizing what will be needed ahead of time saves time and energy. Going in and out of the room can be distressing to the family and other patients.
8. If deceased patient had a room-mate, move that person to another room if possible. the same room. It is also difficult to provide privacy	8. The activities related to caring for the deceased patient may be very upsetting to another patient in for the family to be with the deceased.
9. Provide privacy for the deceased. can show respect. Other patients may also be upset	9. Care of the body to others is the last way the nurse by seeing a dead patient.
10. Remove any valuables and place in envelope and seal. If the family wants the patient to keep a ring on, secure it with tape or according to institutional policy. the patient's chart to protect the nurse.	10. Valuables removed by the nurse should be identified on the envelope and sealed so there is no opportunity for theft or loss. Valuables should be locked in a safe place and this should be documented and signed in
11. Position the body in good alignment in the supine position with the head elevated slightly.	11. This will prevent possible problems with rigor mortis and livor mortis of the face and upper chest.
12. Close eyelids if open by placing fingertips over each eyelid for a few seconds and gradually closing the eyes.	12. When rigor mortis sets in, the eyes will be held open, and this is usually undesirable for an open- casket funeral.

Contd...

Table 33.5: *Contd...*

	Preparations		Rationales
13.	Place dentures in patient's mouth if possible. Send with body to mortician if unable to put in the patient's mouth. to position dentures if not done shortly after death.	13.	Without the teeth in place the patient will have a sun- ken, altered appearance. The teeth are in place for an open-casket funeral. Rigor mortis may make it difficult
14.	Close patient's mouth if open by placing rolled towel under the chin.	14.	The mouth is expected to be closed in death, and rigor mortis may make this difficult later.
15.	Remove all tubes and drains as identified in policies of institution.	15.	This equipment is no longer needed and should be removed and disposed of appropriately.
16.	Soiled areas of the patient's body are washed, hairpins are removed, and the hair is combed. A clean gown is put on the patient if family is to view body. Some institutions do not use a gown under the morgue wrap.	16.	Prevention of contamination and damage to the body by sharp objects. If family views body before it goes to the morgue, a clean gown and combed hair convey respect and optimum care.
17.	Place absorbent pad under buttocks.	17.	Relaxation of sphincters may cause release of stool or urine.
18.	Attach identification tag to body. Leave hospital ID band in place.	18.	Loss of outside tag could cause confusion on patient's identity if no identification is on the body.
19.	Wrap body as described for particular institution.	19.	This serves to protect the body and provide privacy.
20.	Attach outside ID tag to wrapped body.	20.	This is for ease in identification by the morgue and mortuary. Make sure both tags are identical to name on hospital ID band.
21.	Pack all remaining personal belongings in a container for the relatives. Label accurately. Wash hands.	21.	Patient's belongings can easily be forgotten if upset relatives collect them. Accurate labeling is helpful in getting the belongings to the right family members
22.	Arrange for transportation of the body to morgue or mortuary.	22.	This avoids confusion for the relatives and assures that no one arrives to claim the body before the nurse and family are ready for it to be moved.
23.	Document care given in the patient's chart.	23.	Documentation allows others to know what was done to the body and with patient's possessions.
24.	After body is transported, the unit is stripped of linen and utensils. Wash hands. Notify housekeeping or appropriate personnel that the room is ready to be cleaned.	24.	This is done to protect other patients and cleaning personnel from possible contamination.

The patient near death continues to need meticulous nursing interventions. Because of the increased weakness and deterioration of the body, the patient's physical needs are important. Although patients may appear comatose, unconscious, or unresponsible, this appearance is often a result of extreme fatigue, and the nurse will find that patients are aware of those activities occurring around them. Table 33.4 shows signs of approaching death as expressed in physical needs and the appropriate interventions.

Changes in vital signs include: (i) slow, weak, and thready pulse, (ii) lowered blood pressure, and (iii) rapid, shallow, irregular, or abnormally slow respirations. Mouth breathing occurs, which leads to dry oral mucous membranes. The patient often has a detached look in the eyes. There is a diminished sensory and motor function in the lower extremities progressing to the upper extremities. There is diminished touch sensation; pressure and pain sensations remain intact. As death becomes imminent, the pupils will become dilated and fixed, Cheyne-Stokes respirations will occur, the pulse will become increasingly weaker and more rapid, and the blood pressure will continue to fall. There is diminished peripheral circulation. The skin is cool and clammy; profuse diaphoresis may occur. If collection of mucus occurs in the throat, noisy respirations will be heard. The noise is referred to as 'the death rattle'. A period of peace may immediately precede the moment of death. The clinical signs of death are the following:

1. Unreceptivity and unresponsibility.
2. No movement or breathing.

3. No reflexes.
4. Flat encephalogram.
5. Absence of apical pulse.
6. Cessation of respirations.

Postmortem Care

When the patient has been pronounced dead by a physician or professional nurse, the nurse assumes the responsibility of caring for the body (Postmortem care). During this phase of care, the nurse cleans, identifies and positions the body by following the formalities of procedure. At the time of death, the nurse must also make notation of any valuables, such as watch, rings, or money, and secure these articles so that they may be delivered to the family according to facility policy (Table 33.5).

Documentation

Documentation of the care given to the dying patient must be objective, complete, legible, and accurate. As death approaches, documentation should be frequent and include the signs of impending death as they occur. Recording by who was present at the time of the patient's death is important. The nurse should continue to chart until last entry states where and to whom the body was transferred.

Glossary

ABC	Airway; Breathing; Circulation.
Abduction	Movement of a limb away from the body.
Abrasion	Scraping or rubbing away of a surface such as the skin by friction.
Accommodation	Adjustment of the eye to variations in distance.
Accountability	Responsible attitude regarding moral and legal requirements of proper patient care.
Accreditation	Process whereby a professional association or nongovernmental agency grants recognition to a school or institution for demonstrating ability in a special area of practice or education.
Acetabulum	Large, cup-shaped cavity at the juncture of the ilium, the ischium and the pubis; contains the ball-shaped head of the femur.
Acetone	Colorless, aromatic ketone found in small amounts in normal urine and in larger quantities in the urine of patients with diabetes mellitus.
Acetylcholine	Neurotransmitter substance widely distributed in body tissues with a primary function of mediating synaptic activity of the nervous system.
Achalasia	Inability of a muscle to relax, particularly the cardiac sphincter of the stomach.
Achilles tendon	Common tendon of the soleus and gastrocnemius muscles; the thickest and strongest tendon in the body.
Achlorhydria	Abnormal condition characterized by the absence of hydrochloric acid in the gastric juice.
ACLS (advanced cardiac l ife support)	Includes providing basic life support plus using adjunctive equipment for establishing an intravenous line, administering fluid and drugs, monitoring the heart, performing defibrillation, controlling dysrhythmias, and providing postresuscitation care.
Acrocyanosis	Condition characterized by cyanotic discoloration, coldness and sweating of the extremities.
Acromion	Lateral extension of the spine of the scapula, forming the highest point of the shoulder and connecting with the clavicle at a small, oval surface in the middle of the spine; also called the *acromial process*.
Active transport	Movement of materials across the membrane of a cell; chemical activity allows the cell to admit larger molecules than could otherwise enter.
Acuity	Sharpness or acuteness of hearing or sight.
Acute pain	Intense pain of short duration, lasting less than 6 months; a warning of actual or potential tissue damage.
Adaptation	Ability to adjust to change.
Adaptive immunity	Immunity that is acquired, not innate or natural.
Adduction	Movement of a limb toward the axis (center) of the body.
Adenosine triphosphate (ATP)	Compound that stores energy in muscles; the energy is released when it is hydrolyzed to adenosine diphosphate.
Adhesion	Band of scar tissue that binds together two anatomical surfaces that are normally separate.
Adipose tissue	Collection of cells containing stored fat (depot fat).
Adjunct	Additive substance or treatment to increase the effectiveness of a primary procedure or to facilitate its performance.
ADL	Activities of daily living.
Admission	Entry of a patient into a health care facility.
Adolescence	Period that begins with puberty and extends for 8 years or longer, until the person is physically and psychologically mature and ready for adult responsibilities.
Adrenal gland	Either of two secretory endocrine organs located on the superior surface of the kidneys.
Adrenaline	Adrenal hormone and synthetic adrenergic vasoconstrictor.
Adrenocortico-tropic hormone (ACTH)	Hormone of the anterior pituitary gland that stimulates growth of the adrenal gland cortex and the secretion of corticosteroids.
Adverse drug effect	Harmful, unintended reaction to a drug administered at a normal dosage.
Afebrile	Without fever.
Affect	Outward evidence of a person's feelings or emotions.
Afferent	Proceeding toward a center, as applied to arteries, veins, lymphatics, and nerves.
Against-medical-advice (AMA)	Patient leaves a health care facility without a physician's order for discharge.
Ageism	Attitudes, actions or institutional structures that discriminate against individuals on the basis of age.
Agility	Ability to move with quick, easy grace.
Aging	Process of growing old, which begins at conception and ends at death.

Agnosia	Brain damage resulting in total or partial inability to recognize familiar objects or persons.
Agonist	Drug having a specific cellular affinity that produces a predictable response.
AIDS	Acquired immunodeficiency syndrome.
Akinesia	Loss or reduction of the capacity to initiate, maintain, and perform voluntary motor activities.
Al-Anon	International organization that offers guidance and counseling for the relatives, friends and associates of alcoholics.
Albuminuria	Condition of excess serum proteins in the urine; also called *proteinuria*.
Alcohol sponge	Sponge bath using alcohol and water to reduce body temperature.
Alcohol withdrawal syndrome	Clinical signs and symptoms associated with stopping alcohol consumption, including tremor, hallucinations, autonomic nervous system dysfunction and seizures.
Alcoholics anonymous	International nonprofit organization founded in 1935, consisting of abstinence alcoholics whose purpose is to help other alcoholics stop drinking and maintain sobriety.
Alcoholism	Extreme dependence on excessive amounts of alcohol, associated with a cumulative pattern of deviant behaviors.
Alignment	Maintaining of body structures in their appropriate anatomical positions.
Alimentary canal	Musculomembranous tube, about 9 meters (30 feet) long, extending from the mouth to the anus and lined with mucous membrane.
Allergen	Substance that can produce a hypersensitive reaction in the body but is not necessarily harmful.
Alopecia	Partial or complete baldness resulting from aging, endocrine disorder, drug reaction, anticancer medication or skin disease.
Alveoli	Small, saclike structures through which gas exchange takes place in the lungs.
Amenorrhea	Absence of menstruation.
Amino acids	Building blocks of protein; 22 amino acids have been identified as vital for human life. The body can synthesize 13 of these, termed *nonessential* whereas the remaining 9 must be obtained from dietary sources and are called *essential*.
Amniotomy	Rupture of the amniotic sac.
ANA standards of nursing practice	Evaluation that serves as a basis for comparison of similar occurrences, set forth by the American Nurses' Association.
Anabolism	Constructive metabolism characterized by conversion of simple substances into the more complex compounds of living matter.
Analysis	Separation of substances into their constituent parts.
Anaphylaxis	Severe and sometimes fatal hypersensitivity reaction to a sensitizing substance (allergen).
Anaplasia	Change in the structure of cells; a loss of differentiation, characteristic of a malignancy.
Anasarca	Generalized massive edema.
Anastomosis	Surgical joining of two ducts or blood vessels to allow flow from one to the other.
Anatomy	Study of the structure of the human body.
Androgen	Any steroid hormone that produces male physical characteristics.
Anemia	Decrease in hemoglobin in the blood to levels below the normal range.
Anesthesia	Absence of normal sensation, especially sensitivity to pain, induced by an anesthetic substance for surgical purposes.
Animism	Ascribing of human characteristics to nonhuman or inanimate objects.
Anion	Negatively charged ion, atom, or molecule.
Ankylosis	Fixation of a joint, often seen in an abnormal position.
Anomaly	Deviation from what is considered normal.
Anorexia	Lack or loss of appetite, resulting in the inability to eat.
Anorexia nervosa	Psychoneurotic disorder characterized by a prolonged refusal to eat; self-imposed starvation.
Anoxia	Abnormal lack of oxygen.
Answer	Response of a defendant to the complaint of a plaintiff.
Antagonist	Drug that exerts an opposite action to that of another drug.
Anterior	Front of a structure.
Anterior fontanel	Diamond-shaped area at the superior, anterior area of the head.
Antibody	Protein molecule essential to the immune system, produced by lymphoid tissue in response to bacteria, viruses or other antigenic substances an antibody is specific to an antigen.
Anticipatory guidance	Psychological preparation of a patient for an event expected to be stressful, as in the preparation of a child for surgery by explaining what will happen and what it will feel like. It is also used to prepare parents for normal growth and development of their children.
Antigen	Substance, usually a protein, that causes the formation of an antibody and reacts specifically with that antibody, helps form immunity in humans.
Antidiuretic hormone (ADH)	Hormone that decreases production of urine by increasing reabsorption of water by the renal tubules.
Antioxidant	Chemical or other agent that delays or prevents the breakdown of a substance by oxygen.
Anuria	Cessation of urine production, or a urinary output of less than 100 to 250 ml per 24 hours.

Anxiety	Vague sense of impending doom characterized by uneasiness and physiological changes; usually results from a real or perceived threat to the self.
Aorta	Main trunk of the systemic arterial circulation.
Apex	Pertaining to the top, the end or the tip of a structure—as the apex of the heart.
Aphasia	Defective or absent language function caused by injury to certain areas of the cerebral cortex.
Apnea	Absence of spontaneous respiration.
Appeal	Request for review and/or retrial of legal issues.
Approved	Status of a nursing program that meets minimum standards set by the state.
Apraxia	Impairment in the ability to perform purposeful acts or to manipulate objects.
Aqueous humor	Clear, watery fluid circulating in the anterior and posterior chambers of the eye.
Arachnoid membrane	Thin, delicate membrane enclosing the brain and the spinal cord, interposed between the pia mater and the dura mater. The subarachnoid space lies between the arachnoid membrane and the pia; the subdural space lies between the arachnoid membrane and the dura.
ARC	AIDS-related complex.
Areolar gland	One of the large sebaceous glands in the areolae encircling the nipples on women's breasts.
Arrhythmia	See *dysrhythmia*.
Arteriole	Blood vessel in the smallest branch of arterial circulation. Blood flowing from the heart is pumped through the arteries to the arterioles.
Arteriosclerosis	Degenerative thickening, calcification and decreased elasticity of arterial walls.
Artery	One of the large vessels carrying blood away from the heart.
Arthrocentesis	Puncture of a joint with a needle to withdraw fluid.
Arthrodesis	Surgically induced fixation of a joint to relieve pain or to provide support.
Arthroplasty	Surgical reconstruction or replacement of a painful, degenerated joint.
Arthroscopy	Examination of the interior of a joint performed by inserting a specially designed endoscope through a small incision.
Articulation	Gliding, rotation, and angular movement of a joint.
Ascites	Abnormal intraperitoneal accumulation of fluid.
Asepsis	Absence of germs. Surgical asepsis protects against infection before, during or after surgery by the use of sterile techniques.
Asphyxia	Severe lack of oxygen to the blood, leading to hypercapnia, loss of consciousness and, if not corrected, death.
Assessment	Evaluation or appraisal of a patient.
Asthma	Respiratory disorder characterized by recurring episodes of labored breathing, wheezing on expiration, coughing, and viscous, mucoid bronchial secretions.
Astigmatism	Eye condition in which light rays cannot focus clearly on a point in the retina.
Asymptomatic	Without indication of disease, without subjective or objective signs and symptoms.
Ataxia	Impaired ability to coordinate movement; a staggering gait.
Atelectasis	Collapse of lung tissue, preventing respiratory exchange of carbon dioxide and oxygen.
Atheroma	Abnormal mass of fat or lipids deposited on the arterial wall.
Atherosclerosis	Arterial disorder characterized by yellowish plaques of cholesterol, lipids and cellular debris in the walls of the arteries.
Atrioventricular valve	Value in the heart through which blood flows from the atria to the ventricles.
Atrium	Chamber or cavity, such as the right and left atria of the heart.
Atrophy	Decrease in size or physiological activity of a part of the body because of disease or lack of use.
Attachment	Close, mutual relationship between two people that involves contact and proximity and endures through time.
Attitude	Fetal position in the uterus.
Audiometry	Testing of hearing acuity.
Auditor	Person appointed to examine patients' charts and health records to assess the quality of care.
Auditory hallucination	Perception of sound without an external stimulus.
Auscultation	Act of listening for sounds within the body to evaluate the condition of various organs.
Autistic behavior	Self-absorbed, isolated, repetitive behavior and lack of communication with others.
Autograft	Surgical transplantation of any tissue from one part of the body to another in the same individual.
Autoimmunity	Abnormal characteristic or condition in which the body reacts against constituents of its own tissues.
Autonomy	Ability or tendency to function independently.
Axilla	Pyramid-shaped space forming the underside of the shoulder between the upper part of the arm and the side of the chest; also called *armpit*.
Axis	Line that passes through the center of the body or through a part of the body.
Axon	Cylindrical extension of a nerve cell that conducts impulses away from the neuron cell body. Axons may be bare or sheathed in myelin.
Azotemia (uremia)	Excessive nitrogenous compounds in the blood.

B-cell	Type of lymphocyte that responds to stimulation of antigens entering the body, causing an immunological response.
Babbling	Incoherent sounds made by an infant while vocally playing with sounds.
Back rub (massage)	Manipulation of the soft tissue by rubbing and kneading to increase circulation, improve muscle tone, and promote relaxation in the patient.
Basal metabolic rate (BMR)	Amount of energy used by the body at rest to maintain vital functions such as respiration, circulation, temperature, peristalsis, and muscle tone.
Base of support	Stance with the feet slightly apart to provide better stability for work.
Bath basin	Small plastic pan used to hold water for bathing a patient.
Bath mitt	Wash cloth folded over the hand to form a mitt; prevents wet ends of cloth from touching the patient.
Battered woman syndrome	Repeated episodes of physical assault on a woman by a man with whom she has a close relationship.
Bedpan	Shallow pan for use as a toilet by a person confined to bed.
Bedside commode	Chair with a hole in the seat containing a vessel for urination and defecation.
Behavior	Actions that occur intentionally or spontaneously and are observable and measurable.
Beneficence	Bringing about of good.
Benign neoplasm	Localized tumor that has a fibrous capsule, limited potential for growth, and cells that are well differentiated.
Beriberi	Disease of the peripheral nerves caused by deficiency of or inability to assimilate the vitamin *thiamin*.
Bereavement	Common depressed reaction to the loss of a loved one.
Bicarbonate (HCO_3)	Salt of carbonic acid; a base or alka ine.
Biological age	Person's present position with respect to potential life span, which may be younger or older than chronological age and encompasses measures of vital organ functions.
Biological death	Total absence of activity in the brain and central nervous system, the cardiovascular system and the respiratory system as observed and declared by a physician.
Biopsy	Removal of a small piece of living tissue for microscopic examination to confirm or establish a diagnosis.
Birth defect (congenital anomaly)	Abnormality, particularly a structural one, present at birth, which may be inherited genetically, acquired during gestation, or inflicted during parturition.
Blanching	Causing to become pale by applying digital pressure.
Blastocyst	Undifferentiated embryonic cell before germ layer formation.
BLS (basic life support)	Phase of emergency cardiac care that prevents circulatory or respiratory arrest (or insufficiency) by prompt recognition and intervention.
Body mechanics	Field of physiology that studies muscular actions and the function of muscles in maintaining the posture of the body.
Body surface area (BSA)	Total area exposed to the outside environment.
Bolus	Round mass, specifically a masticated lump of food ready to be swallowed.
Bonding	Parent's feeling and attachment behavior toward infant after delivery.
Bony prominence	Area of the body where bones can be easily palpated. Bony areas have greater potential for impaired skin integrity than other areas of the body.
Bowman's capsule	Cup-shaped end of a renal tubule containing a glomerulus.
Bradycardia	Heart rate of less than 60 beats per minute.
Bradykinesia	Abnormal condition characterized by slowness of all voluntary movement and speech, as caused by Parkinsonism and certain tranquilizers.
Bradypnea	Abnormally slow respiratory rate of less than 12 breaths per minute.
Brain death	Irreversible form of unconsciousness characterized by a complete loss of brain function while the heart continues to beat.
Brainstem	Portion of the brain comprising the medulla oblongata, the pons and the mesencephalon. It performs motor, sensory and reflex functions. The 12 pairs of cranial nerves are attached to the base of the brain.
Braxton Hicks contractions	Irregular tightening of the pregnant uterus that begins in the first trimester and increases in frequency, duration and intensity as pregnancy progresses. Contractility of uterine muscle increases in pregnancy. Near term, strong Braxton Hicks contractions are often difficult to distinguish from the contractions of true labor; also called *false labor*.
Bronchiole	Small airway of the respiratory system extending from the bronchi into the lobes of the lung.
Bronchitis	Acute or chronic inflammation of mucous membranes of the tracheobronchial tree.
Bronchopulmonary	Of or pertaining to the bronchi and the lungs of the respiratory system.
Bronchopulmonary dysplasia	Abnormal development of the bronchi and lungs.
Bronchoscopy	Visual examination of the tracheobronchial tree, using the standard metal bronchoscope of the narrower, flexible fiberoptic bronchoscope.
Bronchus	Large passage into the lungs through which pass inspired air and exhaled waste gases.
Bruit	Abnormal sound or murmur heard while auscultating an organ, gland, or vessel, as the liver or an artery.
Buffer	Substance or group of substances that can absorb or release hydrogen ions to correct an acid-base imbalance.

Bulimia	Eating disorder involving an insatiable craving for food, often resulting in episodes of continuous eating followed by periods of depression, self-deprivation, and/or purging.
Burnout	Mental or physical energy loss related to a job, accompanied by feelings of hopelessness or loss of creativity.
Burping	Belching or eructation.
Bursa	Fibrous sac between certain tendons and the bones beneath them. Lined with a synovial membrane that secretes synovial fluid, the bursa acts as a small cushion that allows the tendon, as it contracts and relaxes, to move over the bone.
Cachexia	Ill health, malnutrition, and wasting as a result of chronic disease.
Calcitonin	Hormone produced in the thyroid that participates in regulating the blood level of calcium.
Calcium (Ca++)	White, alkaline earth metal element occurring mainly in the bones of the body.
Callus	Bony deposit formed between and around the broken ends of a fractured bone during healing.
Calyx	Cup-shaped part or organ e.g.: renal calyx.
Candidiasis	Any infection caused by a species of *Candida*, usually *Candida albicans*.
Cannabis or marijuana	Psychoactive drug derived from hemp plants.
Canthus	Angle at the medial (inner) and lateral (outer) margins of the eyelids.
Capillary	One of the tiny blood vessels joining arterioles and venules. Through its walls blood and tissue cells exchange various substances.
Carbohydrate	Any of a group of organized compounds. The most important are sugar, starch, cellulose, and gum.
Carcinoembryonic antigen (CEA)	Antigen present in very small quantities in adult tissue. A greater than normal amount is suggestive of cancer.
Carcinogen	Substance or agent that produces cancer.
Carcinoma	Malignant epithelial neoplasm that tends to invade surrounding tissue and to spread to distant regions of the body.
Carcinoma in situ	Premalignant neoplasm that has not invaded surrounding membranes or tissue but has characteristics of invasive cancer; frequently seen on the uterine cervix.
Cardiac arrest	Sudden cessation of cardiac output and effective circulation. Immediate initiation of cardiopulmonary resuscitation is required to prevent heart, lung, kidney and brain damage.
Cardiac output	Volume of blood expelled by the ventricles of the heart.
Cardiovascular	Of or pertaining to the heart and blood vessels.
Caregiver role	Function of giving care to elderly parents, other elderly family members, or spouse.
Carotid pulse	Pulse of the carotid artery, felt by gently pressing a finger into the groove between the larynx and the sternoecleidomastoid muscle in the neck.
Carrier	Person or animal who harbors and spreads a microorganism causing disease in others but who does not become ill.
Catabolism	Complex, metabolic process in which energy is liberated for use in work, energy storage or heat production by the destruction of complex substances to form simple compounds.
Cataract	Abnormal progressive condition of the lens of the eye, characterized by loss of transparency.
Catatonic state	Extreme immobility and muscular rigidity, usually associated with panic or schizophrenia.
Cation	Positively charged ion, atom or molecule.
CDC	*See centers for disease control.*
Cell	Fundamental unit of all living tissue.
Cellular immunity	Acquired immunity characterized by the dominant role of small T-cell lymphocytes.
Centers for disease control (CDC)	Division of the US Public Health Service, in Atlanta, Georgia; investigates diseases, especially those with epidemic potential.
Center of gravity	Midpoint or center of weight of a body or object. In the standing adult human the center of gravity is in the midpelvic cavity, between the symphysis pubis and the umbilicus.
Centrifuge	Equipment that spins test tubes at high speeds.
Centriole	Intracellular organelle, associated with cell division.
Cerebellum	Part of the brain located in the posterior cranial fossa behind the brainstem. It consists of two lateral cerebellar hemispheres, or lobes, and a middle section called the *vermis*. Its functions are concerned with coordinating voluntary muscular activity.
Cerebral dominance	Specialization of each of the two cerebral hemispheres in the integration and control of different functions.
Cerebrospinal fluid	Fluid that flows through and pro-protects the four ventricles of the brain, the subarachnoid space and the spinal canal.
Cerebrovascular accident	Occlusion of a blood vessel in the brain by a thrombus, an embolus, or cerebrovascular hemorrhage, resulting in decreased blood supply.
Cerebrum	Largest and uppermost section of the brain, divided by a central sulcus into the left and the right cerebral hemispheres.
Certification	Process in which an individual, an institution, or an educational program is evaluated and recognized as meeting certain predetermined standards.

Cerumen	Earwax; a yellow or brown waxy secretion in the external ear canal.
Ceruminous gland	One of a number of tiny structures in the external ear canal, believed to be a modified sweat gland. It secretes a waxy cerumen instead of water sweat.
Cervical cord injury	Spinal injury that may affect upper extremities, trunk, lower extremities, bladder and bowel function.
Chancre	Skin lesion, usually of primary syphilis that begins at the site of infection as a papule and develops into a red, bloodless, painless ulcer with a scooped-out appearance.
Chart or health care record	Patient record that includes all the forms used to document care.
Charting by exception	Process of recording only new data or changes in patient status or care; charting the exceptions to the previously recorded data.
Charting, documenting, or recording	Process of noting data in a patient record, usually at prescribed intervals.
Chemical dependence	Total psychophysical state of one addicted to drugs or alcohol who must receive an increasing amount of the substance to prevent abstinence signs and symptoms.
Cheyne-Stokes respiration	Abnormal respiratory pattern characterized by periods of apnea alternating with deep, rapid respirations.
Child abuse	Attack on a child by an adult caretaker that results in physical, emotional, and/or sexual injury or trauma.
Chlamydia	Microorganism that lives in the epithelium of the urethra and cervix. It is one of the most common sexually transmitted diseases and a frequent cause of sterility.
Chloride (Cl⁻)	Salt compound in which the negative element is chloride.
Cholecystokinin	Hormone produced by the mucosa of the upper intestine; stimulates contraction of the gallbladder and secretion of pancreatic enzymes.
Cholesterol (dietary)	Fat-soluble sterol found in animal fats and oils, organ meats and egg yolk.
Cholesterol (serum)	Fat-soluble sterol found in the blood stream and continuously synthesized in the body, primarily in the liver.
Choroid	Thin, highly vascular membrane covering the posterior five sixths of the eye between the retina and sclera.
Chromatin	Material within the cell nucleus from which the chromosomes are formed. It consists of fine, threadlike strands.
Chronic obstructive pulmonary disease (COPD)	Progressive and irreversible condition characterized by diminished inspiratory and expiratory capacity of the lungs.
Chronic pain	Pain lasting longer than 6 months; may be continuous or intermittent and as intense as acute pain.
Chronological age	Age of an individual expressed as the time that has elapsed since birth.
Chum	Close friend, often of same gender and age.
Chux	Waterproof disposable pad.
Chvostek's sign	Facial spasm occurring when the facial nerve is tapped above the mandibular angle, next to the earlobe in patients who are hypocalcemic (positive sign).
Cilia	Small, hairlike processes on the other surfaces of some cells, aiding metabolism by producing motion, eddies or current in a fluid; most often associated with the respiratory passage way.
Circumcision	Surgical removal of the foreskin of the penis.
Classification	Sorting of objects into groups according to certain attributes such as color, size, or shape.
Claudication	Weakness of the legs with cramplike pains in the calves, caused by poor circulation of blood to the leg muscles.
Cleft lip	Congenital anomaly consisting of one or more clefts in the upper lip, resulting from failure of the maxillary and median nasal processes to close.
Cleft palate	Congenital defect characterized by a fissure in the midline of the palate, resulting from failure of the two sides to fuse during embryonic development.
Climacteric	Cessation of menses; commonly refers to *menopause*.
Clinical death	Total absence of activity in the brain and central nervous system, the cardiovascular system and the respiratory system as observed and declared by a physician.
Clonus (ic)	Abnormal pattern of neuromuscular activity, characterized by rapidly alternating involuntary contraction and relaxation of skeletal muscle.
Closed bed	Hospital bed made with all linens pulled toward the head of the bed.
CMV (cytomegalovirus)	Member of a group of large, species-specific, herpes-type viruses with a wide variety of disease effects.
Co-dependency	Situation in which a person is overly affected by and concerned with controlling other people's behaviors.
Code	Discreet signal used to summon a special team.
Cognitive behavior	Mental processes characterized by knowing, thinking, learning and judging.
Cognitive learning	Learning concerned with problem-solving abilities, intelligence and conscious thought.
Cohabitation	Two people living together in a sexual relationship without marriage.
Coitus	Sexual union of two people of the opposite sex.
Collagen	Tiny protein fibrils that form inelastic fibers of the tendons, ligaments, and fascia.
Colles' fracture	Fracture of the radius at the epiphysis within 1 inch of the joint of the wrist, easily recognized by the resulting dorsal and lateral position of the hand.
Collodion	Clear or slightly opaque, highly inflammable liquid composed of pyroxylin, ether, and alcohol. It dries to a strong transparent film that is used as a surgical dressing.
Color blindness	Inability to distinguish colors of the spectrum.

Colostrum	Fluid secreted by the breast during pregnancy and during the first days of postpartum before lactation begins.
Colporrhaphy	Surgical procedure in which the vagina is sutured, as for the purpose of narrowing or repairing the vagina.
Command hallucination	Imaginary voice commanding the individual to do something.
Communication	Any process in which information is transferred and received.
Community health nursing	Blend of nursing and public health, promoting prevention, education, and maintenance.
Compartment syndrome	Pathological condition caused by progressive development of arterial compression and reduced blood supply.
Compatibility	State in which two or more drugs can be given at the same time without producing undesired side effects or without canceling or changing the therapeutic effects of the other.
Complaint	Pleading by a plaintiff made under oath to initiate a law suit.
Comprehensive rehabilitation plan	Planned, orderly sequence of services for a handicapped individual, designed to help him realize his maximum potential.
Compressor	Individual in two-rescuer cardiopulmonary resuscitation (CPR) who performs external cardiac compressions.
Compulsion	Act carried out, to some degree against a person's conscious will, to avoid anxiety.
Computed tomography	Painless X-ray technique that films a cross section of tissue (CT scan); also called *computerized axial tomography.*
Computer terminal	Machine at a nursing work station used to access the larger main frame computer for data processing.
Concrete stage	Stage of cognitive development that involves reasoning about tangible or familiar situations.
Condyle	Rounded projection at the end of a bone that anchors muscle ligaments and articulates with adjacent bones.
Confidentiality	Process of keeping information and records private or secret.
Conflict	Two incompatible goals occurring at the same time.
Confront	To challenge.
Congruent	In agreement or harmony.
Conjunctiva	Mucous membrane lining the inner surfaces of the eyelids and the anterior part of the sclera.
Conjunctivitis	Inflammation of the conjunctiva.
Connective tissue	Tissue that supports and binds other body structures. The types are *bone, cartilage* and *fibrous tissue.*
Conservation	Mental process of understanding the sameness of a situation or object in spite of a change in some aspect, e.g. that the mass or quantity of an object is the same even if it changes shape or position.
Consumer	One who uses goods or services.
Contact lens	Small, curved glass or plastic lens shaped to fit the eye and to correct refraction or inability of the lens of the eye to focus accurately.
Contamination	Soiling or infection with something undesirable, as bacteria in a wound; also known as *sepsis.*
Context	Meaning of language within a particular setting.
Continuity-of-care	Continuing of care in from one setting to another.
Contracture	Abnormal, usually permanent condition of a joint, characterized by flexion (bending) and fixation caused by atrophy and shortening of muscle fibers.
Convalescence	Period of recovery after an illness, injury or surgery.
Conversion	Unconscious defense mechanism in which repressed emotions are transformed into physical signs and symptoms; also called *conversion hysteria or conversion reaction.*
Cooing	Hum of contentment made by an infant.
Coping	Voluntary pattern of behavior used to relieve stress or anxiety.
Cordotomy	Operation in which an incision is made high in the thoracic area and two laminae are removed; then the pain pathways in the spinothalamic tract (anterior and lateral aspect of the cord) on the side opposite the pain are severed.
Corium	Layer of skin just below the epidermis, containing blood and lymphatic vessels, nerves, nerve endings, glands and hair follicles.
Cornea	Convex, transparent, anterior part of the eye, comprising one sixth of the outermost tunic of the eye bulb.
Coronary (in anatomy)	Of or pertaining to encircling structures, as the coronary arteries of the heart.
Corpuscle	Any cell of the body; a red or white blood cell.
Cortex	Outer layer of a body organ or structure, as distinguished from the internal substance.
Corticosteroid	Antiinflammatory drug for relief of inflammation and pruritus (itching).
Cortisol	Steroid hormone occurring naturally in the body.
Countertraction	Force that counteracts the pull of traction.
Couvade syndrome	Man's physical and emotional reaction to his partner's pregnancy.
Coxsackievirus	Any of 30 serologically different enteroviruses associated with a variety of signs and symptoms and primarily affecting children during warm weather.
Craniotomy	Any surgical opening into the skull, performed to relieve pressure, to control bleeding or to remove a tumor.
Creatinine	Substance formed from the metabolism of creatine, commonly found in blood, urine, and muscle tissue.
Crepitus	Crackling sound heard as a result of bone fragments rubbing together or air in the subcutaneous tissue.

Crisis	Time of change or turning point in life when patterns of living must be modified to prevent disorganization of the person or family.
Cryosurgery	Use of subfreezing temperatures to destroy tissue.
Cryptorchidism	Failure of one or both of the testicles to descend into the scrotum; also called *undescended testis*.
Cue	Word, phrase, or symptom that indicates the nature of something perceived. Cues are grouped to assist the nurse in interpretations of data.
Culdoscopy	Diagnostic procedure to visualize the pelvic organs.
Cultural healing beliefs	Beliefs that reflect a specific culture's orientation to health and illness.
Culture (1)	System of symbols shared by a group of humans and transmitted by them to upcoming generations; also group design for living, i.e. goals, attitudes, roles and values.
Culture (2)	Living cells in a special medium that can support growth of microorganisms.
Cumulative action	Increased activity demonstrated by a drug when repeated doses accumulate in the body.
Curative	Method of combating or preventing; a treatment designed to cure.
Curettage	Scraping of material from the wall of a cavity or other surface with an instrument called a *curet*.
Cushingoid	Having the habitus and facies characteristic of Cushing's disease: fat pads on the upper back and face, striae on the limbs and trunk and excess hair on the face.
Custom	Habitual practice; the usual way of acting under given circumstances.
Cyanosis	Blue discoloration of the skin and mucous membrane caused by inadequate oxygen in the blood.
Cytology	Study of cells; their formation, origin, structure, biochemical activities and pathology.
Cytomegalovirus (CMV)	Member of a group of large, species specific, herpes-type viruses with a wide variety of disease effects.
Damages	Money awarded to a plaintiff by a court as compensation for any loss, detriment or injury to the plaintiff's person, property or rights caused by the wrong doing or negligence of the defendent.
Dander	Dry scales shed from the skin or hair of animals or feathers of birds that may cause an allergic reaction in some individuals.
Data base	Large store of information.
Death	Cessation of life.
Debridement	Removal of dirt, foreign objects, damaged tissue and cellular debris from a wound or burn to prevent infection and to promote healing.
Decentering	Coordination mentally of two or more ideas or characteristics such as space and length.
Decorticate rigidity	Abnormal postural reflex characterized by flexion of the arms, wrists and fingers. The legs may also be flexed.
Decubitus ulcer	Inflammation or sore in the skin over a bony prominence. It results from ischemic hypoxia of the tissue because of prolonged pressure on the part.
Defendant	Party named in a plaintiff's complaint and against whom the accusations are made.
Defense mechanism	Involuntary behavior used to prottect the individual from feeling anxiety.
Dehiscence	Separation of a surgical incision or the rupture of a wound closure.
Delirium tremens (DTs)	Acute and sometimes fatal psychotic and physical reaction caused by withdrawal of alcohol after excessive intake of alcoholic beverages over a long period; characterized by agitation, tremors, excitement, disorientation, mental confusion, vivid hallucinations and other signs and symptoms.
Delusion	False belief, held as true in spite of evidence to the contrary.
Dementia	Progressive, organic mental disorder characterized by confusion and impaired intellectual function, memory and judgment.
Demographics	Statistical study of human populations especially with reference to size, density, distribution, vital statistics and typical characteristics.
Dendrite	Branching process that extends from the cell body of a neuron. Each neuron usually possesses several dendrites, which receive impulses conducted to the cell body.
Denial	Unconscious defense mechanism in which emotional conflict and anxiety are avoided by refusing to acknowledge those thoughts, feelings, desires, impulses or external facts that are consciously intolerable.
Dentin	Chief material of teeth, surrounding the pulp and situated inside the enamel and cementum.
Denture	Artificial tooth or set of teeth not permanently fixed or implanted.
Deposition	Sworn pretrial testimony given by a witness in response to oral or written questions and cross examination.
Despair	Second response to separation from attachment figure, involving quiet hopelessness, sadness and mourning.
Detoxification	Treatment to diminish or remove from a patient'a body the toxic effects of chemical substances such as alcohol or drugs, usually as an initial step in treating a chemically dependent person.
Developmental delay	Preferred term for mental retardadation.
Diabetic retinopathy	Disorder of the retinal blood vessels caused by diabetes mellitus.
Diagnosis related group (DRG)	Designation in a system that classifies patients by age, diagnosis and surgical procedure, producing 300 categories used in predicting use of hospital resources. Cost reimbursement systems by government health plans (Medicare and Medicaid) are based on a patient's DRG.
Diaphragm	Domelike muscular partition between the thoracic and abdominal cavities.

Diaphysis	Shaft of a long bone, consisting of a tube of compact bone enclosing the medullary cavity.
Diarthrosis	Freely movable joint in which contiguous bony surfaces are covered by articular cartilage and connected by ligaments lined with synovial membrane.
Diastole	Time between contractions of the atria or the ventricles during which blood enters the relaxed chambers from systemic circulation and the lungs.
Diencephalon	Division of the brain between the telencephalon and the mesencephalon. It consists of the hypothalamus, thalamus, metathalamus, epithalamus and includes most of the third ventricle.
Diet therapy	Treatment of disease or medical/surgical conditions by diet.
Dietary fiber	Generic term for nondigestible chemical substances in plants.
Differentiation	Process of cellular development in which unspecialized cells or tissues are modified to achieve specific and characteristic physical forms, physiological functions and chemical properties.
Diffusion	Process in which solid, particulate matter in a fluid moves from an area of higher concentration to lower concentration, resulting in even distribution of the particles in the fluid.
Digestion	Conversion of food in the gastrointestinal tract into absorbable substances.
Dilemma	Situation requiring a choice between two equally desirable or undesirable alternatives.
Diplopia	Double vision caused by defective function of the extraocular muscles or by a disorder of the nerves that innervate the muscles.
Disaster-preparedness plan	Formal plan of action, usually prepared in written form, for coordinating the response of the hospital staff in the event of a disaster within the hospital or the surrounding community.
Discharge	Release of a patient from a health care facility.
Discovery	Pretrial procedure allowing one party to examine vital witnesses and/or documents held exclusively by the adverse party.
Disengagement stage	Time in family life when a child or children leave home, leaving the couple or single parent to live alone.
Disinfection	Destruction of disease causing microorganisms.
Disorientation	Mental confusion characterized by inadequate or incorrect perceptions of place, time or identity.
Diuresis	Increased formation and secretion of urine.
Diverticulitis	Inflammation of one or more diverticula (pouchlike herniations through the colon).
Diverticulosis	Presence of pouchlike herniations through the muscular layer of the colon.
Dizygotic	Pertaining to twins from two fertilized ova.
DNR	Do not resuscitate.
Documentation	Written material associated with a computer or a computer program.
Dominant group	Social group that controls the value system and the rewards in a society.
Dorsal (supine)	Pertaining to the back or posterior; the back.
Drainage	Removal of fluids from a body cavity or a wound.
Dramatic play	Play that acts out adult roles.
Drawsheet	Sheet smaller than a bed sheet, usually placed across the middle of the bottom sheet to keep the mattress and bottom linens dry; can also help turn or move a patient in bed.
DRG	See *diagnosis related groups*.
Drip factor	Number of drops an IV tubing set delivers per milliliter; factor needed for determining the drip rate of an IV.
Drug abuse	Use of a drug for nontherapeutic effect, especially one for which it was not prescribed or intended.
Drug addiction	Condition characterized by an overwhelming desire to continue taking a drug in which one has been habituated through repeated consumption. The drug produces a particular effect that is usually an alternation of mental activity, attitude or outlook.
Dumping syndrome	Profuse perspiring, nausea, vertigo, and weakness in some patients who have had a subtotal gastrectomy.
Dura mater	Outermost and most fibrous of the three membranes surrounding the brain and spinal cord.
Duchenne's muscular dystrophy	Abnormal congenital condition characterized by progressive symmetric wasting of the leg and pelvic muscles. It is an X-linked recessive disease that appears insidiously between 3 and 5 years of age and spreads from the leg and pelvic muscles to the involuntary muscles. It usually results in death within 10 to 15 years of the onset of symptoms; also called *pseudohypertrophic muscular dystrophy*.
Dysarthria	Difficult, poorly articulated speech, usually the result of a damaged central or peripheral motor nerve.
Dysmenorrhea	Painful menstruation.
Dysphagia	Difficulty in swallowing.
Dysplasia	Abnormal development of tissue.
Dyspnea	Shortness of breath or difficulty breathing.
Dysrhythmia	Any disturbance or abnormality in normal rhythmic pattern, especially heart or brain waves.
Dysuria	Painful urination.
Eclampsia	Gravest form of toxemia of pregnancy, characterized by grand mal convulsion, coma, hypertension, proteinuria, and edema.

Ectoderm	Outermost of the three primary cell layers of an embryo; gives rise to the nervous system; the organs of the special senses, as the eyes and ears; the epidermis and epidermal tissue as fingernails, hair, skin glands; and the mucous membrane of the mouth and anus.
Ectopic (of an object or organ)	Situated in an unusual place, away from its normal location.
Edema	Abnormal accumulation of fluid in the tissue.
Effacement	Shortening of the vaginal portion of the cervix and the thinning of its walls as it is stretched and dilated by the fetus during labor.
Efferent nerve	Nerve that transmits impulses away or outward from a nerve center such as the brain or spine.
Ego integrity	Feeling of acceptance of life for what it has been, with no wish to relive it.
Egocentric	Self-centered; unable to consider another's viewpoint.
Electrolyte	Element or compound that, when melted or dissolved in water or other solvent, dissociates into ions and can conduct electric current.
Electromyogram (EMG)	Record of the intrinsic electric activity in a skeletal muscle.
Embolism	Abnormal circulatory condition in which an embolus travels through the blood stream and lodges in a blood vessel.
Embolus	Foreign object, tissue, tumor or piece of thrombus that circulates in the blood stream.
Emesis basin	Small, kidney-shaped basin used to collect vomitus.
Empathy	Ability to recognize and to some extent share the emotions and states of mind of another and to understand the meaning and significance of that person's behavior.
Emphysema	Overinflation and other destructive changes of alveolar walls, resulting in loss of lung elasticity and decreased gas exchange.
EMS (emergency medical system)	Network of advanced cardiac life support, usually consisting of a signaling center that receives calls, an ambulance team and a medical facility.
Enface	Position in which the mother's face and the infant's face are approximately 8 inches apart and on the same plane, as when the mother holds the infant up in front of her face or when she nurses the child.
Enamel	Hard, white substance that covers the dentin of the tooth crown.
Endocrine gland	Ductless gland that delivers hormones to specific groups in the body.
Endocrinologist	Physician specializing in the study of the endocrine system and treatment of endocrine disorders.
Endoderm	Innermost of the cell layers that develops from the embryonic disk of the inner cell mass of the blastocyst. From the endoderm arises the epithelium of the trachea, bronchi, lungs, GI tract, liver, pancreas, urinary bladder and canal, pharynx, thyroid, tympanic cavity, tonsils and parathyroid glands.
Endogenous infection	Infection caused by nonpathogenic bacteria.
Endometriosis	Gynecological condition characterized by abnormal growth and function of endometrial (uterine) tissue.
Endorphin	Substance produced by the brain that mimics the effects of opiates, such as morphine.
Endorsement	Statement of recognition of the license of a health practitioner in one state by another state.
Engagement	Fixation of the presenting part of the fetus in the maternal pelvis. The lowest part of the presenting part is at or below the level of the ischial spines.
Engorgement	Swelling of breast tissue caused by an increased flow of blood and lymph preceding true lactation.
Engrossment	Father's initial response to newborn.
Enteral	Pertaining to the intestines.
Enteral nutrition	Administration of nutrients into the GI tract; usually refers to tube feeding.
Enteric	Pertaining to the intestines.
Enucleation	Removal of the eyeball.
Environment	All of the factors that influence the life and survival of a person.
Enzyme	Protein produced by living cells that catalyzes chemical reactions without being changed in the process.
Epidermis	Superficial layers of the skin, made up of an outer, dead portion and a deeper, living, cellular portion.
Epididymitis	Acute or chronic inflammation of the epididymis (sperm duct).
Epiphysis	Head of a long bone, which is separated from the shaft of the bone by the epiphyseal plate until the bone stops growing, the plate is obliterated, the shaft and the head become united.
Epistaxis	Bleeding from the nose.
Epithelium	Covering of the external and internal organs of the body, including the lining of the vessels.
Erythema	Redness or inflammation of the skin or mucous membranes.
Eschar	Scab or dry crust resulting from a burn infection or skin disease.
Essential nutrients	Carbohydrates, proteins, fats, minerals, vitamins, and water necessary for growth, normal function and body maintenance. These substances must be supplied by food—they are not synthesized by the body in the quantities required for normal health.
Estrogens	Hormones that produce female physical characteristics.
Ethics	Science or study of moral values or principles, including ideals of self-determination, kindness and justice.

Ethnic stereotype	Fixed concept or expectation about how members of an ethnic or cultural group act or think.
Ethnicity	Group's sense of belonging associated with its common social and cultural heritage.
Ethnocentrism	Tendency to view members from one cultural or ethnic group in terms of the standards of behavior, values and customs of a person's own group.
Etiology	Study of all factors involved in the development of a disease.
Eustachian tube	Tube that joins the nasopharynx and the tympanic membrane.
Euthanasia	Deliberate bringing about of death in a person who has an incurable disease or condition, either actively by administering a lethal drug or passively by withholding treatment and allowing the person to die.
Evaluation	Judgment of patient and nursing behavior regarding the extent to which the established goals of care have been met.
Evaluation conference	Thorough evaluation of a patient by a medical, nursing, sociological, psychological and spiritual team to establish rehabilitation goals.
Evisceration	Protrusion of an internal organ through a wound or surgical incision, especially in the abdominal wall.
Exacerbation	Increase in the seriousness of a disease or disorder, as marked by greater intensity in the signs and symptoms of the patient.
Excoriation	Injury to the surface layer of skin caused by scratching or abrasion.
Exocrine	Of or pertaining to the process of secreting outwardly through a duct to the surface of an organ or tissue or into a vessel, as a gland that secretes through a duct.
Exocrine gland	Gland that secretes through a series of ducts.
Exogenous infection	Infection caused by microorganisms not present in the human body.
Exophthalmos	Marked protrusion of the eyeball.
Expectant stage	Time in family life when the woman is pregnant, necessitating some changes in lifestyle.
Extended family	Nuclear family plus other relatives who live together.
Extracellular	Occurring outside a cell or cell tissue or in cavities or spaces between cell layers.
Extravasation	Passage or escape into the tissues, usually of blood, serum or lymph.
Exudate	Fluid, cells or other substances that have been slowly exuded or discharged from cells or blood vessels through small pores or breaks in cell membranes. Perspiration, pus, blood and serum are sometimes identified as exudates.
Family	Two or more persons who are related by blood, marriage or adoption and who live together over a period of time.
Family conference	Consultation between the rehabilitation team and the family to discuss the patient's functional status, goals and future.
Family interaction	Total of all roles and behaviors shown in a family at a given time.
Fanfold	Folded like a fan lengthwise, such as the top linen on a hospital bed.
Fasciculation	Localized, uncoordinated, uncontrollable twitching of a single motor muscle group innervated by a single motor nerve.
Fat	Substance composed of lipids or fatty acids, ranging from oil to tallow.
Fatigue	State of exhaustion or a loss of strength or endurance.
Febrile	Having an elevated body temperature above 99.6° F or 37.5°C.
Feces	Waste from the intestine; BM (bowel movement).
Feedback	Cyclic part of the process of communication that regulates and modifies the content of messages.
Feelings	All emotional, physical responses and sensations. Feelings are indicators of well-being.
Fibrin	Stringy, insoluble protein; a product of the action of thrombin on fibrinogen in the clotting process.
Fibroblast	Flat, elongated, undifferentiated cell in connective tissue that forms fibrous, binding and supporting tissue.
Fibromyositis	Any one of a large number of disorders in which the common element is stiffness and joint or muscle pain.
Filtration	Process in which liquid passes through a membrane or partial barrier but the solid particles are too large to pass.
Flaccid	Weak, soft and flabby; lacking normal muscle tone.
Flagella	Hairlike projections that extend from some unicellular organisms and aid in their movement.
Flatus	Air or gas in the intestine that is passed through the rectum.
Flossing	Mechanical cleansing of tooth surfaces with stringlike waxed or unwaxed dental floss.
Fluid	Body fluid either intracellular or extracellular, that is involved in the transport of electrolytes and other vital chemicals to, through, and from tissue cells.
Fluoroscopy	Technique in radiology for visually examining a part of the body or the function of an organ using a fluoroscope.
Focus charting	Expansion of the *data* and *need* columns in nurses' notes to include topics concerning the whole patient such as behavior, treatment and response. The charting format is DAR (data, action, response).
Follicle-stimulating hormone (FSH)	Gonadotropin, secreted by the anterior pituitary gland, that stimulates the growth and maturation of graafian follicles in the ovary.

Fomite	Nonliving material such as bed linens that may convey pathogenic microorganisms.
Fontanel	Space covered by tough membranes between the bones of an infant's cranium. The anterior fontanel, roughly diamond-shaped, remains palpable until about 2 years of age. The posterior fontanel, triangular in shape, closes about 2 months after birth.
Footboard	Board placed at the foot of the patient's bed so the feet rest firmly against the board at right angles to prevent footdrop.
Foramen	Opening or aperture in a membranous structure or bone, such as the apical dental foramen and the carotid foramen.
Foramen magnum	Passage in the occipital bone through which the spinal cord enters the spinal column.
Fossa	Hollow or depression, especially on the end of a bone, such as the olecranon fossa or the coronoid fossa.
Fracture pan	Small bedpan often used for patients with fractures to help prevent pain by reducing the amount of movement required for its placement.
Frustration	Feeling experienced when there is interference with goal-directed activity.
Functional assessment	Admission examination of the patient's functional abilities.
Gait	Manner or style of walking.
Gang	Group whose membership is formed on the basis of skilled performance of some activity; a group of persons having informal and unusually close social relations.
Ganglion	One of the nerve cells, chiefly collected in groups outside the central nervous system.
Gate control theory	Theory proposing that pain impulses transmitted from nerve receptors through the spinal cord to the brain can be altered or blocked in the spinal cord or brain.
Gauge	Measurement that designates space within a needle (lumen).
Generation gap	Conflict between parents and offspring.
Generativity	Concern about providing for others that is equal to the concern of providing for the self.
Geriatrics	Medical and nursing specialty concerned with the physiological and pathological changes of later maturity including study and treatment of health problems.
Gerontology	Study of the individual in later maturity and the aging process from physiological, pathological, psychological, sociological and economic points of view.
Gingiva	Gum of the mouth; a mucous membrane with supporting fibrous tissue that overlies the crowns of unerupted teeth and encircles the necks of teeth that have erupted.
Glasgow coma scale	Standardized system for assessing the degree of conscious impairment in the neurologically impaired patient.
Glaucoma	Elevated pressures within the eye caused by obstruction of the outflow of aqueous humor.
Glioma	Malignant tumor of the brain.
Global cognitive dysfunction	Loss of thinking and reasoning powers caused by severe brain damage.
Glucagon	Hormone produced by the alpha cells in the islets of Langerhans in the pancreas that stimulates the conversion of glycogen to glucose in the liver.
Gluten	Insoluble protein constituent of wheat and other grains.
Glycogen	Polysaccharide that is the major carbohydrate stored in animal cells.
Glycosylated hemoglobin test	Diagnostic test that measures the glucose bound to hemoglobin; used as an index of blood sugar control.
Goal	Purpose toward which an endeavor is directed, as the outcome of diagnostic, therapeutic and educational management of a patient's health problem.
Golgi apparatus	One of many small membranous structures found in most cells, composed of various elements associated with formation of carbohydrate and protein compounds.
Good Samaritan Law	Law that has been enacted in almost every state and province that provides immunity to volunteers at the scene of an accident, provided they are not grossly negligent, do not injure the victim and are acting in good faith.
Graafian follicle	Mature ovarian vesicle that ruptures during ovulation to release the ovum.
Graduated	Container marked with lines that indicate measurement such as number of milliliters, used to measure urine output, for example.
Gravid	Combining form meaning *pertaining to pregnancy or pregnant*.
Gravida	Combining form meaning *pregnant woman with* (specified) *quantity of pregnancies*.
Gray matter	Gray tissue that makes up the inner core of the spinal column, arranged in two large lateral masses connected across the midline by a narrow commissure; also, gray tissue on the surface of the cerebral hemisphere comprising the cerebral cortex.
Grief	Nearly universal pattern of physical and emotional responses to bereavement, separation, or loss.
Grief therapy	Mental treatment aimed at helping a patient deal with the pain of loss.
Grief work	Adaptation process of mourning a loss.
Growth hormone	Hormone released by the anterior pituitary gland that produces normal growth of the body.
Gyrus	One of the tortuous convolutions of the surface of the brain caused by infolding of the cortex.

Habituation	Psychological and emotional dependence on a drug, tobacco or alcohol, resulting from the repeated use of the substance but without the addictive; physiological need to increase dosage.
Hallucinogen	Substance that causes excitation of the central nervous system, characterized by hallucination, mood change, anxiety, sensory distortion, delusion, depersonalization, increased pulse, temperature and blood pressure, and dilation of the pupils.
Handroll	Device, usually a washcloth rolled and placed in the patient's hand, to support the hand while squeezing.
Hazard communication act	Act that requires hospitals to inform employees about harmful exposures, thus reducing the risk of injury or illness to employees.
Head injury	Any traumatic damage to the head resulting from penetration of the skull or from too rapid acceleration or deceleration of the brain within the skull.
Health	Physical, mental and social well-being, and the absence of disease or other abnormal condition.
Health care facility	Agency or institution that provides health care, e.g. hospital, nursing home, clinic or home health agency.
Health care system	Complete network of agencies, facilities and all providers of health care in a specified geographical area.
Health history	Collection of information obtained from a patient and from other sources. The history provides a data base on which a plan for diagnosis, treatment, care and follow-up of the patient may be made.
Hematemesis	Vomiting of bright red blood.
Hematocrit	Measure of the packed cell volume of red cells, expressed as a percentage of total blood volume.
Hematoma	Escaped blood trapped in tissues of the skin or in an organ as a result of trauma.
Hematuria	Blood in the urine.
Hemianopsia	Blindness in one half of the visual field.
Hemiplegia	Paralysis of one side of the body.
Hemoccult	Test for blood in stool.
Hemoglobin	Complex, protein-iron compound in the blood that carries oxygen to the cells from the lungs and carbon dioxide away from the cells to the lungs.
Hemophiliac	Person with an inherited disorder characterized by excessive bleeding caused by a clotting defect.
Hemopoiesis	Formation and development of the various types of blood cells.
Hemoptysis	Expectorating of blood from the respiratory tract.
Heparin lock	Device used with an angiocath or butterfly needle allowing maintenance of an IV route without continuous administration of IV fluid.
Heterograft (xenograft)	Tissue from another species used as a temporary graft, as in treating severe burns with pig skin grafts, when sufficient tissue from the patient is not available.
Heterozygous	Having two different genes for a particular characteristic; an inherited gene from one parent and the alternative gene from the other parent.
Hilum (hilus)	Depression or pit at that part of an organ where vessels and nerves enter.
Hilus	Depression or pit at the part of an organ where vessels and nerves enter.
Hirsutism	Excessive body hair.
HIV	Human immunodeficiency virus.
Holistic health care	System of comprehensive or total patient care that considers the physical, emotional, social, economic, and spiritual needs of the person, the response to the illness and the impact of the illness on the person's ability to meet self-care needs; also called *comprehensive care*.
Home health care	Nursing care provided in the patient's home.
Homeostasis	Relative constancy in the internal environment of the body, naturally maintained by adaptive responses that promote healthy survival.
Homograft (allograft)	Transfer of tissue between two genetically dissimilar individuals of the same species.
Homozygous	Having two identical genes for a particular characteristic, inherited from each parent. An individual homozygous for a genetic disease caused by recessive genes manifests the disorder.
Hormone	Complex chemical substance produced in one part or organ of the body that initiates or regulates the activity of an organ or a group of cells in another part of the body.
Hospice	System of family-centered care provided outside the hospital, designed to assist the dying patient to maintain a satisfactory lifestyle through the terminal phases of dying.
Host	Organism on which a parasite lives and receives nourishment.
Humoral immunity	One of the two forms of immunity that respond to antigens such as bacteria and foreign tissue. It is mediated by the B-cells.
Hydrocephaly	Pathological condition characterized by an abnormal accumulation of cerebrospinal fluid, usually under increased pressure, within the cranial vault and subsequent dilation of the ventricles. In infants the head grows at an abnormal rate with separation of the structures, bulging fontanels and dilated scalp veins. Typical behavior includes irritability with lethargy and vomiting.
Hydronephrosis	Distention of the renal pelvis and calyces of the kidney.
Hydrostatic pressure	Pressure exerted by a liquid.
Hygiene	Practice of cleanliness that is conducive to health.

Hypercalcemia	Abnormally high level of calcium in the blood.
Hypercapnia	Excessive amounts of carbon dioxide in the blood.
Hyperglycemia	Abnormally high level of glucose in the blood.
Hyperkalemia	Abnormally high level of potassium in the blood.
Hyperlipidemia	Excess of lipids in the blood.
Hypermenorrhea	Abnormally heavy or long menstrual periods.
Hyperplasia	Increase in the number of cells of a body part.
Hyperreflexia	Neurological condition characterized by increased reflex reactions.
Hypersensitivity	Excessive reaction to a particular stimulus.
Hypertension	Elevated blood pressure, blood pressure readings consistently elevated above 140/90.
Hyperthermic	Much higher than normal body temperature.
Hypertonic	Having a greater concentration of solute than another solution, hence exerting more osmotic pressure than that solution, as a hypertonic saline solution that contains more salt than is found in intracellular and extracellular fluid.
Hypertrophy	Increase in the size of an organ caused by an increase in the size of the cells rather than the number of cells.
Hyperventilation	Breathing rate that is greater than metabolically necessary for the exchange of respiratory gases.
Hyphema	Hemorrhage into the anterior chamber of the eye, usually caused by a blunt or percusive injury; also called *hyphemia*.
Hypocalcemia	Abnormally low level of calcium in the blood.
Hypoglycemia	Abnormally low level of glucose in the blood.
Hypokalemia	Abnormally low level of potassium in the blood.
Hypotension	Abnormal condition in which the blood pressure is not adequate for tissue perfusion and oxygenation.
Hypothermia	Abnormal condition in which the body temperature is below 95°F (35°C).
Hypotonic	Having a smaller concentration of solute than another solution, hence exerting less osmotic pressure than that solution. Example is a hypotonic saline solution that contains less salt than is found in intracellular or extracellular fluid.
Hypoventilation	Abnormal condition characterized by cyanosis, clubbing of the fingers, Cheyne-Stokes breathing and generally decreased respiratory function.
Hypoxia	Inadequate amount of oxygen available at the cellular level, characterized by cyanosis, tachycardia, hypertension, peripheral vasoconstriction, vertigo and mental confusion.
Hysterosalpingo-oophorectomy	Surgical removal of one or both ovaries and oviduct(s) along with the uterus.
Icterus	Yellow color of the skin, mucous membranes and sclera of the eyes (jaundice).
Ideas of reference	Obsessive delusion that statements or actions of others refer to oneself, seen in paranoid disorders.
Identity	Sense of uniqueness as a person; of internal stability, sameness and continuity, which resist extreme change.
Idiopathic	Without a known cause.
Idiosyncratic	Unique hypersensitivity to a particular drug.
Ileal conduit	Method of urinary diversion in which the ureters are joined to a segment of ileum.
Illness	Abnormal process in which aspects of the social, physical, emotional or intellectual condition and functions of a person are diminished or impaired, compared with that person's previous condition.
Illusion	False perception or experience occurring in response to an environmental stimulus.
Immune response	Reaction of the body to foreign substances.
Immune serum	Serum of an animal or human containing antibodies against a specific disease; used to confer passive immunity to that disease.
Immunity	Quality of being insusceptible to or unaffected by a particular disease condition.
Immunization	Injection of diluted and/or weakened organisms or products produced by organisms to promote resistance to disease.
Immunocompetent	Ability of the immune system to function appropriately.
Immunodeficiency	Abnormal condition of the immune system in which cellular or humoral immunity is inadequate and resistance to infection is increased.
Immunogen	Any agent or substance capable of provoking an immune response or producing immunity.
Immunoglobulins	Proteins capable of acting as antibodies; present in serum, body fluid and body secretions.
Immunosuppressed	Administration of agents that significantly interfere with the ability of the immune system to respond to antigenic stimulation by inhibiting cellular and humoral immunity.
Immunosuppressive	Substance or procedure that lessens or prevents an immune response.
Immunotherapy	Special treatment of allergic responses: administering increasingly large doses of the offending allergens to gradually develop immunity.
Immunotropic	Tendency to have an influence on or be influenced by the immune system.

Implantation	Process involving the attachment, penetration and embedding of the blastocyst in the lining of the uterine wall during the early stages of prenatal development.
Incision	Cut produced surgically by a sharp instrument to create an opening into an organ or space in the body.
Incus	One of the three ossicles in the middle ear, resembling an anvil.
Induration	Hardening of a tissue, particularly the skin because of edema, inflammation or infiltration by neoplasm.
Industry	Interest in doing work of the world, formation of responsible work habits and attitudes and mastery of age-appropriate tasks.
Infant	First 12 to 24 months of life.
Infant mortality	Statistic rate of infant death during the first year after live birth, expressed as the number of such births per 1000 live births in a specific geographical area or institution in a given period.
Infarct	Localised area of necrosis in tissue, a vessel or an organ resulting from tissue anoxia; caused by an interruption in the blood supply to an area.
Infection process cycle	Five-point cycle that enables microorganisms to move from place to place and cause infection. If the cycle is broken, the microorganisms cannot grow, spread or cause disease.
Inferiority	Feeling inadequate, defeated, lazy, unable to learn or do tasks and unable to compete, compromise or cooperate, regardless of actual competence.
Inflammation	Protective response of body tissues to irritation or injury, such as pain, swelling, redness, heat and lack of function.
Inflammatory bowel disease	Refers to both Crohn's disease and ulcerative colitis, involving inflammation and tissue changes in intestinal walls.
Inhibit	To restrain the action or function of an organ or cell as to reduce a physiological activity by an antagonistic stimulation.
Initial/establishment stage	Period when a couple establishes a home.
Innate immunity	Natural and permanent form of immunity to a specific disease.
Inner canthus of the eye	Inner angle at the medial and lateral margins of the eyelid.
Innominate	Without a name. The term is traditionally applied to certain anatomical structures, often identified by their descriptive names, such as hip bone, brachiocephalic artery and brachiocephalic vein.
Insertion	Place of attachment, such as of a muscle to the bone it moves.
Institutionalize	To place a person in an institution for psychological or physical treatment or for the protection of the person or society.
Insulin	Naturally occurring hormone, secreted by the beta cells of the islets of Langerhans in the pancreas as a response to increased levels of glucose in the blood.
Insulin reaction	Adverse effects caused by excessive levels of circulating insulin.
Integument	Covering or skin.
Intelligence	Ability to learn from experience, to acquire and retain knowledge, to solve problems and to respond to a new situation.
Interagency	Between two health care facilities.
Interdisciplinary team	Multiprofessional health team, such as doctors, nurses, social workers and pastors, working together in caring for the terminally ill patient.
Intermittent claudication	Weakness of the legs with cramping pains, occurring usually after an extended period of walking or exercise and normally relieved by rest.
Interrogatories	Series of written questions submitted to a witness or other persons having information of interest to the court.
Interstitial	Of or pertaining to the space between the tissues, as interstitial fluid.
Intervention	Action performed to prevent harm from occurring to a patient or to improve the mental, emotional, physical, or social function of a patient.
Intimacy	Reaching out and using the self to form a commitment to and an intense, lasting relationship with another person or even a cause, an institution or a creative effort.
Intraagency	Within a health care facility.
Intracellular	Located within the cell.
Intraoperative	Occurring during surgery.
Intrathecal	Of or pertaining to a structure, process or substance within a sheath, as the cerebrospinal fluid within the theca of the spinal canal.
Intravascular	Located within the vessel.
Intussusception	Prolapse of one segment of bowel into the lumen of another segment.
Involuntary	Occurring without conscious control or direction.
Iridectomy	Surgical removal of part of the iris.
Iris	Circular, contractile disc suspended in aqueous humor between the cornea and the erystalline lens of the eye and perforated by a circular pupil.
Iron-deficiency anemia	Decrease of hemoglobin in the blood caused by inadequate supplies of iron, characterized by pallor, fatigue and weakness.

Irradiation	Exposure to X-rays.
Ischemia	Deficiency of blood supply caused by circulatory obstruction.
Ischium	One of the three parts of the hip bone, joining the illium and the pubis to form the acetabulum.
Isolation and self-absorption	Inability to be intimate, spontaneous or close with another.
Isolation	Separation of a seriously ill patient from others.
Isotonic	Having the same concentration of solute as another solution, hence exerting the same amount of osmotic pressure as that solution.
Joint	Any of the connections between bones. Each is classified according to structure and movability, as fibrous, cartilaginous or synovial.
Judgment	Final decision of the court regarding a case before it.
Jurisdiction	Power and authority of a constitution of the state and/or local system to pronounce the sentence of the law.
JVD	Jugular vein distention, which reflects increased right arterial pressure.
Kaposi's sarcoma (KS)	Malignant tumor, seen more commonly in men.
Kardex or nursing Rand	Card filing system, usually kept at the nursing station, that allows quick reference to the particular needs of each patient for nursing care.
Kegel's exercises	Also called *pubococcygens exercises*, a regimen of isometric exercises in which a woman executes a series of voluntary contractions of the muscles of her pelvic diaphragm and perineum; may increase the contractility of her vaginal muscles or improve the retention of urine.
Keratoplasty	Surgery to excise an opaque portion of the cornea.
Kernicterus	Abnormal toxic accumulation of bilirubin in central nervous system tissues caused by hyperbilirubinemia.
Ketoacidosis	Abnormal accumulation of ketones in the body, resulting from faulty carbohydrate metabolism, occurring primarily as a complication of diabetes mellitus.
Ketones	Acetone bodies found in diabetes mellitus, breakdown of fatty acids causing increased levels of ketone bodies in the blood called *ketosis*.
Kilocalorie	Unit that denotes the heat expenditure of an organism and the fuel or energy value of food, often abbreviated kcalorie or kcal.
Korotkoff's sounds	Sounds heard when taking a blood pressure using a sphygmomanometer and stethoscope. As air is released from the cuff, pressure on the brachial artery is reduced and blood is heard pulsing through the vessels.
KS	See *Kaposi's sarcoma*.
Kwashiorkor	Malnutrition disease primarily of children, caused by severe protein deficiency and usually occurring when the child is weaned.
Kyphosis	Abnormal, convex curvature of the thoracic spine.
Labia majora	Two large folds of skin, one on each side of the vaginal orifice outside the labia minora.
Labia minora	Two small folds of skin between the labia majora, extending from the clitoris backward on both sides of the vaginal orifice, ending between it and the labia majora.
Labile	Unstable; characterized by a tendency to change or to be altered.
Labyrinthitis	Inflammation of the inner ear canal resulting in vertigo.
Lactation	Synthesis and secretion of milk from the breasts for the nourishment of an infant or child.
Lalling	Infant's movement of tongue with crying and vocalization.
Laminectomy	Surgical chipping away of the bony arches of one or more vertebrae.
Language	Combination of sounds into a meaningful whole to communicate thoughts and feelings.
Lanugo	Soft, downy hair covering a normal fetus. It begins to shed in the fifth month of life and is almost entirely shed by the ninth month.
Lanula	Half-moon structure, such as the crescent-shaped, pale area at the base of the nail of a finger or toe.
Laparoscopy	Any surgical incision into the peritoneal cavity, often performed on an exploratory basis.
Larynx	Organ of voice that is part of the air passage connecting the pharynx with the trachea.
Law	Rule, principle or regulation established and promulgated by a government to protect or to restrict the people affected.
Legg-Calve-Perthes disease	Aseptic (noninfectious) necrosis of the head of the femur, characterized initially by epiphyseal necrosis or degeneration and followed by regeneration or recalcification.
Leisure	Freedom from obligations and formal duties of paid work and opportunity to pursue, at one's own pace, mental nourishment, enlivenment, pleasure and relief from fatigue of work.
Lens	Crystalline lens of the eye; a curved transparent disc that is capable of refracting light.
Lentigo senilis	Irregular areas of dark pigmentation of the skin in the elderly.
Leukemia	Malignant neoplasm of blood-forming organs.
Leukocyte	White blood cell; one of the formed elements of the circulating blood system.
Leukopenia	Abnormal decrease in the number of white blood cells to fewer than 5000 cells per cubic millimeter.
Leukoplakia	Precancerous change in a mucous membrane characterized by thickened, white, firmly attached patches.

Leukorrhea	Normal white vaginal discharge.
Liability	Something one is obligated to do or an obligation required by law, usually financial in nature.
Licensure	Granting of permission by a competent authority to an organization or individual to engage in a practice or activity that would otherwise be illegal.
Lie	Relationship between the long axis of the fetus and the long axis of the mother.
Ligament	One of many predominantly white, shiny, flexible bands of fibrous tissue binding joints together and connecting various bones and cartilages.
Lightening	Subjective sensation reported by many women late in pregnancy as the fetus settles lower in the pelvis, leaving more space in the upper abdomen.
Lipoprotein	Protein and lipid molecule, which facilitates transport of lipids in the blood stream. They are classified according to their composition and density.
Litigate	To carry out a lawsuit or to contest one.
Living will	Instrument by which a dying person makes his wishes known to those who will survive him.
Lochia	Discharge that flows from the vagina after childbirth.
Lordosis	Increased curve in the lumbar region of the spine.
Loss	Any aspect of one's self that is no longer available to that person.
Lumbar cord injury	Spinal injury involving paralysis of the lower extremities.
Lumen	Space within a tube, such as a needle; also, a cavity or channel within an organ, specifically the blood vessels of the cardiovascular system.
Luteinizing hormone	Produced by the anterior pituitary gland, it stimulates the secretion of sex hormones by the ovary and the testes and is involved in the maturation of sperm and ova.
Lymphadenopathy	Disease of the lymph nodes, including hypertrophy and proliferation of lymphoid tissue.
Lymphocyte	Lymph cell or white blood cell; develops in the bone marrow.
Lymphokine	Chemical factor released by the T cell that attracts macrophages to the site.
Lysosome	Cytoplasmic, membrane-bound particle containing hydrolytic enzymes that function in intracellular digestive processes.
Macrophage	Cell that "eats" pathogenic microorganisms.
Macule	Small, flat blemish or discoloration that is flush with the skin surface.
Magical thinking	Belief that merely thinking about an event in the external world can cause it to occur.
Magnesium	Silver-white mineral that is found in combination with other elements in the body.
Magnetic resonance imaging (MRI)	Medical imaging that uses nuclearmagnetic resonance as its source of energy.
Malignant neoplasm	Tumor that progressively spreads to other areas of the body.
Malleolus	Rounded, bony process on each side of the ankle.
Malpractice	Professional negligence that is the most likely cause of injury or harm to a patient, resulting from a lack of professional knowledge, experience, or skill, or from negligence.
Mammography	Radiography of the soft tissues of the breast to identify neoplastic processes.
Management	Act, art, or manner of managing or handling, controlling, or directing: careful, tactful treatment.
Mandatory	Required by a command, order or law.
Manubrium	One of the three bones of the sternum, presenting a broad, quadrangular shape that narrows where it unites with the superior end of the sternum.
Marasmus	Extreme malnutrition and emaciation, occurring chiefly in young children, with wasting of subcutaneous tissue and muscle; results from lack of calories and proteins.
Mastoiditis	Infection of one of the mastoid bones.
Matrifocal/matriarchal family	Family in which a woman has the main authority and power.
Matrix	Basic substance from which a specific type of tissue develops.
Mattress pad (cover)	Material that fits over a mattress to protect it from soiling.
Meconium	Newborn's first fecal material after birth.
Mediastinum	Portion of the thoracic cavity in the middle of the thorax, between the pleural sacs containing the two lungs.
Medicaid	Health insurance program for the indigent and poor passed in 1965 as the Title XIX Amendment to the Social Security Act. It provides payment for certain home care services.
Medical asepsis	Removal or destruction of disease organisms or infected material.
Medical diagnosis	Traditional approach to diagnosis as practiced by physicians focusing on the defect or dysfunction within the patient. Medical diagnosis is focused on the physical and biological aspects of specific diseases and conditions.
Medicare	Health insurance program for the aged and disabled passed in 1965 as the Title XVII Amendment to the Social Security Act. It dramatically changed the delivery of home health services.
Medicated tub bath	Therapeutic bath in which medication is dispersed in water, usually in treating dermatological disorders.
Medicine	Art and science of diagnosis, treatment, prevention of disease and the maintenance of good health.

Medulla	Most internal part of a structure or organ.
Medulla oblongata	Most vital part of the brain; continuing as the bulbous portion of the spinal cord just above the foramen magnum and separated from the pons by a horizontal groove.
Melanin	Black or dark brown pigment that occurs naturally in the hair and skin and in the iris and choroid of the eye.
Melanoma	Malignant neoplasm, primarily of the skin.
Membrane	Thin layer of tissue that covers a surface, lines a cavity or divides a space, such as the membrane that lines the abdominal wall.
Menarche	First menstrual period; physiological marker of puberty in female.
Meninges	Any of the three membranes that enclose the brain and spinal cord, comprising the dura mater, the pia mater and the arachnoid.
Meningomyelocele	Developmental defect of the central nervous system in which a hernial sac containing a portion of the spinal cord, its meninges and cerebrospinal fluid protrudes through a congenital cleft in the vertebral column; also called *myelomeningocele*.
Meniscus	Curved upper surface of a liquid in a container.
Menopause	Permanent ceasing of ovulation and menstruation, which causes loss of reproductive ability.
Menorrhagia	Abnormally heavy or long menstrual periods.
Menstruation	Periodical discharge through the vagina of a bloody secretion from the shedding of the endometrium.
Mental health continuum	Mental health and mental illness can be viewed as opposite ends on a continuum. The point at which the person is deemed mentally ill is determined by behavior, as well as by the circumstances in which the behavior is seen.
Mental illness	Pattern of behavior disturbing to the individual or to the community in which he lives.
Mesentery	Broad, fan-shaped fold of peritoneum connecting the jejunum and ileum with the dorsal wall of the abdomen.
Mesoderm	Middle of three cell layers of the developing embryo, lying between the ectoderm and the endoderm. Bone, connective tissue, muscle, blood, vascular, lymphatic tissue, the membranes of the pericardium and peritoneum are derived from the mesoderm.
Metabolism	Combination of all chemical processes that take place in living organisms, resulting in growth, generation of energy, elimination of wastes, and other body functions as they relate to the distribution of nutrients in the blood after digestion.
Metabolite	Substance produced by metabolic action or necessary for a metabolic process.
Metastasis	Process by which tumor cells spread to distant parts of the body.
Microorganism	Tiny living plant or animal that can be seen only via a microscope; may be pathogenic.
Micturition	Urination.
Middle age	Period of life from mid-40s to mid-60s or 70.
Midlife crisis	Major turning point in one's life related to identity crisis and self-absorption; involves changes in commitments to career and/or spouse and children, as well as emotional turmoil for the individual and others.
Milliequivalent (mEq)	Number of grams of solute dissolved in 1 ml of a normal solution.
Mineral	Inorganic substance ingested as a compound (such as sodium chloride) rather than as a free element. Minerals help regulate many body functions.
Minority group	Group of people who, because of their physical or cultural characteristics, receive unequal and different treatment from others in the society. Minority group members view themselves as victims of collective discrimination.
Miotic	Causing constriction of the pupil of the eye.
Miter	Fold and tuck made on the corner of a sheet; gives hospital bed a finished appearance.
Mitochondria	Powerhouses of the cell. They are bean shaped and convert food to an energy form (ATP) for the cell.
Monocyte	Large, mononuclear leukocyte.
Monozygotic	Pertaining to twins who develop from a single ova; identical twins.
Mood	Particular state of mind of feeling, such as humor or temper.
Morals	Generally accepted customs of conduct and right living in a society.
Morbidity	(1) Illness or abnormal condition or quality; (2) in statistics, the rate at which an illness or abnormality occurs, calculated by dividing the entire number of people in a group by the number in that group who are affected with the illness or the abnormality; (3) the rate at which an illness occurs in a particular area or population.
Mores	Folkways of central importance, accepted without question and embodying the fundamental moral views of a group.
Morphology	Study of physical shape and size.
Morula	Solid, round mass of cells resulting from the cleavage of the fertilized ovum in the early stages of embryonic development.
Motivation	Inner drive that leads an individual to complete a task or meet a goal.
Motor	Pertaining to motion, the body apparatus involved in movement, or the brain functions that direct purposeful activities.
Motor neuron	One of various efferent nerve cells that transmit nerve impulses from the brain or from the spinal cord to muscular or glandular tissue.

Mourning	Reaction activated by a person to assist in overcoming a great personal loss.
Multiaxial system	System used for organizing information in a psychiatric diagnosis.
Multigravida	Woman who has been pregnant more than once.
Multipara	Woman who has been delivered of more than one viable infant.
Multiple myeloma	Malignant neoplasm of the bone marrow.
Muscle tone	Muscle strength; the normal state of balanced tension in muscles.
Myalgia	Diffuse muscle pain, usually accompanied by malaise, occurring in many infectious diseases.
Mydriatic	Causing dilation of the pupil of the eye.
Myelin	Fatty sheath covering neurons.
Myelogram	X-ray film taken after injection of a radiopaque medium into the subarachnoid space; demonstrates any distortions of the spinal cord, spinal nerve roots and subarachnoid space.
Myelosuppression	Inhibition of the production of blood cells and platelets in the bone marrow.
Myocardial infection (MI)	Occlusion of a coronary artery caused by atherosclerosis or an embolus; heart attack.
Myocardium	Thick, contractile, middle layer of uniquely constructed and arranged muscle cells that form the bulk of the heart wall.
Myositis	Inflammation of muscle tissue.
Myringotomy	Surgical incision of the eardrum.
NANDA	North American Nursing Diagnosis Association.
Narcotic abstinence syndrome (NAS)	Affects babies born to narcotic addicted mothers whose addiction is passed onto the child. The baby will demonstrate signs of hyperreflexia, hypertonia, a high-pitched cry, tremors, sneezing and yawning.
Narrative charting	Traditional style of charting in which the nurse documents in story form all pertinent patient observations, care and responses in the nurse's notes section.
Negative feedback	In physiology, a decrease in function in response to a stimulus.
Neglect	Failure of caregivers to provide a child with basic necessities of life.
Negligence	Commission of an act that a prudent person would not have done or the omission of a duty that a prudent person would have fulfilled, resulting in injury or harm to another person.
Neonate	Infant during first 4 weeks of life.
Neoplasia	New and abnormal growth of cells, which may be benign or malignant.
Neoplasm	Any abnormal growth of new tissue, which may be benign or malignant.
Nephron	Structural and functional unit of the kidney, resembling a microscopic funnel with a long stem and two convoluted sections.
Nephrotoxin	Substance destructive to the kidney.
Neurilemma	Layer of cells composed of one or more Schwann cells, which enclose the segmented myelin sheaths of peripheral nerve fibers. The nerve fibers of the brain and the spinal cord are not enclosed by neurilemma.
Neuromuscular junction	Area of contact between the ends of a large myelinated nerve fiber and a skeletal muscle fiber.
Neuropathy	Any abnormal condition characterized by inflammation and degeneration of the peripheral nerves.
Neurotransmitter	Anyone of numerous chemicals that modify or result in the transmission of nerve impulses between synapses.
Neurotropic	Having a tendency to influence or be influenced by the nervous system.
Nocturnal emissions	Ejaculation of semen during sleep; physiological marker of puberty in male.
Nodule	Small, node like structure.
Nonrapid eye movement (NREM)	One of two major stages of sleep; consists of four distinct phases of sleep in which very little movement can be observed.
Nonspecific immunity	Passive immunity; acquired immunity transmitted naturally through the placenta to a fetus or through the colostrum to an infant, or artificially by injection.
Normotensive	Having normal blood pressure.
Nosocomial infection	Infection acquired during hospitalization.
Noxious	Harmful, injurious or detrimental to health.
Nuchal rigidity	Pain and stiffness of the neck.
Nuclear family	Mother, father and child(ren) in the family unit.
Nullipara	Woman who has not been delivered of a viable infant.
Nurse practice act	Outlines the legal scope of nursing within the geographical boundaries of the jurisdiction.
Nurse's notes	Nurse's written documentation of patient observations, care and responses.
Nursing	Practice in which a nurse assists the individual, sick or well, in the performance of those activities contributing to health or its recovery (or to a peaceful death) that he would perform unaided if he had the necessary strength, will, or knowledge.
Nursing assessment	Identification by a nurse of the basis, preferences and abilities of a patient. Assessment provides the scientific basis for a complete nursing care plan.

Nursing care plan	Plan of care based on a nursing assessment and a nursing diagnosis; lists nursing actions necessary to meet a patient's needs.
Nursing diagnosis	Statement of a health problem or a potential problem in the patient's health status that a nurse is licensed and competent to treat.
Nursing process	Process that serves as an organizational framework for the practice of nursing; assists in a systematic approach to nursing assessment of the patient.
Nutrient density	Nutrients relative to calories. Food providing a high quantity of one or more nutrients in a small number of calories is nutrient dense.
Nutrition	All the processes involved in taking in nutrients and in their assimilation and use for proper body functioning and maintenance of health.
Nystagmus	Involuntary, rhythmic movement of the eyes. Oscillations may be horizontal, vertical, rotary or mixed.
Obesity	Abnormal increase in the proportion of fat cells, mainly in the viscera and subcutaneous tissues of the body; overfatness.
Objective data	Data that are both observable and measurable. Vital signs and laboratory reports are examples of objective data.
Objective data collection	Process in which data relating to the patient's problems are obtained through direct physical examination, laboratory analysis, and radiological studies.
Obsession	Thought recognized by the individual as irrational and recurring despite the wish to avoid it.
Occiput	Back of the head; of or pertaining to the occipital region.
Occult	Hidden or difficult to observe.
Occupied bed	Hospital bed that must be made up while it is occupied by a patient.
Olecranon	Projection of the ulna that forms the point of the elbow and fits into the olecranon fossa of the humerus when the forearm is extended.
Oligohydramnios	Abnormally small amount or absence of amniotic fluid.
Oliguria	Diminished capacity to form and pass urine, less than 240 ml in 8 hours.
Oncology	Study of tumors.
Open bed	Fanfolded top linens on a hospital bed, for easy access for patient.
Ophthalmoscope	Device used to examine the interior of the eye.
Opportunistic infection	Infection in a person whose resistance to disease has been decreased by other disorders, such as diabetes mellitus, cancer, or AIDS, or by a procedure, such as surgery or catheterization.
Oral hygiene	Maintenance of tissues and structure of the mouth; includes brushing teeth, dental flossing and cleaning of dentures.
Oral swabs	Swabs impregnated or soaked with various solutions for oral hygiene, such as glycerin and lemon juice.
Orientation	Awareness of one's physical environment with regard to time, place and the identity of other persons; the ability to adapt to such an existing or new environment.
Orifice	Entrance to or outlet of any cavity in the body.
Orthopedic bed	Bed designed to accommodate a patient with fractures.
Orthopnea	Abnormal condition in which a person must sit or stand to breathe.
Ortolani's test	Procedure used to evaluate the stability of the hip joints in newborns and infants. A click or a popping sensation (Ortolani's sign) may be felt if the joint is unstable, because the head of the femur moves out of the acetabulum under pressure from the examiner's hands during rotation and abduction.
OSHA	Occupational Safety and Health Administration.
Osmosis	Movement of a pure solvent, as water, through a semipermeable membrane from a solution with lower solute concentration to one with higher solute concentration.
Osseous	Pertaining to bone.
Ossicle	Small bone, as the malleus, the incus or stapes of the middle ear.
Osteoclasia	Destruction and absorption of bony tissue by osteoclasts, such as during growth or the healing of fractures.
Osteoclast	Large type of multinucleated bone cell that functions in periods of growth or repair, such as the breakdown and resorption of osseous tissue.
Otitis	Inflammation or infection of the ear.
Outer canthus of the eye	Outer angle at the medial and lateral margins of the eyelid.
Ovulation	Release of a mature ovum (egg) from the ovary.
Oxidation	Process in which the oxygen content of a compound is increased.
Oxytocic	Anyone of the numerous drugs that stimulate the smooth muscle of the uterus to contract.
Pain	Unpleasant sensation caused by noxious stimulation of the sensory nerve endings.
Palliation	Therapy to relieve or reduce uncomfortable symptoms but not to cure.
Palliative	To sooth or relieve intensity of uncomfortable symptoms but not to produce a cure.

Palpation	Technique where the examiner feels texture, size, consistency and location of body parts.
Papanicolaou test	Method of examining stained cells obtained from lesions, sputum, urine and other material by aspiration, scraping, a smear, or washings of the tissue. The "pap" test is a vital part of the female pelvic examination to detect cancer of the cervix.
Papule	Small, solid, raised skin lesion, less than 1 cm in diameter.
Para	Combining form meaning woman who has given birth to children in a number of pregnancies.
Parallel play	Playing alongside a peer or same-aged child.
Paralysis	Abnormal condition characterized by loss of muscle function or loss of sensation.
Paranoia	Transitory mental state characterized by illogical thought processes and generalized suspicion and distrust.
Parasympathetic	Of or pertaining to the craniosacral division of the autonomic nervous system, consisting of the oculomotor, facial, glossopharyngeal, vagus and pelvic nerves. The parasympathetic slows heart rate, increases intestinal peristalsis and gland activity and relaxes sphincters.
Parathyroid gland	One of several small structures, usually four, attached to the thyroid gland.
Parathyroid hormone	Secreted by the parathyroid glands; maintains a constant concentration of calcium in the blood.
Parenchyma	Tissue of an organ, as distinguished from supporting or connective tissue.
Parenteral	Not in or through the digestive system; generally refers to needle routes.
Parenteral nutrition	Administration of nutrients by a route other than the alimentary canal, such as intravenously.
Parenthood stage	Stage of family life at birth of a child.
Partial bath	Patient's incomplete bath. A nurse usually must bathe the back, legs and feet.
Passive transport	Movement of small molecules across the membrane of a cell by diffusion.
Patella	Flat, triangular bone at the front of the knee joint, which attaches to the ligamentum patellae also called *kneecap*.
Patent	Condition of being open and unblocked, such as a patent airway.
Pathogen	Any microorganism capable of producing disease.
Patient	Recipient of a health care service.
Patients' rights	Legal and regulatory rights to participate in the planning of care, be informed of services, know by whom and how payment will be made, have privacy and grievance procedures and be shown respect for personal possessions.
Patient-control-led analgesia (PCA)	Method by which a patient can control intravenous analgesia by pressing a button.
Patrifocal/patriarchal family	Family in which a man has the main authority and power.
PCP	*Pneumocystis carinii* pneumonia.
Pediculosis	Infestation of lice; may be of the head, facial hair, skin and pubic region.
Peer	Person deemed an equal for the purpose at hand. A peer is usually about the same age and mental level.
Peer review	Appraisal by professional coworkers of equal status of the way an individual nurse or other health professional conducts practice, education or research; uses accepted standards as measures against which performance is weighed.
Pellagra	Disease resulting from deficiency of the vitamin *niacin*.
Pepsin	Enzyme secreted in the stomach that catalyzes hydrolysis of protein.
Peptic ulcer	Loss of the mucous membrane of the stomach, duodenum or any part of the GI system exposed to gastric juices.
Perception	Understanding based on impressions and feelings.
Percussion	Technique used to evaluate size, border and consistency of some organs and to discover the presence and evaluate the amount of fluid in a body cavity.
Perennial	Present at all seasons of the year; permanent, consistent.
Perinatal death	Death of an infant before, during, or shortly after birth.
Perineal care	Care given the genitalia.
Periodontal disease	Disease of the tissues around the teeth.
Perioperative period	Entire surgical inpatient period, from admission to date of discharge.
Periorbital edema	Swelling around the eyes, which may indicate a pathological condition of the kidney.
Periosteum	Fibrous, vascular membrane covering the bones, except at their extremities; consists of an outer layer of collagenous tissues containing a few fat cells and an inner layer of fine, elastic fibers.
Peripheral nervous system	Motor and sensory nerves and ganglia outside the brain and spinal cord.
Peripheral parenteral nutrition (PPN)	Administration of a nutritionally adequate solution into a peripheral vein.
Pernicious anemia	Progressive decrease in blood hemoglobin, affecting mainly older people and resulting from lack of the factor essential for absorbing vitamin B_{12}.
Personality	Unique pattern of the mental, emotional and behavioral traits of an individual.
PGL	Persistent generalized lymphedema
Phagocytosis	Process by which certain cells engulf and dispose of microorganisms and cell debris.
Phalanges	Any one of 14 tapering bones composing the finger of each hand and the toes of each foot.

Pharynx	Throat; a tubular structure about 13 cm long that extends from the base of the skull to the esophagus.
Phimosis	Narrowing of the prepuce opening so that the foreskin of the penis cannot be retracted.
Phlebothrombosis	Abnormal condition in which a clot forms within a vein.
Phobia	Irrational, exaggerated fear of an object, activity or situation.
Phosphate (HPO4)	Salt element of phosphoric acid.
Physiatrist	Physician who specializes in the field of rehabilitation.
Physician's orders	Specific orders by a physician for a patient's medical care.
Physiology	Study of functions of the various organs and tissues of the body.
Pia mater	Innermost of the three meninges covering the brain and the spinal cord. It is closely applied to both structures and carries a rich supply of blood vessels, which nourish the nervous tissue.
Pica	Craving to eat substances that are not foods, as dirt, clay, chalk, glue, ice, starch or hair.
PIH	Pregnancy-induced hypertension.
Pinocytosis	Process by which extracellular fluid is taken into a cell. The cell membrane develops a saccular indentation filled with extracellular fluid and then closes around it, forming a vesicle or a vacuole of fluid within the cell.
Pituitary gland	Small gland attached to the hypothalamus and couched in the sphenoid bone, supplying numerous hormones that govern many vital processes.
Placebo	Inactive substances, such as saline, distilled water or sugar, prescribed as if it were a needed medication.
Plaintiff	Person who files a lawsuit initiating a legal action.
Pleural effusion	Accumulation of nonpurulent fluid in the space between the visceral and parietal pleura.
Pleural space	Potential space between the visceral and parietal layers of the pleurae.
Pleurisy	Inflammation of the parietal pleura of the lungs, characterized by dyspnea and stabbing pain, leading to restriction of ordinary breathing with spasm of the chest on the affected side.
Pluralistic society	Society in which numerous distinct ethnic, religious or cultural groups coexist within one nation.
Pneumonia	Acute inflammation of the lungs, often caused by inhaled pneumococci.
Poisoning	Condition or physical state produced by the ingestion, injection or inhalation of or exposure to a poisonous substance.
Polydipsia	Excessive thirst.
Polyphagia	Excessive hunger.
Polyuria	Excretion of abnormally large amounts of urine.
Pons	Prominence on the ventral surface of the brainstem, between the medulla oblongata and the cerebral peduncles of the midbrain. The pons consists of white matter and a few nuclei and is divided into a ventral and a dorsal portion.
Portal of entry	Route by which microorganisms enter the human body.
Position	Relationship of a fetal reference point with respect to its location in the maternal pelvis.
Postmortem care	Care of the body after death.
Posterior	Back part of a structure; toward the back.
Posterior fontanel	Triangular-shaped area at center back of head.
Postictal period	Time immediately after a convulsion (usually a grand mal seizure).
Postprandial	After a meal.
Posture	Position of the body with respect to the surrounding space; the sense of balance.
Potassium (K+)	Alkali metal element that is necessary to the life of all plants and animals; the chief intracellular electrolyte.
Potentiation	Synergistic action in which the effect of two drugs given at the same time is greater than the effect of the drugs given separately.
PQRST	Method used when gathering information during a patient interview; P—provocative, palliative; Q—quality, quantity; R—region, radiation; S—severity scale; T—timing.
Preadolescence (Prepubescence)	Period from about age 9 or 10 until the onset of puberty, characterized by an increase in hormone production.
Preeclampsia	Abnormal condition of pregnancy characterized by the onset of acute hypertension after the twenty-fourth week of gestation.
Premenstrual syndrome	Group of signs and symptoms occurring about a week before menstruation, associated with fluid retention.
Presbycusis	Normal loss of hearing, speech and pitch associated with aging.
Presbyopia	Decreasing elasticity of the lens and power of accommodation, so that vision of near objects is blurred or indistinct.
Preschooler	Ages 3 to 5½ years.
Presentation	Part of the fetus that first appears in the pelvis.
Primary caregiver	First or responsible person in decision making or providing care to an ill person.
Primipara	Woman who has given birth to one viable infant.
Prn (pro re nata)	When required.
Problem list for POMR	Prioritized master list of the patient's active, inactive, temporary, potential medical and other problems; serves as an index to the rest of the record.

Problem-oriented medical record (POMR)	Method of recording data about the health status of a patient in a problem-solving system. Parts included are the data base, problem list, initial plan and progress notes.
Procidentia	Downward displacement of an organ; usually applied to a prolapsed uterus.
Progesterones	Female hormones that prepare the uterus to accept a fetus and maintain the pregnancy.
Progress notes	Notes made by a nurse, physician or other team member that describe the patient's condition and the treatments given and planned.
Proliferate	To produce or multiply.
Prone	Lying face down.
Proprioception	Awareness of the position of one's body; pertaining to stimuli originating from within the body regarding spatial position.
Proprioceptor	Any sensory nerve ending, such as those located in muscles, tendons and joints that responds to stimuli originating from within the body regarding movement and spatial position.
Prosthesis	Artificial replacement for a missing body part.
Protein (dietary)	Any large group of naturally occurring, complex, organic nitrogenous compounds necessary for proper growth, development and maintenance of health.
Protest	Initial grief response in separation from attachment figure.
Pruritus	Itching.
PSRO (Professional Standards Review Organization)	Physicians review the services provided under Medicare, Medicaid, and Maternal-Child Health programs to ensure standards are being met and to ascertain the need for the program.
Psychoactive material	Substance that affects mental activity.
Psychological age	Behavioral capacity of the person to adapt to changing environmental demands; includes capacities of memory, learning intelligence, skills, feelings, and motivations for exercising behavioral control or self-regulation.
Psychosocial	Intellectual, emotional and social components of the individual.
Psychotic	State characterized by gross distortion of reality and impaired social functioning.
Ptosis	Drooping of the eyelids.
Pubarche	Beginning development of certain secondary sex characteristics preceding physiological puberty.
Puberty	State of physical development when sexual reproduction first becomes possible with menstruation and spermatogenesis (10 to 14 years for females; 12 to 16 years for males).
Public health nursing	Nursing assessment, identification of high-risk groups, intervention directed at disease prevention and health education and promotion for all ages, groups and individuals.
Puerperium	Time after childbirth approximately 6 weeks, during which anatomical and physiological changes brought about by pregnancy resolve.
Pulmonary edema	Accumulation of extravascular fluid in lung tissues and alveoli, caused most commonly by congestive heart failure.
Pulmonary embolus (PE)	Occlusion of a pulmonary artery by foreign matter, such as fat, air, tumor tissue, or a thrombus, that usually arises from a peripheral vein.
Pulse deficit	Condition that exists when the radial pulse rate is less than the ventricular rate.
Pulse pressure	Difference between systolic and diastolic pressure, usually 30 to 40 mm Hg.
Pulverized	Crushed into a powdered form.
Punctum	Tiny opening in the margin of each eyelid that opens into the tear duct.
Pupillary reflex	Adjustment of the eyes for near vision consisting of pupillary constriction.
Purulent	Producing or containing pus.
Pustule	Small elevation of the skin containing fluid that is usually purulent.
PWA	Person with AIDS.
Pyrexic fever	Having a body temperature above 98.6° F (37°C).
Pyrosis	Heartburn; painful burning centered in the esophagus just below the sternum, often caused by reflux of gastric contents into the esophagus or by gastric hyperacidity.
Quadratectomy	Removal of a quadrant of the breast along with overlying skin.
Quality assurance	Evaluation of services provided and results achieved as compared with accepted standards.
RACE	Rescue patients; sound the Alarm; Confine the fire; and Extinguish or evacuate.
Racism	Any ethnocentric activity—cultural, individual, or institutional, deliberate or not—that is based on a belief in the superiority of one racial group over other racial groups, thus maintaining the oppression and control of these groups.
Radial pulse	Pulse of the radial artery, felt at the wrist over the radium.
Range-of-motion exercise	Anybody action involving the muscles, the joints and natural directional movement.
Rapid eye movement (REM) sleep	Period of sleep when dreams occur, characterized by rapid movement of the closed eyes.
Reagent	Substance producing a chemical reaction.

Receptor	Sensory nerve ending that responds to various kinds of stimulation.
Reconstituted/blended family	Divorced or widowed adult and a new spouse, with each adult's own child(ren) plus the child(ren) of the new partnership, if any, who live together.
Recumbent	Lying down; reclining.
Referred pain	Pain felt at a site other than its origin.
Reflection	Therapist's repetition of statements made by the patient; helps to clarify information.
Reflex	Reflected action, particularly an involuntary action or movement.
Rehabilitation	Process of assisting an individual after a disabling event has occurred.
Remission	Partial or complete disappearance of the clinical and subjective characteristics of a chronic or malignant disease.
Residual urine	Urine left in the bladder after the patient has voided.
Residue	Bulk in the colon that includes undigested food, fiber, bacteria, body secretions and cells.
Respite	Period of relief from responsibilities for the care of a patient.
Responsibility	Moral, legal or mental accountability.
Restraint	Anyone of numerous devices used in aiding the immobilization of patients.
Resume	Summary of one's career and qualifications, prepared typically by an applicant for a position; a brief biography.
Retention	Inability to urinate.
Retraction	Visible sinking of soft tissue of the chest between and around the firmer tissue of the ribs as occurs with increased respiratory effort.
Retrovirus	Member of a family of viruses that alter genetic structure of the host cell by changing RNA to DNA, reversing the usual flow of genetic information.
Reversibility	Performance of opposite mental actions with the same problem or situation, such as addition and subtraction, multiplication and division.
Review of systems (ROS)	System-by-system review of the body functions. ROS is begun during the initial interview.
Rhizotomy	Resection of a posterior nerve root just before it enters the spinal cord, usually performed to control severe pain in the upper trunk or to relieve severe spasms.
Ribosome	Cytoplasmic organelle composed of ribonucleic acid and protein that functions in the synthesis of protein.
Role	Character assigned or assumed; a socially expected behavior pattern usually determined by an individual's status in a particular society.
ROM	Range of motion.
Rubor	Redness, especially when accompanying inflammation.
Rule of nines	Formula for estimating the amount of body surface covered by burns. In the adult 9% is assigned to head and each arm, 18% to each leg, 18% to the anterior and posterior trunk, and 1% to the perineum.
SOAPE charting	Charting format used in POMR. Components include subjective data (S) reported by the patient; objective data (O) acquired by inspection, percussion, auscultation and palpation and by tests, usually measurable findings; assessment (A) of the problem; plan (P) of care; and evaluation (E) of patient's response to the treatment plan.
SOAPIER charting	Same as SOAPE charting except that intervention (I) and revision (R) are added. Interventions are specific actions carried out and revisions are the changes to be made to the original plan.
Sanguineous	Pertaining to blood.
Sarcoma	Malignant neoplasm of connective tissues arising in fibrous, fatty, muscular, synovial, vascular or neural tissue.
Satiety	Feeling of fullness and satisfaction from food.
Scale	Small, thin flake of keratinized (dried-out) epithelium.
Scar	Connective tissue that is avascular, pale, contracted, and firm after the earlier phase of healing.
School age	Period from about six to sixteen years of age.
Sclera	Tough, inelastic, opaque membrane covering the posterior five sixths of the eyeball. It maintains the size and form of the eye and attaches to muscles that move it.
Scoliosis	Lateral or S curvature of the spine.
Scurvy	Condition resulting from lack of ascorbic acid (vitamin C) in the diet.
Sebaceous gland	One of the many small organs in the dermis (skin); secretes oil.
Sebum	Oily secretion from the sebaceous glands.
Secondary gain	Material, emotional or social advantage acquired as a result of a symptom or an illness.
Self-bath	Bath done by the patient in bed or at the bedside.
Self-despair	Feeling that life has not been satisfactory and having a desire to relive it.
Semicircular canals	Any of three bony, fluid-filled loops in the osseous labyrinth of the internal ear, associated with the sense of balance.
Semilunar valve	Valve with half-moon-shaped cusps, as the aortic valve and the pulmonary valve.
Senescence	Mental and physical decline associated with aging.
Sensitivity	Susceptibility to a substance, such as a drug or an antigen.

Separation anxiety	Fear and apprehension caused by separation from familiar surroundings and significant persons.
Septum	Partition, as the interauricular septum that separates the atria of the heart.
Sequela	Any abnormal condition that occurs after a disease, treatment or injury.
Seriation	Mental ordering of objects according to height, weight or strength.
Seroconversion	Point at which a pathogenic organism can be identified in the blood.
Serosanguineous	Composed of serum and blood.
Sex education	Factual teaching about anatomy and physiology related to the sex act and reproduction.
Sex hormones	Biochemical agents that influence structure and function of sex organs and appearance of sexual characteristics.
Sexuality education	Learning about self as a sexual being.
Shearing	Force causing two contacting parts to slide upon one another.
Sibling	Brother or sister.
Sign	Objective finding of an examiner, such as a fever or a rash.
Sims	Position in which the patient lies on the side with the superior knee flexed and the thigh drawn upward toward the chest. The chest and abdomen are allowed to fall forward.
Single parent	One parent who lives with the child(ren).
Sitz bath	Bath in which only the hips and buttocks are immersed in water or saline solution; the time allotted is 20 to 30 minutes.
Skin graft	Portion of skin implanted to cover areas where skin has been lost by burns or injury.
Skin impairment	Irritated skin that breaks open and becomes a decubitus ulcer which can penetrate to the bone.
Smear	Material placed on a microscopic slide or culture medium.
Snellen's test	Chart test used to determine visual acuity.
Social age	Roles and habits of a person with respect to other members of society, resulting from the person's life course through various social institutions.
Social network	Interconnected group of cooperating significant others, related or not, with whom a person interacts.
Sodium	Soft, gray, alkaline metal that is the chief electrolyte in interstitial fluid.
Somatization	Physical manifestation of an individual's feelings, emotional needs, or conflicts.
Souffle cup	Small, white, pleated paper cup used to contain nonliquid oral medications.
Spastic	Of or pertaining to spasms or other uncontrolled contractions of the skeletal muscles.
Specific immunity (or active acquired immunity)	Form of acquired immunity that results from production of anti-bodies in the cells.
Specimen	Small sample, such as of blood or urine.
Speech	Uttering of vocal sounds that form words and express thoughts.
Spermatogenesis	Production of spermatozoa.
Sphygmomanometer	Device for measuring arterial blood pressure.
Spiritual life	That aspect of life involving religious beliefs or value systems.
Spondylolisthesis	Partial forward dislocation of a vertebra over the one below it, most commonly the fifth lumbar vertebra over the first sacral vertebra.
Stagnation or self-absorption	Regression into adolescent or younger behavior, characterized by physical and psychological invalidism.
Stapedectomy	Removal of the stapes of the middle ear and insertion of a graft to restore hearing.
Stapes	One of three tiny ossicles in the middle ear, resembling a stirrup.
Stasis	Disorder in which the normal flow of a fluid through a vessel of the body is slowed or halted.
Statute	Legislative act declaring, commanding or prohibiting something.
Sterile	Free of germs.
Sterilization	Destruction of microorganisms using heat, water, chemicals or gases.
Stethoscope	Device for listening to heart, vascular, lung and bowel sounds.
Stomatitis	Any inflammatory condition of the mouth; may result from drugs used for cancer.
Strabismus	Cross-eye.
Stress	Specific response by the body to a stimulus that disturbs normal functioning.
Stressor	Any factor that causes stress. Common ones include change and loss.
Stridor	Abnormal, high-pitched, musical respiratory sound caused by an obstruction in the trachea or larynx.
Subculture	Large group of people who, although members of a still larger cultural group, has shared characteristics exclusive to its subgroup.
Subjective data	Patient's perceptions and feelings about himself and what is happening to him. Only the patient can give subjective data.
Subjective data collection	Process in which data relating to the patient's problems are elicited from the patient.
Sublingual	Beneath the tongue.
Subluxation	Partial dislocation.
Sudoriferous gland	One of about three million tiny structures within the dermis that produce sweat.

Suicide	Self-inflicted death.
Sulfate (SO4)	Salt of sulfuric acid, which is plentiful in the body.
Summons	Document issued by a clerk of the court on the filing of a complaint.
Supine	Position in which the patient lies horizontally on the back.
Suppression	Cessation of urine production (anuria).
Suppuration	Production of purulent (puscontaining) matter.
Surface tension	Tendency of the surface of a liquid to contract; causes liquids to rise in a capillary tube, affects the exchange of gases in the pulmonary alveoli and alters the ability of various liquids to wet another surface.
Surfactant	Certain lipoproteins that reduce the surface tension of pulmonary fluids, allowing the exchange of gases in the lungs and contributing to the elasticity of pulmonary tissues.
Surgery	Branch of medicine concerned with diseases and trauma requiring operative procedures.
Surgical asepsis	Protection against infection by destruction of all microorganisms and their spores or reproductive cells.
Suture	Surgical stitch taken to repair a tear, incision or wound.
Sweat test	Method for evaluating sodium and chloride excretion from the sweat glands; often the first test performed in the diagnosis of cystic fibrosis.
Sympathetic nervous system	Part of the nervous system that accelerates heart rate, constricts blood vessels and raises blood pressure.
Symptom	Subjective indication of a disease or a change in condition as perceived by the patient.
Synarthrosis	Anyone of many immovable joints, such as those of the skull segments, in which a fibrous tissue or a hyaline cartilage connects the bones.
Syncope	Brief lapse of consciousness; fainting.
Syndrome	Complex of signs and symptoms.
Synovectomy	Excision of a synovial membrane of a joint.
Syntaxic (consensual) communication	Communication in which two people can understand the meaning of their dialogue together, explore and agree on meanings of words used and speak in cause-effect relationships.
Systole	Contractions of the heart, driving blood into the aorta and pulmonary arteries; the first heart sound heard on auscultation during the blood pressure procedure.
T-cell	A small, circulating lymphocyte that participates in cellular immune responses, such as graft rejection and delayed hypersensitivity.
Tachycardia	Abnormally rapid heart rate of more than 100 beats per minute.
Tachypnea	Abnormal rate of breathing, greater than 26 breaths per minute.
Tactile fremitus	Tremulous vibrations of the chest wall felt on palpation.
TBI	Traumatic brain injury.
Tendon	One of many white, glistening, fibrous bands of tissue that attach muscle to bone.
Tenesmus	Persistent, ineffectual spasms of the rectum or bladder, accompanied by the desire to empty the bowel or bladder.
TENS	*See transcutaneous electrical nerve stimulation.*
Tepid	Moderately warm to the touch.
Teratogenic	Any substance, agent or product that interferes with normal prenatal development, causing the formation of one or more developmental abnormalities in the fetus.
Testosterone	Male hormone that contributes to development of male characteristics.
Tetanus toxoid	Active agent prepared from detoxified tetanus toxin that produces an antigenic response in the body, conferring permanent immunity to tetanus infection.
Tetany	Condition characterized by cramps, muscle twitching and possibly convulsions.
Therapeutic	Beneficial, such as a dose of medication that produces a helpful effect.
Therapeutic communication	Process in which a nurse helps the patient to a better understanding through verbal or nonverbal communication.
Third-party-payers	Entities other than the giver or receiver of the service responsible for payment, e.g. medicare or insurance companies.
Thoracic cord injury	Spinal injury that usually involves partial trunk and lower extremity paralysis.
Thrill	Fine vibration felt by the examiner, indicating an organic murmur.
Thrombocytes (platelets)	Smallest cells in the blood. They are disk-shaped, contain no hemoglobin and are essential for clotting of the blood.
Thrombophlebitis	Inflammation of a vein that often accompanies formation of a clot.
Thrombus	Accumulation of platelets, fibrin, clotting factors and the cellular elements of blood, attached to the interior wall of a vein or artery and sometimes occluding the lumen.
Thymus gland	Located in the mediastinum, the primary gland of the lymphatic system.

Thyroid gland	Highly vascular organ at the front of the neck; secretes thyroxin.
Tibia	Second longest bone in the skeleton, located at the medial side of the leg. It articulates with the fibula laterally, the talus distally and the femur proximally, forming part of the knee joint.
Tinnitus	Tingling or ringing in one or both ears.
Tissue	Collection of similar cells that act together in the performance of a particular function.
TMJ	Temporomandibular joint.
Toddler	Ages 1 to 3 years.
Tolerance	Ability to consume ordinarily injurious quantities of such substances as drugs or alcohol without apparent physiological or psychological injury.
Tongue depressor	Wooden blade used to facilitate examination of the throat.
Tonus(ic)	Normal state of balanced tension in the tissues of the body, especially the muscles.
Tophus	Abnormal stone, containing sodium urate deposits that develops in periarticular fibrous tissue, typically in patients with gout.
Tort	Civil wrong, other than a breach of contract.
Total parenteral nutrition (TPN)	Administration of a nutritionally complete solution through a central vein.
Toxicity	Degree to which something is poisonous.
Tracheotomy	Incision made into the trachea through the neck below the larynx, performed to gain access to the airway below blockage with a foreign body, tumor or edema of the glottis.
Tract	In neurology, the neuronal axons grouped together to form a pathway.
Traction	Having a limb, bone or group of muscles under tension with weights and pulleys; aligns or immobilizes the part and relieves pressure on it.
Traditional or block chart	Conventional patient chart broken down into sections or blocks; included are admission data, physicians' orders, history, physical, nursing care plan, nurses' notes graphics, progress notes, and test data.
Transcribing	Making a copy of, in longhand or on a typewriter.
Transcutaneous electrical neural stimulation (TENS)	Alteration of pain sensations by stimulating peripheral nerves; uses application of electric current to the skin.
Transfer	Moving a patient from one unit to another within an institution or moving a patient from one health care facility to another.
Transformation	Shift from one state to another, such as water to ice to vapor.
Transient ischemic attack (TIA)	Episode of cerebrovascular insufficiency, usually owing to partial occlusion of an artery by an atherosclerotic plaque or embolism.
Trauma	Physical injury caused by violent/disruptive action.
Trichomoniasis	Vaginal infection caused by the protozoan *Trichomonas vaginalis*.
Trophic	Having to do with nutritional status.
Trousseau's sign	Test for latent tetany, in which carpal spasm is induced with a sphygmomanometer cuff on the upper arm.
Trust	Risk-taking process whereby an individual's situation depends on the future behavior of another person.
Tube feeding	Administration of nutritionally balanced, liquefied foods or formula into the stomach, duodenum or jejunum by way of a nasoenteric tube or a feeding ostomy.
Turgor	Normal resiliency of the skin caused by outward pressure of cells and interstitial fluid. Decreased turgor indicates dehydration; increased turgor indicates edema.
Tylectomy	Partial mastectomy/lumpectomy; the removal of involved breast tissue (about one fourth or one third of the breast), preserving contour and muscle function.
Tympanic membrane	Thin, semitransparent membrane in the middle ear that transmits sound vibrations.
Tympanoplasty	Surgical procedure performed on the eardrum to restore or improve hearing in patients with conductive deafness.
Tympanostomy tube	Tubes inserted under general anaesthesia to drain accumulated fluid from the middle ear space; also called *pressure equalizer (PE) tubes.*
Type I diabetes mellitus	Insulin-dependent diabetes mellitus.
Type II diabetes mellitus	Non-insulin-dependent diabetes mellitus.
Umbilical cord	Bluish-white, gelatinous structure that transports maternal blood from the placenta to fetus.
Umbilicus	Point on the abdomen at which the umbilical cord joined the fetus. In most adults it is marked by a depression.
Universal donor	Person with type O, Rh factor-negative blood. Such blood may be used for emergency transfusion with minimal risk of incompatibility.
Universal precautions	CDC-recommended "universal blood and body fluid precautions" (prevent injury from needles and sharps; wear protective devices during resuscitation; avoid patient and equipment contact if draining lesion exists in health care worker).
Urate	Any salt of uric acid, as sodium urate.
Ureter	One of a pair of tubes that carry urine from the kidney to the bladder.
Urinal	Metal or plastic receptacle for urine—may be designed for male or female patients.

Urolithiasis	Calculus (stone) formed in any part of the urinary tract.
Urticaria	Itching skin eruption characterized by welts of varying sizes with well-defined, inflamed margins and pale centers (also called *hives*).
Value system	Accepted mode of conduct and set of norms, goals and values binding any social group.
Values	Personal beliefs about the worth of an idea or behavior.
Valve	Combining from meaning a thing that regulates the flow of.
Vegan	Vegetarian whose diet excludes all foods of animal origin.
Vehicle	Fluid or structure in the body that passively conveys a stimulus.
Vein	One of many vessels that convey blood from the capillaries to the heart as part of the pulmonary system.
Vena cava	One of the two large veins returning blood from peripheral circulation to the right atrium of the heart.
Ventilator	Person in two-rescuer CPR who performs rescue breathing technique.
Ventricle	Small cavity, such as the one filled with cerebrospinal fluid in the brain or the right and left ventricles of the heart.
Venule	Anyone of the small blood vessels that gather blood from the capillary plexuses and anastomose to form the veins.
Vertigo	Dizziness; a sensation of faintness or an inability to maintain normal balance in a standing or seated position.
Vesicle	Small, thin-walled, raised skin lesion containing clear fluid; a blister.
Viable	Capable of developing, growing and otherwise sustaining life.
Virulence	Power of a microorganism to produce disease.
Viscus	Internal organs within a body cavity, primarily the abdominal organs.
Visual analog scale	Rating scale using a line to represent a continuum. The ends are marked for two extremes of pain.
Vital signs	Measurements of temperature, pulse, respiration and blood pressure.
Vitamin	Organic compound essential in small quantities for normal physiological and metabolic functioning of the body.
Vitreous humor	Transparent, semigelatinous substance filling the cavity behind the crystalline lens of the eye.
Vomer	Bone forming the posterior and inferior part of the nasal septum, having two surfaces and four borders.
Weaning	(1) Gradually eliminating breast or bottle-feeding, replaced by cup and table feeding, (2) Withdrawing a person from something on which he is dependent.
Wellness	Dynamic state of health in which an individual progresses toward a higher level of functioning, achieving an optimum balance between internal and external environments.
Wernicke's encephalopathy	Inflammatory, hemorrhagic, degenerative condition of the brain caused by thiamine deficiency, seen in association with chronic alcoholism.
Wheal	Elevated lesion; an individual lesion of urticaria.
Whirlpool bath	Immersion of the body or part of the body in a tank of hot water agitated by a jet of equally hot water and air.
White matter	Tissue surrounding the gray matter of the spinal cord, consisting mainly of myelinated nerve fibers but with some unmyelinated nerve fibers, embedded in a spongy network of neuroglia.
Widow (er) hood	Status of the surviving spouse after the death of husband or wife.
Wilms' tumor	Malignant neoplasm of the kidney, occuring in young children. The tumor, an embryonal adenomyosarcoma, is well encapsulated in the early stage, but may later extend into the lymph nodes and the renal vein or vena cava and metastasize to the lungs or other sites.
Withdrawal symptoms	Unpleasant, sometimes life-threatening, physiological changes that occur when certain drugs are withdrawn after prolonged, regular use.
Wound	Any physical injury involving a break in the skin; caused by an act or accident rather than by a disease.
Xerostomia	Dryness of the mouth caused by cessation of normal salivation.
Xiphoid process	Small, fragile bone located at the distal end of the sternum.
Young adulthood	Chronologically a period of life from the mid-20s to the mid-40s.

Appendices

APPENDIX 1
NORMAL REFERENCE LABORATORY VALUES

1. BLOOD, PLASMA, OR SERUM VALUES

Determination	Conventional	Reference Range SI	Minimal mL Required†	Note
Acetoacetate plus acetone	Negative	1-B		
Aldolase	1.3-8.2 U/L	22-137 nmol sec^{-1}/L	2-S	Use unhemolyzed serum
Ammonia	12-55 µmol/L	12-55 µmol/L	2-B	Collect in heparinized tube; deliver *immediately* packed in ice
Amylase	4-25 units/mL	4-25 arb. unit	1-S	
Ascorbic acid	0.4-1.5 mg/100 mL	23-85µmol/L	7-B	Collect in heparinized tube before any food is given
Bilirubin	Direct: up to 0.4 mg/100 mL	Up to 7 µmol/L	1-S	
	Total: up to 1.0 mg/100 mL	Up to 17 µmol/L		
Blood volume	8.5-9.0% of body weight in kg	80-85 mL/kg		
Calcium	8.5-10.5 mg/100 mL (slightly higher in children)	2.1-2.6 mmol/L	1-S	
Carbamazepine	4.0-12.0 µg/mL	17-51 µmol/L		
Carbon dioxide content	24-30 mEq/L	24-30 mmol/L	1-S	Fill tube to top
Carbon monoxide	Less than 5% of total hemoglobin		3-B	Fill tube to top
Carotenoids	0.8-4.0 mg/mL	1.5-7.4 µmol/L	3-S	Vitamin A may be done on same specimen
Ceruloplasmin	27-37 mg/100 mL	1.8-2.5 µmol/L	2-S	
Chloramphenicol	10-20 µg/mL	31-62 µmol/L	0.2-S	
Chloride	100-106 mEq/L	100-106 mmol/L	1-S	
CK isoenzymes	5% MB or less		0.2-S	
Copper	Total: 100-200 µg/100 mL	16-31 µmol/L	1-S	
Creatine kinase (CK)	Women: 10-79 U/L	167-1317 nmol.sec^{-1}/L	1-S	
	Men: 17-148 U/L	283-2467 nmol.sec^{-1}/L		
Creatinine	0.6-1.5 mg/100 mL	53-133 µmol	1-S	
Ethanol	0 mg/100 mL	0 mmol/L	2-B	Collect in oxalate and refrigerate
Glucose	Fasting: 70-110 mg/100 mL	3.9-5.6 mmol/L	1-P	Collect with oxalate-fluoride mixture
Iron	50-150 mg/100 mL (higher in men)	9.0-26.9 mmol/L	1-S	
Iron-binding capacity	250-410 µg/100 mL	44.8-73.4 µmol/L	1-S	
Lactic acid	0.6-1.8 mEq/L	0.6-1.8 mmol/L	2-B	Collect with oxalate-fluoride; deliver immediately packed in ice
Lactic dehydrogenase	45-90 U/L	750-1500 nmol.sec^{-1}/L	1-S	Unsuitable if hemolyzed
Lead	50 mg/100 mL or less	Up to 2.4 µmol/L	2-B	Collect with oxalate-fluoride mixture
Lipase	2 U/mL or less	Up to 2 arb. unit	1-S	
Lipids				
Cholesterol	120-220 mg/100 mL	3.10-5.69 mmol/L	1-S	Fasting
Triglycerides	40-150 mg/100 mL	0.4-1.5 g/L	1-S	Fasting
Lipoprotein electro-phoresis (LEP)			2-S	Fasting, do not freeze serum
Lithium	0.5-1.5 mEq/L	0.5-1.5 mmol/L	1-S	
Magnesium	1.5-2.0 mEq/L	0.8-1.3 mmol/L	1-S	
5'Nucleotidase	1-11 U/L	17-183 nmol.sec^{-1}/L	1-S	
Osmolality	280-296 mOsm/kg water	280-296 mmol/kg	1-S	

Contd...

Contd...

Determination	Conventional	Reference Range SI	Minimal mL Required†	Note
		Reference Range	*Minimal mL*	
	Conventional	*SI*	*Required†*	*Note*
Oxygen saturation (arterial) heparinized syringe	96-100%	0.96-1.00	3-B	Deliver in sealed packed in ice
PCO$_2$	35-45 mm Hg	4.7-6.0 kPa	2-B	Collect and deliver in sealed heparinized syringe
pH	7.35-7.45	Same	2-B	Collect without stasis in sealed heparinized syringe; deliver packed in ice
PO$_2$	75-100 mm Hg (dependent on age) while breathing room air Above 500 mm Hg while on 100% O$_2$	10.0-13.3.kPa	2-B	
Phenobarbital	15-50 µg/mL	65-215 µmol/L	1-S	
Phenytoin (Dilantin)	5-20 µg/mL	20-80 µmol/L	1-S	
Phosphatase (acid)	Men—Total: 0.13-0.63 sigma U/mL Women—Total: 0.01-0.56 sigma U/mL Prostatic: 0-0.5 Fishman-Lerner U/100 mL	36-175 nmol.sec^{-1}/L 2.8-156 nmol.sec^{-1}/L	1-S	Must always be drawn just before analysis or stored as frozen serum; avoid hemolysis
Phosphatase (alkaline)	13-39 U/L; infants and adolescents up to 104 U/L sec^{-1}/L	217-650 nmol.sec^{-1}/L; up to 1.26 µmol	1-S	
Phosphorous (inorganic)	3.0-4.5 mg/100 mL (infants in first year up to 6.0 mg/100 mL)	1.0-1.5 mmol/L	1-S	
Potassium	3.5-5.0 mEq/L	3.5-5.0 mmol/L	1-S	Serum must be separated promptly from cells
Primidone (Mysoline)	4-12 µg/mL	18-55 µmol/L	1-S	
Procainamide	4-10 µg/mL	17-42 µmol/L	1-S	
Protein: Total	6.0-8.4 g/100 mL	60-84 g/L	1-S	
Albumin	3.5-5.0 g/100 mL	35-50 g/L	1-S	
Globulin	2.3-3.5 g/100 mL	23-35 g/L		Globulin equals total protein minus albumin
Electrophoresis	(% of total protein)		1-S	Quantitation by densitometry
Albumin	52-68			
Globulin;				
Alpha$_1$	4.2-7.2			
Alpha$_2$	6.8-12			
Beta	9.3-15			
Gamma	13-23			
Pyruvic acid	0-0.11 mEq/L	0-0.11 mmol/L	2-B	Collect with oxalate fluoride. Deliver immediately packed in ice
Quinidine	1.2-4.0 µg/mL	3.7-12.3 µmol/L	1-S	
Salicylate:	0	2-P		
Therapeutic	20-25 mg/100 mL; 25-30 mg/100 mL to age 10 yr 3 hr post dose	1.4-1.8 mmol/L 1.8-2.2 mmol/L		
Sodium	135-145 mEq/L	135-145 mmol/L	1-S	
Sulfonamide	5-15 mg/100 mL	2-P		
Transaminase, SGOT (AST) (aspartate aminotransferase)	7-27 U/L	117-450 nmol.sec^{-1}/L	1-S	
Transaminase, SGPT (ALT) (alanine aminotransferase)	1-21 U/L	17-350 nmol.sec^{-1}/L	1-S	
Urea nitrogen (BUN)	8-25 mg/100 mL	2.9-8.9 mmol/L	1-S	
Uric acid	3.0-7.0 mg/100 mL	0.18-0.42 mmol/L	1-S	
Vitamin A	0.15-0.6 µg/mL	0.5-2.1 µmol/L	3-S	

2. URINE VALUES

Determination	Conventional	Reference Range SI	Minimal mL Required†	Note
Acetone plus acetoacetate (quantitative)	0	0 mg/L	2 mL	
Amylase	24-76 U/mL	24-76 arb.unit		
Calcium	300 mg/day or less	7.5 mmol/day or less	24-hr specimen	Collect in special bottle with 10 mL of concentrated HCl
Catecholamines	Epinephrine:under 20 μg/day Norepinephrine under 100 μg/day	< 109 nmol/day < 590 nmol/day	24-hr specimen	Should be collected with 10 mL of concentrated HCl (pH should be between 2.0 and 3.0)
Chorionic gonadotropin	0	0 arb. unit	Ist morning void	
Copper	0-100 μg/day	0-1.6 μmol/day	24-hr specimen	
Coproporphyrin	50-250 μg/day Children under 80 Ib (36 kg); 0-75 μg/day	80-380 nmol/day 0-115 nmol/day	24-hr specimen carbonate	Collect with 5 g of sodium
Creatine	Under 100 mg/day or less than 6% of creatinine. In pregnancy: up to 12%. In children under 1 yr: may equal creatinine. In older children: up to 30% of creatinine	< 0.75 mmol/day	24-hr specimen	Also order creatinine
Creatinine	15-25 mg/kg of body weight/day	0.13-0.22 mmol.kg^{-1}/day	24-hr specimen	
Cystine or cysteine	0	0	10 mL	Qualitative
Hemoglobin and myoglobin	0		Freshly voided sample	Chemical examination with benzidine
5-Hydroxyindoleacetic acid	2-9 mg/day (women lower than men)	10-45 μmol/day	24-hr specimen	Collect with 10 mL of concentrated HCl
Lead	0.08 μg/mL or 120 μg/day or	0.39 μmol/L or less	24-hr specimen	
Phosphorus (inorganic)	Varies with intake; average, 1 g/day	32 mmol/day	24-hr specimen	Collect with 10 mL of concentrated HCl
Porphobilinogen	0	0	10 mL	Use freshly voided urine
Protein: Quantitative	< 150 mg/24 hr	< 0.15 g/day	24-hr specimen	
Steroids: 17-Ketosteroids (per day)	Age Boys/Men Girls/Women 10 1-4 mg 1-4 mg 20 6-21 mg 4-16 mg 30 8-26 mg 4-14 mg 50 5-18 mg 3-9 mg 70 2-10 mg 1-7 mg	Boys/Men Girls/Women 3-14 μmol 3-14 μmol 21-73 μmol 14-56 μmol 28-90 μmol 14-49 μmol 17-62 μmol 10-31 μmol 7-35 μmol 8-24 μmol	24-hr specimen	Not valid if patient is receiving meprobamate
17-Hydroxysteroids	3-8 mg/day (women lower than men)	8-22 μmol/day as tetrahydrocortisol	24-hr specimen	Keep cold; chlorpromazine and related drugs interfere with assay
Sugar; Quantitative glucose	0 specimen	0 mmol/L	24-hr or other timed	
Urobilinogen	Up to 1.0 Ehrlich U	To 1.0 arb. unit	2-hr sample (1-3 p.m.)	
Uroporphyrin	0-30 μg/day	< 36 nmol/day	See Coproporphyrin	
Vanillylmandelic acid (VMA)	Up to 9 mg/24 hr	Up to 45 μmol/day	24-hr specimen catecholamines	Collect as for

3. SPECIAL ENDOCRINE TESTS

(i) Steroid Hormones

Determination	Conventional	Reference Range SI	Minimal mL Required†	Note
Aldosterone	Excretion:		5/day	Keep specimen cold
	5-19 µg/24 hr	14-53 nmol/day		
	Supine:		3-S, P	Fasting, at rest, 210-mEq sodium diet
	48 ± 29 pg/mL	133 ± 80 pmol/L		
	Upright (2 hr):			
	65 ± 23 pg/mL	180 ± 64 pmol/L		Upright, 2 hr, 210-mEq sodium diet
	Supine:			
	107 ± 45 pg/mL	279 ± 125 pmol/L		Fasting, at rest, 110-mEq sodium diet
	Upright (2 hr):			
	239 ± 123 pg/mL	663 ± 341 pmol/L		Upright, 2 hr, 110-mEq sodium diet
	Supine:			
	175 ± 75 pg/mL	485 ± 208 pmol/L		Fasting, at rest, 10-mEq sodium diet
	Upright (2 hr):			
	532 ± 228 pg/mL	1476 ± 632 pmol/L		Upright, 2 hr, 10-mEq sodium diet
Cortisol	8 a.m.:		1-P	Fasting
	5-25 µg/100 mL	0.14-0.69 µmol/L		
	8 p.m.:		1-P	At rest
	Below 10 µg/100 mL	0-0.28 µmol/L		
	4-hr ACTH test:		1-P	20 U ACTH, IV per 4 hr
	30-45 µg/100 mL	0.83-1.24 µmol/L		
	Overnight suppression test:		1-P	8 a.m. sample after 0.5 mg dexamethasone by mouth at midnight
	Below 5 µg/100 mL	0.14 nmol/L		
	Excretion:		2/day	Keep specimen cold
	20-70 µg/24 hr	55-193 nmol/day		
Dehydroepiandro-sterone (DHEA)	Men: 0.5-5.5 ng/mL	1.7-19 nmol/L	2-S, P	
	Women:			
	1.4-8.0 ng/mL	4.9-28 nmol/L		Adult
	0.3-4.5 ng/mL	1.0-15.6 nmol/L		Postmenopausal
Dehydroepiandro-sterone sulfate (DHEA-S)	Men:		2-S, P	
	151-446 µg/100 mL	3.9-11.4 µmol/L		
	Women:			
	84-433 µg/100 mL	2.2-11.1 µmol/L		Adult
	1.7-177 µg/100 mL	0.04-4.5 µmol/L		Postmenopausal
11-Deoxycortisol	Responsive:		1-P	8 a.m. sample, preceded by 4.5 g of metyrapone by mouth per 24 hr or by single dose of 2.5 g by mouth at midnight
	Over 7.5 µg/100 mL	> 0.22 µmol/L		
Estradiol	Men: < 50 pg/mL	< 184 pmol/L	5-S, P	
	Women: 23-361 pg/mL	84-1325 pmol/L		Adult
	< 30 pg/mL	< 110 pmol/L		Postmenopausal
	< 20 pg/mL	< 73 pmol/L		Prepubertal
Progesterone	Men: < 1.0 ng/mL	< 3.2 nmol/L	5-S, P	
	Women:			
	0.2-0.6 ng/mL	0.6-1.9 nmol/L		Follicular phase
	0.3-3.5 ng/mL	0.95-11 nmol/L		Midcycle peak
	6.5-32.2 ng/mL	21-102 nmol/L		Postovulatory
Testosterone	Adult men:		1-P	a.m. sample
	300-1100 ng/100 mL	10.4-38.1 nmol/L		
	Adolescent boys:			
	Over 100 ng/100 mL	> 3.5 nmol/L		
	Women:			
	25-90 ng/100 mL	0.87-3.12 nmol/L		
Unbound testosterone	Adult men:		2-P	a.m. sample
	3.06-24.0 ng/100 mL	106-832 pmol/L		
	Adult women:			
	0.09-1.28 ng/100 mL	3.1-44.4 pmol/L		

(ii) Polypeptide Hormones

Determination	Conventional	Reference Range SI	Minimal mL Required†	Note
Adrenocorticotropin (ACTH)	15-70 pg/mL	3.3-15.4 pmol/L	5-P	Place specimen on ice and send promptly to laboratory. Use EDTA tube only
Alpha subunit	< 0.5-2.5 ng/mL	< 0.4-2.0 nmol/L	2-S	Adult men or women
	< 0.5-5.0 ng/mL	< 0.4-4.0 nmol/L		Postmenopausal women
Calcitonin	Men: 0-14 pg/mL	0-4.1 pmol/L	5-S	Test done only on known or suspected
	Women: 0-28 pg/mL	0-8.2 pmol/L		cases of medullary carcinoma of the
	> 100 pg/mL in medullary carcinoma	> 29.3 pmol/L		thyroid
Follicle-stimulating hormone (FSH)	Men: 3-18 mU/mL	3-18 arb. unit	5-S, P	Same sample may be used for LH
	Women: 4.6-22.4 mU/mL	4.6-22.4 arb. unit		Pre- or postovulatory
	13-41 mU/mL	13-41 arb. unit		Midcycle peak
	30-170 mU/mL	30-170 arb. unit		Postmenopausal
Growth hormone	Below 5 ng/mL	< 233 pmol/L	1-S	Fasting, at rest
	Children: Over 10 ng/mL	> 465 pmol/L		After exercise
	Men: Below 5 ng/mL	< 233 pmol/L		
	Women: Up to 30 ng/mL	0-1395 pmol/L		
	Men: Below 5 ng/mL	< 233 pmol/L		After glucose load
	Women: Below 5 ng/mL	< 233 pmol/L		
Insulin	6-26 μU/mL	43-187 pmol/L	1-S	Fasting
	Below 20 μU/mL	< 144 pmol/L		During hypoglycemia
	Up to 150 μU/mL	0-1078 pmol/L		After glucose load
Luteinizing hormone (LH)	Male: 3-18 mU/mL	3-18 arb. unit	5-S, P	Same sample may be used for FSH
	Female:			
	2.4-34.5 mU/mL	2.4-34.5 arb. unit		Pre- or postovulatory
	43-187 mU/mL	43-187 arb. unit		Midcycle peak
	30-150 mU/mL	30-150 arb. unit		Postmenopausal
Parathyroid hormone	< 25 pg/mL	< 2.94 pmol/L	5-P	Keep blood on ice, or plasma must be frozen if it is to be sent any distance; a.m. sample
Prolactin	2-15 ng/mL	0.08-6.0 nmol/L	2-S	
Renin activity	Supine:		4-P	EDTA tubes, on ice, normal diet
	1.1 ± 0.8 ng/mL/hr	0.9 ± 0.6 nmol/L/hr		
	Upright:			
	1.9 ± 1.7 ng/mL/hr	1.5 ± 1.3 nmol/L/hr		
	Supine:			Low-sodium diet
	2.7 ± 1.8 ng/mL/hr	2.1 ± 1.4 nmol/L/hr		
	Upright:			
	6.6 ± 2.5 ng/mL/hr	5.1 ± 1.9 nmol/L/hr		
	Diuretics:			Low-sodium diet
	10.0 ± 3.7 ng/mL/hr	7.7 ± 2.9 nmol/L/hr		
Somatomedin C (Sm-C, IGF-1)	0.08-2.8 U/mL	0.08-2.8 arb. unit	2-P	EDTA plasma
	0.9-5.9 U/mL	0.9-5.9 arb. unit		Prepubertal
	0.34-1.9 U/mL	0.34-1.9 arb. unit		During puberty
	0.45-2.2 U/mL	0.45-2.2 arb. unit		Adult men
				Adult women

(iii) Thyroid Hormones

Determination	Conventional	Reference Range SI	Minimal mL Required†	Note
Thyroid-stimulating hormone (TSH)	0.5-5.0 μU/mL	0.5-5.0 arb. unit	2-S	
Thyroxine-binding globulin capacity	15-25 μg T_4/100 mL	193-322 nmol/L	2-S	
Total triiodothyronine (T_3)	75-195 ng/100 mL	1.16-3.00 nmol/L	2-S	
Reverse triiodo-thyronine (rT_3)	13-53 ng/mL	0.2-0.8 nmol/L	2-S	
Total thyroxine by RIA (T_4)	4-12 μg/100 mL	52-154 nmol/L	1-S	
T_3 resin uptake	25-35%	0.25-0.35%	2-S	
Free thyroxine index (FT_4I)	1-4		2-S	

4. VITAMIN D DERIVATIVES

Determination	Conventional	Reference Range		Minimal mL Required†	Note
		SI			
1, 25 Dihydroxy-vitamin D	26-65 pg/mL	62-155 pmol/L		1-S	
25-Hydroxy-vitamin D	8-55 ng/mL	19.4-137 nmol/L		1-S	

5. HEMATOLOGIC VALUES

Determination	Conventional	Reference Range	Minimal mL Required†	Note
		SI		
Coagulation factors:				
Factor I (fibrinogen)	0.15-0.35 g/100 mL	4.0-10.0 μmol/L	4.5-P	Collect in vacutainer containing sodium citrate
Factor II (prothrombin)	60-140%	0.60-1.40	4.5-P	Collect in plastic tubes with 3.8% sodium citrate
Factor V (accelerator globulin)	60-140%	0.60-1.40	4.5-P	Collect as in factor II determination
Factor VII-X (proconvertin-Stuart)	70-130%	0.70-1.30	4.5-P	Collect as in factor II determination
Factor X (Stuart factor)	70-130%	0.70-1.30	4.5-P	Collect as in factor II determination
Factor VIII (antihemophilic globulin)	50-200%	0.50-2.0	4.5-P	Collect as in factor II determination
Factor IX (Plasma thromboplastic cofactor)	60-140%	0.60-1.40	4.5-P	Collect as in factor II determination
Factor XI (plasma thromboplastic antecedent)	60-140%	0.60-1.40	4.5-P	Collect as in factor II determination
Factor XII (Hageman factor)	60-140%	0.60-1.40	4.5-P	Collect as in factor II determination
Coagulation screening tests:				
Bleeding time (Simplate)	3-9.5 min	180-570 sec		
Prothrombin time	Less than 2-sec deviation from control	Less than 2-sec deviation from control	4.5-P	Collect in vacutainer containing 3.8% sodium citrate
Partial thromboplastin time (activated)	25-38 sec	25-38 sec	4.5-P	Collect in Vacutainer containing 3.8% sodium citrate
Whole-blood clot lysis	No clot lysis in 24 hr	0/day	2.0-whole blood	Collect in sterile tube and incubate at 37°C
Fibrinolytic studies:				
Euglobin lysis	No lysis in 2 hr	0/2 hr	4.5-P	Collect as in factor II determination
Fibrinogen split products	Negative reaction at > 1:4 dilution	0 (at 1:4 dilution)	4.5-S	Collect in special tube containing thrombin and epsilon aminocaproic acid
Thrombin time	Control ± 5 sec	Control ± 5 sec	4.5-P	Collect as in factor II determination
"Complete" blood count:				
Hematocrit	Men: 45-52% Women: 37-48% Men: 13-18 g/100 mL Women: 12-16 g/100 mL	Men: 0.45-0.52 Women: 0.37-0.48 Men: 8.1-11.2 mmol/L Women: 7.4-9.9 mmol/L	1-B	Use EDTA as anticoagulant, the seven listed tests are performed automatically on the Ortho ELT 800, which directly determines cell counts, hemoglobin (as the cyanmethemoglobin derivative), and MCV and computes hematocrit, MCH, and MCHC
Hemoglobin				
Leukocyte count	4300-10,800 mm²	$4.3\text{-}10.8 \times 10^9$/L		
Erythrocyte count	4.2-5.9 million/mm²	$4.2\text{-}5.9 \times 10^{12}$/L		
Mean corpuscular volume (MCV)	86-98 μm³/cell	86-98 fl		
Mean corpuscular hemoglobin (MCH)	27-32 pg/RBC		1.7-2.0 pg/cell	
Mean corpuscular hemoglobin concentration (MCHC)	32-36%	0.32-0.36		

Contd...

Contd...

Determination	Conventional	Reference Range SI	Minimal mL Required†	Note
Erythrocyte sedimentation rate (ESR)	Men: 1-13 mm/hr Women: 1-20 mm/hr	Men 1-13 mm/hr Women: 1-20 mm/hr	5-B	Use EDTA as anticoagulant
Erythrocyte enzymes:				
Glucose-6-phosphate dehydrogenase	5-15 U/g Hb	5-15 U/g	9-B	Use special anticoagulant (ACD solution)
Pyruvate kinase	13-17 U/g Hb	13-17 U/g	8-B	Use special anticoagulant (ACD solution)
Ferritin (serum):				
Iron deficiency	0-12 ng/mL 13-20 ng/mL Borderline	0-4.8 nmol/L 5.2-8 nmol/L Borderline		
Iron excess	> 400 ng/L	> 160 nmol/L		
Folic acid:				
Normal	> 3.3 ng/mL	> 7.3 nmol/L	1-S	
Borderline	2.5-3.2 ng/mL	5.75-7.39 nmol/L	1-S	
Haptoglobin	40-336 mg/100 mL	0.4-3.36 g/L	1-S	
Hemoglobin studies:				
Electrophoresis for abnormal hemoglobin			5-B	Collect with anticoagulant
Electrophoresis for A_2 hemoglobin	3.0%	0.015-0.035	5-B	Use oxalate as anticoagulant
Borderline	0.3-3.5%	0.03-0.035		
Hemoglobin F (fetal hemoglobin)	Less than 2%	< 0.02	5-B	Collect with anticoagulant
Hemoglobin, met- and sulf-	0	0	5-B	Use heparin as anticoagulant
Serum hemoglobin	2-3 mg/100 mL	1.2-1.9 µmol/L	2-S	
Thermolabile hemoglobin	0	0	1-B	Any anticoagulant
Lupus anticoagulant	0	0	4.5-P	Collect as in factor II determination
LE (Lupus erythematosus) preparation:				
Method I	0	0	5-B	Use heparin as anticoagulant
Method II	0	0	5-B	Use defibrinated blood
Leukocyte alkaline phosphatase:			20-Isolated blood leukocytes	Special handling of blood necessary
Qualitative method	Men: 33-188 U Women (off contraceptive pill): 30-160 U	33-188 U 30-160 U	Smear-B	
Muramidase	Serum, 3-7 µg/mL Urine, 0-2 µg/mL	3-7 mg/L 0-2 mg/L	1-S 1-U	
Osmotic fragility of erythrocytes	Increased if hemolysis occurs in over 0.5% NaCl; decreased if hemolysis is incomplete in 0.3% NaCl		5-B	Use heparin as anticoagulant
Peroxide hemolysis	Less than 10%	0.10	6-B	Use EDTA as anticoagulant
Platelet count	150,000-350,000/mm^3	$150-350 \times 10^9$/L	0.5-B	Use EDTA as anticoagulant; counts are performed on Clay Adams Ultraflow; when counts are low, results are confirmed by hand counting
Platelet function tests:				
Clot retraction	50-100%/2 hr	0.50-1.00/2 hr	4.5-P	Collect as in factor II determination
Platelet aggregation	Full response to ADP, epinephrine, and collagen	1.0	18-P	Collect as in factor II determination
Platelet factor 3	33-57 sec	33-57 sec	4.5-P	Collect as in factor II determination
Reticulocyte count	0.5-2.5% red blood cells	0.005-0.025	0.1-B	
Vitamin B_{12}	205-876 pg/mL	150-674 pmol/L	12-S	
Borderline	140-204 pg/mL	102.6-149 pmol/L		

6. CEREBROSPINAL FLUID VALUES

Determination	Conventional	SI	Minimal mL Required†	Note
		Reference Range		
Bilirubin	0	0	2	
Cell count	0-5 mononuclear cells		0.5	
Chloride	120-130 mEq/L	120-130 mmol/L	0.5	
Colloidal gold	0000000000-0001222111	Same	0.1	
Albumin	Mean: 29.5 mg/100 mL	0.295 g/L	2.5	
	± 2 SD: 11-48 mg/100 mL	± 2 SD: 0.11-0.48		
IgG	Mean: 4.3 mg/100 mL	0.043 g/L		
	± 2 SD: 0-8.6 mg/100 mL	± 2 SD: 0-0.086		
Glucose	50-75 mg/100 mL	2.8-4.2 mmol/L	0.5	
Pressure (initial)	70-180 mm of water	70-180 arb. unit		
Protein:				
Lumbar	15-45 mg/100 mL	0.15-0.45 g/L	1	
Cisternal	15-25 mg/100 mL	0.15-0.25 g/L	1	
Ventricular	5-15 mg/100 mL	0.05-0.15 g/L	1	

7. MISCELLANEOUS VALUES

Determination	Conventional	SI	Minimal mL Required†	Note
		Reference Range		
Carcinoembryonic antigen (CEA)	0-2.5 ng/mL	0-2.5 µg/L	20-P	Must be sent on ice
Chylous fluid				Use fresh specimen
Digitoxin	17 ± 6 ng/mL	22 ± 7.8 nmol/L	1-S	Medication with digitoxin or digitalis
Digoxin	1.2 ± 0.4 ng/mL	1.54 ± 0.5 nmol/L	1-S	Medication with digoxin 0.25 mg per day
	1.5 ± 0.4 ng/mL	1.92 ± 0.5 nmol/L	1-S	Medication with digoxin 0.5 mg per day
Duodenal drainage				pH should be in proper range
pH (urine)	5-7	5-7		with minimal amount of gastric juice
Gastric analysis	Basal:			
	Women: 2.0 ± 1.8 mEq/hr	0.6 ± 0.5 µmol/sec		
	Men: 3.0 ± 2.0 mEq/hr	0.8 ± 0.6 µmol/sec		
	Maximal (after histalog or gastrin):			
	Women: 16 ± 5 mEq/hr	4.4 ± 1.4 µmol/sec		
	Men: 23 ± 5 mEq/hr	6.4 ± 1.4 µmol/sec		
Gastrin-I	0-200 pg/mL	0-95 pmol/L	4-P	Heparinized sample
Immunologic tests:				
Alpha-fetoprotein	Undetectable in normal adults		2-S	
Alpha₁-antitrypsin	85-213 mg/100 mL	0.85-2.13 g/L	10-B	
Rheumatoid factor	< 60 IU/mL		10 mL clotted blood	Fasting sample preferred
Antinuclear antibodies	Negative at a 1:18 dilution of serum		2-S	Send to laboratory promptly
Anti-DNA antibodies	Negative at a 1:10 dilution of serum		2-S	
Antibodies to Sm and RNP (ENA)	None detected		10 mL clotted blood	
Antibodies to SS-A (Ro) and SS-B (La)	None detected		10 mL clotted blood	
Autoantibodies to:				
Thyroid colloid and microsomal antigens	Negative at a 1:10 dilution of serum		2-S	Low titers in some elderly normal women
Gastric parietal cells	Negative at 1:20 dilution of serum		2-S	
Smooth muscle	Negative at a 1:20 dilution of serum		2-S	
Mitochondria	Negative at a 1:20 dilution of serum		2-S	
Interstitial cells of the testes	Negative at a 1:10 dilution of serum		2-S	
Skeletal muscle	Negative at a 1:60 dilution of serum		2-S	

Contd...

Contd...

Determination	Conventional	Reference Range SI	Minimal mL Required†	Note
Adrenal gland	Negative at a 1:10 dilution of serum		2-S	
Bence Jones protein	No Bence Jones protein detected in a 50-fold concentrate of urine		50-U	
Complement, total hemolytic	150-250 U/mL		10-B	Must be sent on ice
Cryoprecipitable proteins	None detected	0 arb. unit	10-S	Collect and transport at 37°C
C3	Range, 83-177 mg/100 mL	0.83-1.77 g/L	2-S	
C4	Range, 15-45 mg/100 mL	0.15-0.45 g/L	2-S	
Factor B	12-30 mg/100 mL		5 mL clotted blood	
Cl esterase inhibitor	13.2-24 mg/100 mL		5 mL clotted blood	
Hemoglobin A_{ic}	3.8-6.4%	0.038-0.064	5-P	Sent EDTA tube on ice promptly to laboratory
Hypersensitivity pneumonitis screen	No antibodies to those antigens assayed		5 mL clotted blood	
Immunoglobulins:				
IgG	639-1349 mg/100 mL	6.39-13.49 g/L	2-S	
IgA	70-312 mg/100 mL	0.7-3.12 g/L	2-S	
IgM	86-352 mg/100 mL	0.86-3.52 g/L	2-S	
Viscosity	1.4-1.8 relative viscosity units		10-B	Expressed as the relative viscosity of serum compared with water
Iontophoresis	Children: 0-40 mEq sodium/L	0-40 mmol/L		Value given in terms of sodium
	Adults: 0-60 mEq sodium/L	0-60 mmol/L		
Propranolol (includes bioactive 4-OH metabolite)	100-300 ng/mL	386-1158 nmol/L	1-S	Obtain blood sample 4 hr after last dose of beta-blocking agent
Stool fat	Less than 5 g in 24 hr or less than 4% of measured fat intake in 3-day period	< 5 g/day	24-hr or 3-day specimen	
Stool nitrogen	Less than 2 g/day or 10% of urinary nitrogen	< 2 g/day	24-hr or 3-day specimen	
Synovial fluid:				
Glucose:	Not less than 20 mg/100 mL lower than simultaneously drawn blood sugar	See blood glucose	1 mL of fresh fluid	Collect with oxalate-fluoride mixture
D-Xylose absorption	5-8 g/5 hr in urine; 40 mg/ 100 mL in blood 2 hr after	33-53 mmol/day	5-U	
	ingestion of 25 g of D-xylose	2.7 mmol/L	5-B	

† Abbreviations used: SI, Systeme International d'Unites; P, plasma; S, serum; B, blood; and urine.

APPENDIX 2
CALCULATIONS IN NURSING

The staff nurse must accurately calculate drug dosages to provide safe medication administration to each patient. The review of basic mathematics, "calculations in nursing" will provide the nurses with a review of basic math, three measurement systems, two methods of solving dosage problems, and methods of determining the appropriateness of children's drug orders.

FRACTIONS

Are you afraid of fractions? Many students are. What is a fraction? A fraction is a "part" of a whole number. For example:

Fraction   Whole

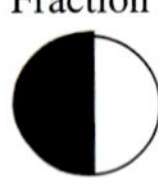   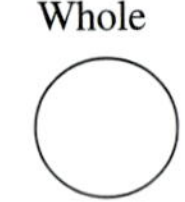

½ of a pie   1 whole pie

Definitions

Numerator The "top" number of a fraction.

Denominator The "bottom" number of a fraction.

Types of Fractions

Proper fractions—the numerator is less than the denominator.

Example: 1 Numerator
                    2 Denominator

Improper fractions—the numerator is larger than the denominator.

Example: 2 Numerator
                    1 Denominator

Mixed fractions—consist of a whole number plus a fraction.

Example: $1\frac{1}{2}$, 1 is the whole number; $\frac{1}{2}$ is the fraction.

Changing an Improper Fraction to a Whole or Mixed Number

Rule 1: Divide the denominator (bottom number) into the numerator (top number).

Example: Change $\frac{10}{5}$ to a *whole* number.

$10 \div 5 = 2$ (a whole number)

Change $\frac{40}{5}$ to a whole number

$40 \div 5 = 8$ (a whole number)

Example: Change $\frac{20}{7}$ (an improper fraction) to a *mixed* number.

$$20 \div 7 = 7 \overline{)20} = 2\frac{6}{7} \quad \text{(a mixed number)}$$

Change $\frac{54}{5}$ to a *mixed* number

$$54 \div 5 = 5\overline{)54}$$

$= 10\frac{4}{5}$ (a mixed number)

Changing a Mixed Number to an Improper Fraction

Rule 1: Multiply the denominator (bottom number) by the whole number.

Rule 2: Add numerator to the product; the sum is now the new number.

Example: change $2\frac{6}{7}$ (a mixed number) to an improper fraction.

Multiply the denominator 7 by the whole number 2.
$7 \times 2 = 14$ (The answer from numbers multiplied is called the *product*).
Add the numerator to the product.
$6 + 14 = 20$ (The answer from numbers added is called the *sum*).
Place the sum, 20, over the original denominator, 7, to have an improper fraction:

$$\frac{20}{7}$$

The mixed number $2\frac{6}{7}$ is now the improper fraction: $\frac{20}{7}$.

Reducing Fractions to the Lowest Term

Fractions are commonly reduced to the lowest term in which they can be expressed, because it is easier to work with smaller numbers.

For example $\frac{20}{80}$ or $\frac{25}{100}$ which

can both be reduced to $\frac{1}{4}$ become more convenient to use in calculation.

Rule 1: Find a number that will evenly divide into the numerator and the denominator.

Example: $\frac{2}{10}$

What number will divide into the numerator, 2?
2 will divide evenly into the numerator, 2, one time.
2 will divide into the denominator, 10, five times.

$\dfrac{2}{10} = \dfrac{1}{5}$ (Reduce all fractions to their lowest terms).

Example: $\dfrac{16}{60}$ or $\dfrac{4}{16}$

Determining which Fraction is Larger

Rule 1: If the denominators are the *same*, the fraction with the *larger numerator* is the largest fraction.

Which is larger? $\dfrac{4}{6}$ or $\dfrac{2}{6}$

$\dfrac{4}{6}$ is larger.

Rule 2: If the denominators are *different*, such as $\dfrac{2}{5}$ and $\dfrac{1}{3}$; you must find a "common denominator". (Finding a common denominator means to find a number into which both denominators can be divided). A common, or equivalent, will also be found.

Problem: Find a common denominator for $\dfrac{2}{5}$ and $\dfrac{1}{3}$

(Try multiplying the denominators to get a common denominator).

Example: $\dfrac{2}{5} = \dfrac{?}{15}$, $\dfrac{1}{3} = \dfrac{?}{15}$

Problem: Which is larger? $\dfrac{2}{3}$ or $\dfrac{6}{8}$

$\dfrac{2}{3} = \dfrac{16}{24}$, $\dfrac{6}{8} = \dfrac{18}{24}$

$\dfrac{6}{8}$ is larger

Rule 3: After the common denominator is found, equivalent numerator for each fraction must be found.

$\dfrac{2}{5} = \dfrac{?}{15}$, $\dfrac{1}{3} = \dfrac{?}{15}$

Find an equivalent numerator by dividing the first denominator into the equivalent denominator, multiply the answer by the first numerator.

Example:

$\dfrac{2}{5} = \dfrac{6}{15}$ $(15 \div 5 = 3; 3 \times 2 = 6)$

$\dfrac{1}{3} = \dfrac{5}{15}$ $(15 \div 3 = 5; 5 \times 1 = 5)$

Rule 4: Compare the two fractions.

Problem: which is larger? $\dfrac{6}{15}$ or $\dfrac{5}{15}$

$\dfrac{6}{15}$ is larger

Multiplying Fractions

Rule 1: Multiply the numerators; multiply the denominators.

Example: $\dfrac{1}{2} \times \dfrac{3}{4} = \dfrac{1 \times 3}{2 \times 4} = \dfrac{3}{8}$

$\dfrac{4}{8} \times \dfrac{1}{3} = \dfrac{4 \times 1}{8 \times 3} = \dfrac{4}{24} = \dfrac{1}{6}$

Multiplying Fractions and Mixed Numbers

Rule 1: Change the mixed number to an improper fraction.
Rule 2: Multiply,

Problem: Multiply $3\dfrac{1}{2}$ by $1\dfrac{2}{3}$

Example: a. Change $3\dfrac{1}{2}$ and $1\dfrac{2}{3}$ to improper fractions.

$3\dfrac{1}{2} = \dfrac{7}{2}$, $1\dfrac{2}{3} = \dfrac{5}{3}$

b. Multiply.

$\dfrac{7 \times 5}{2 \times 3} = \dfrac{35}{6} = 6\overline{)35} = 5\dfrac{5}{6}$

Problem: Multiply $1\dfrac{2}{3}$ by $2\dfrac{3}{4}$

Example: $1\dfrac{2}{3} = \dfrac{5}{3}$ $2\dfrac{3}{4} = \dfrac{11}{4}$

$\dfrac{5}{3} \times \dfrac{11}{4} = \dfrac{55}{12} = 4\dfrac{7}{12}$

Dividing Fractions

Rule 1: Write the problem down *correctly;* invert the second fraction.
Rule 2: Multiply.

Problem: Divide $\dfrac{1}{2}$ by $\dfrac{3}{4}$

Example: a. Write the problem down *correctly.*

$\dfrac{1}{2} \div \dfrac{3}{4}$

b. Invert the second fraction; change the division sign to a multiplication sign; multiply.

$\dfrac{1}{2} \times \dfrac{4}{3} = \dfrac{4}{6}$

c. Reduce to the lowest terms.

$\dfrac{4}{6} = \dfrac{2}{3}$

Dividing Fraction and Whole Numbers

Rule 1: Change the whole number to a fraction.
Rule 2: Divide.

Problem: Divide 4 by $\dfrac{3}{5}$

Example   a. Change 4 to a fraction. Make 4 the numerator and use 1 as the denominator.

$$\dfrac{4}{1}$$

  b. Invert second fraction; multiply.

$$\dfrac{4 \times 5}{1 \times 3} = \dfrac{20}{3}$$

  c. Reduce to lowest terms.

$$\dfrac{20}{3} = 6\dfrac{2}{3} \qquad 3\overline{)\begin{array}{l}20\\ \underline{18}\\ 2\end{array}} \;\; \dfrac{2}{3}$$

DECIMAL FRACTIONS

The decimal fraction is a type of fraction that uses a decimal to indicate the denominator of the fraction. The placement or position of the decimal point determines whether the denominator is 10, multiples of 10, or divisions of 10.

Names of Decimal Places

.00001	One-hundred thousandths
.0001	Ten thousandths
.001	Thousandths
.01	Hundredths
.1	Tenths
1.	Unit (whole numbers)
10	Tens
100	Hundreds
1,000	Thousands
10,000	Ten thousands
100,000	One-hundred thousands.

Rule 1: A decimal point found left of a whole number means that the number is a *fraction* of a whole number.

Example: 0.1 "Point one" is $\dfrac{1}{10}$ of the whole number, 1.

Hint: Place a zero left of the decimal point to avoid mistaking, 1 with 1. Correct placement of decimal points in drug dosages is *critical*.

Rule 2: A decimal point found *after* a number means that it is a whole number.

Example: 5. = 5

Rule 3: A number *without* a decimal point is understood to have an "invisible" decimal point behind it.

Example: 1 = 1.0.

Adding Fractions that have the same denominator

Rule 1: Add the numerators and place the sum of the numerators over the denominator.

Example:

$$\begin{array}{r}\dfrac{1}{6}\\[6pt] +\dfrac{1}{6}\\[4pt]\hline\\[-4pt]\dfrac{2}{6} = \dfrac{1}{3}\end{array}$$

Adding Fractions that have Different Denominators

Rule 1: Find common denominators for all fractions in the problems.

Example:

$$\dfrac{1}{3} = \dfrac{}{12}$$
$$+\dfrac{2}{4} = \dfrac{}{12}$$

(3 and 4 will divide into 12; 12 is the common denominator).

Rule 2: Find the equivalent numerators.

$$\dfrac{1}{3} = \dfrac{4}{12} \quad (12 \div 3 = 4;\; 4 \times 1 = 4)$$
$$+\dfrac{2}{4} = \dfrac{6}{12} \quad (12 \div 4 = 3;\; 3 \times 2 = 6)$$

$$\dfrac{10}{12} = \dfrac{5}{6}$$

$$\dfrac{6}{20} = \dfrac{6}{20}$$

$$+\dfrac{12}{20} = \dfrac{12}{20}$$

$$\dfrac{18}{20} = \dfrac{9}{10}$$

Adding Mixed Numbers

Rule 1: Add the fractions of the mixed number. Then, add the sum of the fractions to the whole numbers.

Example: $1\dfrac{2}{3}$

$$+\,2\dfrac{1}{3}$$

$$3\dfrac{3}{3} = 4$$

$$1\dfrac{3}{5} = 1\dfrac{6}{10}$$

$$+\;\;4\dfrac{5}{10} = 4\dfrac{5}{10}$$

$$5\dfrac{11}{10} = 5 + 1\text{ whole} + \dfrac{1}{10},$$

$$\text{which} = 6\;\dfrac{1}{10}$$

Subtracting Fractions with the Same Denominator

Rule 1: Subtract the numerator and place it over the denominator in the answer.

Example:

$$\dfrac{3}{5} \qquad \dfrac{4}{7}$$
$$-\dfrac{1}{5} \qquad -\dfrac{2}{7}$$
$$\dfrac{2}{5} = \dfrac{2}{7}$$

Subtracting Fractions with Different Denominators

Rule 1: Find a common denominator, then subtract.

Hint: Try multiplying the two denominators as a way to find a common denominator.

Example: $\dfrac{3}{4} = \dfrac{9}{12}$ $\dfrac{1}{2} = \dfrac{3}{6}$

$$\dfrac{1}{3} = \dfrac{4}{12} \qquad \dfrac{2}{3} = \dfrac{4}{6}$$

$$\dfrac{5}{12} \qquad \dfrac{7}{6} = 1\dfrac{1}{6}$$

Subtracting Mixed Numbers

Rule 1: When the numerator of the top fraction is smaller than the bottom fraction, borrow one whole number from the whole number of the mixed fraction and express it as a fraction.

Problem: $3\dfrac{9}{15}$ *Example:* $3 = 2\dfrac{15}{15}$

$-2\dfrac{10}{15}$

Rule 2: Add the fraction of the original mixed number to the new fraction.

$$3\dfrac{9}{15} = 2\dfrac{15}{15} + \dfrac{9}{15} = 2\dfrac{24}{15}$$

Rule 3: Subtract fractions and whole numbers, if any.

$$2\dfrac{24}{15} - 2\dfrac{10}{15}$$
$$\dfrac{14}{15}$$

Example: $5\dfrac{6}{10} = 4\dfrac{10}{10} + \dfrac{6}{10} = 4\dfrac{16}{10}$

$-3\dfrac{8}{10} = 3\dfrac{8}{10} + -3\dfrac{8}{10}$

$-1\dfrac{2}{10}$ or $1\dfrac{1}{5}$

Adding Decimals

Rule 1: Align the decimal point of each decimal fraction in a column.

Rule 2: Add.

Problem: Add 3.34 and 0.6

Example :   3.34   Align decimal point in column; add.
          + 0.6
          ———
          3.94

Make sure that the decimal point is aligned properly in the answer.

Hint: Zeroes may be added to the right of the decimal point if needed to help align the column. The value of the number is *not* changed by adding zeroes.

Example: 1.00 = 1   5.0 = 5

Subtracting Decimals

Rule 1: Align the decimal points of each decimal fraction in a column.

Rule 2: Subract

Problem: Subtract 7.45 from 15.

Example: Align decimal points in column; subtract.

15.00   (Note zeroes used to align the
– 7.45   two columns).
———
7.55

Rounding a Number

Rule 1: Numbers found after the decimal point that are 5 or larger can increase the number before it by one whole number.

Example: 7.55 = 7.6 or 8

Hint: There are times when it is practical to round a volume of medication.

Problem: How can 7.55 minims easily be given?

Example: Round 7.55 to 8; give 8 minims.

Note: Minims are very small units of measurement. Milliliters/cubic centimeters are not rounded in this manner, since drug dosage would be altered.

Multipling Decimals

Rule 1: Multiply. Decimal points in the problem *do not* have to be aligned.

Rule 2: The decimal place in the answer is determined by how many numbers are found right or the decimal points in the numbers multiplied.

Example: 5.50
          ×   2.15   (There are 4 numbers found after
          ———   the decimal points; 2 on the top
            2750   and 2 on the bottom).
            550
          1100
          ————
          11.8250 ×
                    × = 11.8250 or 12 (rounded).

Note: A small "x" hereafter indicates the unexpressed decimal after a whole number or a decimal point that has been moved from one place to another.

Dividing Decimals

Rule 1: Change a decimal fraction in the divisor to a whole number by moving the decimal point *all* the way to the right.

Problem: divide 2.5 by 1.5.

Example: a. (divisor) 1.5 $\overline{\smash{\big)}\ 2.5}$ (dividend)
          b. 1.5 × $\overline{\smash{\big)}\ 2.5}$ (15 $\overline{\smash{\big)}\ 25}$)

Rule 2: Move the decimal point in the dividend the *same number of places* moved in the divisor.

Example: 1.5 x $\overline{\smash{\big)}\ 2.5}$ x. The decimal point in the divisor is unexpressed after it is moved.

Rule 3: Place the decimal point in the answer directly over the decimal point in the dividend after moving the decimal point in the dividend.

Example: 15 $\overline{\smash{\big)}\ 25.}$

Rule 4: If a decimal point is in the divisor, but not in the dividend (such as ·5 $\overline{\smash{\big)}\ 15}$), move it the same number of places as the divisor. Remember there is an unexpressed decimal point at the right of all whole numbers. Add zeroes after the decimal point in the dividend as needed.

Example: .5x $\overline{\smash{\big)}\ 15.0x}$ 5 $\overline{\smash{\big)}\ 150.0}$

Rule 5: If the dividend contains a decimal fraction and the divisor does not, leave the divisor as it is.

Example: 5 $\overline{\smash{\big)}\ 2.5}$ would remain unchanged.

Changing Fractions to Decimals

Rule 1: Divide the numerator (the top number) by the denominator (the bottom number).

Problem: Change $\dfrac{3}{4}$ to a decimal fraction.

Example $\dfrac{3}{4}$ = $4\overline{)3.00}$ = .75
                $\dfrac{28}{20}$
                $\dfrac{20}{}$

Changing a Decimal Fraction to a Common Fraction

Decimal fractions are based on 10's, multiples of 10, and divisions of 10. The position or place of the decimal point indicates the denominator.

Rule 1: To change a decimal fraction to a common fraction, give the decimal fraction a denominator according to the position of the decimal point in the decimal fraction.

Problem: Change .1 to a common fraction.

Example: a. .1 (The decimal point is in the "tens" place;
$\dfrac{}{10}$ 10 is the denominator).

b. Now that the denominator is 10, place the 1 over it to make a common fraction.
$\dfrac{1}{10}$

PERCENTS

The word *percent,* and its symbol, %, mean "hundredths". A hundredth is a fraction of a whole number; therefore a number followed by % is a *fraction.* The denominator of the fraction is understood to be 100.

Example: 25% is the same ase $\dfrac{25}{100}$

$\dfrac{25}{100}$ can be reduced to $\dfrac{1}{4}$

Changing Percent to a Decimal Fraction

Rule 1: Remove %; move the decimal point two places to the left to indicate "hundredths".

Problem: Change 25% to a decimal fraction.

Example: .25.

Changing a Fraction to a Percent

Rule 1: Change a fraction to a percent by dividing the numerator by the denominator.

Rule 2: Multiply the answer by 100.

Rule 3: Label the answer with the percent symbol.

Example: $\dfrac{3}{4}$ = $4\overline{)3.00}$ = .75
                $\dfrac{28}{20}$
                $\dfrac{20}{}$

100
$\times.75$
$\overline{500}$
700
$\overline{75.00x}$

(There are two decimal places in this problem; move the decimal point in the answer 2 places to the left).

75%. Therefore 3/4 = 75%

Multiplying by Percent

Rule 1: Change percent to a decimal (move decimal point 2 places to the left).
Rule 2: Multiply.

Problem: Multiply 80 by 7.5%

Example: 7.5% is .075

80
$\times.075$
$\overline{400}$
560
00
$\overline{6.000x}$

(Move decimal point 3 places to the left = 6).

RATIO

Ratio shows the relationship of one number or quantity to another number or quantity. Numbers of a ratio are separated by a colon. Ratio is also a fraction. The value of a ratio is not changed if both terms are multiplied or divided by the same number.

Example: 2:4 is the same as 1:2 or 4:8

When numbers are written in ratio, they must all be expressed in the same units.

Example: 1 liter, 2 ounces, and 30 milliliters (mL) must all be expressed in the same way, as:

1000 mL: 60 mL: 30 mL

A fraction may be written as a ratio.

Example: $\dfrac{1}{25}$ = 1:25 $\dfrac{3}{4}$ = 3:4

Ratio is an important concept that is used in the following methods of calculating dosages.

PROPORTION

Proportion shows that the relationship between two ratios has equal value.

Example: 1 is 2 as 4 is to 8 or 1:2 :: 4:8

Definitions

Extremes The outer terms of the proportion.

Means The inner terms of the proportion.

$\downarrow$ Extremes $\downarrow$ $\downarrow$ Means $\downarrow$

Example: 1:2   :: 4:8 1:2   ::   4:8

Set up the left side of the proportion as the "known" side using information that is known or given. The known information will be:

Example: a. An equivalent such as 60 milligrams = 1 grain (60 mg:1 gr)
       or
b. A doctor's medication or IV order, such as "give 1000 mL in 8 hr" (1000 mL: 8 hr)
       or
c. A drug dosage you have on hand or available, such as information on a drug label that reads "50 mg/mL (50 mg:1 mL)"

Problem: The doctor orders Demerol 25 mg q 3-4 hr prn for pain. On hand is a vial labeled "50 mg/1 mL."

Rule 1: Set up the known side.

Example: 50 mg: 1 mL (given on the label).

Rule 2: Set up the unknown side. Use x for what you are trying to find, such as "How many milliliters are needed to give 25 mg?"

 *Known* *Unknown*

Example 50 mg: 1 mL   :: 25 mg: x mL.

Rule 3: Set up the units, such as milligrams and milliliters, in the *same position on each side* of the problem.

Example ——   mg: —— mL ::—— mg: —— mL

Rule 4: Multiply the means.

Rule 5: Multiply the extremes.
Problem: 50 mg: 1 mL :: 25 mg:x mL.
Example: Multiply the means.

$$50 \text{ mg}:1 \text{ mL} :: 25 \text{ mg}:x \text{ mL}$$
$$= 25$$

Multiply the extreme

$$50 \text{ mg}:1 \text{ mL} :: 25 \text{ mg}:x \text{ mL}$$
$$50x = 25$$

Rule 6: Solve for x (divide the number with the x into the number on the opposite side of the problem).
Example: 50 mg:1 mL :: 25 mg:x mL

$$50x = 25 \qquad = \qquad 50 \,\big)\, \overline{250}$$
$$x = .5 \qquad\qquad\qquad\qquad 250$$

Rule 7: Label the answer with the unit of measurement that accompanies the x in the problem.
Example: 50 mg:1 mL :: 25 mg:x mL

$$50x = 25$$
$$x = .5 \text{ mL}$$

Review of Proportion Method

1. Set up problems in the *same order* on both sides.
2. Multiply the means; multiply the extremes.
3. The number multiplied with the x is always that number with the x to the right of it.
   Example: 2 mg : mL : 5 mg:x mL
4. Divide the number with the x into the number on the other side of the problem.
5. Label the problem by looking to see what unit of measurement the x is with the proportion.

$$\frac{\text{Desired dosage}}{\text{Available dosage}} \times \text{Amount method}$$

Many nurses use the following method of solving dosage problems.
Rule 1: Place the dose that the doctor wants given over the dose that the nurse has available (on hand).
Problem: The physician orders 40 mg of furosemide (Lasix). The nurse has an ampule of furosemide labeled Lasix 20 mg/mL.

$$\textit{Example: } \frac{\text{(Desired dosage)}}{\text{(Available dose)}} \; \frac{40 \text{ mg}}{20 \text{ mg}} \times \frac{1 \text{ mL}}{1} = \frac{40}{20}$$

$$= 40 \div 20 = 2 \text{ mL}$$

Problem: the physician orders 15 mg of diazepam (Valium). The nurse has valium tablets that contain 5 mg/tablet.
Example:

$$\frac{\text{(Desired dosage)}}{\text{(Available dose)}} \frac{15 \text{ mg}}{5 \text{ mg}} \times \frac{1 \text{ tab}}{x \text{ tab}} = \frac{15}{5x} = x$$

$$= 15 \div 5 = 3 \text{ tablets}$$

Nurse Alert

- There is no room for error in calculating dosages
- Check math work with another nurse
- Work problems systematically and carefully *on paper*
- Reduce distractions while working problems
- Recheck calculations
- Is the answer reasonable?

METRIC SYSTEM

Metric system is the preferred system of weights and measures. It is more accurate and easier to use in calculating dosage problems.

Similar to the US monetary system, which is based on the dollar, the metric system is also based on the decimal system. The decimal system uses division and multiples of a unit, which is always in ratios of tens.
Example:

1 dollar	=	10 dimes
10 dimes	=	20 nickles
20 nickles	=	100 pennies

All of these units are multiples or divisions of tens.

The metric system uses the following basic units of volume, weight, and length:

Liter (L) Volume (amount) of fluids.
Gram (g) Weight of solids.
Meter (m) Measure of length.
Smaller units of the system are designated by the following prefixes:
Deci 0.1 of the unit; tens (liter, gram, meter)
Centi 0.01 of the units; hundredths
Milli 0.001 of the unit; thousandths
Larger units of the system are designated with the following prefixes:
Deka = 10 times the unit (liter, gram, meter)
Hecto = 100 times the unit
Kilo   = 1000 times the unit.

Units of Weight

1 Gram (g) = 1000 milligrams (mg)
0.001 Gram (g) = 1 milligram (mg)
1 Kilogram (kg) = 1000 grams (g)
0.001 Kilogram (kg) = 1 gram (g).

Units of Volume

1 Liter (L) = 1000 milliliters (mL)
0.001 Liter (L) = 1 milliliter (mL)
1 Milliliter (mL) = 1 cubic centimeter (cc).

Approximate Equivalents of the Metric System and the Apothecary System

The apothecary system is a system of measurement that is still used by some physicians and hospitals. It is being replaced slowly by the metric system. Since it continues to be used, the following equivalents are needed to convert dosages from one system to another. The conversions are approximations only but are acceptable equivalents with which to work.

Volume

Metric	Apothecary
1 milliliter (mL)	= 16 minims (m/c XVI)
4 milliliters (mL)	= 1 fluid dram (f3 †)
30 milliliters (mL)	= 1 fluid ounce (3 †)
500 milliliters (mL)	= 1 pint (O †)
1000 milliliters (mL) or 1 Liter (L)	= 1 quart (1 Qt.)

The symbols for the above apothecary units are:

Minim	= m
Fluid dram	= 3
Fluid ounce	= 3
Pint	= O or pt
Quart	= Qt

The symbols appear in front of the number (which is written in roman numerals).
Example: 16 minims is written m/c XVI.

Weight

Metric	Apothecary
60 milligrams (mg)	= 1 grain (the symbol is gr. for grain)
1000 milligrams (mg)	= 15 grains (gr. XV)

4 grains (g or gm)	=	1 dram (3 †)
30 grams (g)	=	1 ounce 3 †
0.45 kilogram (kg)	=	1 pound (lb)
1 kilogram (kg)	=	2.2 pounds (lb)

Convert from one system to another to work dosage problems in the same measurement units.

Metric Measurements of Length

The basic unit of length in the metric system is the meter. The meter is equal to 39.37 inches, about 3½ inches longer than 1 yard (36 inches). Some of the tasks that the nurse will perform using the metric measurements of length will be to:

- Measure area size for topical applications
- Measure results of intradermal skin tests (size of drug or allergen reaction on the skin)
- Measure wound size
- Measure decubiti
- Measure height, length, and head circumference (such as is common in pediatrics)
- Measure abdominal girth (obstetrics)

Length

0.001 meter	=	1 millimeter (mm)
0.01 meter	=	1 centimeter (cm)
0.1 meter	=	1 decimeter (dm)
10 meters	=	1 dekameter (dam)
100 meters	=	1 hectometer (hm)
1000 meters	=	1 kilometer (km)

Most frequently used equivalents are:

1 meter (m)	=	1000 millimeters (mm)
0.001 meter (m)	=	1 millimeter (mm)
1 meter (m)	=	100 centimeters (cm)
1 centimeter (cm)	=	10 millimeters (mm)
1 millimeter (mm)	=	0.1 centimeter (cm)

BIG TO SMALL RULE

Whatever method is used to sole dosage problems, the units of measurement in the problem must *always* be converted to the same unit of measurement.

Some students find it difficult to convert dosages that contain decimal fractions. Discussed here is a quick and easy method called the "big to small" rule. It is useful in converting dosages within the same system (the metric system).

Because there are 1000 mL in 1 L (and 1000 mg in 1 g), milliliters can be converted to liters (and milligrams to grams) by this method. Likewise, liters can be converted to milliliters (and grams to milligrams) by this method.
Converting larger units of measurement to smaller units of measurement (grams to milligrams; liters to milliliters)
Rule 1: Write down BIG → SMALL.
Rule 2: Place the large unit under the word BIG and the small unit under the word SMALL.
Example: BIG → SMALL
2:5 g = ⎯⎯⎯→ mg
Rule 3: Move the decimal point 3 places in the direction of the arrow; add zeroes.
Example: BIG → SMALL
2.5 g = 2 × 500 mg
Converting smaller units of measurement to larger units of measurement (milligrams to grams; milliliters to liters)
Rule 1: Write down the big to small rule formula.
Example: BIG → SMALL
Rule 2: Reverse the direction of the arrow.
Example: BIG ← SMALL

Rule 3: Place the large unit under the word BIG and the small unit under the word SMALL.
Example BIG ← SMALL
× g = 2500 mg
Rule 4: Move the decimal point 3 places in the direction that the arrow points.
Example: BIG ← SMALL
2.5 g = 2500x mg

PEDIATRIC CONSIDERATIONS

Pediatric dosage refers to the determination of the correct amount, frequency, and total number of doses of a medication to be administered to a child or infant.

Age, weight, body surface area, and the ability of the child to absorb, metabolize, and excrete medication must be considered when administering medication to a child.

It is the physician's responsibility to determine medication orders and dosage for a pediatric patient, but the nurse must be able to recognize appropriate and inappropriate drug dosages and orders.

The nurse must be knowledgeable about the four standard formulas for calculating children's dosages. These are Young's rule, Clark's rule, Fried's rule, and the body surface area method.

Young's Rule

Young's rule is as follows:

$$\frac{\text{Age of child}}{\text{Age of child} + 12} \times \text{Average adult dose} = \text{Child's dose}$$

This rule applies to children up to the age of 12.
Problem: The average adult dose of a particular medication is 50 mg. What is an appropriate dose of this medication for an 8-year-old child?
Example:

$$\frac{8 \text{ yr}}{8 + 12} \times 50 \text{ mg} = \frac{8}{20} \times \frac{50}{1} = \frac{400}{20} = 20 \overline{)400}$$

Answer: 20 mg is an appropriate dose.

Clark's Rule

Clark's rule is as follows:

$$\frac{\text{Weight of child}}{150} \text{ in pounds} \times \text{Average adult dose} = \text{Child's dose}$$

This rule uses the child's weight to determine dosage.
Problem: The average adult dose of a particular medication is 25 mg. What is an appropriate dose of this medication for a child who weighs 40 pounds?

Example:

$$\frac{40 \text{ lb}}{150} \times 25 \text{ mg} = \frac{40}{150} \times \frac{25}{1} = \frac{1000}{150} = 150 \overline{)1000.00}$$

Answer: 6.7 mg is an appropriate dose.

Fried's Rule

Fried's rule is as follows:

$$\frac{\text{Age in months}}{150} \times \text{Average adult dose} = \text{Child's dose}$$

This rule is used for infants less than 2 years of age.

Problem: The average adult dose of a particular medication is 25 mg. What is an appropriate dose of this medication for a child who is 22 months of age?

Example:

$$\frac{22\ \text{mon}}{150} \times 25\ \text{mg} = \frac{550}{150} = 150\ \overline{)\ 550.00\ }$$

$$
\begin{array}{r}
3.66 \\
\underline{450} \\
1000 \\
\underline{900} \\
1000
\end{array}
$$

Answer: 3.7 mg is an appropriate dose.

Body Surface Area Method

LaRocca and Otto give the formula and nomogram for determining dosage for a child based on height, weight, and body surface area (Fig. A2.1). Height is correlated with the weight of the child to determine the body surface area of the child. The drug dose is then ordered as mg/m^2.

Example: Child's height = 23 inches; weight = 44 pounds.

Plot the height and weight of the child on the nomogram (which is a graphic representation of a numeric relationship) to determine the body surface area (BSA). Multiply the BSA (which is given in square meters on the nomogram) by mg/m^2.

Example: The drug literature recommends 1 mg/m^2.

$$0.50 \times 1\ \text{mg} = \text{x dose}$$
$$\text{x} = 0.50\ \text{mg of drug.}$$

DILUTION AND MEASUREMENT OF LOTIONS AND DRUGS

1. To make 1 pint of 1 in 80 carbolic lotion from 1 in 20 solution:
    The prepared lotion is to be ¼ as strong as the one from which it is made.
    ∴ ¼ of the pint is of 1 in 20 and the remainder water.
    i.e. 5 oz. of 1 in 20 and 15 oz. water.
    In other words, divide the strength you have into the strength you want and divide the result into the quantity you want, *e.g.*

    $$20\ \overline{)\ 80\ }$$
    $$\underline{4\ 20\ \text{oz.}}$$
    $$5\ \text{oz.}$$

2. To make 1 pint of 1 in 10,000 hydrarg, perchloride from 1 in 2,000 solution:
    The prepared lotion is to be 1/5 as strong as the one from which it is made.
    ∴ 1/5 of the pint is of 1 in 2,000 and the remainder water.
    I.e. 4 oz. of 1 in 2,000 solution and 16 oz. water.

3. To make 1 pint of 1 in 10,000 hydrarg, perchloride from 1 in 500 solution.
    The prepared lotion is to be 1/20 as strong as the one from which it is made.
    ∴ 1/20 of the pint is to be of 1 in 500 and the remainder water.
    i.e. 1 oz of 1 in 500 and 19 oz water.

PERCENTAGE SOLUTIONS

In dispensing solutions of drugs a certain number of grains are dissolved in 100 grains of water, *i.e.* 110 minims. *e.g.*

1. Injection, strychnine 1 percent solution = 1 gr. strychnine in 110 minims.
    ∴ 1/16 gr. (maximum dose) = 7 minims of solution (approximately).

2. Injection, strychnine .75 percent solution = 3/4 gr in110 minims.

    $$\therefore \frac{1}{32}\ \text{gr.} = \frac{110}{32} \times \frac{4}{3}\ \text{minims} = 5\ \text{minims (approximately).}$$

3. Injection, morphia 2 percent solution = 2 gr in 110 minims.

    $$\therefore \frac{1}{4}\ \text{gr.} = \frac{110}{8} \times = 13\ \text{minims (approximately).}$$

Relation of the Grain and the Minim

The chief disadvantage of the English system of weights and measures is that there is no simple relationship between them. A minim is not the volume of a grain of water.

480 minims do not weigh 480 grains but $437\frac{1}{2}$ grains, or 110 minims weight 100 grains.

∴ percentage solutions must be made up to 110 minims.

A 100 percent solution would be 100 gr in 110 minims.

It is useful to remember that 1 oz of a 1 percent solution contains 4.37 gr. Larger quantities and of different concentrations can readily be reckoned from this.

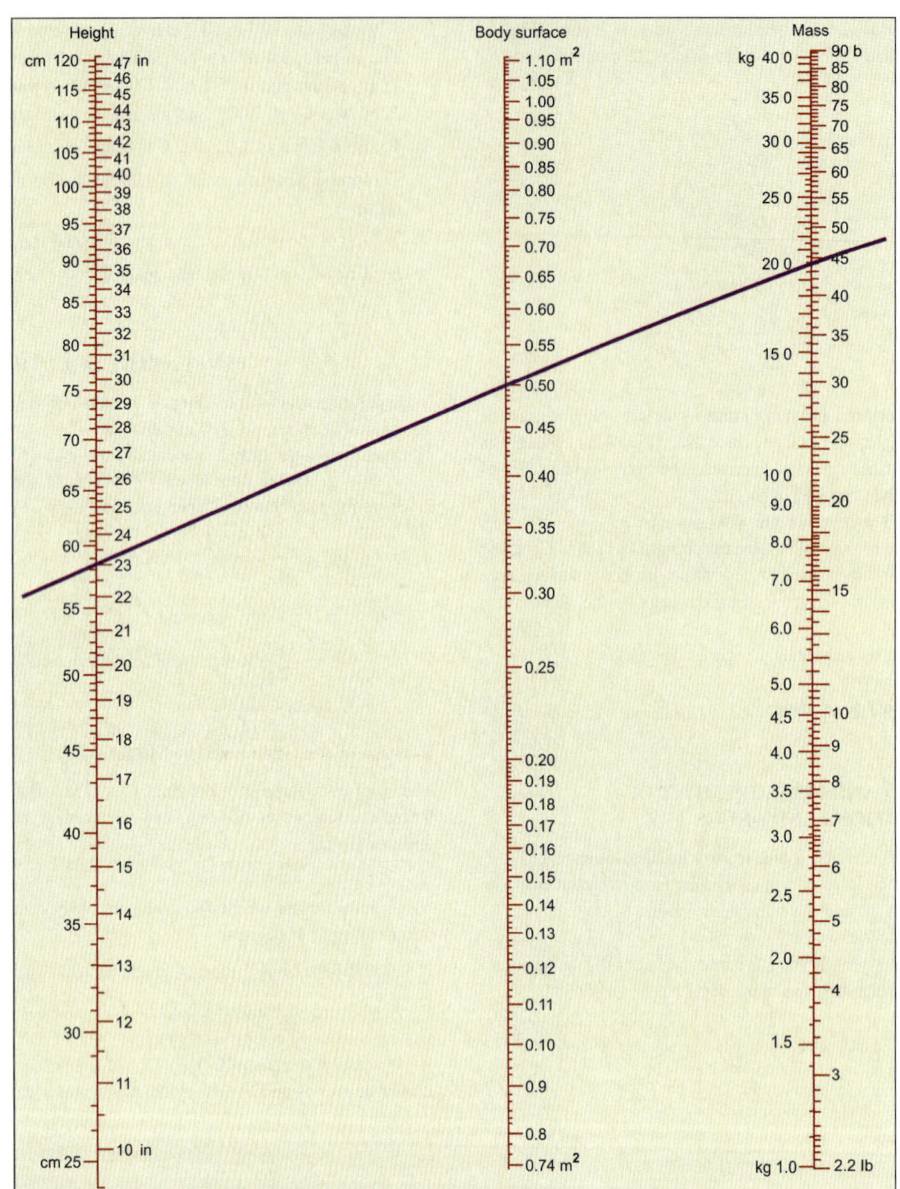

Fig. A2.1: Body surface area of children: Nomogram for determination of body surface from height and mass, based on the formula of DuBois and DuBois, Arch Intern Med 17:863, 1961: $S = M^{0.428} \times H^{0.725} \times 71.84$, or $\log S = \log M \times 0.425 \times \log H \times 0.725 \times 1.8564$ (*S*, body surface in cm^2; *M*, mass in kg; *H*, height in cm). ***Courtesy* CIBA-GEIGY, Ltd, Basel, Switzerland**

APPENDIX 3
GENERAL INSTRUMENTS USED IN NURSING

Cheatles Forcep

Cheatles forcep is a big heavy stainless steel forcep without locking system. It is used to pick up and hold sterilized items like linense instruments, gloves. Also this is known as Transfer forcep as on. Sterilized item is transferred from one place to other by this forcep. It is kept dipped in bottle containing dettol or savlon solution (Fig. A3.1).

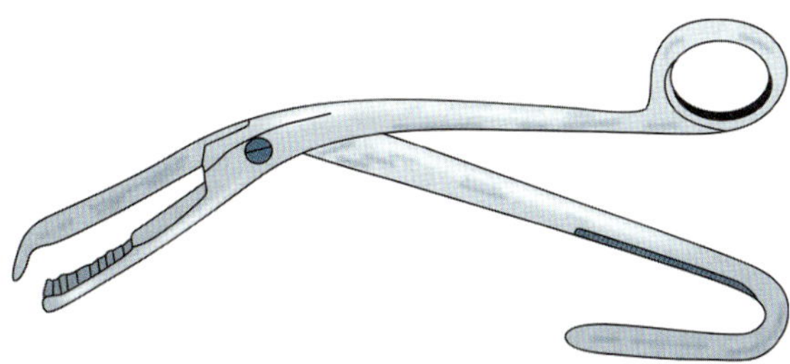

Figure A3.1: Cheatle's forcep

Sponge-holding Forcep

Sponge-holding forcep is a long forcep with locking arrangements. It is used to hold sponge/swabs firmly while dressing, swabbing, cleaning cavities. Also this is used to hold organs like gallbladder, etc. during operation. It can be used to hold cervix in place of ovum forcep (Fig. A3.2).

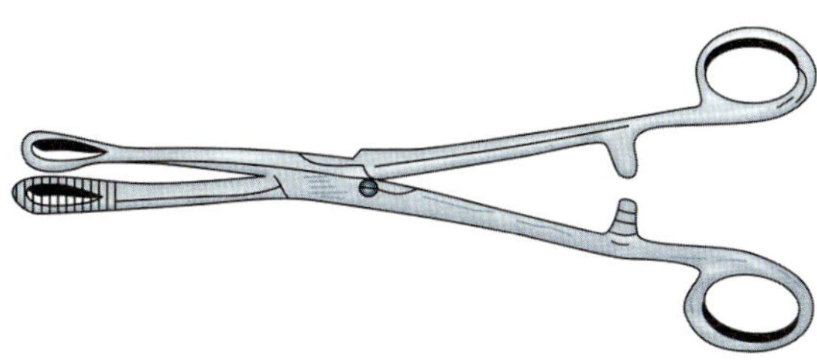

Figure A3.2: Sponge holding forcep

Mayo's Towel Clip

Moyo's towel clip is pointed, stainless steel clip with locking arrangements. The main use of this type of towel clip is during operation to hold drapes to expose only the required area of body (Fig. A3.3).

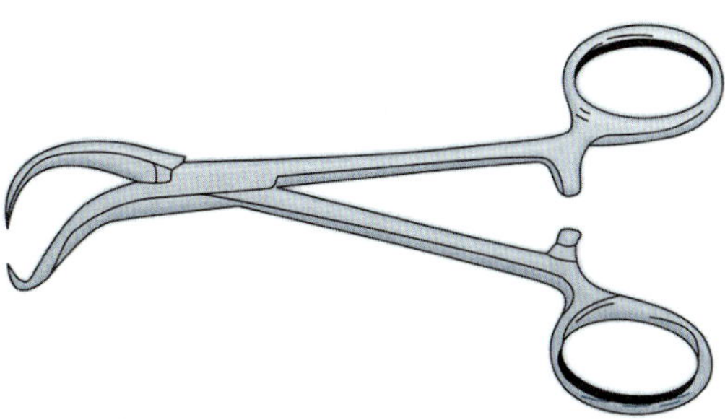

Figure A3.3: Mayo's towel clip

Simple Tourniquet

Simple tourniquet is a belt-like nylon/synthetic on tourniquet. The strip has sticking mechanism. It is used on for making superficial veins prominent during 1 IV therapy/collection of blood samples (Fig. A3.4).

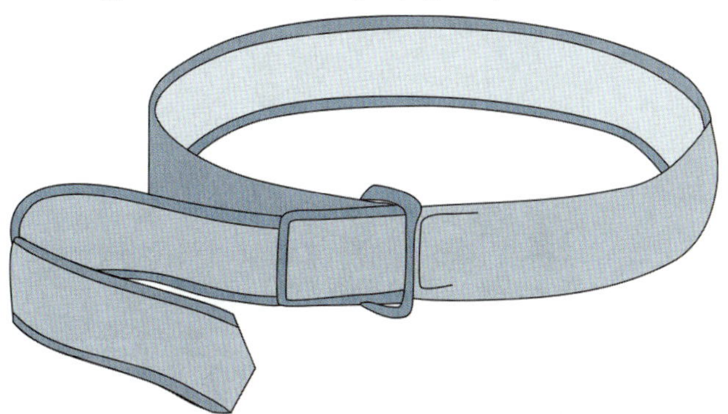

Figure A3.4: Simple tourniquet

Pneumatic Tourniquet

Pneumatic tourniquet is like the cuff of blood pressure instrument. The mechanism of working and application is same as BP instrument (Fig. A3.5).

Uses:

  (i) After snake-bite
  (ii) For bloodless limb surgery
  (iii) For IV therapy
  (iv) For Hess test for capillary fragility
  (v) During pulmonary edema.

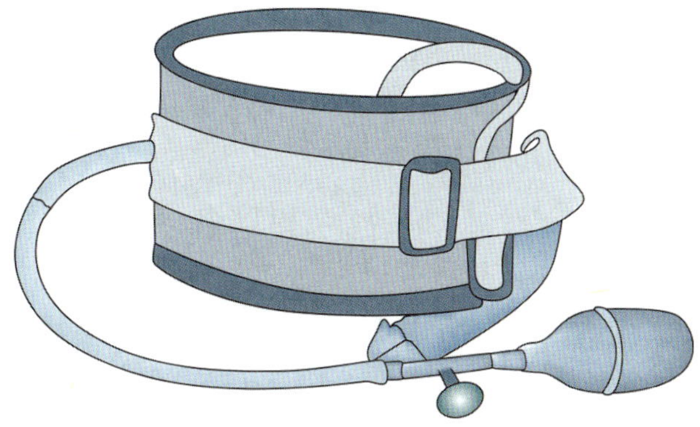

Figure A3.5: Pneumatic tourniquet

Bard-Parker Knife (BP Knife) or Scalpel

Scalpel is a sharp steel cutting instrument used for giving incision. Two types are available. One is single one with sharp cutting blade end. The other has two parts one handle and one blade. The blade is detachable. The later type is more commonly used nowadays as it is convenient to change the blade whenever it is felt. The handle can be used for longtime (Fig. A3.6).

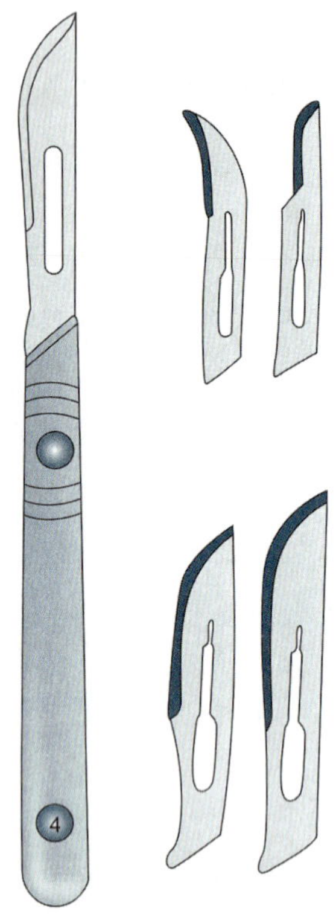

Figure A3.6: Bard-Parker knife with detachable blade

Artery Forceps

Various types of artery forceps are available—straight long, straight medium, mosquito artery forcep, curved artery forcep (Fig. A3.7). Each has locking system. These are used to check bleeding to hold fascia, aponeurosis, peritoneum, pedicles and base of appendix during operation.

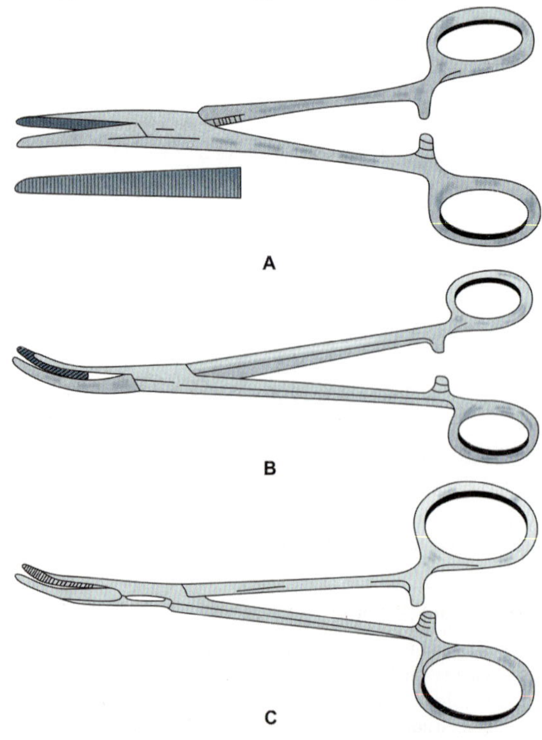

Figures A3.7A to C: Artery forceps

Single-hook Retractor

Single-hook-retractor is a solid sharp instrument without eye at pointed end. It is used to retract skin edges during stitching (Fig. A3.8).

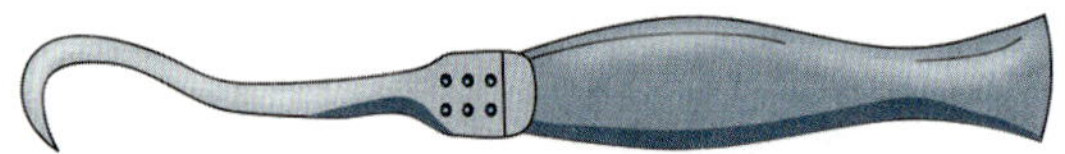

Figure A3.8: Single-hook retractor

Dissecting Forceps

Two types of dissecting forceps are used—plain and toothed (Fig. A3.9). Each type is also available in small and big size. It has no locking system. The plain forceps are used to hold soft delicate structures like peritoneum, vessels, bowel wall where injury to structure may cause harm or problem. The toothed ones are used to hold tough structures like skin, fascia and ligaments.

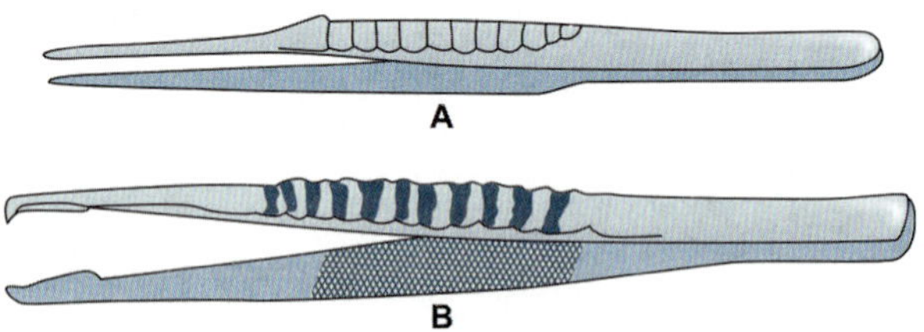

Figures A3.9A and B: Dissecting forceps

Scissors

Various types and forms of scissors are used. The main aim remains the same to cut various structures and sutures. The shape varies according to its use at various places. The curved one is used for cutting deeper structures, adhesion avoiding injury to neighbouring structures. The stitch cutting scissor has serrated ends. It is only used for cutting sutures (Fig. A3.10).

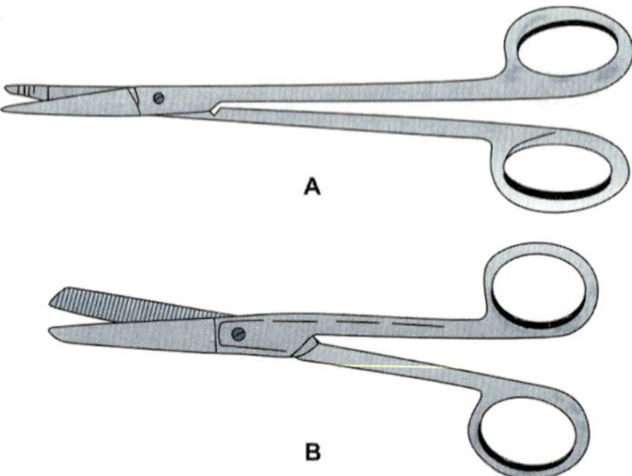

Figures A3.10A and B: Scissors—(A) Fine pointed scissors, (B) Gauze-cutting

Alli's Tissue Forcep

Alli's tissue forcep is a toothed type forcep with locking arrangements to hold tough tissue/structures firmly during operation/incision. While retracting tissue or structure, forceful hold is achieved by this forcep (Fig. A3.11).

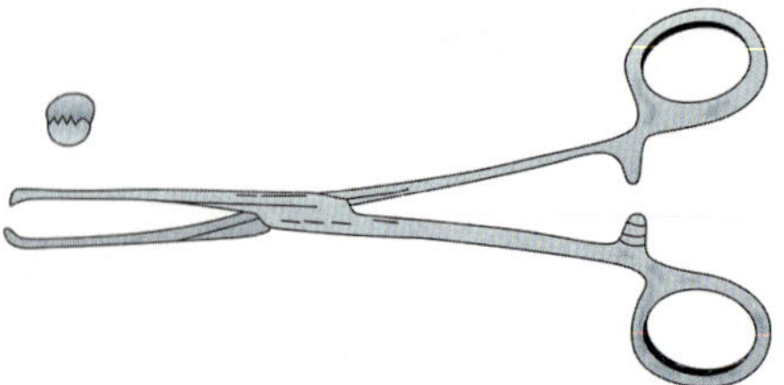

Figure A3.11: Alli's tissue forcep

Lane's Tissue Forcep

Lane's tissue forcep is stronger than Alli's. The blades are curved and stronger with toothed end. It has locking mechanism. It is used to hold still tough or bulky organs—like holding sac-lining for excision, skin for apposition, to hold lymph nodes, appendix during operation (Fig. A3.12).

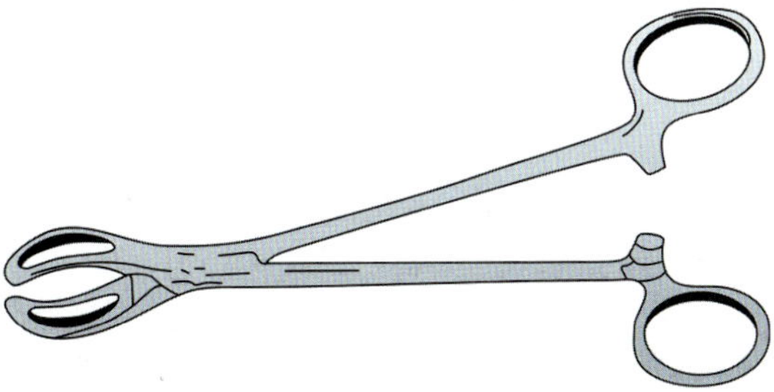

Figure A3.12: Lane's tissue forcep

Valsellum

Valsellum is again one type of tissue forcep. It is mainly used in gynecological and obstetric operations to hold cervix. In stead of pointed and toothed end it has flat toothed end to hold cervix without much injury. It has locking arrangements (Fig. A3.13).

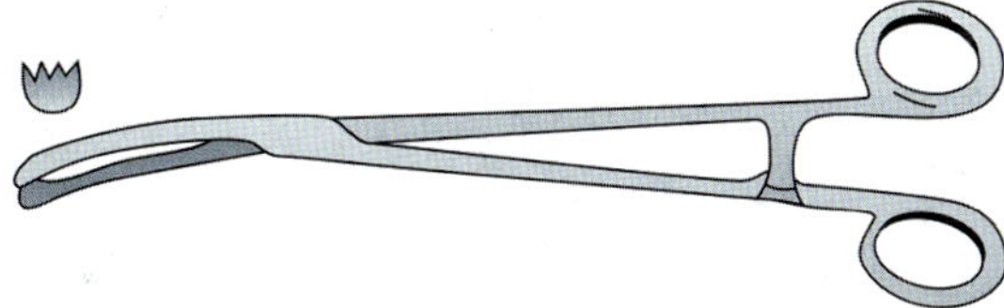

Figure A3.13: Valsellum

Surgical Needles

Various types and forms of surgical needles are used.
(i) Round body, (ii) Cutting needle.
The round may be straight or curved, so also the cutting one may be straight or curved. The curved, may be half-circle curved or full-circle curved. On the basis of eye of the needle it may be traumatic or atraumatic in which the suturing material is swaged by the manufactures. Cutting needle is used for stitching tough structure like skin and fascia. The round body is used for suturing soft delicate structures. Curved one is used in deeper places for convenience where chances of injury to neighboring structure lies. These needles are never sterilized by boiling or autoclaving. It is dipped in cidex or lysol minimum for 12 hours (Fig. A3.14).

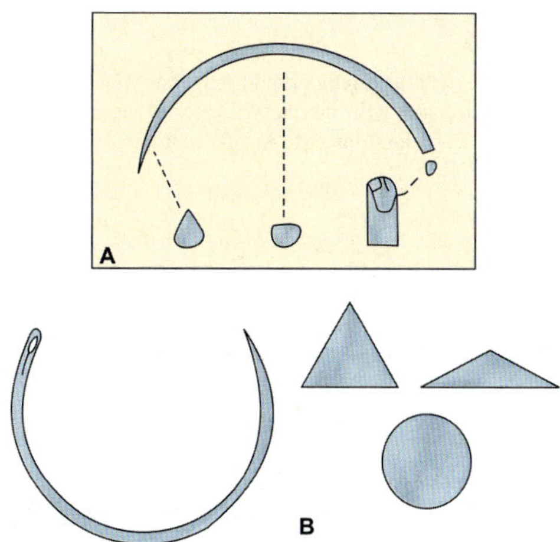

Figures A3.14A and B: Surgical Needles (A) The tip, body and the eye of a needle, (B) Traumatic cutting needle

Needle Holder

Needle holder looks like artery forcep. But the difference lies in shortness of blades and its thickness. It has lock arrangement. The needle is held at junction of posterior 1/3 and anterior 2/3 and then locked. While suturing the needle holder is held between thumb and index finger (Fig. A3.15).

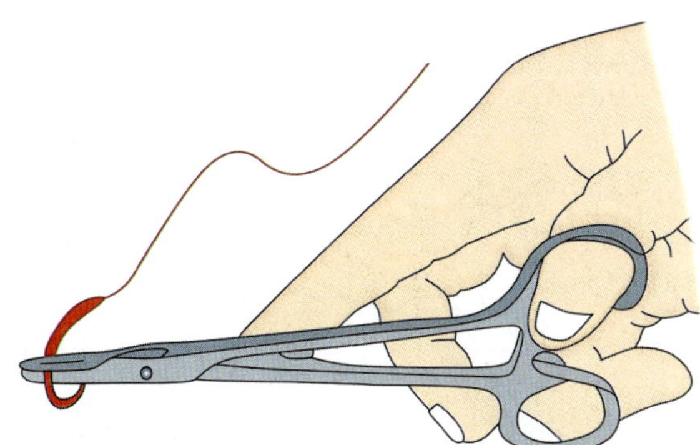

Figure A3.15: Method of using a needle holder

Drainage

Two types of drainages are used—corrugated drainage and closed tube drainage (Fig. A3.16). Closed tube drainage may be penrose type or multiple perforated type. The drainages are given during surgery to encourage removal of pus from abscess, to remove transudate from cavities and to provide warning of leakage of other fluid in drainage fluid. The drainage is always sterilized before use. It is removed by shortest route.

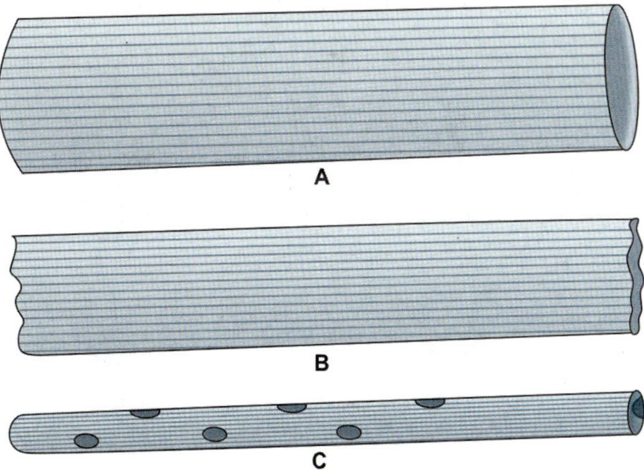

Figures A3.16A to C: Types of drains: (A) Penrose type, (B) Corrugated, (C) Multiple perforated tube drain

Nasogastric Tube

Usually three types nasogastric tubes are available—(i) Ryle's tube, (ii) Levine's tube, (iii) Polythene nasogastric tube. Ryle's tube is a rubber tube of one meter long. The tip is blunt and contains a lead piece for weight and for easy passing of tube. Also the lead shot gives position of tube in X-ray. Short of lead at lower end there are a number of holes for suction of stomach contents or oral feeding. The length of the tube has three markings at various places to indicate the position of tube at various places in stomach. The first mark at 40 cm when remains at tip of nose, indicates, tube at gastroesophageal end. The second mark at 50 cm indicates lower end of tube at body of stomach. The third mark at 60 cm indicates lower end at pylorus.

Infant Feeding Tube

Infant feeding tube is smaller in length and has no lead shot. It has also no marking in the body of tube. It is used for feeding and aspiration purpose in small children or infants.

Doyen's Mouth Gag

Doyen's mouth gag is self-retaining tube retractor with locking system. It is used to keep open mouth during oral surgery, for stomach wash in poisoning cases and for oral toilet in comatous patient (Fig. A3.17).

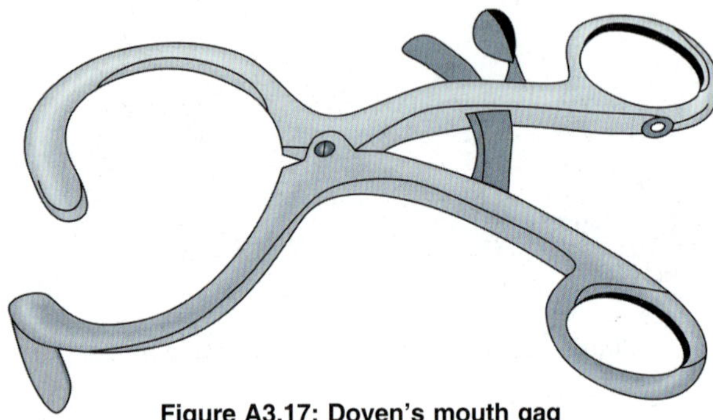

Figure A3.17: Doyen's mouth gag

Scalp-vein Set

Scalp-vein set is a readymade tube with thin needle fixed at end used for fluid therapy in small children. As originally it was used to provide fluid therapy through scalp vein, so it its name. The advantage of the set is if it is used over scalp veins, the movements of limbs of small infants will not dislodge the vein. Also another advantage is that heparin solution can be introduced to the tube for not allowing clotting of blood and so the venous channel can be kept patent when IV fluid is discontinued (Fig. A3.18).

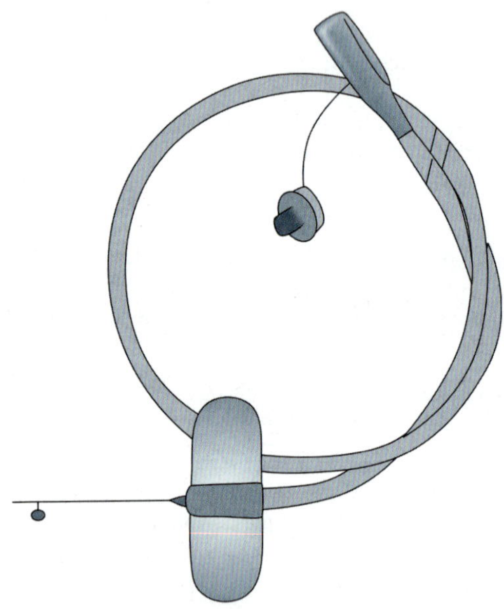

Figure A3.18: Scalp-vein set

Electrical Otoscope

Electrical otoscope is used for visualizing middle ear. It has a aural speculum attached to a lighting arrangement. The whole instrument is handy and separated into three detachable pieces.

Eyelid Retractor

Eyelid retractor is a long handled retractor with spatula like retracting end which is bent over itself. It is used to retract eyelid, conveniently during examination of inner eyelid (Fig. A3.19).

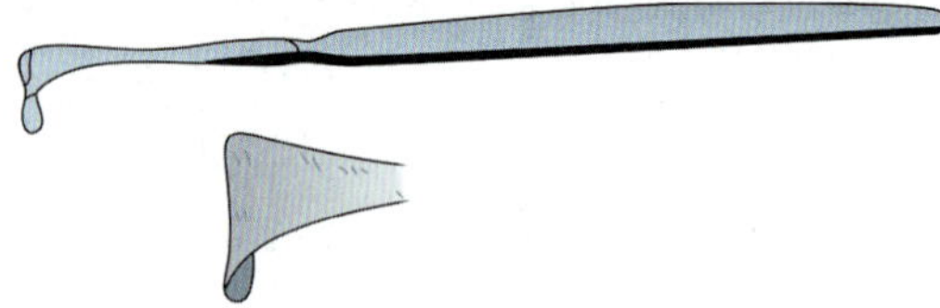

Figure A3.19: Eyelid retractor

Undine

Undine is a retort shape flask with long narrow neck (Fig. A3.20). It has side opening for filling with desired solution. It is used to irrigate conjunctival sac with drugs/cleaning purpose.

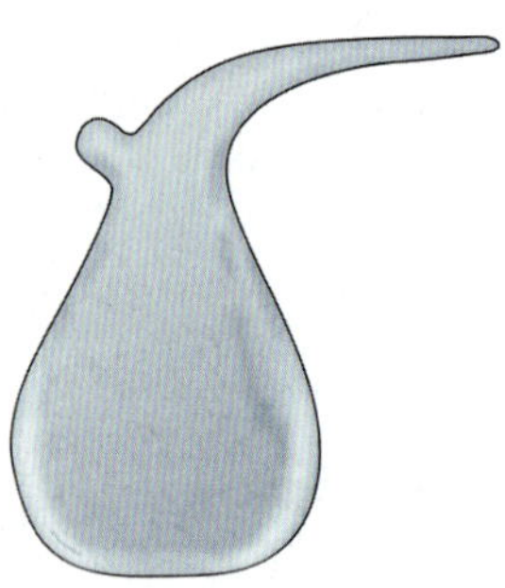

Figure A3.20: Undine

Sims' Speculum

Sims' speculum is single bladed or double bladed. It is a non-retaining type of vaginal speculum used in obstetrics and gynecology. One assistant is required to hold the speculum with pressure while examiner visualizes interior part. It is available in various sizes.

Cusco's Bivalved Speculum

Cusco's bivalved speculum is a vaginal speculum with self-retaining arrangements. The screw is moved for required stretching of vagina. One single examiner can use it without somebody's help.

Hegar's Dilators

Hegar's dilators are metallic dilators used for dilatation of cervix. Various sizes are packed in single pack with numbers. Lesser is the number, lesser is the thickness of dilator. In various obstetric and gynecological purpose these dilators are used.

Uterine Sound

Uterine sound is a graduated metallic rod-like instrument used for measuring length of uterus. It is about 12 inches long. The distal end is curved at angle of 60 and runs 2 inches. The tip is blunt. Before passing cervical dilators, uterine sound is introduced to ascertain uterine size and shape (Fig. A3.21).

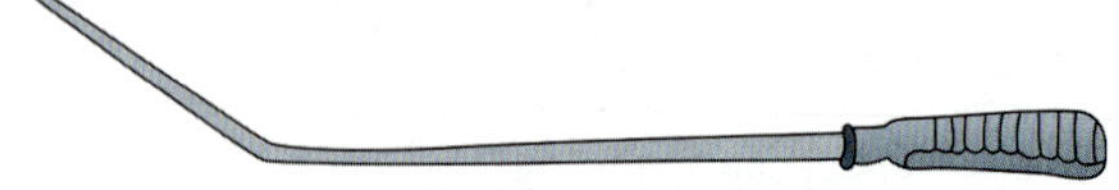

Figure A3.21: Uterine sound

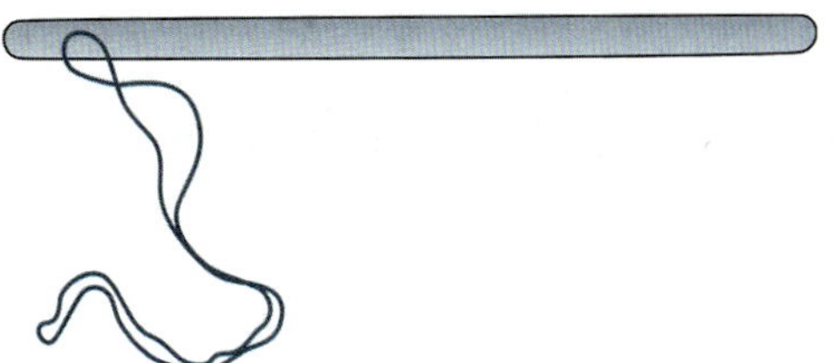

Figure A3.22: Laminoria tent

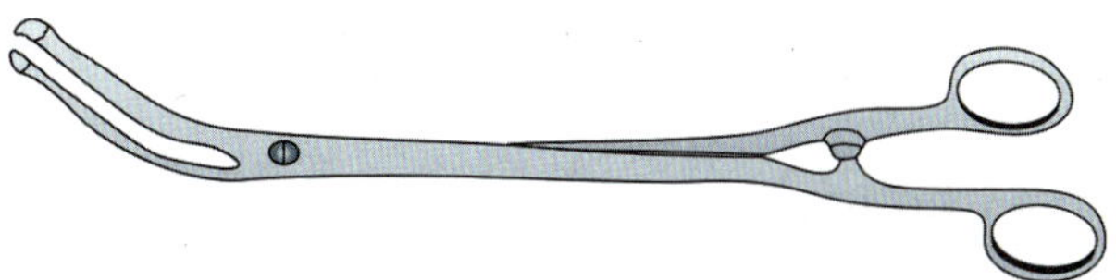

Figure A3.23: Laminoria tent introducer

Laminoria Tent

The name is a misnomer. It is a stick like wooden item. It is derived from sea wood which has high power of absorbing water and to be swollen enormously. At one end one thread is attached for making easy removal by pulling the thread. It is used for cervical dilatation. Sometimes two or three tents are inserted and left for 12-24 hours for its proper action (Fig. A3.22). One laminoria tent introducer is used for its insertion (Fig. A3.23). Laminoria tents, (sticks) are available in packets of 50 or 100 pieces in market.

APPENDIX 4
NURSING TRAYS USED DURING EMERGENCY

For emergency use and quick action various nursing trays are kept ready by nurse. Even for routine use different trays are kept tidy for efficient handling of cases by doctor. It saves time for the doctor and nurse and ensures convenient and efficient care of patients. The various trays used in wards with its contents are enumerated below.

Anaphylactic Tray

(1) Inj Adrenaline, (2) Inj Decadron, (3) Inj Avil, (4) Inj Aminophylline, (5) Inj 25% glucose, (6) Glucose or Glucose-saline infusion bottle, (7) Sterile IV set, (8) Sterile syringe and needle.

Antipoison Tray

(1) Stomach wash tube, (2) Mouth gag, (3) A bottle containing pot permanganate or crystals, (4) Empty bottle with cork for collection of sample of stomach content, (5) Dextrosaline bottle, (6) Sterile IV set, (7) Ryle's tube, (8) 50 cc syringe.

Abdominal Paracentesis Tray

(1) Sterile trocar and cannula, (2) Sterile small rubber tube, (3) Sterile syringe with needle, (4) Sterile cotton balls and dressings, (5) Sterile applicator and artery forcep, (6) Sterile test tube with cotton plug, (7) Sterile towels, (8) Local anesthesia-xylocaine 2%, (9) Bucket, (10) Rubber sheet, (11) Pint measure, (12) Abdominal binder, (13) Triiodine and Tr Benzoin, (14) Transfer forcep (Cheatle forcep), (15) Pulse meter.

Baby's Bath Tray

(1) Oil, (2) Soap and towel, (3) Baby powder, (4) Cotton, (5) Waste receiptacle, (6) Forcep in jar, (7) Applicator.

Breast Care Tray

(1) Breast pump, (2) Nipple shield, (3) Normal saline, (4) Sponge, (5) A bowl.

Catheter Tray

(1) Sterile catheters, (2) Kidney trays, (3) Sponges, (4) Lubricant lotion, (5) Two small bowls, (6) Sterile gloves, (7) Specimen bottle.

Examination Tray

(1) A bottle containing antiseptic lotion with tongue depresser dipped in, (2) Torch, (3) BP instrument, (4) A bottle containing antiseptic lotion with thermometer dipped in, (5) Tuning Fork, (6) Knee hammer, (7) Stethoscope, (8) Pulse meter, (9) Some amount of cotton.

Eye Tray

(1) Lifting forcep, (2) Sterile eye rods, (3) Sterile eye dropers, (4) Sterile cotton balls, (5) Sterile normal saline, (6) Container with water for rinsing dropers, (7) Bowl or kidney tray, (8) Eye medication, (9) Lid retractor.

ENT Examination Tray

(1) Nasal speculum, (2) Aural speculum, (3) Tongue depressor, (4) Two metal applicator, (5) Ear forcep, (6) Laryngeal mirror, (7) Tuning fork, (8) Head mirror, (9) Cotton balls, (10) Slides, (11) Applicator, (12) Cheatle forcep, (13) Dropers, (14) Oto scope, (15) Light arrangement.

Incision or Drainage Tray

(1) Two straight artery forceps, (2) Mosquito forceps, (3) Plain forceps, (4) Suture scissors, (5) Sponge holding forcep, (6) Scalpel with blade, (7) Antiseptic sol, (8) Sinus forcep, (9) Sterile towels, (10) Safety pins, (11) Ethyl chloride, (12) Kidney tray, (13) Drainage tube, (14) Sterile gloves, (15) Sterile test tubes and slides, (16) Sterile dressing liner, (17) Cheatle forcep, (18) Tri iodine.

Rectal Tray

(1) Clean gloves, (2) Clean cotton ball, (3) Lubricant solution, (4) Slides, (5) Long applicator, (6) Waste receiptacle, (7) Rectal speculum or proctoscope.

Spinal Puncture or Lumbar Puncture Tray

(1) Two sterile LP needle with stylets, (2) Artery forcep, (3) Two sterile test tubes, (4) Kidney tray, (5) Sterile syringe with needle, (6) Local anesthesia-xylocaine 2%, (7) Two small enamel bowls, (8) Spinal manometer, (9) Sterile gloves, (10) Sterile towel, (11) Sterile dressing liners, (12) Cheatle forcep, (13) Tri benzoin, (14) Bowl.

Thoracocentesis Set Tray

(1) Sterile aspiration needle No. 18 or No. 15, (2) Sterile 50 cc syringe and 1 cc syringe, (3) Sterile cotton balls, (4) Applicators, (5) Sterile dressing linen, (6) Sterile test tube, (7) Tri iodine, (8) Breast binders with safety pin, (9) Bowl, (10) Local anesthesia.

Venesection or Cut-down Tray

(1) Sterile scalpel with blade, (2) Sterile scissors, (3) Sterile mosquito forcep, (4) Needle holder, (5) Needle curve cutting, (6) Teeth forcep, (7) Cotton suture, (8) Ice syringe, (9) Local anesthesia, (10) Sterile dressing materials, (11) Sterile gloves, (12) Kidney tray, (13) Torch light, (14) Cheatle forcep, (15) Tourniquet, (16) Arm board, (17) Tri iodine.

APPENDIX 5
OPERATION THEATRE INSTRUMENTS

It must be understood that lists of instruments for different operations vary with different surgeons and circumstances, but the following have been found generally satisfactory.

General Set (Plate I)

15 Lane's tissue forceps (I, 1).
9 Spencer Wells' artery forceps (I, 2).
9 Mayo Ochsner's forceps (I, 3).
4 toothed dissecting forceps (I, 4).
2 non-toothed dissecting forceps (I, 5).
2 retractors (I, 6).
2 sponge-holding forceps (I, 7).
4 towel clips (I, 8).
1 small probe (I, 9).
1 long probe.
1 grooved director (I, 10).
1 blunt dissector (I, 11).
1 raspatory (I, 12) 9 extras.
1 sharp spoon (I, 13).
1 aneurysm needle (I, 14).
1 needle holder (I, 15).
1 suture holder (I, 16).
1 pair curved scissors (I, 17).
2 pairs straight scissors (I, 18).
2 scalpels (I, 19).

Bone Set (Plate II)

9 skin clips (II, 1).
2 lion bone-holding forceps (II, 2).
2 small lion bone-holding forceps (II, 2).
1 large straight bone cutting forceps (II, 3).
1 large curved bone cutting forceps (II, 4).
1 small straight bone cutting forceps
1 small curved bone cutting forceps
2 pairs necrosis forceps (II, 5).
1 pair sequestrum forceps (II, 6).
1 awl (II, 7).
1 grooved awl (II, 8).
1 mallet (II, 9).
Langenbeck retractors (II, 10).
1 pair sinus forceps (II, 11).
2 rugines (II, 12).
1 pair large bone levers or spikes (II, 13).
1 pair medium bone levers (grooved) (II, 14).
1 pair small bone levers (or more according to operation).
1 file (II, 15).
1 mechanical drill and drill points (II, 16).

Bone Sharps (Plate IIIA)

1 large saw (III, 1).
1 small saw.

Chisels of varying sizes (III, 2).
Osteotomes of varying sizes (III, 3).
Gouges of varying sizes (III, 4).
Drill points varying sizes (II, 16).

Bone Plating Set (Plate IIIB)

General Set and Bone Set, plus—
2 plate holding forceps (III, 5).
2 plate benders (III, 6).
2 screw holding forceps (III, 7).
2 screwdrivers (III, 8).
Plates (III, 9) and screws (III, 10).

Extralaparotomy Instruments (Plate IIIC)

General set, plus—
1 malleable probe (III, 11).
1 pliable probe (III, 12).
1 malleable spoon or scoop (III, 13).
1 gall-stone forceps (Desjardin's) (III, 14).
2 Moynihan's pedicle forceps (III, 15).
2 straight compression forceps (III, 16).
2 abdominal retractors (III, 17).
2 pairs curved intestinal clamps (III, 18).
2 curved compression forceps (III, 19).

Gastrectomy and Resection of Gut (Plate IVA)

General Set, plus—
2 abdominal retractors (III, 17).
1 self-retaining retractor (IV, 1).
2 straight compression forceps (III, 16).
2 curved compression forceps (III, 19).
2 Moynihan's pedicle forceps (III, 15).
1 double intestinal clamp (IV, 2).
2 large straight intestinal clamps (IV, 3).
2 small straight intestinal clamps
2 curved intestinal clamps (III, 18).
4 Judd's or Allis's basting forceps (IV, 4).
1 large Payr's clamp (IV, 5).
1 small Payr's clamp.

Colostomy (Plate IVB)

General Set, plus—
Abdominal retractors (III, 17).
2 small intestinal clamps (III, 18).
Paul's tube (IV, 6) and colostomy rod (IV, 7).

Empyema (Plate IVC)

General Set, plus—
Rugine (II, 12).

2 rib raspatories (IV, 8).
Rib cutting forceps (II, 3, 4).
Rib shears (IV, 9).
Necrosis forceps (II, 5).

Herniotomy (Plate IVD)

General Set, plus—
Hernia needle (IV, 10).

Hemorrhoids (Plate IVE)

General Set, plus—
Proctoscope (IV, 11).
4 haemorrhoid clamps (IV, 12).

Amputation (Plate IVF)

General Set, plus—
Extra artery forceps (I, 2).
Bone set (II).
Bone sharps (IIIA).
Flat retractor (IV, 13).
Amputation knife (IV, 14).

Tonsillectomy (Plate V)

1 towel clip (I, 8).
4 tongue depressors (V, 1).
1 Davis gag (V, 1).
Suspension apparatus for gag (V, 2).
2 tonsil guillotines (V, 3).
2 Doyen's gags (V, 4).
2 Mayo Ochsner's artery forceps (I, 3).
1 tracheotomy dilator (V, 5).
2 tonsil snares (V, 6).
1 tonsil dissector (V, 7).
2 adenoid curettes (V, 8).
2 pairs toothed dissecting forceps (I, 4).
2 curved tonsil forceps (V, 9).

1 toothed tonsil forceps (V, 10).
4 straight artery forceps (I, 2).
4 curved artery forceps

Some Special Instruments for Gynecological Work (Plate VI)

Vaginal speculae, Auvard's (VI, 1)
Vaginal speculae, Sims' (VI, 2).
Vaginal speculae, Fergusson's (VI, 3).
Pessaries (VI, 5).
Uterine sound (VI, 6).
Playfair's probe (VI, 7).
Ovum forceps (VI, 8).
Vulsellum forceps (VI, 9).
Intrauterine douche nozzle (VI, 10)
Dilators for cervix (VI, 11).
Intrauterine flushing curette (VI, 12).

Some Special Instruments for Ophthalmic Work (Plate VIIA)

Retractor (VII, 1).
Undine (VII, 2).
Ophthalmoscope (VII, 3).
Graefe's knife (VII, 4).
Keratome (VII, 5).
Beer's knife (VII, 6)
Iris scissors (VII, 7)
Elliott's trephine (VII, 8)
Iris forceps (VII, 9).
Roller forceps for trachoma (VII, 10).

Operative Treatment of Fractures (Plate VIIB)

Steinmann's pin, introducer, stirrup (VII, 11).
Apparatus for the insertion of Kirschner's wire (VII, 12).
A Bohler's iron (VII, 13).
A smith-Petersen nail (VII, 14).
(This plate is much reduced from the actual size).
4 gallbladder extras

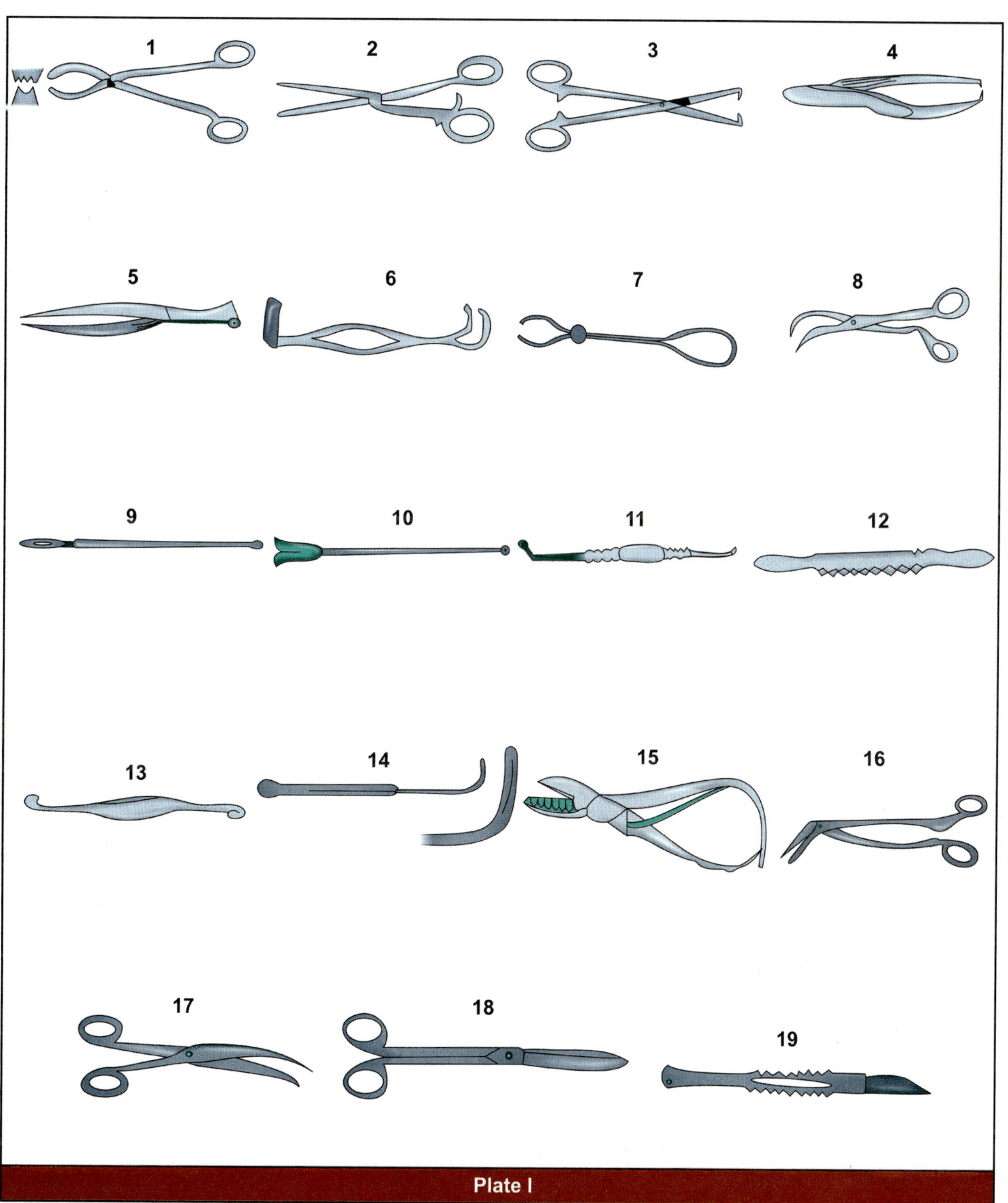

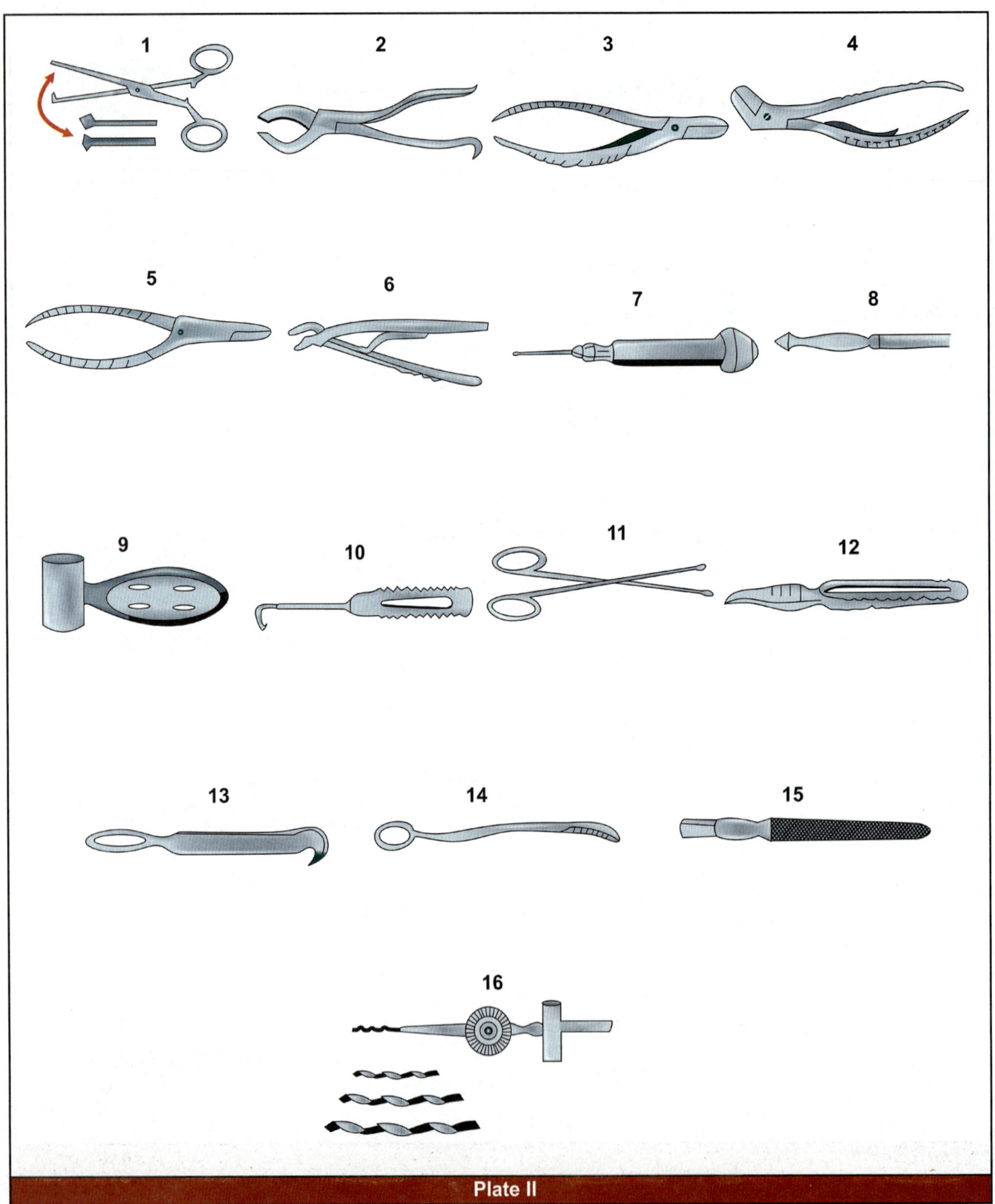

1
2
3
4
5
6
7
8
9
10
11
12
13
14
15
16

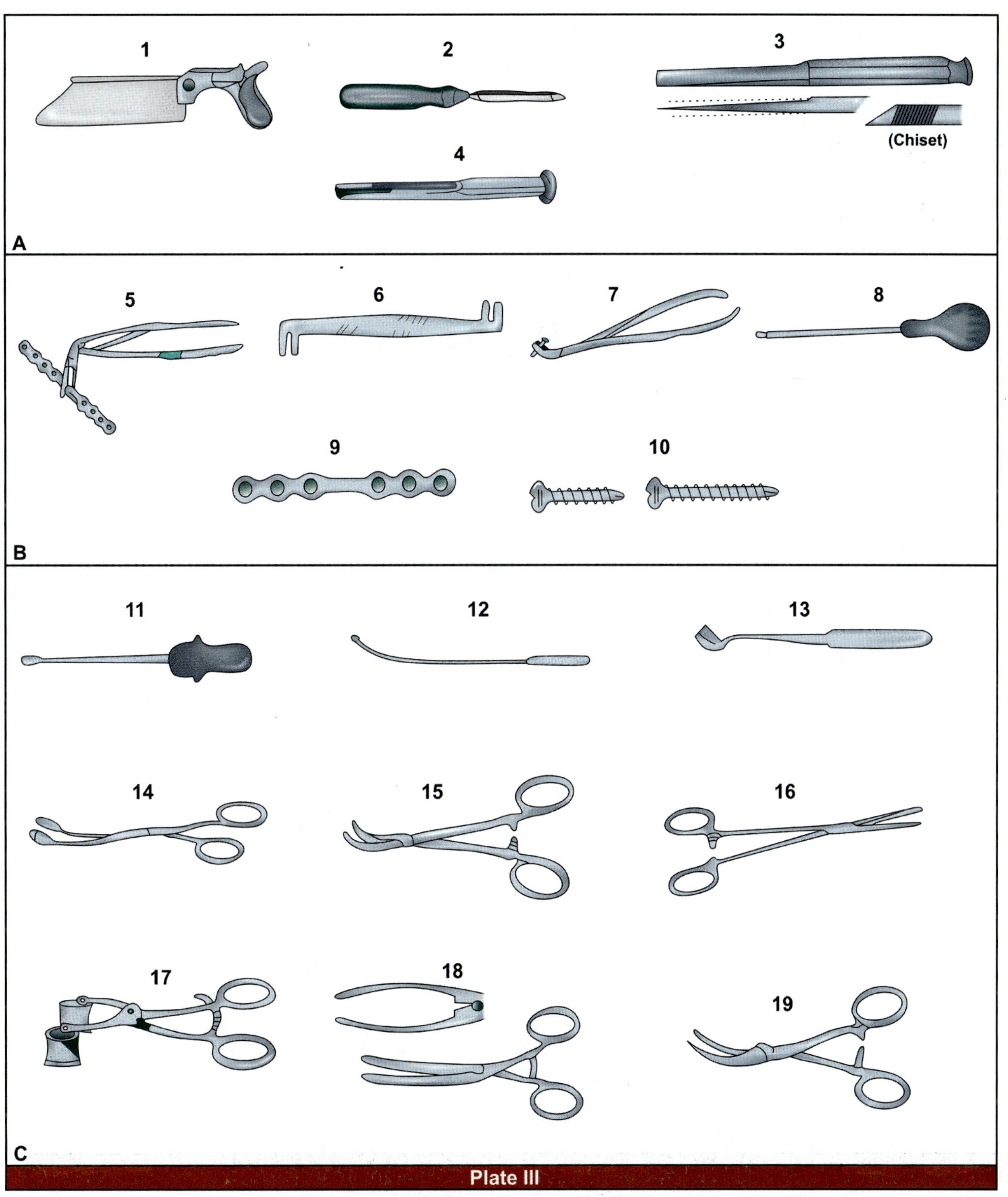
(Chiset)
Plate III

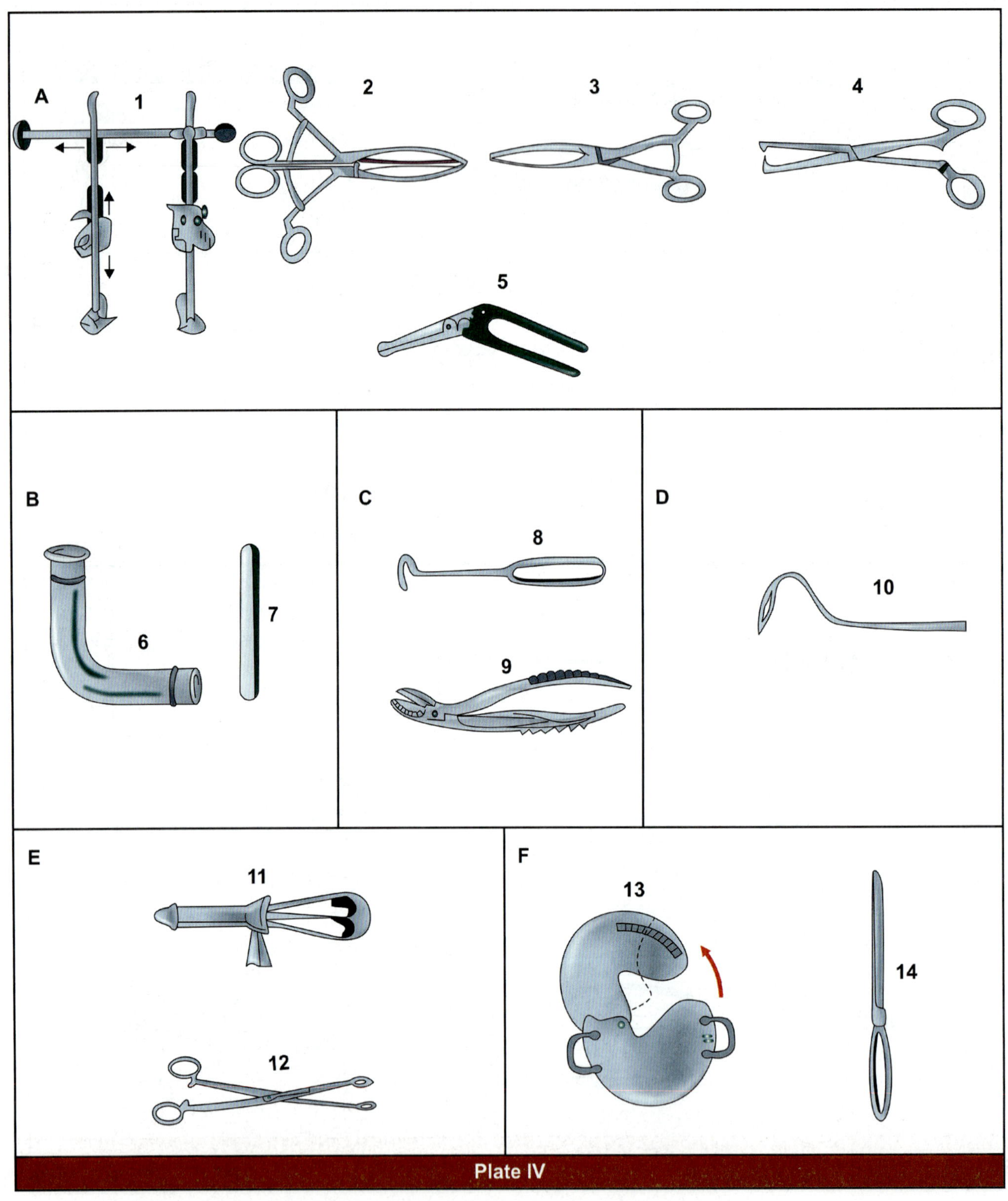

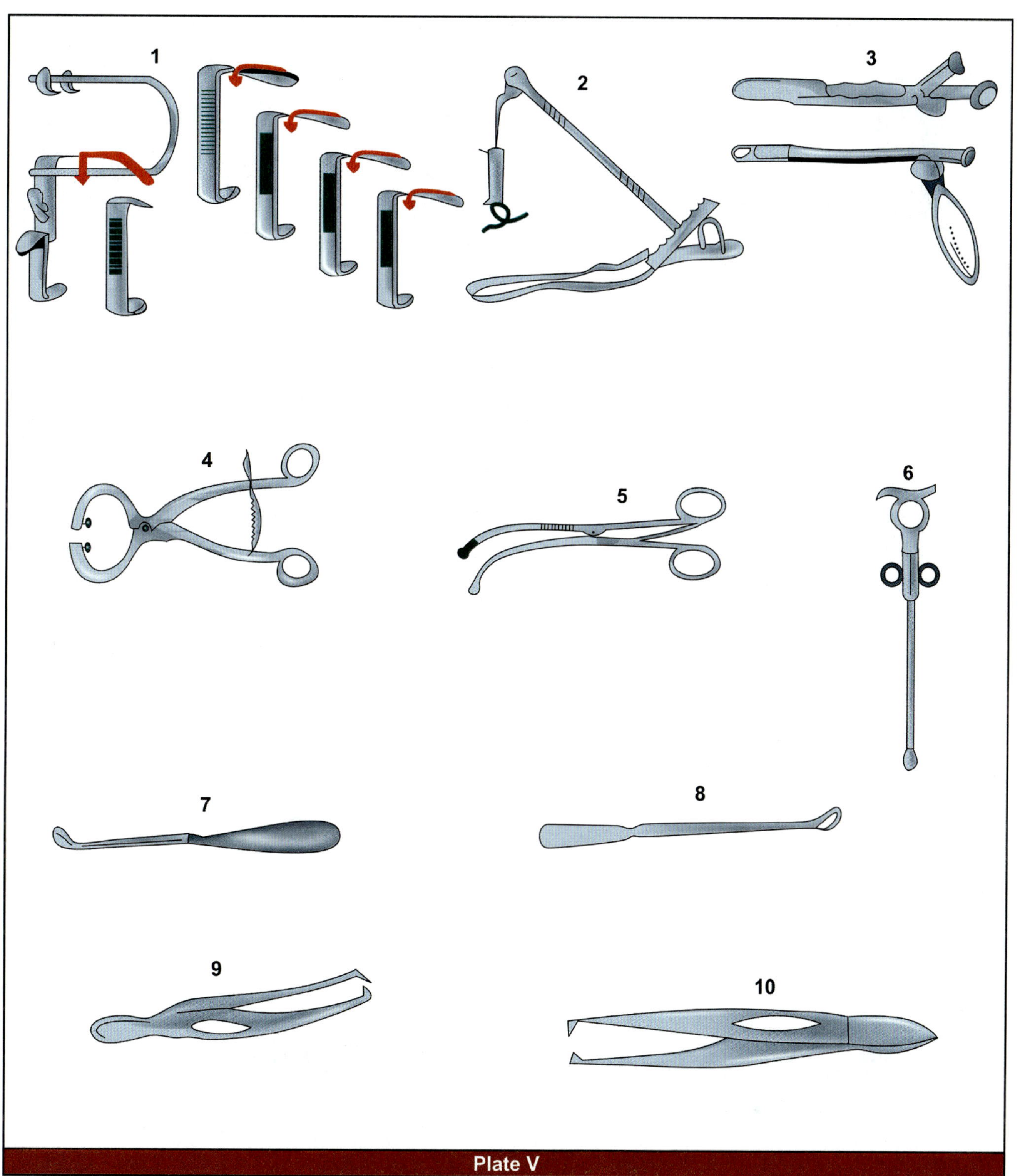

Plate V

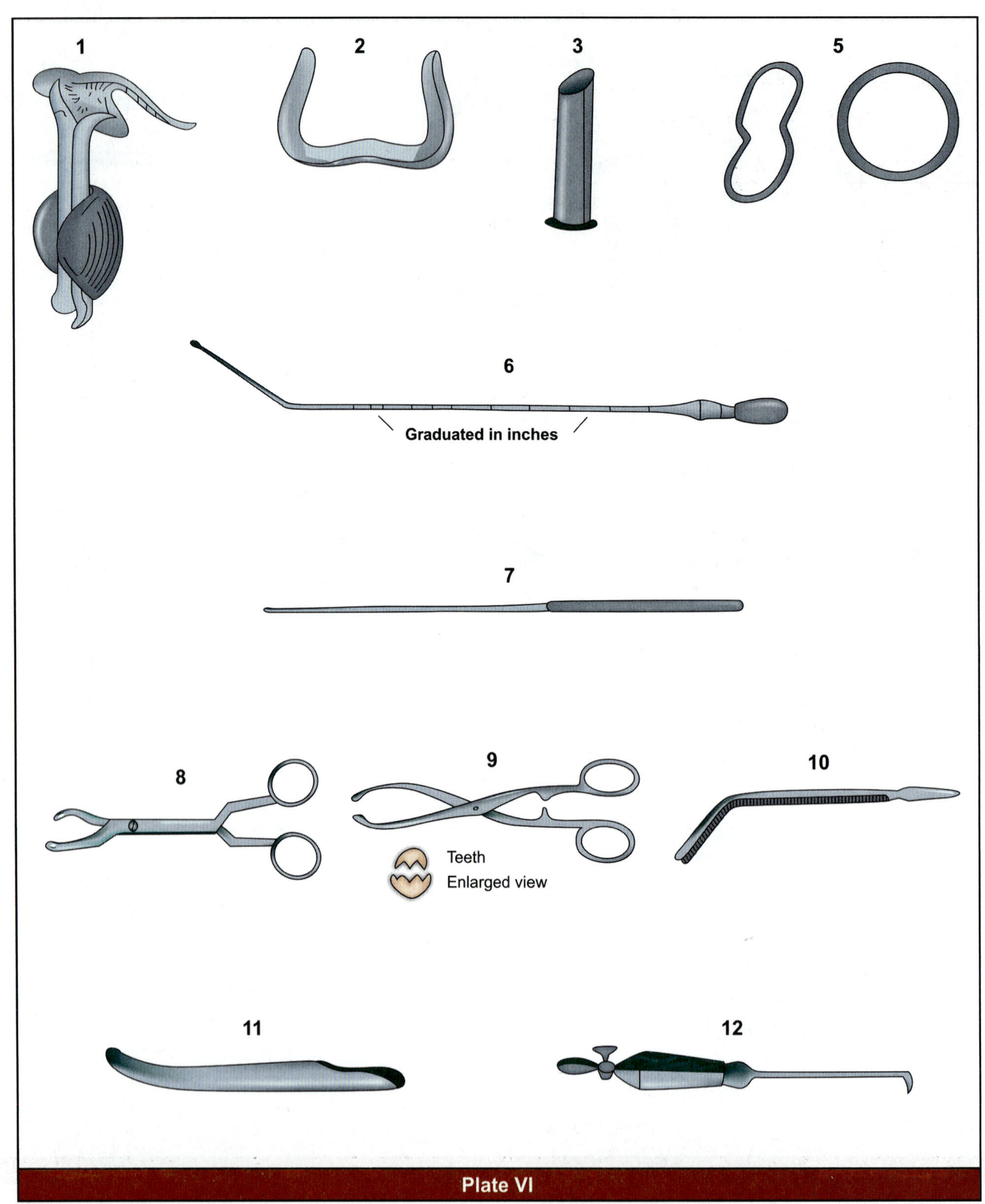
1
2
3
5
6
Graduated in inches
7
8
9
Teeth
Enlarged view
10
11
12
Plate VI

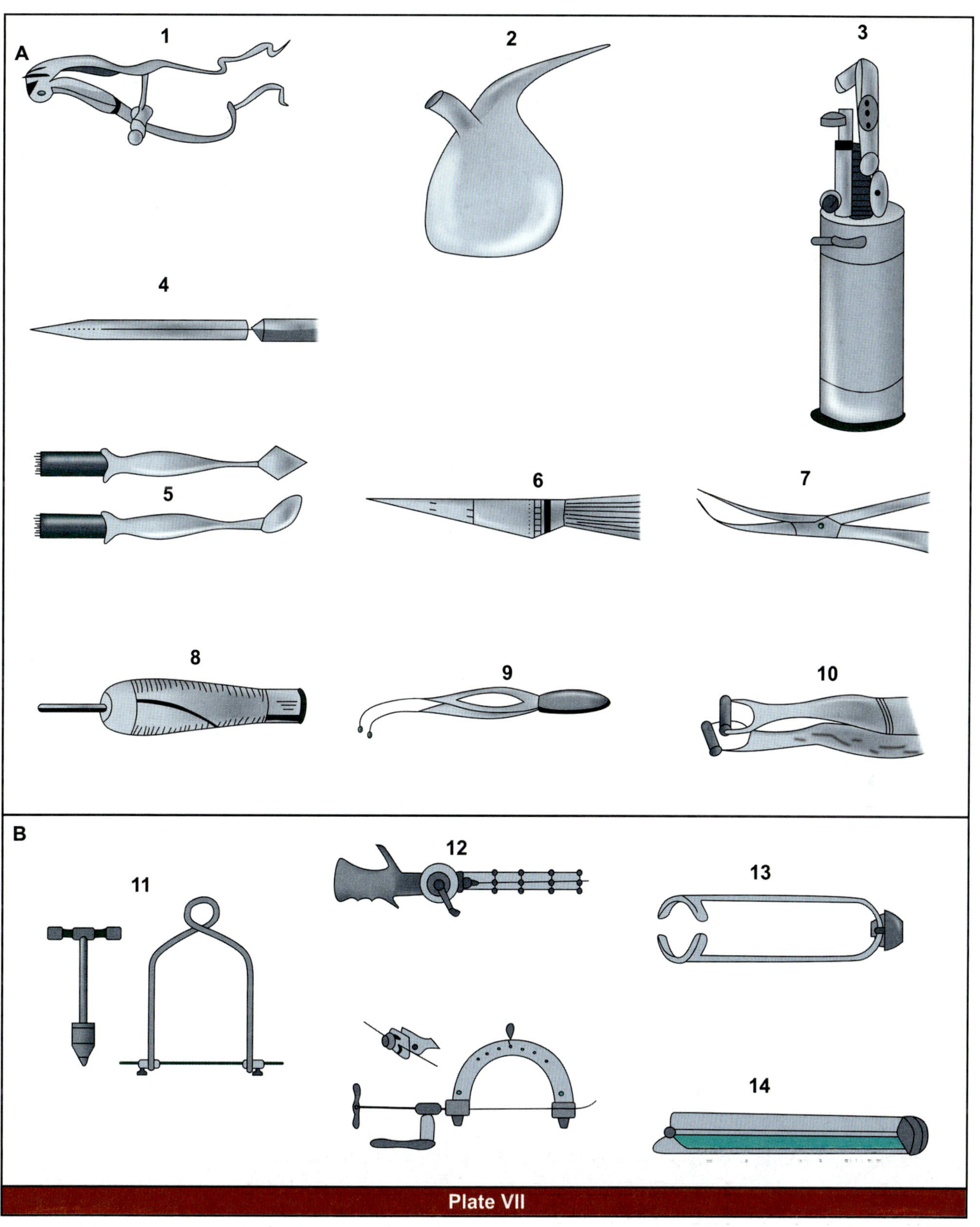
A
1
2
3
4
5
6
7
8
9
10
B
11
12
13
14
Plate VII

Index

A

Abdellah's theory 52
Accident prevention 169,171,175
Acid-base imbalances 564
    metabolic acidosis (base bicarbonate deficit) 566
    respiratory acidosis (carbonic acid excess) 565
    respiratory alkalosis (carbonic acid deficit) 565
Active listening 153
Active transport 548
Actual loss 960
Acute pain 856
Adolescent care 176,355
    developmental tasks 177
    marriage counseling 178
    motor vehicle 178
    nutrition 178
    role of nurse
        in adolescent health promotion 177
    self-esteem 178
    sex education 178
    sources 179
    substance abuse 177
    suicide 178
Adolescents 355
Age 855
Agent-host-environment model 14
Air contamination 695
Airway 820
Alcohol 19
    poisoning 923
Altered nutrition 270
American Nurses Association 79
Ampule 612
Anaphylactic shock 887
Anger 961
    management 796
Anthropometry 477
Anticipatory loss 960
Anxiety 856
Apoplexy 906
Artificial eye 421
Artificial respiration 874
Asphyxia 903
Aspiration/biopsy 739
Atoms 541
Attention 856
Auscultation 213

B

Bandaging materials 834
Basal energy needs 478
Basic human needs 159

Basic nursing skills 312
    advantages 313
    barriers 317
        effective communication 317
        therapeutic communication 321
    cultural considerations 321
    developmental considerations 321
    elements 313
    factors influencing communication 315
    helping relationship skill 312
    intrapersonal communication 313, 314
    level 313
    modes 314
    nurse-patient relationship 312
    phases 312
        helping relationships 312
    principles 317
    public communication 314
    role 312
    therapeutic communication 319
        interview 319
        nursing 318
        techniques 320
Bed linens 357
Bedmaking 357
Behavior control 73
Behavioral responses 787
Beneficence 68
Bicarbonate 557
Bioethical issues 74
Biomedical waste 693
Bland diet 485
Blood chemistry 730
Blood pressure monitoring 345
Blood specimen collection 730
Blood tests/examination 730
Blood transfusion 646
    administering 649
    common sites 647
    complications 648
    contraindications 647
    definition 646
    indications 646
    investigations 647
    method 647
    precaution 647
    prevention 648
    procedure 647
    responsibilities 647
Body defences 677
Body electrolyte component 541
Body fluids 540
Body mechanics 363
    ambulation safety 372
    chair 386
    commode 386

    concepts 364
    equipment needed 365
    moving a client in bed 386
    moving and lifting patient 365
    moving the patient up in bed (one nurse) 372
    performing passive range-of-motion exercises 372
    positioning the patient on bed 365
    principles and techniques of moving and lifting 371
    transferring from bed 386
    transferring from bed to stretcher 391
    turning and positioning a client 380
    using appropriate body mechanics 365
    using proper body mechanics 365
    wheelchair 386
Bone marrow aspiration/biopsy 739
Bowel elimination 502
    administering cleansing enema 512
    administration of enema 507
    changing stone appliance on ileal conduit 513
    enemas 506
    factors 503
    management 502
    physiology 502
Breast self-examination 222
Breathing 820
Buccal medications 608
Buffers 546
Burnout 791
Burns 888

C

Calcium 557
Carbohydrates 468
Cardiopulmonary resuscitation 875
Care giver 46
Central sterile supply services department 30
Cerebral cortex 782
Cerebrospinal fluid aspiration 740
Chemical burns 891
Chemical organization 541
    atoms 541
    compounds 543
    elements 541
    ions 544
    isotopes 543
    molecules 543
Chest compression 879
Chloride 557
Chronic pain 857
Circulation 820
Civil law 101
Clear airway 877
Cognitive responses 787
Cold 902

Comfort 356
  bed linens 357
  bedmaking 357
    occupied bed 358
    unoccupied bed 358
  equipment needed 358
  types of bed linens and their uses 357
Commode 386
Communication 128
  aggressive 148
  aspects 128
  assertive 148
  assessment 150
  barriers 136
  closed questions 136
  communicating with the health care team 142
  congruency of messages 149
  cultural values 148
  diagnosing communication problems 150
  electronic 143
  factors 132
  gestures 147
  goals 134
  guidelines 144
  language development 149
  listening/observing 149
  meaning 148
  methods 129
  non-verbal behavior 149
  non-verbal 130
  nurse-patient relationship 128
  nursing diagnosis 149
  oral 142
  passive 147
  political correctness 148
  psychosocial aspects 147
  style 147, 149
  techniques 136
  telehealth 144
  therapeutic 134
  verbal 129
  written 143
Communicator 46
Community health nursing 125
  legal role 125
  nurse 126
    citizen 126
    employee 126
    provider of care 125
Computerized documentation 197
Concussion 907
Confidentiality 74
Consciousness 820
Consequentialism 69
Contract law 101
Convulsion (epilepsy) 906
Coping enhancement 794
Coping style 856
Counselor 46
Credentialing 106
Criminal law 103
Crisis intervention 798
Critical thinking 239
Cultural change 89
Culture 855
  characteristics 88
  concepts related 89
  cultural change 89

cultural phenomena 91
cultural values 90
culture-bound 89
enculturation 89
environmental control 91
ethnicity 90
ethnocentrism 89
holism 89
meaning 88
religion 90
stereotypes 90

D

Daily requirement 468
Damage 109
Data processing 263
Death 962
Decision maker 46
Decision-making models 82
Deep pain 858
Deep somatic pain 858
Deltoid site 626
Dental department/unit 28
Dental hygiene 174
Dentition 184
Denture care 409
Deontology 66
Depression 962
Dereliction 109
Development 160
  basic concepts 160
  care during pregnancy 165
    first trimester 165
    second trimester 166
    third trimester 167
  factors 163
    external 163
    natural 163
  growth 164
    embryonic stage (4 to 8th week) 165
    fetal stage (9 weeks to birth) 165
    germinal stage (fertilization to 3weeks) 164
    pre-embryonic stage 164
  principles 162
    basic 162
    Elizabeth Hurlock's 162
Dhatura poisoning 923
Diabetes mellitus 487
Diagnostic examination 521
Diagnostic process 262
Diet therapy 481
  carbohydrate modified diets 487
    diabetes mellitus 487
    dumping syndrome 487
    lactose intolerance 488
  fat modified diets 488
    fat-controlled diets 488
    low fat diets 488
  kilocalorie modifications 485
    high kilocalorie 485
    high protein diets 485
    kilocalorie controlled 486
    low kilocalorie diets 486
    very low calorie diet 486
  meal frequency modifications 485

  modified diets 488
    fluid 489
    potassium 489
    protein restricted 488
    sodium restricted 489
  protein 488
  therapeutic diets 484
    bland 485
    high fiber 485
    liquid 484
    soft 485
Dietary department 29
Documentation 194 969
  charting 197
    computerized documentation 197
    confidentiality 197
    cons 197
    pros 197
  documentation systems 194
  focus charting 196
  forms 198
    discharge summary 198
    do's and dont's 198
    flow sheets 198
    kardexes 198
    progress notes 198
    reporting 199
  pie documentation model 196
  problem-oriented medical records 195
  purposes 194
  source-oriented record 195
Doppler 340
Doppler probe 214
Dorsal recumbent position 210
Dorsogluteal site 625
Double bagging 686
Dressing 824
Drug 595
  absorption 595
  action 595
  classification 594
  distribution 597
  excretion 597
  factors 599
  metabolization 597
  names (nomenclature) 594
  preparation/forms 594
Dumping syndrome 487
Duty 109
Dyssomnias 454

E

Education 475
Ego defense mechanisms 788
Elders 356
Electrical burns 892
Electrocardiography 738
Electrodiagnostic studies 737
Electroencephalography 738
Electrolyte imbalances 558
Electrolytes 556
  imbalances 558
    hypercalcemia 561
    hyperkalemia 560
    hypermagnesemia 563

hypernatremia 559
hyperphosphatemia 564
hypocalcemia 560
hypokalemia 559
hypomagnesemia 562
hyponatremia 558
hypophosphatemia 563
main characteristics 558
regulation 556
bicarbonate 557
calcium 557
chloride 557
magnesium 557
phosphate 557
sodium 556
sources 556
Electronic communication 143
Elizabeth Hurlock's principles 162
Emergency childbirth 912
Empathy 151
Employee's rights 104
Enculturation 89
Endocrine system 782
Endocrine system responses 784
End-of-life care 44
Endoscopy 738
Enemas 506
Enhancing therapeutic communication 153
Enteral (nasogastric and gastrostomy) medications 608
Environmental control 91
Environmental dimension 15
Environmental factor 475
Environmental hazards 694
Ethical principles 70
Ethical dilemmas 71
behavior control 73
confidentiality 74
conflicts 72
dilemmas 72
human experimentation 73
informed consent 73
personal value systems 72
right to refuse treatment 73
right 74
treatment 74
truth 73
Ethical principles 76
application 76
autonomy 71
beneficence 71
confidentiality 78
fidelity 78
freedom 77
justice 70
nonmaleficence 77
nursing codes 78
respect 76
rights 77
veracity 71
Ethics 64
Ethnicity 90
Ethnocentrism 89
Euthanasia 964
Evolution 23
Exercise 19
Eye injury hazards 695

F

Facilitate coping 43
Family relationships 9
Fat modified diets 488
Fat-controlled diets 488
Fatigue 856
Fats 467
Feeding and nutrition 172
Feminist ethics 70
Fever 226
Filtration 552
Flail chest injuries 897
Flow sheets 198
Fluid and electrolyte balance 549
body fluids 549
exchange 549
filtration 552
food intake 550
hydrostatic pressure 552
oncotic pressure (colloidal osmotic pressure) 552
osmotic pressure or force 551
regulation 551
regulators 550
thirst 550
Fluid and food intake 550
Fluid imbalances 554
fluid volume deficit 554
fluid volume excess 555
nursing intervention 555
Fluid modified diets 489
Fluid spacing 545
Focus charting 196
Focused nursing assessment 205
assessment tool 229
common signs and symptoms 229
documenting and clustering data 229
auscultation 213
conditions 225
anaphylactic reaction 226
fever 226
heart attack 225
internal bleeding 226
shock 226
stroke or mini-stroke 225
descriptive terminology 210
breast self-examination 222
general constitutional symptoms 224
procedure 222
head-to-toe approach 215
general 215
preliminary evaluation 215
sensory testing 215
palpation 211
percussion 211
physical examination/assessment 205
positions 207
common errors 212
dorsal recumbent 210
knee-chest 210
lateral side lying 210
lithotomy 210
procedure 211
prone 210
semi Fowler's 210
Sims 210
sitting 207
standing 210
supine 207
physical examination instruments 213
doppler probe 214
ophthalmoscope 214
otoscope 215
stethoscope 213
preparation 207
client or patient 207
equipment 207
symptoms analysis 213
techniques 210
inspection 210
observation 210
Food poisoning
Freedom 77

G

Gas poisoning 922
Gases 545
General adaptation syndrome (gas) 783
General anesthesia 819
General approach 215
General care 802
General constitutional symptoms 224
General status 183
Genitourinary 184
Genuineness 151
Geriatric death 963
Gestures 147
GI system 954
Good Samaritan laws 105
Gordon's functional health patterns 278
Grief 960
Grief process (reactions to grief and death) 961
Grooming 19

H

Habit 396
Hall's theory 54
Hand protection 956
Head injuries 907
Headache 858
Health 2
Health assessment 202
evolution 202
functional health patterns 204
types 204
Health belief model 14
Health care delivery system 11
primary 12
secondary 12
tertiary 12
Health hazards 694
Health history 254
Health promotion 44
Health restoration 44
Health-illness continuum model 13
Heat and fire hazards 695
Hematoma (hemorrhage) 831
Henderson's theory 52

Holism 89
Holistic health 4
Homeostasis 540
Homeostatic mechanism 552
Hospital 21
    classification 24
        clinical basis 24
        length of stay of patient 24
        management 25
        objectives 24
        ownership/control 24
        size 25
        system 25
    definitions 21
    evolution 23
    functions 23
    objectives 22
    philosophy 22
    scope 23
Hospital admission 188
    admitting 188
    discharge 193
    discharging a patient 189
        equipment needed 189,191
        nursing process 194
    procedure 489
        admitting 189
        discharging 191
        transferring 189, 190
Hospital departments 25
    central sterile supply services department 30
    children's hospital philosophy 31
    dental department/unit 28
    department 26
        dietary 29
        medicine 26
        nursing 30
        outpatient 25
        pathology/laboratory 28
        pharmacy 29
        psychiatry/mental health 29
        radiology or x-ray department 28
        surgery 26
    laundry 29
    maternity unit 27
    medical unit 26
    OBG unit 27
    patient care 30
    pediatric unit 27
    philosophy 30
    surgical units 26
Host 667
Household poisoning 922
Human experimentation 73
Human response patterns 274
Hydrostatic pressure 552
Hypercalcemia 561
Hyperkalemia 560
Hypermagnesemia 563
Hypernatremia 559
Hyperphosphatemia 564
Hypocalcemia 560
Hypoglycemia 907
Hypokalemia 559
Hypomagnesemia 562
Hyponatremia 558
Hypophosphatemia 563
Hypothalamus 782
Hysteria 906

I

Illness 5
    determinants 5
    stages 5
        assumption 6
        dependent client role 6
        medical care contact 6
        symptoms experience 5
    nature 7
Illness prevention 44
Immune system 783
Infant care 168
    accident prevention 169
    developmental performance 170
    developmental tasks 168
    emotional attachments 170
    feeding methods 169
    hygiene 170
    infections 170
    nutrition 169
    skin care 170
Infection 668
    air contamination 695
    assessment 680
    biomedical waste 693
    body defences 677
    breaking 673
    classification 693
    defenses 669
    double bagging 686
    elements 696
    environmental hazards 694
    evaluation 682
    eye injury hazards 695
    factors 671
    health hazards 694
    heat and fire hazards 695
    ill effects 694
    implementation 681
    isolation technique 687
    maintaining hand hygiene 682
    medical handwashing 687
    noise 695
    nursing diagnosis 680
    nursing process and infection control 680
    planning 680
    preparing for disinfection and sterilization 687
    primary defenses 669
    protective isolation 679
    secondary defenses 669
    stages 668
    standard precautions 678
        deep burial 705
        infection control 678
        liquid waste 704
        microwaving 705
        waste autoclaving 701
    support 671
    teaching 673
    tertiary defenses 669
    transmission-based precautions 679
Injection
    accounting
        for needle "dead space" 616
    administering
        heparin 623
        insulin 623
        intradermal injection 618

        intramuscular injection 627
        parenteral injections 617
        subcutaneous injection 620
    choosing
        deltoid site 626
        intramuscular needle 624
        intramuscular site 624
        subcutaneous needle 620
        subcutaneous site 620
    developmental considerations 618
    dorsogluteal site 625
    drawing up medications 615
    intradermal injections 618
    intramuscular injections 623
    minimizing discomfort 617
    mixing medications 615
    prepacked medications 622
    preventing needlestick injuries 616
    procedures 613
        ampule 613
        subcutaneous injection 622
        vial 614
    recapping 616
        contaminated needles 616
        sterile needles 616
    reconstituting medications 615
    rectus femoris site 627
    reusing 622
        needles 622
        syringes 622
    subcutaneous injections 620
    teaching patient 631
        self-medication 631
    vastus lateralis site 627
    ventrogluteal muscle–site of choice 624
    vial 613
    z-track technique 624
Injury 10
Integumentary system 954
Intractable pain 858
Intradermal injections 618
Intramuscular injections 623
Intrapersonal communication 313
Intravenous medications 631
    adding medications to large-volume (primary)
        infusions 632
    infection control: venipuncture 632
    intermittent infusion 633
    push medications 633
    setting volume 632
    volume-control infusion set 634
Involuntary admission (commitments) 122
Ions 544
Isolation technique 687
Isotopes 543

J

Johnson's theory 55
Judging goal achievement 304
Justice 68

K

Kardexes 198
Kilocalorie modifications 485
King's theory 57
Knee-chest position 210

L

Laboratory tests 730
Lactose intolerance 488
Language development 149
Laundry 29
Law 100
  civil 101
  contract 101
  criminal 103
  definition 100
  elements 102
  functions 100
  sources 100
  tort 101
  vicarious liability 103
  witness 102
Leader/manager 46
Legal issues 964
  absconding 124
  common causes 120
  discharge 124
  discharge on parole 124
  informal admission 122
  involuntary admission (commitments) 122
  maternal and infant nursing 120
  medical-surgical nursing 121
  medicolegal aspects of death 124
  patient's rights 124
  pediatric nursing 121
  psychiatric nursing 122
  records and reports 125
  reports 125
  voluntary admission 122
Legal process 115
  assignment 118
  components and characteristics 115
  legal responsibilities 118
  legal safeguard 115
  purpose 115
  responsibility 120
    appointment 118
    death and dying 120
    equipment 119
    observation and reporting 19
    protect public 119
    quality control 119
    record keeping and reporting 119
    safeguarding public 115
Leininger's theory 60
Leisure activities 795
Levine's theory 55
Licensing 106
Licensing board/council 104
Life-saving technique/resuscitation technique 874
Lifestyle choices 8
Limbic system 782
Liquid diets 484
Listening/observing 149
Lithotomy position 210
Local adaptation syndrome 785
Localised pain 858

M

Magnesium 557
Magnetic resonance imaging 737

Malignant pain 857
Malnutrition 474
  causes 474
  preventive measures 474
Malpractice 107
  abuse 113
  detecting potential chemical dependence 113
  impaired nurses 113
  legal safeguards 113
  nursing student responsibilities 114
  professional liability insurance 114
  safe harbor laws 114
  tips for minimizing 110
  unauthorized practice 113
Mandatory reporting laws 105
Marriage counseling 178
Maslow's hierarchy theory of need 17,159
  love and belonging 17
  physiological 17
  safety and security 17
  self-actualization 18
    self-awareness 18
    development 18
  self-esteem 17
Maternity unit 27
Maturation phase 823
Meal frequency modifications 485
Medical care contact 6
Medical handwashing 687
Medical unit 26
Medical-surgical nursing 121
Medicating children 609
Medicating older adults 609
Medication order 601
  communicating medication orders 602
  legal responsibilities 602
Medications 608
  buccal and sublingual medications 608
  enteral (nasogastric and gastrostomy) errors 661
  medicating children 609
  medicating older adults 609
  pouring liquid medications 608
  special situations 608
  teaching parents 609
Medications errors 661
  agent 665
  host 667
  infection process 664
  modes of transmission 666
  steps 661
  techniques 661
  types 663
Mental health 176
Mental illness 10
Metabolic acidosis 566
Metabolic alkalosis 567
Metered-dose inhalers 610
Middle aged developmental tasks 182
Middle age/middle adulthood 181,356
  adults aged 20 to 40 (female) 183
  adults aged 40 or older 183
  all middle adults 183
  all women 183
  developmental tasks 182
  middle aged developmental tasks 182
  role 182

Minerals 472
Minimizing discomfort 617
Molecules and compounds 543
Moral principles 67
  autonomy 67
  beneficence 68
  fidelity 68
  justice 68
  nonmaleficence 67
  veracity 68
Mouth to nose ventilation 878

N

Nasal instillations 658
Nasal medications 652
Needles 611
Negativism 171
Negligence 107
Neonate care 167
Nervous system 782
Neuman's theory 59
Nightingale's theory (environment model) 50
Noise 695
Nonmaleficence 67
Nonmalignant pain 857
Non-verbal behavior 149
Non-verbal communication 130
Nuclear scans 737
Nurse practice acts 105
Nurse practitioner 46
Nurse-patient relationship 128, 312
Nursing care plan 292
  approaches 308
  collecting data 303
  consulting process 294
  evaluating process 303
  evaluating 308
  evaluation 302
  guidelines 294
  identifying outcome criteria 303
  implementation 295
  judging goal achievement 304
  modifying care plan 306
  process 301
  reexamining 304
  relating nursing actions 304
  tools and methods 309
  types 299
  validating 301
  writing 292
    nursing care plan 294
    nursing orders 292
Nursing codes of ethics 78
Nursing lawsuits 109
Nursing paradigms 245
Nursing process 238
  accountability 249
  advantages 244
  assessment 250
    documenting data 252
    interpreting data 252
    organizing data 251
    sources of data collection 251
    types 251
    validating data 251

characteristics 249
components 246
concepts 240
critical thinking 239
definition 243
diagnosis 260
    advantages 262
    altered nutrition 270
    characteristics 270
    common diagnostic errors 272
    data processing 263
    defining characteristics 267
    diagnosing high-risk states 267
    diagnostic labels 266
    diagnostic process 262
    etiologic/related factors 266
    formulating nursing diagnosis statements 266
    guidelines 267
    health risks and strengths 267
    identifying the client's health problems 267
    nursing diagnosis format 268
    stating wellness diagnoses 270
    writing a diagnostic statement 269
evolution 239
health history 254
    interview proceses 258
    interviewing 255
    planning 257
methods of data collection 254
nature 242
nursing care 250
nursing paradigms 245
nursing process 245
observing 254
organization 244
properties 244
purpose 244
taxonomy 272
    advantages y 274
    Gordon's functional health patterns 278
    grouping on nanda nursing diagnoses 278
    human response patterns 274
Nursing profession 76
Nursing strategies 97
Nursing student responsibilities 114
Nursing theories 50
    Abdellah's theory 52
    Hall's theory 54
    Henderson's theory 52
    Johnson's theory 55
    King's theory 57
    Leininger's theory 60
    Levine's theory 55
    Neuman's theory 59
    Nightingale's theory (environment model) 50
    Orem's theory 56
    Orlando's theory 53
    Paplau's theory 51
    Roger's theory 56
    Roy's theory 59
    Travelebee's theory 58
    Watson's theory 60
    Wiedenbach theory 54
Nutrients
    carbohydrates 468
    causes 465
    classification 472
        mineral 472

nutrients 464
    vitamins 469
daily requirement 468
deficiencies 465
    carbohydrate 468
    proteins/protein-energy malnutrition 465
fats 467
functions 467
    carbohydrates 468
    proteins 465
minerals 472
protein requirement 465
proteins 464
sources 468
    carbohydrate 468
    fats: 468
    proteins 465
sugars 468
vitamins 468
water 468
Nutrition 8,19,178,795
Nutrition support 489
    parenteral nutrition support 497
    tube feedings 483, 489
Nutritional assessment 477
    anthropometry 477
        interpretation 477
        technique 477
        triceps skin fold 477
    biological factors 475
    environmental factor 475
    nutritional assessment 477
    psychological factor 475
    sociocultural factors 475
Nutritional needs/nutrition 462
    classification 464
    meaning 462
    physiology 463

O

Oncotic pressure (colloidal osmotic pressure) 552
Ophthalmic medications 651
Ophthalmoscope 214
Oral communication 142
Oral medication (external route) 636
    bolus iv medication 641
    equipment 645
    heparin or saline lock 642
    iv dressing 642
    iv site and infusion 642
    iv solution container 640
    medications intravenously 636
    primary intravenous 642
    procedures 638
        heparin or saline lock 646
        iv dressing 645
        medication infusion intravenously 638
Orem's theory 56
Organ donations 964
Orlando's theory 53
Osmotic pressure or force 551
Otic medications 652
Otoscope 215
Outpatient department (OPD) 25
Overweight 478
Oxygen cylinder and fittings 570

Oxygen therapy administration 570
Oxygenation 570
    clean dressing and tape 590
    disposable inner cannula 590
    factors 570
    indications 570
    mask 583
    modes 571
    nasal cannula 585
    naso/oropharyngeal areas 586
    nasopharyngeal and oropharyngeal suctioning 575
    oxygen administration 572
    oxygen cylinder 571
    oxygen cylinder and fittings 570
    oxygen therapy administration 570
    pulse oximeter 584
    tent 583
    tracheostomy 588
    tracheostomy care 577
    tracheostomy suctioning 580
    Wolff's humidifier bottle 591

P

Pain 856
    acute pain 856
    age 855
    anxiety 856
    artificial respiration 874
    assessment 859
    attention 856
    cardiopulmonary resuscitation 875
    chest compression 879
    chronic pain 857
    clear airway 877
    conduction 852
    constipation and opioids 866
    coping style 856
    cultural norms 852
    culture 855
    deep pain 858
    deep somatic pain 858
    effects of meperidine (demerol) 866
    factors influencing pain 855
    family and social support 856
    fatigue 856
    first aid 874
    guidelines 869
    headache 858
    intractable pain 858
    invasive intervention 864
    life-saving technique/resuscitation technique 874
    localised pain 858
    malignant pain 857
    meaning 856
    mouth to nose ventilation 878
    nature 850
    noninvasive interventions 867
    nonmalignant pain 857
    nonopioid drugs 865
    nursing diagnosis 862
    nursing intervention 870
    nursing management 859
    objectives 874
    opioid analgesia 866
    perception 854

physiology 850
planning 863
process 852
psychogenic 859
purpose 850
reaction 855
reception 852
recovery position 879
referred pain 858
restore circulation 878
resuscitation 876
sex 856
situation 855
splanchnic 858
stimulation 850
superficial 857
TENS contraindications 869
transduction 853
transmission 854
types 856
Pain transduction 853
Pain transmission 854
Paplau's theory 51
Papnicolaou test 733
Paracentesis 739
Parasomnias 456
Parenteral medications 610
injectable medications 611
injections 611
Parenteral nutrition support 497
Passive transport 547
Patient care 30
Patient education 830
Patient's rights 124
Pediatric death 963
Pediatric nursing 121
Pediatric unit 27
Percussion 211
Perinatal death 963
Perineal care 432
applantiembolic stockings 438
back rub 437
bedpan or urinal 441
equipment needed 432
perineal care 436
routine catheter care 432
Personal hygiene 396
artificial eye 421
bathing 401
care 409
cleanliness 399
denture care 409
equipment 404
habit 396
maintenance 427
shaving 430
tepid sponge bath 407
Personal protection 956
Personal value systems 72
Pharmacodynamics 599
primary effects 599
secondary effects 599
Philosophy 22
Phosphate 557
Physical care 966
Physical disease 10
Physical examination instruments 213
Physical examination/assessment 205
Physical fitness 176

Physical wellness 18
Physiological needs 160
Pie documentation model 196
Planning 150,280
alternative nursing interventions 290
barriers 154
asking too many questions 154
asking why 154
changing the subject inappropriately 154
expressing approval or disapproval 155
failing to listen 155
failing to probe 155
offering advice 155
providing false reassurance 155
stereotyping 156
using patronizing language 156
components 284
enhancing therapeutic communication 153
active listening 153
being assertive 153
clarifying 153
establishing trust 153
exploring issues 154
interpreting body language 153
restating 153
sharing observations 153
summarizing 154
using silence 154
validating messages 153
establishing goals 287
guidelines 289
helping groups 152
implementation 151
phases 283
planning nursing interventions 289
selecting nursing interventions 290
setting priorities 284
therapeutic communication 151
concreteness 151
confrontation 151
conveying acceptance 156
empathy 151
genuineness 151
respect 151
Planning nursing interventions 289
Planning patient care 929
Play habits 172
Poisoning 921
Political correctness 148
Portable wound suction 830
Postmortem care 969
Postoperative nursing 820
Post-traumatic stress disorder 791
Posture 19
Potassium modified diets 489
Pouring liquid medications 608
Pouring sterile liquids 809
Precordial thump 878
Preoperative nursing care 802
Prepacked medications 622
Preschoolers (3 to 6 years) care 172,355
accident prevention and safety 173
dental hygiene 174
infections 173
play habits 174
role 173
self-esteem 174
sleep disorders 173
Primary defenses 669

Primary health care 12
Primary nursing 33
Problem identification 82
Problem-oriented medical records 195
Professional liability insurance 114
Professional nursing 104
Professional versus personal values 92
Progress notes 198
Progressive patient/client care 33
Prone position 210
Protective isolation 679
Protective measures of accidental poisoning 924
Protein requirement 465
Protein restricted diets 488
Proteins 464
Psychiatric nursing 122
Psychogenic pain 859
Psychological wellness 20
Public communication 314
Pulse 336
Pulse-monitoring techniques 340
assessment 343
blood pressure 343
respirations 343
auscultation 340
blood pressure monitoring 345
counting 344
doppler 340
equipment needed 341
factors 347
palpation 340
respiration monitoring 341
respiratory rate 344
vital signs flow sheet 352
weighing 350
Push medications 633

R

Radiological studies 737
Recapping contaminated needles 616
Recapping sterile needles 616
Reconstituting medications 615
Recording vital signs flow sheet 352
Rectal applications 660
Rectal medications 653
Rectus femoris site 627
Referred pain 858
Reflex pain response 786
Regional anesthesia 819
Rehabilitation team 926
Rehabilitator 46
Relaxation 19
Relaxation techniques 797
Relieving anxiety 796
Religion 90
Reporting 199
Respiration monitoring 341
Respiratory acidosis (carbonic acid excess) 565
Respiratory alkalosis (carbonic acid deficit) 565
Respiratory inhalations 609
metered-dose inhalers 610
teaching 610
types of nebulizers 610
Rest 19
Restorative care 932
Reticular formation 782

Rights 77
Roger's theory 56
Roller bandages 838
Routine catheter care 432
Roy's theory 59

S

Safe harbor laws 114
Safety 354
    adolescents 355
    elders 356
    factors affecting safety 354
    middle-aged adults 356
    newborns and infants 355
    preschoolers 355
    preventive measures 356
    safety measures during the life span 355
    school-age children 355
    toddlers 355
    young adults 356
Saline lock 642
School age child (six to eleven years) care 174
    accident prevention 175
    communicable diseases 175
    developmental tasks 174
    mental health 176
    nurse's role 175
    physical fitness 176
    self-esteem 176
    substance abuse 176
Secondary defenses 669
Secondary health care 12
Self-actualization needs 160
Self-esteem needs 160
Selye's stages 783
Semi Fowler's position 210
Sensory testing 215
Sex 856
Sex education 178
Simple dressing 829
Sims position 210
Six rights 635
Skull fracture 907
Sleep 19,448
    common sleep disorders 454
    dyssomnias 454
    factors 453
    medications 458
    nursing management 457
    nursing measures 459
    parasomnias 456
    physiology 449
    regulation 450
    sleep requirements 449
Sleep disorders 173
Slings 836
Smoking 19
Snake bite 908
Sociocultural wellness 20
Sodium 556
Sodium restricted diets 489
Soft diets 485
Somatoform disorders 790
Source-oriented record 195
Special senses 184
Specimen collection 713

Spiritual dimension 15
Spiritual wellness 20
Splanchnic pain 858
State laws 105
    credentialing 106
    damage 109
    dereliction 109
    disciplinary procedure 106
    duty 109
    failure
        assess and diagnose 109
        evaluate 110
        implement 110
        plan 110
    good samaritan laws 105
    issues 107
    licensing 106
    malpractice 107
    mandatory reporting laws 105
    negligence 107
    negligence 108
    nurse and law 106
    nurse practice acts 105
    nursing lawsuits 109
Stereotypes 90
Stereotyping 156
Sterile dressing change 809
Stethoscope 213
Stool tests/ examination 726
Stress management techniques 796
Stress test 738
Stress-induced organic responses 789
Stress-induced psychological responses 791
Stressors 778
Strict isolation 816
Stroke 906
Stump bandaging 837
Style 147
Subcutaneous injections 620
Substance abuse 176
Sugars 468
Suicide 178, 963
Superficial pain 857
Supine position 207
Surgical asepsis 804
Surgical dressings 829
Surgical handwashing 804
Surgical skills/techniques/procedures 804
Surgical units 26
Symptoms analysis 213
Symptoms experience 5
Syringes 611
System review 820

T

Teacher/client family educator 46
Teaching 930
    principles 324
    role 325
    media 325
    modes 324
    strategies 324
    theory 323
Team nursing/modular nursing 32
Telehealth 144
Temperature monitoring 326

    assessment 328
    character 337
    equipment needed 330
    factors 327
    pulse 336
    pulse/monitoring pulse 336
Tepid sponge bath 407
Tertiary health care 12
Thallium test 738
Therapeutic communication 134
Therapeutic diets 484
Therapeutic relationship 134
Thirst 550
Thoracocentesis 740
Time management 796
Toddlers 355
    accident prevention 171
    feeding and nutrition 172
    hygiene and dental care 172
    infections 172
    negativism 171
    play habits 172
    roles 171
    toilet training 171
Toilet training 171
Topical medications 650
    creams 651
    ear instillations 656
    ear irrigation 658
    equipment 653
    eye applications 650
    eye drops 653
    eye drops ointment 655
    eye irrigation 655
    instillation 656
    irrigations 652
    lotions 651
    nasal instillations 658
    nasal medications 652
    ointments 651
    ophthalmic medications 651
    otic medications 652
    rectal applications 660
    rectal medications 653
    skin applications 650
    transdermal medications 651
    vaginal applications 659
    vaginal medications 652
    vaginal suppository or creams 660
Tort law 101
Total energy requirements 478
Total patient care 31
Tracheostomy care 577
Tracheostomy suctioning 580
Transdermal medications 651
Travelebee's theory 58
Triangular bandage 836
Triceps skin fold 477
Tube feedings 489

U

Ultrasonography 737
Unauthorized practice 113
Unconscious patient 936
Unconsciousness 905
Underweight 479

Urine analysis 714
    blood chemistry 730
    blood specimen collection 730
    blood tests/examination 730
    clean catch urine collection 724
    culture and sensitivity tests 731
    laboratory tests 730
    Papnicolaou test 733
    stool tests/ examination 726
    type and crossmatch 730
    urine collection 719
Urinary elimination 518
    common urinary problems 522
    condom catheter 534
    diagnostic examination 521
    equipment needed 534
    factors 519
    instructions 530
    measuring intake and output 536
    physiology 518
    role 522
Urine analysis 714
Urine collection 719
Utilitarianism 65

V

Vaginal medications 652
Values transmission 93

Vastus lateralis site 627
Ventrogluteal muscle 624
Veracity 68
Verbal communication 129
Very low calorie diet 486
Vial 613
Vitamins 468
Volume-control infusion set 634
Voluntary admission 122

W

Water 468
    body size 544
    body water 544
    fluid spacing 545
Watson's theory 60
Weight management 478
    basal energy needs 478
    overweight 478
    total energy requirements 478
    underweight 479
Wellness 18
    intellectual 20
    physical 18
        alcohol 19
        body mechanics 19
        drugs 19
        exercise 19
        grooming 19
        nutrition 19
        posture 19
        relaxation 19
        rest 19
        sleep 19
        smoking 19
    psychological 20
    sociocultural 20
    spiritual 20
    tips 21
Wheelchair 386
Wiedenbach theory 54
Wolff's humidifier bottle 591
Wound classification 822
Wound complications 831

Y

Young adult care 180,355
    developmental tasks 180
    roles 181

Z

Z-track technique 624

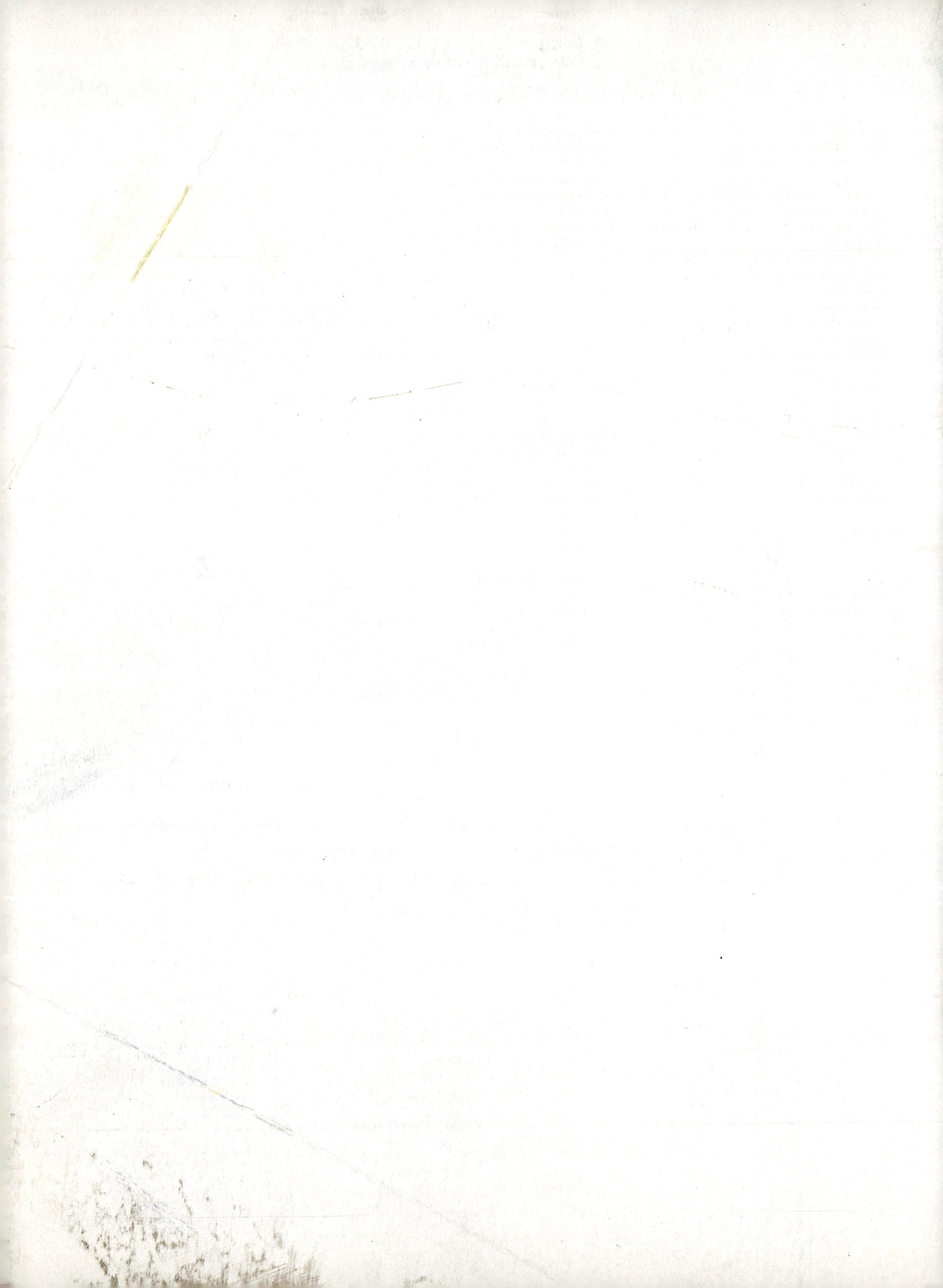